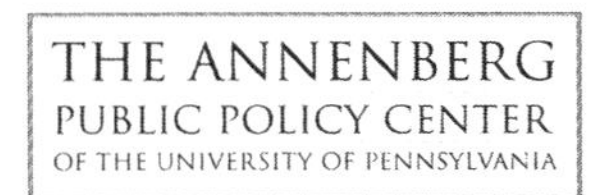

Daniel Romer, PhD, Director of Research

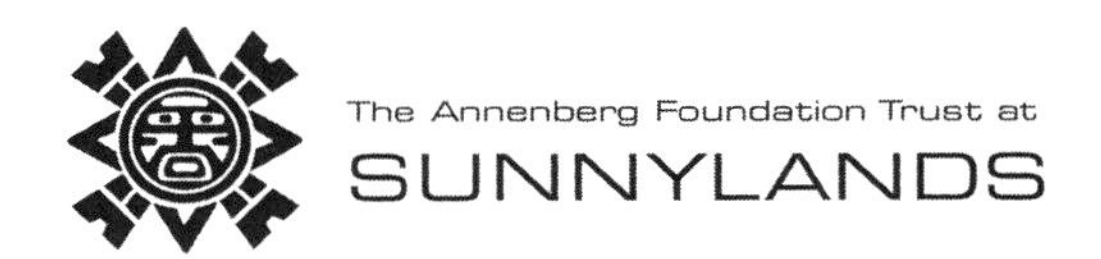

The Adolescent Mental Health Initiative of the
Annenberg Public Policy Center and the Sunnylands Trust

COMMISSIONS	COMMISSION CHAIRS
Anxiety Disorders	Edna B. Foa, PhD
Depression and Bipolar Disorder	Dwight L. Evans, MD
Eating Disorders	B. Timothy Walsh, MD
Positive Youth Development	Martin E. P. Seligman, PhD
Schizophrenia	Raquel E. Gur, MD, PhD
Substance and Alcohol Abuse	Charles P. O'Brien, MD, PhD
Suicide Prevention	Herbert Hendin, MD

Treating and Preventing Adolescent Mental Health Disorders

EDITED BY

Daniel Romer, PhD, Director of Research
Annenberg Public Policy Center
University of Pennsylvania

and

The Commission Chairs of The Adolescent
Mental Health Initiative of the Annenberg
Public Policy Center and the Sunnylands Trust

Dwight L. Evans, MD
Edna B. Foa, PhD
Raquel E. Gur, MD, PhD
Herbert Hendin, MD
Charles P. O'Brien, MD, PhD
Daniel Romer, PhD
Martin E. P. Seligman, PhD
B. Timothy Walsh, MD

Treating and Preventing Adolescent Mental Health Disorders

What We Know and What We Don't Know

A RESEARCH AGENDA FOR IMPROVING THE MENTAL HEALTH OF OUR YOUTH

SECOND EDITION

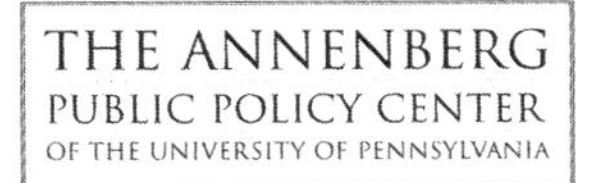

The Adolescent Mental Health Initiative of the Annenberg Public Policy Center and the Sunnylands Trust

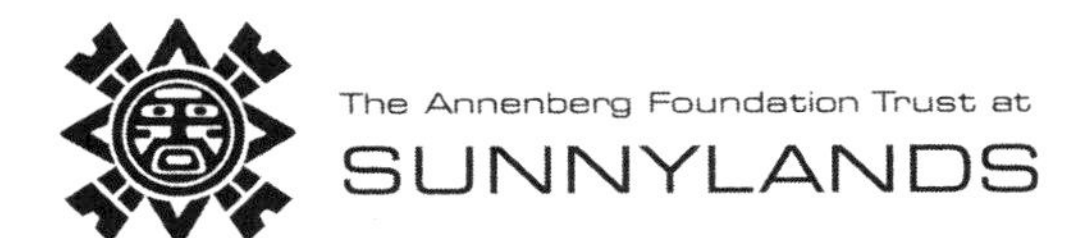

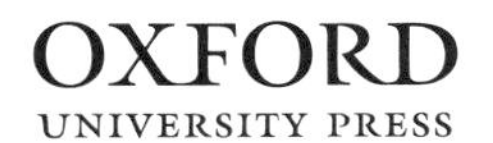

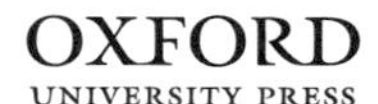

Oxford University Press is a department of the University of Oxford. It furthers the University's objective of excellence in research, scholarship, and education by publishing worldwide. Oxford is a registered trade mark of Oxford University Press in the UK and certain other countries.

Published in the United States of America by Oxford University Press
198 Madison Avenue, New York, NY 10016, United States of America.

First Edition published in 2005
Second Edition published in 2017

Library of Congress Cataloging-in-Publication Data
Names: Romer, Daniel, editor. | Annenberg Public Policy Center, issuing body. |
Annenberg Foundation Trust at Sunnylands, issuing body.
Title: Treating and preventing adolescent mental health disorders :
what we know and what we don't know : a research agenda for improving
the mental health of our youth / edited by the Commission Chairs of
the Annenberg Foundation Trust at Sunnylands' Adolescent Mental Health Initiative,
Dwight L. Evans, Edna B. Foa, Raquel E. Gur, Herbert Hendin,
Charles P. O'Brien, Daniel Romer, Martin E.P. Seligman, B. Timothy Walsh.
Other titles: Annenberg Foundation Trust at
Sunnylands' adolescent mental health initiative.
Description: Second edition. | New York, NY : Oxford University Press, [2017] |
Series: Annenberg Foundation Trust at Sunnylands' adolescent mental
health initiative | Includes bibliographical references and index.
Identifiers: LCCN 2016059220 (print) | LCCN 2016059949 (ebook) |
ISBN 9780199928163 (hardcover : alk. paper) | ISBN 9780199928170 (UPDF) |
ISBN 9780190685836 (EPUB) | ISBN 9780190923198 (custom paperback)
Subjects: | MESH: Mental Disorders—diagnosis | Mental Disorders—therapy |
Adolescent | Psychology, Adolescent | Adolescent Health Services—organization &
administration | United States
Classification: LCC RJ503 (print) | LCC RJ503 (ebook) | NLM WS 463 |
DDC 616.8900835—dc23
LC record available at https://lccn.loc.gov/2016059220

1 3 5 7 9 8 6 4 2

Printed by Sheridan Books, Inc., United States of America

Contents

Adolescent Mental Health Initiative

Project Director **Kathleen Hall Jamieson, PhD**
Professor, Annenberg School for Communication, University of Pennsylvania
Director, Annenberg Public Policy Center, University of Pennsylvania

Part I: Commission on Adolescent Depression and Bipolar Disorder

Commission Chair **Dwight L. Evans, MD**
Roerhoff Rickels Professor of Psychiatry, Professor of Psychiatry, Medicine, and Neuroscience, Department of Psychiatry, Perelman School of Medicine, University of Pennsylvania
Department Chair, Psychiatry, University of Pennsylvania
Chief of Psychiatry, Hospital of the University of Pennsylvania, Presbyterian Medical Center, Pennsylvania Hospital

Commission Members (Second Edition)

William Beardslee, MD
Psychiatrist-in-Chief and Chairman, Psychiatry, Children's Hospital Boston
Professor, Child Psychiatry, Harvard Medical School

Tami Benton, MD
Associate Professor, Psychiatry and Pediatrics, University of Pennsylvania

David Brent, MD
Academic Chief, Child & Adolescent Psychiatry, Western Psychiatric Institute and Clinic
Professor, Child Psychiatry, Pediatrics & Epidemiology, University of Pittsburgh School of Medicine

W. Edward Craighead, PhD
J. Rex Fuqua Professor and Director, Child and Adolescent Mood Program, Department of Psychology, Emory College

Paul Crits-Christoph, PhD
Professor, Psychology in Psychiatry, University of Pennsylvania
Director, Center for Psychotherapy Research, University of Pennsylvania

Marivel Davila, MD
Postdoctoral Fellow, Columbia University College of Physicians and Surgeons

Robert Findling, MD
Leonard and Helen R. Stulman Professor in Child and Adolescent Psychiatry, Director of Child and Adolescent Psychiatry, and a Vice Chair in the Department of Psychiatry and Behavioral Sciences at Johns Hopkins
Vice President of Psychiatric Services and Research at the Kennedy Krieger Institute

Robert Johnson, MD
Dean, Professor, Pediatrics and Director of the Division of Adolescent and Young Adult Medicine, New Jersey Medical School, University of Medicine and Dentistry of New Jersey
Director, Division of Adolescent and Young Adult Medicine, University of Medicine and Dentistry of New Jersey

Charles Nemeroff, MD
Professor & Chairman, Department of Psychiatry and Behavioral Sciences and Director, Center on Aging, University of Miami Miller School of Medicine

Rachel Neuhut, MD
Professor, Psychiatry and Behavioral Sciences, University of Miami Miller School of Medicine

Moira Rynn, MD
Professor, Implementation of Science for Child and Adolescent Mental Health in Psychiatry, Columbia University Medical Center
Director of the Division Child and Adolescent Psychiatry, New York State Psychiatric Institute/Columbia University

Karen Dineen Wagner, MD, PhD
Professor and Chair, Psychiatry and Behavioral Sciences, University of Texas Medical Branch, Galveston

Myrna Weissman, PhD
Diane Goldman Kemper Family Professor of Epidemiology and Psychiatry, Columbia University College of Physicians & Surgeons
Chief, Division of Epidemiology, New York State Psychiatric Institute

Commission Members (First Edition)

William Beardslee, MD
Joseph Biederman, MD
David Brent, MD
Dennis Charney, MD
Joseph Coyle, MD
W. Edward Craighead, PhD
Paul Crits-Christoph, PhD
Robert Findling, MD
Judy Garber, PhD
Robert Johnson, MD
Martin Keller, MD
Charles Nemeroff, MD, PhD
Moira A. Rynn, MD
Karen Wagner, MD, PhD
Myrna Weissman, PhD
Elizabeth Weller, MD

Part II: Commission on Adolescent Schizophrenia

Commission Chair

Raquel E. Gur, MD, PhD
Professor, Psychiatry, Neurology, and Radiology, University of Pennsylvania
Director, Neuropsychiatry Section in Psychiatry, University of Pennsylvania

Commission Members (Second Edition)

Ruben C. Gur, PhD
Professor, Psychiatry, Neurology, and Radiology, University of Pennsylvania
Director, Neuropsychology and the Brain Behavior Laboratory, University of Pennsylvania

Matcheri S. Keshavan, MD
Professor, Department of Psychiatry, Beth Israel Deaconess Medical Center

Christian Kohler, MD
Associate Professor, Psychiatry and Neurology, Hospital of the University of Pennsylvania

Judith Rapoport, MD
Chief, Child Psychiatry Branch, National Institute of Mental Health

Elaine Walker, PhD
Professor, Psychology and Neuroscience, Emory University

Commission Members (First Edition)

Nancy Andreasen, MD, PhD
Robert Asarnow, PhD
Ruben Gur, PhD
Peter Jones, MD
Kenneth Kendler, MD
Matcheri Keshavan, MD
Jeffrey Lieberman, MD
Robert McCarley, MD
Robin Murray, MD
Judith Rapoport, MD
Carol Tamminga, MD
Ming Tsuang, MD, PhD
Elaine Walker, PhD
Daniel Weinberger, MD

With Contributions From **Kristin Lancefield, MBBS, MRCPsych**

Commission Coordinator **Stacy L. Moore III, BA**

Part III: Commission on Adolescent Anxiety Disorders

Commission Chair

Edna B. Foa, PhD
Professor, Clinical Psychology in Psychiatry, University of Pennsylvania
Director, Center for the Treatment and Study of Anxiety, University of Pennsylvania

Commission Members (Second Edition)

Martin Franklin, PhD
Associate Professor, Clinical Psychology in Psychiatry, University of Pennsylvania
Director, Child and Adolescent OCD, Tic, Trich & Anxiety Group (COTTAGe), University of Pennsylvania School of Medicine

Carmen McLean, PhD
Assistant Professor, Psychiatry, University of Pennsylvania

Richard J. McNally, PhD
Professor, Psychology, Harvard University

Daniel Pine, MD
Chief, Section on Development and Affective Neuroscience, National Institute of Mental Health
Chief, Child and Adolescent Research Mood and Anxiety Disorders Program, National Institute of Mental Health

Commission Members (First Edition)

E. Jane Costello, PhD
Martin Franklin, PhD
Jerome Kagan, PhD
Philip Kendall, PhD
Rachel Klein, PhD
Henrietta Leonard, MD
Michael Liebowitz, MD
John March, MD, MPH
Richard McNally, PhD
Thomas Ollendick, PhD

Daniel Pine, MD
Robert Pynoos, MD
Wendy Silverman, PhD
Linda Spear, PhD

Part IV: Commission on Adolescent Eating Disorders

Commission Chair

B. Timothy Walsh, MD
William and Joy Ruane Professor of Pediatric Psychopharmacology, College of Physicians and Surgeons, Columbia University
Director of the Division of Clinical Therapeutics, New York State Psychiatric Institute

Commission Members (Second Edition)

Evelyn Attia, MD
Professor of Psychiatry at Columbia University Medical Center
Professor of Clinical Psychiatry at Weill Cornell Medical College
Director, Eating Disorders Research Program, New York State Psychiatric Institute
Director, Columbia Center for Eating Disorders, Columbia University Medical Center

Anne E. Becker, MD, PhD, SM
Maude and Lillian Presley Professor of Global Health and Social Medicine, Harvard Medical School
Founding Director, Eating Disorders Clinical and Research Program, Department of Psychiatry, Massachusetts General Hospital

Cynthia M. Bulik, PhD, FAED
Distinguished Professor, Eating Disorders, Department of Psychiatry, University of North Carolina at Chapel Hill
Founding Director, Center of Excellence for Eating Disorders, University of North Carolina at Chapel Hill
Professor, Department of Medical Epidemiology and Biostatistics, Karolinska Institutet, Stockholm, Sweden

Alison E. Field, ScD
Professor and Chair, Department of Epidemiology, Brown University School of Public Health
Director, Center for Population Health and Clinical Epidemiology
Professor of Pediatrics, Department of Pediatrics, Hasbro Children's Hospital

Neville H. Golden, MD
The Marron and Mary Elizabeth Kendrick Professor of Pediatrics, Chief, Division of Adolescent Medicine and Director of the Adolescent Medicine Fellowship Program, Stanford University School of Medicine

Richard E. Kreipe, MD, FAAP, FSAM, FAED
Dr. Elizabeth R. McAnarney Professor in Pediatrics funded by Roger and Carolyn Friedlander, Division of Adolescent Medicine, Department of Pediatrics, Golisano Children's Hospital, University of Rochester Medical Center
Rochester Director, New York State ACT for Youth Center of Excellence
Medical Director, Western New York Comprehensive Care Center for Eating Disorders

Daniel Le Grange, PhD
Benioff UCSF Professor in Children's Health, Eating Disorders Director, Department of Psychiatry and UCSF Weill Institute for Neurosciences, University of California, San Francisco

James E. Mitchell, MD
Chester Fritz Distinguished University Professor Emeritus University of North Dakota

Kathleen M. Pike, PhD
Professor of Psychology, Departments of Psychiatry and Epidemiology
Director, Global Mental Health Program & Associate Director, Health and Aging Policy Fellowship
Columbia University Medical Center

Robyn Sysko, PhD
Assistant Professor of Psychiatry, Icahn School of Medicine at Mount Sinai, Mount Sinai Hospital, New York

C. Barr Taylor, MD
Professor of Psychiatry (Emeritus), Stanford University
Research Professor, Palo Alto University
Director, Center for m2Health, Palo Alto University

With Contributions From
Patricia E. Dunne
Department of Counseling and Clinical Psychology, Columbia University, USA

Commission Members (First Edition)
Cynthia M. Bulik, PhD, FAED
Christopher G. Fairburn, DM, FRCPsych, FMedSci
Neville H. Golden, MD
Katherine A. Halmi, MD
David B. Herzog, MD
Allan S. Kaplan, MD, FRCP
Richard E. Kreipe, MD, FAAP, FSAM, FAED
James E. Mitchell, MD
Kathleen M. Pike, PhD
Eric Stice, PhD
Ruth H. Striegel-Moore, PhD
C. Barr Taylor, MD
Thomas A. Wadden, PhD
G. Terence Wilson, PhD

With Contributions From
Meghan L. Butryn, MS
Eric B. Chesley, DO
Michael P. Levine, PhD
Marion P. Russell, MD

Commission Coordinator
Robyn Sysko, PhD

Part V: Commission on Adolescent Substance and Alcohol Abuse

Commission Chair
Charles P. O'Brien, MD, PhD
Kenneth E. Appel Professor of Psychiatry, Department of Psychiatry, University of Pennsylvania
Founding Director, Center for Studies of Addiction, University of Pennsylvania

Commission Members (Second Edition)

James Anthony, PhD
Professor, Epidemiology and Biostatistics, Michigan State University

Hui Cheng
Doctoral Candidate, Michigan State University

Brian Fairman, PhD
Fellow, Department of Mental Health, Johns Hopkins Bloomberg School of Public Health

Daniel Romer, PhD
Director of Research, Annenberg Public Policy Center, University of Pennsylvania

Claudia Szobot, MD, PhD
Child and Adolescent Psychiatric Service, Hospital de Clínicas de Porto Alegre, Brazil

Gary L. Wenk, PhD
Professor, Departments of Psychology & Neuroscience and Director, Neuroscience Undergraduate Programs, The Ohio State University

With Contributions From

Richard Spoth, PhD
F. Wendell Miller Senior Prevention Scientist, and Director, Partnerships in Prevention Science Institute at Iowa State University

Commission Members (First Edition)

James C. Anthony, PhD
Kathleen Carroll, PhD
Anna Rose Childress, PhD
Charles Dackis, MD
Guy Diamond, PhD
Robert Hornik, PhD
Lloyd D. Johnston, PhD
Reese Jones, MD
George F. Koob, PhD
Thomas Korsten, MD
Caryn Lerman, PhD
A. Thomas McLellan, PhD
Howard Moss, MD
Helen Pettinati, PhD
Richard Spoth, PhD

Part VI: Commission on Adolescent Suicide Prevention

Commission Chair

Herbert Hendin, MD
CEO and Medical Director, Suicide Prevention Initiatives

Commission Members (Second Edition)

Ann P. Haas, PhD
Senior Consultant, American Foundation for Suicide Prevention

Jill Harkavy-Friedman, PhD
Vice President of Research, American Foundation for Suicide Prevention
Associate Professor of Clinical Psychology (in Psychiatry), Columbia University

Maggie G. Mortali, MPH
Director, Interactive Screening Program, American Foundation for Suicide Prevention

Commission Members (First Edition)

David A. Brent, MD
Jack R. Cornelius, MD, MPH
Tamera Coyne-Beasley, MD, MPH
Ted Greenberg, MPH
Madelyn Gould, PhD, MPH
Ann Pollinger Haas, PhD
Jill Harkavy-Friedman, PhD
Richard Harrington, MD, FRC Psych
Gregg Henriques, PhD
Douglas G. Jacobs, MD
John Kalafat, PhD
Mary Margaret Kerr, EdD
Cheryl A. King, PhD
Richard Ramsay, MSW
David Shaffer, FRCP, FRC Psych
Anthony Spirito, PhD
Howard Sudak, MD
Elaine Adams Thompson, PhD, RN

Commission Coordinator

Ann Pollinger Haas, PhD

Part VII: Commission on Positive Youth Development

Commission Chair

Martin E. P. Seligman, PhD
Zellerbach Family Professor of Psychology, University of Pennsylvania
Director, Positive Psychology Network
Scientific Director, Values-in-Action Classification of Strengths and Virtues Project, Mayerson Foundation

Commission Members (Second Edition)

Margaret L. Kern, PhD
Senior Lecturer, Centre for Positive Psychology, Melbourne Graduate School of Education, University of Melbourne, Australia

Nansook Park, PhD
Professor, Psychology, University of Michigan
Director, Michigan Positive Psychology Center

Daniel Romer, PhD
Director, Adolescent of Research, Annenberg Public Policy Center, University of Pennsylvania

Commission Members (First Edition)

Marvin W. Berkowitz, PhD
Richard F. Catalano, PhD
William Damon, PhD
Jacquelynne S. Eccles, PhD
Jane E. Gillham, PhD
Kristin A. Moore, PhD
Heather Johnston Nicholson, PhD
Nansook Park, PhD
David L. Penn, PhD
Christopher Peterson, PhD
Margaret Shih, PhD
Tracy A. Steen, PhD
Robert J. Sternberg, PhD
Joseph P. Tierney, MA
Roger P. Weissberg, PhD
Jonathan F. Zaff, PhD

Commission Coordinator **Tracy Steen, PhD**

Part VIII: Other Behavioral Disorders

Amy Bleakley, PhD, MPH
Senior Research Scientist, Annenberg School for Communication, University of Pennsylvania

Jeffrey L. Derevensky, PhD
Chair, Department of Educational and Counselling Psychology, International Centre for Youth Gambling Problems and High-Risk Behaviors, McGill University

Lynette Gilbeau, BEd
International Centre for Youth Gambling Problems and High-Risk Behaviors, McGill University

Sunhee Park, PhD, MPH, RN
Associate Professor, College of Nursing Science, Kyung Hee University

Daniel Romer, PhD
Director of Research, Annenberg Public Policy Center, University of Pennsylvania

Part IX: Summary of Conclusions, Recommendations, Priorities

John Cacciola, PhD
Treatment Research Institute, Philadelphia, Pennsylvania

Ka Ho Brian Chor, PhD
Chapin Hall at the University of Chicago

Kimberly E. Hoagwood, PhD
Cathy and Stephen Graham Professor of Child and Adolescent Psychiatry, Center for Mental Health Implementation and Dissemination Science in States for Children, Adolescents, and Families (IDEAS Center), New York University Child Study Center, Department of Child and Adolescent Psychiatry, New York University School of Medicine
New York State Office of Mental Health

Patrick E. Jamieson, PhD
Director, Adolescent Risk Communication Institute, Annenberg Public Policy Center, University of Pennsylvania

Kathleen Meyers, PhD
Treatment Research Institute, Philadelphia, Pennsylvania

Su-Chin Serene Olin, PhD
Center for Mental Health Implementation and Dissemination Science in States for Children, Adolescents, and Families (IDEAS Center), New York University Child Study Center, Department of Child and Adolescent Psychiatry, New York University School of Medicine

Daniel Romer, PhD
Director of Research, Annenberg Public Policy Center, University of Pennsylvania

Suzanne Ward
Treatment Research Institute, Philadelphia, Pennsylvania

Abigail Woodworth
Treatment Research Institute, Philadelphia, Pennsylvania

Preface

We are pleased to present this updated version of our award-winning volume. Thanks go to the editors who organized this update, and the many others who contributed to it. We also thank Timothy Walsh, who reviewed the entire volume and provided a new introduction to this edition.

We originally intended to release the volume in 2014, but with the introduction of the new *Diagnostic and Statistical Manual of Mental Disorders* (DSM-5) in 2013, we felt it wise to incorporate the changes that were made to that important resource. This volume takes note of those changes while also keeping a focus on the most recent advances in the treatment and prevention of common and difficult disorders of adolescence. We hope this updated volume continues to fulfill our aim of informing practitioners and researchers of the successes achieved and the challenges that remain in ensuring the well-being and health of the nation's youth.

We wish to thank the Sunnylands Trust. It was the Trust's generous funding and its president Leonore Annenberg's vision that originally enabled the Annenberg Public Policy Center to organize the seven commissions that are represented in this volume. That commitment by Mrs. Annenberg and Sunnyland trustees Diana and Lee Deshong to furthering the mental and behavioral health of our youth inspires us as we continue this effort. In addition, to this volume, we have also released four trade books for parents and six for youth regarding best practices for treating and preventing many of the disorders discussed here. We plan on introducing new volumes in that series as well as updating the ones previously released.

Finally, we thank Oxford University Press, and in particular Joan Bossert and Lynnee Argabright, who coordinated the many activities that went into orchestrating this revision. It is their talents, perseverance, and good humor that brought forth the hundreds of pages in this new volume. We also note that this volume will be freely available online after one year, so that no barriers will stand in the way of its dissemination. We thank Oxford's leadership for agreeing to this arrangement.

Kathleen Hall Jamieson
Director, Annenberg Public Policy Center
University of Pennsylvania

Daniel Romer
Research Director
Annenberg Public Policy Center
University of Pennsylvania

Introduction

B. Timothy Walsh

Adolescence is a critical developmental period biologically, psychologically, and socially. It is also a time of life during which many of the most serious mental disorders emerge—about one quarter of youth will experience a mental illness over the course of a year (Merikangas, Nakamura, & Kessler, 2009). This high rate underscores the critical need to understand the origins of mental disorders and to develop effective treatment and prevention interventions. As did the first edition, this second edition of *Treating and Preventing Adolescent Mental Health Disorders* aims to provide, in a single volume, a comprehensive review of current knowledge of serious mental health problems affecting adolescents, as well as efforts to enhance positive youth development. We again focus on six specific problem areas—mood disorders, anxiety disorders, substance abuse, eating disorders, suicide, and schizophrenia—as these typically first emerge during adolescence and, among many individuals, continue into adulthood. In the 10-plus years since the publication of the first edition, several developments have altered how these disorders are characterized and understood. The final section of the book describes emerging information on gambling and excessive Internet use, phenomena that have been termed "behavioral addictions," and provides updated reviews of policy areas and broad recommendations for change that have the potential to improve adolescent mental health on a wide scale.

The sections focused on specific disorders review the major impact of the publication of the fifth edition of the *Diagnostic and Statistical Manual of Mental Disorders* (DSM-5) in 2013 on the description and conceptualization of these disorders. Among a number of important changes, DSM-5 eliminated the opening section of DSM-IV, Disorders Usually First Diagnosed in Infancy, Childhood, or Adolescence, in recognition of the fact that *most* psychiatric illnesses begin early in life and frequently continue into adulthood. The disorders in that section were distributed to thematically relevant sections in DSM-5. For example, the Feeding and Eating Disorders of Infancy or Early Childhood of DSM-IV (i.e., Pica, Rumination Disorder, and Feeding Disorder of Infancy or Early Childhood) were combined with the Eating Disorder section of DSM-IV to make up Feeding and Eating Disorders in DSM-5. Similarly, Separation Anxiety Disorder and Selective Mutism were moved into the section on Anxiety Disorders. In contrast, Posttraumatic Stress Disorder (PTSD) was relocated to a new section, Trauma- and Stress-Related Disorders, and Obsessive-Compulsive Disorder (OCD) to another new section, Obsessive-Compulsive and Related Disorders. One of the potentially most important changes in DSM-5 relevant to youth was the addition of a newly described disorder, Disruptive Mood Dysregulation Disorder, to the Depressive Disorders section of DSM-5, in hopes of providing clarity about presentations in some ways resembling Bipolar Disorder. In the DSM-5 section on Substance-Related and Addictive Disorders, the distinction between substance abuse and substance dependence was eliminated because of strong evidence that the relevant phenomena are more usefully viewed as occurring on a continuum. These and other changes to the diagnostic nomenclature are reviewed in this edition.

The years since the first edition have witnessed dramatic growth in investigators' ability to safely and noninvasively observe brain structure and function in awake adolescents and adults, using magnetic resonance imaging

(MRI), functional MRI, magnetic resonance spectroscopy, and electrophysiology. Emerging findings from these techniques are highlighted in this edition. For example, neuroimaging studies of young people with mood disorders have documented alterations in areas of the brain known to be involved in emotional regulation. Studies of youth with anxiety disorders have begun to explore changes in activity in areas that process information related to potential threats in the environment. Given the profound and clinically impairing neurocognitive deficits characteristic of schizophrenia, substantial effort has been devoted to assessing brain activity during the performance of cognitive tasks, such as those assessing attention and working memory, and to understanding how such changes evolve during adolescence among individuals at high risk.

At least arguably, our fundamental understanding of pathophysiological mechanisms and of disturbances in neural circuitry is clearest for substance use disorders. Research in this area has benefited from the availability of useful animal models and from extensive research in both animals and humans on the brain reward mechanisms, especially those involving mesolimbic dopamine. Recent work, examining both psychological and biological characteristics, aims at elucidating the impact of substance use on the developing brain and understanding why some individuals are more vulnerable; notably, although many adolescents experiment with drugs, relatively few develop substance use disorders.

Other new information relevant to investigators, clinicians, and policymakers has emerged. Epidemiological studies published in the past decade convincingly document that mood disturbances—which were once thought simply *not* to impact children and adolescents—affect a substantial minority, and that evidence of vulnerability may be observed before puberty. Recent studies continue to document a substantial frequency among adolescents of syndromes resembling adult bipolar disorder, but the nature and characteristics of bipolar disorder, as it appears during adolescence, remain subjects of some controversy and considerable debate. Recent treatment research has buttressed prior evidence regarding the efficacy of selective serotonin reuptake inhibitors (SSRIs) and of psychotherapy, especially cognitive-behavioral therapy and interpersonal therapy, for mood disturbances. There has been increasing focus on more complicated questions such as when and how they should be combined and on identifying what factors predict response to which treatments. Similarly, for many of the anxiety disorders, rigorous randomized trials have documented the benefits of specific forms of psychotherapy and of SSRIs, benefits that, at the time of the first edition, had been assumed to occur but had not been documented. Strong evidence has been developed since the first edition demonstrating that the active involvement of the family can be a critical therapeutic element in the treatment of adolescents with eating disorders and also for adolescents with substance abuse.

The identification and treatment of substance use disorders among adolescents remain high priorities, given that most affected adults began to abuse drugs as youths. Important epidemiological shifts are occurring in the United States. Likely related to the increasing legalization of marijuana, and to decreases in use of both alcohol and cigarettes, marijuana use among youth is now more prevalent than cigarette smoking. An increased number of emergencies associated with marijuana use and a decline in concerns about the risks of marijuana emphasize a need for better education and early intervention.

There is growing evidence that preventive interventions are of use. Universal prevention, aiming to benefit an entire population and reduce or even eliminate the initial development of clinical symptoms, is the ultimate goal. However, the resources required to develop and test such programs are daunting, and, from a theoretical perspective, it is not clear that a universal approach is best suited to the prevention of disorders that, while all too common, affect a minority of adolescents. Therefore, many prevention efforts are selective or indicated, focusing on high-risk youth and/or individuals who have already begun to develop symptoms. Growing evidence suggests that such targeted strategies, particularly those based on cognitive and familial interventions, have promise for the prevention of mood, eating, and anxiety disorders. In addition, there is intense and growing interest in the identification of individuals with prodromal psychosis, and the development of psychotherapeutic and pharmacological interventions to prevent progression to schizophrenia or, for those who have experienced a psychotic episode, recurrence.

Suicide among youth has increased markedly in the past 50 years and is the third leading cause of death among adolescents. The origins of suicidal behavior are multifactorial and include the presence of psychiatric disorders; recent evidence has also documented links to bullying and harassment by peers. The past decade has witnessed increased involvement of schools and school personnel in prevention efforts as well as the development of programs to identify previously unidentified youth at risk. However, many challenges persist, such as the expense of such programs and relatively poor rates of follow-through with treatment recommendations once individuals at high risk have been identified.

A novel and important element of the first edition was the inclusion of a chapter on positive youth development. As described in this edition, this approach has been increasingly studied and implemented in the past decade. While the problem-focused chapters review prevention efforts aimed at specific disorders, the chapter on positive youth development notes that targeting a single problem may miss an opportunity for a more integrated and more broadly effective approach. Evidence acquired since the first edition documents growing support for the utility of this approach, and its potential value in enhancing both physical and psychological health and educational achievement. However, clear challenges remain, for example in successful implementation in economically disadvantaged communities.

New to this edition are chapters on gambling disorder and on Internet addiction. These reflect an emerging interest in "behavioral addictions," patterns of behavior that bear strong similarities to substance use disorders (e.g., persistent and excessive time committed to the behaviors, leading to interference with other activities; reluctance to disclose the level of involvement to others, including parents). It has been suggested that such behavioral addictions engage and distort the central reward-processing networks in a similar fashion to abused substances. We do not know precisely how to understand such phenomena and how they fit into the range of behaviors that individuals may find rewarding and to which they may devote substantial time and money (e.g., sex, exercise, shopping, work). Reflecting such uncertainties and the amount of peer-reviewed research, Gambling Disorder was officially recognized in DSM-IV (as Pathological Gambling) and was moved to the section retitled Substance-Related and Addictive Disorders in DSM-5, but Internet Gaming Disorder is included only in the DSM-5 section on Conditions for Further Study.

As did the first edition, this volume focuses not only on "what do we know?" but, importantly, also on "how do we implement change?" A thoroughly updated chapter on policy and practice highlights the impact of rapid changes that are under way in the delivery of healthcare in the United States. Major efforts are occurring at the state level to ensure that the mental health care of children and adolescents uses established evidence-based practices. At the federal level, groundbreaking legislation, including the Affordable Care Act, is producing profound changes in the infrastructure and financing of mental health care. The Affordable Care Act, combined with the passage of the Mental Health Parity and Addiction Equity Act, has the potential to have a major impact on the availability of treatment services for youth with mental disorders. In addition, standalone mental health centers are being replaced by facilities providing both medical and behavioral treatment. Research funding, for example from the recently established Patient-Centered Outcomes Research Institute, is increasingly focused on issues surrounding dissemination. These major shifts in healthcare policy and delivery have potentially profound implications regarding the mental health care of adolescents. As this volume goes to press in 2017, the implications of the recent national U.S. elections regarding these policies and developments are unclear but worrisome.

Finally, we note that there have been a number of changes to the list of contributors to this volume. Many of the contributors were re-enlisted, including all of the Annenberg Commission Chairs who provided leadership for the first edition. However, recent developments in the field, the inclusion of new topics, and the need for additional expertise led to some alterations in the contributors. We hope that the extensive efforts and hard work of all who contributed to the first and/or to the second edition will provide a foundation for advancing our understanding of, and enhance our ability to treat and to prevent, adolescent mental health disorders.

Depression and Bipolar Disorder

COMMISSION ON ADOLESCENT DEPRESSION AND BIPOLAR DISORDER

Dwight L. Evans, *Commission Chair*

Second Edition

William Beardslee
Tami Benton
David Brent
W. Edward Craighead
Paul Crits-Christoph
Marivel Davila
Robert Findling
Robert Johnson
Charles Nemeroff
Rachel Neuhut
Moira Rynn
Karen Dineen Wagner
Myrna Weissman

First Edition

William Beardslee
Joseph Biederman
David Brent
Dennis Charney
Joseph Coyle
W. Edward Craighead
Paul Crits-Christoph
Robert Findling
Judy Garber
Robert Johnson
Martin Keller
Charles Nemeroff
Moira A. Rynn
Karen Wagner
Myrna Weissman
Elizabeth Weller

part

Defining Depression and Bipolar Disorder

Rachel Neuhut
Tami Benton
Paul Crits-Christoph
Marivel Davila
Myrna Weissman
Charles Nemeroff

chapter 1

INTRODUCTION

The etiology of mood disorders involves a complex, multifactorial model (e.g., Akiskal & McKinney, 1975; Cicchetti & Toth, 1998; Kendler, Gardner, & Prescott, 2002). No single risk factor accounts for all or even most of the variance. The most likely causal model will include individual biological and psychological diatheses that interact with various environmental stressors. There is little question that early-onset, like adult-onset, major depressive disorder (MDD) is highly recurrent, whether the data derive from clinical samples (Kovacs, 1994), long-term population studies (Kessler & Walters, 1998), studies of high school students (Lewinsohn et al., 1998), or depressed patients (Garber et al., 1988; Rao et al., 1995). Over 50% of depressed adolescents had a recurrence within 5 years (Birmaher et al., 1996; Lewinsohn et al., 2000), although only small portions continue to have significant psychopathology in any one year. The few studies of depressed adolescents followed into adulthood show strong continuity between adolescent and adult depression (Frombonne et al., 2001; Harrington et al., 1990, 1998; Weissman et al., 1999a, 1999b), as well as an increased rate of suicide attempts and psychiatric and medical hospitalization, and studies of prepubertal depression show continuity onto adolescence (Kovacs, 1994). The most serious outcome is suicide, which is the third leading cause of death among adolescents. The recent *Healthy People 2020: A Report Card on the Health of the Nation* described how major depressive episodes in adolescents predict worsening outcomes and suicide deaths in adolescents; the rates have been increasing over time (2014).

Other outcomes include lack of social development and skills, withdrawal from peers, poor school performance, less-than-optimal career and marriage choices, and substance abuse (Frost et al., 1999; Rao et al., 1995, 1999; Weissman et al., 1999a).

This first chapter reviews the epidemiology, the definition of the disorder, psychological factors, social factors, and biological factors that have been shown to increase the risk of mood disorders in children and adolescents. Two major developments have taken place since the publication of the previous edition of this volume, which include new population-based studies as well as the publication of the DSM-5. The previous edition of this book reported epidemiologic data based on studies of adults and extrapolated rates for youth from retrospective reports of age of onset. Since the preparation of the original report, a number of large-scale, population-based studies of children and adolescents have been conducted.

The DSM-5 was published in May 2013, and therefore no epidemiologic studies have yet used DSM-5 criteria. This chapter will present these new data directly derived from U.S. epidemiologic studies of youth either nationally or based on a selected community/school and will update risk factors and speculate on the implications of DSM-5 changes.

Table 1.1 lists the relevant national and community/school-based studies reviewed in this chapter.

MAJOR DEPRESSION

Overview

For many years, children and adolescents were considered theoretically incapable of experiencing depression due to the psychoanalytic concept of the underdeveloped superego. Thus, depression was considered "an adult disease." However, case reports as early as the 17th century have described adolescents exhibiting symptoms resembling those observed in adults with depressive disorders. The National Institute of Mental Health (NIMH) convened a meeting of thought leaders in 1975, followed by a book published by Shulterbrant and Ruskin, that finally made the diagnosis of depression acceptable in this population.

The past two decades have produced a radical change in understanding the age of onset of mood disorders. MDD is no longer seen primarily as a disorder of the middle-aged and elderly. Epidemiologic and clinical research from the United States and elsewhere has clearly documented that the age of first onset of major

Table 1.1 National and Community/School-Based Studies (Children and Adolescents)

Study Authors	*Location*	*N*	*Age*	*Diagnostic Interview*	*Period*
National Health and Nutrition Examination Survey (NHANES) (Merikangas et al., 2010a)	National	3,042	8–15	Diagnostic Interview Schedule for Children, Version IV, based on DSM-IV criteria	12-month prevalence
National Comorbidity Survey Replication—Adolescent Supplement NCS—A (Kessler et al., 2012)	National	10,123 (6,483 adolescent–parent pairs)	13–18	Composite International Diagnostic Interview Version 3.0—DSM-IV	Lifetime and 12-month prevalence
Costello et al., 1996, 2003; Great Smoky Mountains Study	North Carolina	1,420 at baseline assessed annually until age 16 over eight waves	9–13	Child and Adolescent Psychiatric Assessment (CAPA)—DSM-III-R; Child and Adolescent Psychiatric Assessment—DSM-IV	3-month prevalence
Lewinsohn et al., 2000; Oregon Adolescent Depression Project Study	Oregon	1,709 (Time 1) 1,507 (Time 2)	14–18	Schedule for Affective Disorders and Schizophrenia for School-Age Children; Longitudinal Interval Follow-up Evaluation	Lifetime and point prevalence
Angold et al., 2002; Caring for Children Study	North Carolina	920	9–17	Child and Adolescent Psychiatric Assessment—DSM-IV	3-month prevalence
Canino et al., 2004	Puerto Rico	1,886	4–17	Diagnostic Interview Schedule for Children, Version IV, based on DSM-IV criteria	12-month prevalence
Roberts et al., 2007; Teen Health 2000 Study	Texas	4,175	11–17	Diagnostic Interview Schedule for Children, Version IV, based on DSM-IV criteria	12-month prevalence

depression is commonly in adolescence and young adulthood and that prepubertal onsets, while less common, do occur. There may be symptoms of depression that manifest as early as preschool age. In a recent longitudinal prospective study of preschool children, the authors concluded that preschool-onset depression is a significant predictor of MDD in later childhood, even after accounting for the effect of maternal history of depression and other risk factors (Luby et al., 2014).

It is also clear that adolescent depression is a chronic, recurrent, and serious illness. The offspring of depressed, as compared to nondepressed, parents have over a twofold to fourfold increased risk of depression. Depressions occurring in adolescents share similar features to depression at other ages, including symptom patterns; a higher rates in females (twofold risk); high comorbidity with anxiety disorders, substance abuse, and suicidal behaviors; and high social, occupational, and educational disability. In contrast, childhood MDD tends to be male predominant and mood reactive and is commonly associated with high levels of irritability and dysphoria and high rates of comorbidity with the disruptive behavior disorders (Biederman et al., 1995; Leibenluft et al., 2003).

The epidemiologic data on bipolar disorder in childhood and adolescence are considerably sparser than for MDD. This is in part based on the earlier beliefs that bipolar disorder begins in adulthood; that it is difficult to assess boundaries between normal mood and mood irritability in youth, especially in community studies; and that the first signs of bipolar disorder are uncertain (Nottelman & Jensen, 1998). Most evidence on juvenile bipolar disorder comes from clinical samples where efforts, especially recently, have been made to characterize early clinical presentations of bipolar disorder.

Unfortunately, until recently, persons under age 18 have been excluded from epidemiologic studies, so empirically based information on prevalence, risk factors, course, and treatment are scanty, especially for bipolar disorder. This situation is changing, but not rapidly enough, because mood disorders in youth have a long-term effect on school, work, marriage, and the next generation. This chapter will highlight the empirical basis for understanding the epidemiology, phenomenology, course, and comorbidity of youth with MDD and bipolar disorder. Because a sharp distinction between childhood and adolescent onset cannot be readily made, information on childhood (prepubertal)-onset disorder will be included when relevant.

Diagnosis: Prepubertal- and Adolescent-Onset Depressive Disorders

Evidence suggests that depressive disorders often present during childhood and that there are distinct differences in depressive disorders that present in prepubertal youth and adolescents (Harrington et al., 1990; Weissman et al., 1999). Evidence further suggests that they may be distinctly different conditions rather than continuous (Kauffman, 2001). While some studies have demonstrated continuity of depression among preschoolers through the early school years (Luby, 2010), and continuity through adolescence (Kovacs et al., 1994), other studies of prepubertally depressed children have not found continuity into adulthood (Copeland et al., 2009; Harrington et al., 1990; Weissman et al., 1999a). As many as 1% to 5% of children and 3% to 8% of adolescents are estimated to be affected by a depressive disorder, with a lifetime prevalence of approximately 20% by the end of adolescence (Costello et al., 2003; Lewinsohn et al., 1998; Reinherz et al., 1993).

In contrast to adolescent-onset disorders, childhood-onset depressive disorders are characterized by male predominance, or gender equivalence, and are commonly comorbid with other neurodevelopmental disorders and disruptive impulse control disorders (Biederman et al., 1995; Birmaher et al., 1996; Costello et al., 1996; Egger & Angold, 2006; Rutter, 1996). Pubertal status has been shown to be a strong predictor for the emergence of major depression in girls (Angold et al., 1998).

Another feature of pediatric-onset depression that differs from adult-onset depression is the frequent presentation of irritable rather than depressed mood. The occurrence of irritability associated with disruptive behaviors among prepubertal youths with depression is so common that it has been a focus of much investigation. In the recent past, many practitioners viewed the persistent irritability present in prepubertal depression as characteristic of bipolar disorder, despite requirements for a discrete manic or hypomanic episode as defined by the DSM-IV and DSM-5. By combining these two distinct presentations (persistent, nonepisodic irritable mood and the discrete episodes of mania occurring with classical bipolar disorder), excessively high rates of pediatric bipolar disorder were reported. To strengthen diagnostic clarity and discrimination from bipolar disorder, a new diagnostic category, disruptive mood dysregulation disorder (DMDD), was established in DSM-5. This new category will capture children who present with the hallmark symptoms of severe, nonepisodic irritability. Although the prevalence estimates of this disorder in the community are unclear, the overall 6-month to 1-year period prevalence rates among children and adolescents are estimated to be 2% to 5%. It appears to be male predominant, persistent, impairing, and associated with later development of depression and anxiety disorders in adulthood (DSM-5; Axelson, Birmaher, Strober, et al., 2011; Axelson et al., 2012; Liebenluft, 2011).

DMDD is typified by the following:

- Chronic, severe, persistent irritability manifesting as frequent verbal or behavioral outbursts (aggression against others, self or property) occurring at least three times per week, over the course of one year.
- The outbursts must be developmentally inappropriate and occur in at least two settings such as home or school. The other required manifestation of severe irritability is its persistence between the severe temper outbursts. The angry or irritable mood must be present most of the day, nearly every day and evident to others.
- The onset of this disorder must occur prior to 10 years of age and should not be applied to children whose developmental age is less than 6 years or after 18 years.
- There cannot be more than one day during which mania/hypomania has been present or during an episode of depression or another mental disorder and cannot co-occur with oppositional defiant disorder, intermittent explosive disorder, or bipolar disorder.

This diagnosis should not be given if the criteria for a manic/hypomanic episode have ever been met and it cannot be explained by another medical condition or substance. If DMDD occurs in the presence of oppositional defiant disorder (ODD) or intermittent explosive disorder, then the diagnosis of DMDD should be given. Distinguishing features of DMDD in comparison to intermittent explosive disorder are the absence of disruptive mood between episodes and duration of only 3 months compared with the 12 months required for DMDD.

The prevalence of dysthymic disorders, now classified as persistent depressive disorder, has been less well studied among children and adolescents. The few existing studies suggest a prevalence of 0.6% to 1.7% among prepubertal children and 1.6% to 8.0% among adolescents (Birmaher, 1996).

Studies examining prepubertally affected youths with depression are conflicting. While some studies demonstrate higher rates of MDD among prepubertal boys compared with girls, other studies (Spencer et al., 1999) suggest that higher male than female representation in prepubertal MDD was due to the comorbidity with attention-deficit/hyperactivity disorder (ADHD); youth without this comorbidity had a similar gender representation before and after puberty. Studies suggest that prepubertally depressed children often grow up to have a variety of psychiatric disorders, especially increased rates of bipolar, anxiety, and substance use disorders (Kovacs et al., 1996; Weissman et al., 1999).

Among preschoolers, comorbidities of ADHD, ODD, and anxiety have been found with depression (Eggar & Angold, 2006). These findings add to a growing literature that suggests that the observed associations between disorders may in fact represent overlap among disorders. Investigation has focused upon understanding whether depressive disorders among prepubertal children represent a state of pervasive emotional and behavioral dysregulation that might represent a different syndrome from the syndrome of depression seen later in development (Egger & Angold, 2006).

Diagnostic Criteria for Depressive Disorders

MDD

The same criteria defined in the DSM-5 for adults are used for adolescents, as follows:

> Five or more of the following symptoms must be present nearly every day during the same 2-week period, representing a marked change in function in order to diagnose an adolescent with a major depressive episode:
>
> - Depressed or irritable mood most of the day
> - Markedly diminished interest or pleasure in almost all activities, most of the day
> - Weight loss or weight gain or increase/decrease in appetite or for children, failure to make weight gains
> - Insomnia or hypersomnia
> - Psychomotor agitation or retardation
> - Fatigue or loss of energy
> - Feelings of inappropriate guilt or hope lessness
> - Indecisiveness or diminished ability to concentrate
> - Recurrent thoughts of death or suicidal ideation, suicide attempt or a specific plan
>
> Depressed or irritable mood or markedly diminished interest or pleasure in almost all activities must be present, and must represent a clear change in affect, cognition and neurovegetative functions from the adolescent's usual state. The symptoms must cause clinical impairment in important areas of functioning and cannot be due to the direct physiological effect of substance abuse or a general medical condition. There cannot ever have been a manic/hypomanic episode and it cannot be accounted for by bereavement or schizoaffective disorder. A major depressive episode cannot be superimposed on schizophrenia, schizophreniform disorder, delusional disorder, specified and unspecified schizophrenia spectrum, and other psychotic disorders. When recording the diagnosis of depression, one should include whether it is a single or recurrent episode and a severity specifier, mild, moderate or severe. When describing depressive disorders, greater specificity and clarity of risk and prognostic factors may be obtained by specifying accompanying features. For example, "with melancholic features" applies if there is an almost complete loss of pleasure in almost all activities, including previous highly desired events that would normally generate brightened mood, in addition to at least three of the following:
>
> - Depressed mood characterized by profound despondency, despair, or moroseness or by "empty mood"
> - Depression is typically worse in the morning
> - Morning waking at least 2 hours before usual waking (early morning)
> - Change in psychomotor activity (retardation or agitation)
> - Weight loss or anorexia
> - Guilt that is inappropriate or excessive
>
> If hallucinations or delusional thoughts are present, then the "psychotic features" specifiers should be used in reference to the mood congruency (consistent with depressive themes) or incongruency (not involving typical themes of inadequacy) of those psychotic features. In addition to psychotic features, catatonia may be associated with depressive disorders, and is defined by three or more of the following psychomotor symptoms:
>
> - Waxy flexibility, catalepsy, or stupor
> - Motor overactivity that is purposeless and not in response to external stimuli

- Negativism or mutism
- Peculiarities of movement (posturing, grimacing, stereotypy, and mannerisms)
- Echolalia or echopraxia

When depression is accompanied by high levels of anxiety, the specifier "with anxious distress" should be used. In addition, the following must be present:

- Feeling tense or keyed up
- Feeling unusually restless
- Difficulty concentrating because of worry
- Fear that something awful may happen
- Feeling that the individual might lose control of himself or herself

"With mixed features" should be used if manic or hypomanic symptoms are present with at least three of the following:

- Elevated or expansive mood
- Inflated self-esteem or grandiosity
- More talkative than usual or pressure to keep talking
- Flight of ideas or subjective experience that thoughts are racing
- Increase in energy or goal-directed activities that have a high potential for painful consequences
- Decreased need for sleep

When mood brightens during positive events, called "mood reactivity," the "atypical features" specifier should be used. Two or more of the following must be present:

- Significant weight gain or increase in appetite
- Heavy leaden feeling in arms and legs
- A longstanding pattern of interpersonal rejection, not occurring exclusively during the mood episode, that results in occupational and social impairment
- Hypersomnia

Depressive disorders may also present in a seasonal pattern in children and adolescents. Diagnostic challenges may be imposed by the frequent predictable seasonal stressors that occur during particular times of the year, for adolescents, such as the start of the new school year. Furthermore, a major depressive episode can present initially as seasonal affective disorder in children and adolescents. To establish the presence of a seasonal mood disorder, there must be a regular temporal relationship between the mood disorder (depression or mania) and a particular time of the year. A full remission or switching from depression to mania must occur within that particular time of the year. There must be at least two episodes of mood disturbance during the last 2 years and the seasonal episodes must outnumber nonseasonal episodes. This specifier does not apply when a predictable psychosocial stressor, such as the start of the school year, is an explanatory factor.

The specifier "with peripartum onset" should be considered in female adolescents when the onset of depression occurs during pregnancy or within 4 weeks of giving birth.

Dysthymia

Persistent depressive disorder (dysthymia) is a chronic illness often beginning insidiously during childhood, adolescence, and young adulthood. It is commonly comorbid with ADHD and conduct disorder. Predisposing factors are early parental loss or separation, and a chaotic home environment. Kovacs et al. (1984) report that children with persistent depressive disorder (dysthymic) are at risk for developing depression and mania on follow-up. Adolescents who have persistent depressive disorder and who subsequently develop a major depressive episode should be diagnosed with persistent depressive disorder with the specifier "intermittent major depressive episode." Several features distinguish persistent depressive disorder from major depression in children and adolescents.

Dysthymia, a diagnosis that was often undetected in adolescents, has been consolidated with chronic major depressive disorder into a new diagnostic category, Persistent Depressive Disorder. This disorder is defined in adolescents as depressed or irritable mood which must be present for a year or longer and the youth must never be symptom-free for more than 2 months. During the depressive episode, two or more of the following symptoms must be present:

- Increase or decrease in appetite
- Increased or decreased sleep
- Decrease in energy or fatigue
- Low self-esteem
- Poor concentration or difficulty with decision making
- Hopelessness

With this disorder, criteria for a major depressive episode may be continually present for 1 year. Major depressive episode may precede Persistent Depressive Disorder and may occur during persistent depressive disorder. Persistent Depressive Disorder (dysthymia) should not be diagnosed if it is a direct result of a substance or medication, is a general medical condition, or is occurring during the course of a psychotic disorder. Persistent Depressive Disorder utilizes the same specifiers as depressive disorders. Specifiers exclusive to this disorder are:

1. with pure dysthymic syndrome, suggesting that full criteria for a major depressive episode have not been met in at least the preceding 1 year;
2. with persistent major depressive episode: MDE criteria have been met in the preceding 1-year period;
3. with intermittent major depressive episodes, with current episode, meaning that full criteria for major depression are currently met, but there have been subthreshold symptoms for at least 8 weeks in the preceding year;
4. with intermittent major depressive episodes, without current episode, meaning that full MDE criteria are not currently met but there has been an episode of MDD in the preceding 1 year.

It should be further specified if onset is early (before 21 years) or late (after 21 years).

Premenstrual Dysphoric Disorder

The core features of this disorder are the occurrence of irritability, mood lability, anxiety, and dysphoric mood, occurring consistently during the premenstrual phase of the menstrual cycle and remitting proximal to the period of menses. The symptoms must have occurred in most of the cycles during the past year and must impact social and occupational functioning. Prevalence estimates for 12 months suggest that 1.8% to 5.8% of women are affected by this disorder. Limited data exist regarding the prevalence of this disorder among adolescents. MDD is the most commonly associated premorbid condition among women presenting with premenstrual dysphoric disorder.

Bereavement Exclusion

Depressive symptoms lasting less than 2 months after the death of a loved one (referred to as the *bereavement exclusion*) was excluded in DSM-5 for a number of reasons, including the recognition that bereavement usually lasts 1 to 2 years. A comprehensive footnote has replaced the DSM-IV exclusion to assist clinicians in deciding whether symptoms are consistent with normal bereavement versus those of MDD. Specific to children and adolescents, this change is not expected to impact rates of depression greatly.

Summary of Implications of DSM-5 Changes in Criteria

A number of changes specific to depressive disorders were made in DSM-5, but as noted above no epidemiologic studies have yet included these changes. We can only speculate on the changes their incorporation will make on rates.

1. Due to concern about overdiagnosis of bipolar disorder in children, disruptive mood dysregulation disorder has been included for children up to age 18 years who report frequent episodes of extreme behavioral dyscontrol and persistent irritability.
2. Premenstrual dysphoric disorder has been moved from Appendix B, "Criteria Sets and Axes Provided for Further Study," to the main body of DSM-5.
3. Persistent depressive disorder replaces what was referred to as dysthymia, a mild but chronic form of depression in DSM-IV.
4. Within a major depressive episode, the presence of at least three manic symptoms has now been recognized by the specifier "with mixed features."
5. The bereavement exclusion was excluded in DSM-5.
6. A new specifier signifying the presence of mixed symptoms has been included across both bipolar and depressive disorders.

Epidemiology

Previously, epidemiologic data from community surveys directly studying children and adolescents were sparse due to the long-held view that MDD was rare before adulthood or a self-limiting and normal part of growing up. There are now a number of national as well as community studies specific to depression and dysthymia in children and adolescents.

Major Depression

National Studies

Table 1.2 reports the results from national samples of studies conducted among children and adolescents specific to depression.

The 2001–2004 National Health and Nutrition Examination Survey (NHANES) reported 12-month prevalence estimates for 3,042 participants ages 8 to 15 years based on DSM-IV criteria (Merikangas, He, Brody, Fisher, Bourdon, & Koretz, 2010a), with results broken down by gender and age. Specific to major depression, girls had a significantly higher prevalence than boys (3.7% vs. 1.8%, respectively, $\chi^2 = 4.65$, $p = .04$). Children ages 12 to 15 years also had a significantly higher 12-month prevalence than children ages 8 to 11 years (3.8% vs. 1.6%, respectively, $\chi^2 = 10.00$, $p = .004$). The 12-month prevalence estimate for major depression with severe impairment was 2.4% (see Table 1.2).

Kessler, Petukhova, Sampson, Zaslavsky, and Wittchen (2012), using the National Comorbidity Survey Replication—Adolescent Supplement (NCS-A) sample, compared lifetime prevalence rates of major depressive episodes and MDD, further broken down into single and recurrent episodes based on DSM-IV-TR criteria, among youth ages 13 to 17 years. Among youth, 16.8% of females met the criteria for lifetime major depressive episode compared to 8.5% of males. On the other hand, 14.2% of females met the criteria for lifetime MDD compared to 7.2% of males. Further lifetime prevalence estimates for single and recurrent episodes are also reported in Table 1.2. In addition, a lifetime morbid risk (LMR), defined as the proportion of individuals who are expected to experience a major depressive episode, using a survival model for projections irrespective of whether or not they report a lifetime history of the disorder at the time of interview, were also presented. In this analysis, the adolescent sample (NCS-A) was combined with the adult sample of the National Comorbidity Survey Replication (NCS-R) in order to project LMR as of age 75 based on age-of-onset distributions (Kessler et al., 2012). While results for LMR were reported for the entire sample (adults and adolescents), the ratio of lifetime prevalence to morbid risk (LT/LMR) of major depressive episode among 13- to 17-year-olds was reported as 0.4 (see Table 1.2).

Table 1.2 Rates of DSM Major Depression and Dysthymia in National Samples of Children and Adolescents

National Studies	*Prevalence Rates/100 (SE)*
NHANES, 2001–2004, Merikangas et al., 2010a	
12-Month Prevalence of Major Depression (without Impairment)	**2.7 (0.6)**
Females	3.7** (0.8)
Males	1.8** (0.6)
8–11 years	1.6** (0.5)
12–15 years	3.8** (0.8)
12-Month Prevalence of Major Depression (with Severe Impairment)	**2.4 (0.5)**
Females	3.2 (0.7)
Males	1.6 (0.5)
8–11 years	1.4** (0.4)
12–15 years	3.2** (0.7)
12-Month Prevalence of Dysthymia (without Impairment)	**1.0 (0.3)**
Females	1.2 (0.4)
Males	0.7 (0.3)
8–11 years	0.8 (0.4)
12–15 years	1.1 (0.3)
12-Month Prevalence of Dysthymia (with Severe Impairment)	**0.5 (0.2)**
Females	0.9** (0.4)
Males	0.1** (0.1)
8–11 years	0.4 (0.2)
12–15 years	0.7 (0.3)

*** Significant difference*

National Study Based on NCS-A	*Prevalence Rates/100 (SE)*
NCS-A, Kessler et al., 2012	
Total Major Depressive Disorder—Lifetime Prevalence	**10.6 (0.8)**
Females	14.2* (1.2)
Males	7.2* (0.8)
Single episode—females	3.4 (0.5)
Single episode—males	2.4 (0.5)
Recurrent episodes—females	10.8* (1.1)
Recurrent episodes—males	4.8* (0.7)
Lifetime morbid risk (LMR) and ratio of lifetime prevalence to morbid risk (LT/LMR) of Major depressive episode among 13- to 17-year-olds	0.4

** Significant gender difference within subsample*

A previous analysis, also using the NCS-A sample, reported lifetime prevalence of MDD or dysthymia (Merikangas, He, Burstein, Swanson, Avenevoli, Cui, Benjet, Georgiades, & Swendsen, 2010b), which differed slightly from the results shown above by Kessler et al. (2012). While the lifetime prevalence for MDD or dysthymia was 11.7%, 15.9% of adolescent females met criteria for DSM-IV MDD or dysthymia compared to 7.7% of adolescent males. Broken down by age group, 8.4% of youth ages 13 or 14 years met the criteria, compared to 12.6% of 15- and 16-year-olds, and 15.4% of 17- and 18-year-olds. In this analysis (results not shown), the lifetime prevalence of MDD or dysthymia with severe impairment was 8.7%. As noted by Kessler et al. (2012) in their analysis using the same dataset, minor discrepancies in results are most likely due to changes in data coding and weighting in an effort to improve estimates.

Community Studies

Table 1.3 presents the rates of depression in community samples of studies conducted among children and adolescents.

Costello et al. (1996) reported 3-month weighted prevalence estimates using DSM-III-R diagnoses in the baseline results for the Great Smoky Mountains Study of Youth (longitudinal) conducted among children ages 9, 11, and 13 years. In this study, three cohorts of children ages 9, 11, and 13 years at baseline were assessed annually over the course of eight waves. In the baseline results, among all children, 1.52% met the criteria for any depressive disorder, with 1.68% and 1.36% of females meeting the criteria. Specific to depression not otherwise specified, 1.45% of all children met the criteria, with 1.68% of males and 1.22% of females meeting the criteria. In this sample, 0.03% of all children met the criteria for DSM-III-R major depression. In the 2003 analysis, Costello et al. (2003) reported the results from all eight waves up to age 16 from the three age cohorts with results broken down by each age (9–10 through 16). Results were also presented by gender. The 3-month prevalence estimate for any depressive disorder was 2.2% among all respondents (2.8% among female children and adolescents and 1.6% among male children and adolescents). Three-month prevalence estimates for major depression and depression not otherwise specified, further broken down by age group and gender, are presented in Table 1.3, including results from the 1996 baseline analysis.

Angold et al. (2002), in the Caring for Children in the Community Study, reported the prevalence of DSM-IV psychiatric disorders, including depression, among 920 youth ages 9 to 17 years, further broken down by gender and ethnicity. A significantly higher prevalence of depressive disorder (odds ratio [OR] = 3.4, 95% confidence interval [CI], 1.6–7.4) was found among white youth. Three-month prevalence estimates are presented in Table 1.3, with results broken down by gender and white versus African-American youth.

Canino et al. (2004) sampled 1,886 child–caretaker dyads in Puerto Rico and conducted Spanish-language interviews among children ages 4 to 17 years. DSM-IV last-year prevalence rates for any depressive disorder, including major depression, were reported. Results were further broken down four ways: (1) Diagnostic Interview Schedule for Children (DISC) criteria for any depressive disorder met in either parent or child reports excluding the DISC impairment criteria (4.1%); (2) met DISC criteria for any depressive disorder including the DISC-specific impairment criterion in either parent or child reports (3.4%); (3) met the DISC criteria for any depressive disorder including significant impairment based on a cutoff less than 69 on the impairment rating scale, Parent-Interview—Children's Global Assessment Scale (PIC-GAS) (2.1%); and (4) met full DISC criteria including the DISC-specific impairment criterion in either parent or child reports and a cutoff score less than 69 on the PIC-GAS (1.7%). Results are also presented for major depression in Table 1.3. In logistic regression analyses, girls were found to have significantly more depressive disorders in general (specifically major depression). Rates for depressive disorders and major depression increased significantly with

Table 1.3 Rates of DSM Depression in Community Samples of Children and Adolescents

AUTHORS	*Major Depression*	*Dysthymia*	*Minor Depression*	*All Depression*	*Depression NOS***
Great Smoky Mountains Study (Baseline Results) Three-Month Prevalence Estimates—DSM-III-R	**Prevalence Rate/100 (SE)**	**Prevalence Rate/100 (SE)**	**Prevalence Rate/100 (SE)**	**Prevalence Rate/100 (SE)**	**Prevalence Rate/100 (SE)**
Costello et al. (1996)	0.03 (0.03) §	0.13 (.07) §	–	1.52 (0.46)	1.45 (.46)
Female	0.07 (.07) §	0.07 (.07) §		1.36 (0.65)	1.22 (.65)
Male	0 §	0.20 (.12) §		1.68 (0.66)	1.68 (.66)
Caring for Children in the Community Study Three-Month Prevalence Estimates—DSM-IV	**Prevalence Rate/100 (95% CI)**	**Prevalence Rate/100 (95% CI)**	**Prevalence Rate/100 (95% CI)**	**Prevalence Rate/100 (95% CI)**	**Prevalence Rate/100 (95% CI)**
Angold et al. (2002)	1.0 (0.5–1.8)	0.3 (0.1–0.6)	1.7 (1.0–2.8)	2.9 (2.0–4.2)	–
White	1.5 (0.7–3.1)	0.3 (0.1–1.0)	2.8 (1.5–5.3)	4.6 (2.9–7.3)	
African-American	0.5 (0.2–1.5)	0.2 (< 0.1–0.9)	0.7 (0.3–1.5) *	1.4 (0.8–2.5) *	
Female	1.2 (0.5–2.8)	0.2 (<0.1–0.9)	1.4 (0.7–2.7)	2.8 (1.7–4.6)	
Male	0.7 (0.3–1.6)	0.3 (0.1–1.0)	2.0 (0.9–4.1)	3.0 (1.7–5.1)	
Great Smoky Mountains Study Three-Month Prevalence Estimates—DSM-IV	**Prevalence Rate/100 (95% CI)**	**Prevalence Rate/100 (95% CI)**	**Prevalence Rate/100 (95% CI)**	**Prevalence Rate/100 (95% CI)**	**Prevalence Rate/100 (95% CI)**
Costello et al. (2003)	0.4 (0.2–0.7)	0.3 (0.1–0.6)	–	2.2 (1.6–3.0)	1.5 (1.1–2.2)
Females	0.5 (0.2–0.9)	0.3 (0.1–0.8)		2.8 (1.8–4.3)	2.1 (1.3–3.4)
Males	0.4 (0.2–0.9)	0.3 (0.1–0.8)		1.6 (1.0–2.5)	1.0 (0.6–1.5)

* $p < .01$ significant difference between white and African-American youth

** Not otherwise specified

[§] <5 cases in interviewed sample

(**Table 1.3** Rates of DSM depression in community samples of children and adolescents – Continued)

Authors	*Any Depressive Disorder*	*Major Depression*	*Dysthymia*
Child–Caretaker Dyads in Puerto Rico Last-Year Prevalence Estimates—DSM-IV	**Prevalence Rate/100 (95% CI)**	**Prevalence Rate/100 (95% CI)**	**Prevalence Rate/100 (95% CI)**
Canino et al. (2004)			
Partial DSM-IV/DISC-IV		3.6 (2.5–5.1)	0.6 (0.30–1.2)
Full DSM-IV/DISC-IV	4.1 (2.9–5.6)	3.0 (2.0–4.5)	0.5 (0.23–1.0)
Partial DSM-IV/DISC-IV + PIC-GAS < 69	3.4 (2.4–4.9)		
Full DSM-IV/DISC-IV + PIC–GAS < 69		1.8 (1.0–3.0)	0.4 (0.16–0.97)
	2.1 (1.3–3.4)		
		1.4 (0.75–2.8)	0.3 (0.10–0.87)
	1.7 (0.92–3.0)		
Teen Health 2000 Past-Year Prevalence Estimates—DSM-IV	**Prevalence Rate/100 (95% CI)**	**Prevalence Rate/100 (95% CI)**	**Prevalence Rate/100 (95% CI)**
Roberts et al. (2007)			
Prevalence of Disorder	–	1.70 (1.27–2.12)	0.33 (0.13–0.52)
Prevalence with DISC Impairment		1.54 (1.14–1.95)	0.29 (0.11–0.48)
Prevalence with CGAS ≤ 69		0.67 (0.41–0.93)	0.20 (0.04–0.39)

age. Children whose parents were not married were significantly more likely to meet criteria for MDD.

Roberts et al. (2007), in the Teen Health 2000 Study of 4,175 youths ages 11 to 17 years in the Houston area, also reported prevalence estimates based on the DISC. The past-year prevalence of major depression was 1.70%, past-year prevalence of major depression with DISC impairment was 1.54%, and past-year prevalence of major depression with a CGAS score less than or equal to 69 was 0.67% (see Table 1.3).

Dysthymia

National Studies

Tables 1.2 and 1.3 also report the results from national and community samples of studies conducted among children and adolescents that assessed dysthymia.

Twelve-month prevalence estimates for dysthymia, with and without severe impairment, were included in the 2001–2004 NHANES (Merikangas et al., 2010a). There were no statistically significant differences in prevalence estimates between males and females, or between older and younger children: 1.2% of females and 0.7% of males met the criteria for 12-month dysthymia (χ^2 = 1.53, p = .225). Likewise, 1.1% of children ages 12 to 15 years and 0.8% of children ages 8 to 11 years met the criteria for 12-month dysthymia without impairment (χ^2 = 0.28, p = .601). The 12-month prevalence estimate for dysthymia with severe impairment was 0.5% (see Table 1.1).

As previously noted, Merikangas et al. (2010b) assessed the prevalence of MDD or dysthymia together as one entity (results not presented in tables).

Community Studies

Table 1.3 reports the results from community studies that included dysthymia in their assessments.

Costello et al. (1996), in the Great Smoky Mountains Study, reported 3-month weighted prevalence estimates using DSM-III-R diagnoses for dysthymia at baseline. Among children ages 9, 11, and 13 years, 0.13% of children met the criteria for dysthymia. Broken down by gender, 0.20% of males and 0.07% of females met the criteria (see Table 1.3). In 2003, Costello et al. (2003) presented 3-month prevalence estimates for dysthymia. Results were also presented by gender. The 3-month prevalence estimate for dysthymia was 0.3% among all respondents (0.3% among female children and adolescents and 0.3% among male children and adolescents). Three-month prevalence estimates for dysthymia further broken down by age group and gender are presented in Table 1.3.

Angold et al. (2002), in the Caring for Children in the Community Study, reported the prevalence of DSM-IV psychiatric disorders, including dysthymia, among 920 youth ages 9 to 17 years. The 3-month prevalence estimate for dysthymia among all youth was 0.3%; it was 0.3% in white youth and 0.2% in African-American youth. The 3-month prevalence estimate was 0.2% in female youth and 0.3% in male youth (see Table 1.3).

Canino et al. (2004) reported DSM-IV last-year prevalence rates for dysthymia among Puerto Rican children. Results were further broken down four ways: (1) DISC criteria for dysthymia met in either parent or child reports excluding the DISC impairment criterion (0.6%); (2) met DISC criteria for dysthymia including the DISC-specific impairment criterion in either parent or child reports (0.5%); (3) met the DISC criteria for dysthymia including significant impairment based on a cutoff less than 69 on the PIC-GAS (0.4%); and (4) met full DISC criteria including the DISC-specific impairment criterion in either parent or child reports and a cutoff score less than 69 on the PIC-GAS (0.3%). Results are presented in Table 1.3.

Roberts et al. (2007), in the Teen Health 2000 Study, reported past-year prevalence of dysthymia (0.33%), past-year prevalence of dysthymia with DISC impairment (0.29%), and past-year prevalence of dysthymia with CGAS score less than or equal to 69 (0.20%) (see Table 1.3).

Comparison of Rates Based on Age of Onset to Rates Based on Child/Adolescent Samples

Specific to depression, the lifetime prevalence for 15- to 18-year-olds based on the National Comorbidity Survey (NCS; Kessler & Walters, 1998) was found to be roughly 14%, with an additional 11% having a lifetime history of minor depression. Using the NCS-A adolescent sample, the lifetime prevalence of MDD or dysthymia was found to be 11.7% (Merikangas et al., 2010b). Kessler et al. (2012), also using the NCS-A sample of adolescents, reported a lifetime prevalence of MDD to be 10.6%. These statistics are consistent with data derived from clinical samples documenting that more that 30% of children referred to clinical centers have major depression and that, in many of these cases, the disorder starts in the preschool years. Moreover, reports from student health services on college campuses note a marked increase in requests for counseling for depression over the past decade and list suicide as the second leading cause of death among students (American College Health Association, 2008).

In summary, there is increasing evidence that the first onset of MDD frequently occurs during adolescence and is not uncommon in childhood.

Comorbidity

Depressive disorders among youth are commonly comorbid with other psychiatric and medical conditions. Prevalence estimates across varied treatment settings suggest that 40% to 90% of depressed youths have another psychiatric condition, with as many as 50% having two or more comorbid conditions. The most common comorbid conditions are anxiety disorders, estimated to occur in as many as 60% of youths with depression (Angold et al., 1999; Birmaher et al., 1996, 2002; Pine et al., 1998).

Disruptive behavior disorders and ADHD follow anxiety disorders in frequency, often emerging before puberty. Among adolescents, substance use disorders are common. Depressive disorders presenting during childhood are often preceded by another psychiatric condition such as an anxiety disorder or ADHD. Furthermore, the presence of a depressive disorder increases the risks for the onset of other nonaffective psychiatric disorders. Depressive disorders are also highly comorbid with pediatric diseases across many conditions, suggesting potential shared etiologies for these illnesses, including epilepsy (Caplan, 2012; Caplan et al., 1998; Davies et al., 2003; Weisbrot & Ettinger, 2001), end-stage renal disease (Bakr et al., 2007), obesity (Pine et al., 2001), headaches (Pine et al., 1996), asthma (Katon et al., 2007; Mrazek et al., 1998), HIV disease (Mellins et al., 2009; Pao et al., 2005), cancer (Kersun & Elia, 2007), and diabetes (Kovacs, 1997; Lustman, 2000).

Risk Factors

Information on risk factors for adolescent MDD comes both from epidemiologic and clinical studies. The two most consistent risk factors for MDD in studies of adolescents and adults are female gender (twofold to threefold increased risk) and a family history of MDD. The offspring of depressed parents are at a twofold to fourfold increased risk of experiencing MDD and show an earlier age of onset and recurrent episodes (Rice et al., 2002). The risk is transmitted across generations to grandchildren (Weissman et al., 2016). One large-scale longitudinal study has identified age 12.5 as the developmental point at which a significant gender difference in risk emerges (Hankin et al., 2015).

Other risk factors that contribute both to the onset and recurrence of adolescent MDD are adverse family environments characterized by absence of supportive interactions; poor parental bonding; poor primary attachments; and harsh discipline (Fendrich et al., 1990; Garber & Little, 1999; Hakim, Larson, & Essau, 1999; Sheeber et al., 2001). A recent study involving a Norwegian community sample of 345 adolescents found that adolescent depression was significantly linked to financial concerns, physical illness or disability, and internalizing and externalizing issues among mothers but not fathers (Agerup, Lydersen, Wallander, & Sund, 2015).

Of these maternal risk factors, only internalizing issues significantly predicted adolescent depression after controlling for the other maternal characteristics. Separating out the effects of parental MDD from other risk factors is problematic because parental MDD is frequently associated with other risk factors (e.g., divorce, poor parental bonding). One study of offspring at high and low risk of depression found that parental depression was the strongest risk factor for offspring depression, over and above other family risks, such as divorce or poor parental bonding. The rates of MDD were considerably lower in the offspring of nondepressed parents (low risk), but when MDD was present in the low-risk offspring it was associated with poor parental bonding, parent–child conflict, and parental divorce (Fendrich et al., 1990; Nomura et al., 2002).

Although initial attempts to link childhood adversity (such as early parental death, poverty, and single-parent households) specifically to MDD using twin and epidemiologic data yielded disappointing results (Kendler et al., 1992; Kessler et al., 1997), recent evidence suggests that childhood adversity may elevate MDD risk among adolescents and/or adults. The influence of childhood adversity may be limited to particular developmental stages and may depend on the nature and severity of the adverse experiences. In one study, severe and hazardous adverse experiences during the preschool years had a significant impact on age 14 depressive symptoms in both boys and girls, but by age 17, these effects were only present in girls (St. Clair et al., 2015). In boys, maturational effects may be partially responsible for dampening the effects of severe early childhood adversity after age 14. Another study found that adult MDD was significantly associated with both prospective and retrospective reports of childhood adversity (Patten et al., 2015).

Notwithstanding the significant impact of involuntary risk factors (including gender, family history, family environment, and adversity), numerous studies have also pointed to an array of risk and protective factors that adolescents themselves may have the power to modify. In a recent meta-analysis of self-modifiable traits and behaviors, substance use, dieting, negative coping strategies, and unhealthy weight were identified as significant risk factors for depression in adolescents, while healthy eating and sleep habits were found to have protective effects (Cairns, Yap, Pilkington, & Jorm, 2014).

Personality/Temperament

Several theorists have hypothesized a heritable trait vulnerability factor common to most, if not all, emotional disorders. This trait has been defined slightly differently and given various labels by different theorists, including harm avoidance (Cloninger, 1987), neuroticism (Eysenck, 1947), trait anxiety (Gray, 1982), behavioral inhibition (Kagan, Reznick, & Snidman, 1987), and negative affectivity (Watson & Tellegen, 1985), though the conceptual and empirical overlap among these constructs far outweighs the differences. Each implies a trait disposition to experience negative affect. The term *neuroticism* often is used to refer to this trait, and is consistent with the emergence of the "Big 5" model of personality as the dominant model of personality structure in children (e.g., Digman & Inouye, 1986; Digman & Shmelyov, 1996), adolescents (e.g., Digman, 1989; Graziano & Ward, 1992) and adults (e.g., Goldberg, 1992; John, 1990; McCrae & Costa, 1987).

Longitudinal studies have shown that neuroticism predicts later negative affect and symptoms of emotional distress (Costa & McCrae, 1980; Larson, 1992; Levenson, Aldwin, Bosse, & Spiro, 1988), even after controlling for initial symptom levels (Gershuny & Sher, 1998; Jorm, Christensen, Henderson, & Jacomb, 2000). Clark, Watson, and Mineka (1994) reviewed several longitudinal studies showing that neuroticism predicts both subsequent diagnoses and chronicity of major depression. Since this review, studies reported by Hayward, Killen, Kraemer, and Taylor (2000), Kendler and colleagues (Kendler et al., 1993, 2002; Roberts & Kendler, 1999), and Krueger et al. (1996) have each obtained results consistent with the conclusions of Clark et al. (1994). For example, in a large adult female twin sample, Kendler et al.

(1993) found that neuroticism predicted the onset of MDD over a 1-year period, and Kendler et al. (2002) tested a multifactorial model and showed that after stressful life events, neuroticism was the strongest predictor of the onset of major depression.

The relation between neuroticism and depression may vary somewhat by age. Hirschfeld et al. (1989) found that whereas among older individuals (31–41 years old) neurotic-like characteristics of decreased emotional strength, increased interpersonal dependency, and increased thoughtfulness predicted the first onset of depression, this was not the case for younger individuals (17–30 years old). Similarly, Rohde, Lewinsohn, and Seeley (1990) found that adult participants who experienced a first episode of MDD had exhibited elevated levels of dependent traits 2 to 3 years earlier, whereas Rohde, Lewinsohn, and Seeley (1994) found no differences with regard to prior levels of dependency between adolescents who later developed a first MDD and adolescents who were depression-free during a 1-year follow-up period.

In contrast, studies using other measures of neurotic-like traits in children have found evidence of a link with vulnerability for depression. Elevated levels of behavioral inhibition have been observed in laboratory tasks with young offspring of depressed parents (Kochanska & Kuczynski, 1991; Rosenbaum et al., 2000). Caspi, Moffit, Newman, and Silva (1996) reported that children who had been rated as inhibited, socially reticent, and easily upset at age 3 had elevated rates of depressive disorders at age 21. Similarly, van Os, Jones, Wadsworth, and Murray (1997) found that physicians' ratings of behavioral apathy at ages 6, 7, and 11 predicted both adolescent mood disorders and chronic depression in middle adulthood. St. Clair et al. (2015) identified higher overall emotionality in childhood as a direct predictor of depressive symptoms at age 14 and an indirect predictor of depressive symptoms at age 17, with stronger associations in girls than boys. Finally, Gjerde (1995) reported that gender may moderate the relation between temperament and mood disorders. Whereas females with higher levels of chronic depression during young adulthood had been described as shy and withdrawn at ages 3 to 4, males with chronic depression had exhibited higher levels of undercontrolled behaviors as young children. Thus, there is some evidence of an association between neurotic-like traits during childhood and subsequent depression, although it may depend on gender as well as how these traits are measured.

Neuroticism also has been found to be a risk factor for other forms of psychopathology, however, and thus it is not specific to mood disorders. For example, neuroticism has been shown to be a risk factor in the development of posttraumatic stress disorder (PTSD; e.g., Breslau & Davis, 1992; Breslau et al., 1995; Helzer et al., 1987). Behaviorally inhibited children are at greater risk for the development of multiple phobias and various anxiety disorders in later childhood (Biederman et al., 1990; Hirshfeld et al., 1992), and social phobias in adolescence (Hayward et al., 1998). Hayward et al. (2000) also found that neuroticism predicted the development of panic attacks in a 4-year prospective study in adolescents. Thus, neuroticism appears to be a significant predictor of depression, although it might not be a specific vulnerability marker. Moreover, it is still difficult to distinguish among common cause, precursor, predisposition, and scar models of the relation between neuroticism and mental disorders (Klein, Durbin, Shankman, & Santiago, 2002; Ormel et al., 2013).

General negative emotionality (rather than neuroticism per se) has also been targeted as a vulnerability factor in several recent studies. In particular, exaggerated emotional responses to negative stimuli have been explored in relation to depression heritability. In one study, boys ages 7 to 13 with high familial risk for depression exhibited elevated sensitivity to sadness in a facial emotion recognition task (Lopez-Duran, Kuhlman, George, & Kovacs, 2013). This effect was specific to sadness (boys in the high-risk group were no different than their low-risk peers in their responses to angry faces) and did not appear to be present in girls at high familial risk. However, these trends have not been consistent across all studies of emotion recognition: in a sample of youth ages 7 to 16, including currently depressed, never depressed, and remitted depressed participants, Jenness, Hankin, Young, and Gibb (2015) found that those with current depression more often mistook happy and sad faces for angry faces. This finding suggests a potential bias toward threat detection, but no apparent difference in terms of sensitivity to sadness or happiness.

Notably, the vulnerability conferred by negative emotionality may depend on other cognitive and affective traits. Vasey et al. (2013) found that a three-way interaction among high negative emotionality, low positive emotionality, and low self-regulation significantly predicted depressive symptoms in four out of five independent youth samples. This interaction did not predict levels of anxiety, suggesting potential diagnostic specificity.

Cognitive Vulnerability

According to cognitive theories of depression (Abramson, Metalsky, & Alloy, 1989; Abramson, Seligman, & Teasdale, 1978; Beck, 1967), depressed individuals have more negative beliefs about themselves, the world, and their future, and tend to make global, stable, and internal attributions for negative events. These negative cognitions are expected to be concurrently associated with depression and to contribute to the onset and exacerbation of depressive symptoms. Cognitive theories of depression are inherently diathesis-stress theories. When confronted with stressful life events, individuals who have such negative cognitive tendencies will appraise the stressors and their consequences negatively and hence are more likely to become depressed than are individuals who do not have such cognitive styles

Several types of cognitions have been proposed to be related to depression, including low self- esteem, negative automatic thoughts, dysfunctional attitudes, and cognitive distortions (Beck, 1967), self-control (Rehm, 1977), control-related beliefs (Weisz & Stipek, 1982), self-efficacy (Bandura, 1977), depressive attributional style (Abramson et al., 1978), hopelessness (Abramson et al., 1989), and a ruminative response style (Nolen-Hoeksema, 2000). Cross-sectional studies with clinic and community samples of children consistently have shown a significant relation between negative cognitions, particularly low self-esteem and a pessimistic attributional style, and depression (Garber & Hilsman, 1992). A recent study of 647 Mexican-origin adolescents ages 10 to 12 supported the conceptualization of low self-esteem as a vulnerability factor rather than a product of depression. A vulnerability effect was present across genders and developmental stages, even after controlling for social support, maternal depression, life stress, and other risk factors (Orth, Robins, Widaman, & Conger, 2014). Meta-analyses of studies reporting on attributional style and depression have demonstrated moderate to large effect sizes in cross-sectional studies, suggesting a strong concurrent association between negative attributional style and higher levels of depressive symptoms in children and adolescents (Gladstone & Kaslow, 1995; Joiner & Wagner, 1995).

Neurocognitive studies point to altered response to reward in adolescent depression. Potential neural correlates of this altered response include disrupted corticostriatal circuit function and high medial prefrontal activity in the presence of reward stimuli (as reviewed by Forbes & Dahl, 2012). Different types of rewards may have differential relevance to the altered neural responses associated with depression. Among boys, status-related rewards appear to be most provocative of depressotypic neural responses, while among girls, social rewards are most associated with these responses (Morgan, Olino, McMakin, Ryan, & Forbes, 2013). Developmental status also appears to moderate the relationship between altered reward response and depressive symptom severity, with the strongest association evident among pubertal adolescents (Morgan et al., 2013). Longitudinal investigations of the role of cognitions in the prediction of childhood depression have yielded varying results. Global self-worth (Allgood-Merton et al., 1990; Garber, Martin, & Keiley, 2002; Vitaro, Pelletier, Gagnon, & Baron, 1995) and perceived self-competence in specific domains (Hoffman, Cole, Martin, Tiam, & Seroczynski, 2001; Vitaro et al., 1995) have predicted child and adolescent depressive symptoms (e.g., Allgood-Merton et al., 1990; Vitaro et al., 1995) and diagnoses (Garber et al., 2002), controlling for prior levels of depression. On the other hand, these same cognitive constructs also have failed to predict depressive symptoms (Dubbis, Felner, Brand, & George, 1999) and onset of new episodes (Goodyer & Kyte, 2008). However, in one of these null studies (Robertson & Simons, 1989), participants were selected from a drug and alcohol treatment clinic. The mean depression score, in this sample, was lower at the second assessment. Treatment procedures may have reduced depression levels during the assessment interval, making it difficult to predict maintenance or exacerbation of depression.

Attributional style generally has been investigated in the context of stress, although several studies have tested main effects models or reported main effects in the absence of interactions. Significant prospective relations have been observed between attributional style and later depressive symptoms in children and young adolescents (Nolen-Hoeksema, Girgus, & Seligman, 1986; 1992; Panak & Garber, 1992), although a few studies have failed to find this relation (Bennett, Pendley, & Bates, 1995; Hammen et al., 1988). In a longitudinal study of the developmental trajectories of negative attributions and depressive symptoms, Garber, Keiley, and Martin (2002) showed that attributional styles that were increasingly negative across time were associated with significantly higher initial levels and increasing growth of depressive symptoms during adolescence.

Prospective studies in children and adolescents also have found support for the cognitive diathesis-stress model of depression (Dixon & Ahrens, 1992; Hilsman & Garber, 1995; Lewinsohn, Joiner, & Rohde, 2001; Nolen-Hoeksema et al., 1992; Panak & Garber, 1992; Robinson et al., 1995). Garber and colleagues showed in three different short-term longitudinal studies, using different stressors (grades, peer rejection, and school transition) and different time periods, that cognitions (attributions, self-worth) measured before the stressors occurred moderated the effect of the stressors on depressive symptoms in children. Among children who experienced high levels of stress, the relation between negative cognitions about the self or causes of events and depressive symptoms was stronger compared to those without such negative cognitions. Lewinsohn et al. (2001) found that among adolescents who had experienced negative life events, intermediate levels of dysfunctional attitudes predicted the onset of depressive disorders a year later.

Developmental theorists (Cole & Turner, 1993; Nolen-Hoeksema et al., 1992; Weisz, Southam-Gero, & McCarty, 2001) have suggested that negative cognitions emerge over time and that their relation with depression becomes stronger with development. For example, in a longitudinal study of children in grades three through eight, Nolen-Hoeksema et al. (1992) showed that attributional style alone and in conjunction with stress significantly predicted depressive symptoms in the older but not in the younger children. Similarly, in a cross-sectional comparison of children in grades four, six, and eight, Turner and Cole (1994) found that negative cognitions contributed to the prediction of depressive symptoms for the oldest children, but not for the two younger groups. Thus, the relation between the cognition–stress interaction and depressive symptoms may increase from middle childhood to early adolescence. However, a more recent study found that cognitive vulnerability factors measured in early childhood (including self-referent encoding and depressotypic attributional style) demonstrated modest stability over time and predicted depressive symptoms in middle childhood (Hayden et al., 2013).

If negative cognitions contribute to the development of mood disorders, then "high risk" offspring of depressed parents should be more likely to exhibit a cognitive vulnerability than children whose parents have not experienced mood disorders. Indeed, children of depressed mothers report significantly lower perceived self-worth and a more depressive attributional style than do children of well mothers (Garber & Robinson, 1997; Goodman, Adamson, Riniti, & Cole, 1994, Jaenicke et al., 1987). Hayden et al. (2013) similarly report that parental depression and maternal criticism are predictive of cognitive vulnerability in early childhood. Thus, children who are at risk for depression, but who have not yet experienced depression themselves, have been found to report a more negative cognitive style, which might be a vulnerability to later depression.

In summary, correlational, predictive, and offspring studies have provided evidence that there is a cognitive style that may be a vulnerability to depressive symptoms and disorders in children. This cognitive style involves beliefs about the self and explanations about the causes of negative events. Future studies need to examine the development of this cognitive vulnerability over time (Cole & Turner, 1993) and whether or not it needs to be primed in children (Ingram, Miranda, & Segal, 1998).

Stress

Common to all definitions of stress is a focus on environmental conditions that threaten to harm the biological and/or psychological well-being of the individual (Grant et al., 2003). Stress may occur either as an acute event or as chronic adversity, and as a major life event or as minor events with accumulated effects (either additive or multiplicative) (Grant et al., 2003; Monroe & Simons, 1991). Stressful events may be normative (e.g., school transition) or atypical (e.g., abuse) and may be independent of, or directly related to and thus dependent on, an individual's actions. Objective environmental consequences of a stressor (i.e., can be reliably rated by objective observers) are hypothesized to have a direct effect on the development of depression. The subjective threat of a stressor involves individuals' appraisals of an event as stressful, which then may impact their psychological well-being (Lazarus, DeLongis, Folkman, & Gruen, 1985). Finally, there may be specificity in the relation between stress and psychopathology such that certain subdomains of stressors may be more highly related to depression than others (Beck, 1967; Grant et al., 2003; Hammen, Ellicott, & Gitlin, 1989; Monroe & Simons, 1991).

Stress plays a prominent role in most theories of depression, and a clear empirical link exists between stressful life events and depression in children and adolescents (Compas, 1987; Compas, Grant, & Ey, 1994). In infants, depressive symptoms have been associated with stressful life circumstances and often are responsive to changes in the environment. One stressor particularly linked with depression in infants is separation. Spitz and Wolf (1946) noted that a common feature in depressed infants ages 6 to 8 months is separation from the mother. Separation in young children has been found to be associated with grief responses characterized by negative changes in sleep patterns, activity, heart rate, temperature, monoamine systems, immune function, and endocrine function (Kalin & Carnes, 1984). Spitz (1945) noted the phenomenon of hospitalism, referring to evidence that infants subjected to long hospital stays experienced a number of psychological difficulties. Longer and more frequent hospital stays and earlier age of entering the hospital were associated with more depressive symptoms in infants (Moreau, 1996).

In school-aged children, cross-sectional studies using either life events checklists or interview methods consistently have shown that depressive symptoms and disorders are significantly associated with both minor and major undesirable life events in children, particularly cumulative or chronic stressors, and negative life events are more prevalent among depressed compared to nondepressed children (e.g., Compas, 1987; Goodyer, Wright, & Altham, 1988). Cross-sectional studies, however, are not informative about the direction of the relation between stress and depression. Given the association between dependent stressors and depression (Garber, Martin, & Keiley, 2002), it is possible that depression contributes to the occurrence of stressors. Depressed individuals have been found to generate many of the stressors they encounter, and these stressors then serve to exacerbate and maintain the depressive symptoms (Bennett & Bates, 1995; Coyne, Kessler, Tal, Turnbull, Wortman, & Greden, 1987; Hammen, 1991).

Among both adolescents and adults, self-reported stressful life events have been found to longitudinally predict an increase in rumination, which is a known risk factor and clinical feature of MDD (Michl, McLaughlin, Shepherd, & Nolen-Hoeksema, 2013). In adults, rumination appears to mediate the relationship between stressful live events and depressive symptoms; however, in adolescents, rumination has acted as a mediator between stress and anxiety but not depression (Michl et al., 2013).

Animal studies that manipulate stress in the laboratory have shown that antenatal stress impacts the developing physiology of the fetus and later physiological and behavioral outcomes in the offspring of stressed rat and primate mothers. Henry, Kabbaj, Simon, Le Moal, and Maccari (1994) showed that prenatally stressed rat pups had an elevated corticosterone response to novel environments and reduced corticosteroid receptors in the hippocampus, suggesting that prenatal stress may affect the neurobiological development of systems associated with depression (i.e., the hypothalamic–pituitary–adrenal [HPA] axis). Behaviorally, rat pups stressed in utero had greater distress and defensive behavior (Fride & Weinstock, 1988; Takahashi, Baker, & Kalin, 1990), and reduced environmental exploration when they were exposed to aversive or stressful conditions (Fride, Dan, Feldon, Halevy, & Weinstock, 1986; Poltyrev, Keshet, Kay, & Weinstock, 1996).

Prepartum exposure to stress also may result in hyperresponsiveness to later stressors. Clarke and Schneider (Clarke & Schneider, 1993; Clarke, Wittwer, Abbott, & Schneider, 1994) randomly assigned pregnant rhesus monkeys to stress and control conditions. The prenatally stressed offspring were less likely than control offspring to play and explore the environment and more likely to engage in clinging, which is associated with distress in primates. In addition, the prenatally stressed monkeys had significantly higher levels of cortisol and tended to have higher levels of adrenocorticotropin (ACTH) when blood levels were taken while the monkeys were anesthetized. In stressful situations while awake, the prenatally stressed offspring had marginally higher levels of ACTH but did not differ significantly from control offspring on levels of cortisol. Clarke and Schneider suggested that HPA axis functioning is implicated in the hyperresponsiveness to later environmental stressors of prenatally stressed rhesus monkeys.

Thus, animal models indicate that stress that occurs as early as conception can influence outcomes that have been associated with depression in humans. In human infants, stress during pregnancy is associated with negative outcomes for offspring (e.g., Lou et al., 1994). Although the mechanisms by which stress impacts the developing fetus are still unknown, Glover (1997) hypothesized that fetal neurophysiological development may be sensitive to the intrauterine hormonal environment, and neurophysiological vulnerability (e.g., HPA axis dysregulation) may make these offspring more sensitive to stress and thereby predispose them to depression as they mature. One study has found that mothers with more total lifetime anxiety have children with higher morning cortisol levels at age 6, suggesting an effect on the physiological stress response, and lifetime maternal depression may also interact with children's positive affectivity at age 3 (a protective factor) to predict morning cortisol levels at age 6 (Dougherty et al., 2013).

Other studies have further elucidated the role of stress, the HPA axis, and psychiatric disorders in human subjects (Goldman-Mellor et al., 2012; Heim & Nemeroff, 2001; Heim et al., 2010). This concept will be discussed in more detail in the biology section of the chapter.

Longitudinal studies in which stressors are assessed prior to the onset of symptoms can be informative about the temporal relation between stress and depression. Prospective studies have found that stress predicts depressive symptoms, controlling for prior symptom levels in children (Goodyer, Herbert, & Altham,1998; Hammen, 1991; Nolen-Hoeksema et al., 1992;

Panak & Garber, 1992; Velez, Johnson, & Cohen, 1989) and adolescents (e.g., Allgood-Merten, Lewinsohn, Hops, 1990; Aseltine, Gore, & Colten, 1994; Garrison et al., 1990; Ge, Conger, Lorenz, & Simons, 1994; Leadbeater, Kuperminc, Blatt, & Hertzog, 1999). The relations tend to be stronger predicting children's self-reports compared to parents' reports of children's depressive symptoms (Compas, Howell, Phares, Williams, & Giunta, 1989; Stanger, McConaughy, & Achenbach, 1992).

Fewer studies have examined the contribution of negative life events to the first onset of depressive disorders in children. Stress has predicted the onset of depressive symptoms in previously asymptomatic children (Aseltine et al., 1994) and the onset of clinically significant depressive episodes, controlling for prior symptom levels in samples comprising both children and adolescents (Hammen, 1991) and adolescents alone (Garber et al., 2002; Monroe, Rohde, Seeley, & Lewinsohn, 1999). Only three of these studies (Aseltine et al., 1994; Monroe et al., 1999) controlled for lifetime history of MDD to rule out the possibility that earlier depressive disorder contributed to onset.

Reports of stressful life events have been shown to increase for both boys and girls from childhood through adolescence, with increases being greater for girls (Ge et al., 1994), paralleling increases in rates of depression for boys and girls (Hankin et al., 1998). Cohen et al. (1987) reported that negative events predicted depressive symptoms in girls who had experienced minimal positive events in the same time interval, and Ge et al. (1994) showed that growth of stressful life events over time predicted growth in depressive symptoms for girls but not boys.

Although no one specific type of stressful event invariably leads to depression in children and adolescents, certain stressors consistently have been found to be associated with depression. Childhood abuse/maltreatment is an especially potent predictor of depression (Andrews, 1995; Bifulco, Brown, & Adler, 1991; Browne & Finkelhor, 1986; Levitan et al., 1998; McCauley et al., 1997; Pribor & Dinwiddie, 1992; Trad, 1994), and this is particularly true for women (Weiss, Longhurst, & Mazure, 1999; Whiffen & Clark, 1997). Childhood maltreatment has also been linked to more recurrent and persistent depressive episodes across 16 studies, as well as greater treatment nonresponsiveness across 10 studies (Nanni, Uher, & Danese, 2012). Sexual assault during childhood or adulthood has been found to increase the risk of depression by 2.4 in women (Burnam et al., 1988). Poverty also has been shown to be a significant correlate of depression (Bruce, Takeuchi, & Leaf, 1991; Grant et al., 2003; McLoyd, 1998). For example, the rates of depression among low-income mothers are about twice as high as in the general population (Bassuk, Buckner, Perloff, & Bassuk, 1998; Brown & Moran, 1997). Caspi et al. (2003) demonstrated a relationship between a genetic variable, polymorphism of the serotonin transporter (SERT), and the development of depression after exposure to child abuse.

Events such as disappointments, loss, separation, and interpersonal conflict or rejection also are particularly linked with depression (Aseltine et al., 1994; Monroe et al., 1999; Panak & Garber, 1992; Reinherz et al., 1999; Rueter, Scaramella, Wallace, & Conger, 1999; Shirk, Boergers, Eason, & Van Horn, 1998). This is especially probable for individuals who tend to be more socially dependent or sociotropic. According to the specific vulnerability hypothesis (Beck, 1983; Blatt, Quinlan, Chevron, McDonald, & Zuroff, 1982), individuals whose self-esteem is derived from interpersonal relationships (sociotropy) are at increased risk for depression when they experience stressors within the social domain; in contrast, those who derive their self-worth from achievement-related goals are at greater risk for depression when they encounter failure. Studies investigating this specific vulnerability hypothesis in children have been supportive (Little & Garber, 2000).

In summary, a clear link exists between stress and depression. But by what mechanisms does stress increase an individual's vulnerability to depression? Although stressors often precede mood disorders, not all individuals exposed to stressors become depressed. There is no perfect correspondence between exposure to negative life events and the onset of depressive symptoms or disorders. Rather, how individuals interpret and respond to events differentiates who does and does not become depressed. Much of the individual variability is due to differences in appraisals of the meaning of the events with regard to the self and future.

Interpersonal Relationships

Interpersonal perspectives on depression emphasize the importance of the social environment and the development of secure attachments (Gotlib & Hammen, 1992). Vulnerability to depression presumably arises in early family environments in which the children's needs for security, comfort, and acceptance are not met. Bowlby (1980) argued that children with caretakers who are consistently accessible and supportive will develop cognitive representations, or "working models," of the self and others as positive and trustworthy. In contrast, caretakers who are unresponsive or inconsistent will produce insecure attachments, leading to working models that include abandonment, self-criticism, and excessive dependency. Such working models may contribute to the development of negative cognitions about the self and others, and presumably increase individuals' vulnerability to depression, particularly when exposed to new interpersonal stressors. Although most studies of the family process as it relates to depression have focused on dyadic interactions, a recent study found that triads involving depressed adolescents also display a variety of affective differences compared to healthy triads, including less time spent in matched affective states (particularly during problem-solving interactions) and more time spent in mismatched affective states (Hollenstein, Allen, & Sheeber, 2016). Thus, multiple types of family structures involving adolescents and caretakers may be impacted in depression and may in turn have a negative impact on the working model.

Reviews of the literature on the relation between the family environment and depression (e.g., Beardslee et al., 1998; Downey & Coyne, 1990; Rapee, 1997) indicate that families of depressed individuals are characterized by problems with attachment, communication, conflict, cohesion, and social support, as well as poor childrearing practices. Security in attachments help infants cope with the environment, and a lack of such attachments may lead infants to seek protection by withdrawing from the environment altogether (Bowlby, 1980; Trad, 1994). Two-year-old children with secure attachments have been found to be more cooperative, persistent, and enthusiastic, to show more positive affect, and to function better overall than those with insecure attachments (Matas, Arend, & Sroufe, 1978). In adolescents, depression has been linked with less secure attachments to parents (Kenny, Moilanen, Lomax, & Brabeck, 1993). Moreover, adolescents undergoing stressful life events are more likely to become depressed if they had insecure attachments to their parents than adolescents with more secure attachments (e.g., Kobak et al., 1991).

Beyond attachment, other kinds of dysfunctional family patterns have been found to be associated with depression in children (Kaslow et al., 1994; Rapee, 1997). Serious abuse and neglect interfere with normal expressions of infants' emotions and lead to avoidant or resistant attachments, especially if the mother is the perpetrator of the abuse. Maltreatment also leads to withdrawal behaviors in infants and self-esteem deficits later in childhood (Gaensbauer & Sands, 1979; Trad, 1987). The parent–infant relationship is inevitably worsened from such abuse, which in turn puts the infant in higher danger of being abused again (Trad, 1987).

Two main parenting dimensions particularly associated with depression in children are acceptance/rejection and psychological control/autonomy (e.g., Barber, 1996; Parker, Tupling, & Brown, 1979; Schwarz, Barton-Henry, & Pruzinsky, 1985). In retrospective studies, currently depressed adults recalled their parents to have been critical, rejecting, controlling, and intrusive (Parker, 1993). Currently depressed children have described their parents as authoritarian, controlling, rejecting, and unavailable (Stein et al., 2000), and they tend to perceive their families to be less cohesive and more conflictual than do nondepressed youth (e.g., Stark, Humphrey, Crook, & Lewis, 1990; Walker, Garber, & Greene, 1993; although see

Asarnow, Carlson, & Guthrie, 1987 for contrary findings). A meta-analysis of 164 studies involving adolescent depression identified deficient warmth, high interparental conflict, overinvolvement, aversiveness, insufficient autonomy granting, and monitoring as parental characteristics that increase the risk of depression for adolescents ages 12 to 18 (Yap, Pilkington, Ryan, & Jorm, 2014).

Mothers of depressed children describe themselves as more rejecting, less communicative, and less affectionate than do mothers of both normal and psychiatric controls (Lefkowitz & Tesiny, 1985; Puig-Antich et al., 1985), and in observational studies, mothers of depressed children have been described as less rewarding (Cole & Rehm, 1986) and more dominant and controlling (Amanat & Butler, 1984) than mothers of nondepressed children. Conversely, maternal warmth may act as a protective factor. Among boys who are at socioeconomic risk for depression and are exposed to maternal depression, maternal warmth and affection during adolescence may reduce depressotypic neural responses to reward during young adulthood (Morgan, Shaw, & Forbes, 2014). Several longitudinal studies have found a significant relation between the family environment and subsequent depressive symptoms (e.g., Barber, 1996; Garrison et al., 1990; Ge, Best, Conger, & Simons, 1996; Rueter et al., 1999; Sheeber, Hops, Alpert, Davis, & Andrews, 1997), although others have reported only cross-sectional analyses despite having longitudinal data available and others have reported null findings (Burge & Hammen, 1991; Burge et al., 1997). Barber (1996) showed that children's ratings of parents' psychologically controlling behavior predicted their depressive symptoms, controlling for prior levels of depression, although children's prior depressive symptoms also predicted their ratings of their parents' behavior. Burt, Cohen, and Bjorck (1988) found that for girls, ratings of family expressiveness predicted depression after controlling for prior depressive symptoms. Other studies have shown that adolescents' reports of family adaptability and cohesion (Garrison et al., 1990; McKeown et al., 1997) and perceptions of family support (McFarlane et al., 1995) made significant prospective contributions to adolescent depressive symptoms, controlling for prior symptom levels. In addition, maternal hostile childrearing attitudes have been found to significantly predict increases in children's depressive symptoms (Katainen, Raikkonen, Keskivaara, & Keltikangas-Jarvinen, 1999). Using observational data of parental warmth, hostility, and disciplinary skills, Ge et al. (1996) reported that increases in adolescent internalizing symptoms were predicted by lower levels of parental warmth and higher levels of maternal hostility. In this same sample, Rueter et al. (1999) found that escalating parent–adolescent conflict predicted increases in adolescent internalizing symptoms, which in turn increased the risk of the onset of internalizing disorders. However, the effects of depressogenic parenting may differ by gender, and some evidence suggests that they subside by late adolescence. In one study that examined "aberrant parenting" as a form of childhood adversity, negative parenting styles were associated with elevated depression risk in girls but not boys, and for girls, the effect was present at age 14 but not age 17 (St. Clair et al., 2015).

Depressed children also have significant peer difficulties and social skills deficits (e.g., Altmann & Gotlib, 1988). Self-reported depression significantly correlates with teachers' reports of peer rejection in children (Rudolph, Hammen & Burge, 1994). In laboratory studies, children with depressive symptoms were rated by their peers more negatively than were children without symptoms (Peterson, Mullins, & Ridley-Johnson, 1985). French, Conrad, and Turner (1995) noted that rejection by peers predicted higher levels of self-reported depressive symptoms among antisocial but not among non-antisocial youth. Panak and Garber (1992) found a significant relation between peer-rated rejection and self-reported depression, and this relation was mediated by perceived rejection. Kistner, Balthazor, Risi, and Burton (1999) similarly found that perceived rejection predicted increases in depressive symptoms during middle childhood. Finally, in a longitudinal study of children in sixth grade, Nolan, Flynn, and

Garber (2003) found that a composite measure of rejection by peers, family, and teachers significantly predicted depressive symptoms across 3 years. Thus, depression in children is generally associated with high levels of interpersonal conflict and rejection.

However, the effects of interpersonal stress—particularly peer stress—may differ according to gender and depend significantly on gene–environment interactions. In a recent longitudinal study of 665 youth, female adolescents reported significantly greater peer stress than their male counterparts, and gender interacted with peer stress such that chronic peer stress was significantly more predictive of depression in female adolescents than in males (Hankin et al., 2015). There was also an interaction between chronic peer stress (lasting at least 3 years) and genetic vulnerability from the 5-*HTTLPR* serotonin transporter polymorphism among older adolescents, even after controlling for depression history and other (non-peer) forms of chronic stress. Notably, gender did not moderate the interaction between 5-*HTTLPR* vulnerability and chronic peer stress.

Finally, relationships between depressed parents and their children also consistently have been found to be disrupted (Goodman & Gotlib, 1999). Depressed parents report more conflict and less coherence in their families (Billings & Moos, 1983), are less involved and affectionate with their children, and experience poorer communication in parent–child relationships than nondepressed parents (Weissman, Paykel, Siegal, & Klerman, 1971). Moreover, depressed mothers tend to feel more hostile toward their children and less positive and competent about their parenting than do well mothers (Webster-Stratton & Hammond, 1988).

Observations of depressed mothers interacting with their children reveal that these mothers are more negative (Garber et al., 1991; Lovejoy, 1991), more controlling (Kochanska, Kuczynski, Radke-Yarrow, & Welsh, 1987), and less responsive and affectively involved (Cohn & Tronick, 1989), and use less productive communications (Gordon et al., 1989). Depressed mothers spend less time talking to and touching their infants, and show more negative affect in their interactions with their infants, who themselves show less positive affect, less activity, and more frequent protests (Field, 1995). Parental depression also can lead to disturbed attachment behavior and an inability by the infant to regulate emotions, thereby putting the infant at greater risk for developing depression (Gaensbauer, Harmon, Cytryn, & McKnew, 1984). Offspring of depressed parents have more insecure attachments compared to offspring of well mothers (DeMulder & Radke-Yarrow, 1991; Teti, Gelfand, Messinger, & Isabella, 1995). Moreover, insecurely attached offspring of depressed mothers tend to have difficulties in their relationships with peers (Rubin, Booth, Zahn-Waxler, Cummings, & Wilkinson, 1991). Finally, negative reciprocal interaction patterns have been observed between depressed mothers and their children. The quality of parental relationships may moderate adolescents' responses to other forms of stress. For example, in adolescents with positive parental relationships, the depressogenic effects of peer stress appear to be substantially reduced (Hazel, Oppenheimer, Technow, Young, & Hankin, 2014).

In summary, two important findings emerge regarding the link between interpersonal vulnerability and depression. First, families with a depressed member tend to be characterized by less support and more conflict, and such family dysfunction increases children's risk of developing depression. Second, depressed individuals are themselves more interpersonally difficult, which results in greater problems in their social network. Thus, the link between interpersonal vulnerability and depression likely is bidirectional (Gotlib & Hammen, 1992). Longitudinal studies examining the contribution of family dysfunction, parent–child conflict, peer difficulties, and interpersonal rejection to increases in and maintenance of depressive symptoms in children have shown both that social problems temporally precede depression, and that depression contributes to interpersonal difficulties. Moreover, interpersonal difficulties appear to persist after depressive symptoms have remitted (Puig-Antich et al., 1985). In addition, social adversities such as persistent poor friendships, low involvement of fathers, negative attitudes by family members, and stressful family environments can contribute to the maintenance or relapse of depressive disorders in youth (e.g., Asarnow, Goldstein, Tompson, & Guthrie, 1993; Goodyer, Germany, Gowrusankur, & Altham, 1991; McCauley et al., 1993).

The interpersonal environment clearly is an important and sometimes stressful context in which children develop schema about themselves and others, which then can serve as a vulnerability to depression. In addition, children's own reactions to these environments can exacerbate and perpetuate negative social exchanges, which furthers the interpersonal vicious cycle, thereby resulting in more rejection and depression (Coyne, 1976). Thus, a transactional model of mutual influence probably best characterizes the association between depressed individuals and their social environment.

Socioeconomic Status

A relationship between low socioeconomic status (SES) and increased depression risk has been well documented in children and adolescents (Bird et al., 1988; Costello et al., 1996; Gilman et al., 2003; Reinherz et al., 1993). In a sample of 875 youth ages 19 to 21, the relationship between low SES and depressive symptoms was fully accounted for by family-related stress and emotional support (Miller & Taylor, 2012). Similarly, another study reported that parental support (particularly on the part of the mother) mediated the relationship between socioeconomic status and depression in adolescents, possibly by influencing the degree of optimism transmitted through the parenting style (Piko, Luszczynska, & Fitzpatrick, 2013).

Some studies have failed to document a consistent relationship between SES and depression, however (Costello et al., 1988, 2003; Whitaker et al., 1990), and one meta-analysis of 310 child samples found no association between social class and depression based on the Children's Depression Inventory (CDI) (Twenge & Nolen-Hoeksema, 2002). Mixed findings may be the result of a temporary equalization effect in middle adolescence. A longitudinal study of 14,000 North American youth showed that family SES during early adolescence substantially impacted depressive symptoms during the same timeframe (Wickrama, Noh, & Elder, 2009). The effects of early adolescent SES faded during middle and late adolescence and re-emerged during early adulthood. SES has also displayed a reliable relationship with depression among adults: a meta-analysis of 60 adult studies found that both education level and income displayed a dose–response relationship with depression odds (Lorant et al., 2003).

Race/Ethnicity

Due to differences in samples, reporting techniques, and measures used to assess depressive disorders, comparisons across racial/ethnic groups have been difficult (Merikangas & Nakamura, 2011). There is evidence to suggest that both African- and Latino-American youth may experience more symptoms of depression than their white counterparts (Guiao & Thompson, 2004; McLaughlin, Hilt & Nolen-Hoesksema, 2007; Merikangas & Nakamura, 2011; Roberts & Chen, 1995; Roberts, Roberts & Chen, 1997; Twenge & Nolen-Hoeksema, 2002), including two studies that specifically found African-American males reporting higher rates of depressive symptoms than European-American males (Schoenbach et al., 1982). In the period following high school, African-American and Hispanic youth appear to experience significantly more depression than Caucasian and Asian-American youth, with differences explained partly by underrepresentation in universities and partly by conflict in peer and family relationships (Gore & Aseltine, 2003). However, some studies have reported lower rates of depression among African-American and Latino youth (Angold et al., 2002; Roberts, Roberts & Chen, 1995; Roberts, Roberts & Chen, 1997). Interactions between race, family stress, and emotional support may help to explain discrepant findings. Miller and Taylor (2012) reported that in a large sample of young adults, depressive symptoms were significantly more prevalent among African-Americans than among Caucasians, and this difference was partly mediated by family-related stress. In addition, Caucasians experienced more depressive symptoms when family support was lacking, suggesting greater resilience among African-Americans, but African-Americans experienced more depressive symptoms when family support was high, indicating that family support did not have as much of a protective effect as it did for Caucasians.

BIPOLAR DISORDER

Overview

The view that mania in younger people is extremely rare or nonexistent has been increasingly challenged by many case reports and by large-scale community surveys of adults. For example, Akiskal et al. (1985), in a case history of adolescent relatives of "classic" adult bipolar patients, found that despite frank symptoms of depression and mania, and frequent mental health contacts, none of these youth had been diagnosed with an affective disorder. Weller et al. (1986) reviewed over 200 articles published between 1809 and 1982 and identified 157 cases that would likely be considered manic by modern standards. However, 48% of those subjects retrospectively diagnosed as manic according to DSM-III criteria were not considered so at the time of referral. Wozniak et al. (1999) reported that 16% of psychiatrically referred prepubertal children satisfied diagnostic criteria for bipolar disorder. Biederman et al. (1996) reported that a sizeable minority of children with ADHD has bipolar disorder. These reports suggested that pediatric mania may not be rare, but is difficult to diagnose. Despite continued debate and controversy over the validity of the diagnosis of mania in children (Biederman, 1998; Klein et al 1998), there is a growing consensus that many seriously disturbed children are afflicted with severe affective dysregulation and high levels of agitation, aggression, and dyscontrol that may be early bipolar disorder. These children have received increased scientific attention, as is evident in the multiple NIMH workshops on bipolar disorder in children and adolescents and in exhaustive reviews that have supported the validity of the disorder in youth (Faedda et al., 1995; Geller & Luby 1997; Weller et al., 1995). The NIMH Strategic Research Plan for Mood Disorder Research recommended the establishment of multisite network programs on pediatric-onset bipolar disorder (Costello et al., 2002).

Agreement about what is the first presentation of bipolar illness is critical for epidemiologic studies to obtain the true age of onset and estimate of prevalence and risk. The questions include: Does juvenile bipolar disorder differ from the adult form? What are the early signs and symptoms? What is the relationship of ADHD and other disruptive disorders to juvenile-onset bipolar disorder? Answers to these questions are complicated by the uncertainty regarding the appropriate duration of a manic episode, since youth more frequently report manic symptoms that last only a few hours or days (Carlson & Kelly, 1998; Geller et al., 1995) and therefore do not meet adult criteria.

Studies suggest that bipolar disorder may be more accurately characterized as a spectrum disorder, as many people with the illness are not receiving appropriate treatment due to subthreshold symptoms and inappropriate diagnosis. Three subtypes of the illness have been identified: bipolar type I disorder, bipolar type II disorder, and bipolar disorder not otherwise specified (BD-NOS), which includes patients who have manic and depressive symptoms but do not meet strict criteria for type I or type II. The results of the 2007 Merikangas et al. study, which analyzed data from the NCS-R, indicate that bipolar I and bipolar II each occur in about 1% of the population, while BD-NOS occurs in about 2.4% of the population. Only 69% of BD-NOS patients receive treatment, and they are often prescribed inappropriate medications; in contrast, 89% to 95% of those with bipolar type I or type II are in treatment. These findings suggest that bipolar disorder may be better characterized as bipolar spectrum disorder (BPSD), which will include these individuals with subthreshold symptoms.

As part of the Longitudinal Assessment of Manic Symptoms (LAMS) Study, Findling et al. (2010) found that although elevated symptoms of mania (+ESM) were associated with higher rates of bipolar spectrum disorder than those without ESM, 75% of children with ESM did not meet criteria for bipolar spectrum disorder. This study suggests that longitudinal assessment is needed to examine which factors are associated with diagnostic evolution to bipolar spectrum disorder in children with ESM.

Another study resulting from the LAMS data has shown that in many cases, obtaining repeated parent report of mania symptoms significantly altered the probability of a bipolar spectrum disorder diagnosis being made and may be a useful adjunct in forming a clinical diagnosis (Frazier et al., 2011).

As a part of the Course of Subthreshold Bipolar Disorder in Youth (COBY) study, Axelson et al. (2011) found that children and adolescents presenting with mood symptoms who meet criteria for BD-NOS, particularly those with a family history of bipolar disorder, frequently progress to bipolar disorder type I or bipolar disorder type II. Identifying these children and effectively intervening may have the potential to alter the progression of mood disorders in this high-risk population.

In February 2009 the NIMH convened a meeting of experts to discuss diagnostic issues regarding classification of bipolar disorder in children and adolescents. Suggestions for defining a subthreshold diagnosis of bipolar disorder included the following:

- The patient meets DSM-IV Criterion B for manic or hypomanic episode (i.e., all the symptoms), except for duration criteria (<4 consecutive days).
- Four hours/day of manic symptoms to count as a day; require lifetime occurrence of >20 days meeting DSM-IV criteria for mania or hypomania
- There is a distinct change in functioning (but not necessarily functional impairment).
- The episode is not substance or medication induced and symptoms are not better accounted for by other disorders.
- The patient does not meet DSM-IV criteria for cyclothymic disorder.

The group agreed that future studies need to further explore subthreshold bipolar disorder and other BD-NOS subgroups. Investigators need to explicitly document how BD-NOS is defined in their studies.

Diagnosis

Despite the growing body of evidence demonstrating that bipolar disorder can be diagnosed in children and adolescents, the diagnosis continues to evoke controversy. Further complicating this problem is that experts around the world disagree about the criteria and symptoms of pediatric mania and hypomania (Dubicka et al., 2008). Most investigators agree that pediatric mania can be diagnosed using current DSM criteria for adults (Axelson et al., 2006; Birmaher et al., 2007; Carlson, 2011; Findling et al., 2010; Kowatch et al., 2005; Youngstrom et al., 2008). Although the majority of studies have shown that mania in youth presents episodically, as with adults, other studies suggest that pediatric bipolar disorder is characterized by chronic continuous symptoms, continuous cycling, and long-duration episodes (Geller, 2000; Mick et al., 2003; Wozniak et al., 1995) and fewer episodes of remission (Carlson et al., 2000). Findings from other studies suggest that children with bipolar disorder have high rates of rapid cycling and low interepisode recovery rates (Findling et al., 2001). Taken together, the existing studies suggest that children and adolescents have more mixed presentations and rapid shifts in polarity of their mood episodes than bipolar adults, although continuity between pediatric mania and adult mania has not been confirmed (Harrington & Maat, 2003; Judd & Akiskal, 2003). There has been general consensus among experts that adult criteria may be used to diagnose bipolar disorder among youths. The DSM-5 criteria for bipolar disorders in youth specify the following:

A. A distinct period of abnormally and persistently elevated, expansive, or irritable mood, and abnormally and persistently increased goal-directed activity or energy lasting at least one week (or any duration if hospitalization is necessary).

B. During the period of mood disturbance, three (or more) of the following symptoms have persisted (four if the mood is only irritable) and have been present to a significant degree representing a noticeable change in behavior:

- Inflated self-esteem or grandiosity
- Decreased need for sleep
- More talkative than usual or pressure to keep talking
- Flight of ideas or subjective experience that thoughts are racing
- Distractibility
- Increase in goal-directed activity
- Excessive involvement in pleasurable activities that have a high potential for painful consequences

In addition, the symptoms do not meet the criteria of a Mixed Mood Episode, where both criteria for a manic episode and for MDD (except for duration) are met with symptoms nearly every day during at least a 1-week period. For hypomania the elevated or irritable mood lasts for four days. The mood disturbance must cause significant impairment and is not better accounted for by other psychiatric disorders or medical conditions.

As with adults, children and adolescents with bipolar disorder can meet criteria for bipolar I disorder, bipolar II disorder, mixed-manic episodes, cyclothymia, and specified/unspecified bipolar and related disorders (Axelson et al., 2006; Birmaher et al., 2004, 2007; Findling et al., 2010; Youngstom et al., 2008). While youth may present initially with either a manic or depressive episode, pediatric bipolar individuals most frequently present with depression (Birmaher, 2007). Furthermore, bipolar youths present with more mixed episodes and are more likely to present with psychotic symptoms (delusions or hallucinations) (Axelson et al., 2006; Birmaher et al., 2012).

Although the diagnostic criteria for adults and youths are the same, making the diagnosis in youth can be challenging. Difficulties differentiating manic symptoms from normative mood and behaviors, and overlap with symptoms of other pathologies can confound diagnosis. Difficulties expressing mood states due to cognitive and developmental immaturity may also complicate diagnosis (Birmaher et al., 2013). Thus, the criteria must be used considering the following when diagnosing mania or hypomania:

- The symptoms must exceed those expected for normal developmental age and stage. This can be challenging. For example, it can be difficult to distinguish grandiosity from the normative overestimation of abilities that occurs among children and young adolescents.
- The symptoms should cluster in episodes so that their onset and intensity increase with the onset of the abnormal mood
- If other psychiatric comorbidities are present, as is commonly the case with ADHD and ODD, the symptoms must worsen during the episode of mania or hypomania.
- The symptoms cannot be better explained by environmental or cultural context, medical illnesses, or use of medications or substances.

Summary of Implications of Changes in Criteria

The diagnostic criteria for bipolar disorders in DSM-5 now include changes in both mood and activity or energy. More specifically, a new specifier "with mixed features" replaces the diagnosis criteria for bipolar I disorder, mixed episodes, which required that an individual meet full criteria for both mania and major depressive episode.

Individuals with a past history of MDD whose symptoms meet all criteria for hypomania, with the exception of the duration criteria (e.g., an episode lasts less than the required 4 consecutive days or more) are now diagnosed under the "other specified bipolar and related disorder." For individuals with too few symptoms of hypomania present to meet the criteria for full bipolar II syndrome, a second category of "other specified bipolar and related disorder variant" has been created.

As in the depressive disorders category, an anxious specifier has been defined.

Longitudinal studies will track how these changes to criteria impact rates of psychopathology among children and adolescents.

Epidemiology

Epidemiology data on juvenile bipolar disorder must be seen within these diagnostic uncertainties. The 1980s Epidemiologic Catchment Area (ECA) study, based on over 18,000 adults age 18 and over in five U.S. communities, provided the first epidemiologic clue about the youthful onset of bipolar disorder (Robins & Price, 1991). The lifetime prevalence of bipolar disorder was about 1/100, with little sex differences in rates and an overall median age of onset of 18 years.

The 1990 National Comorbidity Survey (NCS) included a representative national sample in the United States of over 8,000 subjects ages 15 to 54 (Kessler et al., 1994) and provided the best epidemiologic information at the time. The younger age included in the NCS was based on the ECA findings that many psychiatric disorders have a youthful age of onset. The overall lifetime prevalence of bipolar I was 1.7% in the full sample and 1.3% in the sample ages 15 to 17, with equal sex rates and a median age of onset of 21 years. Both the ECA and the NCS suggested that the onset of bipolar disorder often occurs during adolescence and childhood.

In the 1990s, the Cross National Collaborative Group was formed to directly compare rates and risk of psychiatric disorders by standardizing analysis to overcome the problem of disparate presentation of data between studies. Seven countries (United States, Canada, Puerto Rico, Germany, Taiwan, Korea, and New Zealand) provided data on bipolar disorder. The lifetime prevalence rates for bipolar I ranged from 0.3% in Taiwan to 1.5% in New Zealand (Weissman et al., 1996), with equal sex ratios across sites (with the exception of Korea) and median ages of onset of 18 to 25 years.

More recent studies include national and community samples.

More Recent Studies Include National and Community Samples

National Studies

Table 1.4 reports the results from national studies specific to bipolar disorder among children and adolescents.

Kessler, Petukhova, Sampson, Zaslavsky, and Wittchen, (2012), combining results from the NCS-R (Kessler & Merikangas, 2004) and the NCS-A (Merikangas et al., 2009), also compared lifetime prevalence rates of bipolar I or II based on DSM-IV-TR criteria. Among youth ages 13 to 17 years, 0.3% of females and 0.1% of males met the criteria for bipolar I disorder. However, 2.8% of both sexes met the criteria for bipolar II disorder. The overall lifetime prevalence estimates for either bipolar I or II was 3.0%, with 3.1% of females and 2.8% of males meeting the criteria for bipolar I or II (see Table 1.4).

In this analysis, Kessler et al. (2012), also reported an LMR for bipolar I disorder, bipolar II disorder, and bipolar I or II disorder (see previous discussion regarding calculation). Among 13- to 17-year-olds, the LT/LMR ratio was 0.1 for bipolar I disorder; 1.0 for bipolar II disorder, and 0.7 for bipolar I or II disorder (see Table 1.4).

Merikangas, He, Burstein, Swanson, Avenevoli, Cui, Benjet, Georgiades, and Swendsen (2010b), also using the NCS-A sample, reported a lifetime prevalence of bipolar I or II disorder of 2.9%. Presented by gender, 3.3% of adolescent females and 2.6% of adolescent males met criteria for DSM-IV bipolar I or II. Broken down by age group, 1.9% of youth ages 13 and 14 met the criteria, compared to 3.1% of 15- and 16-year-olds and 4.3% of 17- and 18-year-olds (results not reported in Table 1.4).

Community Studies

Table 1.5 reports the results from community studies of children and adolescents.

The Great Smoky Mountains Study of Youth (Costello et al., 1996) reported a 3-month

Table 1.4 Rates of Bipolar Disorders in National Samples of Children and Adolescents

National Study	*Prevalence Rates/100 (SE)*
NCS-A, Kessler et al., 2012	
Bipolar Disorder I or II—Lifetime Prevalence	**3.0 (0.4)**
Females	3.1 (0.5)
Males	2.8 (0.5)
Bipolar Disorder I—Lifetime Prevalence	0.2 (0.1)
Females	0.3 (0.2)
Males	0.1 (0.0)
Bipolar Disorder II—Lifetime Prevalence	2.8 (0.4)
Females	2.8 (0.5)
Males	2.8 (0.5)
Lifetime morbid risk (LMR) and ratio of lifetime prevalence to morbid risk (LT/LMR) of:	
Bipolar Disorder I among 13- to 17-year-olds	0.1
Bipolar Disorder II among 13- to 17-year-olds	1.0
Bipolar Disorder I or II among 13- to 17-year-olds	0.7

prevalence for hypomania (0.10%), with 0.07% of females and 0.13% of males meeting the DSM-III-R criteria (see Table 1.5). In the 2003 report that followed the same subjects, the 3-month prevalence of bipolar disorder was less than 0.01% among all respondents, using DSM-IV criteria (Costello et al., 2003).

Lewinsohn et al. (2000), in the Oregon Adolescent Depression Project based on a school sample of adolescents, reported lifetime and point prevalence results for bipolar disorder (see Table 1.5). At Time 1, the lifetime prevalence for bipolar disorder was 0.9%; at Time 2 (approximately 1 year later), it was found to be 1.0%.

Roberts et al. (2007) reported past-year prevalence of mania and hypomania in the Teen Health 2000 Study. While the past-year prevalence of mania was 0.39%, the past-year prevalence of hypomania was 0.81% (see Table 1.5).

Differences in Reporting Prevalence

Among both national and community studies, differences in how rates are reported render it difficult to compare across such studies. While 12-month and lifetime prevalence rates are common, 3-month prevalence rates were used among community studies. Such differences in reporting have been noted in the literature, in turn leading to a lack of synthesis across studies (Kessler et al., 2012).

Comparison of Rates Based on Age of Onset to Rates Based on Child/Adolescent Samples

The lifetime prevalence of bipolar I disorder in the full sample, ages 15 to 54 (Kessler et al., 1994), of the 1990 NCS was 1.7%; in the younger sample (ages 15–17) it was found to be 1.3%. The ECA (Robins & Price, 1991), based on more than 18,000 adults age 18 and over in five U.S. communities, reported a lifetime prevalence of 0.9% for bipolar I disorder. In comparison, based on the NCS-A sample, the lifetime prevalence of bipolar I or II disorder was reported to be 2.9% (Merikangas et al., 2010). Kessler et al. (2012) reported a lifetime prevalence rate of 0.2% for bipolar I disorder, also based on the NCS-A sample.

Table 1.5 Rates of Bipolar Disorders in Community and School-Based Samples of Children and Adolescents

Authors	*Mania*	*Hypomania*	*Bipolar*
Great Smoky Mountains Study, Three-Month Prevalence Estimates—DSM-III-R	**Prevalence Rate/ 100 (SE)**	**Prevalence Rate/ 100 (SE)**	**Prevalence Rate/ 100 (SE)**
Costello et al. (1996)	—	0.10 (0.06)§	—
Females		0.07 (0.07)§	
Males		0.13 (0.09)§	
Great Smoky Mountains Study, Three-Month Prevalence Estimates—DSM-IV	**Prevalence Rate/ 100 (95% CI)**	**Prevalence Rate/ 100 (95% CI)**	**Prevalence Rate/100 (95% CI)**
Costello et al. (2003)	—	—	< 0.1 (< 0.1–0.1)
Females			< 0.1 (< 0.1–0.1)
Males			< 0.1 (< 0.1–0.1)
Oregon Adolescent Depression Project, Lifetime Prevalence Estimates—DSM-III-R	**Prevalence Rate/ 100**	**Prevalence Rate/100**	**Prevalence Rate/100**
Lewinsohn et al., 2000	—	—	0.9% (T1, LT) 0.6% (T1, Point) 1.0% (T2, LT) 0.5% (T2, Point)
Teen Health 2000 Past-Year Prevalence Estimates—DSM-IV	**Prevalence Rate/ 100 (95% CI)**	**Prevalence Rate/ 100 (95% CI)**	**Prevalence Rate/100 (95% CI)**
Roberts et al. (2007)			
Prevalence of Disorder	0.39 (0.18–0.61)	0.81 (0.50–1.12)	—
Prevalence with DISC Impairment	0.31 (0.12–0.51)	—	
Prevalence with CGAS ≤ 69	0.22 (0.05–0.39)	0.09 (0–0.20)	

§ <5 cases in interviewed sample

In summary, the epidemiologic studies of adolescents and adults show an early age of onset of bipolar disorder and prevalence in adolescents close to what is found in studies of adults.

Risk Factors

Among risk factors, family history has been demonstrated to be one of the strongest and most consistent risk factors for the development of bipolar disorder. Family studies of bipolar disorder have found adult relatives of probands with bipolar disorder to have a 10-fold increased risk of the disorder when compared to family members of control subjects (Merikangas & Yu, 2002). Further evidence for the role of genetic factors in the development of bipolar disorder among family members have come from a small number of twin studies that have found a an aggregate estimate of threefold risk among monozygotic versus dizygotic twins (Smoller & Gardner-Schuster, 2007). However, inheritance of bipolar disorder appears to be complex, as results from twin studies have found an average concordance rate of 40% for monozygotic twins compared to 5% for dizygotic twins (Smoller & Finn, 2003).

Despite these findings, there are few data on susceptibility genes that have been shown to have a consistent, significant predictive value for developing bipolar disorder (Merikangas & Pato, 2009). Thus, while family history of bipolar disorder represents a risk factor due to either genetics or environment, it remains an important predictor for the development of bipolar disorder among youth (Merikangas & Pato, 2009).

No sex differential in rates of bipolar disorder among youth has been found (Soutullo et al., 2005), mirroring findings from U.S. population surveys conducted among adults (Grant et al., 2005; Jonas et al., 2003; Merikangas et al., 2007); however, some studies have reported that women are more likely to exhibit the bipolar II subtype (Benazzi, 2006). Caution regarding conclusions specific to the lack of a sex differential among youth is warranted because females may be more likely to exhibit depression whereas males may be more likely to present with mania (Duax, Youngstrom, Calabrese, & Finding, 2007).

Among adults, individuals with lower educational and income levels have been found to be at higher risk for bipolar disorder (Grant et al., 2005; Jonas et al., 2003; Merikangas et al., 2007). In the three U.S. population surveys (NHANES, NCS-R, and the National Epidemiological Survey on Alcohol and Related Conditions [NESARC]), only the NESARC had a large enough sample to compare across several ethnic subgroups. In this survey, Native Americans were found to report higher rates of the bipolar I subtype when compared to other ethnic groups (Grant et al., 2005).

Similar to depression, early life trauma and stressful life events have been shown to be a major risk factor for bipolar disorder, and many studies have examined this correlation (Horesh et al., 2011; Romero et al., 2009; Tillman et al., 2003). Gilman et al. (2014) further investigated the role of childhood adversities and adulthood stressors in liability for bipolar disorder using NESARC data (n = 33,375). Risk was analyzed for initial-onset and recurrent DSM-IV manic episodes during a 3-year follow-up period. Childhood physical abuse and sexual maltreatment were associated with significantly higher risks of both first-onset mania and recurrent mania. Stressors within the past year in the domains of interpersonal instability and financial hardship were associated with a significantly higher risk of incident and recurrent mania.

Comorbidity

Studies of bipolar disorders in youth report high rates of comorbidities with other psychiatric disorders. Estimates suggest that 20% to 80% of bipolar youths have comorbidities, with variations due to different clinical populations and methods of ascertainment (Birmaher, 2013). The most common comorbidities are ADHD; disruptive, impulse control, and conduct disorders; anxiety disorders; and substance use disorders (Axelson et al., 2006; Goldstein et al., 2008; Kowatch & Youngstrom, 2005; Sala et al., 2010). Among adolescents, conduct disorders and substance use disorders are more common.

ADHD

ADHD is the psychiatric disorder of childhood most often confused with mania due to overlapping symptoms. Bipolar spectrum disorder and ADHD share symptoms of impulsivity, distractibility, hyperactivity, and overproductive, rapid speech (Milberger et al., 1995). Further complicating diagnostic clarity are the high rates of reported comorbidity of these two disorders. Estimates suggest that 11% to 98% of pediatric patients with mania will also have ADHD (Biederman, 1996; Geller, 1997; Kowatch, 2005; Lewinsohn, 1995; Wozniak, 1995). Several research groups suggest that ADHD is associated with an earlier onset of bipolar spectrum disorder (Egeland, 2003; Henin, 2007; Masi et al., 2006; Tillman, 2003), consistent with previous studies demonstrating higher rates of ADHD among children presenting with mania (90%) compared with 57% of adolescents with mania (West et al., 1995; Wozniak, 1995a).

The Longitudinal Assessment of Manic Symptoms Study (LAM) attempted to clarify some of the diagnostic issues relating to ADHD and bipolar spectrum disorder. The researchers compared a sample of 6- to 12-year-olds (n = 621) whose parents reported manic symptoms, with a lower-scoring comparison group (n = 86). Among the 707 children in the sample, 59.5% met criteria for ADHD without bipolar spectrum disorder; 6.4% had bipolar spectrum disorder without ADHD; 16.5% had ADHD and bipolar spectrum disorder, and 17.5% did not meet criteria for either disorder. For those meeting criteria for bipolar spectrum disorder, the sample was evenly divided between type I and NOS. Seventy-two percent of the sample who had bipolar spectrum disorder (n = 162) also had ADHD. Comorbidities with other psychiatric disorders were highest for the children with ADHD and bipolar spectrum disorder; the rate was higher for those who had only ADHD than for those who had only bipolar spectrum disorder. The authors found no difference in age of symptom onset between the children who had both ADHD and bipolar spectrum disorder and those who had bipolar spectrum disorder alone. The dually affected group exhibited more impaired functioning than those with either diagnosis (Arnold et al., 2011). The authors concluded that most children presenting with manic symptoms did not have bipolar spectrum disorder, consistent with prior studies (Carlson & Blader, 2011), and that children presenting with both disorders suffer greater functional impairment and disability than those having either disorder alone.

Retrospective studies of adults with bipolar disorder suggest that childhood anxiety disorders and ODD are more common among adults with bipolar spectrum disorder (Hennin & Biederman, 20007). Other studies focused on the developmental aspects of pediatric mania have found associations between anxiety disorders in youth and elevated rates of bipolar spectrum disorder in adulthood (Goldstein, 2007). Several studies have found comorbid ADHD and bipolar spectrum disorder in adults who had the onset of bipolar spectrum disorder during childhood and adolescence (Chang et al., 2000; Sachs, 2000), suggesting that the onset of mania rather than the chronological age at diagnosis might be a predictor for a subtype of bipolar spectrum disorder that is highly comorbid with ADHD and that might have a worse prognosis (Chang et al., 2000).

To further understand the relationship between ADHD and bipolar spectrum disorder, family studies have been used to study this comorbidity in youth. These findings suggest that offspring of parents with bipolar spectrum disorder have higher rates of ADHD (Faraone et al., 1999). Relatives of children with mania were at higher risk for ADHD, similar to the risk in relatives of children with ADHD without bipolar spectrum disorder (Wozniak, 1995b). Moreover, mania, and mania with ADHD, aggregated among relatives of manic youth compared with ADHD and controls (Faraone et al., 1998; Wozniak, 1995), suggesting that mania in children might be a distinct subtype of either bipolar disorder or ADHD.

Goldstein and colleagues approached the question of bipolar spectrum disorder and comorbidities from another perspective in the Bipolar Offspring Study (BIOS). They studied 388 offspring (ages 7–17 years) of 233 parents with bipolar spectrum disorder (type I/II) using structured diagnostic interviews for diagnostic accuracy. A cohort of 41 offspring were identified with bipolar spectrum disorder (type I, n = 9; type II, n = 5; NOS, n = 27). They identified several clinical, demographic, and familial correlates of bipolar spectrum disorder. They found a significantly greater prevalence of ADHD, anxiety disorders, ODD, and conduct disorders among offspring with bipolar spectrum disorder than those without bipolar spectrum disorder (Goldstein, 2010).

Some investigators suggest that disruptive disorders (ADHD and ODD) are early manifestations of bipolar spectrum disorder and not separate diagnoses (Goldstein, 2009). Tillman et al. (2006) reported a 28.5% rate of conversion from ADHD to bipolar disorder during a 6-year prospective follow-up study, whereas other studies have found no conversion during longitudinal follow-up (Biederman et al., 1996; Mannuza, 1993), suggesting that children with ADHD and ODD who go on to develop bipolar spectrum disorder may represent a different diagnostic group.

Many factors contribute to the challenges for studies of ADHD and bipolar spectrum disorder in youth. Many of the existing studies use differing definitions for bipolar disorder. Some research groups, for example, use a technique of counting overlapping symptoms, while other groups do not (Biederman et al., 1996; Geller et al., 2006). Some groups require episodes to make the diagnosis of bipolar spectrum disorder, while others do not. Furthermore, three of the seven criteria for a manic episode are also criteria for ADHD: distractibility, excessive talkativeness, and physical hyperactivity.

Conduct Disorder

Studies of pediatric bipolar disorder document high rates of comorbidity with conduct disorder, similar to those studies that suggest higher rates of ADHD.

Kutcher et al. (1989), in a study of hospitalized youth with mania, reported that 42% also met diagnostic criteria for conduct disorder. Similarly, Wozniak et al. (1995) found that prepubertal children with mania exhibited high rates of comorbid conduct disorder.

A growing number of studies demonstrate elevated risks for conduct disorder among youth with bipolar disorder (Biederman, Faraone, Chu, & Wozniak, 1999; Carlson, 1999; Kovacs & Pollock, 1995). Kovacs and Pollack (1995) suggest an episode prevalence of conduct disorder of 54% for bipolar youths and a 69% lifetime comorbidity. Lewinsohn et al. (1995) have also shown strong associations between pediatric bipolar disorder and disruptive behavior disorders.

In the only empirical study to date investigating the overlap between mania and conduct disorder, Biederman et al. (1999) studied a sample of consecutively referred youth who met diagnostic criteria for either mania (n = 186), conduct disorder (n = 192), or both (n = 76). The investigators found that 40% of youth with conduct disorder and 41% of youth with mania had both disorders, demonstrating that they met the criteria for two distinct disorders, true comorbidities and not disorders that mimic each other.

On further examination of the sample, distinct phenotypic characteristics for each disorder persisted regardless of comorbidity. For example, among children with conduct disorder and mania, both groups demonstrated primarily irritable mood, chronicity, and a mixed presentation (Biederman et al., 1999, 2003). Characteristics that were identified as unique among the comorbid (mania + conduct disorder) group included physical restlessness and poor judgment. In comparison with the conduct disorder group, the comorbid group exhibited higher rates and levels of aggressiveness. Overall, the comorbid groups were found to have more severe and impairing symptoms than those with either conduct disorder or mania alone (Biederman et al., 1999). Along these same lines, Biederman et al. (2003) synthesized the findings of their prior pediatric bipolar disorder and comorbidities studies, suggesting that overall, children with comorbid pediatric bipolar disorder and conduct disorder experience an increased risk for poor outcomes, including increased psychiatric hospitalizations and drug and alcohol dependence.

Evidence suggests that pediatric bipolar disorder can be distinguished from disruptive behavior disorders using existing diagnostic criteria; other studies, however, suggest that this is not conclusive, specifically as it relates to distinguishing manic symptoms from the symptoms of disruptive behavior disorders (Carlson, Loney, Salisbury, & Volpe, 1998). Though complex, efforts should be made to clarify the diagnosis, as both disorders are distinct clinical conditions that require different interventions. When both conditions exist together, treatment of both is indicated to optimize outcomes.

Anxiety Disorders

Anxiety disorders are common comorbidities among youth with bipolar spectrum disorders. While many studies exist documenting the high rates of comorbid anxiety disorders in adult bipolar spectrum disorder, few studies have examined these comorbidities in pediatric populations. Existing studies of this comorbidity for pediatric bipolar spectrum disorder have shown lifetime prevalence rates of 14% to 56%, with a weighted average of 27% (Axelson, 2006; DelBello, 2007; Biederman, 1997; Dickstein, 2005; Kowatch, 2005; Tillman, 2003). Furthermore, family studies of offspring of parents with bipolar spectrum disorder consistently find high rates of anxiety disorders (Birmaher et al., 2009; Henin et al., 2005;

Simeonova et al., 2009). In a retrospective study of adults with bipolar spectrum disorder, those reporting the onset of bipolar spectrum disorder prior to 13 years of age had a 70% rate of a comorbid lifetime anxiety disorder diagnosis, compared with 54% for those with onset between 13 and 18 years of age and 38% for those with onset after 18 years of age (Perliss et al., 2004).

To determine the prevalence and correlates of comorbid anxiety disorders among youth with bipolar spectrum disorder, investigators studied 446 youth ages 7 to 17 who met criteria for bipolar spectrum disorder as part of the COBY study. The sample consisted of 260 subjects with type I, 32 with type II, and 154 with NOS. They found that 44% of the sample met the criteria for at least one lifetime anxiety disorder, primarily separation anxiety disorder and generalized anxiety disorder. Approximately 18% of the sample met the criteria for two or more lifetime anxiety disorders. The onset of anxiety generally predated the onset of bipolar spectrum disorder, after adjusting for demographics and subtypes. After adjusting for significant demographic factors and bipolar subtypes, bipolar youth with anxiety showed significantly higher rates of type II disorder, longer duration of mood symptoms, higher current depression scores, lower likelihood of reporting an index episode of the mania, and higher rates of familial depression and reported a worst lifetime depressive episode, characterized by greater severity of hopelessness, and aches and pains.

These findings are consistent with prior studies in which anxiety disorders have been found at high rates among youth and adults with bipolar spectrum disorder, along with the higher prevalence rates of type II bipolar disorder in bipolar youths with anxiety. These findings have important implications for treatment and deserve increased clinical and scientific study.

Substance Use Disorders

Epidemiologic and clinical studies suggest higher rates of substance use disorders among youth with bipolar spectrum disorders when compared with adolescents without bipolar spectrum disorder (Lewinsohn et al., 1995; Wilens et al., 1999, 2004). Evidence further supports the bidirectional overlap between pediatric mania and substance use disorders (Biederman et al., 1997c; West et al., 1996; Wilens et al., 1997b, 1999, 2000, 2004). Pediatric mania may be a risk factor for substance use disorders; several studies have demonstrated overrepresentation of bipolar youth among youth with these disorders (Biederman et al., 1997c, 2000; West et al., 1995; Wilens, 1997a, 1999). Investigators have further demonstrated that mania significantly increases the risk for substance use disorders, independent of conduct disorder and ADHD (Wilens, 1999; Biederman, 1997, 2000).

Wilens et al. (2004), as part of an ongoing, controlled family-based study of adolescents with bipolar spectrum disorder, examined risks for substance use disorders among adolescents with bipolar spectrum disorder (n = 57; mean age 13.3 ± 2.4) compared with adolescents without bipolar spectrum disorder (n = 46; mean age 13.6 ± 2.2). Bipolar spectrum disorder was associated with a highly significant risk for substance use disorders in comparison to the non-mood-disordered group, even after controlling for conduct disorder. Furthermore, adolescent-onset bipolar spectrum disorder was associated with a higher risk of substance use disorder than for youths with childhood-onset bipolar spectrum disorder. Some investigators suggest that developmental heterogeneity may be relevant in juvenile bipolar spectrum disorder based upon onset in childhood or adolescence (Faraone et al., 1997). The authors suggested that further study of the developmental relationships between substance use and mood disorders is needed.

A study aimed to document the prevalence and correlates of substance use disorders among youths with bipolar spectrum disorder. The COBY study is a long-term naturalistic study of youth with bipolar spectrum disorder consisting of 446 children and adolescents, ages 7 to 17 years. The investigators sought to determine the prevalence of substance use disorders in this cohort and to identify clinical and demographic factors associated with substance use disorders. For this study, ages were restricted to 12 to 17 years due to absence of substance use disorders among children (n = 249). Subjects met criteria for type I or type II bipolar disorder or NOS. Lifetime prevalence rates of substance use disorders were 16% among the 249 adolescent subjects. Eighteen (45%) met full criteria for an active substance use disorder at intake. Cannabis use disorders were most common, with a lifetime prevalence of 12% among all adolescents and 73% among adolescents with substance use disorders. Eight percent of all adolescents had a lifetime alcohol use disorder compared with 50% of subjects with any substance use disorder. There was a trend, yet not statistically significant, toward an increased prevalence of substance use disorder among those with adolescent-onset bipolar disorder (20%) versus childhood-onset bipolar disorder (12%). The presence of substance use disorders among youth with bipolar disorder was associated with significant health risks, including suicide attempts, police involvement, teen pregnancy, and abortion. Identification and intervention may have important public health implications.

BIOLOGY OF CHILD AND ADOLESCENT MOOD DISORDERS

Overview

There has been an exponential increase in our understanding of the pathophysiology of mood disorders in adults, and initially we were largely dependent on extrapolating from these adult findings to inform us about the biology of childhood and adolescent mood disorders. Recently, considerably more research on the biology of depression and bipolar disorder in children has been conducted.

Genetics

Serious mood disorders are known to have their onset in childhood and adolescence and to persist into adulthood. Thus, much of the information that has accrued concerning the pathophysiology of mood disorders in adulthood would appear to be applicable to the childhood-onset mood disorders. One important difference, however, is the apparent lack of efficacy of tricyclic antidepressants in youth as compared to the selective serotonin reuptake inhibitors, whereas both classes are effective in adults (Wagner & Ambrosini, 2001).

As highlighted earlier, heritable factors appear to be the most consistent predictors of risk, though environmental factors also play an important role. Thus, twin, family, and adoption studies have shown that heritable factors are substantial predictors of risk, especially with regard to bipolar disorder. Studies of children and adolescents with depression show a twofold increase in risk to first-degree relatives and a threefold to fourfold increased risk for offspring of depressed parents (Rice et al., 2002). Overall heritability estimates for depression have been shown to be about 35% throughout one's lifetime (Uher, 2014).

Studies have also consistently shown a higher rate of bipolar disorder among first-degree relatives of youths with bipolar disorder, and the offspring of parents with bipolar disorder have up to a 25-fold increase in rates of bipolar disorder (Birmaher et al., 2009). This increased risk in offspring of bipolar parents also extends to other psychiatric disorders, including MDD, anxiety, ADHD, and behavioral problems, as well as earlier onset of mood symptoms (Wozniak et al., 2012). Heritability estimates have been shown to be about 80% (Uher, 2014).

While considerable research has focused on genetic contributions in adult-onset mood disorders, much less is known about the genetic influences on early-onset bipolar disorder and depression. Genetic studies have mainly focused on the allelic associations found in adult studies, such as brain-derived neurotrophic factor (BDNF) val66 alleles, and the serotonin transporter-linked promoter region short and long alleles (SERT) in bipolar disorder (Geller & Cook, 1999; Geller et al., 2004; Ospina-Duque et al., 2000) and also in major depressive disorder (Goodyer et al., 2009; Kaufman et al., 2006). Unlike adult studies, which have shown correlations (Craddock et al., 2001), results in the pediatric population reveal conflicting evidence. Some studies show a relationship between risk of childhood depression conferred by BDNF and SERT genetic vulnerability combined with stressful life events (Gutierrez et al., 2015), while others do not show a correlation (Rimay et al., 2015).

In one study, the catechol-O-methyltransferase (COMT), a dopamine metabolizing enzyme, lacked linkage disequilibrium with ultradian rapid cycling pediatric bipolar disorder (Geller & Cook, 2000), which also differs from adult data (Craddock et al., 2001) These discrepancies between pediatric and adult populations may be the result of phenotypic differences or developmental influences on gene expression over time. These genes of interest are mainly expressed in limbic areas and represent areas of future study (Faraone et al., 2003)). There is also some evidence indicating that early-onset bipolar disorder may be associated with genetic anticipation, as evidenced by trinucleotide repeats (CAG/CTG) coding for polyglutamine tracts (Schürhoff et al., 2000; Vincent et al., 2000) and the fact that genotypes in FKBP5 that encodes subsensitivity of the glucocorticoid receptor are associated with suicidal events and behavior in adolescent depression (Brent et al., 2010; Tatro et al., 2009). Studies have also found that pediatric bipolar disorder, along with other affective and psychotic disorders, is significantly associated with microdeletion of chromosome 22 based on data from patients with velo-cardio-facial syndrome (Jolin et al., 2012; Scambler et al., 1992).

One study found the familial transmission of mania and major depressive episodes to be independent of each other, despite common comorbidity of mood states. This suggests that bipolar disorder may have its own distinct biological pathway, which is separate from that of MDD and even bipolar type II disorder, rather than representing a more severe manifestation of other mood disorders (Merikangas, 2014).

Longitudinal studies of community and high-risk groups are needed to further explore the genetic influences on childhood depression and bipolar disorder. Genetic influences affect neurobiological processes that modulate susceptibility to environmental risk via gene–environment interaction.

Early Life Stress

Despite the preeminent significance of genetic influences, environmental factors are clearly substantial in the development of mood disorders. Consistent with predictions from early psychoanalytic models, losses early in life, shameful experiences, maternal deprivation, and physical and sexual abuse appear to be major risk factors for the development of mood disorders. Research has highlighted the seminal importance of early adverse life events into the mainstream of the neurobiological processes thought to underlie the pathophysiology of mood disorders (Heim et al., 2010). The pronounced adverse effects of early life stress are believed to be mediated by the substantial plasticity of the developing central nervous system as a function of experience. It has been proposed that stress and emotional trauma during development permanently shape the brain regions that mediate stress and emotion, leading to altered emotional processing and heightened responsiveness to stress, which in the genetically vulnerable individual may then evolve into syndromal psychiatric disorders, such as depression and bipolar disorder (Gilman et al., 2014; Heim & Nemeroff, 2001).

HPA Axis

The system that has been most closely scrutinized in depression is the HPA axis. Upon stress exposure, neurons in the hypothalamic paraventricular nucleus (PVN) secrete corticotropin-releasing factor (CRF) into the hypothalamic-hypophyseal portal circulation, which stimulates the production and release of ACTH from the anterior pituitary. ACTH in turn stimulates the release of glucocorticoids from the adrenal cortex. Glucocorticoids have marked effects on metabolism, immune function, and the brain, adjusting physiological functions and behavior in response to the stressor. Glucocorticoids exert negative feedback control on the HPA axis by regulating hippocampal and PVN neurons. Persistent glucocorticoid exposure exerts adverse effects on hippocampal neurons, including reduction in dendritic branching, loss of dendritic spines, and possibly impairment of neurogenesis. Such damage might progressively reduce inhibitory control of the HPA axis. CRF neurons integrate information relevant to stress not only at the hypothalamic PVN but also in a widespread circuit throughout the limbic system and brain stem. Direct central nervous system administration of CRF to laboratory animals produces integrated endocrine, autonomic, and behavioral responses that parallel signs of stress, depression, and anxiety, including loss of appetite, sleep disruption, decreased sexual behavior, despair, increased motor activity, neophobia, and enhanced startle reactivity.

Laboratory animal studies have provided direct evidence that early life stress leads to heightened stress reactivity and alterations in the aforementioned neural circuits that persist into adulthood. For example, adult rats that were separated from their dams for 180 minutes a day on postnatal days 2 through 14 exhibit up to threefold increases in ACTH and corticosterone responses to a variety of psychological stressors when compared to control rats (Ladd et al., 2000; Plotsky & Meaney, 1993). Maternally separated rats also develop marked behavioral changes, including increased anxiety-like behavior, anhedonia, alcohol and cocaine preference, sleep disruption, decreased appetite, and cognitive impairment. Subsequent studies revealed multiple central nervous system changes that likely underlie physiological and behavioral sensitization to stress after maternal separation or lack of maternal care. These findings include increased activity (increased CRF mRNA expression) and sensitization of CRF neurons in hypothalamic and limbic regions, decreased glucocorticoid receptor density in the hippocampus and prefrontal cortex, increased mineralocorticoid receptors in the hippocampus, decreased mossy fiber development and neurogenesis in the hippocampus, as well as alternations in norepinephrine, GABA, oxytocin sensitization of the norepinephrine system, and behavioral sensitization to fear stimuli in nonhuman primates reared by mothers exposed to unpredictable conditions with respect to food access over 3 months (Coplan et al., 1996). Taken together, early life stress induces manifold changes in multiple neurologic circuits that are involved in neuroendocrine, autonomic, and behavioral responses to stress. If similar changes also occurred in humans exposed to early life stress, these changes likely confer an enhanced risk for depression.

As noted earlier, several retrospective clinical studies have evaluated the long-term consequences of early life stress in adult humans. In an astonishing parallel to findings in rodents, women who were abused as children, including those with and those without current depression, exhibit greater plasma ACTH responses than controls. The increase was more pronounced in abused women with current depression, and these women also showed greater cortisol and heart rate responses than controls (Heim et al., 2000). Several studies have reported similar neuroendocrine and neurochemical changes in abused children (Harkness et al., 2011; Heim & Nemeroff, 2001, Heim et al., 2010). A more recent study found two divergent patterns of cortisol activity in adults with a history of childhood maltreatment. Those exposed to early life stress with a history of recurrent psychological distress during adulthood had significantly blunted cortisol reactivity, while subjects who were exposed to early life stress but who had no notable distress during adulthood had significantly elevated baseline cortisol levels, prolonged responses, and greater total cortisol production (Goldman-Mellor et al., 2012).

One recent study showed that young daughters of depressed mothers had shorter telomere length than those of never-depressed mothers, putting them at higher risk of developing MDD and other age-related medical illnesses. This shorter telomere length is a sign of accelerated biological aging, and it is also associated with greater cortisol reactivity to stress (Gotlib, 2015). Cortisol reactivity has proven to be a crucial part of the diathesis-stress model in the development of MDD.

Neuroimaging of Childhood Mood Disorders

Brain imaging studies are beginning to provide replicable findings of informative differences between controls and those with early-onset mood disorders. Similar to adult neuroimaging, pediatric depression and bipolar disorder appear to involve abnormalities in the prefrontal cortex, hippocampus, and amygdala networks. Neuroimaging of pediatric MDD has revealed multiple findings. Volumetric studies have highlighted anatomic changes such as significant reductions in frontal lobe volume, overall gray matter volume loss and thinning, and increased ventricular volume in large cohorts of children and adolescents with depressive disorders (Luby et al., 2016; Steingard et al., 2002).

Magnetic resonance imaging (MRI) studies have reported decreased hippocampal volumes in adults exposed to various types of early life stress (Vythilingam et al., 2002). Because hippocampal volume loss is not observed in abused children or young adults (Teicher, 2002) (although corpus callosum, amygdala, and cortical development seems to be impaired), some have suggested that repeated bursts of cortisol secretion over the course of time may eventually result in smaller hippocampi. Enhanced CRF secretion during development may also contribute to progressive hippocampal volume loss (Brunson et al., 2001). The fact that adult patients with major depression exhibit HPA axis hyperactivity and profound CRF hypersecretion, as evidenced in studies of cerebrospinal fluid and postmortem brain tissue (Flores et al., 2004; Merali et al., 2004), and that these findings are also observed after early life stress, may provide additional evidence that this critical stress system plays a role in the pathogenesis of childhood mood disorders.

One review paper examined functional MRI findings in 28 different studies focusing on five functional imaging domains in depressed youth: emotional processing, cognitive control, affective cognition, reward processing, and resting-state functional connectivity. The findings illuminated differences in activation of the ventromedial frontal regions, the anterior cingulate, and the amygdala of depressed and control youths across all five domains (Kerestes et al., 2013). Another review compared functional MRI differences between bipolar youths (12 studies) and bipolar adults (73 studies) and found significantly greater convergence of hyperactivation of the amygdala, inferior frontal, gyrus, and precuneus when using emotional stimuli among bipolar youths versus bipolar adults. This review also showed greater hypoactivation in the anterior cingulate cortex when employing nonemotional cognitive tasks among bipolar youths versus bipolar adults. These developmental differences may represent more emotional dysfunction in bipolar youths caused by amygdala, prefrontal, and visual system hyperactivation and more cognitive deficits related to anterior cingulate cortex hypoactivation when compared to bipolar adults (Wegbreit et al., 2014).

A preliminary diffusion tensor imaging study found lower fractional anisotropy in white matter tracts between the amygdala and subgenual anterior cingulate cortex in depressed youth (Cullen, Klimes-Dougan, et al., 2010). A similar functional circuit also involving the subgenual ACC was identified using functional connectivity methods acquired at rest (Cullen, Gee, et al., 2009).

A review of 12 magnetic resonance spectroscopy studies in children with depression showed changes in glutamate and choline levels in areas of emotional regulation, though there are discordant findings (Kondo et al., 2014).

Neuroimaging studies examining pediatric bipolar disorder have also explored similar areas of the brain involved in mood regulation. Volumetric studies have revealed a decrease in total cerebral volume in youths with pediatric bipolar disorder (DelBello et al., 2004; Frazier et al., 2005). Studies have also shown decreased volume of the amygdala, hippocampus, and nucleus accumbens compared to healthy controls (DelBello et al., 2004; Dickstein et al., 2005; Frazier et al., 2005). One recent study showed depressed left hippocampal volume in pediatric bipolar disorder when associated with low family cohesion and the BDNF val66met polymorphism (Zeni et al., 2016).

A review of 26 magnetic resonance spectroscopy studies in children with bipolar disorder has shown changes in glutamate neurons and mitochondrial functioning in areas of emotional regulation (Kondo et al., 2014).

Neuroimaging in children with mood disorders has shown changes in the areas of the brain that control emotional regulation. Spectroscopy has also revealed possible impaired cellular function in these areas. Similar to genetic studies of pediatric mood disorders, further investigation of the neuroimaging findings is warranted.

Gender

Gender is well known to be an important but poorly understood factor influencing the risk of mood disorders. The prevalence of MDD, while equal between boys and girls prior to puberty, doubles in young women after puberty. This same phenomenon occurs across many different nations, cultures, and ethnicities (Weisman et al., 1996). This increase in females has been hypothesized to be secondary to hormonal changes occurring during puberty, exposure to different stressors, and gender differences in the stress response. One hypothesis is that women are more likely than men to have a dysregulated HPA response to stress, which makes them more likely to develop depression in response to stress (Weiss et al., 1999). Women may be more likely to have a dysregulated HPA response because they are more likely to have suffered traumatic events, which are known to contribute to HPA dysregulation (Heim et al., 2000). Twin studies also suggest that the impact of genetic risk factors becomes more prominent as girls pass through puberty and enter adolescence (Silberg et al., 1999). While these changes may influence brain function, the attendant social/psychological factors of puberty may also play an important role.

The prevalence of bipolar disorder has consistently been shown to be equal in males and females, yet some clinical differences have been noted. A cohort study of 604 subjects showed that bipolar women are more likely than men to show a predominance of depressive polarity as well as a depressive onset while bipolar men are more likely to have comorbid substance use disorders. Women have a significantly higher lifetime prevalence of psychotic depression and a higher prevalence of Axis II comorbid disorders. Bipolar women are also more likely to have a family history of suicide and a lifetime history of attempted suicide (Nivoli et al., 2011).

Another major distinction between men and women with regard to bipolar disorder is the impact of reproductive life events, particularly during the postpartum period (Diflorio & Jones, 2010).

CONCLUSION

Accurate epidemiologic data are useful for determining the magnitude of the problem, identifying risk factors, monitoring changes in rates (epidemics), and identifying the underserved. There are no data yet available on how the new DSM-5 criteria will affect rates, because DSM-5 was only released in May 2013; longitudinal studies will track how these changes to criteria impact rates of psychopathology among children and adolescents. Accurate estimates rest on accurate diagnosis, yet another challenge is stigma and underreporting in this population. In a recent *New York Times* article, two high school students wrote about the stigma of psychiatric problems among their classmates and how school administrators did not allow them to publish articles revealing personal accounts of mental health issues in their school district. They reported that students are not comfortable discussing mental health issues, despite the fact that many of them are receiving psychiatric treatment (Halpert & Rosenfeld, 2014). Stigma of mental illness must be decreased in this population in order to accurately identify the rates of these disorders and to improve treatment-seeking behavior; this topic will be discussed in further detail in a later chapter.

The explosive developments in neurosciences, genetics, and neuroimaging will undoubtedly help refine the diagnostic process of these complex mood disorders afflicting the young. Such advances can shed light on the etiology and underlying pathophysiology, including the identification of dysfunctional brain circuits and ultimately treatment of afflicted youth and their families. These data will also likely identify subtypes of depression and bipolar disorder, and ideally this will allow us to predict treatment response. Longitudinal studies focusing on the biology and treatment response of childhood and adolescent mood disorders are sorely needed.

Treatment of Depression and Bipolar Disorder

Moira Rynn
David Brent
Paul Crits-Christoph
Robert Findling
Karen Dineen Wagner

chapter 2

Although it is clear that adolescent mood disorders exist and lead to significant immediate and lifelong impairment for the child, as shown in Chapter 1, as compared to the adult treatment literature there exists limited treatment research in this special population. This has led clinicians to consult with the adult literature to provide guidance in their treatment approaches. In fact, the adult research studies have provided the template for the present interventions being explored in adolescent treatment studies. To appreciate how the adult literature informs the field of adolescent mood disorder treatments, the current status of the adult literature for both psychosocial and psychopharmacologic treatments will be reviewed. This will be followed by an appraisal of the same treatment areas for adolescents.

PSYCHOSOCIAL TREATMENTS FOR MAJOR DEPRESSIVE DISORDER

In 2014, an estimated 15.7 million adults aged 18 or older in the United States (6.7% of all adults) had one or more episodes of major depressive disorder in the past year (Center for Behavioral Health Statistics and Quality, 2015). There is now substantial evidence that major depressive disorder (MDD) can be treated successfully with certain targeted psychotherapies. This literature is briefly reviewed below.

Psychosocial Treatment of Major Depression in Adults

The strongest empirical evidence exists for three manual-based psychotherapies for the treatment of MDD (behavior therapy, cognitive-behavioral therapy, and interpersonal therapy) with less but still substantial evidence existing for two other forms of psychotherapy (brief psychodynamic therapy and problem-solving therapy). Initial evidence (not reviewed here) exists for humanistic-experiential therapy (Elliot et al., 2013).

Cognitive Therapy

The most widely studied psychotherapy for MDD is cognitive therapy, also known as cognitive-behavioral therapy (CBT) (Beck, Rush, Shaw, & Emery, 1979). This treatment is based on the model that the cognitions (conscious or readily accessible to consciousness) of depressed individuals are negatively biased. This negative bias is evident in negative beliefs about the self, the world, and the future. Such negative cognitions are one factor that plays a role in the initiation and maintenance of depressive symptoms. Cognitive therapy, typically consisting of 16 to 20 sessions over a period of 12 to 16 weeks, involves the application of both behavioral and cognitive techniques. The behavioral techniques serve to help patients engage in activities that give them pleasure, while cognitive techniques are used to help patients recognize negative cognitions and to evaluate the veracity of their beliefs.

The most recent meta-analytic review of CBT for depression covered a total of 115 studies (Cuijpers et al., 2013). This meta-analysis revealed a mean effect size (ES) for 94 comparisons from 75 studies of CBT and control groups of Hedges' g = 0.71 (95% confidence interval [CI] 0.62–0.79) (number needed to treat = 2.6). However, there was no evidence CBT was more or less effective than other psychotherapies or pharmacotherapy, but combined CBT and medication was found to be significantly more effective than pharmacotherapy alone (g = 0.49). Another recent meta-analysis (N = 11 studies) of comparisons of CBT and second-generation antidepressants for MDD found no statistically significant difference in effectiveness between second-generation antidepressants and CBT for response (risk ratio 0.91, 95% CI 0.77–1.07), remission (0.98, 0.73–1.32), or change in the 17-item Hamilton Rating Scale for Depression score (weighted mean difference, –0.38, –2.87 to 2.10) (Amick et al., 2015).

Even among those with recurrent depression, and among those with moderate to severe MDD, cognitive therapy has been found to be similar in efficacy as antidepressant medication (Blackburn & Moore, 1997; DeRubeis et al., 2005). Moreover, a direct examination of the comparative effects of cognitive therapy and medication across four studies revealed no evidence of a difference among those with moderate to severe depression (DeRubeis, Gelfand, Tang, & Simons, 1999). However, a meta-analysis examining studies comparing cognitive therapy to treatment as usual concluded that cognitive therapy may not be superior to treatment as usual (Jakobsen, Hansen, Storebø, Simonsen, & Gluud, 2011a, 2011b).

Despite the lack of evidence that CBT is uniquely efficacious as compared to other psychotherapies in the treatment of MDD, the overall weight of the evidence is that CBT is an efficacious acute-phase treatment for MDD.

Behavior Therapy

The original behavioral model of MDD treatment was Lewinsohn's (1974) approach. In this model, the primary goal is to increase the frequency of pleasant activities in the patient's life. Derived from Lewinsohn's model is a newer version that has been labeled behavioral activation (BA) treatment of depression (Lejuez et al., 2011; Martell, Dimidjian, & Herman-Dunn, 2013).

A meta-analysis of 17 efficacy studies reported that behavior therapy was superior to control (Cohen's d effect size = 0.70), brief psychotherapy (d = 0.56), and supportive therapy (d = 0.75) and equal to standard CBT (d = –0.08) in the treatment of depression (Ekers et al., 2008). However, 12 of these 17 trials were done in the 1970s or 1980s, prior to the advent of current BA treatment methods; 12 of the 17 trials were very small (N's per group of 15 or less); and many of the studies did not diagnose patients.

There have been two major efficacy trials of a modern form of BA for MDD completed to date. In the first study (Jacobson et al., 1996), there was no evidence that a full cognitive therapy produced better outcomes than BA at either termination or 6-month follow-up, despite excellent adherence to treatment protocols by the therapists and an allegiance of the therapists and supervisor to full cognitive therapy. In the second study (Dimidjian et al., 2006), patients (N = 241) were randomized to BA, standard CBT, antidepressant medication, and pill placebo. No significant differences between treatments were evident among low-severity patients. In the high-severity group, BA was significantly better than cognitive therapy. Furthermore, remission rates strongly favored BA (56%) compared to antidepressant medication (23%) and CBT (36%) in the more severe subgroup. The response rate for BA in the more severe group was 76%.

As with CBT, there appears to be evidence that behavior therapy is an efficacious, but not uniquely effective, acute treatment for MDD. The possibility that BA may be more efficacious than both CBT and pharmacotherapy among more severely depressed patients awaits replication.

Interpersonal Therapy for Depression

Klerman and Weissman's (1989) interpersonal psychotherapy (IPT) for depression assumes that although depression is caused by a number of factors (genetic, biological, social) interacting in complex ways, it is usually triggered by problems in four interpersonal domains: role transition, grief, interpersonal deficits, and interpersonal disputes. In IPT, the interpersonal problem that triggered the current depressive episode is addressed and the person is helped to build communication and interaction skills to resolve it. The acute phase of IPT typically lasts for 16 to 20 sessions.

IPT is generally recognized as an evidence-based treatment for depression. A meta-analysis of IPT for depression reported an overall effect size (Cohen's d) for 16 studies that compared IPT and a control group of 0.63 (95% CI 0.36–0.90), corresponding to a number needed to treat of 2.91 (Cuijpers, Geraedts, van Oppen, Markowitz, & van Straten, 2011). Ten studies that compared IPT and other psychological treatments showed a nonsignificant differential effect size of 0.04 (95% CI –0.14 to 0.21). However, based on nine studies (removing one outlier), pharmacotherapy was more effective than IPT (d = –0.19, 95% CI –0.38 to –0.01; number needed to treat = 9.43), but combination treatment was not more effective than IPT alone, although the small number of studies precluded drawing definite conclusions.

IPT has also been used to treat antepartum and postpartum depression. Treatment with IPT was superior to a parenting education program for women with antepartum depression in all measures of mood at termination (Spinelli & Endicott, 2003). Also, for symptomatic relief and social adjustment, IPT was superior to a waitlist control for women with postpartum depression (O'Hara, Stuart, Gorman, & Wenzel, 2000). In a different study, IPT for postpartum depression was found to be as effective as a mother–infant therapy group and superior to a waitlist control (Clark, Vittengl, Kraft, & Jarrett, 2003). Finally, in the only randomized clinical trial (RCT) of a Western psychotherapy adapted for Africa, group IPT was better than treatment as usual for depressed people in rural Uganda for depressive symptomatology and social functioning (Bolton et al., 2003).

Brief Dynamic Therapy

Psychodynamic psychotherapy comes in many forms. Brief versions of this treatment typically have a clear interpersonal or intrapsychic focus and use therapist interpretations as the key intervention designed to increase self-understanding about interpersonal or intrapsychic issues that might be contributing to or maintaining depressive symptoms.

The empirical status of dynamic therapy for MDD is supported by the results of a meta-analytic review of 54 studies (33 RCTs) (Driessen et al., 2015). Brief dynamic therapy was found to be significantly more effective than control groups at posttreatment on depression, general psychopathology, and quality-of-life measures (d = 0.49–0.69). No significant differences were evident between brief dynamic therapy and other psychotherapies at posttreatment (d = −0.14) or follow-up (d = −0.06). There was evidence, however, that brief dynamic therapy was significantly more efficacious than other psychotherapies on anxiety measures at both posttreatment (d = 0.35) and follow-up (d = 0.76).

Recently, two large-scale randomized noninferiority trials evaluated whether brief dynamic therapy was inferior to CBT in the treatment of MDD. Both studies, one conducted in the Netherlands (Driessen et al., 2013) and one conducted in a community mental health center in the United States (Connolly Gibbons et al., 2016), found that brief dynamic therapy was statistically not inferior to CBT in change in depressive symptoms.

Two controlled studies have demonstrated the efficacy of dynamic psychotherapy in combination with antidepressant medication. Both de Jonghe, Kool, van Aalst, Dekker, and Peen (2001) and Burnand, Andreoli, Kolatte, Venturini, and Rosset (2002) found that combined dynamic psychotherapy and medication interventions were statistically and clinically superior to medication alone in the treatment of MDD. In addition, the Burnand et al. (2002) investigation implemented a supportive session with a nurse in the medication condition, and therefore the results of this study indicate that the between-group effects may be due to the specific interventions of the dynamic treatment rather than the nonspecific relationship effects of a purely supportive intervention.

The evidence base for brief dynamic therapy as an efficacious acute standalone treatment of MDD is now reasonably strong, though more studies comparing brief dynamic therapy to pharmacotherapy and credible control groups are needed.

Problem-Solving Therapy

Problem-solving therapy (PST) is a particular form of CBT for depression that has a specific focus on training in adaptive problem-solving attitudes and skills. In PST, the therapist attempts both to foster the adoption of a positive problem orientation and to facilitate the acquisition and real-life application of a rational problem-solving style. To instill a positive problem orientation, the therapist will encourage the patient to appraise problems as opportunities for benefit, to adopt the belief that problems are solvable and that he or she has the ability to solve problems effectively, and to recognize that effective problem solving takes time and effort.

A meta-analysis of 21 independent studies concluded that PST was equally effective as other psychosocial therapies and medication treatments and significantly more effective than no treatment and support/attention control groups in the treatment of depression (Bell & D'Zurilla, 2009). Effect sizes (Cohen's d) were 0.45 for the comparison to supportive therapy/attention control groups and 2.38 for the comparison to no treatment (waitlist control groups).

PST also appears to be promising for the acute treatment of MDD. Limitations of the existing literature are that several studies focus on minor depression rather than MDD, and that follow-up data are more limited, with heterogeneous results across studies. In addition, larger studies are needed, as are more comparisons to other standard psychotherapies for MDD.

Prevention of Relapse and Recurrence

From the literature reviewed in the sections on CBT, BA, IPT, PST, and brief dynamic therapy, it is apparent that the efficacy of short-term acute-phase treatment of MDD is similar across these various psychotherapy modalities. However, CBT has a particular focus on the prevention of relapse and recurrence of depressive episodes. To address this important question, controlled relapse/recurrence prevention studies involving CBT have been conducted. A meta-analysis of 28 such studies documented that responders to CBT have a relapse or recurrence at a rate of 29% within 1 year and 54% within 2 years (Vittengl et al., 2007). These relapse/recurrence rates were similar to those associated with other depression-specific psychotherapies. Across seven studies, relapse/recurrence rates were lower for CBT (39%) compared with pharmacotherapy (68%).

In an effort to achieve even lower relapse/recurrence rates, investigators have examined continuation therapy (i.e., additional therapy sessions after an acute-phase response has been achieved). One form of CBT, mindfulness-based cognitive therapy (MBCT; Segal, Williams, & Teasdale, 2012), was developed specifically to prevent relapse and is delivered after a person has recovered from depression following acute treatment. MBCT is delivered in a group format over 3 months. The treatment encourages patients to process experience without judgment through mindfulness and meditation techniques. A meta-analysis of six MBCT studies found that MBCT has a 34% reduction in risk of relapse compared to controls, with an even higher reduction in relapse rates (43% reduction) among patients who have had three or more previous episodes of depression (Piet & Hougaard, 2011).

A recent meta-analysis of 29 studies of continuation treatments examined the recurrence of new episodes for CBT, MBCT, and IPT (Clarke et al., 2015). The reductions in relapse rates at 12 months were similar for CBT (25%), MBCT (21%), and IPT (22%). The effect was maintained at 24 months for CBT, but not for IPT (no 24-month MBCT studies were available). In relation to comparator groups, CBT, MBCT, and IPT reduced the risk of relapse compared to treatment as usual (relative risk [RR] = 0.79, 95% CI 0.70–0.91) and active comparators (RR = 0.77, 95% CI 0.68–0.87), but there was no significant difference among CBT, MBCT, and IPT.

Less research has been conducted on the prevention of relapse/recurrence of MDD following BA treatment. However, one study found BA to be at least as effective as CBT and continuation medication in the prevention of relapse of MDD (Dobson et al., 2008).

Conclusion

A relatively large and growing body of literature has substantiated the efficacy of targeted psychotherapies in the treatment of MDD in adults. Research evidence from controlled clinical trials in particular supports the efficacy of CBT, IPT, BA, and brief dynamic therapy. Acute-phase CBT and IPT reduce the risk of relapse or recurrence of MDD, and continuation treatment with CBT, IPT, or MBCT reduces such risks further. CBT, BA, and IPT generally have been found to be equally efficacious to medications, even with more severely depressed patients.

Although many of the psychotherapeutic interventions studied in adults have been adapted to the treatment of adolescents, including IPT, CBT, and BA, the adult literature is characterized by a much broader set of studies than in the child and adolescent MDD treatment literature. Even with the relatively large number of MDD studies conducted to date, numerous questions remain about psychotherapy for MDD in adults. Despite the success of certain psychotherapies in the treatment of adult MDD, it may be risky to assume such treatments are likely to be the best psychosocial treatments for childhood and adolescent MDD. The biological, developmental, cognitive, and experiential differences between children and adolescents and adults raise the question of whether wholly different intervention strategies may be most effective with children and adolescents (Mueller & Orvaschel, 1997). For example, psychodynamic psychotherapy, especially variants that rely heavily on symbolic interpretations, may not be appropriate for younger individuals who lack the cognitive maturity to understand such interventions. Treatments that have been little studied in adults, such as family therapy, may have much greater relevance among children and adolescents. New treatments that incorporate developmental issues may be needed. Although it may be hazardous to export treatment modalities developed for adults to children and adolescents, research on children and adolescents can benefit greatly from the methodological developments in the treatment of MDD in adults, particularly the study of prevention of relapse or recurrence. Ongoing dialog and interchange among investigators in the adult and child areas is likely to facilitate the continued development of literature on treatment of children with MDD.

Psychosocial Treatment of Child and Adolescent Major Depression

In this overview of psychosocial treatments for early-onset depression, we review the RCTs in children and adolescents with depressive disorders and symptomatology. Both CBT and IPT have been shown in several trials to be efficacious in the treatment and prevention of adolescent depression. In addition, other promising psychosocial treatments are described that have positive but unreplicated results. Finally, given the frequent interrelationship between depression and suicidal behavior, we review the published clinical trials that show some evidence with regard to the treatment of adolescent suicide attempters, suicidal ideation, and nonsuicidal self-injury (NSSI).

CBT of Youth Depression

CBT approaches for youth depression are quite heterogeneous, but all have two key components: a focus on identifying and modifying negative cognitive bias that leads to distress and depression, and the employment of behavioral activation, in which the depressed individual is encouraged to participate in activities that are likely to be associated with a sense of mastery or pleasure. Other common techniques used in CBT include problem solving, emotion-regulation strategies, and social skills to improve interpersonal effectiveness, since all of these domains can be impaired in depression (Kaslow & Thompson, 1998, Kazdin & Weisz, 1998, Weersing & Brent, 2006). CBT, when compared to alternative treatments for youth depression, shows consistently positive but modest effects (d = 0.35) (Weisz et al., 2006). This result was more recently validated in a network meta-analysis that found that CBT for depression was significantly more effective at posttreatment than control conditions, play therapy, and problem-solving therapy in children and adolescents (Zhou et al., 2015). Below we discuss the highest-quality studies conducted in settings most relevant to clinical practice.

Wood et al. (1996) compared the impact of a five- to eight-session CBT intervention with a comparable dose of relaxation training in the treatment of early- to middle-adolescent outpatients with depressive disorders, with 54% of the CBT group and 26% of the relaxation group remitting by the end of treatment. Similar results were obtained on self-report measures of depressive symptoms, self-esteem, and general psychosocial adjustment. At 6-month follow-up, the outcomes of the two treatment groups converged because of continued improvement in the relaxation group and relapse in the CBT group. Younger age of diagnosis and higher level of functioning at intake were associated with better outcome (Jayson et al., 1998). The addition of a median of six monthly booster CBT sessions after acute treatment resulted in a much lower relapse rate than acute treatment alone in a quasi-experimental study (20% vs. 50%) (Kroll et al., 1996).

Brent et al. (1997) tested a version of CBT adapted for adolescents from Beck et al. (1979) against systemic behavioral family therapy (SBFT) and a nondirective supportive therapy (NST), using a primarily clinically referred sample (2/3 vs. 1/3 from newspaper advertisements) of depressed adolescents. In comparison to the treatment used by Wood et al. (1996), these treatments consisted of more sessions (12–16 weekly sessions).

At posttreatment assessment, significantly fewer of the subjects receiving CBT (17%) than NST (42%) continued to have diagnosable MDD. Remission, as defined by the absence of MDD and at least three consecutive Beck Depression Inventory (BDI) scores of less than 9, was more common in the CBT group (60%) than in either SBFT (38%) or NST (39%). Reductions in suicidality and improvements in general psychosocial adjustment were not different across groups. CBT resulted in a greater change in cognitive distortions compared to either SBFT or NST, although changes in depressive symptoms were not mediated by changes in cognitive style (Kolko et al., 2000).

Moderators of a favorable response to CBT relative to the other two treatments were comorbid anxiety and the total number of adverse predictors to overall treatment response (Brent et al., 1998). On the other hand, a history of sexual abuse and current maternal depressive symptoms both eliminated the advantage that CBT had over alternative treatments (Barbe et al., 2004; Brent et al., 1998). At 2-year follow-up, differences between treatment groups were not significant (Birmaher et al., 2000). Recurrence of depression over the 2-year follow-up period was predicted by greater severity of depression symptoms at intake, higher levels of parent–child conflict, and a lifetime history of sexual abuse (Barbe et al., 2004; Birmaher et al., 2000).

CBT has been adapted to be delivered via the Internet. One brief (four or five sessions) intervention that primarily emphasized problem solving was not superior to a waitlist control (van der Zanden et al., 2012), but two RCTs with CBT have shown quite significant effects compared to waitlist control, including one for symptomatic youth excluded from mainstream education (Fleming et al., 2012; Hoek et al., 2012).

Weisz et al. (2009) conducted a community-based effectiveness trial comparing CBT to treatment as usual, and CBT was found to produce similar outcomes to community treatment, but in fewer sessions, with fewer additional services, lower costs, and great parent satisfaction.

There have been no treatment trials of CBT in preadolescent depressed patients in clinical settings, but one form of CBT, Positive and Secondary Control Enhancement Therapy (PASCET), has been shown to be superior to no intervention in reducing depressed symptoms in nonreferred, symptomatic youth, and has also been tested in clinically depressed youth with inflammatory bowel disease (Thompson et al., 2012; Weisz et al., 1997).

The Treatment of Adolescent Depression Study (TADS) compared 439 depressed adolescents randomized to placebo, CBT, fluoxetine, and a combination of CBT and fluoxetine (combination). At 12 weeks, the response rate for CBT alone was no different than placebo (43% vs. 35%) and inferior to fluoxetine (61%) and combination (71%) (March et al., 2004). By 18 weeks, the CBT-alone group had caught up with the other active treatment groups. Positive predictors of CBT response were high levels of cognitive distortions and higher family income (Curry et al., 2006). Combination treatment resulted in the highest rates of remission and fastest reduction in symptoms of suicidal ideation and depression (Kennard et al., 2006; March et al., 2004).

The Antidepressant and Psychotherapy trial (ADAPT) randomized 208 depressed adolescents to either fluoxetine alone or a combination of CBT and fluoxetine, and in contrast to TADS, did not find a benefit from the addition of CBT (Goodyer et al., 2007). The ADAPT sample was clinically severe, and these findings were consistent with TADS, in which combination treatment did not outpace fluoxetine alone for more severely ill youth (Curry et al., 2006).

Clarke et al. (2005) randomized 152 depressed youth treated in primary care to either medication treatment as usual, or medication treatment plus a structured, individual form of CBT based on the Coping With Depression for Adolescents (CWD-A) intervention. Although the combination was superior to medication alone in some secondary measures, there were no differences in the rate of diagnosable depression at the end of the trial, or upon follow-up.

The Treatment of SSRI-Resistant Depression in Adolescents (TORDIA) study examined four strategies for the management of 334 depressed youth who had not responded to an adequate trial with a selective serotonin reuptake inhibitor (SSRI): switch to another SSRI, switch to venlafaxine, switch to SSRI plus CBT, or switch to venlafaxine plus CBT. The combination of CBT and either medication was superior to medication monotherapy at 12 weeks (55% vs. 41%), although the outcomes among groups converged over longer-term follow-up (Brent et al., 2008). Similar to earlier studies of CBT alone (Brent et al., 1997, 1998), combination treatment was superior to medication monotherapy for those with comorbidity (most commonly attention-deficit/hyperactivity disorder [ADHD] or anxiety), whereas a history of abuse predicted a greater advantage of medication monotherapy over combination treatment (Asarnow et al., 2009).

Two meta-analyses have been conducted to see if CBT in addition to medication is superior to medication monotherapy for adolescent depression. The first, which focused on adolescents with primary depression, found that while combination treatment was superior to medication monotherapy for improving functional status, it was not superior to medication monotherapy in the reduction of depression or suicidal events (Dubicka et al., 2010). The second, which included studies of depression comorbid with substance abuse, for which CBT focused on substance abuse, found an advantage of combination treatment over medication alone for depression and with respect to the incidence of suicidal events (Cox, Callahan, Churchill, et al., 2012).

Interpersonal Psychotherapy for Adolescent Depression

Interpersonal psychotherapy for adolescents (IPT-A), an adaptation of IPT, is a time-limited, focused psychotherapy that addresses common adolescent developmental issues that are closely related to depression: separation from parents, authority and autonomy issues in the parent–teen relationship, development of dyadic interpersonal relationships, peer pressure, loss, and issues related to single-parent families (Mufson et al., 1994, 1999). Summarizing all available literature, a network meta-analysis found that IPT for depression was significantly more effective than control conditions, play therapy, and problem-solving therapy in adolescents (Zhou et al., 2015). Specific higher-quality studies are discussed below.

In a controlled, 12-week, clinical trial of IPT-A, 48 adolescents with major depression were randomly assigned to either weekly IPT-A or biweekly to monthly 30-minute sessions of clinical monitoring (Mufson et al., 1999). The sample was largely Hispanic and female. At termination, a much lower proportion of those in IPT-A still met criteria for major depression (12.5% vs. 41.6%) and a greater proportion were remitted (75% vs. 46%). Patients who received IPT-A reported a significant decrease in depressive symptoms and a greater improvement in overall social functioning, functioning with friends, and problem-solving skills.

Mufson et al. (2004) assessed the effectiveness of IPT-A in school-based mental health clinics in New York City: they randomized 63 depressed adolescents referred for a mental health intake visit to IPT-A or treatment as usual, both performed by the clinic staff. At termination, the adolescents in the IPT-A treatment experienced significantly greater symptomatic relief than the treatment-as-usual group. IPT has been shown to be especially effective compared to clinical management or usual care in depressed adolescents with poorer interpersonal functioning, high levels of conflict with parents, greater depressive severity, and comorbid anxiety (Gunlicks-Stoessel et al., 2010; Young et al., 2009).

Rossello and Bernal (1999) compared the efficacy of a 12-week, individually administered CBT program to IPT and waitlist control in adolescents with diagnosed MDD and/or dysthymia referred by school personnel. Although the study was limited by poor attendance in both treatment arms, 59% of adolescents in the CBT condition and 82% of those receiving IPT achieved clinically significant improvement in depression symptoms by posttreatment; data were not provided for the waitlist control condition. In a subsequent study, participants were randomized to group or individual IPT or CBT (four cells) versus treatment as usual. Counter to the previous study, either form of CBT resulted in greater functional improvement and reduction in depressive symptomatology than either form of IPT (Rossello et al., 2008).

Attachment-Based Family Therapy

Diamond, Reis, Diamond, Siqueland, and Isaacs (2002) conducted a randomized clinical trial comparing attachment-based family therapy (ABFT) with a waitlist control in 32 clinically referred, depressed adolescents in a largely (69%) African-American, poor, inner-city sample. On average, subjects received eight sessions of ABFT, which focused on strengthening family bonds, reducing conflict, improving trust, and communication. Those in the waitlist condition received 15 minutes of weekly telephone monitoring of their clinical condition as well as a face-to-face assessment at week 6, at which point those still meeting criteria for major depression were offered ABFT (the treatment data from these latter cases were not included in the primary outcome analyses). At posttreatment, 81% of those treated with ABFT no longer met criteria for depression, compared to 47% in the waitlist control group. A significantly greater number of those assigned to ABFT reported a BDI score of less than 9 (62% vs. 19%). A significant treatment-by-time interaction favoring ABFT was found for interview-rated depression, self-reported anxiety, and child-reported parent–child conflict, with nonsignificant trends favoring ABFT for attachment to mother, suicidal ideation, and hopelessness.

A replication of these effects in suicidal adolescents in discussed below (Diamond et al., 2010). One other study of adolescent self-harm, in which the participants were also depressed, showed a positive effect on depression using mentalization-based therapy and is described below (Rossouw and Fonagy, 2012).

Fine, Forth, Gilbert, and Haley (1991) compared two forms of short-term group therapy, either social skills training or therapeutic support, for depressed adolescents in an RCT. Subjects in the therapeutic support group showed significantly greater reductions in clinical depression and significant increases in self-concept, although there were no group differences by 9-month follow-up. Subjects in the support group maintained their gains, and those who attended the social skills group caught up.

Prevention

A wellness-oriented CBT offered along with continuation medication for adolescents who responded to fluoxetine treatment was found to prevent depressive relapse compared to medication alone (15% vs. 37%, hazard ratio [HR] = 0.11; Kennard et al., 2008). This result was replicated in a subsequent larger trial (9% vs. 26.5%, HR = 0.31; Kennard et al., 2014). In a four-site study of the offspring of depressed parents, the majority of whom had had a previous depressive episode, a version of the CWD-A has been shown to prevent the onset or recurrence of depression compared to ordinary care at 8 and 33 months after the end of the intervention (21% vs. 33%, HR = 0.63 at 8 months) (Beardslee et al., 2013; Garber et al., 2009). A family group CBT has been shown to prevent the onset of depression in the offspring of depressed parents compared to usual care even 2 years after the intervention (odds ratio [OR] = 0.34; Compas et al., 2011), with effects mediated by improvements in youth coping and positive parenting. CBT, in combination with motivational interviewing, was more efficacious than CBT alone in preventing the incidence of depression in primary care (Saulsberry et al., 2013; Van Voorhees et al., 2009). Group IPT and individual IPT were found to be equally efficacious as group CBT and individual CBT for the prevention of depression in at-risk adolescents (Horowitz et al., 2007).

Suicide Attempters, Suicidal Ideation, and Self-Harm

Depression is the most significant psychiatric risk factor for adolescent suicide (Brent et al., 1993, 1999; Shaffer et al., 1996). We first review the interventions that focus on depression that also examined the impact of treatment on suicidal events (attempters or emergency referral for suicidal ideation), and then turn to studies that have examined impact on suicidal ideation, suicide attempts, or self-harm (including suicidal behavior and NSSI). NSSI is an important treatment target because of evidence that nonsuicidal self-harm is a stronger predictor of a suicide attempt than a previous attempt in some studies (Asarnow et al., 2011a; L.J. Cox et al., 2012; Wilkinson et al., 2011) and is also a predictor of completed suicide (Hawton et al., 2012). In the studies reviewed below, the term "self-harm" refers to behavior that is self-injurious regardless of suicidal intent.

In the TADS study, it was reported that the combination of medication and CBT was protective against suicidal events relative to medication alone (March et al., 2004, 2007), but this was not found in two other studies of combination therapy in adolescent depression (Goodyer et al., 2007), or in an overall meta-analysis of treatment of primary depression (Dubicka et al., 2010). However, in a meta-analysis that included studies of adolescents with depression comorbid with substance abuse, and including CBT treatments aimed at substance abuse, combination treatment did seem to protect against suicidal events relative to medication monotherapy (G.R. Cox et al., 2012).

Suicidal Ideation

A meta-analysis (N = 13 studies) of CBT found that CBT was significantly better than control groups in reducing suicidal ideation (Hedges' $g = 0.40$, 95% CI 0.30–0.49, $p < .001$) (Labelle et al., 2015).

Diamond et al. (2010) found that ABFT was four to six times more efficacious than clinical management in reducing suicidal ideation to below a clinical cutpoint in 66 suicidal adolescents; among adolescents in the study with significant depression, similar effects were found on reduction in depressive symptomatology. Similar to the first study, one weakness is the imbalance in duration and the intensity of the treatments (10 sessions for ABFT vs. three sessions for clinical management). The effects appeared to be mediated by improvement in family climate (Shpigel et al., 2012).

King et al. (2006, 2009) conducted two clinical trials in suicidal adolescents recruited from inpatient units using the Youth-Nominated Support Team intervention (YST). This brief intervention helped the youth to identify possible supportive adults and coach those adults on how to respond to the adolescent's request for support. Although there were no main effects on reattempts or on suicidal ideation, subgroups in each of these two studies (girls in the first, and multiple attempters in the second) showed greater reductions in suicidal ideation than usual care. The studies had relatively low participation of eligible subjects, and, at least in the second study, the intervention may have been overpowered by the intensity of treatment as usual, which in both intervention arms was over 30 sessions.

Tang et al. (2009) randomized 73 adolescents with high suicidal ideation, hopelessness, depression, or anxiety to either an intensive modification of IPT (IPT-A-IN) or supportive counseling in a school-based intervention. Participants in IPT-A-IN received 12 sessions over 6 weeks plus a weekly 30-minute follow-up call, whereas the counseling group received 30 to 60 minutes of support once or twice a week. The focus on IPT-A-IN was on interpersonal problems that precipitated suicidality or urges for self-harm, and included dyadic sessions with teachers or peers where relationships were problematic. The active treatment resulted in much greater reductions in ideation, hopelessness, anxiety, and depression, although its impact on suicidal behavior or self-harm was not reported. Limitations include the imbalance in attention between groups, lack of report on suicidal or self-harm activity, and exclusion of adolescents with a recent attempt from the study.

Suicide Attempts

Esposito-Smythers et al. (2011) compared integrated CBT (iCBT) to treatment as usual (consisting of "usual CBT" and medication management in 36 suicidal, alcohol- or substance-abusing adolescents). iCBT, in addition to the components of standard CBT, included motivational interviewing for substance abuse, and intensive family work to improve monitoring, supervision, and positive parenting. Despite its small size, this is the only study that has reported a difference in suicide attempts upon 18-month follow-up, which was paralleled by a decrease in alcohol/substance abuse, hospitalizations, and arrests. In the Labelle et al. (2015) meta-analysis, there was no significant effect for CBT compared to control groups for suicide attempts, possibly because of a low baseline prevalence of suicide attempts in most studies.

Huey et al. (2004) reported that Multi-Systemic Therapy (MST) compared to hospitalization resulted in a decreased incidence of suicide attempts. However, the treatment groups were not distinct, as 44% of those in the MST group were also hospitalized, and the rate of reattempt was the same in both groups, but the rate of previous attempts was higher in the MST group, making the results difficult to interpret.

Self-Harm (Includes Both Attempts and NSSI)

The Labelle et al. (2015) meta-analysis reported that, across eight studies, CBT was significantly better than control groups in reducing self-harm (Hedges' g = 0.27, 95% CI 0.17–0.38).

Rossouw and Fonagy (2012) compared mentalization-based therapy (MBT) to usual care in 80 mostly depressed and borderline personality–disordered adolescents who had engaged in self-harm. MBT, consisting of around 20 sessions (vs. 17 sessions in usual care) had weekly individual and monthly family sessions and aimed at helping the patient and family to understand action in terms of thoughts and feelings. MBT compared to usual care showed a dramatic reduction in the frequency of self-harm and also a very strong effect on depression and borderline personality symptoms. The effect of the treatment on self-harm was mediated by a decrease in avoidant attachment and improved self-reported ability to mentalize.

Pineda and Dadds (2013) randomized 48 adolescents with self-harm to either the Resourceful Adolescent Parenting Program (RAP-P) plus treatment as usual versus treatment as usual alone. RAP-P consisted of four 2-hour, biweekly, didactic sessions aimed at augmenting parental strengths. RAP-P was associated with a much greater reduction in self-harm and symptomatic improvement, and these effects were mediated by improvement in parent-reported family functioning.

A number of large trials for adolescent self-harm have been negative, including treatments that used a brief home-based family therapy and a group skills psychotherapy intervention, termed developmental group therapy (DGP) (Green et al., 2011; Harrington et al., 1998; Hazell et al., 2009). These three studies may have had too low a dose of treatment, especially relative to the intensity of treatment as usual. For example, in the Green et al. study, participants in the experimental condition received about nine DGP group sessions plus 10 treatment-as-usual sessions, versus 10 treatment-as-usual sessions in the comparison treatment. There are no definitive findings that support any specific intervention for suicidal or self-harming youth, but we review those that had some positive findings.

Treatment Engagement

Asarnow et al. (2011b) found that a one-session emergency department–based session for adolescent suicide attempters was successful in increasing attendance at subsequent sessions but not in reducing the incidence of suicidal events or attempts. Similarly, Ougrin et al. developed a brief 30-minute intervention for adolescents engaging in self-harm and found that it increased engagement, but this increased attendance to treatment did not translate into a reduction in recurrent self-harm (Ougrin et al., 2011, 2012, 2013).

Conclusion

Both CBT and IPT-A are effective in reducing depressive symptoms compared to comparator treatments as well as in preventing the onset of depression in at-risk youth. CBT can be successfully delivered over the Internet for either treatment or prevention. In addition, there is evidence that both interventions can be delivered in community settings with good results. Although IPT has not been studied in combination with medication, CBT when added to medication improves the outcome for treatment-resistant depression over medication monotherapy, and functional outcomes across studies of depressed youth. CBT does particularly well in patients with comorbidity (e.g., anxiety, ADHD, and conduct disorder), whereas IPT-A does well in patients with greater severity, interpersonal dysfunction, and high levels of parent–child discord. Although not studied in IPT-A, abuse and parental depression appear to be negative moderators for CBT. The combination of CBT and fluoxetine continuation treatment may be superior to fluoxetine continuation alone for the prevention of depressive recurrence. Both CBT and IPT may be promising interventions for preadolescents, but further work is needed. Both CBT and IPT have been shown to be efficacious in preventing the onset of depression in high-risk youth.

In addition to CBT and IPT-A, ABFT appears to be a promising treatment for depression, and perhaps MBT as well. With regard to suicidal risk in depressed adolescents, CBT alone is effective in reducing suicidal ideation and self-harm behaviors. The addition of CBT to medication, however, does not appear to convey additional protection for primary depression. There are some promising, albeit unreplicated other treatments for suicidal ideation (ABFT, IPT-A-IN; perhaps YST), self-harm (MBT, RAP-P), and suicide attempt (iCBT).

Pharmacologic Treatment of Adult Major Depression

Monotherapy

At this time the first-line medications for treating adult MDD are the SSRIs, which include fluoxetine (Prozac), sertraline (Zoloft), paroxetine (Paxil), fluvoxamine (Luvox), citalopram (Celexa), and escitalopram (Lexapro). They have a greater affinity for the serotonin transporter than for the noradrenergic transporter, and each compound selectively inhibits 5-hydroxytryptamine (5-HT) reuptake and has unique secondary binding properties. This class of drug is rarely associated with fatalities and given its safety profile provides an easy treatment option for the clinician (Farvolden, Kennedy, & Lam, 2003).

Also approved in the United States for the treatment of adult MDD are the selective serotonin and noradrenaline reuptake inhibitors (SNRIs), which include venlafaxine (Effexor), desvenlafaxine (Pristiq), duloxetine (Cymbalta), and levomilnacipran (Fetzima). Another SNRI, milnacipran (Savella), is not approved in the United States but is approved in other countries for the treatment of MDD. It appears that venlafaxine possesses a selective high affinity for the noradrenergic and serotonergic reuptake sites; however, it is only at higher doses (150–225 mg) that its noradrenergic reuptake becomes activated. This dual reuptake inhibition may contribute to the high rates of remission of depressive symptoms compared to those with SSRIs (Thase, Entsuah, & Rudolph, 2001). Although venlafaxine's side-effect profile is similar to that of SSRIs, at 200 mg there is a 5.5% clinically significant elevation of blood pressure and at 300 mg the incidence of hypertension reaches 13%. Duloxetine reportedly has dual reuptake inhibition that is equal at clinical doses.

Reboxetine is a selective norepinephrine reuptake inhibitor not approved in the United States for the treatment of major depression. Mirtazapine, which belongs to the piperazine–azepine group of compounds, has not been investigated in the treatment of pediatric depression.

A more recent (2013) approved agent for adult MDD is vortioxetine (Brintellix), a serotonin modulator and stimulator. A meta-analysis of studies evaluating vortioxetine concluded that although it was more effective than placebo for acute treatment of MDD, it was potentially less effective than SNRIs (Meeker et al., 2015). The most common adverse events with vortioxetine, relative to placebo, are nausea and vomiting (Meeker et al., 2015).

Another compound used for the treatment of adult depression is bupropion, which works by blocking noradrenergic and dopamine reuptake (Dong & Blier, 2001). It has the side effects of insomnia, nausea, increased anxiety, and restlessness. Another potential side effect is an increased incidence of seizures, which occur at a rate of 0.4% with daily doses below 450 mg and 2.4% with daily doses between 450 and 600 mg (Johnston et al., 1991).

Older classes of antidepressants efficacious in treating adult MDD, such as the tricyclic and heterocyclic antidepressants (amitriptyline, amoxapine, clomipramine, desipramine, doxepin, imipramine, maprotiline, nortriptyline, and protriptyline), inhibit different combinations of serotonin, noradrenergic, and dopamine receptors. Their antagonism at other receptor types causes difficult side effects such as dry mouth, confusion, orthostatic hypotension, tachycardia, weight gain, urinary retention, and constipation. In addition, doses outside of the therapeutic range may be lethal because of conduction abnormalities. The monoamine oxidase inhibitors (MAOIs; phenelzine and tranylcypromine) irreversibly inhibit the MAO isozymes A and B. It is thought that the blockade of the isozyme A lends these compounds their clinical efficacy (Mann et al., 1989). One major issue with this class of antidepressants is the required tyramine-restricted diet; if the diet is not adhered to, dangerous and possibly fatal elevation of the blood pressure can occur. Also, drugs that increase synaptic monoamines must be avoided, such as over-the-counter cold medications, tricyclic antidepressants, SSRIs, stimulants, and cocaine. There is also a risk of lethal, rare hyperthermic reactions that occur with meperidine and other opiates. Given these issues of tolerability and potentially serious adverse events, tricyclics and MAOIs have been more often reserved as second- and third-line agents for patients who have failed to respond to treatment with one of the newer antidepressant classes.

Pharmacologic Combination and Augmentation Therapy

Combination and augmentation strategies have been used when there is an inadequate response to an initial antidepressant and for treatment-resistant depression. The definition of treatment-resistant depression is the failure to clinically respond to one or two antidepressant trials with an adequate amount of time and dosage. There are several strategies for treating adults with an inadequate response or treatment-resistant depression: maximize the dose and duration of treatment; switch to another antidepressant within a class or another class; use a combination of antidepressants; and augment with other compounds.

By far the most ambitious attempt to examine the effects of switching and augmentation was the Sequenced Treatment Alternatives to Relieve Depression (STAR*D) trial (Rush et al., 2004). In STAR*D, patients with MDD (N = 3,671) were initially treated with citalopram. Those who did not achieve remission or could not tolerate citalopram were then randomly assigned using an equipoise stratified randomized design (allowing patients to decline treatment options) to four switch treatment options (sustained-release bupropion, cognitive therapy, sertraline, or extended-release venlafaxine) and three augmentation options (citalopram plus bupropion, buspirone, or cognitive therapy). Those who did not achieve remission at this second step were offered a third step consisting of two medication switch strategies (mirtazapine or nortriptyline) or two medication augmentation strategies (lithium or triiodothyronine [T_3, 25 mg]). A fourth step consisted of a single randomization to either tranylcypromine or extended-release venlafaxine plus mirtazapine. Remission rates were 36.8%, 30.6%, 13.7%, and 13.0% for the first, second, third, and fourth acute treatment steps, respectively, with an overall cumulative remission rate of 67% (Rush et al., 2006). Switching and augmentation appear to achieve similar remission rates (Gaynes et al., 2012). Thus, an initial one or two attempts at augmentation/switching appear useful for achieving remission, but additional (three or more) treatment changes do not yield meaningful further improvements.

Earlier studies supported the efficacy of lithium and triiodothyronine augmentation with patients who did not respond to SSRIs (one study with citalopram and one with fluoxetine) and newer antidepressants (Baumann, 1996; Katona et al., 1993). Other evidence supports the use of lithium and triiodothyronine as augmentation treatment for patients who do not respond to tricyclics (Aronson, Offman, Joffee, & Naylor, 1996; Freemantle, Anderson, & Young, 2000).

Several approaches are now approved by the U.S. Food and Drug Administration (FDA) for adjunctive (augmentation) therapy in the treatment of MDD. These include the atypical antipsychotics aripiprazole, quetiapine, brexpiprazole, and olanzapine (the latter in combination with fluoxetine). A meta-analysis of 17 trials of augmentation of MDD treatment with atypical antipsychotics found that the remission rate and overall response rate of adjunctive treatment were significantly higher than placebo treatment (remission: 32.6% for adjunctive groups vs. 18.2% for placebo; response: 43.8% for adjunctive groups vs. 28.7% for placebo), although there was a higher discontinuation rate due to adverse effects with the atypical antipsychotics (Wen et al., 2014).

Although effective, the approval of atypical antipsychotics for augmentation therapy has generated concern about the metabolic effects of these agents. The concept of metabolic syndrome is used to evaluate these risks. Metabolic syndrome has been defined by a combination of high blood pressure, low levels of high-density lipoprotein cholesterol, elevated triglycerides, and central obesity (Expert Panel, 2001). Depression itself is believed to be an independent risk factor for cardiovascular disease (Niranjan et al., 2012), so it is important to separate out the effects of the disorder from the influence of treatment on metabolic syndrome. This was done in a meta-analysis of studies that assessed metabolic parameters in MDD patients and found that use versus non-use of atypical antipsychotics was significantly associated with metabolic syndrome (Vancampfort et al., 2014).

Prevention of Relapse and Recurrence

Although multiple antidepressant agents are effective for short-term treatment of acute episodes of MDD in adults, if treatment is not continued relapse/recurrent rates have been found to range from 1.56% to 17.8% per month across 45 studies (Baldessarini et al., 2015). Given high rates of relapse/recurrence, longer-term treatment (beyond 1 year) has been evaluated to reduce such rates. In a meta-analysis of 72 trials, antidepressants were found to be more effective than placebos in preventing relapses (relative response rates [RR] = 1.90, number needed to treat = 4.4; $p < .0001$) and recurrences (RR = 2.03, number needed to treat = 3.8; $p < .0001$), with only minor differences evident among drug types (Sim et al., 2015).

Conclusion

SSRIs remain a first-choice option for pharmacologic therapy for adult MDD, with SNRIs also widely used. Longer-term treatment (>1 year) with SSRIs/SNRIs has been successful in reducing relapse/recurrence rates. For those who do not achieve remission with (or fail to tolerate) a first agent, switching or augmenting, particularly with an approved atypical antipsychotic, is a viable option for improving the likelihood of achieving remission of symptoms, at least through a second switch/augmentation trial. However, the possibility that atypical antipsychotics may contribute to metabolic syndrome raises concerns about longer-term use.

Pharmacologic Treatment of Adolescent Major Depression

The only antidepressants that have demonstrated efficacy in double-blind placebo-controlled trials for children and adolescents with major depression are the SSRIs. Two SSRIs have FDA approval for acute and maintenance treatment of major depression in children and adolescents: fluoxetine (>8 years old) and escitalopram (>12 years old). Three double-blind placebo-controlled trials demonstrated the efficacy and safety of fluoxetine in the treatment of children and adolescents with major depression (Emslie et al., 1997, 2002; Treatment for Adolescents with Depression Study [TADS] Team 2004). Fluoxetine doses ranged from 10 to 40 mg in these studies. Clinical Global Impressions-Improvement (CGI-I) scores of less than 2 (much or very much improved) were 56%, 52%, and 61% for the fluoxetine groups compared to 33%, 37%, and 43% respectively for the placebo groups. The efficacy and safety of escitalopram for the treatment of major depression in adolescents has been demonstrated in two double-blind placebo-controlled multicenter trials. In the first (Emslie et al., 2009), 157 adolescents were randomly assigned to escitalopram (dose range 10–20 mg/day) or placebo for an 8-week trial. A statistically significant greater improvement in depression (CDRS-R scores) was found for escitalopram compared to the placebo: 64% of patients treated with escitalopram were much or very much improved versus 53% of patients treated with placebo. In the second trial (Findling et al., 2013), improvement in CDRS-R scores was significantly greater for escitalopram than for placebo, with response rates also significantly different (63.6% for escitalopram; 47.1% for placebo).

Although not FDA approved for pediatric depression, two other SSRIs have demonstrated efficacy for the treatment of major depression in youth. In a double-blind placebo-controlled 8-week trial, 174 youths ages 7 to 17 years were randomized to citalopram (dose range 20–40 mg/day) for an 8-week trial (Wagner et al., 2004). The citalopram-treated group showed statistically significant greater improvement in depression (CDRS-R scores) than did the placebo group. The efficacy of sertraline for the treatment of children and adolescents with major depression was demonstrated in two a priori combined pooled analyses of identical double-blind placebo-controlled multicenter studies (Wagner et al., 2003). Three hundred seventy-six youth were randomized to sertraline (dose range 50–200 mg/day) or placebo for 10 weeks. The sertraline group showed a statistically significant greater improvement in depression (CDRS-R scores) compared with the placebo group. Negative double-blind placebo-controlled SSRI trials include citalopram for adolescent depression (von Knorring et al., 2006), paroxetine (Berard et al., 2006; Emslie et al., 2006; Keller et al., 2001), and an escitalopram study that included children and adolescents (Wagner et al., 2006).

Adverse events among children and adolescents treated with SSRIs are a particular concern. One study reported that 74% of children/adolescents experienced an adverse event to an SSRI over the course of their treatment (Wilens et al., 2004). Some differences in adverse events are evident in relation to age. Using adverse events from all double-blind placebo-controlled trials of SSRIs in children and adolescents that separated findings by age group, Safer and Zito (2006) found that activation and vomiting were twofold to threefold more prevalent in children than in adolescents, but rates of these events were low in adults. Furthermore, while somnolence was not common in children, rates of this adverse event increased with advancing age. Both insomnia and nausea were common adverse events across the full age span from children to adults. The most frequent reason for discontinuation from SSRI clinical trials in children was activation; in contrast, somnolence, nausea, and insomnia were the most common reasons for discontinuations in adults (Safer & Zito, 2006).

Of particular concern is the possibility that SSRIs increase suicidality in children and adolescents. Following up on reports of suicidal behavior in case reports and clinical trials of SSRI treatment in children and adolescents, the FDA conducted an analysis of 23 placebo-controlled trials of antidepressants in children/adolescents. Results indicated an overall statistically significant ($p < .05$) relative risk increase in suicide-related adverse events of 1.66 in MDD trials, and 1.95 when all trials were pooled, for SSRIs compared to placebo (Hammad, Laughren, & Racoosin, 2006). The data were interpreted as indicating that for every 100 treated child/adolescent patients treated with an SSRI, one to three patients will have an increase in suicidality beyond the risk that occurs with depression itself. There were no completed suicides reported in the data reviewed by the FDA (Hammad, Laughren, & Racoosin, 2006).

The FDA's response to these results was to implement a "black box" label warning in 2004 for SSRI use in children and adolescents. The warning states that SSRIs may increase the risk of suicidal thinking and behavior in children and adolescents with MDD and other psychiatric disorders. A recommendation is given in the black box warning that children and adolescents taking SSRI medications should be closely monitored for any worsening in depression, emergence of suicidal thinking or behavior, or unusual changes in behavior. During the first 4 weeks of treatment monthly monitoring is stated to be especially important. The warning also adds that adults should be similarly closely monitored during the initial few months of drug therapy.

The data on suicidality risk with SSRIs in children and adolescents need to be weighed against the benefits of treating MDD with SSRIs. Despite the rare suicide-related adverse events that occur, studies indicated that treatment with SSRIs overall decreases suicidal ideation and suicide attempts in children/adolescents (Kutcher & Gardner, 2008; March et al., 2004). Moreover, population studies have found that regions of the United States with increased antidepressant use have shown a decrease in suicides in children and adolescents (Gibbons, Hur, Bhaumik & Mann, 2006; Olfson, Shaffer, Marcus & Greenberg, 2003). Consistent with such studies, postmortem studies have failed to find a link between SSRI use and youth suicide (Isacsson, Holmgren, & Ahlner, 2005; Leon et al., 2006). Thus, in general, SSRI use appears to decrease suicide rates rather than increase them. In 2007, the FDA modified the black box warning to include young adults ages 18 to 24, but also to include a statement that depression itself was associated with an increased risk of suicide, thereby highlighting the balance between the small risk associated with antidepressant treatment and the proven efficacy of such treatments. Initiation of antidepressants at high therapeutic doses has been associated with an increased risk of self-harm behavior in patients ages 10 to 24 years (Miller et al., 2014).

Other classes of antidepressants have not demonstrated superiority of medication to placebo in RCTs for the treatment of children and adolescents with major depression, including desvenlafaxine (ClinicalTrials.gov Identifier:NCT01372150), duloxetine (Atkinson et al., 2014; Emslie et al., 2014), mirtazapine (FDA, 2004), nefazodone (Rynn et al., 2002; FDA, 2004), venlafaxine (Emslie et al., 2007), and selegiline transdermal system (DelBello et al., 2011). Bupropion has not been evaluated in controlled studies for major depression in children and adolescents.

Overall, rates of response for depressed youth treated with antidepressants are 61% and for placebo are 50% in treatment trials (Bridge et al., 2007), Remission rates in trials of acute treatment with antidepressants ranged from 30% to 40%. Clinical response by week 12 of treatment increased the likelihood of clinical remission (Curry et al., 2011; Emslie et al., 2010). The number needed to treat to benefit is 10, whereas the number needed to harm is 112. Therefore, the benefits of the antidepressants outweigh the potential harm from suicidal ideation or attempt.

Consensus guidelines recommend that antidepressants be continued for 6 to 12 months after symptom remission (Birmaher et al., 2007; Hughes, 2007). There is one maintenance study of antidepressant treatment for adolescent depression (Cheung et al., 2008). In this study, 93 adolescents with major depression received sertraline for 12 weeks, and responders were enrolled in a 24-week continuation study. At the end of the continuation phase, responders were randomized to sertraline or placebo for a 52-week maintenance phase. Thirty-eight percent of the adolescents in the sertraline group maintained response (i.e., no recurrence), whereas none of the placebo-treated patients maintained response. This study suggests that treatment of depression in adolescents should continue for a minimum of 1 year following 9 months of adequate treatment response.

Since approximately 40% of youths do not respond to initial treatment with an SSRI, the clinician is faced with a decision regarding selection of another antidepressant. The findings from the TORDIA trial provide guidance about the next antidepressant choice (Brent et al., 2008), as described earlier. Of note, adverse events of increased diastolic blood pressure and pulse and skin problems were more frequent in the venlafaxine group compared to the SSRI group. On the basis of these findings, approximately 50% of adolescents who do not respond to initial treatment with an SSRI will respond to treatment with an alternate antidepressant. Since adverse events were lower in the SSRI-treated patients, it is recommended that adolescents who fail to respond to an initial SSRI switch to a different SSRI. If a depressed youth fails to respond to two SSRI trials, then it would be reasonable to switch to an alternate class of antidepressants such as venlafaxine, duloxetine, bupropion, or mirtazapine.

Some depressed youth have a partial response to an antidepressant. Unfortunately, there are no controlled data to guide treatment-augmentation strategies for depressed children and adolescents. In a small case series, augmentation with an atypical antipsychotic (quetiapine) improved treatment response for depressed adolescents (Pathak et al., 2005). Based upon extrapolation from adult data, augmentation of SSRIs with lithium, bupropion, or mirtazapine has been recommended (Hughes et al., 2007).

Repetitive transcranial magnetic stimulation (rTMS) has been studied in a small open-label trial for treatment-resistant depression. Nine adolescents received rTMS for 14 days (10 Hz, 2-second trains given 20 minutes per day). One third of the adolescents responded to treatment (response defined as a >30% reduction in CDRS-R score). In a 3-year follow-up of rTMS for eight adolescents, improvement in depression was maintained.

Conclusion

Pharmacologic treatment of MDD in children and adolescents requires a careful consideration of potential risks and benefits. Unlike in adults, only fluoxetine and escitalopram have shown efficacy and are approved for acute and maintenance treatment in the United States for pediatric patients. The data on rare suicide-related adverse events and the black box warning regarding SSRI use in children and adolescents led to a subsequent decrease in the use of such drugs in the pediatric population (Friedman, 2014). This was likely an overreaction, given that the studies that emerged demonstrated that, on balance, antidepressant use was associated with reduced suicidality among youth and that no actual suicides were present in the clinical trials database involving SSRI use in children/adolescents. Nevertheless, close monitoring for clinical worsening and any suicidal ideation or behaviors is critical when SSRIs are prescribed in both youth and young adults.

BIPOLAR DISORDER

Mood disorders by definition disrupt functioning in several areas of an individual's life, including school, family, and peer relationships. Practice guidelines for the treatment of bipolar disorder in adults recognize both pharmacotherapy and psychotherapy as essential components of optimal treatment (American Psychiatric Association, 1994). From a developmental standpoint, research supports the notion that early psychosocial impairment tends to promote later impairment, as the individual arrives at each progressive stage of development with inadequate resources available to meet the challenges unique to the ensuing developmental period (Cicchetti, Rogosch, & Toth, 1998). Thus, it is crucial that treatment be provided promptly and effectively to maintain a normal developmental trajectory as much as possible, and minimize the effects that symptoms have on functioning.

Given the recognition of bipolar disorder in childhood, there is a growing body of evidence supporting treatment strategies, both pharmacologic and psychotherapeutic, for this population. Potentially promising treatment approaches for pediatric bipolar disorder build upon the literature for treatment of adult bipolar disorder. In the next section we review the literature on the psychosocial treatment of adult bipolar disorder.

Psychosocial Treatment of Adult Bipolar Disorder

Several different manualized psychosocial treatments have been applied to the treatment of bipolar disorder in adults; although they are based on different theoretical orientations, they share the goal of diminishing relapse to ultimately improve quality of life. Common areas of treatment focus include increasing treatment compliance, enhancing protective factors (e.g., support, self-care routines), and decreasing risk factors associated with relapse (e.g., stress, substance use).

CBT

CBT conceptualizes mood swings as a function of negative thought and behavioral patterns. These maladaptive patterns are then targeted in the therapy. Three RCTs with bipolar adults (for a review see Craighead, Miklowitz, Frank, & Vajk, 2002) suggest that adjunctive CBT leads to increased medication compliance, fewer hospitalizations, and improved social and occupational functioning.

IPT and Social Rhythm Therapy

Interpersonal therapy, as discussed earlier, is a short-term, present-oriented, problem-focused individual therapy developed and supported for the alleviation of symptoms of major depression (Klerman et al., 1984). In IPT, the onset of the depressive episode is placed in the context of interpersonal relationships, and current interpersonal difficulties are addressed. With the knowledge that circadian rhythm disturbances are linked to bipolar disorder (Ehlers, Frank, & Kupfer, 1988), Frank et al. (1997) supplemented IPT with social rhythm therapy (SRT) to create IPSRT for bipolar disorder. The focus of IPSRT is on the regularization of both social and circadian rhythms to control mood cycling. Results of a controlled trial with bipolar adults indicate that IPSRT is most effective in controlling the depressive symptoms of bipolar disorder, and also affects greater stabilization of sleep–wake cycles than case management treatment.

Family-Based Therapies

Several RCTs of family-based treatments have been documented in the literature. Inpatient family intervention (Clarkin et al., 1990), a nine-session intervention focused on psychoeducation, aims to modify negative family patterns and increase coping skills. Results indicate that female patients had better global and symptomatic functioning than those receiving standard hospital treatment (Clarkin et al., 1990).

Miklowitz and Goldstein (1990) developed family-focused therapy (FFT), a 9-month treatment incorporating psychoeducation, communication skills training, and problem-solving skills training. In a randomized trial, patients receiving FFT experienced fewer depressive symptoms, showed increased compliance with medication regimens, had fewer hospitalizations, and experienced a longer period to mood relapse than patients in a case management condition (Miklowitz et al., 2000).

FFT has been adapted and studied in adolescents in several studies by Miklowitz et al. (2004, 2006, 2008). The results suggest this form of therapy helps by shortening the duration of symptoms but must be used as adjunctive treatment to pharmacotherapy. We know that familial climate is related to relapse in bipolar adults (Miklowitz, Goldstein, Nuechterlein, Snyder, & Mintz, 1988). Therefore, family-based interventions among the families of bipolar children and adolescents should assist with improved long-term outcome.

Group Psychotherapy

Among adults with bipolar disorder, several different group approaches have been successful. For example, Colom et al. (2003) demonstrated increased time to relapse of mood symptoms, as well as lower rates of hospital readmission among remitted bipolar adults attending a psychoeducational group, compared with those receiving standard treatment (medications alone). Another structured group approach, The Life Goals Program (Bauer, McBride, Chase, Sachs, & Shea, 1998), consists of psychoeducation, behavioral skills, and individually tailored goals; at present, no data are available on outcome.

Psychosocial Treatment of Adolescent Bipolar Disorder

In adapting existing adult psychosocial treatments used with bipolar disorder for children and adolescents, several considerations should be made. For example, modifications should take into account the developmental level of the patient. Thus, information provided within an age-appropriate context may be more understandable and more widely accepted by the patient and family members; this may include the use of age-appropriate language rather than medical terminology. Psychoeducation conducted against the backdrop of a normal developmental trajectory may help distinguish normal childhood tantrums and adolescent moodiness from bipolar disorder (Fristad et al., 2009). Given the high rate of comorbidity in pediatric bipolar disorder (Findling et al., 2001; Goldstein, 2012), information about comorbid conditions may be included as part of psychoeducation. Comparative risks and benefits of psychotropic medications used with this population should be included. Psychoeducation may also focus on the manner in which early-onset bipolar disorder differs from adult bipolar disorder—childhood bipolar disorder often manifests in less discrete episodes and more frequent mood episodes (Findling et al., 2001; West & Pavuluri, 2009). Additionally, the manner in which symptoms manifest may need to be considered within a developmental framework, as children exhibit several affective symptoms differently than adults (Goldstein, 2012). Furthermore, age-specific issues may be targeted, including substance use, suicide prevention, family conflict, teasing, and academic concerns that may not be relevant in an adult population. Finally, because bipolar disorder is highly familial, it is likely that at least one of the parents of a child with pediatric bipolar disorder has either unipolar or bipolar mood disorder (Findling et al., 2001). The course of a parent's mood disorder is likely to be intimately related to the child's presentation, compliance, and management. Given that parental depression may interfere with a mood-disordered child's response to treatment (Brent et al., 1998), it is particularly important that the parent's own affective illness be addressed when treating a bipolar child or adolescent.

Conclusion

The empirical literature on psychosocial treatment of adult and adolescent bipolar disorder suggests that several forms of therapy, including FFT-A, CBT, IPT supplemented with SRT, family-based treatments, and group therapy, may be adjunctive treatments (Weinstein et al., 2013; West & Pavuluri, 2009). These treatments have been reported to produce better medication compliance, fewer hospitalizations, and improved social and occupational functioning.

Pharmacologic Treatment of Adolescent Bipolar Disorder

Compared with what is known about the pharmacotherapy of bipolar disorder in adults, relatively little is known about the medication management of bipolar disorder in young people. This is unfortunate, as there has been an increased appreciation over the past few years that bipolar disorder is a chronic, debilitating condition when it occurs in children and adolescents. Until recently, most prospective pharmacotherapy studies in pediatric bipolar disorder were uncontrolled and methodologically limited. However, over the past several years, more definitive treatment studies have been conducted.

The manic and mixed phases of bipolar disorder are more prevalent in teenagers compared to the depressed phase of illness. This may explain why more methodologically stringent work has been done in patients with manic and mixed states compared to adolescents with bipolarity who are depressed. It should be noted that most recently conducted studies are acute treatment studies, often only a few weeks in duration. As such, there is still a substantive need for longer-term controlled trials.

Fortunately, there has been a substantial increase in the number of methodologically stringent medication studies within this patient population over the past few years (Table 2.1). These data can provide practicing clinicians practical information on rational treatment approaches to the pharmacotherapy of this illness.

Monotherapy

Despite lithium's role as a benchmark treatment in adults (Severus et al., 2014), there is a limited research base in regard to adolescents. Some studies have focused on characterizing lithium's pharmacokinetics (Findling et al., 2010) and dosing for youths (Findling et al.,

Table 2.1 Selected Double-Blind, Placebo-Controlled Acute Monotherapy Studies in Adolescent Bipolar Disorder

Study	*Agent*	*Mood State(s)*	*Age (years)*	*Study Length (wks)/ Sample Size*	*Comments*
Wagner et al., 2006	Oxcarbazepine	Manic or mixed	7–18	7/116	Oxcarbazepine not superior to placebo
Tohen et al., 2007	Olanzapine	Manic or mixed	13–17	3/161	Olanzapine superior to placebo ($p < .001$); mean weight gain with olanzapine = 3.7 kg
Findling et al., 2009	Aripiprazole	Manic or mixed	10–17	4/296	Aripiprazole superior to placebo ($p < .0001$); MCA = extrapyramidal disorder, sedation
Haas et al., 2009	Risperidone	Manic or mixed	10-17	3/169	Risperidone superior to placebo ($p < .001$); MCA = somnolence, headache
Wagner et al., 2009	Extended-release divalproex	Manic or mixed	10–17	4/150	Extended-release divalproex not superior to placebo ($p = .604$)
Findling et al., 2013	Ziprasidone	Manic or mixed	10–17	4/237	Ziprasidone superior to placebo ($p = .0005$); MCA = sedation, somnolence, headache
Pathak et al., 2013	Quetiapine	Manic	10–17	3/277	Quetiapine superior to placebo ($p < .001$); MCA = somnolence, sedation
Findling et al., 2015	Lithium	Manic or mixed	7–17	8/81	Lithium superior to placebo ($p = .03$); MCA = vomiting, nausea

MCA = most common adverse event

2011). One large randomized trial evaluated monotherapies in adolescent bipolar disorder. The Treatment of Early Age Mania study targeted 6- to 15-year-old children and adolescents (N = 279) with manic or mixed-phase bipolar disorder and randomized them to receive lithium, divalproex sodium, or risperidone (Geller et al., 2012). In this study, risperidone was found to be significantly more efficacious than lithium or divalproex sodium for the initial treatment of childhood mania but was associated with potentially serious metabolic effects.

Only one placebo-controlled trial has been published. This recent study randomized youth ages 7 to 17 years with bipolar I manic or mixed episodes to lithium or placebo for up to 8 weeks of treatment (Findling et al., 2015). Results indicated that lithium was associated with significantly greater manic symptom improvement compared to placebo, but was not associated with weight gain. Response rates were 32% for lithium and 21% for placebo.

Carbamazepine has historically been given as a treatment to young people with a variety of neuropsychiatric conditions. Most reports describing the use of this drug in young people with neuropsychiatric conditions lack methodological rigor. However, one prospective open-label treatment study examined the effectiveness of an extended-release formulation of carbamazepine (CBZ-ERC) in 157 youths between the ages of 10 and 17 years. The CBZ-ERC was administered in divided doses with flexible total daily dosing ranging between 200 and 1.200 mg/day. The results of that prospective clinical trial provide preliminary data to suggest that CBZ-ERC may be effective in this patient population (Findling & Ginsberg, 2012). However, more definitive studies are needed to ascertain whether the efficacy that CBZ-ERC has in adults also is present in pediatric patients.

At present, one published placebo-controlled study has examined the efficacy of extended-release divalproex sodium (Depakote-ER) in the treatment of pediatric mania; it was not found to be superior to placebo (Wagner et al., 2009). However, in an unpublished 8-week study that compared divalproex sodium (Depakote) to placebo in the treatment of pediatric manic or mixed states, divalproex was found to be superior to placebo (Kowatch et al., 2007). The specific reason for the divergent results between these two studies is not known.

Topiramate does not appear to have efficacy in the treatment of mania in adults, but preliminary data suggest that it might be of benefit for bipolar youths (DelBello et al., 2005). However, a double-blind, randomized trial of 120 Iranian youths with manic or mixed-episode bipolar disorder (ages 12–18 years) found that sodium valproate was superior to topiramate (Hebrani, Behdani, & Manteghi, 2009).

Another anticonvulsant medication that has been studied in this patient population is oxcarbazepine. In a multisite, placebo-controlled study, oxcarbazepine was shown not to be effective in the treatment of youth with mania (Wagner et al., 2006).

Several other agents have been examined in the context of acute prospective placebo-controlled monotherapy treatment trials (see Table 2.1). Most of these published placebo-controlled trials have focused on the atypical antipsychotics. These larger-scale studies have examined risperidone, olanzapine, quetiapine, aripiprazole, and ziprasidone. In addition, results from an 8-week open-label study of 15 patients provide preliminary data that paliperidone monotherapy might be of benefit for pediatric patients with bipolar illness (Joshi et al., 2013). For youth in a manic or mixed state, risperidone, olanzapine, quetiapine, and aripiprazole are FDA approved for treatment. As with MDD, there are ongoing concerns about risks for metabolic syndrome with antitypical antipsychotic use for those with bipolar disorder. The overall rate of metabolic syndrome in those with bipolar disorder was estimated in a meta-analysis of 37 studies to be about 37% (Vancampfort et al., 2013). The rate was 45.3% for those taking antipsychotics compared to 32.4% among those not taking antipsychotics (Vancampfort et al., 2013).

Asenapine has also been shown to be effective in the treatment of manic or mixed states in adults. No articles on the use of asenapine in the treatment of bipolar adolescents have been published.

As mentioned previously, most medication monotherapy trials in pediatric bipolar disorder have focused on patients either in the manic or mixed phase of illness. At present, only one published placebo-controlled study has examined the efficacy of medication monotherapy in youths with bipolar disorder who are currently in a depressive episode. In that clinical trial, 32 depressed youths between the ages of 12 and 18 who also met diagnostic symptom criteria for bipolar I disorder were administered either quetiapine or placebo for up to 8 weeks in a double-blind fashion (Delbello et al., 2009). The patients who were treated with active medication received between 300 and 600 mg/day of quetiapine. Quetiapine was found to have no greater efficacy in reducing depressive symptoms than placebo. More than two thirds of both placebo- and quetiapine-treated patients responded during study participation.

The atypical antipsychotic lurasidone has been shown to have efficacy in the treatment of the depressed phase of bipolar illness in adults. At present, there are no data regarding lurasidone's use in adolescents with bipolar illness.

Psychopharmacologic Combinations

A substantial number of patients do not appear to derive optimal clinical response from acute treatment with a single drug. As a result, investigators have begun to explore whether pharmacotherapy with more than one agent may be useful in the acute treatment of symptomatic bipolar youth. The majority of these studies have explored intervention with (1) an atypical antipsychotic combined with a traditional mood stabilizer or (2) combined treatment with lithium and divalproex sodium.

Data show that the combination of olanzapine and fluoxetine (Symbyax) is effective in the treatment of the depressed phase of bipolar illness in teenagers (Detke et al., 2012). In that study 291 depressed youths between the ages of 10 and 17 were randomized to receive placebo or flexible doses of olanzapine/fluoxetine. Reductions in depressive symptomatology with active treatment were superior to those seen with placebo. The most common side effects noted in the patients receiving olanzapine/fluoxetine were weight gain and increased appetite. Olanzapine/fluoxetine is FDA approved for the treatment of depressed pediatric patients with bipolar I disorder.

Data from chart reviews suggest that clozapine may serve as a useful adjunct to traditional mood stabilizers for treatment-resistant patients (Emslie, Kennard, & Kowatch, 1995). Preliminary reports have noted that the antipsychotics haloperidol and risperidone might be helpful when combined with a traditional mood stabilizer in the treatment of teenagers with mania, particularly those with psychotic symptoms (Frazier et al., 1999; Kafantaris, Coletti, Dicker, Padula, & Kane, 2001; Pavuluri et al., 2004, 2006). Similarly, a case series reported that adjunctive olanzapine may provide benefit to pediatric patients who do not receive satisfactory benefit from lithium or anticonvulsants (Emiroglu et al., 2006).

Data from case series have described the potential usefulness of topiramate as an adjunct to antipsychotics and/or traditional mood stabilizers in this population (Barzman et al., 2005). In addition, preliminary data from a prospective trial suggest that adjunctive topiramate might be an effective way to reduce the weight gain associated with olanzapine use in this population (Wozniak et al., 2009).

One published study rigorously examined quetiapine treatment as an adjunct in patients ages 12 to 18 with bipolar I disorder (DelBello et al., 2002). In that 6-week trial, 30 hospitalized adolescents with mania or mixed presentations were treated with divalproex sodium at an initial dose of 20 mg/kg per day. Half of the subjects were randomized to receive adjunctive quetiapine and half were randomized to receive adjunctive placebo. The quetiapine was titrated to a total daily dose of 450 mg. Results showed greater reductions in manic symptomatology in the youths receiving combination therapy, but sedation was also more common in these youths.

Another prospective trial that examined combination pharmacotherapy in pediatric bipolar disorder described the response of 90 outpatients (mean age ~11 years) who were treated with combination lithium and divalproex sodium therapy for up to 20 weeks (Findling et al., 2003). Response rates were larger than those seen in other prospective trials in this population. Response rates were higher than those described in adults using a similar combination treatment paradigm. Combination treatment was well tolerated. Of particular interest was the observation that residual depressive symptomatology was not manifest after combination lithium plus divalproex treatment in this population. This is in direct contrast to adults, in whom depression was often seen as a problematic residual mood state.

Conclusion

On the basis of available evidence, it appears that combination pharmacotherapy with more than one mood-stabilizing agent may be a rational approach for some youth who have manic, hypomanic, or mixed states. Whether treatment should begin with drug monotherapy or combination pharmacotherapy should be a topic of further study.

Maintenance Trials

The first data to suggest that lithium maintenance therapy might be useful in the treatment of adolescents with bipolar disorder were published in 1990. That report described the results of a naturalistic, prospective, 18-month follow-up study of 37 youth with bipolar I disorder who had responded to lithium treatment (Strober et al., 1990). In the 13 youth who discontinued lithium maintenance therapy, the relapse rate was 2.5 times greater than in those who continued lithium treatment. Despite methodological limitations inherent in this study design, these data suggest that maintenance lithium treatment in young people who respond to this compound may be beneficial.

In one prospective trial of maintenance pharmacotherapy in pediatric bipolar disorder, 60 youths who had responded to acute treatment with combination therapy using both lithium and divalproex sodium were randomized to receive monotherapy treatment with either lithium or divalproex for up to 76 weeks in a double-blind fashion (Findling et al., 2005). The overall median survival time in the study was approximately 100 days. Lithium and divalproex sodium had similar effectiveness as monotherapy.

In another study, Findling et al. (2013) conducted a double-blind continuation study in a group of youths who had completed a 4-week, double-blind, placebo-controlled trial of aripiprazole. At the time of initial randomization, patients were between the ages of 10 and 17 years and received 10 mg/day or 30 mg/day of active treatment or placebo. Subsequently, 210 patients continued on their same blinded treatment assignment for up to 26 more weeks. Continued pharmacotherapy with aripiprazole was found to be more effective during this 26-week period than treatment with placebo. However, the rates of study completion were low: 45.3% for aripiprazole 10 mg/day; 31.0% for aripiprazole 30 mg/day; 18.8% for placebo.

Finally, lamotrigine has been shown to be an effective maintenance treatment in adults with bipolar illness. Currently, there are no published data about whether lamotrigine has efficacy either as a maintenance therapy or as an acute treatment for pediatric patients.

Conclusion

There are only limited data from methodologically rigorous trials in pediatric bipolar disorder. Evidence suggests that monotherapy with lithium, carbamazepine, divalproex sodium, or olanzapine may be useful in the treatment of young patients with mania and related mood states. Risperidone was found in one large trial to be superior to lithium and divalproex sodium for the initial treatment of childhood mania, but metabolic adverse effects were apparent. A consistent theme from the literature is that a substantial number of patients do not respond to monotherapy with these agents. For this reason, investigators have begun to explore combination pharmacotherapy. It seems that simultaneous treatment with more than one agent may be a rational form of intervention for some patients. The combination of divalproex sodium and quetiapine has shown efficacy compared to divalproex plus placebo, though sedation was a common adverse event with quetiapine. Beyond this study, circumstances in which combination drug therapy might be most rationally employed have not been identified. Because pediatric bipolar disorder is a chronic condition, it appears that young people with this illness will need long-term treatment. Although maintenance pharmacotherapy data are lacking, patients who respond to a given acute pharmacotherapy regimen may continue to benefit from ongoing treatment with the drug(s) that led to symptom amelioration. Concerns about long-term treatment with atypical antipsychotics suggest that other agents may have a potentially better risk/benefit balance for maintenance treatment.

In summary, pediatric bipolar disorder is a chronic condition associated with substantial dysfunction and suffering. There are few methodologically sound pharmacologic treatment studies; thus, more research on this topic is sorely needed.

Prevention of Depression and Bipolar Disorder

W. Edward Craighead
William Beardslee
Robert Johnson

chapter 3

The prevention of an individual's first episode of depression is worthy of greater study among investigators concerned with mood disorders. Not only is the first episode devastating for individuals and those around them, but depression is among the top three major causes of societal and economic disease burden across the globe (Ferrari et al., 2013; Mathers & Loncar, 2006; World Health Organization, 2008). The sequelae following the first episode of major depressive disorder (MDD) are substantial. The probability of subsequent episodes is significantly increased, even to the point that most now consider MDD to be a chronic disease (e.g., Pettit, Hartley, Lewinsohn, Seeley, & Klein [2013] recently reported that approximately 73% of those teens who experienced a first episode before age 18 had a recurrence within the next 12 years). As noted in Chapter 1, the sequelae to MDD are numerous and include more life stress, poorer social relationships, increased substance abuse, increased use of medical services, interference with long-term cognitive functioning, significant comorbidity with major health problems, and younger ages of death (when deaths by suicide are taken into account). Most investigators of mood disorders believe that the first episode lays down neural pathways (especially among those with relevant genetic vulnerabilities) that are difficult to overcome and, without modification via medications or psychosocial interventions or their combination, are likely to be lasting pathways that impact individuals' lives.

Even though prevention of MDD is an urgent and timely topic (England & Sim, 2009; see O'Connell, Boat, & Warner, 2009), empirical work regarding prevention is difficult and has been slow to progress. Considerably more work has been conducted on the prevention of second and subsequent episodes (Cox et al., 2012; Sheets et al., 2013), but the work designed to prevent the first episode of MDD remains meager. Prior to describing the empirical work on prevention of MDD, it is important to note the conceptual and historical context in which general prevention research has been defined.

HISTORICAL CONTEXT AND DEFINITIONS

A Brief History of Prevention in Mental Health

During the 1990s three reports established an historical context and defined the mental health prevention classification system:

1. *Reducing Risk for Mental Disorders: Frontiers for Prevention Intervention Research*, Institute of Medicine (1994)
2. *Priorities for Prevention Research at NIMH: A Report by the National Advisory Mental Health Council Workgroup on Mental Disorders Prevention Research*, National Institutes of Health, National Institute of Mental Health (1998)
3. *Mental Health: A Report of the Surgeon General*, U.S. Department of Health and Human Services (US-DHHS), Substance Abuse and Mental Health Services Administration, Center for Mental Health Services, National Institute of Health, National Institute of Mental Health (1999)

In 1998, the National Institute of Mental Health (NIMH) established an ad hoc committee to review the progress of mental health prevention research. The committee's report, *Priorities for Prevention Research at NIMH: A Report by the National Advisory Mental Health Council Workgroup on Mental Disorders Prevention Research*, traced the history of prevention in mental health and proposed the following generational taxonomy.

The first generation of efforts to prevent mental disorder began in the 1930s when, as an outgrowth of the turn-of-the-century mental hygiene movement, the focus gradually expanded beyond ameliorating the plight of those in asylums to include the prevention of many forms of social and emotional maladjustment. The new goal was to ensure the well-being and "positive mental health" of the general population through primary-prevention interventions aimed at creating health-promoting environments for all. These efforts were based on humanitarian concern, but had minimal research underpinnings.

Beginning in the late 1960s, the second generation of interventions to prevent mental disorders reflected the impact of a growing health and mental health research knowledge base. Some scientists retained their broad-based emphasis on primary prevention, while others began to target specific "at-risk" groups for study and intervention. During the 1960s there had been a burgeoning of research on the causes, mechanisms, and effects of stress on bodily and mental functioning. "At-risk" persons were defined as those who would predictably experience periods of substantial life stress, such as domestic violence, divorce, bereavement, or unemployment as precursors of mental distress or disorder. During the same time period, prevention and changing behavior for health also became active areas of investigation; those studies placed a strong emphasis on preventing lung cancer and heart disease through programs to prevent or reduce smoking, obesity, high cholesterol intake, and sedentary lifestyles.

The NIMH committee observed that over the next decade mental health preventive interventions continued to proliferate. After reviewing progress in this field, however, the 1978 President's Commission on Mental Health determined that previous investigations had been "unfocused and uncoordinated." As a remedy the commission recommended the establishment of a Center for Prevention at NIMH to coordinate and enhance research in mental health primary prevention. The NIMH report determined that "during the last 20 years The NIMH Center for Prevention Research and its programmatic successors have stimulated considerable progress in building the scientific foundation of an interdisciplinary field of prevention research in areas of epidemiology, human development, and intervention research methodology" (NIMH, 1998). The committee concluded that sufficient progress had been made in establishing the scientific basis for mental health prevention to declare that we were then in a third generation of prevention activity. Thus, prevention research could build on accomplishments of prior preventive interventions and integrate these with advances in the biomedical, behavioral, and cognitive sciences.

Despite the described significance and need for prevention research and this sanguine view of the 1998 NIMH committee, the amount of work studying the prevention of an initial episode of depression has remained meager. In contrast, considerable progress has been made in the development of a nomenclature for prevention research. In order for the field to progress, it was necessary to develop a clear terminology for investigators to follow.

Early Classification Systems

The Commission on Chronic Illness (1957) developed the original public health classification system of disease prevention. Three types of preventive interventions were identified: primary, secondary, and tertiary. During the last 40 years the definitions of these types of prevention have expanded to include an array of nuanced but related meanings.

Gordon's Definitions

In 1983 and in 1987, Robert Gordon proposed an alternative prevention classification system that was based on the empirical relationships found in practically oriented disease prevention and health-promotion programs. He labeled prevention programs as universal, selective, and indicated.

Although Gordon's classification system was distinct from that of the Commission on Chronic Health, the use of these two classification systems slowly deteriorated into a confusing merging and mixing of definitions (e.g., "universal primary prevention"). This confusion was particularly problematic when this terminology was applied to the classification of the prevention of psychiatric disorders, because the classic public health prevention classification system and Gordon's reclassification were both designed for use in the description of the prevention of other diseases, not of interventions to prevent psychiatric and psychological disorders. The 1994 Institute of Medicine (IOM) report, *Reducing Risk for Mental*

Disorders: Frontiers for Prevention Intervention Research, presented a cogent discussion of the inherent pitfalls in applying general prevention classifications to problems in mental health.

One of the main problems has been the concept of "caseness" that is used in public health. It is often more difficult to document that a "case" of mental disorder exists than it is to document a physical health problem. Agreement regarding the occurrence of a case of psychiatric disorder varies with time, with the instruments and diagnostic systems employed, and with the theoretical perspective of the evaluators. Also, symptoms and dysfunctions may exist even though criteria for a DSM-IV or 5 diagnoses are not met. Finally, the outcomes in very young children (birth to age 5) are often not diagnosable as "psychiatric caseness" but rather as impairments in cognition and psychosocial development.

IOM's Definitions of Prevention

The IOM report (1994) chose to resolve the confusion in terminology by using the term *prevention* to refer only to interventions that occur before the initial onset of a disorder. In this system, prevention included all three elements of Gordon's system (1983, 1987). Efforts to identify cases and provide care for known disorders were called treatment, and efforts to provide rehabilitation and reduce relapse and recurrence of a disorder were called maintenance/interventions. Further distinctions were made within the prevention category. We have employed these definitions throughout this chapter. The definitions are described in the following paragraphs.

Universal mental health prevention interventions are defined as efforts that are beneficial to a whole population or group. They are targeted to the general public or a whole population group that has not been designated or identified as being at risk for the disorder being prevented. The goal at this level of prevention is the reduction of the occurrence of new cases of the disorder.

Selective mental health prevention interventions are defined as those efforts that target individuals or a subgroup of the population whose risk for developing the mental health disorder is significantly higher than average. The risk may be immediate or lifelong. Biological, psychological, or social risk factors associated with or related to the specific mental health disorder are used to identify the individual or group level of risk. Those with the identified risk factors make up one group of those referred to as "at risk."

Indicated prevention interventions are defined as those efforts that target high-risk individuals who are identified as having minimal but detectable signs or symptoms that predict the mental disorder or biological markers indicating predisposition to the disorder. For example, individuals who have some symptoms of MDD but do not yet meet criteria for the disorder would fall into this group; such individuals represent the second group of individuals referred to as "at risk." Indicated prevention excludes individuals whose signs and symptoms meet diagnostic criteria for the disorder.

The IOM identified three aims or desired outcomes for mental health prevention: (1) reduction in the number of new cases of the disorder; (2) delay in the onset of illness; and (3) reduction in the length of time the early symptoms continue as well as halting the progression of severity so that individuals ultimately do not meet diagnostic criteria. The 1999 *Mental Health: A Report of the Surgeon General* agreed with the IOM and defined prevention as the "prevention of the initial onset of a mental disorder or emotional or behavioral problem, including prevention of comorbidity" (U.S. Department of Health and Human Services, 1999). Additionally, the report defined other terms that were often imprecisely used in discussions of prevention:

- First (initial) onset: the initial point in time when an individual's mental health problems meet the full criteria for a diagnosis of a mental disorder
- Risk factors: "characteristics, variables, or hazards that, if present for a given individual, make it more likely that this individual, compared to someone selected at

random from the general population, will develop a disorder" (US-DHHS, 1999). Although risk factors precede the first onset of a disorder, they may change in response to an episode of the disorder, development, or stressors.
- Protective factors: These factors "improve a person's response to some environmental hazard resulting in an 'adaptive outcome.' These factors can be found within the individual or within the family or community. They do not necessarily cause normal development in the absence of risk factors, but they may make an appreciable difference in the influence exerted by risk factors" (US-DHHS, 1999). Individuals with high levels of protective factors are frequently referred to as "resilient."
- Risk of onset versus risk of relapse: The terms that refer to the risk of the development of a disorder are often used without specification of the risk of onset versus the risk of relapse. This is a key distinction because "the risks for onset of a disorder are likely to be somewhat different from the risks involved in relapse of a previously diagnosed condition" (US-DHHS, 1999). Undoubtedly, this same distinction is true for factors that protect against onset or relapse. As will be noted later, not all "prevention" projects have made this distinction between initial and second or subsequent episodes of MDD.

Goals of Prevention Programs

In addition to the IOM's goals of reducing the number of new cases and delaying the onset of MDD and the insidious nature of the onset and course of MDD, there are other ancillary and associated goals of prevention programs. For example, prevention of initial MDD is likely to have an impact on school and work performance, social skills, and quality of life; to reduce the need of medical services; and to reduce MDD-related substance abuse disorders. In the long run, prevention programs may actually extend the lives of individuals who were at risk but did not develop the disorder, by reducing both the risk of suicide completion and the social, behavioral, and biological sequelae of an initial episode of the disorder.

Another goal of prevention programs is to teach resiliency to the program participants. Individuals at risk for MDD are likely to experience negative and traumatic events, as are other individuals in our society. Prevention programs have a goal of teaching at-risk individuals to become more resilient—to develop skills and abilities to recover from or adapt to adversity.

A further goal of prevention programs is to enhance and enrich the positive aspects of living. By changing cognitive processes, enhancing social skills, and increasing resiliency, individuals who otherwise might live a marginally happy life may have the opportunity to develop greater self-esteem and self-efficacy and live a more flourishing, successful, and adaptive life. This positive adaption in life may lead to the development of more adaptive neural pathways. Emotional intelligence (Goleman, 1995) may be enhanced by successful preventive programs.

The societal goals of depression prevention programs are also numerous. For example, even a modest reduction in new cases of MDD would reduce the economic burden of the disorder. The disorder itself would not have to be treated so frequently, nor would the associated (sometimes self-treatment) problems of alcohol, tobacco, and other forms of substance abuse. Each prevented case of MDD would increase the limited resources available to other health initiatives. Productivity would be increased in the workplace. Thus, the call for effective programs to prevent the first episode of MDD is a forceful and significant one—significant for individuals, families, and society as a whole (England & Sim, 2009).

RISK FACTORS FOR MAJOR DEPRESSION

To develop programs for individuals "at risk" for MDD, it is necessary to develop knowledge and understanding of factors and their interactions that render one likely to develop MDD. Chapter 1 provided evidence for many of the risk factors for MDD, so the details will not be reiterated here. These risk factors include dysfunctional parenting and family interactions; gender; personality, and temperament; cognitive vulnerabilities; internal and external stress, including negative life events; and poor interpersonal relationships.

In addition to the preceding risk factors, the following risk factors that have implications for prevention of MDD are important and worthy of further detailed review. These include subsyndromal depression, poverty, violence, and cultural factors.

Subsyndromal Depression

Among adults, subsyndromal depression (two or more symptoms for 2 weeks or longer) appears to cause as much health impairment and economic burden as MDD, and these individuals are at increased risk for developing subsequent MDD (Fava, 1999; Johnson, Weissman, & Klerman, 1992; Judd, Akiskal, & Paulus, 1997). In longitudinal studies, subsyndromal depression among adolescents predicted poorer functioning when these individuals became adults (Devine, Kempton, & Forehand, 1994; Pettit, Hartley, Lewinsohn, Seeley, & Klein, 2013; Pettit, Lewinsohn, & Joiner, 2006). Subsyndromal depressive symptoms among adolescents predict MDD later on in adolescence and young adulthood (Pine, Cohen, Cohen, & Brook, 1999; Rao et al., 1995; Weissman, Warner, Wickramaratne, Moreau, & Olfson, 1997; see also Monroe & Harkness, 2011). Lewinsohn, Solomon, Seeley, and Zeiss (2000) found that increasing levels of depressive symptoms among a large sample of nondepressed adolescents (average age of 16.5) predicted increased levels of social dysfunction and incidence of MDD, as well as increased substance abuse at age 24. These data indicate that subsyndromal depression renders adolescents at risk for a first episode of MDD, and they are prime candidates for depression prevention programs.

Poverty

Poverty has been linked with an early onset of depression. It is not clear whether this represents an independent risk factor or can be grouped among the more general examples of diversity that are associated with depression. Results from epidemiologic studies have linked lower socioeconomic status with depression and a multitude of other mental health problems (Robins, Locke, & Regier, 1991). This vulnerability is particularly strong for families living at poverty levels (Bruce, Takeuchi, & Leaf, 1991). This relationship may be explained in part by a phenomenon of selection, whereby those with mental health problems are more inclined to drift toward economic disadvantage and remain there (Dohrenwend et al., 1992). Longitudinal data have also demonstrated that socioeconomic disadvantage is largely a cause of higher vulnerability to psychiatric disorder, particularly for depression (Dohrenwend et al., 1992; Gilman, Kawachi, Fitzmaurice, & Buka, 2002; Johnson, Cohen, Dohrenwend, Link, & Brook, 1999; Kiely & Butterworth, 2013). In a study of over 4,000 Australian families, poverty caused a small but significant increase in risk when other sociologic variables were controlled (Spence, Najman, Bor, O'Callaghan, & Williams, 2002); this effect was more pronounced in girls than in boys.

If poverty is a generator for a variety of stressors, the possible mechanisms driving poverty-induced vulnerability appear boundless. A number of mediators between socioeconomic disadvantage and depression have been studied empirically. These include external mediators such as access to healthcare, quality of social networks and resources, quality of parenting and parent availability, and, of course, level of exposure to violence. Children of families who are of lower socioeconomic status are most likely to witness violence and to be the victims of abuse (Buka, Stichik, Birdthistle, & Earls, 2001; Sedlak & Broadhurst, 1996).

Internal individual mediators include self-esteem, health-risk behaviors, cognitive deficits, interpersonal skills, and academic achievement. Several comprehensive reviews on the consequences of poverty and mediating factors demonstrate the vast amount of knowledge we have accumulated on the relation between poverty and depression (Aber, Bennett, Conley, & Li, 1997; Leventhal & Brooks-Gunn, 2000; Turner& Lloyd, 1999). This literature highlights the importance of two larger factors: (a) the need for universal healthcare with parity for mental illness and physical illness and parity for services for adults and children and (b) the need to address large-scale public health risk factors that have a strong effect on the occurrence of adolescent depression (i.e., exposure to violence).

Violence

Exposure to violence during childhood is a potent risk factor for future psychological and psychiatric disorders (Kilpatrick et al., 2003; MacMillan et al., 2001) and also a risk factor for poor physical health (Felitti et al., 1998), in both the short and long term. The violence to which children are exposed has many forms. This includes being a victim of sexual or physical abuse as well as witnessing violence in the home (Devries et al., 2013; Heim et al., 2010; Kilpatrick et al., 2003). A large number of children also frequently witness violence in the community (Buka et al., 2001). Children who are exposed to violence are most often exposed to more than one type, and evidence suggests that the amount of violence-related adversities a child encounters has a substantial impact on the severity of the outcome (Felitti et al., 1998). The most disturbing illustration of this accumulation phenomenon is the gradation effect of violence-related adversities on risk for suicide attempt. Results from the Adverse Childhood Experiences Study demonstrated that for every additional adversity experienced as a child, the risk of suicide attempts increased from twofold to fivefold, such that children or adolescents who encounter seven or more adversities are 50 times as likely to attempt suicide as those without violence exposure (Dube et al., 2001). Although the mental health consequences of violence exposure are diverse, the most prevalent and commonly studied are posttraumatic stress disorder (PTSD) and major depression. This makes sense, particularly if violence exposure is viewed as a form of trauma.

Violence-related trauma experienced during childhood can have particularly devastating effects, because the trauma is inflicted during a critical period of development. Neurobiological and neuroendocrine studies of depressed women, which look at the volume of certain brain regions and at hormonal stress-response mechanisms, provide evidence that violence-related trauma experienced during childhood can have profound and lasting effects on brain structure and function (Heim et al., 2008; Klengel & Binder, 2013; Klengel et al., 2013). These alterations, in turn, increase vulnerability to stress-related disorders like depression.

Depression that is comorbid with PTSD or other disorders, as well as depression that has an established neurobiological etiology like that seen in childhood victims of trauma, are forms of the disorder that are particularly resistant to treatment and are associated with increased levels of impairment (Mervaala et al., 2000; Petersen et al., 2001). Thus, it is important that prevention strategies attend to violence exposure.

Cultural Factors

The role of ethnocultural factors has been understudied. Some ethnic groups appear to have higher rates of adolescent depression than others. For example, Mexican-Americans and African-American adolescents appear to have a higher risk for depression, whereas American adolescents of Chinese descent may be at lesser risk (Chentsova-Dutton & Tsai, 2009; Roberts, Roberts, & Chen, 1997). The rates of depression and the economic burden vary across countries around the world (Ferrari et al., 2013).

It appears that depression rates for some groups (e.g., African-American or Hispanic adolescents) may not show the gender disparity following puberty that is seen among those for Caucasian adolescents (Hayward, Gotlib, Schraedley, & Litt, 1999). Furthermore, some prevention or prevention of recurrence programs (reviewed later) have reported differential effectiveness for different ethnic groups within the United States (Cardemil et al., 2002).

In sum, there appear to be cultural and ethnic differences in both the prevalence of depression and in the symptomatology indicative of depression (Chentsova-Dutton & Tsai, 2009). Clearly this is a topic in great need of further study.

DEPRESSION PREVENTION PROGRAMS FOR ADOLESCENTS

During the past two decades, a number of promising strategies for the prevention of childhood depression have emerged. The overarching principles of these programs are similar, and the specifics of preventive interventions for children and adolescents have taken into account the development level of the participants. The evaluated preventive strategies are based primarily on cognitive-behavioral and family-educational approaches that seek to reduce risk factors and enhance protective and resiliency factors relevant to depression in youth.

In general, progress in the field of prevention science has been made through the introduction of rigorous standards for the development and evaluation of manualized preventive strategies that are based on well-established theoretical frameworks and proceed through a series of orderly stages. This is best described in the 1994 IOM's *Report on the Prevention of Mental Disorder*. The IOM suggested that prevention development and evaluation proceed through five stages. The first and second stages are identifying risk factors and describing the relative contributions of different factors to the disorder. The third stage is applying strategies developed in pilot studies and completing efficacy trials to evaluate the overall outcomes of these approaches. The fourth stage, carrying out effectiveness trials, involves the examination of such strategies in multiple sites in large-scale investigations under non-ideal, real-world conditions. The final stage consists of implementing such strategies in large-scale public health campaigns. Following this sequence and the articulation of a set of rigorous empirical standards by which to test preventive intervention approaches, a number of important strategies for prevention of depression have emerged. These have begun to be tested in randomized trial designs according to the recommended guidelines.

Consideration of the prevention of depression also must take place in the context of the remarkable progress in developmental neuroscience, the sequencing of a human genome, and psychiatric epidemiology. As these important scientific advances unfold, they will offer significant opportunities for future prevention programs. These findings will need to be integrated with adolescents' developmental, social, cultural, and family contexts in the development of preventive interventions. Within the context of personalized medicine, the larger question becomes one of identifying which characteristics of "at risk" individuals indicate which treatment will work for which subgroups of "at risk" youth.

To date, two major conceptual frameworks have guided most of the development of the prevention studies. First, cognitive-behavioral programs have been used and show considerable promise (e.g., the Penn Group, Clarke and Garber and colleagues in the United States, Shochet and Spence in Australia, and Arnarson and Craighead in Iceland). The second conceptual framework is exemplified by Beardslee and colleagues, who have developed and evaluated a program designed to prevent depression in the family intervention context. All of these programs have in common a strong theoretical orientation—an orientation toward building strengths and resiliency; they have all been written into manuals for dissemination; and they have been or are being tested with randomized trials designs. It is important to note that these are programs for "at risk" individuals, and as noted earlier universal programs have limited supporting evidence. Further, the studies included in this review are for prevention programs; at the end of this review, data regarding those programs that combine prevention and prevention of relapse or recurrence programs will be noted. In the sections that follow, we first describe and evaluate studies designed to prevent initial episodes of depression; these include the Penn Prevention Program, the findings from groups working in Australia, the work in Iceland, and the work of Beardslee and associates. These descriptions of programs designed to prevent initial episodes of depression are followed by presentations of programs that were designed to prevent initial episodes of depression AND relapse and recurrence of depression; these latter studies include the work of Garber, Beardslee, Clarke, and their associates.

Prevention of Initial Episode of Depression

Penn Prevention Program

In the Penn Prevention Program (PPP), Seligman and colleagues (Gillham & Reivich, 1999; Gillham, Reivich, Jaycox, & Seligman, 1995; Jaycox, Reivich, Gillham, & Seligman, 1994) developed and evaluated a school-based "indicated" prevention program targeting 10- to 13-year-old children in school districts in the Philadelphia suburbs. The youth were defined as at risk for depression on the basis of elevated self-reported depressive symptomatology, self-reported parental conflict, or both. The PPP was based on a model of explanatory style introduced by Seligman and colleagues (Nolen-Hoeksema, Girgus, & Seligman, 1992) and on research identifying core cognitive deficits associated with youth depression, including negative self-evaluation, dysfunctional attitudes, poor interpersonal problem solving, and low expectations for self-performance (Garber, Weiss, & Shanley, 1993; Kaslow, Rehm, & Siegel, 1984; Quiggle, Garber, Panak, & Dodge, 1992). Participants recruited for the treatment group were assigned to one of three treatment programs: a cognitive training program, a social problem-solving program, or a combined program. Eighty-eight students, whose scores were matched to prevention participants, were recruited from nearby schools and made up the no-participation control group. Assessments included child self-report, teacher-report, and parent-report questionnaires.

Results indicated that relative to control participants, children who participated in any of the treatment groups reported significantly fewer depressive symptoms immediately following the program and at the 6-month and 2-year follow-ups, but not at the 12-month and 3-year follow-ups. Moreover, teacher reports at follow-up revealed better classroom behavior in treatment participants than in control participants. Finally, overall treatment effects were more significant for children who, at the screening phase of the study, reported more significant depressive symptomatology and more significant parental conflict at home. The major limitations of the study are the lack of randomization to intervention conditions, the use of only self-report measures, attrition of approximately 30% of participants during follow-up, and the failure to include diagnoses for clinical depression.

Over the past few years, this program has been slightly revised and is now referred to as the Penn Resiliency Program (PRP; Gillham, Reivich, & Jaycox, 2008); it added problem solving and coping skills to the more cognitive behavioral focus of PPP. The PPP/PRP program has been evaluated in multiple meta-analyses (e.g., Horowitz & Garber, 2006; Stice, Shaw, Bohon, Marti, & Rhode, 2009), and there has been at least one additional study since those meta-analyses (Gillham et al., 2012). As is typical of meta-analyses, the context, sample size, constituency of interventionists, and so forth have varied considerably. In sum, the PPP or PRP has been found to reduce depressive symptoms and depressive disorders relative to control groups, and these effects have been largely sustained at 12 months of follow-up. As has been found with other programs, when the PPP/PRP has been applied in a universal manner rather than in an indicated context, the program has only been effective with those "at risk" by way of baseline hopelessness or elevated depressive symptoms. Interestingly, the program has been effective with Latino adolescents but less so with African-American adolescents (Cardemil, 2002; Cardemil, Reivich, Beevers, Seligman, & James, 2007). This calls attention to the significance of possible ethnic and cultural differences that need to be noted in the development of prevention programs. Effects have varied considerably across studies, with universal programs and programs administered by less well-trained individuals having less immediate and lasting effects. Adding parental participation has had minimal additional effects to those achieved by the adolescent program, but it has been difficult to gain parental involvement and participation has been minimal. This may have precluded an enhanced effect from the inclusion of parents in the program (Gillham et al., 2012).

More recently, Seligman and his group at Penn have focused on "positive psychology" programs, which are likely to have an indirect effect of preventing episodes of MDD. These programs are included in Part VII of this book.

Programs in Australia

Several prevention programs (mostly universal) in Australia have been described and evaluated. Shochet and colleagues (2001) evaluated a "universal" prevention program applied in a school setting. This was a skills-based program of 11 sessions offered by a psychologist and based on a downward extension of principles of cognitive-behavioral therapy (CBT) and interpersonal therapy (IPT). The student sessions could be supplemented with three parental sessions, but not many parents took advantage of this offer. There were 242 12- to 15-year-old subjects, who were assigned to assessment-only control, prevention without parental sessions, or prevention with parental sessions.

No differences were found between the two prevention groups, but students who completed either prevention program showed fewer depressive symptoms than controls on one measure of depression (but not another). The prevention program subjects also reported less hopelessness at the end of the project. All of these effects were maintained at a 10-month follow-up. The limitations of this program include the lack of random assignment of subjects (controls participated in one academic year, and intervention subjects in the next academic year), a small sample size, and the fact that assessments were conducted at different times of the year in different conditions. The findings, though limited, were encouraging for such a short program and short follow-up period.

A very sophisticated study evaluated the long-term impact of a universal, teacher-implemented, and school-based prevention program that was developed by Spence, Sheffield, and Donovan (2003). The program, Problem Solving for Life, is a combination of cognitive restructuring and problem-solving approaches, and it is designed to prevent a first episode of depression. Subjects were 1,500 eighth-graders (ages 12–14; mean = 12.9) attending 16 participating high schools in the Brisbane region of Queensland, Australia. The program of eight 1-hour classroom sessions was implemented by 28 teachers in eight randomly assigned schools (N = 751), while the control subjects (N = 749) attended the other eight schools. There were approximately equal numbers of girls and boys.

Appropriate data analyses indicated that the program significantly decreased depressive symptoms between the beginning and end of the program. This finding, however, was only true for those adolescents who had elevated ("high risk," defined as 13 or higher on the Beck Depression Inventory) depression scores at the beginning of the study. Unfortunately, this difference was not maintained at a 12-month follow-up.

Sawyer and colleagues (2010) implemented the "beyondblue" extensive universal program designed to prevent symptoms of depression but also to address some environmental variables that may affect depression onset and extend beyond those typically addressed in depression prevention programs. Beginning in 2003, the group randomly assigned 25 schools to the prevention program and 25 schools to the assessment-only and treatment-as-usual control condition (except they were allowed to participate in the community forum aspects of the program). Participants were 5,633 students beginning eighth grade, and they participated in the program for 3 years and were then followed for 2 more years. This remains the largest, most comprehensive, and best designed universal program to date. Because of the magnitude of the study, all outcome measures were self-report and included measures of depression, anxiety, well-being, and parental support. In addition to classroom educational programs broadly based on CBT interventions, this study included attempts to improve the environment in the school (e.g., social relationships, safety) as well as outside-of-school programs (e.g., community forums) that provided information for students and families regarding possible clinical services for those who might need them. Adherence measures showed that the program was successfully implemented as described. The program materials can be downloaded at http://www.beyondblue.org.au/index.aspx?link_id=4.1305.

Unfortunately, the end-of-treatment data (3 years; Sawyer et al., 2010) and the follow-up data (5 years; Sawyer et al., 2010) showed no significant effects of the program on clinical symptoms (e.g., depression or anxiety) or well-being. Similar to those of most other universal programs, the outcomes were nonsignificant (Merry et al., 2011; Spence & Shortt, 2007; Stice et al., 2009). Even with a large sample size, the effect sizes of the program were small, even with a broadly based CBT program, and even with school environmental changes.

In an effort to understand the failure to find significant effects for the extensive universal "beyondblues" study, Spence and her colleagues (personal communication, Feb. 18, 2014) conducted an informative follow-up on secondary analyses of the previous outcome data. Namely, they evaluated the effects of family relationship support as a moderator of the outcomes of the program. Significant differences, including lower levels of depression and anxiety and higher levels of well-being, were found supporting the effectiveness of the program relative to the control group among those youth who had low levels of family support in eighth grade at the beginning of the program. No differences between prevention program and control groups were obtained for those who had higher levels of family support at the beginning of the program. Thus, level of family relationship support was a moderating variable affecting the outcome of this universal program.

The findings by Spence and colleagues (2014) highlight the importance of absent or limited effects of universal programs that fail to take into account moderator variables such as family support, level of depressive symptoms before the intervention (see Spence et al., 2003), or presence of a depressed parent (see below, Garber et al., 2009). Despite the conclusions by Merry and colleagues (2012) that a limited number of universal programs have some impact, these effects are minimal for prevention of depression for the reasons highlighted earlier: the effect sizes are very small even with large sample sizes, and the programs are largely applied to individuals who do not need them (e.g., no depressive symptoms, no prior depression, no depressed family member) and do not profit from them (no increase in resiliency or well-being, as these individuals are already high-functioning at baseline). It seems that the limitations and warnings noted by Spence and Shortt (2007) still accurately describe the universal prevention program outcomes.

Arnarson and Craighead (Iceland)

Because of the stable population of Iceland and because most of the citizens live in one city, Reykjavik, Arnarson and Craighead spent several years translating and standardizing assessment instruments and developing a manualized, developmentally based, behavioral and cognitive program designed to prevent depression in Iceland. The primary aim of this study was to evaluate the effectiveness of a program designed to prevent an initial episode of major depression or dysthymia among adolescents "at risk" for depression. The initial participants in a screening process were 1,920 ninth-grade Icelandic adolescents who were 14 or 15 years old at the beginning of the study. Following the selection procedures and exclusion and inclusion criteria described in detail in Arnarson and Craighead (2009), study participants were 171 14-year-old "at risk" but never previously depressed Icelandic adolescents who were randomly assigned to a prevention program or a treatment-as-usual assessment-only control group. They were identified as "at risk" by reporting the presence of depressive symptoms *or* a negative attributional style.

The program was based on a developmental psychosocial model of enhancement of resilience to factors associated with the occurrence of mood disorders. It is called the "Thoughts and Health" program and includes a student workbook as well as a group leader's manual. It was administered in a school setting by trained school psychologists. The program comprised 14 sessions with groups of six to eight adolescents. Diagnostic clinical interview and self-report data were collected at baseline, posttest, 6-month follow-up, and 12-month follow-up sessions. There were no significant differences between the prevention and treatment-as-usual groups for dropout rates or for "dropouts" compared to the "completers" on any of the screening measures.

At posttest, diagnoses of new (initial) episodes of depression and/or dysthymia were reported in 2.5% of the control group but 0% of the prevention group. By the 6-month follow-up, the diagnosis for initial episodes of depression and/or dysthymia had occurred in 13.3% of the control group but only 1.6% in the prevention group; data for 12-month follow up were similar (21% for the control group and 4% for the prevention group). Twice as many girls as boys experienced an initial episode of depression/dysthymia (Arnarson & Craighead, 2009).

Survival curves for initial episode rates were separately estimated at 6- and 12-month follow-ups using the Cox proportional hazards model. Students not available for follow-up were treated as censored observations. At 6-month follow-up, the prevention program relative to treatment as usual significantly reduced the risk of development of a first episode of depression and/or dysthymia ($\chi^2 = 4.03$, $p = .0448$; odds ratio [OR] = .122). Survival analysis for the 12-month follow-up data indicated continued group differences ($\chi^2 = 5.02$, $p = .025$; OR = .182); at the end of 1-year follow-up a student who participated in the prevention program was only 18.2% as likely to have developed an initial episode of depression/dysthymia as a student who was in the control group. Stated differently, the prevention program relative to treatment as usual decreased the likelihood of having a first episode by 81.8%.

A logistic regression model was estimated for the control subjects in order to determine if the screening CDI, CASQ-NEG, and CASQ-POS predicted either the diagnosis of depression or dysthymia. Only the CDI significantly predicted the diagnosis of depression or dysthymia (estimate = .0997, standard error = .0467, Wald $\chi^2 = 4.55$, $p = .0330$).

The program was originally drafted in English but was then adapted to the Icelandic culture and rewritten in Icelandic. As the program was pilot testing, the illustrations and examples were modified to reflect more accurately teen culture in Iceland. Subsequent to the completion of the study, the manuals have been translated into English, back-translated to Icelandic, and then retranslated into English, and they are available for research purposes. Most recently the manuals have been translated into Portuguese, and the program is being replicated by A.P. Matos and her colleagues in Coimbra, Portugal. Again, the examples, cartoons, classroom posters, and so forth have been adapted to Portuguese youth culture. Preliminary data, including baseline descriptive information, are available from A.P. Matos (see Matos et al., 2013).

Beardslee and Associates

Beardslee and associates, following the IOM stages, first studied risk and resilience, then developed pilot interventions and conducted a large efficacy trial, and then moved to effectiveness and programmatic interventions. Their prevention programs were designed to be public health interventions and useful to all families in which a parent is depressed. The programs (Family Talk and adaptations of this intervention) can be used by a range of health practitioners, including internists, pediatricians, school counselors, and nurses, as well as by mental health practitioners such as child psychiatrists, child psychologists, and family therapists. Moreover, this approach includes a strong emphasis on treatment, given that so much depression is undiagnosed and untreated, so in that sense they are not limited to prevention of depression.

Rates of depression are two to four times higher in children of depressed parents than for children of parents with no illness (Beardslee, Gladstone, & O'Connor, 2011; Beardslee, Versage, & Gladstone, 1998). To understand the transmission of depression, it is important to recognize that in many instances, depression in parents serves as an identifier of a constellation of risk factors that, taken together, result in poor outcomes. In Rutter's classic epidemiological studies, six factors were identified, including maternal psychiatric disorder. When only one was present, there was no increased risk to the child, but when two or more were present, the risk increased dramatically. In a random health maintenance organization sample over a 4-year period, Beardslee and associates (1996) demonstrated that the same principles were evident in predicting who became depressed. They devised an adversity index consisting of parental major depression, parental nonaffective illness, and a prior history of disorder in the child. When no risk factors were present, less than 10% of the children became depressed. When all three were present, 50% of the children became depressed, with a gradation in between. A recent review of the effects of parental depression again highlighted the substantial risk and stressed the importance of both familial genetic factors and of current and past adversities in leading to depression. It further highlighted that epigenetic phenomena and developmental plasticity are important in weighing the balance of risk and protective factors. As is true throughout this chapter, they advocate addressing both specific risk factors for depression (e.g., having a parent who is depressed) and nonspecific risk factors (e.g., poverty and exposure to violence) (Beardslee et al., 2011).

In studying resilience, Beardslee and associates identified three characteristics that described resilient children of depressed parents (Beardslee & Podorefsky, 1988). The three characteristics, which were incorporated into the preventive intervention, were (a) support for activities and accomplishment of developmental tasks outside of the home; (b) a deep involvement in human relationships; and (c) the capacity for self-reflection and self-understanding, in particular, in relation to the parent's disorder. Resilient youth repeatedly said that understanding that their parent was ill, that the disorder had a name, and that they were not to blame for it contributed substantially to their doing well. Correspondingly, parents who raised children resilient in the face of parental depression were deeply committed to parenting despite depression and to openness and communication. These principles became central parts of the preventive intervention strategy devised by this group.

Family Talk is a six-session intervention conducted by a clinician in collaboration with the parents. The clinician takes a history and provides psychoeducation to the parents. A child meeting with the clinician precedes the family meeting, and a follow-up meeting is conducted 6 months after the family discussion. This intervention is designed to prevent depression in offspring of depressed parents by improving family communication, relationships, and functioning; acknowledging the impact of parental depression; and encouraging parental and child resilience by building on family strengths. The program is specified within a manual. It has proved possible to train large numbers of people with fidelity, and Beardslee and associates made web-based training available through the FAMpod.org website.

Initial studies of Family Talk and adaptations of the program revealed that they were safe and feasible, and that families believed them to be helpful. A comparison active condition—two lectures about depression and resilience in families—has been compared to Family Talk. In an initial random-assignment study of the first 20 families enrolled, promising effects were observed 6 months after intervention, and a further follow-up study of parents' reports showed sustained effects over 3 years. In addition, pilot studies revealed that greater benefits were associated with the clinician-facilitated intervention than with the lecture condition.

Beardslee, Gladstone, Wright, and Cooper (2003) presented findings from follow-up interviews conducted with their entire sample of families at the fourth data point, nearly 2.5 years after intervention. They followed 100 families of over 300 individuals. They chose the interval of 2.5 years postintervention because it was long enough to begin to see substantial, sustained changes in several main domains hypothesized to be affected by participation in the prevention programs. They focused on effecting change in a mediating variable that they described as parental child-related behavior and attitude change.

Results revealed several important findings about the primary prevention of depression and other forms of psychopathology in children at risk for dysfunction due to parental mood disorder. They found that these programs did have longstanding effects in how families problem solve about parental depression (i.e., behavior and attitude change). There was evidence that the clinician-facilitated program was more beneficial than the lecture program, and that the amount of change in parent's child-related behaviors and attitudes increased over time. More importantly, the intervention was targeted to increase the children's understanding of the disorder in their parents. Children's understanding increased significantly in both groups, with greater change in the clinician-facilitated program. They found a significant relation between the amount of child-related behavior and attitude change manifested by parents and the amount of change in understanding manifested by children, even though change was rated entirely separately by assessors blind to the knowledge of the other subjects' reports. Finally, they found that children who participated in the intervention programs reported decreased internalizing symptomatology over time.

After the success of the randomized trial, Beardslee and associates (2003) examined the mechanisms by which change took place. Briefly, they found that when families did make changes, they talked repeatedly about depression. Often, breaking the silence about depression led the families to talk and strategize successfully about many other things. This process was named the "emergence of the healer within." Similarly, they found that what works for a child at 12 does not work for the same child at 16. In this sense, understandings of depression change both as the course of parental illness changes and as children grow and mature. Finally, many parents, despite the negativism and self-doubt of depression, end up functioning effectively as parents. In essence, they made peace with their disorder and moved on.

As part of a dissemination effort, Beardslee and associates then examined the effectiveness of the intervention in different populations and worked with colleagues to examine it in different systems. They first adapted the intervention for use with single-parent, multiple-risk, African-American families in Dorchester, MA. In a randomized trial, the intervention led to behavior and attitude changes, it was well tolerated, families were satisfied, and more change occurred in families receiving the clinician-based intervention. They then adapted the intervention for use with Latino families using a bicultural, bilingual team and demonstrated in an open trial that the same kinds of effects were obtained in these families. Beardslee and associates have argued that adapting an intervention to a different cultural group often transforms it for the better, as occurred in these two adaptations.

Family Talk has been used as part of countrywide programs for children of the mentally ill as systematic efforts to improve the health of families with mental illness (Solantaus & Toikka, 2006). Solantaus has led the effort in Finland, which is an entirely Finnish program. In developing the countrywide program, she used three strategies:

1. *Development of a family of interventions.* The most widely used intervention is the Let's Talk About It Intervention that uses books written about parental mental illness and is administered by the clinician treating the parents. She also developed a group intervention.
2. *Strong investment in master trainers.* Solantaus spent several years training them.
3. *Adaptation of approaches to be used with a wide variety of risk conditions such as parental alcoholism or severe medical illness.*

Using this approach, her program is now widely disseminated in Finland and used in all health districts. She conducted a randomized trial comparing a lecture intervention to the Family Talk Intervention with generally similar results, although follow-up on the children found more pro-social behavior in the group receiving the lectures.

Family Talk has been used in countrywide programs in Holland, Sweden, and Norway, and an extensive adaptation in Costa Rica has led it to be part of the national health service there.

At the request of Federal Head Start, Beardslee developed a program based on these principles to be used in Head Start and Early Head Start, where the rates of depression in mothers can exceed 50%. This program is a teacher training and empowerment program designed to increase the staff's ability to deal with parental adversity and to encourage resilience. Evaluations of the program have been favorable. These materials are available for free on the Head Start website (Beardslee et al., 2011).

Mix of Prevention of Initial Episode and Recurrence

Investigators have implemented several interventions designed to prevent the *recurrence* of MDD. These include maintenance treatment (Frank et al., 1990; Paykel et al., 1999), booster sessions (e.g., Jarrett et al., 2001), and specific programs for previously depressed individuals (Sheets et al., 2013) who are not currently depressed.

Several programs labeled "prevention programs" are largely prevention of recurrence programs because such a large percentage of the participants have experienced a previous depressive episode. Some of the findings, as noted below, have been impressive, but the designs of the studies preclude one from determining whether the program actually prevented an initial MDD or the recurrence of the disorder. Indeed, it may eventually be determined that the most effective programs are the same prevention programs for initial episodes and recurrences, but at the present time that conclusion is premature. Data indicate that causal factors may be different for initial episodes and recurrent episodes; for instance, both parental depression and minor depressive symptoms predicted the initial episode of MDD, but life events were also predictive of further occurrences over a 12-year longitudinal study (Pettit et al., 2013). Further, both epigenetic and neural pathways affected by an initial episode of MDD may render individuals subsequently more vulnerable to external stressors than are the pre-episode brains of "at risk" youth. It may also be that the first episode of MDD produces social, behavioral, and cognitive changes that result in individuals creating greater stress or being more reactive to stressors that occur in their lives following the first episode. Currently, we do not have adequate data to argue strongly that the interventions that prevent initial episodes also prevent recurrence; conversely, we do not know that they will fail to prevent second episodes.

Clarke and Colleagues

Clarke and colleagues (1995) in Oregon were among the first to study prevention of MDD among adolescents, and they focused on the prevention of diagnosed clinical depression rather than the presence of depressive symptoms via self-report measures that have been used by many other prevention programs. In an excellent, well-designed study, 150 adolescent students from ninth and tenth grades were assigned randomly to either a "prevention" or "usual-care" group. The prevention program, entitled Adolescent Coping with Stress Course, was delivered in groups and was a prevention-focused adaptation of this group's Adolescent Coping with Depression Course (Clarke, Lewinsohn, & Hops, 1990). The 5-week intervention was conducted within the adolescents' school setting and comprised fifteen 45-minute group sessions (three after-school meetings per week). The usual-care youngsters were free to continue with preexisting treatment or seek new treatment. This program employed both behavioral and cognitive coping techniques designed to reduce vulnerability to future depressive episodes.

Participants were followed for 1 year, and the results were positive. Namely, significantly ($p < .05$) fewer prevention group subjects (14.5%; 8 of 55) were diagnosed with MDD or dysthymia than control group subjects (25.7%; 18 of 70). The major strengths of this study included random assignment of subjects, adequate sample sizes, diagnoses of clinical mood disorders, and encouraging outcomes. It is important to note, however, that approximately 36% of their participants had suffered a prior episode of MDD. Because 30% to 50% of adolescents who have had a prior episode can be expected to have a relapse or recurrence of the disorder during the time (18 months) of this study (Hart, Craighead, & Craighead, 2001; Lewinsohn, Rohde, Seeley, & Fischer, 1993; Rao et al., 1995), it very well may be that Clarke and colleagues actually had their biggest impact on preventing relapse or recurrence rather than on preventing a first episode of MDD. In addition, there was differential dropout between conditions (Clarke et al., 1995), but as the authors suggested, this probably operated against their favorable outcomes.

In an expansion of this program, Clarke and associates (2001) applied this approach to a health maintenance organization population of adolescents of parents with diagnosed depression and youngsters already manifesting symptoms. They screened all those at risk and divided them into three groups: low or no depressive symptomatology, medium symptomatology, and those already in episode. Those already meeting criteria for MDD were referred for treatment, and those with no depressive symptomatology were excluded. In this trial, those adolescents (ages 13–18) with moderate symptomatology were randomized into a usual-care condition ($N = 49$) or their cognitive-behavioral intervention group ($N = 45$). As in their previous study, prevention group subjects participated in 15 group sessions.

This intervention yielded substantial preventive effects, with significant treatment-by-time effects in the expected direction on the Center for Epidemiological Studies–Depression (CES-D) and the Global Assessment of Functioning scales; in other words, adolescents in the prevention condition did much better than those in the usual-care condition. Survival analysis indicated that over a 15-month follow-up period, there was a cumulative rate of major depression of only 9% in the experimental group in contrast to 28% in the usual-care condition (Clarke et al., 2001). Even though this is the most sophisticated prevention study to date, its specific implications for prevention are limited by the choice to include adolescents who had previously had an episode of depression; these subjects made up 67% of the adolescents in this study. Thus, as with the prior study, it is impossible to determine if the study prevented first episodes or relapse and recurrence of prior episodes of MDD.

Garber, Beardslee, and Colleagues

Building upon the work of Clarke and his colleagues, Garber and colleagues (2009) reported the results of a multisite study that evaluated the Coping with Depression Course written into a prevention format (copies available at http://www.kpchr.org/research/public/acwd/acwd.html). Participants were identified by the presence of a parent with MDD currently or in the past (about 40% of participants), the adolescent having a history of prior MDD (about 80% of participants), and/or the presence of some current symptoms of MDD in the adolescent (sometimes referred to as minor depressive symptoms). Across four sites spread across the United States, 316 participants ages 13 to 17 were randomly assigned to participate in the treatment program or an assessment-only program (essentially a treatment-as-usual control group). The prevention group participated in eight weekly 90-minute group sessions that focused on cognitive restructuring and problem-solving skills. Data were reported for baseline, end of treatment, and 9-month follow-up; six continuation sessions focusing on behavioral activation, relaxation training, and assertiveness were conducted between the end of the 8-week intervention and the 9-month follow-up assessment (Beardslee et al., 2013; Garber et al., 2009).

The primary finding was that the program resulted in the prevention group experiencing significantly fewer depressive episodes (21.4%) than the control group (32.7%). There was, however, an interaction between treatment and "presence of active parental depression at enrollment" such that the prevention program resulted in significantly fewer depressive episodes among those adolescents who did not have a parent with active MDD at baseline, but the program was not significantly more beneficial than treatment as usual when parental MDD was present.

The strengths of the study include the sample size, the multiple sites and multiple investigators, the fact that intervention offered by a wide range of interventionists, the sophistication of the design and statistical analyses, and the sustainability of the findings. The delivery of the program was state-of-the-art, and the findings strongly support the effectiveness of the program to prevent initial and recurrent episodes of MDD. The interaction findings further highlight the previous work of Beardslee and his colleagues demonstrating the importance of parental depression in the development and prevention of MDD among adolescents. This study suggests that future prevention studies may need to address current depression in parents in order for offspring to benefit from preventive interventions. As noted in the work of Gillham and colleagues (2012), this is very difficult to do, but it remains extremely important. Indeed, it may be necessary to treat the parental depression or offer recurrence prevention programs separately for the parents of adolescents who are "at risk" for MDD.

Beardslee and colleagues (2013) reported a 33-month follow-up to the 2009 study by Garber and colleagues—that is, data for the 24 months following the 9-month follow-up previously reported. Impressively, the investigators were able to evaluate almost 85% of the adolescents at the 33-month follow-up. The primary outcome measure was the presence of MDD at any time during the follow-up period; the prevention group had a slower and lower rate (36.8%) of onset of MDD compared to the control condition (47.7%), corresponding to a number needed to treat of 10. As in the 9-month follow-up, there was a significant parental-depression-by-group interaction: among adolescents whose parents were not depressed at baseline, the prevention program participants' rate of MDD was 32.1% versus 51.9% in the control group, corresponding to a number needed to treat of 6. On the other hand, among adolescents who had at least one parent who was depressed at baseline, the prevention program had virtually no impact (41.6% vs. 43.4%), with an estimated number needed to treat of 54. The findings were further complicated by a treatment-by-parental-depression-by-site interaction. The parental-depression-by-treatment-condition interaction varied such that the effects of parental depression on the treatment outcomes varied by site; however, the sample sizes within sites were small relative to the overall findings, precluding an interpretation of the cause of this finding (see Beardslee et al., 2013).

Brent and colleagues (2015) reported 6-year follow-up data for the preceding prevention cohort (Garber et al., 2009). They retained a remarkable 88% of the participants from the original prevention sample. The rate of depression remained significantly lower than the treatment-as-usual group, and as with the original finding, this was true for those participants who did not have a depressed parent in the house. As with the 3-year follow-up, the differential preventive effects of the prevention program were obtained by the end of the 9 months of intervention and did not increase further over the 6-year period; however, the positive 9-month effects were maintained at the 6-year follow-up. The new findings that emerged in the 6-year follow-up were that the successful participants (those in the program but without a depressed parent in the house) evinced greater developmental competence and functional adaptivity than did the other groups of participants.

In summary, the work of Clarke, Garber, Beardslee, and their associates indicates that the modified Coping with Depression Course can be used to prevent MDD among youth at risk for a first episode of depression or to prevent the recurrence of MDD among those who have previously had an episode. However, the program does not appear to have a positive preventive impact on adolescents who have a parent who currently has MDD. The program effects were maintained at 33 months, the longest follow-up to demonstrate a preventive program effectiveness. However, the moderating effects of parental depression and the three-way interactions with sites indicate that the program may only have its preventive effects for adolescents who have some symptoms of depression or who have been previously depressed but not for those with one or both parents with MDD.

PREVENTION OF BIPOLAR DISORDER

Miklowitz and his colleagues have manualized his family-focused therapy (FFT; Miklowitz, 2008) for use as a prevention program for youth at risk for bipolar disorder (Miklowitz et al., 2013). The program was evaluated with 40 high-risk youth ages 9 to 17. "At risk" for bipolar disorders was defined as having a family member with a history of mania and a first-degree relative with bipolar I or bipolar II disorder. Participants were currently diagnosed with MDD, bipolar disorder not elsewhere classified, or cyclothymic disorder. Forty participants were randomly assigned to the FFT program or a two-session education control group; about 60% of the participants were receiving psychotropic medications. During this 1-year randomized clinical trial, FFT participants recovered more rapidly from their initial diagnosed symptoms, spent more weeks in remission of mood symptoms, and showed greater improvement in hypomania symptoms than did the participants in the education control group. As with clinical trials of FFT with bipolar patients, the treatment was most efficacious for youth from families with higher levels of Expressed Emotion. Despite the small sample sizes and other limitations of this study, it is encouraging in that a treatment with demonstrated efficacy with bipolar patients might be modified and employed in a preventive manner for youth at risk for bipolar disorders.

FUTURE DIRECTIONS AND RECOMMENDATIONS

Based on the preceding summaries of outcomes, we should begin to disseminate CBT and family-based programs as a major public health initiative. Both the international consortium on the prevention of depression (Cuijpers, Beekman, & Reynolds, 2012) and others (Muñoz, Beardslee, & Leykin, 2012) have strongly suggested such an effort, with the outcome being population-level change in the incidence of major depression in the groups targeted. Based on the studies reviewed here, it seems likely that wider use of programs aimed at "indicated" or "at risk" populations will yield the greatest public health benefits.

1. The number of empirical studies of effectiveness of preventive interventions for initial episodes of depression needs to be dramatically increased.
2. We need to continue to expand the study of cognitive-behavioral and educational approaches based on public health principles. The promising interventions described here need much further study, but the core principles are likely to be highly applicable.
3. A number of methodological issues need to be clarified: (1) how to increase retention of participants in prevention studies and (2) how to identify who drops out of prevention studies (dropouts may be those at highest risk [e.g., high family conflict, more negative life events, and greater depressive symptoms]).
4. The optimal timing of prevention interventions needs to be established. Current data suggest that ages 13 and 14 may be the best time, because this is the age just before a sharp upturn (ages 15–18) in initial episodes of MDD and bipolar disorder.
5. The low rate of "caseness" of mood disorders must be taken into account in calculating the sample sizes necessary for prevention studies. At-risk samples are likely to result in 40% to 50% of individuals (ages 13 and 14) with MDD during

a 3-year follow-up, whereas universal programs are more likely to see a control group caseness in a very much lower range essentially equal to the prevalence rates for MDD.

6. We need continually to expand the science base of depression, particularly regarding the question of its heterogeneity. It is important to identify robust subtypes of depression because specific programs for some of these subtypes are likely to be more effective than general prevention programs for a heterogeneous overall MDD. Robust subtypes of MDD are also likely to yield important genetic information. It is likely that certain vulnerabilities to depression are conveyed by multiple genes acting in concert and expressed in stressful situations. Promising leads include the work of Garber (Garber, Kieley, & Martin, 2002) on the diathesis-stress hypothesis, work by Goodman and associates (Goodman & Gotlib, 1999) on ways in which genes and the environmental and internal stressors in families with parental depression interact, and work by Reiss and colleagues (Reiss, Neiderhiser, Hetherington, & Plomkin, 2000) on behavioral genetics. Other work points to other subtypes and suggests that depression may represent an underlying dysregulation of emotion (Dahl, 2001), or that it may be part of a general phenomenon of inhibition (Kagan & Snidman, 1991). Recent work on differential responses to CBT and antidepressants in patients with differing patterns of baseline neural activation and connectivity suggests that identifying subtypes of depression via neuroimaging or genetic biomarkers may be an efficient approach to the study of prevention of depression (see McGrath et al., 2013, 2014). The more we understand the risk factors and risk mechanisms (i.e., how risks come together) of heterogeneous MDD, the better we will be able to mount successful and efficient preventive interventions.
7. It is also very important to remember that better treatments make a huge difference in the lives of families (e.g., quicker recoveries, less misunderstanding). And, as better interventions are found, they will contribute to the prevention of depression among other family members.
8. We need more study of prevention programs in different contexts with an awareness of cultural, racial, and ethnic differences.
9. The occurrence of depression in either a parent or a child requires educational support from the other family members (see England & Sim, 2009). Important opportunities exist for prevention in these situations. Some groups have found that adult family members with MDD do not want their children to know of the disorder; this attitude needs to be overcome by reducing stigma associated with mood disorders. It has become increasingly clear that the presence of a depressed parent in the home affects the outcome of prevention programs designed to prevent depression among "at risk" adolescents. It remains to be determined whether this impact is primarily a genetic or environmental risk, or their interaction.
10. Prevention of depression is closely related to other preventive efforts—in particular, the prevention of suicide and the consideration of victimization by violence. The work by Marikangas and colleagues suggests the possibility that MDD may be prevented by preventing the development of anxiety, which is a risk factor for subsequent development of MDD (Marikangas, Avenevoli, Dierker, & Grillon, 1999). It is also possible that programs that prevent depression simultaneously prevent or ameliorate anxiety in "at risk" groups.
11. Although the prevention of adolescent depression is a common goal in adolescent health, it is rarely approached in a comprehensive and systematic manner that includes continuous attention to all aspects of prevention. Most often, adolescent depression rises to the attention of

the local or national health agenda after a series of well-publicized adolescent suicides. National and local advocacy groups have been effective in raising the public visibility of issues such as teenage pregnancy and drug abuse; similar community and political approaches are needed for the prevention of adolescent depression. Three specific approaches are needed:

a. Campaigns to educate local and national governmental agencies and institutions and to assist them with developing policies and programs that ensure the use of effective and comprehensive models that prevent adolescent depression at all stages
b. Advisory groups that work with national professional organizations to assist them in developing protocols and professional standards that place a higher priority on the prevention of adolescent depression. These efforts should include all professionals who interact with youth—in the fields of healthcare, education, social service, and juvenile justice.
c. Self-help groups that work on the local level with families, communities, and youth development agencies to assist them in developing effective prevention interventions.

Research Agenda for Depression and Bipolar Disorder

Rachel Neuhut
W. Edward Craighead
Charles Nemeroff
Moira Rynn
Dwight L. Evans

chapter 4

MAJOR DEPRESSIVE DISORDER

The Disorder

What We Know

Basic knowledge about major depressive disorder (MDD) in adolescence has begun to accumulate over the past three decades. Most importantly, MDD is now no longer seen primarily as a disorder of the middle-aged and elderly. It is clear that MDD often begins in adolescence and has a serious impact on the adolescent's development into adulthood. In contrast, prepubertal onset is less common, with a higher proportion of males who experience mood reactivity, irritability, dysphoria, and comorbidity with disruptive disorder. Adolescent MDD is chronic and recurrent, sharing diagnostic features with those of adult MDD, including high comorbidity with anxiety and substance abuse disorders, and risk for suicide. Adolescent MDD is associated with a lack of social development and skills, withdrawal from peers, and poor school performance.

Information on risk factors for the development of adolescent MDD has also begun to emerge. The most consistent risk factors for MDD in both adolescents and adults are female gender (twofold to threefold increased risk) and a family history of MDD. Offspring of depressed parents are at increased risk (twofold to fourfold) for depression. A previous episode is a major risk factor for the occurrence of additional episodes; over 50% of adolescents with MDD have a recurrence within 5 years and 70% within 10 years, with MDD episodes often continuing into adulthood. This confers an increased risk of suicide attempts and psychiatric and medical hospitalizations. Adverse family environments, especially childhood maltreatment (abuse and neglect) as well as the absence of supportive interactions, poor parental bonding, poor primary attachments, and harsh discipline, are also risk factors that contribute to both the onset and recurrence of adolescent MDD. Negative cognitions about oneself appear to mediate the relation between stressful life events and the occurrence of depressive symptoms.

Biologically, there are abnormalities in hypothalamic–pituitary–adrenal (HPA) axis activity in adolescence similar to those found in adults, as well as a higher rate of thyroid dysfunction.

Adolescent depression exhibits similar levels of heritability to adult depression. The limited data from twin studies suggest a heritability estimate of approximately 37% for adolescent depression.

What We Do Not Know

We have only begun to characterize the possible adverse effects of depression on brain structure, function, and development. We have limited data on brain plasticity and neurogenesis. In addition, the way in which treatment interventions (psychosocial and/or psychopharmacologic) impact brain plasticity and neurogenesis is unknown. No specific genes have yet been identified that are unequivocally associated with MDD, regardless of age of onset. We have gained some knowledge about which patterns of neural connectivity respond to psychotherapy versus pharmacology.

Although there appears to be a clear link between life events and depression, we do not know the mechanisms by which stress increases an individual's vulnerability to depression or the genetic and environmental factors that influence vulnerability or resilience. Furthermore, it is known that various forms of stressors often precede mood disorders, but it is not known why only some individuals exposed to these stressors become depressed. There is some evidence that a patient's response to an external stressor may be moderated by the individual's genetic constitution, as a result of possessing a functional polymorphism in the promoter region of the serotonin transporter gene, though these data remain a source of considerable debate in adults and adolescents. A number of other candidate genes have been explored as mediating risk for MDD in adolescents exposed to adverse early life stress, following up on promising findings in adults. These include FKBP5 genotypes associated with adolescent suicidal events and BDNF Val66Met polymorphism possible interaction with the environment leading adolescent depressive symptoms, to name two. Some evidence has pointed to negative cognitive appraisals of the self and life events as mediators of the relation between stress and depression, but these factors do not appear to tell the whole story. Thus, other mediators are likely. Moreover, we know little about the ways in which such negative cognitions develop in adolescence, and whether they can be prevented, although recent school-based preventive interventions provided encouraging outcomes.

The biological mechanisms that mediate the relation between life events and risk of MDD in adolescents are also not known. We do not know whether the presence of adolescent depression is a risk factor for the development of other medical diseases and how its presence may affect the course of the medical illness. In addition, we do not know if treatment and/or prevention of depression decreases the potential impact and severity of the expressed medical illness.

Research Priorities: What We Need to Know

Research on adolescent MDD needs to proceed on many fronts. To facilitate research across broad aspects of the disorder, we propose that highest priority be given to the following areas:

- Studies of the prodromal phase of child and adolescent mood disorders. Such research would allow for better identification of the illness and how it evolves over time to its full clinical course.
- Integrative studies of the range of possible psychological, sociological, familial, and biological variables that contribute to the development of adolescent depression. By identifying which variables are most important and contribute the most to the development of adolescent MDD, we can target treatment and prevention efforts to such risk factors and yield the best outcomes.
- Examination of the mediational links among environmental stressors, cognitive and personality variables, genetics, biological systems, and depressive symptoms. Uncovering these links will provide information on the causal chain of events that leads to the clinical disorder, and suggest avenues for the development of new treatments and preventive programs.
- We are no closer to having a large enough cohort to conduct a well-powered genome-wide association study of adolescent depression.
- Considerable progress has been made in recent years on defining unique adult MDD endophenotypes, including increased inflammation, shortened telomeres, and altered mitochondrial DNA, as well as several epigenetic modifications. None of these have been explored in adolescent MDD.
- Investment in designing developmentally informed longitudinal brain imaging studies that identify potential biological markers that inform risk, provide prevention targets, and direct treatment pathways.

Treatment

What We Know

As found in the adult depression treatment literature, cognitive-behavioral treatment (CBT) and interpersonal therapy (IPT) for youth depression appear to be more efficacious than no treatment, waitlist control, or attention placebo controls. In addition, preliminary evidence suggests that attachment-based family therapy and behavioral activation may be useful for the treatment of adolescent depression. To date, the only medications that have demonstrated safety and efficacy in double-blind placebo-controlled trials for children and adolescents with major depression are the selective serotonin reuptake inhibitors (SSRIs). Fluoxetine was the first SSRI and received federal Food and Drug Administration (FDA) approval for the treatment of pediatric depression (age 8 and greater); escitalopram received FDA approval for ages 12 and greater. The National Institute of Mental Health (NIMH)–funded study called the Treatment of Adolescents with Depression Study (TADS) showed that 71% of patients responded well to acute (12-week) combination treatment of CBT with fluoxetine compared with 61% of those who received fluoxetine alone, 43% of those who received CBT alone, and 35% of those treated with placebo. At the end of acute and sustained treatment (36 weeks), all treatments showed equal treatment effects, with remission rates of 60% for the combination of fluoxetine and CBT, 55% for fluoxetine, and 64% for CBT, yielding an overall remission rate of 60% (Kennard et al., 2009). The study also reported that patients became significantly less suicidal regardless of the treatment they received, but CBT alone or in combination produced greater reductions than medications. The TADS team reported a 1-year naturalistic follow-up; data were available for 66.6% of the participants, and the improvements reported at the end of active treatment were sustained for both the depression and suicidality measures. In addition, after reviewing 24 double-blind placebo-controlled pediatric trials using antidepressants, an FDA panel has determined that SSRIs may carry an increased risk of suicidal ideation or behaviors for a small proportion of users (perhaps 2% or 3%). The FDA has labeled all SSRI antidepressants with a warning about the potential risk of increased suicidal thinking and behavior and the need for close medical monitoring, particularly in the first month of treatment and when the medication dose is adjusted. The FDA expects physicians to educate patients and families about the risks and benefits of these medications and to watch for behavioral changes in the child, such as irritability, aggression, and impulsivity. In spite of these concerns, antidepressants can be very effective in treating mood and anxiety disorders in this group.

What We Do Not Know

Although initial treatment studies have been promising, many patients continue to have clinically significant levels of depression after psychotherapy and medication treatment, most patients experience at least one recurrence of depression within 5 years of treatment termination, and about half seek subsequent treatment. More importantly, we do not know which specific psychosocial or pharmacologic treatments are most efficacious for which patients. In addition, little is known about the efficacy of sequencing or combining various treatments. Even though combinations of CBT and medications appear to provide slightly more efficient treatments, the burden and costs of such combinations may outweigh the increased efficiencies in general clinical practice. There is little information regarding the management of partial response and nonresponse in the treatment of adolescent depression. We have limited information about the optimal length of time for any of these treatments and how to maintain the treatment response once achieved by using such options as booster sessions and/or varying the length of medication treatment. However, the increased efficacy of the longer TADS treatment protocol of 36 weeks as compared to 12 or 16 weeks suggests that longer treatments may be somewhat more effective and their effects may be more durable. There is also little information on how our present treatments that target adolescent depression impact comorbid psychiatric disorders such as substance abuse, disruptive disorders, and anxiety disorders that affect the outcomes of standard first-line treatments among adults. Perhaps the most pressing unanswered questions that need to be addressed among adolescents is the identification of predictors of clinical outcome (which treatments work for which patients) and clarification of the differential mechanisms of change with each evidence-based intervention (i.e., moderators and mediators of treatment outcomes).

Research Priorities: What We Need to Know

We have identified a number of high-priority topics for treatment research on MDD in adolescence:

- There is a need for more research into the safety and efficacy of SSRIs. The benefits versus risks of using SSRIs with adolescents should be carefully assessed in such studies.

- Future studies need to have adequate statistical power to determine the efficacy and safety of antidepressants in both child and adolescent populations.
- There is a particular need to investigate the use of antidepressant treatment in suicidal adolescents. Independent, federally funded centers should be established to evaluate treatment to prevent suicide.
- Long-term studies of antidepressants are required to evaluate their safety profile in children. This information will enable a risk/benefit analysis of extended antidepressant use. In addition, maintenance studies are needed to guide the optimal duration of medication treatment.
- There is a need for antidepressant studies focusing on remission of symptoms and full functional recovery, rather than just treatment response.
- The development and testing of interventions that focus on maternal depression and family discord might be an effective way of preventing adolescent depression.
- Additional treatment research such as the TADS program is needed to explore further the acute efficacy of combination treatment, with a focus on determining which subpopulation of patients will do best with monotherapy versus combined treatment.
- Treatment research is needed on refractory and chronic conditions, such as "double depression" in adolescence. These chronic disorders may respond better to combinations of medication and CBT than to either monotherapy alone, as suggested by comparable data on adults with chronic depression.
- Interventions designed to improve outcome in patients with poor prognostic risk factors need to be examined.
- Studies need to be undertaken to identify the genetic and other biomarkers of treatment outcome so we can know which patients respond to which treatments.
- There is little in the literature about the transportability of manualized treatments to community settings; this important issue needs to be addressed.

Prevention

What We Know

A number of promising strategies for the prevention of childhood and adolescent depression have emerged. Of special significance is the fact that these emerging prevention strategies make a point of taking into account the developmental level of participants. The evaluated preventive strategies are based primarily on cognitive-behavioral and family-educational approaches, with the focus of reducing risk factors and enhancing protective and resiliency factors associated with depression in youth. Rigorous standards for the development and evaluation of manual-based preventive approaches have been introduced, and these innovations have greatly facilitated research in this area.

To date, we have initial evidence that these prevention programs are more effective than both no treatment and usual care (staying in existing treatment or patients seeking treatment on their own) in reducing future episodes of MDD. These effects are particularly evident for those at highest risk of MDD and for those with the greatest severity of depressive symptoms.

What We Do Not Know

Despite the promising studies on prevention of depression, much remains to be learned. There are not enough data about the timing of preventive interventions or about the appropriate setting for such interventions to be assured that the expected outcomes occur for the targeted population. Most studies have used samples that include adolescents who have had previous episodes of MDD (high-risk samples). Only one study has studied prevention among "at risk" but specifically never previously depressed youth, so we know little about the prevention of first episodes of MDD. Long-term follow-up data are scarce but crucial to understanding whether preventive interventions have an impact on the occurrence of MDD episodes into adulthood.

Research Priorities: What We Need to Know

Prevention research is in its infancy; therefore, a number of basic studies are sorely needed. These include the following:

- Creating prevention programs based on the full range of risk factors for MDD need to be developed and tested.
- Comparisons among existing preventive programs need to be conducted.
- Studies on the active ingredients of preventive programs and the mediators of change should be performed.
- Examination of prevention programs in different contexts with an awareness of cultural, racial, and ethnic differences.
- Dissemination of prevention programs so that they reach the families most at need and at risk. This is especially a challenge because of the lack of sophisticated delivery systems of prevention programs.
- Evaluation of the impact of prevention programs for individuals with different types of risk factors for MDD.

BIPOLAR DISORDER

The Disorder

What We Know

We now know that variants, or precursors, of bipolar disorder may be more common in adolescence than previously thought. There is a growing consensus that youth who are afflicted with severe affective dysregulation, high levels of agitation, aggression, and dyscontrol may have an early form of bipolar disorder. Approximately 65% of individuals who are ultimately diagnosed with bipolar disorder experience their first episode during adolescence. This issue has received increased scientific attention, as is evident in the scheduling of two NIMH workshops on bipolar disorder in children and adolescents and in exhaustive reviews that have supported the validity of the disorder in youth.

Bipolar disorder is highly heritable. There are several loci of the human genome that have been identified with the disorder in association or linkage studies. More recently, adult BPD has been scrutinized in a well-powered, large-scale genome-wide association study that yielded multiple novel candidate genes, including several components of the inflammatory cascade.

What We Do Not Know

We know little about how to accurately identify the early signs and symptoms of bipolar disorder in youth. There is still controversy over the definition of early-onset mania; this is complicated by the fact that this disorder is highly comorbid with other psychiatric disorders.

We also do not know whether pediatric bipolar disorder differs from the adult form of the disorder. Related to this, there is little information on the adult course of pediatric-onset mania. Other than a likely genetic contribution, little is known about the risk factors for the development of bipolar disorder in youth.

Research Priorities: What We Need to Know

Several priorities for research can be suggested:

- Most importantly, additional epidemiologic studies are needed to determine the prevalence of pediatric and adolescent bipolar disorder.
- Additional long-term longitudinal studies are needed to clarify the relation of adolescent onset of symptoms to the course of bipolar disorder in adulthood. These data would assist with informing us about the clinical course and acute and long-term treatment outcome.
- The relationship of comorbid disorders such as ADHD and conduct disorder to juvenile-onset bipolar disorder needs to be further evaluated.

- Genetic and epigenetic studies in childhood-onset and adolescent bipolar disorder are needed.
- Structural and functional brain imaging studies are few in bipolar disorder in adolescence.

Treatment

What We Know

As learned from treatment of adults diagnosed with bipolar disorder, the complexity of this illness in adolescents requires a combination of medication and psychosocial interventions to reduce and sustain that reduction in the burden of the illness. We also know that patients who respond to a given acute pharmacotherapy regimen continue to benefit from ongoing treatment with the medication that led to symptom amelioration. There are some well-controlled studies of specific psychosocial and pharmacologic interventions for pediatric bipolar disorder. Psychosocial interventions, which are used adjunctively with appropriate medical regimens and target adolescent bipolar disorder, include group psychoeducation, CBT, IPT, and family-focused therapy. The psychosocial interventions seem to have their impact primarily on the depressive symptoms and less on the manic/hypomanic symptoms of the disorder. The maintenance effects of acute treatment with mood stabilizers and antidepressants are enhanced by the adjunctive use of the psychosocial interventions.

What We Do Not Know

It may be that combination pharmacotherapy with more than one mood-stabilizing agent may be a rational approach for some youth who have manic, hypomanic, depressed, or mixed states. There are virtually no studies regarding the prevention of bipolar disorder, despite good knowledge regarding who is at risk for development of the disorder during adolescence.

There are also limited data on the impact of long-term exposure to psychotropic compounds on the developing brain. We also do not have studies of the side effects that arise from medication treatment over a long period of time.

Research Priorities: What We Need to Know

Treatment studies of highest priority would include the following:

- More, and larger, efficacy studies that include evaluation of the mechanisms of change produced by medications and psychosocial treatments are urgently needed.
- Whether treatment should begin with drug monotherapy or a combination of medications, or medication plus psychotherapy, should be a topic of further study.
- Treatment of those who do not respond to standard bipolar treatment should be evaluated.
- Studies of long-term maintenance pharmacotherapy and psychotherapy are sorely needed.
- Given the chronicity of this disorder and the high risk for these patients to die from suicide, there needs to be research on the development of prevention programs that would target patients at risk for this disorder that have an impact on prevention of suicide, the most serious consequence of the illness.

Prevention

What We Know and Do Not Know

Unfortunately, we know almost nothing about the prevention of bipolar disorder in youth. One factor hindering prevention research is the challenge of making an accurate diagnosis. Not until we can accurately identify high-risk cases and the emergence of the actual disorder in adolescence can studies on prevention begin. At this point, even if we could properly identify a target population and clinical endpoint, we do not yet know how best to design and evaluate preventive strategies for this disorder.

Research Priorities: What We Need to Know

As mentioned above, scientific advancement in accurately characterizing the early signs and full emergence of bipolar disorder in youth is a crucial first step. The next step is further research on risk factors for the development of bipolar disorder in youth. Once these goals have been accomplished, we need to design and evaluate preventive programs that target such risk factors. Although such preventive studies are in the future, they represent one of the more important directions for alleviating the burden of this serious and potentially debilitating disorder in adulthood.

Schizophrenia

COMMISSION ON ADOLESCENT SCHIZOPHRENIA

Raquel E. Gur, *Commission Chair*

Second Edition

Ruben C. Gur

Matcheri S. Keshavan

Christian Kohler

Judith Rapoport

Elaine Walker

First Edition

Nancy Andreasen

Robert Asarnow

Ruben Gur

Peter Jones

Kenneth Kendler

Matcheri Keshavan

Jeffrey Lieberman

Robert McCarley

Robin Murray

Judith Rapoport

Carol Tamminga

Ming Tsuang

Elaine Walker

Daniel Weinberger

With contributions from

Kristin Lancefield

part II

Defining Schizophrenia

Raquel E. Gur
Ruben C. Gur
Matcheri S. Keshavan
Christian Kohler
Elaine Walker

chapter 5

OVERVIEW

Schizophrenia is a chronic and severe mental disorder with a typical onset in adolescence and early adulthood and a lifetime prevalence of about 1%. On average, males have their illness onset 3 to 4 years earlier than females. Onset of schizophrenia is very rare before age 11, and prior to age 18 the illness has been called early-onset schizophrenia, while onset before age 13 has been termed very-early-onset schizophrenia (Werry, 1981).

Prior to examining topics in schizophrenia, we must address a basic question as to the definition of "adolescents" and "adults." The way these groups will be defined is partly related to the question being asked. That is, research studies that emphasize the study of neural development or finding links between endocrine changes and onset of schizophrenia are likely to place more emphasis on defining adolescence in terms of body or brain maturation. For example, adolescence could be defined as the period between the onset and offset of puberty. Alternatively, it could be defined based on our current knowledge of brain development, which suggests that maturational processes accelerate around the time of puberty but that they continue on into what is often considered "young adulthood." Most recent studies of normal brain development suggest that brain maturation continues to the early 20s. If this rather extended definition of adolescence is used, then the appropriate "adult" contrast groups are likely to be somewhat older—people in their late 20s, 30s, or even 40s.

Under the general rubric of phenomenology, four major topics need to be considered as we explore the relevance of research on adults to the understanding of adolescents: diagnostic criteria, "phenomenology," the relationship of phenomenology to neural mechanisms, and the use of phenomenology to assist in identifying the phenotype for genetic studies.

Diagnostic Criteria

Two different sets of diagnostic criteria are currently used in the world literature. For most studies that emphasize biological markers, and for almost all of those conducted in the United States, the standard diagnostic criteria were from DSM-IV. However, international epidemiologic studies are likely to use the World Health Organization's *International Classification of Diseases, Tenth Revision* (ICD-10). Differences in the choice of diagnostic criteria may affect the results of studies, and the research highlighted here is based on the above classifications.

There are many similarities between the ICD and DSM, largely as a consequence of efforts by the ICD and DSM workgroups to achieve as much concordance as possible. Both require 1 month of active symptoms and the presence of psychotic symptoms such as delusions or hallucinations. There are, however, important differences between the ICD and DSM. In most respects, the DSM provides a slightly narrower conceptualization of schizophrenia than does the ICD. For example, the ICD only requires 1 month of overall duration of symptoms, while the DSM requires 6 months. In addition, the ICD includes schizotypal disorder and simple schizophrenia within its nomenclature under the general heading of the diagnosis of schizophrenia. In the DSM, simple schizophrenia is excluded, and schizotypal disorder is placed among the personality disorders. Other less significant differences include a greater emphasis on first-rank symptoms in the ICD, as well as a much more specific and complex system list.

How important is the choice of diagnostic criteria for research on adolescents? It could be very important. Setting criteria boundaries more broadly or more narrowly will have a significant impact on the groups of adolescents chosen for study. Furthermore, although the developers of these criteria paid close attention to examining their reliability and, when possible, their validity, it was assumed almost without question that the criteria could and should be the same for children, adolescents, and adults. This decision was not based on any published empirical data; rather, it was based primarily on "clinical impressions." The DSM is now in its fifth edition, with further changes introduced, and the ICD is in revision as well.

A frequently expressed clinical impression among those who study schizophrenia or psychosis in children and adolescents, however, is that making a diagnosis in these younger age ranges is much more difficult than diagnosing individuals in their 20s. Multiple issues arise for a diagnosis in the adolescence age range. One important issue is comorbidity: teenagers frequently may meet criteria for multiple diagnoses, such as conduct disorder or attention-deficit/hyperactivity disorder (ADHD). Although the DSM tends to encourage the use of multiple diagnoses, this policy also has no empirical basis. An alternative approach that might be considered from research on adolescents is to try to identify a single "best" diagnosis that would summarize the child parsimoniously. However, the high rate of neurodevelopmental disorders seen in childhood-onset patients years before psychosis onset precludes this solution for many cases.

Many adolescents also abuse substances of many different kinds. This is important in the diagnosis of adults who may have schizophrenia, but it poses even greater problems among adolescents. Abuse of substances such as amphetamines may potentially induce a psychotic picture that is very similar to schizophrenia. We do not know whether young people who continue to meet the criteria for schizophrenia after discontinuing amphetamine use should be considered "typical schizophrenics" or whether they should in fact be given another diagnosis, such as substance-induced psychotic disorder. However, given the fact that amphetamines have a significant effect on the dopamine system—a key neurotransmitter implicated in the neurochemical mechanisms of schizophrenia—it is at least plausible that amphetamines (and perhaps other substances as well) may be considered to be triggers or inducers of schizophrenia. According to this view, substance abuse could be one of the many factors that rank among the nongenetic causes of schizophrenia. However, there is still no strong consensus on this issue.

In summary, there are many unanswered research questions under the heading of "diagnosis." More studies are needed to explore how well existing diagnostic criteria actually work in children and adolescents. Specifically, studies of both their reliability and validity are needed, as well as studies examining issues of comorbidity and longitudinal studies examining changes in both diagnosis and phenomenology in cohorts of adolescents and of adults.

Phenomenology

The concept of "phenomenology" can be relatively broad, describing clinical symptoms, psychosocial functioning, cognitive functioning, and "neurological" measures such as soft signs. Here we will focus primarily on clinical symptoms and psychosocial functioning.

For the assessment of clinical symptoms in schizophrenia, choosing the appropriate informant is a key issue. Whatever their age, patients with schizophrenia frequently have difficulty in reporting their symptoms and past history accurately. Optimally, one gets the best information from several informants—usually a parent plus the patient. In the case of adolescents, a friend may be a good additional informant. Another critical issue in phenomenology when assessing adolescents is to determine the distinction between "normal" adolescent behavior and psychopathology. Again, this can be difficult in assessing adults, but it is even more difficult in adolescents. It can be hard to draw the line between "teenage scruffiness" and disorganization, or a withdrawal to seek privacy versus avolition. As discussed above, drug use or abuse can also confound the picture. For example, when an adolescent known to be using marijuana regularly exhibits chronic apathy and avolition, is this due to marijuana use or is it a true negative symptom? At the moment, no data are available to help us address any of these issues pertaining to the assessment of clinical symptoms in adolescents versus adults. This is clearly an area where more information is needed.

Another issue is the identification of appropriate developmental milestones and needs that are appropriate to the adolescent age range for the assessment of psychosocial functioning. For example, when we assess peer relationships in young or older adults with schizophrenia, we are evaluating the extent to which they have a circle of friends with whom they get together socially. In the case of adolescents, peer relationships are far more important and are more intensely driven by a need to establish independence from the family setting and to bond with others from the same age range. Likewise, the assessment of family relationships among adolescents is guided by quite different conditions than in mature adults. Finally, the "work" of an adolescent is quite generally to do well in school, while the "work" of an adult is normally to find a paying job. Again, assessment tools have simply not been defined for assessing these aspects of psychosocial functioning in adolescents.

Box 5.1 Prodromal Features in First-Episode Psychosis Frequently Described in Adolescent Patients

Unusual perceptual experiences
Unusual ideas
Suspiciousness
Reduced concentration, attention
Decreased motivation, drive, and energy
Mood changes: depression, anxiety
Sleep difficulties
Social withdrawal
Suspiciousness
Irritability
Decline in role functioning (e.g., academic performance, social and recreational activities, neglecting appearance)

Expression of Early Symptoms and Illness Course

Prior to the onset of the clinical syndrome of schizophrenia and other psychotic disorders, there is typically a period of functional decline and gradual emergence of symptoms (Addington & Heinssen, 2012; Cannon et al., 2008). This period, referred to as the *prodrome*, is the transitional stage from the premorbid state to the point at which the patient meets criteria for clinical psychosis. The prodrome can last from months to years, and the first signs usually appear during adolescence, even when the clinical onset does not occur until early adulthood. With respect to functional impairment, there is often a decline in academic and work performance and interest in social and recreational activities, as well as problems with memory and concentration.

A range of symptoms is associated with the prodromal period (Box 5.1), and the symptom pattern and sequence of emergence of symptom subtypes vary among patients (Neumann et al., 1995; Yung & McGorry, 1996). Included among the early prodromal signs are mood changes, and many who are subsequently diagnosed with psychosis display depression before they have psychotic symptoms (Fusar-Poli et al., 2013a). Positive symptoms initially present in an attenuated form during the prodrome (Cannon et al., 2008). For example, the individual might report unusual perceptual experiences, such as hearing voices when no one else is around or seeing some unidentifiable object out of the corner of his eye. In the prodrome, such experiences are attributed by the individual to "imagination" or "error," thus lacking the conviction that is required to meet DSM criteria for hallucinations. In fact, these "psychotic-like" symptoms increase in frequency through the course of normal adolescence, then diminish for most by early adulthood (Kelleher & Cannon, 2011). But for those who eventually develop a psychotic disorder, the unusual sensory experiences and ideas become more compelling, and eventually the individual is convinced they are real. When this threshold of conviction is crossed, and the symptoms persist, the individual is likely to meet diagnostic criteria for a psychotic disorder. If there are accompanying symptoms of mood disorder, such as depression or mania, the individual may meet criteria for a diagnosis of schizoaffective disorder or major depression with psychotic features. If mood disturbances are not pronounced, then schizophrenia is likely to be the diagnosis.

The prodromal phase has been the subject of increasing research interest because it may be the optimal period for identifying neuropathological processes and, ultimately, for preventive intervention. While the initial research on the prodrome relied on retrospective data obtained from diagnosed patients, investigators are now studying the prodrome prospectively by using assessments aimed at measuring the presence and severity of prodromal signs. Several structured approaches for prospective assessment of prodromal syndromes have been developed and are currently being used in longitudinal studies (Addington & Heinssen, 2012; Correll et al., 2010). These measures focus on *subclinical* manifestations of the perceptual, ideational, and behavioral symptoms of psychosis. In the research literature, individuals who manifest symptoms that meet predetermined severity and duration criteria are designated as "clinical high risk," "ultra-high risk" or "prodromal." Because the term "prodromal" may be taken to imply the inevitability of a subsequent illness, most in the field use the term "clinical high risk" (CHR) to refer to individuals who are manifesting putative prodromal syndromes.

In the United States, the Structured Interview for Prodromal Syndromes (SIPS; Miller et al., 2003) has been the most widely used measure. Like other prodrome assessment tools, it rates the presence and severity of subclinical positive (e.g., suspiciousness, unusual ideas and perceptual experiences) and negative (e.g., social withdrawal, decreased emotional expression and role functioning) symptoms, as well as mood and vegetative symptoms. Based on SIPS ratings, individuals who meet CHR criteria can manifest several different syndromes, most often an "attenuated positive symptom" syndrome and/or schizotypal personality disorder. Using such measures to identify CHR samples enhances positive predictive power above the population prevalence of 1% to 2%, as well as the risk rate (i.e., about 12%) for first-degree relatives of patients with psychosis (Sørensen et al., 2009). Specifically, among those who meet the criteria for CHR status based on the SIPS, the rate of subsequent "conversion" to psychosis is between 25% and 35% within 2 to 4 years (Addington & Heinssen, 2012; Cannon et al., 2008). Ongoing prospective CHR studies are aimed at boosting predictive power beyond this level in order to reduce false positives. In addition, these studies are concerned with elucidating neural mechanisms involved in the emergence of psychosis. In pursuit of these goals, the North American Prodrome Longitudinal Study (NAPLS) project, the largest such investigation in the United States, is tracking biobehavioral development in CHR individuals (Cannon et al., 2008).

The modal course of schizophrenia and other psychotic disorders, with prodromal signs typically appearing as the individual enters adolescence, has led investigators to assume that postpubertal neurodevelopmental mechanisms are playing an important role in triggering illness expression. At the same time, the observation of more subtle signs of dysfunction in early and middle childhood suggest that for some patients earlier developmental periods are also characterized by deviation from normal developmental trajectories (Walker et al., 2008).

While the clinical features of adolescent-onset and adult-onset schizophrenia are overall quite similar, the initial clinical presentation does vary as a function of age at onset (Fig. 5.1). In general, adolescent-onset schizophrenia patients manifest more premorbid behavioral deficits and higher levels of depression and suicidal behavior than adult-onset patients (Langeveld et al., 2012). They also have more severe negative symptoms and cognitive impairments, less structured delusions, and a lower frequency of hallucinations and are less responsive to treatment (Clemmensen, Vernal, & Steinhausen, 2012; Holmen et al., 2012; Levine & Rabinowitz, 2010; Nicolson & Rapoport, 1999; Werry et al., 1991). As would be expected with an earlier illness onset, when compared to adult-onset patients, adolescents with schizophrenia tend to have lower levels of academic achievement and interpersonal adjustment. Very-early-onset cases tend to have an insidious onset, while adolescent-onset cases tend to have a more acute onset. Early-onset and very-early-onset patients also are more often diagnosed with an undifferentiated subtype, although well-formed delusions and hallucinations are very frequent in childhood-onset cases and more often multimodal than adult-onset cases (David et al., 2011; Nicolson & Rapoport, 1999).

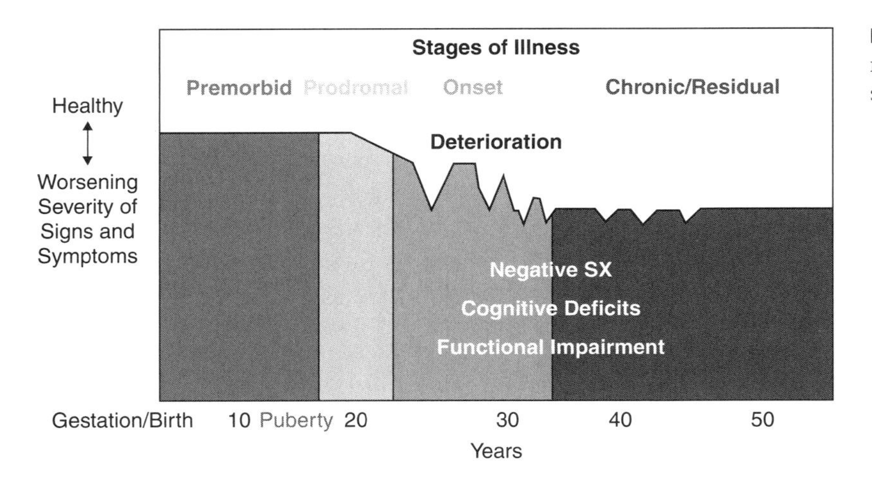

Figure 5.1 The natural history of schizophrenia.

In summary, functional decline and a range of subthreshold symptoms precede the onset of schizophrenia and other psychotic disorders in adolescents. Identifying clinical signs of risk so that youth can be identified prior to, or soon after, their first psychotic episode will enhance our opportunities for reducing illness-associated disability and functional impairment. Moreover, the longitudinal study of youth who manifest CHR syndromes has the potential to shed light on the developmental trajectories that lead to schizophrenia, as well as the neuropathological processes involved in symptom expression. As described below, advances in our understanding of normal adolescent brain development have provided a framework for a clearer view of the abnormalities that give rise to psychosis. This, in turn, will provide a firmer base for the development of more effective treatments and, in the long run, preventive interventions.

Some of the key research questions in the area of the clinical phenomenology of adolescent schizophrenia are as follows:

- Are there identifiable subtypes of patients who differ in premorbid indicators and/or in the nature and sequence of emergence of prodromal and early psychotic symptoms?
- Can we enhance the sensitivity and specificity of prediction of risk for illness onset by refining CHR criteria?
- Are there biomarkers that can be reliably measured and combined with indices of clinical phenomenology to enhance prediction?

These questions are currently under intense investigation by research teams throughout the world who are conducting longitudinal studies of CHR youth (Addington & Heinssen, 2012). As findings from these studies emerge, we can expect significant improvements in both risk identification and early intervention.

Linking Phenomenology to Its Neural Basis

Through the use of neuroimaging, neuropathology, and neurogenetics, substantial progress in understanding the neural underpinnings of schizophrenia is being made. Excellent work has recently been done that examines the relationship between brain development and the occurrence of schizophrenia in children and adolescents, as described in other chapters (Andreasen et al., 2011; Brent et al., 2013; DeLisi et al., 1997; Fusar-Poli et al., 2012; Giedd et al., 1999; Gur et al., 1998b, 1999; Ho et al., 2003; Hollis & Rapoport, 2011; Jacobsen et al., 1998; Kumra et al., 2000; Lieberman et al., 2001a; Rapoport et al., 1997; Thompson et al., 2001). As this work continues to mature, however, more work needs to be done to examine precisely how the specific symptoms of schizophrenia arise in the human brain, and whether imaging and other tools can be used to assist in diagnosis, treatment planning, and ultimately prevention.

This work must also address several questions in the realm of phenomenology. Specifically, how should we proceed as we attempt to link phenomenology to neural mechanisms? As discussed above, the phenomenology has multiple levels and aspects—symptoms, outcome, cognitive function, and psychosocial function. Which of these should be linked to imaging and other "biological" measures?

Most work to date has taken several different approaches. At the simplest level, investigators have conducted studies linking specific symptoms to neural measures. For example, studies have used positron emission tomography (PET) to identify brain regions active during auditory hallucinations (e.g., Silbersweig et al., 1995). Other investigators have examined symptoms such as thought disorder in relation to brain measures (e.g., Shenton et al., 1992; Whitford et al., 2015). One of the critical conceptual issues, however, is the fact that the phenomenology of schizophrenia is complex. That is, the illness cannot be characterized on the basis of a single symptom. Although auditory hallucinations are common in schizophrenia, they are not omnipresent. Therefore, other investigators have proceeded by examining groups of symptoms that are correlated with one another, or "dimensions." Many factor analytic studies have examined the factor structure of the symptoms of schizophrenia; nearly all find that the symptoms group naturally into three dimensions: psychoticism, disorganization, and negative symptoms (Andreasen et al., 1982, 1986, 1995b; Arndt et al., 1991, 1995; Bilder et al., 1985; Gur et al., 1991; Kulhara et al., 1986; Lenzenweger et al., 1989; Liddle et al., 1987). Some studies have used the dimensional approach to examine brain–behavior relationships. Several studies also suggest that these three dimensions may have different functional neural substrates, as seen with PET, or different structural or functional brain correlates, as evaluated with magnetic resonance imaging (MRI), and may also have different and independent longitudinal courses (Andreasen et al., 1995a, 1996, 1997; Arndt et al., 1995; Flaum et al., 1995, 1997; Gur et al., 1991; Miller et al., 1993; O'Leary et al., 2000).

In concert with this work examining the symptoms of schizophrenia, other investigators have pursued the study of relationships between cognition and brain measures. Some have argued that some form of cognitive dysfunction may ultimately provide the best definition of the phenotype of schizophrenia, and that ultimately cognitive measures may replace symptom measures in defining the phenomenology of schizophrenia (Andreasen, 1999). Again, however, a consensus has not been achieved.

Defining the Phenotype for Genetic Studies

Contemporary geneticists applying the tools of modern genetics have become very much aware of how important it is to have good definitions of complex disorders such as schizophrenia. In fact, reflecting this awareness, they are beginning to speak about a new (but actually old) field, referred to as "phenomics," the genetic underpinnings of phenomenology. The emergence of this term reflects the fact that the definition of the phenotype of illnesses like schizophrenia may be the single most important component of modern genetic studies.

Here the issues are very similar to those discussed above, involving the relationship between clinical presentation and neural mechanisms. At what level should the phenotype be defined: the symptom level? Dimension level? Diagnosis level? Cognitive level? Or should we abandon these more superficial clinical measurements and attempt to find more basic definitions, often referred to as endophenotypes (or intermediate phenotypes), "measurable components unseen by the unaided eye along the pathway between disease and distal genotype"(Gottesman & Gould, 2003)? The criteria for endophenotypes include association with the disease, presence in unaffected relatives, heritability, co-segregation with the illness within families, and state-independence.

Many investigators believe that endophenotypic definitions may provide a better index of the presence of this disorder than classic symptom-based definitions, such as those created by the DSM or ICD. While there is no strong consensus yet, some candidates that have been proposed include problems with working memory, eye tracking, or prepulse inhibition. To date most of this work has been conducted with adults. The application of this approach to defining and identifying the schizophrenia endophenotype in children and adolescents is another important future direction, as is the search for additional new candidate endophenotypes.

ETIOLOGY

Two complementary approaches have emerged as providing much-needed insight into the causes and underlying substrates of schizophrenia: neurobiology and genetics. Current efforts in neurobiology are to integrate data from behavioral measurements with the increasingly informative data from work with neuroimaging and electrophysiology. Neurobiological studies were stimulated by the well-documented neurobehavioral deficits that are present in schizophrenia. Some of the impairments are evident at the premorbid phase of illness and progress in adolescence, with onset of symptoms. These have become targets for therapeutic interventions. The application of structural and functional neuroimaging has enabled researchers to obtain in vivo measures and highlight the brain circuitry affected in schizophrenia. Progress in genetics has moved the field from earlier efforts relying on family studies of the phenotype to molecular studies that probe the underlying biology. In this section, we will review neurobehavioral measures, proceed to describe studies of brain structure and function, review the impact of hormones critical during adolescence, describe the implicated brain circuitry, and conclude by presenting the genetics of schizophrenia.

Neurobehavioral Deficits

Cognitive deficits have been recognized since early descriptions of schizophrenia, when it was called "dementia praecox." More recent evidence confirms that cognitive deficits are evident in vulnerable individuals, are present at the onset of illness, and predict outcome (Barch & Ceaser, 2012; Gur & Gur, 2013; Kahn & Keefe, 2013). Furthermore, as summarized in the sections on treatment and prevention, early detection and efforts at intervention may hold a key for ameliorating the ravages of schizophrenia later in life. Here we will describe evidence for deficits in neuromotor and neurocognitive functioning, with special emphasis on early presentation.

Neuromotor Functions

Prior to the advent of antipsychotic medications, there were reports in the scientific literature of elevated rates of movement abnormalities in patients with schizophrenia (Huston & Shakow, 1946; Walker, 1994; Yarden & Discipio, 1971). After the use of antipsychotics became widespread, attention shifted to drug-induced abnormalities in motor behavior. Because these drug-induced movement abnormalities were of such great concern, they temporarily eclipsed research on naturally occurring motor dysfunction in schizophrenia. Nonetheless, there is an extensive body of research on motor functions in adults with schizophrenia, both medicated and nonmedicated, and these studies have revealed deficits in a wide range of motor measures, from simple finger tapping to the execution of complex manual tasks (Manschreck et al., 1982; Walker, 1994; Wolff & O'Driscoll, 1999). In addition, when compared to healthy comparison subjects, schizophrenia patients manifest more involuntary movements and postural abnormalities.

Research has shown that motor deficits predate the onset of schizophrenia, and for some patients are present early in life. Infants who later develop schizophrenia show delays and abnormalities in motor development (Fish, Marcus, Hans, & Auerbach, 1993; Walker, Savoie & Davis, 1994). They are slower to acquire coordinated patterns of crawling, walking, and bimanual manipulation. They also manifest asymmetries and abnormalities in their movements, such as abnormal postures and involuntary movements of the hands and arms. It is important to note, however, that these early motor signs are not specific to schizophrenia; delays and anomalies in motor development are present in children who later manifest a variety of disorders, as well as some who show no subsequent disorder. Thus, motor signs are not diagnostic, but the presence of motor deficits in infants who subsequently manifest schizophrenia suggests that the congenital vulnerability to the disorder can involve brain systems that play a role in movement.

Deficits in motor function have also been detected throughout the premorbid period, including adolescence (Dickson et al., 2012). Retrospective studies of the school and medical records of individuals diagnosed with schizophrenia in late adolescence or early adulthood reveal an elevated rate of motor problems, such as deficits in coordination (Cannon et al., 1999a). Similarly, prospective research has shown that youth who later develop schizophrenia score below normal controls on standardized tests of motor proficiency (Marcus et al., 1993; Niemi et al., 2003; Schreiber et al., 1992). Motor abnormalities have also been detected in adolescents who manifest CHR syndromes, including schizotypal personality disorder. Compared to healthy adolescents, CHR youth show more involuntary movements and coordination problems (Nagy & Szatmari, 1986; Walker et al., 1999). Longitudinal research has compared CHR individuals who develop psychosis to those who do not, and the results indicate that CHR adolescents with motor abnormalities are more likely to show worsening of symptoms and to transition to a psychotic level of symptom severity (Mittal & Walker, 2007; Mittal et al., 2008).

Because the neural circuitry subserving motor functions is well documented, motor behaviors are particularly informative with respect to the neuropathophysiology of schizophrenia (Walker, 1994). In clinical practice, neurologists are often able to identify the locus of brain lesions based on the nature of motor impairments. To date, the motor signs observed in schizophrenia have generally been too subtle and nonspecific to suggest a lesion in a particular brain structure. Nonetheless, there is growing evidence that motor dysfunction may offer some clues about the nature of the brain dysfunction associated with the disorder.

The nature of the motor deficits observed in schizophrenia and CHR adolescents suggests abnormalities in subcortical brain areas, in particular a brain region referred to as the striatum (comprising the caudate nucleus and putamen) (Walker, 1994). This brain region is a part of the neural circuitry that connects subcortical with higher cortical areas of the brain. The dorsal striatum is the larger area of the caudate and putamen and is often referred to as the *nigrostriatal pathway*. The dorsal striatum primarily receives dopamine input from the substantia nigra and is known to play an important role in motor functions because it has projections leading to the premotor, supplementary, and primary motor cortices. In addition, it has projections to areas of the cortex that are involved in higher-level cognitive functions such as the dorsolateral prefrontal, somatosensory, and parietal association cortices. As described below, the cognitive functions governed by these brain regions are also impaired in schizophrenia.

Several lines of investigation, extending from the 1970s, have implicated elevated dopamine activity in the dorsal striatum in schizophrenia patients (Kuepper, Skinbjerg, & Abi-Dargham, 2012). More recently, investigators have reported elevated dopamine synthesis in the dorsal striatum of CHR youth compared with healthy controls, and this was most pronounced in CHR youth who transitioned to psychosis (Bauer et al., 2012; Egerton et al., 2013; Howes et al., 2011). Another neuroimaging study showed that a higher synaptic dopamine concentration, measured globally in the striatum, was associated with more severe positive symptoms in CHR patients and a greater reduction of these symptoms following dopamine depletion (Bloemen et al., 2013). Finally, providing a link between environmental factors and dopamine activity, both CHR individuals and schizophrenia patients were found to show greater stress-induced dopamine release in dorsal regions of the striatum, including the associative striatum (i.e., the predorsal putamen, predorsal and postdorsal caudate) and the sensorimotor striatum (i.e., postdorsal putamen) when compared to healthy participants (Mizrahi et al., 2012). In contrast, there was no group difference in dopamine in the ventral striatum. This emerging evidence of more pronounced dopamine activity in the dorsal striatum of CHR and psychotic patients is consistent with the findings of motor abnormalities in CHR youth.

As our understanding of brain function and motor circuitry expands, we will have greater opportunities for identifying the origins and significance of motor dysfunction in schizophrenia. Some of the important questions that remain to be answered are as follows:

Is the presence of motor dysfunction in schizophrenia linked with a particular pattern of neurochemical or brain abnormalities?

When combined with ratings of CHR symptoms, can the presence of motor abnormalities aid in predicting which individuals with prodromal syndromes will develop schizophrenia?

Would neuromotor assessment aid in the prediction of treatment response?

Neurocognition

Early studies examining cognitive function in schizophrenia focused on single domains, such as attention or memory, and preceded developments in neuroimaging and cognitive neuroscience that afford better linkage between cognitive aberrations and brain circuitry. Neuropsychological batteries, which have been initially developed and applied in neurological populations, attempt to link behavioral deficits to brain function. When applied in schizophrenia, such batteries have consistently indicated diffuse dysfunction, with relatively greater impairment in executive functions and in learning and memory (Bilder et al., 2000; Censits et al., 1997; Elvevag & Goldberg, 2000; Green, 1996; Gur et al., 2001; Saykin et al., 1994).

It is noteworthy that the pattern of deficits is already observed at first presentation and is not significantly changed by treatment of the clinical symptoms. Therefore, studying adolescents at risk or at onset of illness avoids confounding by effects of treatment, hospitalization, and social isolation that may contribute to compromised function. While the literature evaluating the specificity of cognitive deficits in schizophrenia is limited, the profile and severity are different from bipolar disorder. Thus, early evaluation during adolescence may have diagnostic and treatment implications. Given the evidence on cognitive deficits at the premorbid stage it would be important to evaluate whether a pattern of deficits in adolescents at risk can predict the onset and course of illness. The executive functions impaired in adults with schizophrenia are the very abilities that are essential for an adolescent to make the transition to young adulthood, where navigation through an increasing complexity of alternatives becomes the issue.

In addition to the cognitive impairment, emotion-processing deficits in identification, discrimination, and recognition of facial expressions have been observed in schizophrenia (Kohler et al., 2003; Kring et al., 2003). Such deficits may contribute to the poor social adjustment already salient before the disease onset. Emotional impairment in schizophrenia is clinically well established, manifesting in flat, blunted, inappropriate affect and in depression. These affect-related symptoms are notable in adolescents during the prodromal phase of illness preceding the positive symptoms. While these may represent a component of the generalized cognitive impairment, they relate to symptoms and neurobiological measures that deserve further research.

Several brain systems are implicated by these deficits. The attention-processing circuitry includes brainstem-thalamo-striato-accumbens-temporal-hippocampal-prefrontal-parietal regions. Deficits in working memory implicate the dorsolateral prefrontal cortex, and the ventromedial temporal lobe is implicated by deficits in episodic memory. A dorsolateral-medial-orbital prefrontal cortical circuit mediates executive functions. Animal and human investigations have implicated the limbic system, primarily the amygdala, hypothalamus, mesocorticolimbic dopaminergic systems, and cortical regions including orbitofrontal, dorsolateral prefrontal, temporal, and parts of parietal cortex. These are obviously complex systems, and impairment in one may interact with dysfunction in others. Studies with large samples are needed to test models of underlying pathophysiology.

The link between neurobehavioral deficits and brain dysfunction can be examined both by correlating individual differences in performance with measures of brain anatomy, and through the application of neurobehavioral probes in functional imaging studies. With these paradigms, we can investigate the topography of brain activity in response to engagement in tasks where deficits have been noted in patients. Thus, there is "online" correlation between brain activity and performance in a way that permits direct examination of brain–behavior relations (Gur et al., 1997; Gur & Gur, 2010).

Neuroanatomic Studies

The availability of methods for quantitative structural neuroimaging has permitted examination of neuroanatomic abnormalities in schizophrenia. Because the onset of schizophrenia takes place during a phase of neurodevelopment characterized by dynamic and extensive changes in brain anatomy, establishing the growth chart is necessary to interpret findings. Two complementary lines of investigation have proved helpful. Examining the neuroanatomic differences between healthy people and individuals with childhood-onset and first-episode schizophrenia, as well as individuals at risk, permits identification of regional abnormalities early in the course of illness. Complementary efforts are needed to examine changes associated with illness progression. Understanding the neuroanatomic changes in the context of the dynamic transitions of the developing brain during adolescence, however, requires careful longitudinal studies during this critical period. A brief introduction to the methodology of quantitative MRI and its application to examine neurodevelopment is needed to appreciate findings in schizophrenia.

Several approaches developed in the early 1990s have now become standard and have been shown to produce reliable results (e.g., Filipek, Richelme, Kennedy, & Caviness, 1994; Kohn et al., 1991). These methods have provided data on the intracranial composition of the three main brain compartments related to cytoarchitecture and connectivity: gray matter (GM; the somatodendritic tissue of neurons [cortical and deep]), white matter (WM; the axonal compartment of myelinated connecting fibers), and cerebrospinal fluid (CSF).

In one of the first studies examining segmented MRI in children and adults, Jernigan and Tallal (1990) documented the "pruning" process proposed by Huttenlocher's (1984) work. They found that children had higher GM volumes than adults, indicating loss of GM during adolescence. This group replicated these results using advanced methods for image analysis (Sowell et al., 1999). The newer study also demonstrated that the pruning is most "aggressive" in prefrontal and temporo-parietal cortical brain regions. As a result of this work we now recognize that both myelination and pruning are important aspects of brain development.

In a landmark 1996 paper, the NIH group reported results of a brain volumetric MRI study on 104 healthy children ranging in age from 4 to 18. While they did not segment the MRI data into compartments, they observed developmental changes that clearly indicated prolonged maturation beyond age 17. In a later report on this sample, where segmentation algorithms were applied, they were able to pinpoint the greatest delay in myelination, defined as WM volume, for frontotemporal pathways (Paus et al., 1999). This finding is very consistent with the Yakovlev and Lecours (1967) projections. The NIH group went on to exploit the ability of MRI to obtain repeated measures on the same individuals. Using such longitudinal data they were able to better pinpoint the timing of the preadolescent increase in GM that precipitated the pruning process of adolescence. Of importance to the question of maturation as defined by myelogenesis, the results indicated that the volume of WM continued to show increases up to age 22 years (Giedd et al., 1999).

The Harvard group developed a sophisticated procedure for MRI analysis (Filipek et al., 1994), which they applied to a sample of children ranging in age from 7 to 11 years and compared to adults (Cavines et al., 1996). They found sex differences suggesting earlier maturation of females, and generally supported the role of WM as an index of maturation. Their results also indicated that WM shows a delay in reaching its peak volume until early adulthood.

Another landmark study, published by the Stanford group, examined segmented MRI on a "retrospective" sample of 88 participants ranging in age from 3 months to 30 years and a "prospective" sample of 73 healthy men aged 21 to 70 years (Pfefferbaum et al., 1994). The retrospective sample used scans available from the clinical caseload, although images were carefully selected to include only those with a negative clinical reading, while the prospective sample was recruited specifically for research and medically screened to be healthy. The results demonstrated a clear neurodevelopmental course for GM and WM, the former showing a steady decline during adolescence and the latter showing increased volume until about age 20 to 22 years.

The Hopkins group used a similar approach in a sample of 85 healthy children and adolescents ranging in age from 5 to 17 years (Reiss et al., 1996). Consistent with the postmortem and the other volumetric MRI studies, they reported a steady increase in WM volume with age that did not seem to peak by age 17. They did not have data on older individuals. Their results are consistent with those of Blatter et al. (1995) from Utah, although the extensive Utah database combined ages 16 to 25 and therefore would not permit evaluation of changes during late adolescence and early adulthood.

In an early study that examined segmented MRI volumes from a prospective sample of 28 healthy children aged 1 month to 10 years, as well as a small adult sample, Matsuzawa et al. (2001) applied the segmentation procedures developed by the Penn group. They demonstrated increased volume of both GM and WM in the first postnatal months, but whereas GM volume peaked at about 2 years of age, the volume of WM, which indicates brain maturation, continued to increase into adulthood (Fig. 5.2). Furthermore, consistent with the postmortem and other MRI studies that have examined this issue, the frontal lobe showed the greatest

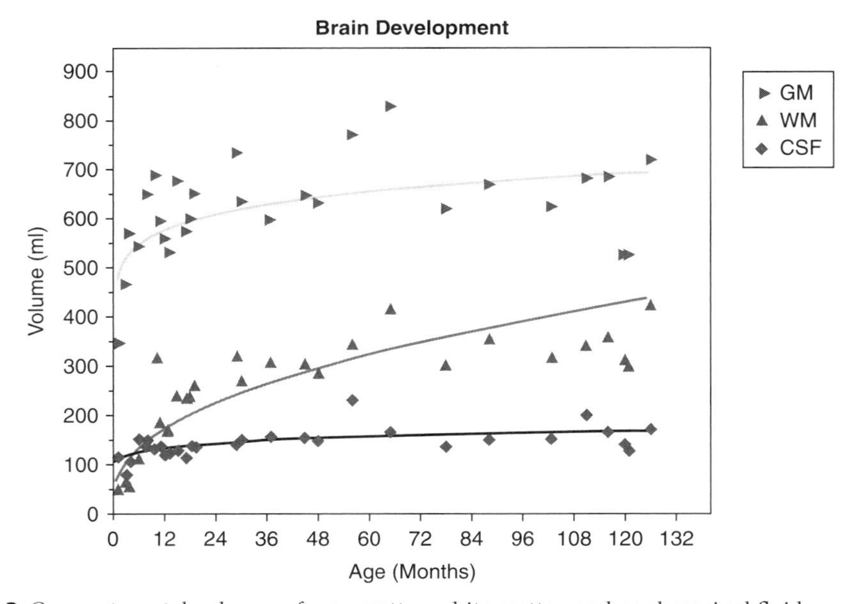

Figure 5.2 Compartmental volumes of gray matter, white matter, and cerebrospinal fluid.

maturational lag and its myelination is unlikely to be completed before young adulthood.

MRI studies in first-episode patients have indicated smaller brain volume and an increase in CSF relative to healthy people. The increase is more pronounced in ventricular than in sulcal CSF. Brain and CSF volumes have been related to phenomenological and other clinical variables such as premorbid functioning, symptom severity, and outcome. Abnormalities in these measures are likely to be more pronounced in patients with poorer premorbid functioning, more severe symptoms, and worse outcome. The concept of brain reserve or resilience may apply to schizophrenia as well, with normal brain and CSF volumes as preliminary indicators of protective capacity. As our understanding of how brain systems regulate behavior in health and disease improves, we can take advantage of neuroimaging to examine specific brain regions implicated in the pathophysiology of schizophrenia.

GM and WM tissue segmentation can help determine whether tissue loss and disorganization in schizophrenia are primarily the result of a GM deficit or whether WM abnormalities are also involved. Several studies using segmentation methods have indicated that GM volume reduction characterizes individuals with schizophrenia, while the WM volume is normal. The GM reduction is apparent in first-episode, never-treated patients and supports the growing body of work that schizophrenia is a neurodevelopmental disorder.

In evaluating specific regions, the most consistent findings are of reduced volumes of prefrontal cortex and temporal lobe structures. Other brain regions have also been noted to have reduced volumes, including the parietal lobe, thalamus, basal ganglia, cerebellar vermis, and olfactory bulbs. Relatively few studies have related sub-lobar volumes to clinical or neurocognitive measures. Available studies, however, support the hypothesis that increased volume is associated with lower severity of negative symptoms and better cognitive performance.

The question of progression of tissue loss has been addressed in relatively few studies and in small samples, reflecting the difficulty of recruiting for study patients in the early stages of illness. Longitudinal studies applying MRI have examined first-episode patients. One group of investigators found no ventricular changes in a follow-up study, conducted 1 to 2 years after the initial study, of 13 patients and eight controls. Another study evaluated 16 patients and five controls, studied 2 years after a first psychotic episode. Patients showed no consistent change in ventricular size with time, although there were individual increases or decreases. With a slightly larger group of 24 patients and six controls, no significant changes were observed in ventricular or temporal lobe volume at follow-up. Subsequently, 20 of these patients and five controls were rescanned over 4 years, and greater decreases in whole-brain volume and enlargement in left ventricular volume was observed in patients. The authors concluded that subtle cortical changes may occur after the onset of illness, suggesting progression in some cases.

In a longitudinal study with a larger sample, 40 patients (20 first-episode, 20 previously treated) and 17 healthy participants were rescanned an average of 2.5 years later. Volumes of whole brain, CSF, and frontal and temporal lobes were measured (Gur et al., 1998a). First-episode and previously treated patients had smaller whole-brain, frontal, and temporal lobe volumes than controls at intake. Longitudinally, reduction in frontal lobe volume was found only in patients, and was most pronounced at the early stages of illness, whereas temporal lobe reduction was seen also in controls. In both first-episode and previously treated patients, volume reduction was associated with decline in some neurobehavioral functions.

The question of specificity of neuroanatomic findings to schizophrenia was addressed in a study that evaluated 13 patients with first-episode schizophrenia, 15 patients with first-episode affective psychosis (mainly manic), and 14 healthy comparison subjects longitudinally, with scans separated by 1.5 years (Kasai et al., 2003). The patients with schizophrenia had progressive decreases in GM volume over time in the left superior temporal gyrus compared with both other groups. The existence of neuroanatomic abnormalities in first-episode patients indicates that brain dysfunction occurred before clinical presentation. However, the longitudinal studies suggest evidence of progression, in which anatomic changes may impact some clinical and neurobehavioral features of the illness in some patients. There is also evidence that progression is significantly greater in early-onset patients during adolescence than it is for adult subjects (Sporn et al., 2003).

MRI findings have been most consistent for GM volume reduction, but the availability of diffusion tensor imaging (DTI) has enhanced the efforts to examine compartmental abnormalities (Kubicki & Shenton, 2014; Roalf et al., 2013). To date the growing understanding of brain development and MRI data obtained from children suggest that the neuroanatomic neuroimaging literature in schizophrenia is consistent with diffuse disruption of normal maturation. Thus, there is clear evidence for structural abnormalities in schizophrenia that are associated with reduced cognitive capacity and less clearly with symptoms. With the shift to study earlier stages in the psychosis process, MRI technology has been applied to people at risk for psychosis, enabling examination of brain integrity as psychosis unfolds. Measures obtained include structural parameters such as GM and WM volumes, cortical thickness and DTI measures of structural connectivity, as well as functional parameters such as functional connectivity and activation in response to neurobehavioral tasks designed to probe a specific circuitry. The neuroimaging literature on clinical risk for psychosis is growing, although it is still relatively limited in size of samples examined and follow-up (Fusar-Poli et al., 2013a).

Electrophysiology

Electroencephalography, Event-Related Potentials, and the Place of Electrophysiology in the Neuroimaging Spectrum

The electroencephalogram (EEG) measures the electrical activity of the brain; it originates from the summated electrical potentials generated by inhibitory and excitatory inputs onto neurons. The main source of the scalp-recorded EEG is in the cortex of the brain, which contains the large and parallel dendritic trees of pyramidal neurons whose regular ordering facilitates summation. One of the important advances in EEG-based research was the development of a technique to isolate the brain activity related to specific events from the background EEG; this activity related to specific events is termed event-related potentials (ERPs). Using averaging techniques, it is possible to visualize events related to one of the many different brain operations reflected in the EEG. Typically these ERPs are related to the specific processing of certain sensory stimuli.

In recent years many new means of measuring brain structure and function have been developed, each with its advantages in study of the brain. EEG and ERP measures are unsurpassed in providing real-time, millisecond resolution of normal and pathological brain processing, literally at the speed of thought, while functional MRI and PET have temporal resolutions some thousand-fold less. Moreover, functional MRI and PET only indirectly track neural activity through its effects on blood flow or metabolism. However, the ability of EEG and ERP techniques to localize sources of activity is much less than fMRI and PET, and these methods, together with structural MRI, are needed to supplement EEG/ERP information.

Current ERP Research in Schizophrenia

Space limitations preclude discussion of all ERPs and we here provide a sample of current work designed to illuminate a fundamental question in schizophrenia research, namely how the brains of patients with this disorder differ from those of healthy subjects. ERPs provide a functional window on many aspects of brain processing. These include the most elementary, likely involving cellular circuitry (gamma band activity), early, simple signal detection and gating (P50), automatic detection of changes in the environment (MMN activity), and on to more complex activity such as conscious updating of expectations in view of unusual events (P300).

In this section we will first briefly review studies of ERP processes in adults with schizophrenia that illustrate the potential of these measures to provide clues about the cellular circuitry that may be impaired in schizophrenia. The auditory modality plays a special role because it is severely impacted in schizophrenia, as evinced in the primacy of auditory hallucinations and speech/language pathology. The data presented here support the hypothesis that schizophrenia involves abnormalities in brain processing from the most simple to the most complex level, and that the anatomic substrates of auditory processing in the neocortical temporal lobe, most carefully investigated in the superior temporal gyrus, themselves evince reduction in GM volume. Next, we summarize a series of studies of adolescents with schizophrenia where ERPs are recorded while the youngsters perform poorly on cognitive tasks that make extensive demands on processing resources. These studies use ERPs to attempt to identify the earliest stage of cognitive processing at which deficits emerge in adolescents with schizophrenia.

Gamma Band Activity and Neural Circuit Abnormalities at the Cellular Level

The first ERP we will consider is the steady-state gamma band response. Gamma band refers to a brain oscillation at and near the frequency of 40 Hertz (Hz) or 40 times per second, while "steady-state" refers to its being elicited by a stimulus of the same frequency. At the cellular level, gamma band activity is an endogenous brain oscillation thought to reflect the synchronizing of activity in several columns of cortical neurons, or between cortex and thalamus, with this synchronization facilitating communication. At the cognitive level, work in humans suggests that gamma activity reflects the convergence of multiple processing streams in cortex, giving rise to a unified percept. A simple example is a "fire truck," where form perception, motion perception, and auditory perception are melded to form this percept. Gamma activity at its simplest, however, involves basic neural circuitry composed of projection neurons, usually using excitatory amino acid neurotransmission, linked with inhibitory GABAergic interneurons. Studies of gamma activity in schizophrenia aim to determine if there is a basic circuit abnormality present, such as might arise from a deficiency in recurrent inhibition, postulated by a number of workers (see review in McCarley et al., 1996), although gamma band studies themselves cannot reveal any specific details of neural circuitry abnormality.

Kwon and colleagues (1999) began the study of gamma in schizophrenia using an exogenous input of 40-Hz auditory clicks, leading to a steady-state gamma response. The magnitude of the brain response was measured by power, the amount of EEG energy at a specific frequency, with the degree of capability of gamma driving being reflected in the power at and near 40 Hz. Schizophrenia patients had, compared with healthy controls, a markedly reduced power at 40-Hz input, although they showed normal driving at slower frequencies, indicating this was not a general reduction in power but one specific to the gamma band.

Spencer et al. (2003) took the next logical step and evaluated the gamma band response to visual stimuli in schizophrenia, determining whether high-frequency neural synchronization associated with the perception of visual Gestalts is abnormal in schizophrenia patients. Previous studies of healthy individuals reported enhancements of gamma band power (Tallon-Baudry & Bertrand, 1999) and phase locking (Rodriguez et al., 1999) when Gestalt objects are perceived. In the Spencer et al. study, individuals with schizophrenia and matched healthy people discriminated between square Gestalt stimuli and non-square stimuli. Schizophrenia patients demonstrated an absence of the early visual system gamma band response to Gestalt square stimuli. There were also abnormalities in gamma band synchrony between brain regions, with schizophrenia patients showing decreasing rather than increasing gamma band coherence between posterior visual regions and other brain regions after perceiving the visual Gestalt stimuli. These findings support the hypothesis that schizophrenia is associated with a fundamental abnormality in cellular neural circuitry evinced as a failure of gamma band synchronization, especially in the 40-Hz range.

Sensory Gating and the P50

Several ERPs have been related to the search for an electrophysiological concomitant of an early sensory gating deficit in schizophrenia. These include, for example, the startle response, where the size of a blink to an acoustic probe is measured. Schizophrenia patients appear to be unable to modify their large startle response when forewarned that a probe is coming, by contrast with controls (e.g., Braff et al., 1978).

Another ERP thought to be sensitive to an early sensory gating abnormality in schizophrenia is the P50. In the sensory gating paradigm, an auditory click is presented to a subject, eliciting a positive deflection about 50 msec after stimulus onset, the P50 component. After a brief interval (about 500 msec), a second click elicits a much smaller amplitude P50 in normal adult subjects, who are said to show normal gating: the first stimulus inhibits, or closes the gate, to neurophysiological processing of the second stimulus. Patients with schizophrenia, on the other hand, show less reduction in P50 amplitude to the second click, which is referred to as a failure in gating (Freedman et al., 1983). This gating deficit occurs in about half the first-degree relatives of a schizophrenic patient, suggesting that it may index a genetic factor in schizophrenia in the absence of overt psychotic symptoms (Waldo et al., 1991). While patients with affective disorder may show a gating deficit, the deficit does not persist after successful treatment, whereas in patients with schizophrenia the deficit occurs in both medicated and unmedicated patients and persists after symptom remission (Adler & Waldo, 1991; Freedman et al., 1983).

The gating effect is thought to take place in temporal lobe structures, possibly the medial temporal lobe (Adler et al., 1985). P50 gating is enhanced by nicotinic cholinergic mechanisms, and it is possible that smoking in patients with schizophrenia is a form of self-medication. Freedman et al. (1994) have shown that blockade of the alpha 7 nicotinic receptor, localized to hippocampal neurons, causes loss of the inhibitory gating response to auditory stimuli in an animal model. The failure of inhibitory mechanisms to gate sensory input to higher-order processing might result in "sensory flooding," which Freedman suggests may underlie many of the symptoms of schizophrenia.

Mismatch Negativity and Post-Onset Progression of Abnormalities

The mismatch negativity (MMN) is a negative ERP that occurs about 0.2 sec after infrequent sounds (deviants) are presented in the sequence of repetitive sounds (standards). Deviant sounds may differ from the standards in a simple physical characteristic such as pitch, duration, intensity, or spatial location. MMN is primarily evoked automatically (that is, without conscious attention). Its main source is thought to be in or near primary auditory cortex (Heschl gyrus) and to reflect the operations of sensory memory, a memory of past stimuli used by the auditory cortex in analysis of temporal patterns.

There is a consistent finding of a reduction in amplitude of the MMN in chronically ill schizophrenia patients that appears to be trait-like and not ameliorated by either typical (haloperidol) or atypical (clozapine) medication (Umbricht et al., 1998). A point of particular interest has been the finding that the MMN elicited by tones of different frequency (the pitch MMN) is normal in patients at the time of first hospitalization (Salisbury et al., 2001, confirmed by Umbricht et al., 2002), whereas the MMN elicited by the same stimuli is abnormal in chronic schizophrenia. This suggests that pitch MMN might be indexing a post-onset progression of brain abnormalities. Indeed, the prospective longitudinal study by Salisbury et al. now has preliminary data showing that schizophrenia subjects without an MMN abnormality at first hospitalization develop an abnormality over the next 1.5 years.

In the same group of patients, the Heschl gyrus, the likely source of the MMN, demonstrates a progressive reduction in GM volume over the same time period (Kasai et al., 2003).

In participants with both MRI and MMN procedures, the degree of GM volume reduction was found to parallel the degree of MMN reduction, although the number of subjects examined is currently relatively small and this conclusion is tentative. While the presence of post-onset progression of abnormalities is controversial in the field, it is of obvious importance to our understanding of the disorder and particularly important in adolescents with onset of schizophrenia, since it would prompt a search for possible medication and/or psychosocial treatment that might ameliorate progression.

Multimodal imaging (Wible et al., 2001) has demonstrated the presence of a deficiency of functional MRI activation (BOLD) in schizophrenia to the mismatch stimulus within the Heschl gyrus and nearby posterior superior temporal gyrus. Because MMN may reflect, in part, NMDA-mediated activity, a speculation about the reason for progression is that NMDA-mediated excitotoxicity might cause both a reduction in the neuropil (dendritic regression) and a concomitant reduction in the MMN in the months following first hospitalization. Only further work will tell if this speculation is valid. Of note, the MMN abnormalities present in schizophrenic psychosis are not present in manic psychosis.

P300 and the Failure to Process Unusual Events

The P300 is an ERP that occurs when a low-probability event is detected and consciously processed. Typically, subjects are asked to count a low-probability tone that is interspersed with a more frequently occurring stimulus. The P300 differs from the typical MMN paradigm in that the stimuli are presented at a slower rate (typically around 1 per second) and the subject is actively and consciously attending and processing the stimuli, whereas the MMN stimuli are not consciously processed. P300 is larger when the stimulus is rare. Whereas MMN is thought to reflect sensory memory, by definition preconscious, P300 is thought to reflect an updating of the conscious information-processing stream and of expectancy.

Reduction of the P300 amplitude at midline sites is the most frequently replicated abnormality in schizophrenia, although P300 reduction is also found in some other disorders. This widespread P300 reduction also appears to be trait-like and an enduring feature of the disease. For example, Ford et al. (1994) demonstrated that although P300 showed moderate amplitude increases with symptom resolution, it did not approach normal values during these periods of remission. Umbricht et al. (1998) reported that treatment with an atypical antipsychotic led to a significant increase of P300 amplitudes in patients with schizophrenia.

In addition to the midline P300 reduction, both chronically ill and first-episode schizophrenic subjects display an asymmetry in P300, with smaller voltage over the left temporal lobe versus right. The more pronounced this left temporal P300 amplitude abnormality, the more pronounced is the extent of psychopathology, as reflected in thought disorder and paranoid delusions (e.g., McCarley et al., 1993, 2002). It is possible the increased delusions reflect a failure of veridical updating of cognitive schemata. This left temporal deficit is not found in affective (manic) psychosis.

There are likely several bilateral brain generators responsible for the P300, with a generator in the superior temporal gyrus likely underlying the left temporal deficit, since, in schizophrenia, the greater the reduction in GM volume in the posterior superior temporal gyrus, the greater the reduction in P300 amplitude at left temporal sites in both chronic and first-episode schizophrenia patients. It is of note that the posterior superior temporal gyrus, on the left in right-handed individuals, is an area intimately related to language processing and thinking (it includes part of Wernicke's area), and an area where volume reductions are associated with increased thought disorder and severity of auditory hallucinations.

ERP Measures in Children and Adolescents with Schizophrenia

Event-Related Indices of Information-Processing Deficits

Brain activity reflected in ERPs recorded during performance of information-processing tasks can be used to help isolate the component or stage of information processing that is impaired in schizophrenia. A series of ERP studies of children and adolescents with schizophrenia conducted by the UCLA Childhood Onset Schizophrenia program are summarized below (see Strandburg et al., 1994a, and Asarnow, Brown & Strandburg, 1995, for reviews). These studies examined ERP components while children and adolescents with schizophrenia performed tasks like the span of apprehension (Span; Strandburg et al., 1984) and a continuous performance test (CPT; Strandburg et al., 1990). Several decades of studying mental chronometry using ERPs has produced a lexicon of ERP components with well-established neurocognitive correlates (Hillyard & Kutas, 1983). These ERP components can be used to help identify the stages of information processing that are impaired in schizophrenia.

The UCLA ERP studies have focused primarily on four components: contingent negative variation (CNV), hemispheric asymmetry in the amplitude of the P1/N1 component complex, processing negativity (Np), and a late positive component (P300). The CNV measures orienting, preparation, and readiness to respond to an expected stimulus. There are at least two separate generators of the CNV: an early frontal component believed to be an orienting response to warning stimuli, and a later central component associated with preparedness for stimuli processing and response (Rohrbaugh et al., 1986).

Healthy individuals typically have larger visual P1/N1 components over the right cerebral hemisphere. Many of the UCLA studies compared hemispheric laterality between healthy and schizophrenic individuals. Differences in lateralization during visual information-processing tasks could reflect either differences in the strategic utilization of processing capacity of the hemispheres or a lateralized neural deficit.

The Np is a family of negative components that occur within the first 400 msec after the onset of a stimulus, indicating the degree to which attentional and perceptual resources have been allocated to stimulus processing. Because the Np waves occur contemporaneously with other components (P1, N1, and P2), they are best seen in difference potentials resulting from the subtraction of non-attend ERPs from attend ERPs (Hillyard & Hansen, 1986; Naatanan, 1982). Finally, as described above, the P300 is a frequently studied index of the recognition of stimulus significance in relation to task demands.

ERP Results in Child and Adolescent Schizophrenia

Table 5.1 summarizes by component the ERP results from six UCLA studies of children or adults with schizophrenia. In all the studies summarized in this table, there were large and robust performance differences between groups in both the accuracy and reaction times of signal detection responses. Thus, the behavioral paradigms were successful in eliciting information-processing deficits in these patients.

CNV differences between normal subjects and schizophrenics were not consistently found across studies. In the Span task (which includes a warning interval) all possible results have been obtained (normals > schizophrenics; normals = schizophrenics; and normals < schizophrenics). For the CNV-like negative wave occurring in the CPT task, no group differences were found in either experiment. Because the warning interval was short and the wave was largest frontally, the CNVs in both tasks were most likely the early wave related to orienting. Thus, differences in prestimulus orienting do not seem to reliably account for the poor performance of schizophrenics on these tasks. There are mixed results in CNV experiments on adults with schizophrenia, although most studies found smaller CNVs in schizophrenics (Pritchard, 1986). A longer warning interval than used in the UCLA experiments (500 msec in the Span and 1,250 msec interstimulus interval [ISI] in the CNV) may be required to detect preparatory abnormalities in schizophrenia.

In every study summarized in Table 5.1 where processing negativities were measured, Np's have been found to be smaller in schizophrenics. This deficit has been seen in both

Table 5.1 Information-Processing Tasks in Child/Adolescent- and Adult-Onset Schizophrenia: Summary of Evoked Potential Studies

Paper[a]	*Task*	*Group Tested*	*CNV*	*P1/N1*	*Np*	*P300*
Asymmetry						
1984	Span	Schizophrenic children	Norm > schiz	Norm > schiz	Norm > schiz[b]	Norm > schiz
1990	CPT	Schizophrenic children	Norm = schiz	Norm > schiz	—	Norm > schiz
1991	Span	Schizophrenic children	Norm = schiz	Norm > schiz	Norm > schiz	—
1994a	Span	Schizophrenic adults	Schiz > norm	Norm > schiz	Norm > schiz	Norm > schiz
1994b	CPT	Schizophrenic children	Norm = schiz	Norm > schiz	Norm > schiz	Norm > schiz[c]
1997	Idiom	Schizophrenic adults	Norm > schiz	—	—	Norm > schiz

[a] Authors of all papers are Strandburg et al.
[b] Larger task-difficulty increase in N1 amplitude in normals than schizophrenics
[c] Normals had larger P300 than schizophrenics for targets in the single-target CPT.
CPT = continuous performance task; CNV = contingent negative variation; Np = processing negativity; P300 = late positive component

children and adults, with both the Span and CPT (Strandburg et al., 1994c) tasks. In contrast, a group of children with ADHD studied while they performed a CPT task showed no evidence of a smaller Np. Diminished Np amplitude is the earliest consistent ERP index of schizophrenia-related information-processing deficit in the UCLA studies. These results suggest impaired allocation of attentional and perceptual resources.

Most studies of processing negativities during channel selective attention tasks (Nd) find that adults with schizophrenia produce less attentional-related endogenous negative activity than do normal controls (see reviews by Cohen, 1990, and Pritchard, 1986). The UCLA results complement this finding in adults by using a discriminative processing task and extend these findings to childhood/adolescent-onset schizophrenia. Reductions in the amplitude of processing negativity in schizophrenia result from impairments in executive functions responsible for the maintenance of an attentional trace (Baribeau-Braun et al., 1983). Baribeau-Braun and colleagues (1983) observed normal Nd activity with rapid stimulus presentation rates but reduced amplitudes with slower rates, suggesting that the neural substrates of Nd are intact but improperly regulated in schizophrenia. Individuals with frontal lobe lesions resemble individuals with schizophrenia in this regard: both groups do not show increased processing negativity to attended stimuli in auditory selection tasks (Knight et al., 1981).

As noted earlier, reduced-amplitude P300 in schizophrenic adults has been consistently found using a wide variety of experimental paradigms (Pritchard, 1986). As can be seen in Table 5.1, the UCLA studies also consistently observed a smaller P300 amplitude in studies of both schizophrenic children and adults in the Span, CPT, and idiom recognition tasks. P300 latency was also measured in two of these studies. Although prolonged P300 latency was found in one study (Strandburg et al., 1994c), no differences were found in another (Strandburg et al., 1994b). The majority of ERP studies have reported normal P300 latency in schizophrenics (Pritchard, 1986).

Absence of right-lateralized P1/N1 amplitude in visual ERPs was a consistent finding in all five of the UCLA studies that used the CPT and Span tasks. Abnormal lateralization of electrophysiological responses, related either to lateralized dysfunction in schizophrenia or a pathology-related difference in information-processing strategy, is a consistent aspect of both adult- and childhood-onset schizophrenia. These results are consistent with abnormal patterns of hemispheric laterality in schizophrenics (e.g., Tucker & Williamson, 1984).

In summary, ERP studies of schizophrenia adults and children performing discriminative processing tasks suggest that the earliest reliable electrophysiological correlate of impaired discriminative processing in schizophrenia is the Np component. It appears that children and adolescents with schizophrenia are deficient in the allocation of attentional resources necessary for efficient and accurate discriminative processing. Although diminished-amplitude processing negativities have been observed in ADHD in auditory paradigms (Loiselle et al., 1980; Satterfield et al., 1990), Np was found to be normal in ADHD children during the UCLA CPT task (Strandburg et al., 1994a). Diminished Np visual processing may be specific to schizophrenic pathology. Later ERP abnormalities in schizophrenia (e.g., diminished-amplitude P300) may be a "downstream" product of the uncertainty in stimulus recognition created by previous discriminative difficulties, or may be additional neurocognitive deficits. Abnormalities in later ERP components are not specific to schizophrenia, having been reported in studies of ADHD children (reviewed by Klorman, 1991).

The absence of P1/N1 asymmetry in the visual ERPs of schizophrenics is contemporaneous with diminished Np. However, the fact that Np amplitude varies with the processing demands of the task, whereas P1/N1 asymmetry does not, suggests that the Np deficit plays a greater role in the information-processing deficits manifested by children and adolescents with schizophrenia.

Magnetoencephalography: A Complement to EEG

Magnetoencephalography (MEG) is the measure of magnetic fields generated by the brain. A key difference in the physical source of the MEG as contrasted to the EEG is that the MEG is sensitive to cells that lie tangential to the brain surface and consequently have magnetic fields oriented tangentially. Cells with a radial orientation (perpendicular to the brain surface) do not generate signals detectable with MEG. The EEG and MEG are complementary in that the EEG is most sensitive to radially oriented neurons and fields. This distinction arises, of course, because magnetic fields are generated at right angles to electrical fields. One major advantage magnetic fields have over electrical potentials is that, once generated, they are relatively invulnerable to intervening variations in the media they traverse (i.e., the skull, GM, WM, and CSF), unlike electrical fields, which are "smeared" by different electrical conductivities. This has made MEG a favorite for use in source localization, where attention has been especially focused on early potentials.

Perhaps because of the expense and nonmobility of the recording equipment needed for MEG, there has been relatively little work using MEG in schizophrenia to replicate and extend the findings of ERPs. A search of Medline in 2000 revealed only 23 published studies using MEG measures of brain activity in schizophrenia. The extant studies have shown interesting results. Reite et al. (1999) demonstrated that the M100 component (the magnetic analog to the N100) showed less interhemispheric asymmetry in male schizophrenics and had different source orientations in the left hemisphere. The review by Reite et al. (1999) should be consulted for more details of the work on MEG in schizophrenia.

In summary, electrophysiology has the advantage of providing real-time information on brain processing, with a resolution in the millisecond range. In schizophrenia, it shows abnormalities of processing from the very earliest stages (Np, MMN, P50, gamma activity) to later stages of attentive discrepancy processing (P300) and semantic processing (N400). This suggests a model of disturbance that encompasses a wide variety of processing and is most compatible with a brain model of circuit abnormalities underlying processing at each stage, particularly in the auditory modality. This is also compatible with MRI studies of abnormal GM regions associated with abnormal ERPs.

One of the more intriguing potential applications to schizophrenia in adolescence is using ERPs to track the progression of brain abnormalities. The MMN ERP is normal at the onset (first hospitalization) of schizophrenia but becomes abnormal in the course of the disorder (this developing abnormality is associated with a loss of GM in auditory cortex). The MMN is thus potentially of use in tracking the ability of therapeutic interventions to minimize brain changes. Likewise, gamma abnormalities are evident early in the course of schizophrenia as well as in CHR individuals (Tada et al., 2016).

Neuroendocrinology

The postpubescent period has received increasing attention from researchers in the field of schizophrenia (Stevens, 2002; Trotman et al., 2013). This interest stems largely from the fact that adolescence is associated with a significant rise in the risk for psychotic symptoms, particularly prodromal signs of schizophrenia (Addington & Heinssen, 2012; Walker, 2002). Further, rates of other psychiatric syndromes, including mood and anxiety disorders, escalate during adolescence. It has been suggested that hormonal changes may play an important role in this developmental phenomena, making adolescence a critical period for the emergence of mental illness (Walker, 2002).

Puberty is associated with increased activation of the hypothalamic–pituitary–gonadal axis and a rise in secretion of sex hormones (e.g., estrogen and testosterone) by the gonads in response to gonadotropin secretion from the anterior pituitary. There is also an augmentation of activity in the hypothalamic–pituitary–adrenal (HPA) axis during adolescence. This neural system governs the release of several hormones and is activated in response to stress. Cortisol is among the hormones secreted by the HPA axis, and researchers can measure it in body fluids to index the biological response to stress. Beginning around age 12, there is an age-related increase in baseline cortisol levels in normal children. The change from prepubertal to postpubertal status is linked with a marked rise in cortisol (Walker, Mittal, & Tessner, 2008).

The significance of postpubertal hormonal changes has been brought into clearer focus as researchers have elucidated the role of steroid hormones in neuronal activity and morphology (Peper et al., 2011; Strelzyk et al., 2012). Neurons contain receptors for adrenal and gonadal hormones. When activated, these receptors modify cellular function and impact neurotransmitter function. Short-term effects of steroid hormones on cellular function are believed to be mediated by membrane receptors. Longer-term effects can result from the activation of intraneuronal or nuclear receptors. These receptors can influence gene expression. Brain changes that occur during normal adolescence may be regulated by hormonal effects on the expression of genes that govern brain maturation.

Both gonadal and adrenal hormone levels are linked with behavior in adolescents. In general, levels outside the normal range, both elevated and reduced, are associated with greater adjustment problems (Berenbaum & Beltz, 2011). For example, children with an earlier onset of puberty have significantly higher concentrations of adrenal androgens, estradiol, and cortisol, and they also manifest more psychological disorders, self-reported depression, and parent-reported behavior problems (Lee & Styne, 2013).

Although there has been only limited research on gonadal hormones and schizophrenia, a comprehensive review of the literature by Markham (2012) concluded that both estrogen and testosterone may be linked with psychosis risk. With respect to estrogen:

1. Women with schizophrenia manifest reduced estrogen levels compared to healthy same-sex controls.
2. Peak bone mass, an indicator of cumulative estrogen exposure, is significantly lower in women with first-episode schizophrenia than in matched controls.

3. Risk for psychosis is higher during periods of low estrogen.
4. There is evidence that adjunctive estradiol may reduce symptom severity in women with psychotic disorders.

These findings are consistent with the notion that estrogen has antidopaminergic and neuroprotective effects, thus contributing to the later onset and milder course in females than males (Arad & Weiner, 2009).

In contrast, the preponderance of studies find lower testosterone levels in men with schizophrenia, especially those with negative symptoms. Lower testosterone levels were also reported in a study of CHR male adolescents, suggesting that lower levels may precede illness onset (van Rijn et al., 2011).

The role of the HPA axis in schizophrenia has received greater attention. In part, this is because a large body of research literature suggests a link between exposure to psychosocial stress and symptom relapse and exacerbation in schizophrenia (Holtzman et al., 2013; Walker, Mittal, & Tessner, 2008). It has been suggested that activation of the HPA axis mediates this effect. Dysregulation of the HPA axis, including elevated baseline cortisol and cortisol response to pharmacological challenge, is often found in schizophrenia patients, especially prior to treatment with antipsychotics (Walker, Mittal, & Tessner, 2008).

Basic research has demonstrated that cortisol affects the activity of several neurotransmitter systems and has an augmenting effect on dopamine activity (Niwa et al., 2013; Shansky & Lipps, 2013). Thus, it has been suggested that, when individuals are exposed to stress, and elevations in cortisol ensue, dopamine activity increases and psychotic symptoms are triggered or exacerbated.

Although we are aware of no published reports on cortisol secretion in adolescents diagnosed with schizophrenia, elevated cortisol levels have been observed in CHR adolescents (Weinstein et al., 1999). When compared to healthy adolescents, CHR youth show elevated baseline levels of cortisol (Weinstein et al., 1999) and a more pronounced developmental increase in cortisol when measured over a 2-year period (Walker, Walder, & Reynolds, 2001). A study of 56 CHR youth (ages 12–18) found that those who go on to develop a psychotic disorder showed significantly higher cortisol levels (Walker et al., 2010). Thus, when compared with the CHR subjects who did not develop a psychotic disorder within the 4-year period, the 14 later diagnosed with psychosis manifested higher cortisol levels over the first year following baseline. As in previous studies of adolescent HPA activity, an age-related increase in cortisol secretion was also observed, suggesting that the developmental period of heightened risk for prodromal symptom onset may also be characterized by greater stress sensitivity. Using similar methods, a recent investigation of baseline cortisol levels from the ongoing NAPLS project reported significantly higher salivary cortisol levels in CHR subjects (n = 260) than healthy controls matched on age and sex (Walker et al., 2013). Cortisol levels were also predictive of progression in CHR youth, with those who subsequently developed psychosis manifesting higher baseline cortisol than CHR youth whose clinical symptoms remitted. This suggests that increased activation of the HPA axis may contribute to the worsening of symptoms as the child progresses through adolescence.

Research on the role of neurohormones in schizophrenia, especially the gonadal and adrenal hormones, should be given high priority in the future. In particular, it will be important to study hormonal processes in youth at risk for schizophrenia. There are several key questions to be addressed in clinical research:

- Are hormonal changes linked with the emergence of the prodromal phases of schizophrenia?
- Is there a relationship between hormonal factors and the brain changes that have been observed in the prodromal phase of schizophrenia?
- If so, are changes in gene expression mediating this effect?

The answers to these questions may shed light on mechanisms underlying the emergence of psychosis.

BRAIN CIRCUITRY IN SCHIZOPHRENIA

Information processing in the brain is a complex task, and even simple sensory information, such as recognizing a sight or a sound, engages circuits of cells in multiple regions of the brain. Scientists early in the 20th century imagined that brain function occurred in discrete steps along a linear stream of information flow. However, the recent emergence of brain imaging as an important tool for understanding the neuroscience of cognition and emotion has demonstrated that the brain operates more like a parallel processing computer, with feed-forward and feedback circuitry that manages information in distributed and overlapping processing modules working in parallel. Thus, abnormal function in one brain region will have functional ripple effects in other regions, and abnormal sharing of information between regions, perhaps because of problems in the connectional wiring, can result in abnormal behavior even if individual modules are functionally intact.

In light of the elaborate and complex symptoms of schizophrenia, it is not surprising that researchers have increasingly focused on evidence of malfunction within distributed brain circuits rather than within a particular single brain region or module. Most of this work has been based on in vivo physiological techniques, such as imaging and electrophysiology. At the same time, basic research in animals and to a lesser extent in humans has shown that the elaboration of brain circuitry is a lifelong process, especially the connection between cells in circuits within and between different regions of the cortex. This process of development and modification of connections between neurons is particularly dynamic during adolescence and early adult life. In this section, we will review some of the recent evidence that local and distributed abnormalities of brain circuitry are associated with schizophrenia and their implications for adolescent psychosis.

Intracortical Circuits

Among the most often cited areas of the brain said to be abnormal in schizophrenia are the cortices of the frontal temporal and parietal lobes. Indeed, damage to these regions caused by trauma, stroke, or neurological disease is more likely to be associated with psychosis than is damage to other brain regions. Studies using neuroimaging techniques have suggested that malfunction at the systems level—that is, the relationship of processing in the frontotemporal and frontoparietal circuits combined—best characterizes the problem in patients with schizophrenia (Kyriakopoulos & Frangou, 2009). For example, in a study of identical twins discordant for schizophrenia, differences within each twin pair in volume of the hippocampus predicted very strongly the difference in the function of the prefrontal cortex assayed physiologically during a cognitive task dependent on the function of the prefrontal cortex (Weinberger et al., 1992).

A peculiar disturbance in the use of language, so-called thought disorder, is one of the cardinal signs of schizophrenia. Language is highly dependent on frontotemporal circuitry, which is disturbed in schizophrenia. When patients are asked to generate a list of words beginning with a specific consonant, instead of activating the frontal lobes and deactivating the temporal lobes as seen in healthy subjects, they do the opposite. More detailed analyses have examined declarative memory encoding, storage, and retrieval as related to language. Encoding is manipulated by instructing subjects to process material more deeply, as for example to make semantic judgments about to-be-remembered words, such as whether the words represent living or nonliving, or abstract or concrete words. This deeper, more elaborate encoding is compared with a shallower, more superficial level of encoding, such as having subjects judge the font (uppercase vs. lowercase) of each word presented. Compared with healthy controls, patients with schizophrenia show different patterns of functional MRI activation for semantically encoded words, showing significantly reduced left inferior frontal cortex activation but significantly increased left superior temporal cortex activation (Kubicki et al., 2003).

During tests of word retrieval, patients with schizophrenia tend to show reduced engagement of the hippocampus, but at the same time their prefrontal cortex is overactive (Heckers et al., 1998). On the other hand, during performance of effortful tasks, people with schizophrenia show increased activity in hippocampus and an alteration in the connection between hippocampus and anterior cingulate cortex (Holcomb et al., 2000; Medoff et al., 2001). These studies suggest that the information-processing strategy for encoding and retrieving learned information, which depends on an orchestrated duet between frontotemporal brain regions, is disturbed in patients with schizophrenia.

Similar results have been found in studies focused on prefrontal mediated memory, so-called working memory, in which the normal relationships between prefrontal activation and hippocampal deactivation are disrupted in schizophrenia (Callicott et al., 2000). Finally, statistical approaches to interpreting functional imaging results based on patterns of intercorrelated activity across the whole brain have demonstrated that abnormalities in schizophrenia are distributed across cortical regions. In particular, the pattern based on the normal relationships between prefrontal and temporal cortical activity is especially abnormal (Gur & Gur, 2010). This apparent functional abnormality in intracortical connectedness has been supported by anatomic evidence from DTI, which has pointed to an abnormality in the WM links between frontal and temporal lobes (e.g., Fitzsimmons et al., 2013).

The evidence for abnormal function across distributed cortical circuitry is quite compelling in schizophrenia, and other regions representing other circuits are also implicated (Tamminga et al., 2002; Weinberger et al., 2001). Indeed, it is not clear that any particular area of cortex is normal under all conditions. This may reflect simply the interconnectedness of the brain or it may suggest that schizophrenia is especially characterized by a "dysconnectivity." It is impossible at the current level of our understanding of the disease to differentiate between these possibilities.

Schizophrenia disrupts not only circuitry linking brain regions but also the microcircuitry within brain regions, as shown by abnormal electrophysiological activity during simple, early-stage "automatic processing" of stimuli, processing relatively independent of directed, conscious control. For example, healthy subjects automatically generate a robust EEG response in and near primary auditory cortex to tones differing slightly in pitch from others in a series ("mismatch" response), whereas the processing response in schizophrenia to the mismatch is much less pronounced (Wible et al., 2001).

Corticostriatal Circuitry

Neurophysiological studies have focused largely on function of the cerebral cortex, but the pharmacological treatment of schizophrenia targets principally the dopamine system, which has long implicated the striatum and related subcortical sites such as the thalamus. In fact, cortical function and activity of the subcortical dopamine system are intimately related, consistent with circuitry models of brain function. Animal studies have demonstrated conclusively that perturbations in cortical function, especially prefrontal function, disrupt a normal tonic brake on dopamine neurons in the brain stem, leading to a loss of the normal regulation of these neurons and to their excessive activation (Weinberger et al., 2001). It is thought that the prefrontal cortex helps guide the dopamine reward system toward the reinforcing of contextually appropriate stimuli. In the absence of such normal regulation, reward and motivation may be less appropriately targeted.

Neuroimaging studies of the dopamine system in patients with schizophrenia, particularly those who are actively psychotic, have found evidence of increased presynaptic dopamine synthesis capacity in the striatum (Fusar-Poli et al., 2012a). This apparent overactivation of the subcortical dopamine system may be related to abnormal prefrontal cortical function (Bertolino et al., 2000; Meyer-Lindenberg et al., 2002). Moreover, reducing dopaminergic transmission with dopamine antagonists in subcortical dopamine-rich regions is associated with substantial alterations in frontal cortex function (Holcomb et al., 1996), presumably mediated through circuits connecting the striatum to the frontal cortex (Alexander & Crutcher, 1990). These data indicate that the behavioral disturbances of schizophrenia involve impaired interactions between cortical and subcortical brain systems.

Brain Circuitry and Implications for Adolescence

Contrary to long-held ideas that the brain was mostly grown-up after childhood, it is now clear that adolescence is a time of explosive growth and development of the brain (Giedd & Rapoport, 2010; Satterthwaite et al., 2013). While the number of nerve cells does not change after birth, the richness and complexity of the connections between cells do, and the capacity for these networks to process increasingly complex information changes accordingly. Cortical regions that handle abstract information and that are critical for learning and memory of abstract concepts—rules, laws, codes of social conduct—seem to become much more likely to share information in a parallel processing fashion as adulthood approaches. This pattern of increased cortical information sharing is reflected in the patterns of connections between neurons in different regions of the cortex. Thus, the dendritic trees of neurons in the prefrontal cortex become more refined (pruned) during adolescence, indicating that the information flow between neurons becomes more efficient, with the emergence of executive function and abstract thinking during this period (Selemon, 2013). The possibility that schizophrenia involves molecular and functional abnormalities of information flow in these circuits suggests that such abnormalities may converge on the dynamic process of brain maturation during adolescence and increase the risk of a psychotic episode in predisposed individuals (Paus et al., 2008).

PATHOPHYSIOLOGY OF SCHIZOPHRENIA IN ADOLESCENCE

Despite over a century of research, we only have a limited understanding of what causes schizophrenia and related psychotic disorders. Early studies of the biological basis of schizophrenia mostly relied either on postmortem studies of brains of people with this illness, or brain imaging studies typically of older patients with chronic schizophrenia, many of whom were treated with medications. It was therefore difficult to know to what extent the observed changes were the results of aging, illness chronicity, or medication effects. One can avoid such difficulties by conducting studies of individuals in the early phases of schizophrenia (Keshavan & Schooler, 1992). First, these studies allow us to clarify which of the biological processes may be unique to the illness and which ones might be a result of medications or of persistent illness. Second, first-episode studies allow us to longitudinally evaluate the course of the brain changes, and how such changes can help us predict outcome with treatment. Follow-up studies suggest that fewer than half of early psychosis patients go on to develop a chronic form of schizophrenia with a poor level of functioning and intellectual deficits (Harrison et al., 2001). An understanding of which patients may have such an outcome will greatly help treatment decisions early in the illness. Finally, not all who have features of the prodromal phases of the illness go on to develop the psychotic illness (Fusar-Poli et al., 2013; Yung et al., 2003). Studies of the prodromal and early course of psychotic disorders provide an opportunity to elucidate the neurobiological processes responsible for the transition from the prodromal to psychotic phase of the illness.

Several conceptual models of the biology and causation of schizophrenia have been suggested and serve to guide research into the early phase of this illness. One view, which dates back to the late 1980s, is the so-called early neurodevelopmental model (Murray & Lewis, 1987; Weinberger, 1987). This model posits abnormalities early during brain development (perhaps at or before birth) as mediating the failure of brain functions in adolescence and early adulthood. Several lines of evidence, such as an increased rate of birth complications, minor physical and neurological abnormalities, and subtle behavioral difficulties in children who later developed schizophrenia, support this view. However, many nonaffected persons in the population also have these problems; their presence cannot inform us with confidence whether or not schizophrenia will develop later in life. The fact that the symptoms typically begin in adolescence or early adulthood suggests that the illness may be related to some biological changes related to adolescence occurring around or prior to the onset of psychosis. Childhood is characterized by proliferation of synapses and dendrites, and normal adolescence is characterized by elimination or pruning of unnecessary synapses in the brain, a process that serves to make nerve cell transmission more efficient (Huttenlocher et al., 1982). However, this process could go wrong, and an excessive pruning before or around the onset phase of illness (Feinberg, 1982a, 1982b; Keshavan, Anderson, & Pettegrew, 1994) has been thought to mediate the emergence of psychosis in adolescence or early adulthood. Consistent with this view, there is evidence for reductions in dendrite density in cortical brain regions in schizophrenia; these may be related to molecular mechanisms, perhaps glutamatergic, that underlie spine formation, pruning, and/or maintenance (Glausier & Lewis, 2013). However, our understanding of the underlying neurobiology of this phase of illness remains poor.

Another view is that active biological changes could occur after the onset of illness, during the commonly lengthy period of untreated psychosis. This model proposes progressive neurodegenerative changes (Lieberman et al., 2001b). It is possible that all three processes or "hits" are involved in schizophrenia (Keshavan & Hogarty, 1999); additionally, environmental factors such as drug misuse (Addington & Addington, 1998) and psychosocial stress (Erickson et al., 1989) may trigger the onset and influence the course of schizophrenia. Careful studies of the early phase of schizophrenia can shed light on these apparently contrasting models. The three proposed pathophysiological models might reflect different critical periods for prevention and therapeutic intervention.

THE GENETICS OF SCHIZOPHRENIA

Remarkable progress has been made in understanding genetic factors related to schizophrenia. We will summarize this work in the following section. Since almost no work has been done specifically on the genetics of adolescent-onset schizophrenia, we focus on studies of typical samples of adult-onset cases.

Is Schizophrenia Familial?

The most basic question in the genetics of schizophrenia is whether the disorder aggregates (or "runs") in families. Technically, familial aggregation means that a close relative of an individual with a disorder is at increased risk for that disorder compared to a matched individual chosen at random from the general population. Twenty-six early family studies, conducted prior to 1980 and lacking modern diagnostic procedures and appropriate controls, consistently showed that first-degree relatives of schizophrenia patients had a risk for schizophrenia that was roughly 10 times greater than would be expected in the general population (Kendler, 2000). Since 1980, 11 major family studies of schizophrenia have been reported that used blind diagnoses, control groups, personal interviews, and operationalized diagnostic criteria. The level of agreement in results is impressive: every study showed that the risk of schizophrenia was higher in first-degree relatives of schizophrenic patients than in matched controls. The mean risk for schizophrenia in these 11 studies was 0.5% in the relatives of controls and 5.9% in the relatives of schizophrenics. Modern studies suggest that, on average, parents, siblings, and offspring of individuals with schizophrenia have a risk of illness about 12 times greater than the general population—a figure close to that found in the earlier studies.

Results of the first methodologically rigorous family study of child-onset schizophrenia have been reported. Compared to parents of matched normal controls and children with ADHD, parents of patients with childhood-onset schizophrenia had over a 10-fold increased risk for schizophrenia, supporting the hypothesis of etiologic continuity between childhood-onset and adult-onset schizophrenia (Asarnow et al., 2001).

To What Extent Is the Familial Aggregation of Schizophrenia Due to Genetic Versus Environmental Factors?

Resemblance among relatives can be due to either shared or family environment (nurture) and/or genes (nature). A major goal in psychiatric genetics is to determine the degree to which familial aggregation for a disorder like schizophrenia results from environmental versus genetic mechanisms. While sophisticated analysis of family data can begin to make this discrimination, nearly all of our knowledge about this problem in schizophrenia comes from twin and adoption studies.

Twin studies are based on the assumption that "identical" or monozygotic (MZ) and "fraternal" or dizygotic (DZ) twins share a common environment to approximately the same degree. However, MZ twins are genetically identical, while DZ twins (like full siblings) share on average only half of their genes. Results are available from 13 major twin studies of schizophrenia published from 1928 to 1998 (Kendler, 2000). While modest differences are seen across studies, overall the agreement is impressive. Across all studies, the average concordance rate for schizophrenia is 55.8% in MZ twins and 13.5% in DZ twins. When statistical models are applied to these data to estimate heritability (the proportion of variance in liability in the population that is due to genetic factors), the average across all 13 studies is 72%. This figure, which is higher than that found for most common biomedical disorders, means that, on average, genetic factors are considerably more important than environmental factors in impacting the risk of schizophrenia.

Adoption studies can clarify the role of genetic and environmental factors in the transmission of schizophrenia by studying two kinds of rare but informative relationships: (1) individuals who are genetically related but do not share their rearing environment and (2) individuals who share their rearing environment but are not genetically related. Three studies conducted in Oregon, Denmark, and Finland all found significantly greater risk for schizophrenia or schizophrenia-spectrum disorders in the adopted-away offspring of schizophrenic parents compared to the adopted-away offspring of matched control mothers. The second major adoption strategy used for studying schizophrenia begins with ill adoptees rather than with ill parents and compares rates of schizophrenia between groups of biological parents and groups of adoptive parents. In two studies from Denmark using this strategy, the only group with elevated rates of schizophrenia and schizophrenia-spectrum disorders were the biological relatives of the schizophrenic adoptees (Kety et al., 1994).

Twin and adoption studies provide strong and consistent evidence that genetic factors play a major role in the familial aggregation of schizophrenia. Although not reviewed here, evidence for a role of nongenetic familial factors is much less clear. While some studies suggest they may contribute modestly to risk for schizophrenia, the majority of studies find no evidence for significant nongenetic familial factors for schizophrenia.

What Psychiatric Disorders Are Transmitted Within Families of Individuals with Schizophrenia?

Since the earliest genetic studies of schizophrenia, a major focus of such work has been to clarify more precisely the nature of the psychiatric syndromes that occur in excess in relatives of schizophrenic patients. To summarize a large body of evidence, relatives of schizophrenia patients are not only at increased risk for schizophrenia but also are at increased risk for schizophrenia-like personality disorders (best captured by the DSM-IV categories of schizotypal and paranoid personality disorder) and other psychotic disorders (Kendler, 2000). However, there is good evidence that relatives of schizophrenic patients are not at increased risk for other disorders, such as anxiety disorders and alcoholism. The most active debate in this area is the relationship between schizophrenia and mood disorders. Most evidence suggests little if any genetic relationship between these two major groups of disorders, but some research does suggest a relationship, particularly between schizophrenia and bipolar disorder (Craddock & Owen, 2010).

The evidence that other disorders in addition to schizophrenia occur at greater frequency in the close relatives of individuals with schizophrenia has led to the concept of the schizophrenia spectrum—a group of disorders that all bear a genetic relationship with classic or core schizophrenia.

What Is the Current Status for Identifying Specific Genes That Predispose to Schizophrenia?

Given the evidence that genetic factors play an important role in the etiology of schizophrenia, a major focus of recent work has been to apply the increasingly powerful tools of human molecular genetics to localize and identify the specific genes that predispose to schizophrenia. Two strategies have been employed in this effort: linkage and association. The goal of linkage studies is to identify areas of the human genome that are shared more frequently than would be expected by relatives who are affected. If such areas can be reliably identified, this suggests strongly that those regions contain one or more specific genes that influence the liability to schizophrenia. The method of linkage analysis has been extremely successful in identifying the location of genes for simple, usually rare medical genetic disorders (termed Mendelian disorders) where there is a one-to-one relationship between having the defective gene and having the disorder. This method, however, has had more mixed results when applied to disorders like schizophrenia that are genetically "complex." Such complex disorders are likely to be the result of multiple genes, none of which have a very large impact on risk, interacting with a range of environmental risk factors.

The number and the sample size of genome-wide association studies (GWAS) studies in schizophrenia have increased substantially over the past decade. In a recent paper from the Schizophrenia Working Group of the Psychiatric Genomics Consortium (PGC), 128 independent associations from 108 loci met criteria for genome-wide significance. Of these loci, 83 were novel and not reported previously (2014). Kendler and O'Donovan (2014) highlight several lessons from the growing genomic literature in schizophrenia, including the contribution of multiple loci with small effects across the genome and the need to apply network analyses to elucidate emerging disease pathways—glutamatergic transmission, calcium channels, and immune function. There is no evidence for a single gene with a large impact on risk for schizophrenia. Indeed, these results suggest that the existence of a single susceptibility locus that accounts for a large majority of the genetic variance for schizophrenia can now be effectively ruled out.

A brief highlight of progress provides a sense of how much has been accomplished. Earlier, the most pressing scientific issue in the interpretation of linkage studies of schizophrenia was whether there is agreement at above-chance levels across studies on which individual regions of the genome contain susceptibility genes for schizophrenia. The across-study agreement had not been very impressive. Two findings have increased our confidence that linkage studies of schizophrenia may be producing reliable results. First, in a large-scale study of families containing two or more cases of schizophrenia conducted in Ireland, the sample was divided, prior to analysis, into three random subsets (Straub et al., 2002b). When a genome scan was performed on these three subsets, three of the four regions that most prominently displayed evidence for linkage (on chromosomes 5q, 6p, and 8p) were replicated across all three subsets. Interestingly, one region, on chromosome 10p, was not replicated even within the same study. Probably more important, Levinson et al. were able to obtain raw data from nearly all major published genome scans of schizophrenia to perform a meta-analysis—a statistical method for rigorously combining data across multiple samples (Lewis et al., 2003). Ten regions produced nominally significant results, including 2q, 5q, 6p, 22q, and 8p. Continued data sharing is critical for progress.

On the Cusp of Gene Discovery in Schizophrenia

The evidence for replicated linkages in schizophrenia represents an important step toward the ultimate goal of identifying susceptibility genes and characterizing their biological effects. Because the human genome contains within its 23 pairs of chromosomes over 3 billion nucleotides (i.e., "letters" in the genetic alphabet) and 30,000 genes (i.e., protein-encoding units), it is a large territory to explore. Linkage is a strategy to narrow the search and to provide a map of where the treasure (i.e., the genes) may lie. The linkage results in schizophrenia so far have highlighted several regions of the genome for a more thorough search. Association (also called linkage disequilibrium) is the next critical step in this search for the treasure. Linkage represents a relationship between regions of the genome shared by family members who also share the phenotype of interest, here schizophrenia. It provides a low-resolution map because family members share relatively large regions of any chromosome. Association, however, represents a relationship between specific alleles (i.e., specific variation in a gene or in a genetic marker) and illness in unrelated individuals. It provides a high-resolution map because unrelated people share relatively little genetic information. For a given allele to be found more frequently in unrelated individuals with a similar disease than it is in the general population, the probability that this specific allele is a causative factor in the disease is enhanced. If the frequency of a specific allele (i.e., a specific genetic variation) is greater in a sample of unrelated individuals who have the diagnosis of schizophrenia than it is in a control population, the allele is said to be associated with schizophrenia. This association represents one of three possibilities: the allele is a causative mutation related to the etiology of the disease; the allele is a genetic variation that is physically close to the true causative mutation (i.e., in "linkage disequilibrium" with the true mutation); or the association is a spurious relationship reflecting population characteristics not related to the phenotype of interest. This latter possibility is often referred to as a population stratification artifact, meaning that differences in allele frequencies between the cases and control samples are not due to disease but rather are due to systematic genetic differences between the comparison populations.

Association has become the strategy of choice for fine mapping of susceptibility loci and for preliminary testing of whether specific genes are susceptibility genes for schizophrenia. The strategy involves identifying variations ("polymorphisms") in a gene of interest and then performing a laboratory analysis of the DNA samples to "type" each variation in each individual and determine its frequency in the study populations. Genetic sequence variations are common in the human genome, and public databases have been established to catalog them. The most abundant sequence variations are single nucleotide polymorphisms (SNPs), which represent a substitution in one DNA base. Common SNPs occur at a frequency of approximately one in every 1,000 DNA bases in the genome, and over 2 million SNPs have been identified. While SNPs are relatively common, most SNPs within genes either do not change the amino acid code or are in noncoding regions of genes ("introns") and are, thus, not likely to have an impact on gene function.

Early association studies in schizophrenia focused on genes based on their known function and the possibility that variations in their function might relate to the pathogenesis of the disease. These so-called functional candidate gene studies had no a priori probability of genetic association. A number of studies compared frequencies of variations in genes related to popular neurochemical hypotheses about schizophrenia, such as the dopamine and glutamate hypotheses, in individuals with schizophrenia in comparison to control samples. In almost every instance the results were mixed, with some positive but mostly negative reports. Many of the positive studies were compromised by potential population stratification artifacts. However, because the effect on risk of any given variation in any candidate gene (e.g., a dopamine or glutamate receptor gene) is likely to be small (less than a twofold increase in risk), most studies have been underpowered to establish association or to rule it out.

Recent association studies have been much more promising, primarily because of the linkage results. By using the linkage map regions as a priori entry points into the human genetic sequence databases, genes have been identified in each of the major linkage regions that appear to represent at least some of the basis for the linkage results. Moreover, confirmation of association in independent samples has appeared, which combined with the linkage results represent convergent evidence for the validity of these genetic associations.

In the August and October 2002 issues of the *American Journal of Human Genetics*, the first two papers appeared claiming to identify susceptibility genes for schizophrenia starting with traditional linkage followed by fine association mapping. Both of these were in chromosomal regions previously identified by multiple linkage groups: dysbindin (DTNBP1) on chromosome 6p22.3 (Straub et al., 2002a) and neuregulin 1 (NRG1) on chromosome 8p-p21 (Stefansson et al., 2002). Both groups identified the genes in these regions from public databases and then found variations (SNPs) within the genes that could be tested via an association analysis. In both papers, the statistical signals were strong and unlikely to occur by chance. In the January 2003 issue of the same journal, two further papers were published replicating, in independent population datasets also from Europe, association to variations in the same genes (Schwab et al., 2003; Stefansson et al., 2003). In the December 2002 issue of the same journal, a large population sample from Israel reported very strong statistical association to SNPs in the gene for catechol-O-methyltransferase (COMT), which was mapped to the region of 22q that had been identified as a susceptibility locus in several linkage studies (Shifman et al., 2002). Positive association to variation in COMT had also been reported in earlier studies in samples from China, Japan, France, and the United States (Egan et al., 2001). Starting with the linkage region on chromosome 13q34, a group from France discovered a novel gene, called G72, and reported in two population samples association between variations in this gene and schizophrenia (Chumakov et al., 2002). SNP variations in G72 have recently been reported to be associated with bipolar disorder as well.

In addition to these reports based on relatively strong linkage regions, several other promising associations have emerged from genes found in weaker linkage regions. For example, a weak linkage signal was found in several genome scans in 15q, a region containing the gene for the alpha-7 nicotine receptor (CHRNA7; Raux et al., 2002). This gene has been associated with an intermediate phenotype related to schizophrenia, the abnormal P50 EEG evoked response. Preliminary evidence has been reported that variants in CHRNA7 are associated with schizophrenia as well. DISC-1 is a gene in 1q43, which was a positive linkage peak in a genome linkage scan from Finland. A chromosomal translocation originating in this gene has been found to be very strongly associated with psychosis in Scottish families having this translocation (Millar et al., 2000). Finally, in a study of gene expression profiling from schizophrenic brain tissue, a gene called RGS4 was found to have much lower expression in schizophrenic brains than in normal brain. This gene is found in another 1q region that was positive in a linkage scan from Canada, and SNPs identified in RGS4 have now been shown to be associated with schizophrenia in at least three population samples (Chowdari et al., 2002). This convergent evidence from linkage and association implicates at least seven specific genes as potentially contributing risk for schizophrenia.

From Genetic Association to Biological Mechanisms of Risk

Genetic association identifies genes, but it does not identify disease mechanisms. Most of the genes implicated so far are based on associations with variations that are not clearly functional, in the sense that they do not appear to change the integrity of the gene. Most are SNPs in intronic regions of genes, which (as far as we know) do not have an impact on traditional aspects of gene function, such as the amino acid sequence or regulation of transcription. Thus, the associations put a flag on the gene but do not indicate how inheritance of a variation in the gene affects the function of the gene or the function of the brain. More work is needed in searching for variations that may have obvious functional implications and in basic cell biology to understand how gene function affects cell function.

In two of the genes implicated to date, there is evidence of a potential mechanism of increased risk. Preliminary evidence suggests that SNPs in the promoter region of the CHRNA7 gene that are associated with schizophrenia affect factors that turn on transcription of the CHRNA7 gene, presumably accounting for the lower abundance of CHRNA7 receptors reported in schizophrenic brain tissue (Leonard et al., 2002). This receptor is important in many aspects of hippocampal function and in regulation of the response of dopamine neurons to environmental rewards. Both hippocampal function and dopaminergic responsivity have been prominently implicated in the biology of schizophrenia. The COMT valine allele, which has been associated with schizophrenia in the COMT studies, translates into a more active enzyme that appears to diminish dopamine in the prefrontal cortex. This leads to various aspects of poorer prefrontal function, in terms of cognition and physiology, which are prominent clinical aspects of schizophrenia and also intermediate phenotypes associated with risk for schizophrenia (Weinberger et al., 2001). The COMT valine allele also is associated with abnormal control of dopamine activity in the parts of the brain where it appears to be overactive in schizophrenia (Akil et al., 2003). Thus, inheritance of the COMT valine allele appears to increase risk for schizophrenia because it biases toward biological effects implicated in both the negative and positive symptoms of the illness.

Schizophrenia-Susceptibility Genes and Adolescence

It is not obvious how the genes described would specifically relate to adolescence and the emergence of schizophrenia during this time of life. The evidence so far suggests that each of the candidate susceptibility genes affects fundamental aspects of how a brain grows and how it adapts to experience. Each gene may affect the excitability of glutamate neurons, either directly or through GABA neuron intermediates, and indirectly the regulation of dopamine neurons by the cortex. These are fundamental processes related to the biology of schizophrenia. These are also processes that may be especially crucial to adolescence because cortical development and plasticity are changing dramatically during this period. Thus, it is conceivable that the variations in the functions of these genes associated with schizophrenia lead to compromises and bottlenecks in these processes. In keeping with this, a recent study has shown childhood-onset schizophrenia to be associated with a higher rate of rare copy number variants (CNVs) than seen for adult-onset patients, and these CNVs are nonspecific, being associated with a range of other neurodevelopmental disorders, including intellectual disability, autism, and epilepsy (Ahn et al., in press).

The Potential Gene-Finding Utility of Endophenotypes

Despite encouraging results from recent linkage and association studies, the literature also contains prominent failures and inconsistencies. Failures to replicate linkage and association signals for schizophrenia suggest that genomic strategies may benefit from a redirection based on our current understanding of the pathophysiology of schizophrenia. For example, the power of genetic studies may be increased by examining linkage with quantitative traits that relate to schizophrenia rather than with a formal diagnosis itself. The concept of using intermediate phenotypes, or endophenotypes, is not new (Gottesman & Gould, 2003) but has only recently started to enjoy widespread popularity among those seeking genes for schizophrenia. Gottesman and Shields suggested over 30 years ago that features such as subclinical personality traits, measures of attention and information processing, or the number of dopamine receptors in specific brain regions might lie "intermediate to the phenotype and genotype of schizophrenia" (Gottesman & Shields, 1973). Today, other traits, such as eye-movement dysfunctions, altered brain-wave patterns, and neuropsychological and neuroimaging abnormalities, are under consideration as potentially useful endophenotypes of schizophrenia, because all of these are more common or more severe in schizophrenia patients and their family members than in the general population or among control subjects (Faraone et al., 1995). These deficits may relate more directly than the diagnosis of schizophrenia to the aberrant genes. At the biological level, this is a logical assumption, as genes do not encode for hallucinations or delusions; they encode primarily for proteins that have an impact on molecular processes within and between cells. Thus, endophenotypes may serve as proxies for schizophrenia that are closer to the biology of the underlying risk genes.

Early Findings from Molecular Genetic Studies of Endophenotypes

While much recent work has been dedicated toward establishing the heritability of endophenotypes, only a handful of molecular genetic studies of endophenotypes have emerged. Results observed to date have been encouraging. Some chromosomal loci that have been found to harbor genes for schizophrenia have also shown evidence for linkage with an endophenotype, and the Consortium on the Genetics of Schizophrenia (COGS) study examining associations between heritable neurophysiological and neurocognitive endophenotypes has revealed several previously implicated genes of potential functional and neurobiological significance (Greenwood et al., 2011). The Bipolar-Schizophrenia Network for Intermediate Phenotypes (B-SNIP) study has shown substantive phenotypic overlap (Hill et al., 2013; Tamminga et al., 2013) between schizophrenia and schizoaffective and psychotic bipolar disorders, consistent with observations of genetic overlaps between these disorders (Smoller et al., 2013). However, the greater potential of endophenotype studies is that genes might be identified that would not be implicated from regions of the genome highlighted in linkage regions. This is because minor genes for schizophrenia may turn out to be major genes for some index of central nervous system dysfunction. The proof of this has been supported by evidence that COMT, which is a weak susceptibility gene for schizophrenia, is a relatively strong factor in normal human frontal lobe function (Weinberger et al., 2001).

Whether classical criteria or quantitative phenotypes are used to further study schizophrenia, refining the definition of an "affected" individual is a top priority for genetic studies. Given the overlap between symptom-based diagnostic categories, a more useful approach will be to map genes to phenotypic dimensions *across* diagnostic categories (Keshavan et al., 2013). This diagnostically agnostic approach is central to a recent paradigm shift in psychiatry, the research domain criteria (RDoC) (Cuthbert & Insel, 2010). RDoC offers a framework for acquiring and organizing new knowledge across translational units of analyses (genes, molecules, circuits, behavior) and across domains (e.g., cognition, salience, arousal states) to transform the approach to the nosology of mental disorders. Finally, since not all individuals with schizophrenia-susceptibility genes develop the actual disorder, understanding the measurable effects of these aberrant genes is a critical step in tracking their passage from preclinical to clinical expression and in identifying their clinical biology. In the not-too-distant future, the amount and types of expressed protein products of these disease genes may be used as the ultimate endophenotypes for schizophrenia. To the extent that we can reduce measurement error and create measures that are more closely tied to individual schizophrenia genes, we will greatly improve our understanding of the genetics of schizophrenia.

Genetic Counseling Issues

With increasing attention in the media to issues relating to genetics and particularly the role of genetic factors in mental illness, an increasing number of individuals will likely be seeking genetic counseling in the future for issues related to schizophrenia. In our experience, by far the most common situation is a married couple who are contemplating having children and the husband or wife has a family history of schizophrenia. They typically ask any combination of three questions:

1. Is there a genetic test that can be performed on us to determine whether we have the gene for schizophrenia and so may pass it on to our children?
2. Is there an in utero test that can be given that would determine the risk of that fetus to develop schizophrenia later in life?
3. What is the risk for schizophrenia to our children?

Unfortunately, given the current state of our knowledge, answers to the first two questions are both "No, we are not yet in the position of having a genetic test that can usefully predict risk for schizophrenia." We would often add something like, "This is a very active area of research, and there is hope that in the next few years, some breakthrough might occur that would allow us to develop such a test, but right now we really do not know when or even if that will be possible."

By contrast, useful information can be provided for the third question. Most typically, the husband or wife has a parent or sibling with schizophrenia but himself or herself has been mentally healthy. Therefore, the empirical question is this: What is known about the risk of schizophrenia to the grandchild or niece/nephew of an individual with schizophrenia? Interestingly, this is a subject that has not been systematically studied since the early days of psychiatric genetics in the first decades of the 20th century. The results of these early studies have been summarized in several places, most notably by Gottesman (Gottesman & Shields, 1982), with aggregate risk estimates for schizophrenia of 3.7% and 3.0%, respectively, in grandchildren or niece/nephews of an individual with schizophrenia. However, this is a considerable overestimate if the parent with the positive family history remains unaffected. That is, the risk to a grandchild or nephew of an individual with schizophrenia when the intervening parent never develops the illness is probably less than 2%. Most individuals find this information helpful and broadly reassuring.

Future Work

By the time this chapter is read, a great deal more information is likely to have accumulated about the scientific status of these findings. At this early stage, several trends are noteworthy:

1. At least some of these potential gene discoveries have now been replicated enough times that it is increasingly unlikely that they are false-positive findings (due, for example, to the performance of many statistical tests).
2. We can expect that the biochemical pathways represented by these genes will be explored at the level of basic cell biology and new leads about pathogenesis and potential new targets for prevention and treatment will be found.
3. We can expect a number of studies to emerge that will try to understand whether the expression of these genes is changed in the brains of schizophrenic patients.
4. Efforts are already under way to try to understand how these genes influence psychological functions such as attention, sensory gating, and memory that are disturbed in schizophrenia.
5. Intense efforts will be made to try to determine whether these different genes are acting through a common pathway as, for example, has been postulated for the known genes for Alzheimer's disease.

Treatment of Schizophrenia

Raquel E. Gur
Ruben C. Gur
Matcheri S. Keshavan
Christian Kohler
Judith Rapoport
Elaine Walker

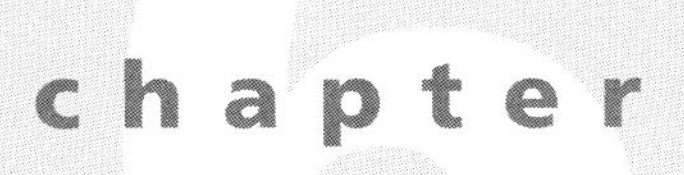

PSYCHOLOGICAL TREATMENTS

Interest in psychological treatments for schizophrenia has increased, particularly in Europe and Australia, driven by understandable patient dissatisfaction with purely pharmacological approaches. The recognition that 40% of patients do not achieve symptom resolution with drug treatment (Kane et al., 1996) has added impetus to the search for alternatives and adjuncts. Unfortunately, the paucity of data concerning the application of such approaches to adolescents with schizophrenia means that, at least for the time being, inferences have to be drawn mainly from studies of adult populations.

Nevertheless, the similar lack of data regarding efficacy and safety of antipsychotic drug treatment in adolescents, and the observation that adolescents may be especially sensitive to the adverse effects of typical antipsychotics (e.g., extrapyramidal side effects; Lewis, 1998) and clozapine (e.g., neutropenia and seizures; Kumra et al., 1996) mean that there is a real need for alternative or supplementary interventions. Indeed, one could hypothesize that psychological treatments might be more effective in adolescents than adults. Adolescents represent a group who have a greater degree of neural plasticity and a still evolving personality, and who are especially likely to have an ongoing system of support in the form of family and educational input; furthermore, they present opportunities for early detection. Alongside early treatment with antipsychotics, there is potential for psychotherapeutic interventions to lessen the impact of positive symptoms, to improve coping strategies, and potentially to reduce the cognitive deficits, which so impair psychosocial function.

Early and Educational Interventions

In common with those who go on to develop other serious mental disorders, individuals who develop schizophrenia in later life often, but not invariably, demonstrate interpersonal and emotional difficulties during childhood and adolescence. However, Cannon et al. (2002) reported that schizophrenia was specifically predicted by the presence of deficits in receptive language, neuromotor function, and cognitive development between 3 and 11 years of age.

Schools

Since such abilities are already observed and assessed, to an extent, as part of a child's schooling, there is potential for the development of predictors and the identification of targets for psychological intervention. Studies examining the ability of teachers and other educational professionals in day-to-day contact with adolescents to predict future sufferers of schizophrenia do show some statistical power, but this is at the cost of many false positives and even more false negatives (Murray et al., 2003) unless restricted to high-risk populations (Kravariti et al., 2004). One possible exception was the study by Davidson et al. (1999) linking the Israeli Draft Board Registry with the National Psychiatric Hospitalization Case Registry. Adolescent boys underwent preinduction assessments at age 16 and 17 years to determine suitability for military service. Those admitted to a psychiatric hospital with schizophrenia 4 to 10 years later were matched with control individuals from their school class at the time of the original assessment. Identified predictors for schizophrenia in the male adolescents included deficits in social and intellectual functioning and organizational activity. The predictive model derived by the authors had 75% sensitivity, 100% specificity, and a positive predictive value of 72%. However, as highlighted in a commentary by Jones and van Os (2000), the predictive power of this model was achieved by excluding from the sample those school classes without individuals who later became schizophrenic.

So far the best prediction has come not from teachers but from a psychiatric interview. In the Dunedin study (Poulton et al., 2000), 11-year-old children were asked about experiences of quasi-psychotic symptoms. The questions were as follows:

1. Do you believe in mind reading or being psychic? Have other people ever read your mind?

2. Have you ever had messages sent just to you through the television or radio?
3. Have you ever thought that people are following you or spying on you?
4. Have you heard voices other people can't hear?
5. Has something ever gotten inside your body or has your body changed in some way?

Those who answered positively to one of the five questions or possibly positively to two were 16 times more likely to develop a schizophrenia-like psychosis by age 26. Teachers or school nursing staff could be advised of the value of such questions. However, according to Murray et al. (2003), little work aiming at primary prevention (i.e., preventing progression from premorbid abnormalities to prodrome) is in progress.

Early Treatment Projects

Falloon initiated an early intervention for "prodromal" symptoms in adolescents and adults in the form of the Buckingham Project, a "shared care model" between primary and secondary care (using low doses of medication, interventions designed to reduce stress, psychoeducation, and follow-up for 2 years after the symptoms had occurred). He claimed that this reduced the annual incidence of first-episode psychosis from 7.4 per 100,000 per year, as measured by the same group in 1989, to 0.75 per 100,000, per year during the 4-year study period (Falloon et al., 1996).

Unfortunately, adolescents developing schizophrenia suffer the same delays as their older counterparts, often not receiving diagnosis or treatment for a prolonged period. In consequence, a number of projects have been developed to reduce this unnecessary period of untreated psychosis.

Projects such as the Personal Assessment and Crisis Evaluation (PACE) clinic in Melbourne, Australia, and the Early Treatment and Intervention in Psychosis (TIPS) project in Norway aim at secondary prevention (i.e., preventing progression from prodrome into syndrome) in adolescents and adults. Such programs are motivated by the belief that the chronicity of schizophrenia may develop in the early stages of the illness and that long-term outcomes may be linked to the "duration of untreated psychosis" (DUP)—that is, the period between onset of symptoms and initiation of treatment. However, the latter remains theoretical. Norman and Malla (2001) reviewed the concept of DUP, and while they confirmed that there was evidence to suggest a relationship between DUP and the ease with which first remission of symptoms is achieved, they could not find evidence to support a link with disease progression. Although the concept of DUP focuses on initiation of pharmacological treatment, de Haan et al. (2003) suggest that delay in initiating intensive psychosocial treatment may have similar implications for outcome, particularly in relation to negative symptoms at follow-up.

The TIPS project is a prospective clinical trial, which started in Norway in 1997, comparing an experimental sector with two other control sectors (age range 15–65 years). The experimental sector developed a system for early detection and also established a comprehensive information, service, and education program aimed at both the general public and professionals involved in healthcare and education (Johannessen et al., 2001). In the 2 years after the initiation of the TIPS project, mean DUP decreased from 1.5 years to 0.5 years.

The PACE clinic was established in Melbourne in 1994; the aim was to evaluate the prodromal phase, develop interventions that prevent further deterioration and maximize function, and set up a clinical service to identify and engage young people experiencing potential early psychosis. Preliminary results, which are further discussed in the following section on cognitive-behavioral therapy, show that early intervention in the prodrome can at least delay the onset of first-episode psychosis.

It seems likely that the wider-ranging public and educative measures in the TIPS project and PACE clinic are vital to any health service initiatives or collaboration, especially in view of adolescents' poor primary-care attendance.

However, it is important to note that while a number of the early intervention services cover the adolescent age range, their remit is actually to intervene in an "early stage" of the disorder rather than to specifically target those who develop schizophrenia in adolescence.

Cognitive-Behavioral Therapy

Cognitive-behavioral therapy (CBT) addresses problems in the "here and now" by targeting dysfunctional thoughts and behaviors within a collaborative therapeutic relationship. The efficacy of CBT and its acceptability in disorders such as depression and anxiety have been demonstrated (Beck et al., 1992; Kovacs et al., 1981). In support of the growing (but relatively underevaluated) practice of CBT in adults with schizophrenia, Rector and Beck (2002) suggest that since the inferential errors and faulty logic in hallucinations and delusions are similar to those seen in other disorders, CBT should also work in schizophrenia. They describe CBT for psychosis as an active, structured therapy, usually with a duration of 6 to 9 months, given individually.

Adolescent Studies

We could not find any reports of the use of definitive CBT in specifically adolescent individuals. However, data are beginning to accumulate from the early intervention programs, reporting on the use of CBT in early-onset psychosis. McGorry et al. (2002a) conducted a randomized controlled trial (RCT) with 14- to 30-year-olds at the Early Psychosis Prevention and Intervention Centre, Melbourne, which is associated with the PACE clinic discussed earlier. This study compared interventions designed to reduce the risk of progression to first-episode psychosis in a clinical sample aged 14 to 30 years, termed ultra-high risk (first-degree family history of schizophrenia and subthreshold symptoms). The interventions comprised a needs-based intervention and a specific preventive intervention (low-dose risperidone and CBT) for 6 months, with assessments at baseline and 6 and 12 months, using a defined threshold outcome rather than a formal diagnosis of schizophrenia. Ten of 28 in the needs-based intervention versus 3 of 31 in the specific intervention had reached the defined outcome by the end of treatment; however, there was no significant difference at 6-month follow-up. When the data were assessed taking into account drug adherence, a significant difference was found between the fully adherent specific intervention group versus the needs-based group. It seemed as though the specific intervention delayed onset.

Adult Studies

Dickerson (2000) reviewed all studies investigating CBT in schizophrenia in adult populations (though age data are not supplied) between 1990 and 1999. She examined the available data for seven different CBT approaches—some focusing on acute psychosis, others on persisting positive symptoms. Her conclusion was that there were some CBT strategies that reduced positive symptomatology, especially in individuals with clearly defined symptoms that they themselves viewed as problematic. The most beneficial outcome appeared to be in reducing conviction in, and distress about, delusions; there was little evidence to suggest that CBT was efficacious in negative symptoms or social functioning. The overall superiority of CBT was reduced when the control condition was matched for therapist input.

Even more disappointing, a Cochrane meta-analysis of CBT in schizophrenia (Cormac et al., 2002) found no evidence that CBT, in addition to standard care, reduces the relapse and readmission rate in the short term or longer term (1 year) any more than standard care alone. Moreover, there was no overall difference between CBT and supportive psychotherapy with respect to relapse rate or improvements in mental state.

Pilling et al. (2002) conducted a systematic review of RCTs of CBT (and family interventions, social skills training, and cognitive remediation). The trials reviewed compared CBT with supportive therapies and standard care in predominantly chronic psychosis. There was no evidence for increased effectiveness of CBT during treatment, though CBT showed a clear advantage over the comparison treatment at follow-up when measured continuously in terms of "important improvement." This superiority persisted for up to 18 months after treatment. Furthermore, the CBT group had lower dropout rates. It was not possible to identify any particular responder characteristics or the optimal frequency or length of treatment.

The Study of Cognitive Reality Alignment Therapy in Early Schizophrenia (SoCRATES; Lewis et al., 2002) was conducted in individuals with an average age of 27, but it is one of the more relevant adult studies to this discussion since the patients recruited were in the early phases of their illness. The RCT compared (1) CBT with routine care, (2) supportive counseling and routine care, and (3) routine care alone, all for a duration of 5 weeks, in individuals experiencing their first or second episode of schizophrenia. CBT showed only transient advantages over the other two intervention conditions in speeding remission from acute symptoms in this group of individuals.

In summary, the adult literature suggests that although CBT might have some beneficial effects, questions such as defining the length of treatment required, which patients would benefit, and at which stages in their illness it should be implemented remain unanswered. Until these questions are answered in adult populations, it would be foolish to commence large trials in adolescents, especially without adequately defined aims. This caution should not prevent CBT techniques from being borrowed in part in the development of specific interventions targeted at the special needs of adolescents with schizophrenia.

Cognitive Remediation Therapy

Deficits in cognitive function such as working memory, attention, and executive functioning are core features of schizophrenia. Cognitive remediation therapy (CRT) aims to teach people "thinking skills." More specifically, it uses material that is not personal to the individual and targets the specific domains affected in schizophrenia. CRT can be characterized into three generic approaches (Bellack & Brown, 2001):

1. Practice and brief training on neurocognitive tests or computer tasks to improve a single domain of functioning
2. Repetitive practice on a battery of computer tasks aimed at multiple domains
3. Strategies to improve cognitive functioning in general by increasing self-confidence, interest, and initiative

The assessment of CRT's efficacy has again been hampered by methodological constraints, in particular the heterogeneity of intervention packages used and then inappropriately compared. Wykes et al. (2001) have made attempts to reduce this phenomenon by describing a typology for classification of methods.

Adolescent Populations

Techniques targeting cognitive differentiation, attention, memory, and social perception are being evaluated in adolescent populations by Borg Rund and colleagues in Oslo. Ueland et al. (2004a) carried out an RCT comparing the effects of psychoeducation and cognitive training versus psychoeducation in a small group of adolescents with early-onset psychosis. They did not detect any significant between-group differences in any of their treatment scores, though there were some specific significant improvements in visual long-term memory and early visual information processing and Brief Psychiatric Rating Scale (BPRS) scores, limited to the remediation group. This group has also focused on the remediation of more specific cognitive deficits. Ueland et al. (2004b) assessed the effect of enhanced instructions and contingent monetary reinforcement on attentional skills. A group of adolescents with early-onset psychosis received the Span of Apprehension Performance (SPAN) at baseline, three times as an intervention, and then after testing and at 10-day follow-up. Improvements in performance were evident at the end of the intervention, diminishing slightly after testing but recovering at 10-day follow-up.

Adult Populations

Research into CRT in adults, based on the third category listed above, has found an effect on memory durable to 6 months of follow-up, which, if large enough, gave rise to associated improvement in social performance (Wykes et al., 2001). We await with interest the ongoing study this group is conducting in patients between 16 and 21 years of age. Furthermore, a study involving "cognitive enhancement therapy" in early-course patients, some of whom will be within the adolescent age range, is being undertaken by Hogarty's team in Pittsburgh (personal communication).

Interpersonal Psychotherapy

Very little evaluative work has been published in the area of interpersonal therapy since the 3-year trial conducted by Hogarty et al. (1997). Though this study was aimed at reducing the "late relapse" observed to occur in the second year after psychotherapeutic intervention, and it was conducted in a mixed adult and adolescent cohort (16–55 years old), it warrants discussion because its conclusions seem particularly pertinent to the adolescent population. This study examined relapse and noncompliance in outpatients with schizophrenia and schizoaffective disorder in two concurrent trials. One trial studied individuals who lived with their families who were randomly assigned to (1) personal therapy, (2) family therapy, (3) personal therapy and family therapy, or (4) supportive therapy; the other trial studied individuals who lived alone and who were randomly assigned to either personal or supportive therapy.

Personal therapy occurred in three stages, and though it focused on internal, personal responses to stress as opposed to the regulation of external triggers, it did not use symbolic interpretation or analysis of unconscious factors. It aimed, more specifically, to identify and manage the "affect dysregulation" that might mediate relapse or inappropriate behavior. All patients were on the minimum effective dose of medication. The overall rate of relapse over the 3-year period was 29% over all groups, which was lower than expected. For individuals living with their family, the group receiving personal therapy relapsed less than the other groups, though this was only significant for family intervention. For individuals living alone, personal therapy significantly increased relapse rates compared to supportive treatment, though the latter was particularly rich in its provisions. The authors suggested that the group living away from their family may not have reached a stable independence; they may have been too distracted to prioritize the therapy or the intervention itself may have overloaded them. Perhaps this conclusion should serve as a more global caution: full assessment of levels of independence and subjective perceptions of stability may be required before initiating any form of psychotherapy.

Social Skills

Social skills training is a structured educative program that involves modeling, role play, and reinforcement (Bellack & Mueser, 1993). It is based on the hope that the improved social skills generalize to real-life situations and might even improve symptomatology and reduce relapse. Such interventions are targeted at the profound impairments in social functioning that characterize schizophrenia and affect life in the workplace, family, and the wider community. There are three forms of social skills training as detailed by Bellack and Mueser (1993): the basic model, the social problem-solving model, and the cognitive remediation model (considered in the previous section).

The basic model involves breaking down complex social interactions into smaller elements. The patients are therefore taught the steps and then the combined elements using role play and targeting areas such as self-care, medication management, and conversation. Bustillo et al. (2001) reviewed reports from between 1996 to 2001 and found that the basic model was repeatedly efficacious in improving social skills and that this effect continued for up to 12 months. However, there was not much to suggest that this affected overall social performance. Evidence from studies of the problem-solving approach suggests modest benefits on very discrete areas of social functioning that appear to have some durability.

Though such research seems old-fashioned and potentially out of sync with the dilemmas and challenges facing an adolescent with schizophrenia, the approach may have merits. For a child, the transition into adolescence and then adulthood is a difficult process requiring support and structure. Developing schizophrenia during this process disrupts personal development in an infinite number of ways. Therefore, there is a real need for research, in groups of adolescents with schizophrenia, into developing ways to teach them social skills that generalize to real life.

Family Therapies

Successful family therapies have psychoeducation at their heart, taking the form of a collaborative and respectful relationship with the family, provision of information, and teaching family members less stressful ways of communicating and solving problems. It seems intuitive that family interventions, in a nonspecific sense, would be particularly beneficial in adolescents with schizophrenia, especially those who remain dependent on their parents.

The need for intervention is supported by reports that children with schizotypal personality disorder or schizophrenia, and the parents of such children, tend to show increased rates of thought disorder during direct family interactions (Tompson et al., 1997). Some reports claim that the parents also show increased communication deviance (an index of difficulties associated with a failure to establish and maintain a shared focus of attention; Asarnow, 1994). It is not possible to know at this stage whether this represents a shared genetic vulnerability to psychosis or a parental response to the child's illness.

Additional support comes from the work on expressed emotion (EE), and though this was originally investigated in adult populations, the majority of data assessing family interventions in adolescents is based around it. The concept of EE, which encompasses critical comments, hostility, and overinvolvement, arose out of a body of research focused on the effect of the family environment in the maintenance of schizophrenia and other severe mental disorders (Brown et al., 1962). Family interventions evolved, again targeted at adults, that aimed to reduce high EE and thus reduce relapse rates (Leff et al., 1982).

Adolescents

The applicability of therapies directed at high EE in adolescent schizophrenia is hampered by three problems.

First, adolescent families have less EE or different EE. Asarnow et al. (1994) found relatively low parental EE (compared to the families of adults with schizophrenia) when measuring criticism and overinvolvement on the Five-minute Speech Sample Expressed Emotion (FMSS-EE): 23% families of adolescents with schizophrenia or schizotypal personality disorder were rated as having high EE compared to 44% families of adults with schizophrenia in a similar study by Miklowitz et al. (1989).

The second problem is stability over time and lack of response to treatment. Lenior et al. (2002) conducted a longitudinal study to analyze the stability of parental EE in individuals with recent-onset schizophrenia ages 15 to 26 years in the 8 years following discharge from two interventions from inpatient care: community care alone and with additional family intervention according to the model of Falloon et al. (1984). The families were stratified according to high and low EE before allocation, and EE was measured over the follow-up period using the FMSS. EE, according to these measurements, does change over time, though this study failed to detect any overall treatment effect on EE levels. In addition, this group found no intervention effect on number of months of psychosis during 5-year follow-up.

Nugter et al. (1997) studied individuals, ages 16 to 25, with recent-onset schizophrenia and related disorders who were randomly allocated to individual treatment with or without a family intervention (modeled on Falloon et al., 1984). At the end of treatment (1 year), there were no significant between-group differences in EE (as assessed by the FMSS). There were no detectable relationships between EE and relapse, except that in the individual group, changeable EE (in whichever direction) was correlated with relapse rate.

The final problem is the lack of specificity to schizophrenia. A meta-analysis of EE-outcome relationships in mental disorders (Butzlaff et al., 1998), though confirming EE as a significant predictor of relapse in schizophrenia, found significantly larger effect sizes for EE in mood and eating disorders. This study did not specify the age ranges covered by the reviewed studies.

Thus, attempts to evolve therapies targeted at underlying problems, particularly in younger populations, has been complicated.

Linszen et al. (1996) found that adding a behavioral family intervention (modeled after Falloon et al., 1984) to an individual psychosocial intervention in patients ages 15 to 26 years made no difference to rates of psychotic relapse in the 15 months following first-episode psychosis. In fact, Linszen's group found a near-significant increase in relapse rate in low-EE families who participated in the intervention, possibly due to the families' perception of the therapy as artificial, critical, or interfering in their reactions to their offspring's illness. However, during that 15-month intervention period, the relapse rate was 15%, suggesting that early intervention improved outcome. The cohort was then referred for care by other agencies and, at 5-year follow-up, the low relapse rate had not been maintained. The authors suggest that sustained intervention above and beyond regular services might be required to improve outcome in the longer term. This result, taken in conjunction with the increase in relapse of low-EE families, calls into question the value and possibly the ethics of using this intervention in early psychosis.

Asarnow et al. (2001) concluded that though available data support the use of family interventions in the treatment of adolescents with schizophrenia, it is not yet possible to determine which model is most effective. There is, however, an encouraging shift from reducing putative risk factors to empowering and channeling this "resource." We concur with this viewpoint but would welcome more work into alternative means of monitoring response to family therapy.

Adult Studies

The preliminary results from the multicenter NIMH Treatment Strategies Study (Schooler et al., 1997), which compared variable medication strategies in conjunction with "supportive family management" (psychoeducational workshop for relatives with a monthly support group for 2 years) and "applied family management" (which included the former and an intensive at-home family intervention based on the Falloon et al. behavioral program), suggest that the latter, more intensive program does not yield better results and does not permit the use of lower or intermittent medication regimes.

McFarlane et al. (1995) conducted a pilot study looking at the application of psychoeducation administered in single-family compared to multiple-family groups in individuals ages 18 to 45 years. There were lower relapse rates (12.5% at 12 months and 25% at 24 months) with the multiple-family groups (compared to 23.5% and 47.1%, respectively). Both of these programs resulted in lower relapse rates compared to a multiple-family program without a psychoeducational model.

Pilling et al. (2002), in the aforementioned systematic review, also analyzed family intervention data. The mean age of studied individuals was 31 years, and the mean number of admissions per individual was 2.7. All family interventions (single and multiple) were more effective at reducing relapse in the first 12 months of treatment than the control condition, especially where that was standard care. Only single-family interventions reduced readmission during this time. At 1 to 2 years only, single-family interventions were still reducing relapse, though all treatments were effective at reducing readmission. Interestingly, all family interventions studied had higher rates of treatment compliance both to the family intervention and to concurrently prescribed medication. It is important to note, however, that not all the studies included in this review used a supportive individual program as the control condition. Some control conditions actually represented a family intervention itself, as noted in a response to the review (Bentsen, 2003).

The Family to Family Education Program developed by the National Alliance for the Mentally Ill, and detailed on their website (http://www.nami.org), involves a highly structured program conducted by trained family members for 2- to 3-hour sessions over 12 weeks. Participants report decreases in family members' "worry and displeasure," as well as "subjective burden," with increased empowerment, knowledge, and improved coping strategies. This program is cheap, it is popular with family members, and it can be widely disseminated, thus aiding implementation.

Compliance Therapy

Compliance therapy is a brief pragmatic intervention using cognitive-behavioral techniques, very closely linked with motivational interviewing, that focuses on improving treatment adherence. It evolved out of initial work in programs using psychoeducational and behavioral techniques (e.g., Eckman et al., 1992), and its further development was encouraged by the UK National Health Service, which declared noncompliance a research priority. It was tested in a pilot study, modified, and then used in an RCT in adult inpatients with psychotic illnesses by Kemp et al. (1996) with follow-up to 6 months. Eighteen-month follow-up was reported (Kemp et al., 1998) using an expanded sample. The therapy itself takes place over four to six sessions, of 20 to 60 minutes each, approximately biweekly. It involves the following:

1. Reviewing the individual's treatment history and his or her views and understanding of the illness and treatment
2. Exploring symptoms and side effects and thus evaluating pros and cons of treatment
3. Discussing stigma

Despite the fact that the therapy was biased to encourage only positive attitudes to treatment, the therapy also aimed to reframe the use of medication as a decision, freely chosen to enhance quality of life, referred to as an "insurance policy" or "protective layer." Immediately after the intervention, the compliance therapy had significantly improved insight and compliance compared to supportive counseling matched for therapist time, with the same therapists. This effect was maintained at 6-month follow-up with a 23% difference between groups, with those with higher IQ achieving better results. It was not possible to determine whether these gains resulted in increased function or diminished relapse rate. The 18-month follow-up confirmed that compliance therapy improved compliance and insight in the intervention group compared to the control condition, by 19%, and improved global functioning, especially as time progressed. It had no overall effect in improving symptomatology or reducing time spent in the hospital over the follow-up period.

The positive effects on compliance were not replicated by O'Donnell et al. (2003) in an RCT in adult inpatients with schizophrenia. Compliance therapy, administered according to Kemp et al. (1996/1998), conferred no advantage in compliance, symptomatology, or overall function outcomes at 1 year after therapy, compared to a control condition of equivalent duration with nonspecific counseling. Furthermore, one struggles to see how such a therapy could exert such a persuasive effect in a teenager in the throes of puberty and a battle for independence. Yet again, there is a real need for adaptation of such techniques to adolescent populations followed by RCTs evaluating their effect.

Summary of Psychological Treatments

Studies attempting to assess the efficacy of psychological treatments have been hampered by a multitude of methodological problems. Often very different versions of a treatment model are described as one and the same. They are often applied to heterogeneous populations (e.g., different ages or illness stages) and compared with a control condition unmatched for therapist time and attention.

Debate also continues as how best to assess the outcome of such interventions. Bellack and Brown (2001) felt that judging psychosocial treatments on the same outcome measures as pharmacological intervention might not be appropriate. Rather than evaluating therapies on whether they reduce symptoms, induce remission, or prevent relapse, they recommended focusing on their effect in reducing impairments in social role functioning and improving overall quality of life and treatment adherence. Thus, they recommend rehabilitation rather than treatment—taking into account the confounding effect of cognitive deficits and the need for newly learned skills to generalize to real life in the community. They liken psychosocial therapies to the use of Braille in visually impaired individuals.

Outcome studies in schizophrenia tend to focus on categorical measures such as hospital admission, and on professional observations of relapse, symptomatology, or cognitive impairment. Very few assess psychosocial outcome or quality of life, especially as rated by users of services and their caregivers. Such measures of outcome are particularly important for adolescent populations. Lay et al. (2000) conducted a 12-year follow-up study of 96 consecutively admitted individuals with schizophrenia (ages 11–17). Of the 68% reassessed at 12 years, 66% had serious social disability, which was predicted by severity of positive symptoms in the early stages and by admissions numbering more than two; 75% were financially dependent. Jarbin et al. (2003) conducted a 10-year follow-up of adolescents (<19 years old) who were diagnosed with first-episode early-onset psychosis in the 1980s and early 1990s; 79% of those with early-onset schizophrenia spectrum disorders suffered a chronic course with poor outcome.

The collaborative and empowering nature of many of the psychotherapeutic options, though incompletely evaluated and not always available, switches our focus from such sobering outcomes and inflicted choices to a more patient-driven framework. It is encouraging to see that the quest for alternatives and adjuncts to pharmacological treatments has been stepped up, and that attempts are being made to improve the methodological quality of their evaluation.

However, a clinician faced with an adolescent newly diagnosed with schizophrenia would find it extremely difficult to tease out which interventions might be helpful and, of these, which might be a cost-effective use of available resources. Adolescents continue, as before, to fall between child and adult services in terms of service provision (National Institute of Clinical Excellence, 2002). Perhaps mental health initiatives, building on the continuing outcomes of early intervention programs, can shape devoted services, targeted at problems that beset adolescents with schizophrenia by virtue of their developmental stage, that are designed specifically for young minds and hearts.

ILLICIT DRUG USE

Though many illicit substances are used by individuals with psychosis, this account will be limited to cannabis, which is by far the most common illicit substance used by adolescents.

Treatment

There is much evidence to suggest that cannabis consumption among those already schizophrenic has a detrimental effect, though the strength of this effect is not yet certain (Johns, 2001). There is less evidence concerning what can be done about it.

Prevention

Zammit et al. (2002) conducted an analysis of the Swedish conscript data for 1969–1970 (>97% of the country's male population ages 18–20). They separated the cohort into those with psychosis onset more than or less than 5 years after data collection to rule out the possibility of prodrome at the time of conscription. They found a significant dose-related relationship between cannabis and increased risk of developing schizophrenia, strongest in those who had onset of psychosis within 5 years of conscription and present in both those who used cannabis alone and cannabis with other drugs. Similar results were obtained when only those with onset of more than 5 years were analyzed. However, this study could not determine whether cannabis use in adolescence was as a result of preexisting psychotic symptomatology rather than a cause in itself for psychosis. This issue was addressed by the Dunedin study (Arseneault et al., 2004), a longitudinal, prospective study that allowed assessment of preexisting psychotic symptoms at age 11, drug use at 15 and 18 years of age, and psychiatric outcome measures at 26 years. This study showed that adolescents who used cannabis at 15 and 18 years of age had significantly more symptoms of schizophrenia than controls at 26 years of age. Furthermore, these results remained significant when quasi-psychotic symptoms at 11 years were controlled for. Use of cannabis at 15 years increased adult risk of schizophreniform disorder by a factor of four, though these results did not remain significant when psychotic symptoms at age 11 were controlled for.

Thus, cannabis use, especially earlier in life, increases the risk of schizophrenia symptoms. This effect is not explained by use secondary to psychosis, and this effect appears to be specific to cannabis use. Though cannabis is not thought to be necessary or sufficient to cause the onset of psychosis, it was estimated that 8% of schizophrenia cases in New Zealand could be prevented by the cessation of use in the general population (Arsenault et al., 2003).

Therefore, as well as discouraging the legalization and supply of cannabis, mental health initiatives are needed to educate adolescents on the previously unrecognized risks of cannabis misuse. Potentially, such initiatives could occur concurrently with the campaigns already implemented by early intervention services.

PHARMACOLOGICAL MANAGEMENT

As noted in Chapter 5, schizophrenia is a severe mental illness characterized by abnormalities of thought and perception that affects about 1% of the population worldwide over the course of a lifetime (Bourdon et al., 1992; Eaton, 1985; Hare, 1987; Helgason, 1964; Jablensky, 1986; Kramer, 1969; Robins et al., 1984). The optimal time to treat this illness with the currently available therapeutic agents is as early in the course and as close to the onset as possible. Often the onset of the illness precedes, by a considerable period of time, the manifestation of symptoms that are diagnosable at the syndromal level. As also summarized in Chapter 5, the onset of the formal symptoms of schizophrenia is generally preceded by a prodromal phase. So-called prodromal symptoms and behaviors (i.e., those that herald the approaching onset of the illness) include attenuated positive symptoms (e.g., illusions, ideas of reference, magical thinking, superstitiousness), mood symptoms (e.g., anxiety, dysphoria, irritability), cognitive symptoms (e.g., distractibility, concentration difficulties), social withdrawal, or obsessive behaviors, to name a few (McGlashan, 1996; Yung & McGorry, 1996). Because many of these prodromal phenomena extensively overlap with the range of mental experiences and behaviors of persons in the ages of risk who do not subsequently develop schizophrenia, prodromal symptoms cannot be considered diagnostic. It is precisely their nonspecificity and lack of high predictive validity that limits their utility for the purposes of early intervention (Gottesman & Erlenmeyer-Kimling, 2001; Schaffner & McGorry, 2001).

The development of frank psychotic symptoms marks the formal onset of first-episode schizophrenia, although this is usually not diagnosed for some time until the patient seeks or is brought to medical attention. Indeed, the duration of psychotic symptoms prior to diagnosis and treatment averages about 1 year, and if time since prodromal symptoms first appeared is considered, the average duration is about 3 years (McGlashan, 1996). Despite this, most individuals recover symptomatically from the first episode. However, the majority of patients proceed to have one or more subsequent episodes in the form of psychotic relapses, from which some proportion fail to recover, at least to the same degree as they had during their first or prior episode (Lieberman et al., 1993, 1996; Robinson et al., 1999a). This process of psychotic relapses, treatment failure, and incomplete recovery leads many patients to a chronic course of illness. Finally, persistent disturbances and deficits in perceptions, thought processes, and cognition affect development (Lieberman, 1999; McGlashan, 1988). In this way, patients accumulate morbidity in the form of residual or persistent symptoms and decrements in function from their premorbid status.

The process of accruing morbidity in the context of exacerbations and (relative) remissions has been attributed to progression of the illness (Kraepelin, 1919) and described as "clinical deterioration" (Bleuler, 1980). Interestingly, the deterioration process predominantly occurs in the early phases of the illness, in the prepsychotic prodromal period and during the first 5 to 10 years after the initial episode. For these reasons early intervention is highly indicated. In this context treatment serves two purposes: first, it is remedial for active symptoms of whatever level of severity or syndromal criteria; second, it may be preventive of the deterioration that can occur and is the most devastating consequence of the illness.

However, there are several challenges for treating patients optimally in the earliest stages of schizophrenia:

1. Patients usually do not seek (or are brought in for) treatment until they have had the symptoms for often lengthy periods of time.
2. The symptoms that identify persons in the prodromal stage and at imminent risk for psychosis are not highly specific or sufficiently validated to use in clinical practice.
3. The optimal treatment agents and strategies for prodromal patients have not been determined.
4. Patients in the prodromal stages and experiencing first episodes of schizophrenia are reluctant to take medications for sustained periods of time, as they have limited insight into the nature of their illness and are sensitive to, and object to, side effects.

Acute Treatment

There have been relatively few studies on first-episode schizophrenia and very few on patients in the prodromal phase. There are currently two published studies that used controlled or standardized acute treatment of patients with prodromal symptoms of schizophrenia and eight published studies that used controlled or standardized acute treatment of patients with first-episode schizophrenia (Tables 6.1 and 6.2; Emsley, 1999; Kopala et al., 1996; Lieberman et al., 1993; May et al., 1976; Sanger et al., 1999; Scottish Schizophrenia Research Group, 1987; Szymanski et al., 1994). From these data, as well as the results of some uncontrolled studies and secondary analyses, several principles can be derived to provide guidance for the treatment of patients experiencing a first episode of schizophrenia and also for future research to improve the standard of care for this critical stage of psychotic disorders. With such limited data regarding the management of prodromal and first-episode schizophrenia, practice is guided by a hybrid of clinical trials evidence, real-life studies, and clinical experience.

Dosing and Selection of Pharmacological Agents for Early Stages of Schizophrenia

The pharmacology of treating the prodromal stages of schizophrenia and related psychotic disorders has not been sufficiently well developed. Many agents have been suggested (by theories of pathogenesis) as preventive agents for schizophrenia to be used in the prodromal stage. These include a wide variety of treatments: antioxidants, benzodiazepines, phospholipids, lithium and mood stabilizers, antidepressants, glutamatergic and nicotinic agents, selective DRD 1, 3, 4 dopamine receptor antagonists, and antipsychotic drugs. For both prodromal and first-episode patients, if an antipsychotic drug is to be used, the general consensus is that this be one of the second-generation antipsychotics (Addington 2002; Bhana et al., 2001; Bustillo, Lauriello, & Keith, 1999; Green & Schildkraut, 1995; Lieberman, 1996; NICE, 2002; Sartorius et al., 2002).

Table 6.1 Studies of Acute Treatment in Prodromal Stages of Schizophrenia

Reference	*Population*	*Inclusion/Exclusion*	*Design/Protocol*	*Response Criteria*	*Response Rates*
McGorry et al., 2002	59 patients at incipient risk of progression to first-episode psychosis ("high risk")	Age 14–30, living in Melbourne metropolitan area, meets criteria for 1 or more of 3 operationally defined "high-risk" categories	Single-blind RCT with blinded interviews. Subjects were randomized to need-based intervention (based on presenting or existing problems) and specific preventive intervention, which included 1–2 mg risperidone and a modified CBT.	Progression to psychosis at 6 months (post-intervention) and 12 months (follow-up) after study entry, defined by a predetermined threshold of positive symptoms sustained for 1 week or more (based on Brief Psychiatric Rating Scale and comprehensive assessment of symptoms and history)	Needs-based intervention: 36% postintervention, 36% at 12 months; specific prevention intervention: 10% postintervention, 19% at 12 months
Woods et al., 2002	60 patients from four North American centers diagnosed using the Structured Interview for Prodromal Symptoms	Not available in published abstract	Randomized to 5–15 mg/day olanzapine or placebo	Scale of Prodromal Symptoms score at 8 weeks; weight gain	Olanzapine: least squares Scale of Prodromal Symptoms score mean = −14.0 ± 3.3 versus −2.1 ± 3.4. Olanzapine patients gained significantly more weight (p = .001).

Currently, there are no specific guidelines or sufficient evidence to determine which second-generation antipsychotic to use. Side effects are the primary distinguishing features among the various drugs.

Young patients without prior exposure to antipsychotic drugs may be more sensitive to the antipsychotic side effects than patients in other stages of the illness. In a sample of 70 treatment-naïve patients who received fluphenazine at 20 to 40 mg/day for the first 10 weeks of treatment, 34% developed parkinsonism, 18% developed akathisia, and 36% developed dystonia (Chakos et al., 1992). Lower doses of antipsychotics may be adequate to achieve remission of positive symptoms but less likely to cause side effects (Cullberg, 1999; Zhang-Wong et al., 1999). For example, in a post hoc analysis, low-dose risperidone (maximum of 6 mg/day or less) was more effective and better tolerated than high-dose risperidone (maximum of more than 6 mg/day; Emsley, 1999). Another study of 49 acutely psychotic, neuroleptic-naïve patients with schizophrenia, schizophreniform disorder, or schizoaffective disorder treated with either 2 mg or 4 mg daily of risperidone showed the two doses to be comparable in efficacy, with an advantage for the lower dose in fine motor functioning (Merlo et al., 2002).

Table 6.2 Studies of Acute Treatment in First-Episode Schizophrenia

Reference	*Population*	*Inclusion/Exclusion*	*Design/Protocol*	*Response Criteria*	*Response Rates*
May et al., 1976	228 patients selected from consecutive admissions to a state psychiatric hospital between 1959 and 1962	Inclusions: First-admission patients with a diagnosis of schizophrenia and "no significant prior treatment." Exclusions: Those who were judged unlikely to be discharged and those who remitted fairly quickly (within 18 days).	Randomization to either individual psychotherapy, trifluoperazine, psychotherapy in combination with trifluoperazine, electroconvulsive therapy, or milieu therapy only	Release from the hospital after a "fair trial" (6–12 months) of the assigned treatment	Individual psychotherapy (65%), trifluoperazine (96%), psychotherapy in combination with trifluoperazine (95%), electroconvulsive therapy (79%), and milieu therapy only (58%)
Scottish Schizophrenia Research Group, 1987	46 patients with first-episode schizophrenia admitted to the hospital	Inclusion: Diagnosis of first-episode criteria on the clinician's *International Classification of Diseases*, Ninth Revision	5-week, double-blind, randomized trial of flupenthixol versus pimozide. Adjunctive medications allowed.	"Responders": able to enter maintenance treatment on their assigned drug therapy. "Nonresponders": those who received further treatment, either electroconvulsive treatment or another antipsychotic. "Noncompleters": those who did not proceed to maintenance therapy but were not clearly "nonresponders."	63% were "responders" overall. Positive symptoms improved significantly ($p < .01$) for both drug groups during the study period, but negative symptoms did not change.
Lieberman et al., 1993; Robinson et al., 1999	70 Research Diagnostic Criteria (RDC)-diagnosed patients with schizophrenia (N = 54) and schizoaffective disorder (N = 16)	1. No prior psychotic episodes 2. Age 16–40 3. No history of neurological or general medical illness that could influence diagnosis or the biological variables being studied	Open, prospective study using a standardized antipsychotic protocol of sequential trials until response criteria were met of fluphenazine, haloperidol, molindone, and clozapine.	Operationally defined as a Clinical Global Impression (CGI) rating of "much" or "very much" improved and a rating of mild or less on specified Schedule for Affective Disorders and Schizophrenia SADS — Change Version With Psychosis and Disorganization Items rating scale (SADS-C+ PDI) items with response sustained for at least 8 weeks	83% of the patients remitted by 1 year, with mean and median times to remission of 35.7 weeks and 11 weeks, respectively.

Szymanski et al., 1994	10 patients in the Lieberman et al. (1993) study	Patients in the above study who had failed to respond to treatment with a standardized protocol of 3 typical antipsychotics	After a 2-week washout period, patients were treated for 12 weeks on clozapine.	20% reduction in their Brief Psychiatric Rating Scale (BPRS) score and a CGI Severity of Illness score of 3 or less	30% (3/10)
Kopala et al., 1996	22 neuroleptic-naïve patients consecutively admitted for the first time. Mean age = 25 years.	DSM-IV diagnosis of a first episode of schizophrenia	Open trial of risperidone monotherapy for a mean duration of treatment of 7.1 weeks (SD = 3.2, range 1.8–14.1). Benztropine for extrapyramidal symptoms and lorazepam or clonazepam for insomnia were the only adjunctives allowed.	20% reduction in the total Positive and Negative Syndrome Scale (PANSS) score	59%; negative symptoms improved less than positive symptoms.
Sanger et al., 1999	83 first-episode patients out of 1,996 patients who were enrolled in a multicenter trial of olanzapine versus haloperidol in psychotic disorders	1. First episode of psychosis with a DSM-II-R diagnosis of schizophrenia, schizophreniform disorder, or schizoaffective disorder 2. Duration of episode of less than 5 years 3. No more than 45 years old at their episode onset 4. Minimum BPRS score of 18 or intolerant to current antipsychotic therapy	6-week, double-blind, randomized trial of olanzapine (N = 59) or haloperidol (N = 24) at mean modal doses of 11.6 (SD = 5.9) and 10.8 (SD = 4.8) mg/day, respectively	Defined a priori as a 40% or greater reduction in total BPRS from baseline, also calculated for a 20% reduction	40% BPRS reduction in total BPRS: olanzapine 67.2% response rate, haloperidol 29.2% (Fisher's exact p = .003). 20% BPRS reduction: olanzapine 82.8% response rate, haloperidol 58.3% (Fisher's exact p = .03).
Emsley et al., 1999	183 patients recruited in multiple international sites	1. Ages 15–40 2. Diagnosis of provisional schizophreniform disorder or schizophrenia according to DSM-III-R 3. No prior treatment beyond 3 days of emergency antipsychotics 4. No clinically relevant medical abnormalities	6-week, double-blind study of risperidone versus haloperidol 2–16 mg/day. Antiparkinsonian drugs or benzodiazepines administered only if essential.	A 50% improvement in total PANSS score was defined a priori as clinical response.	Risperidone 63% response; haloperidol 56% response

(*continued*)

Table 6.2 Continued

Reference	*Population*	*Inclusion/Exclusion*	*Design/Protocol*	*Response Criteria*	*Response Rates*
Yap et al., 2001	24 patients recruited from Woodbridge Hospital and Geylang Psychiatric Outpatient Clinic	Previously untreated male and female patients aged 18–65 with DSM-IV schizophreniform disorder or DSM-IV schizophrenia for no longer than 12 months	Open-label, 8-week study of risperidone	20% reduction in total PANSS score; response for 50% reduction in total PANSS score was also calculated.	The responder rate (> or = 20% reduction in the total PANSS score) was 87.5%. 13 patients (54.2%) exhibited a 50% or greater reduction in total PANSS score.
Lieberman et al., 2003	160 Chinese patients with a first episode of schizophrenia	1. Ages 16–45 2. Diagnosis of provisional schizophreniform disorder or schizophrenia according to DSM-IV 3. No prior antipsychotic treatment 4. No clinically relevant medical abnormalities	52-week, double-blind RCT of clozapine and chlorpromazine and trihexyphenidyl.		
Lieberman et al., 2003	263 patients recruited from 14 sites in North America and Western Europe	1. Ages 16–40 2. Diagnosis of provisional schizophreniform disorder, schizophrenia, or schizoaffective disorder according to DSM-IV 3. Prior lifetime treatment < 16 weeks 4. No clinically relevant medical abnormalities	12-week, acute treatment results of 2-year double-blind RCT of olanzapine (5–15 mg/day) and haloperidol (2–20 mg/day). Antiparkinsonian drugs or benzodiazepines administered only if essential.	Total PANSS response defined as 30% reduction of PANSS and CGI severity < 4 (moderately ill)	Significantly greater reduction in total PANSS and PANSS Negative Scale with olanzapine on mixed models but not last observation carried forward (LOCF) analysis. 55% of olanzapine and 46% of haloperidol patients met response criteria by week 12.

The greater sensitivity to side effects of first-episode patients compared to chronic patients was dramatically demonstrated by McEvoy et al. (1991) in comparing their neuroleptic thresholds for extrapyramidal symptoms. In the context of a gradual dose titration paradigm, first-episode patients exhibited lower thresholds to develop signs of extrapyramidal symptoms than previously treated, more chronic patients. Younger patients are also more susceptible to other side effects such as weight gain (Kumra et al., 1998; Lieberman et al., 2003).

Consistent with these studies, the Schizophrenia Patient Outcomes Research Team recommended that patients in a first psychotic episode should be treated with relatively lower doses (300–500 mg chlorpromazine equivalents per day) of antipsychotics than for patients with schizophrenia in general (300–1,000 mg chlorpromazine equivalents per day; Lehman & Steinwachs, 1998). Clinical experience and available research findings suggest that lower doses of antipsychotics are as effective as higher doses in patients experiencing a first episode of schizophrenia, with superior tolerability.

Since the first episode is a time when patients form their attitudes about treatment, efforts to minimize unpleasant side effects may influence the patient's willingness to take medications long term. In a study of first-episode patients, the only variable that predicted whether patients would attend a follow-up assessment was antipsychotic dose, with those on higher doses less likely to comply (Jackson et al., 2001).

Treatment of Positive Symptoms

Available data indicate that in prodromal and first-episode patients, positive symptoms, including hallucinations and delusions, will usually remit with antipsychotic treatment. Thus, clinicians should expect remission of positive symptoms in these patients. A series of adequate trials of available agents should be employed with this goal in mind. If residual symptoms persist, a trial of clozapine or the addition of adjunctive treatments should be considered.

Treatment of Negative and Cognitive Symptoms

While positive symptoms in first-episode patients tend to respond well to antipsychotic treatment, negative and cognitive symptoms generally take longer to respond or are less responsive to antipsychotics (Kopala et al., 1996; Sanger et al., 1999; Scottish Schizophrenia Research Group, 1987). This indicates that negative and cognitive symptoms may have a different time course for response than positive symptoms, or that the relative refractoriness of negative and cognitive symptoms may contribute to the less-than-optimal functional recovery often observed in first-episode patients. Improving treatments for negative and cognitive symptoms in the first episode of schizophrenia is an area of major importance in future research and drug development efforts, especially since these symptoms likely affect these patients' functional abilities.

Adjunctive Treatments of Residual Symptoms and Comorbid Syndromes

Often antipsychotics are insufficient by themselves to achieve full symptom remission and functional recovery in early-stage schizophrenia patients. For these reasons, a variety of adjunctive treatments, both pharmacological and nonpharmacological, can be used to enhance and optimize treatment response. Adjunctive treatments have different roles in the management of first-episode schizophrenia, targeting residual symptoms and treating comorbid syndromes. A clinical approach to treatment-refractory, first-episode schizophrenia, as described in a manual on first-episode schizophrenia should include strategies that promote medication adherence, attention to substance abuse, sequential trials of antipsychotic agents, or dose adjustment if clinical improvement is not seen by 6 to 12 weeks of treatment, and consideration of clozapine even early in the course of treatment (Edwards & McGorry, 2002).

While not yet systematically studied in prodromal or first-episode patients, data from studies in chronic patients suggest that cognitive therapy also may benefit residual symptoms

(Cormac, Jones, & Campbell, 2002). Even given the lack of specific trials in first-episode patients, it is likely that CBT may have a role in the treatment of prodromal and first-episode schizophrenia, especially in helping patients to comply with treatment and the transition to outpatient care.

Adjunctive treatments that have been studied in the treatment of schizophrenia include benzodiazepines, anticonvulsants, and antidepressants. Benzodiazepines are often used as adjuncts to antipsychotics in acute schizophrenia. There have been no controlled studies of benzodiazepines in groups of first-episode patients with schizophrenia. Literature on mixed populations of patients with schizophrenia suggest overall that benzodiazepines have a role in treating agitation, anxiety, and aggression in patients with acute psychosis (Barbee et al., 1992; Battaglia et al., 1997; Kellner et al., 1975; Salzman et al., 1991) and in preventing an impending psychotic relapse (Carpenter et al., 1999).

Mood stabilizers, including anticonvulsants and lithium, are widely used in patients with schizophrenia (Citrome, Levine, & Allingham, 2000), and there is some evidence that they may also have a role in reducing aggression and agitation (Christison, Kirch, & Wyatt, 1991; Ko et al., 1985; Leucht et al., 2002; Linnoila & Viukari, 1979; Wassef et al., 2000). Although there is no evidence as to their efficacy in early-stage patients, mood stabilizers should be considered for patients who have mood symptoms of excitement and mood lability during residual to the prodromal and first episodes of schizophrenia.

Depressive syndromes are common in prodromal and first-episode patients. Patients who ultimately manifest symptoms of schizophrenia often report a previous depressive episode (Hafner et al., 1999) or suicide attempt in their prodromal period (Cohen et al., 1994). On presentation with an acute psychotic episode, first-episode patients often have mood symptoms (Addington, Addington, & Patten, 1998). Depressive symptoms will often resolve as psychotic symptoms remit (Koreen et al., 1993); however, in some cases they may persist or occur in the episode's aftermath (postpsychotic depression). Antidepressants should be used cautiously in prodromal and first-episode schizophrenia patients as they could provoke or exacerbate psychotic symptoms. In addition, negative symptoms that persist after the stabilization of the acute episode may respond to antidepressant treatment (Berk, Ichim, & Brook, 2001; Hogarty et al., 1995; Silver & Nassar, 1992; Silver et al., 2000).

Suicidal behavior can occur in prodromal and first-episode schizophrenia patients (Steinert, Wiebe, & Gebhardt, 1999). While depression in the presenting psychotic episode or in the postpsychotic period is an important risk factor for suicide (Axelsson & Lagerkvist-Briggs, 1992), prodromal and first-episode patients may attempt suicide in the absence of prominent depressive symptoms as a result of hallucinations, paranoia, disorganization, or other symptoms considered more primary to psychosis or other factors. Some literature supports the use of clozapine (Meltzer & Okayli, 1995; Meltzer et al., 2003; Reid, Mason, & Hogan, 1998; Sernyak et al., 2001) in patients with psychotic disorder and suicidal behaviors. Though its use in first-episode schizophrenia has been studied (Lieberman, 2003), clozapine is not considered at this time as a first-line drug for first-episode schizophrenia. It should be considered early in the course of treatment only in patients who are unresponsive to other second-generation antipsychotics.

Another important comorbid syndrome in the treatment of first-episode schizophrenia is substance abuse, with its possible role in lowering initial vulnerability to the onset or recurrence of psychosis (Chouljian et al., 1995; DeQuardo, Carpenter, & Tandon, 1994; Gupta et al., 1996; Hambrecht & Hafner, 2000; Linszen, Dingemans, & Lenior, 1994; Rabinowitz et al., 1998). Thorough evaluations of substance abuse habits in prodromal and first-episode schizophrenia patients are critical to directing appropriate clinical attention to this issue throughout care of the patient.

Treatment After Symptom Remission

As the symptomatic response to treatment of young early-stage patients is generally very good, clinicians should expect and aim for achieving maximal remission of symptoms, recognizing that psychosis may resolve first and then negative and cognitive symptoms. Residual symptoms should be targeted with adjunctive therapies as needed.

After achieving optimal treatment response, the next goal of treatment is to maximize the functional recovery of patients. To some extent this depends on the resolution of symptoms, but it may not necessarily occur fully concurrent with symptom remission. Maximizing functional recovery involves the use of adjunctive pharmacological treatments for any residual symptoms and then various nonpharmacological treatments to enhance functional recovery. These may include psychoeducation about the nature of the illness, supportive psychotherapy, supported employment, social and vocational rehabilitation, and case management. We think of many of these psychosocial interventions as being associated with the care of chronic patients; however, they can and should also be adapted to young early-stage patients. Clinicians must be patient and not rush patients prematurely into the activities with which they may have been previously engaged.

The need for interventions aimed at achieving functional recovery is reflected by the results of outcome studies in first-episode patients. While patients typically recover from a first episode of schizophrenia, the long-term course for most patients is still characterized by chronic illness, disability, and relapse. Studies report that a minority of patients, about 15% to 20%, will maintain good symptomatic and functional recovery from a first episode. For example, in a study of 349 patients followed up to 15 years after their first onset of schizophrenia, 17% had no disability at follow-up, while 24% still had severe disability, and the remaining 69% had varying degrees of disability (Wiersma et al., 1998, 2000). The long-term prognosis of patients in the pre-antipsychotic era was similar, with about 20% of patients having good symptomatic and functional recovery (Bleuler, 1978). In a study of first-episode patients with operationally defined criteria for recovery (a period of 2 years of remission of positive and negative symptoms, fulfillment of age-appropriate role expectations, performance of daily living tasks without supervision, and engagement in social interactions), 16.8% of the 118 patients achieved full functional recovery (Robinson et al., 1999b). However, a study of 1,633 patients with psychotic disorders from diverse cultures found more optimistic rates of favorable outcome, with nearly half of the patients with schizophrenia considered to be recovered (Harrison et al., 2001).

The next question in the clinical management of prodromal and first-episode patients is after achieving maximal therapeutic response, how long treatment (particularly pharmacological treatment) should be continued. There are not sufficient data to answer that question in prodromal patients. Thus, treatment of prodromal symptoms should be considered as time-limited and aimed at alleviating current symptoms and stabilizing the patient. On the other hand, a growing body of evidence in first-episode patients suggests the value of continuing medication for a sustained and possibly indefinite period. Ideally, this decision would be informed by data from prospective, controlled studies answering the following questions:

1. How likely is relapse with and without antipsychotic medication?
2. Is it possible to predict who will relapse after remission of a first episode?
3. Will antipsychotic therapy improve the course and long-term outcome of the illness or merely suppress symptoms in the short to medium term?

Table 6.3 summarizes six controlled studies of maintenance antipsychotic treatment of remitted first-episode schizophrenia (Crow et al., 1986; Gitlin et al., 2001; Kane et al., 1982; McCreadie et al., 1989; Nuechterlein et al., 1994).

The risk of eventual relapse after recovery from a first psychotic episode is very high and is greatly diminished by maintenance antipsychotic treatment. However, even with strong evidence of the risk of relapse without antipsychotic medication, there is still no clear

Table 6.3 Studies of Maintenance Treatment in First-Episode Schizophrenia

Reference	*Population*	*Inclusion/Exclusion*	*Design/Protocol*	*Relapse Criteria*	*Relapse Rates*
Kane et al., 1982	28 patients referred for aftercare with a diagnosis of a single episode of schizophrenia; 19 of the 28 patients met Research Diagnostic Criteria (RDC) for schizophrenia.	1. At least 4 weeks of remission 2. 1 year or less since hospitalization 3. No treatment prior to 3 months before hospitalization 4. No evidence of drug abuse, alcoholism, or important medical illness	Double-blind, 1-year duration. Random assignment to fluphenazine hydrochloride (5–20 mg/day), fluphenazine decanoate (12.5–50 mg/2 weeks), or placebo. Only patients thought to have possible compliance problems were randomized to decanoate. Procyclidine hydrochloride for all patients, with substitution of placebo in 2nd month for the placebo patients.	Substantial clinical deterioration with a potential for marked social impairment. Patients considered dropouts only if they showed no clinical deterioration at the time they left the study.	For all patients: 0% (0/11) on fluphenazine and 41% (7/17) on placebo relapsed. Of those with RDC schizophrenia: 0% (0/6) on fluphenazine and 46% (6/13) on placebo relapsed. Follow-up with 26 patients (mean interval of 3.5 years): 69% had a 2nd relapse; 54% had a 3rd relapse.
Crow et al., 1986	120 patients diagnosed with first-episode schizophrenia recruited from both psychiatric and district general practices in Harrow, England	1. Age 15–70 2. Suffering from a first psychotic episode that was "not unequivocally affective" 3. Admission to an inpatient psychiatric unit for at least 1 week 4. Clinical diagnosis of schizophrenia 5. Absence of organic disease of probable etiological significance	Drugs (fluphenthixol [40 mg/ month intramuscularly], chlorpromazine [200 mg/day orally], haloperidol [3 mg/day orally], pimozide [4 mg/day], or trifluoperazine [5 mg/day]) chosen by clinicians, then patients randomized to either drug or placebo 1 month after remission of their initial episode. Adjunctive medications allowed.	Psychiatric readmission for any reason; readmission deemed necessary by treating clinician, but not possible; or active antipsychotic medication considered to be essential because of features of imminent relapse. Relapse determinations made by treating clinicians.	Actuarial relapse rates: 6 months, placebo 43% vs. drug 21%; 12 months, placebo 63% vs. drug 38%; 18 months, placebo 67% vs. drug 46%; 24 months, placebo 70% vs. drug 58%
Scottish Schizophrenia Research Group, 1989	15 patients who had suffered a first episode of schizophrenia	Patients had to respond to acute treatment and then be relapse-free for an additional year of treatment on either once-weekly pimozide or intramuscular fluphenthixol decanoate.	Double-blind trial of active medication (either once-weekly pimozide or intramuscular fluphenthixol decanoate) or placebo for 1 year	Deterioration in schizophrenia symptoms or behavior sufficient to warrant the patient's withdrawal from the study	0% (0/8) of the patients who received active drug but 57% (4/7) of those who received placebo were readmitted in the second year of the study treatment.

Nuechterlein et al., 1994	106 patients from four public hospitals and an outpatient clinic of an academic medical center. 66% had never taken antipsychotic medication, and the remainder had a mean duration of treatment of 2.7 months (SD = 3.1)	Inclusion: Recent-onset psychotic symptoms lasting at least 2 weeks and not more than 2 years, age 18–45 years, and RDC diagnosis of schizophrenia or schizoaffective disorder (mainly schizophrenia). Exclusions: Known neurological disorder, recent significant substance abuse, or African-American descent*	Phase I: Stabilized patients were treated with 12.5 mg fluphenazine decanoate every 2 weeks for 12 months. Phase II: Those who remitted in Phase I were recruited into Phase II, where they were treated for 12 weeks with either placebo or fluphenazine, followed by crossover to the opposite treatment.	Operationally defined as: a two-point worsening on any three Brief Psychiatric Rating Scale (BPRS) psychotic items, excluding changes where the scores remained at nonpsychotic levels; a score of 6 or 7 was obtained on any three items; or clinical deterioration warranting a change in treatment as judged by treating psychiatrist	Phase I: 11 patients needed to have their dose lowered due to side effects and 6 were prescribed antidepressants. Phase II: 6% (3/53 subjects) had a relapse while on active medication and 13% (7/53) relapsed on placebo.
Robinson et al., 1999	104 patients who responded to treatment of their index episode of schizophrenia and were at risk for relapse	1. RDC-defined diagnosis of schizophrenia or schizoaffective disorder 2. Total lifetime exposure to antipsychotic medications of 12 weeks or less 3. Rating of 4 (moderate) or more on at least 1 psychotic symptom item on the Schedule for Affective Disorders and Schizophrenia SADS —Change Version With Psychosis and Disorganization Items rating scale (SADS-C + PDI)	Patients were treated openly according to a standard algorithm, progressing from one phase of the algorithm to the next until they met response criteria. The sequence was initial treatment with fluphenazine, then haloperidol, then lithium augmentation, then molindone hydrochloride or loxapine, then clozapine.	At least "moderately ill" on the Clinical Global Impression (CGI) Severity of Illness Scale, "much worse" or "very much worse" on the CGI Improvement Scale, and at least "moderate" on 1 or more of the SADS-C+PD psychosis items listed above; these criteria had to be sustained for at least 1 week.	5-year overall relapse rate- 81.9%. By 4 years after recovery from a 2nd relapse, the cumulative 3rd relapse rate was 86.2%. Discontinuing antipsychotic drug therapy increased the risk of relapse by almost 5 times.

(*continued*)

Table 6.3 Continued

Reference	*Population*	*Inclusion/Exclusion*	*Design/Protocol*	*Relapse Criteria*	*Relapse Rates*
		4. No medical contraindications to treatment with antipsychotic medications 5. No neurological or endocrine disorder or neuromedical illness that could affect diagnosis or the biological variables in the study			
Gitlin et al., 2001	53 patients with RDC schizophrenia or schizoaffective disorder who had been stabilized for 1 year on fluphenazine decanoate	Patients who completed Phase II of the Nuechterlein et al. study above and did not relapse	Open-label discontinuation of drugs	Two-point worsening on any three BPRS psychotic items, excluding changes where the scores remained at nonpsychotic levels, a score of 6 or 7 was obtained on any 3 items, or the treating psychiatrist deemed that there was a clinical deterioration warranting a change in treatment	78% relapsed by 1 year and 96% by 2 years with a low threshold for relapse. Only 13% required hospitalization.

*Excluded because of differences in electrodermal conductivity from other groups since this was a biological variable being studied.

consensus on the recommended duration of treatment for patients who have recovered from a first episode of schizophrenia. Clinicians may have a difficult time convincing patients who have recovered from one episode of schizophrenia that indefinite and possibly lifelong antipsychotic treatment is indicated because of (1) the diagnostic uncertainty and instability associated with a first psychotic episode (Amin et al., 1999), (2) limited patient understanding and awareness of the illness (Thompson, McGorry, & Harrigan, 2001), and (3) the risks of long-term antipsychotic therapy. Most practice guidelines for the treatment of patients with schizophrenia recommend that patients who have had only one episode of positive symptoms and have been symptom-free during the subsequent year of maintenance therapy can be considered for a trial period without medication, provided that dose reductions are made gradually over several months with frequent visits (Rose, 1997). Similarly, the Schizophrenia Patient Outcomes Research Team (Lehman & Steinwachs, 1998) recommended in their report that patients should continue treatment for at least 1 year after remission of acute symptoms, with continual reassessment of the maintenance dose for possible reduction. The draft consensus statement of 26 international consultants (Addington, 2002) recommends taking into consideration the severity of the first episode when deciding how long to continue maintenance treatment. They suggest that patients who achieve full remission be offered gradual withdrawal of medication after 12 months of maintenance treatment, but patients who experienced more severe episodes and who are slow to respond be maintained on medication for 24 months. This panel further suggests that patients who respond incompletely to medication but clearly benefit from treatment be maintained for 2 to 5 years on medication.

Conclusion

Patients in the prodromal phase or first episode of schizophrenia respond very favorably to antipsychotic treatment in terms of their positive symptoms. However, cognitive and negative symptoms are often slower to respond or refractory to treatment, leaving many of these individuals with significant social disability. Sequential trials of adequate dose and duration of antipsychotics and adjunctive treatments should be employed to help patients achieve their optimal response. Psychosocial therapies such as CBT and education groups may be helpful in addressing residual symptoms and helping patients to adhere to their medication regimens.

In addition to lessening the morbidity of the presenting episode, early intervention in prodromal and first-episode schizophrenia may improve the long-term course of the disorder, as evidenced by studies showing an inverse correlation between the duration of untreated psychosis and outcome. The outcome of schizophrenia is variable, and despite a large literature, we know relatively little about the predictors of outcome. Duration of untreated illness in various studies also varies widely, ranging between 22 and 166.4 weeks (Norman & Malla, 2001). Several studies have suggested that prolonged duration of untreated illness may predict poor outcome, as evidenced by longer time to and level of remission. Based on such findings, it has been suggested that decreasing the duration of untreated illness, perhaps by early identification and intervention, might lead to a more favorable outcome. It has also been argued that prolonged untreated illness might be causally related to poor outcomes, perhaps as a result of a neurotoxic process. However, controversy has shrouded this literature, as some studies have not found an association between the duration of untreated illness and outcome.

Prevention of schizophrenia through presymptomatic treatment is an exciting possibility, but future research is needed to develop the methodology by which to reliably identify those at risk before this strategy can become part of routine clinical practice. Once remission from the first episode is reached, maintenance with antipsychotic treatment is indicated for at least 1 year. The overwhelming majority of individuals who do not remain on antipsychotic therapy eventually experience a relapse. This raises the question of the optimal length of continuation and maintenance treatment for patients who have recovered from a first episode of schizophrenia or related psychosis. Clinically useful predictors of the small minority who maintain remission without pharmacotherapy have not yet been identified.

Atypical antipsychotics represent an advance in the treatment of first-episode schizophrenia, with strong evidence for greater tolerability with equal or better therapeutic efficacy. While future research will help to characterize their efficacy relative to one another and define the effect of their use on the long-term outcomes of schizophrenia, available evidence and consensus expert opinion support their use as first-line treatment in first-episode schizophrenia.

Prevention of Schizophrenia

Raquel E. Gur
Ruben C. Gur
Matcheri S. Keshavan
Christian Kohler
Elaine Walker

chapter 7

OVERVIEW

There are currently recognized precursors of schizophrenia that are apparent during adolescence. A wide variety of early intervention techniques have been developed that draw on the knowledge of these precursors to identify individuals at risk for the illness and to prevent the predisposition toward schizophrenia from developing into the full disorder. Most of the research that enabled the identification of these precursors and the development of these intervention techniques was performed retrospectively in adults with schizophrenia, with little specific research attention directed toward forms of schizophrenia that manifest during adolescence. In addition, prevention efforts have necessarily lagged behind studies of the risk factors, detection, and early intervention of the disease. Yet a great deal has already been learned about risk-profiling and early intervention in schizophrenia generally, and those aspects that may be useful in understanding the adolescent forms of the illness are discussed below.

Traditionally, prevention efforts have been classified into three levels: (1) primary prevention, which is practiced prior to the onset of the disease, (2) secondary prevention, which is practiced after the disease is recognized but before it has caused suffering and disability, and (3) tertiary prevention, which is practiced after suffering or disability has been experienced, in order to prevent further deterioration. This classification scheme is attractive and simple, but it does not distinguish between preventive interventions that have different epidemiological justifications and require different strategies for optimal utilization. For example, it focuses on intended outcomes rather than on target populations or prevention strategies.

The terms *universal, selective*, and *indicated* have been adopted as a valuable way to distinguish preventive interventions. All three of these strategies refer to the target population. Universal preventive interventions are applied to whole populations and aim at reducing risk and promoting protective factors. Because obstetric complications have been linked to the subsequent onset of schizophrenia in several studies (Zornberg et al., 2000), one potentially effective universal prevention strategy would be to focus on lowering the incidence of such complications through improved prenatal, perinatal, and postnatal care.

In contrast to universal prevention strategies, selective and indicated interventions target specific subgroups for intervention. Selective interventions target those who are at elevated risk based on group-level characteristics that are not directly related to etiology. Because schizophrenia is a familial and heritable disorder (Gottesman, 1991), a selective prevention program for schizophrenia might focus on asymptomatic children with first-degree affected relatives or, more specifically, on those with particular combinations of schizophrenia-risk-specific gene variants, as they become known.

Finally, an indicated intervention involves targeting individuals who either have signs of the disorder but are currently asymptomatic, or are in an early stage of a progressive disorder. Because there are no universal signs of schizophrenia, indicated interventions for this disorder have a somewhat broad definition. Two lines of research that may lead to indicated interventions for schizophrenia include the study of individuals with prodromal signs of schizophrenia (Eaton et al., 1995) and the characterization of individuals with schizotaxia, which can be defined as the underlying predisposition to schizophrenia that may or may not be expressed as prodromal symptoms (Tsuang et al., 2002).

To develop and refine selective and indicated prevention efforts for schizophrenia, the disorder itself (as well as its precursors) must be thoroughly understood. Some of the risk factors for schizophrenia, such as birth complications and a family history of the disorder, are widely recognized. Others are just becoming known or are still being validated. When a wide variety of schizophrenia-specific precursors are available, these features can be used to maximize the efficiency and effectiveness of preventive efforts by narrowly specifying the characteristics of at-risk individuals, allowing only those who would benefit from intervention to be selected to receive it.

PREMORBID ASPECTS OF SCHIZOPHRENIA

The etiology of schizophrenia is complex, most likely involving a range of genetic and gene–environment interactions that are well summarized as the "epigenetic puzzle" (Gottesman & Shields, 1982; Plomin et al., 1994), as discussed in Chapter 5. The schizophrenia syndrome, the delusions, hallucinations, thought disorder, negative features, and cognitive dysfunction, is manifest at some stage during the lives of around 1 in 100 people. Figure 7.1 shows that the occurrence begins to take off in the early teenage and adolescent years, being rare before puberty and becoming less common in the second half of life.

However, important events may be occurring in the period leading up to illness and in the early years of development, the so-called prodromal and premorbid periods.

Prodromal and Premorbid Phases of Schizophrenia

In most cases, schizophrenia does not come totally out of the blue; there are important changes that occur before the psychotic syndrome. Fragmentary psychotic symptoms, depression, changes in behavior, attenuated general functioning, and other nonspecific features commonly occur in the weeks, months, and sometimes years before the first psychotic break. This period before the schizophrenia syndrome is established is known as the prodrome, and it represents a change that can frequently be identified by either the affected individual or his or her family members.

The prodrome is a period of considerable interest from a clinical and theoretical point of view because it may be possible to intervene early during this time and so prevent the onset of psychosis or improve its outcome. This exciting prospect of early intervention, considered in Chapter 6, is technically complex because of the nonspecific nature of some of the symptoms in the prodrome. Schizophrenia or other psychoses are by no means inevitable in a group of adolescents who show apparently prodromal features. Looking back to adolescents who have developed schizophrenia, the psychological difficulties are, of course, much more difficult. Much research is aiming to understand the biology underlying this period just before and around the onset of schizophrenia when important neuropsychological and structural changes may be occurring (Pantelis et al., 2003; Wood et al., 2003). There is general agreement, however, that earlier-onset cases such as these occurring in childhood or adolescence are likely to have more severe premorbid abnormalities (Nicolson & Rapoport, 1999; Nicolson et al., 2000).

There are other differences and abnormalities that occur well before the period of risk shown in Figure 7.1 begins. They are not only in a psychological domain and show no obvious continuity

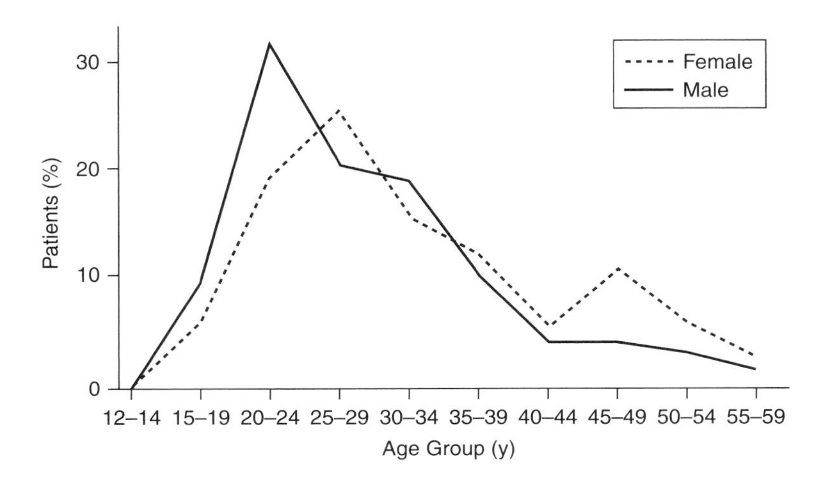

Figure 7.1 Age at onset distribution of schizophrenia. From Häfner et al. (1993).

with the schizophrenia syndrome. Rather than changes from the preexisting state that herald the illness during a prodrome, these differences are more a long-term part of the person, his or her personality and early development.

These differences are known as premorbid features. The distinction from the prodrome is not always clear, particularly in younger people, but may have theoretical importance because they seem to point toward early vulnerability or predisposing factors, rather than to events that occur as an illness is triggered or precipitated. The existence of premorbid abnormalities and differences in those who will, years later, develop schizophrenia suggests that parts of the epigenetic puzzle are put in place in very early life.

In childhood-onset cases, the distinction may be almost impossible because of the severity and insidious onset of schizophrenia before age 13 (Alaghband-Rad et al., 1995). However, it does seem that the variety of premorbid neurodevelopmental impairments in childhood-onset schizophrenia are striking compared to adolescent- and adult-onset populations (Addington & Rapoport, 2009). Why look in early life for premorbid differences and causes of schizophrenia?

From its first descriptions, schizophrenia has had a longitudinal dimension. Thomas Clouston (Clouston, 1892; Murray, 1994; Murray & Jones, 1995) recognized a syndrome that he called "developmental insanity" in which developmental physical abnormalities were associated with early-onset psychotic phenomena, particularly in adolescent boys. When defining the schizophrenia syndrome more clearly, both Kraepelin (1896) and Bleuler (1908, 1911) noted that many of the people who developed the psychotic syndrome had been different from their peers long before the psychosis began. Here is a quotation from one of Bleuler's early accounts of what has become known as schizophrenia:

> It is certain that many a schizophrenia can be traced back into the early years of the patient's life, and many manifest illnesses are simply intensifications of an already existing character. . . . All ten of my own school comrades who later became schizophrenics were quite different from the other boys. (Bleuler 1911/1950)

If some of the seeds of schizophrenia are sown in early life, then there ought to be other evidence. The excess of minor physical abnormalities (Green et al., 1989; Gualtieri et al., 1982; Guy et al., 1983; Lane et al., 1997; Lohr & Flynn, 1993; Sharma & Lal, 1986), and the dermatoglyphic or fingerprint abnormalities in people with schizophrenia (Bracha et al., 1992; McGrath et al., 1996) are seen as "fossilized" reminders of insults very early in life, during the first or second trimester of pregnancy, such as infections and nutritional problems (reviewed in Tarrant & Jones, 1999). These factors and some of the neuropathological data are probably best explained in terms of developmental processes having gone awry (Weinberger, 1995).

However, these processes are difficult to observe directly. Genetic high-risk studies, where the offspring of people with schizophrenia are followed up, have shown subtle differences in the neurological development of these children at special risk, and in those not known to be so (Erlenmeyer-Kimling et al., 1982; Fish, 1977; Fish et al., 1992; Walker & Lewine, 1990). Genetic studies such as these are discussed in Chapter 5.

What Are the Premorbid Differences Seen in Schizophrenia?

Bleuler wasn't very precise when he mentioned that many of the people he'd known who developed schizophrenia as adults were different from other boys as children. It's certainly interesting that he mentions boys, specifically, because tightly defined schizophrenia does seem to be more common in men than in women, and the early developmental differences are often more obvious in boys than in girls. This may be partly an artifact of some research designs, as well as an effect of differences in the wiring of male and female brains.

Many aspects of development can be seen to be slightly different in children who will later develop schizophrenia. Often these differences are subtle and would not be noticed at the time by parents or professionals. Usually, differences can be noted in characteristics that are developing rapidly according to the age of the child, things that are on the cusp of the developmental wave, and the child appears to catch up later on. Here are some examples.

Early Milestones and Motor Development

Direct evidence of neurodevelopmental differences is available (Weinberger, 1995). One source is a remarkable piece of opportunistic research by Walker and colleagues (1990, 1993). They studied "home movies" of families in which one child later developed schizophrenia. Facial expression of emotion and general motor functions were rated blind to that child's identity among the siblings. The pre-schizophrenic children were distinguished on both accounts, some with fairly gross but transitory motor differences. These may point to the basal ganglia of the brain as being involved in the underlying mechanism, reminding us that subtle motor disturbances are apparent at the beginning of schizophrenia, before any treatment (Gervin et al., 1998).

Such developmental differences have now been demonstrated in large, population-based or epidemiological samples. In the British 1946 birth cohort, a group of several thousand people born in one week in March 1946 have been studied regularly throughout their lives. Their mothers were asked about development when the children were age 2 years, before anyone knew what would happen later on. All the milestones of sitting, standing, walking, and talking were slightly though clearly delayed in those who developed schizophrenia as adults, but there was nothing that would have alarmed parents at the time. There were other indications that language acquisition was different before onset of schizophrenia. Nurses were more likely to notice a lack of speech by 2 years in the children who developed schizophrenia as adults, and school doctors noted speech delays and problems in them throughout childhood.

Developmental differences have been replicated in similar cohort studies in other domains, such as bladder control, fine motor skill, and coordination during late childhood and adolescence (Cannon et al., 1999; Crow et al., 1995). The motor and language delays were replicated and extended in a birth cohort study from Dunedin, New Zealand (Cannon et al., 2002), where over a thousand children have been followed during childhood. Those who indicated in their mid-20s that they had experienced symptoms suggestive of schizophrenia, mania, and other disorders were compared with those who said that they had never had such phenomena.

Figure 7.2 shows how a summary motor performance score was lower through most of

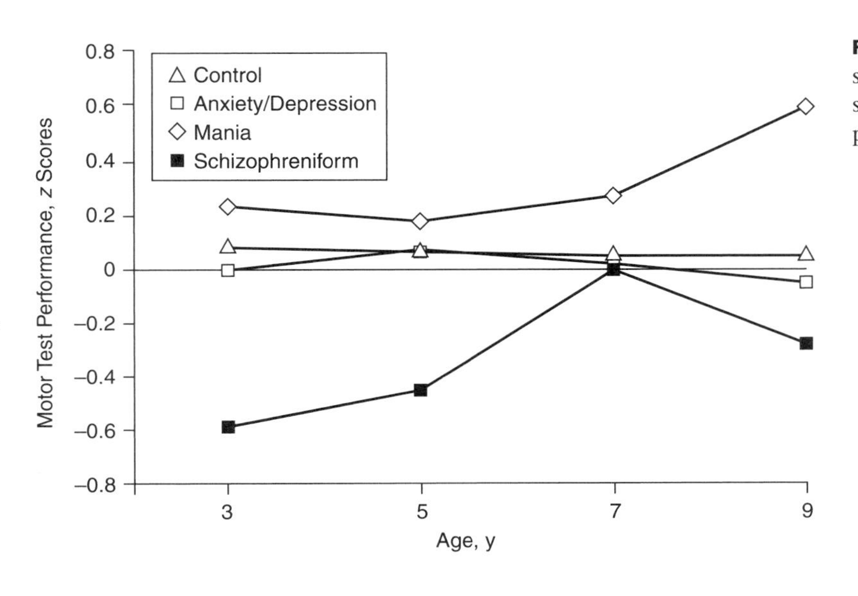

Figure 7.2 Mean standardized scores for motor performance.

childhood for those who experienced a schizophreniform disorder compared with the other groups; Figure 7.3 indicates that there was also a receptive language problem in those who later had hallucinations, delusions, and thought disorders.

Developmental differences before the onset of schizophrenia have been observed during the first year of life in the North Finland 1966 birth cohort. This comprises about 12,000 babies due to be born in this geographic area during 1966 (Rantakallio, 1969). Their early development was charted in the first year of life and later linked to information about who had developed schizophrenia through adolescence and into the early 30s (Isohanni et al., 2001). Figure 7.4 shows the incidence of schizophrenia in male subjects according to how quickly the little boys had learned to stand without support or "toddle" during the first year. The figure for girls was similar.

It is clear that not only was there an effect whereby the later a boy learned to toddle, the greater was his chance of developing schizophrenia in later life, but also that this effect seemed to hold true throughout the range of variation in reaching this milestone, all of which might be considered normal. If one were looking only for very late developers, then one might be more likely to find them within the pre-schizophrenia group than in those who did not develop the illness. However, this approach would completely obscure the widespread nature of this association, the meaning of which is considered later on.

There is another finding apparent from Figure 7.4. For the boys who passed the milestone early, in the 9-month and 10-month categories, the relatively few individuals who developed schizophrenia all did so in their mid-teens to mid-20s; their period of risk seemed fairly short. For those who were later developers, the period of risk was longer; these groups are still accruing cases of schizophrenia into their early 30s and beyond. It may be that the overall risk period for schizophrenia is shorter where neurodevelopment is more efficient, and longer where it is less efficient.

Behavioral Development

Bleuler's quotation above most obviously implies differences in behavior and temperament. Studies in this area have also moved on through retrospective research methodologies to cohort designs. Sophisticated rating scales for the retrospective assessment of behavior and personality demonstrate differences prior to psychosis, with the most common being characteristics of a shy, "schizoid" habit (Ambelas,

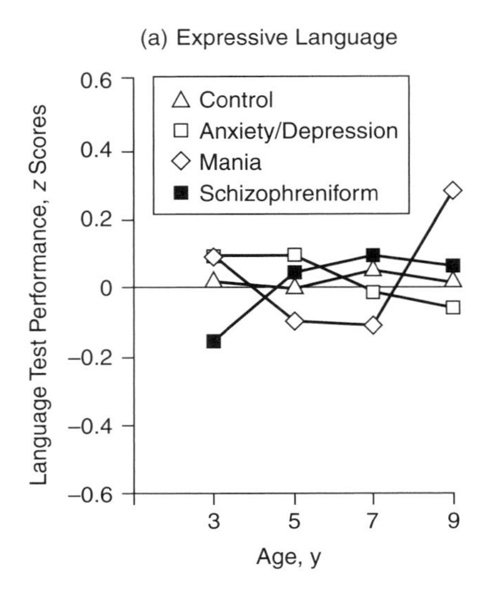

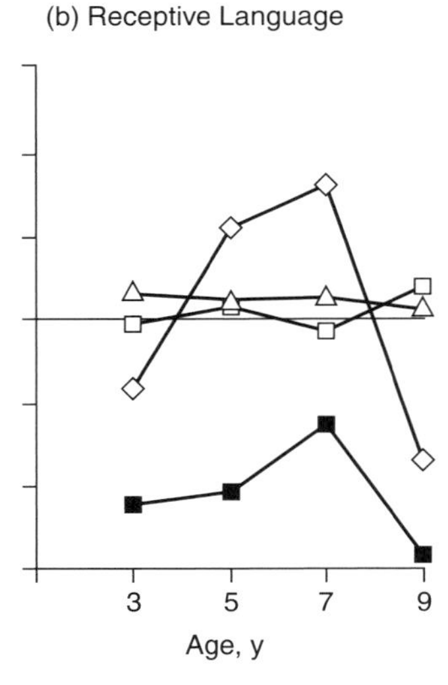

Figure 7.3 Mean standardized scores for expressive and receptive language performance.

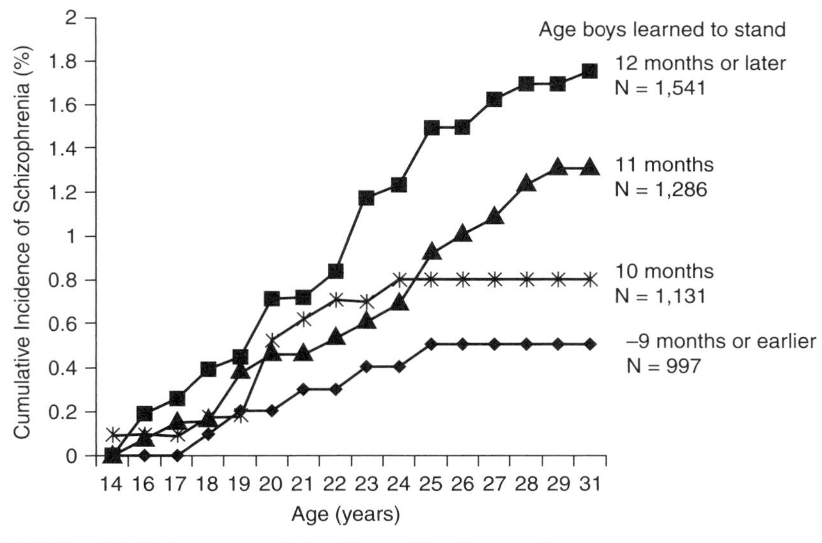

Figure 7.4 Relationship between age at standing without support.

1992; Cannon-Spoor et al., 1982; Foerster et al., 1991; Gittleman-Klein & Klein, 1969).

Robins (1966) undertook a pioneering, historical cohort study in which she followed a group of boys who had been referred to a child guidance clinic in St. Louis, Missouri. Here antisocial behavior was associated with later schizophrenia. Watt and Lubensky (1976; Watt, 1978) traced the school records of people with schizophrenia who came from a geographically defined neighborhood in Massachusetts. Girls who were to develop schizophrenia were introverted throughout kindergarten into adolescence. Boys who were to become ill were more likely to be rated as "disagreeable," but only in the later school grades (seven to 12). This pattern has been identified (Done et al., 1994) in a British cohort using a similar set of behavioral ratings, and in the Dunedin cohort mentioned above (Cannon et al., 2002). The 1946 British birth cohort contained children's own ratings of their behavior at age 13 years, and teachers' ratings 2 years later. These data showed no evidence of antisocial traits in the pre-schizophrenia group but a strong association with shy, "schizoid" behaviors at both ages. The two views gave a very similar picture; the shyer someone seemed as a child, the greater the risk. Other studies do, however, remind us of the varied childhood psychiatric conditions that predate schizophrenia (Kim et al., in press).

The behavioral differences seem to persist toward the prodrome but are independent from it. Malmberg et al. (1998) studied a sample of some 50,000 men conscripted into the Swedish army at age 18 to 20 years when they underwent a range of tests and assessments. Four behavioral variables at age 18 were particularly associated with later schizophrenia: having only one or no friends, preferring to socialize in small groups, feeling more sensitive than others, and not having a steady girlfriend. Cannon et al. (1997) also noted the same relationship.

Another twist to the story about premorbid behavioral differences comes from the recognition that some of the individual parts of the schizophrenia syndrome, such as hallucinations or delusions, can exist in otherwise well-functioning individuals in the population. However, they are indeed associated with a greater risk of occurrence of subsequent schizophrenia whether they occur in early adolescence (Poulton et al., 2000) or adulthood (Myin-Germeys et al., 2003a, 2003b).

Thus, there seems to be a consistency over childhood and adolescence, and across several types of study, regarding the presence of premorbid behavioral differences. People who will develop schizophrenia as adolescents and adults are different from their peers in terms of behavior in childhood, just as Bleuler noted a century ago; the effects may be even more widespread than he thought.

Cognitive Function and IQ

This aspect of psychological function also shows differences in the premorbid period. Aylward, Walker, and Bettes (1984) have provided a comprehensive review of intelligence in schizophrenia. They concluded that intellectual function is lower in pre-psychotic individuals than in age-matched controls. Linking the pre-psychotic deficit to outcome, they raised the question as to whether IQ may be an independent factor that can protect otherwise vulnerable individuals, or whether the deficits are part of that vulnerability.

Once again, the birth cohort studies shed light on the question. Cannon et al. (2002) showed that mean IQ test scores were consistently lower during childhood in those children who developed schizophreniform disorder (Fig. 7.5). This mean shift in premorbid IQ had also been seen in two British cohorts (Jones & Done, 1997). When the childhood IQ data from the 1946 cohort (Pidgeon, 1964, 1968) are studied in greater detail, it is clear that the lower mean premorbid IQ is not due to a subset of people with very low scores; rather, the whole distribution of those who will develop schizophrenia when they reach adolescence or adulthood is shifted down—the majority or most children seem not to be doing as well as they might have been expected to perform (Jones et al., 1994). This is a similar situation to the motor findings in the Finnish cohort. It is not that there is a group of very abnormal individuals driving the findings; the effects are seen across the normal range.

David et al. (1997; see above) replicated this result in the Swedish conscript study, although the measures were later in life, at age 18. There was no evidence of a threshold effect below or above which this relationship did not hold. Very bright individuals can develop schizophrenia, but they are less likely to than those who are less able. Put another way, any individual is more likely to develop schizophrenia than someone who is more able in terms of IQ, although the effect is small. Interest in the cognitive aspects of schizophrenia (David & Cutting, 1994; Green, 1998) suggests a parsimonious conclusion that pre-psychotic IQ deficits (and perhaps social characteristics) may be manifestations of the same abnormal cognitive processes that later result in psychosis.

WHAT DO PREMORBID ABNORMALITIES MEAN?

The range of differences in the developmental histories of people who will develop schizophrenia when they are older suggests that something

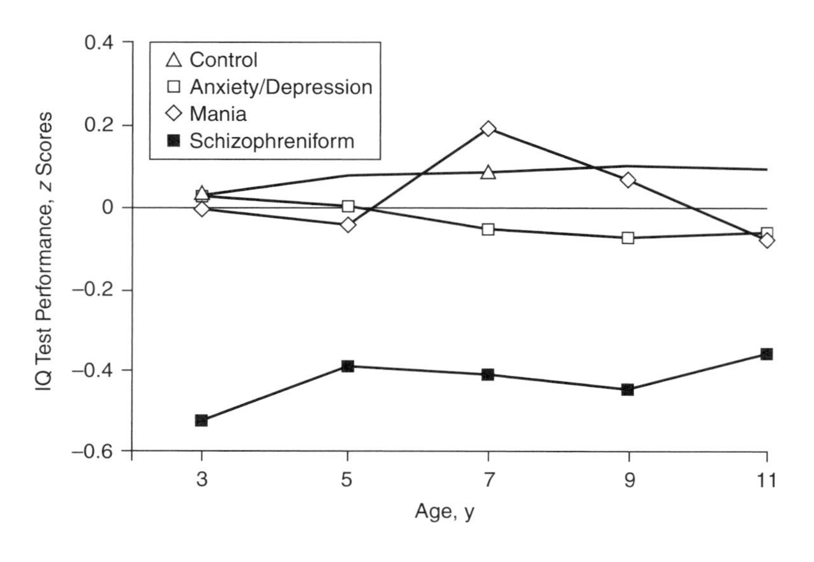

Figure 7.5 Mean standardized scores for IQ performance.

to do with the causes of this syndrome is active long before the characteristic features begin (Marenco & Weinberger, 2000). There is evidence for many such early factors, including genetic effects (Fish et al., 1992; Jones & Murray, 1991), obstetric complications (Cannon et al., 2002), psychosocial stresses, famine, infections, and other toxic events during brain development (see Jones, 1999, for review).

It seems that many events that may lead to early brain development being suboptimal may increase the risk of later schizophrenia. There may be specific causes or combinations of causes, such as gene–environment interactions, that make people vulnerable to developing the schizophrenia syndrome, perhaps after later, necessary events that act as triggers. These may include normal (Weinberger, 1987, 1995) or abnormal brain development (Feinberg, 1982a, 1982b, 1997; Pogue-Geile, 1997), as well as traditional precipitants such as psychosocial stressors or drugs (see Chapter 6).

The behavioral, motor, language, and cognitive differences shown in the premorbid period may be manifestations of vulnerability or predisposition to schizophrenia; they may not be risk modifiers in themselves. These indicators seem remarkably homogeneous—in retrospect, like a final common pathway. The idea of only a subgroup of individuals having this manifest vulnerability as suggested in the seminal views of developmental aspects of schizophrenia (Murray & Lewis, 1987) is not supported by research. Most or even every person who develops the syndrome may have had a degree of developmental vulnerability, although this will not have been obvious at the time.

The early motor findings in the Finnish birth cohort (see Fig. 7.4) are consistent with the vulnerability being due to developmental processes being generally less efficient—the formation or enhancement of functional neural networks, for instance. The greater the inefficiency, the greater the risk of schizophrenia when that same inefficiency is played out in the formation of complex and integrative systems later in adolescence and adult life (see Chapter 5).

There are several candidates to explain this unifying vulnerability. These include hormonal events (Walker & Bollini, 2002) that are able to tie together motor and other system abnormalities in early life and links with psychosocial stress in models of predisposition and precipitation (Walker et al., 1999). Molecular biology and the investigation of not only the presence but also the functional activity of genes and the proteins for which they code may yield other dimensions of vulnerability. For instance, Tkachev et al. (2003) showed that expression of genes associated with glial cells that are associated with the nutritional support of nerve cells (oligodendrocytes), and with myelin, the insulating sheaths they provide for these neurons, were downregulated in the frontal cortex of brains of people who had died having suffered schizophrenia in life. This seems a very good candidate for the homogeneous vulnerability factor posited in this account of premorbid abnormalities before schizophrenia, and may be an endophenotype or hidden manifestation of the disorder. The deficient gene expression remains to be demonstrated before the onset of schizophrenia and will, itself, have its own prior causes.

As mentioned at the beginning of this section, premorbid features of schizophrenia are, in our current understanding, not yet of use in terms of prediction and early intervention. They occur in multiple domains, but many of the effects we can measure are subtle and leave individuals remaining well within the wide range of normality. Premorbid features tell us a great deal about what we should be looking for in terms of underlying mechanisms and causes of schizophrenia, and when these may operate; they are signposts toward these. As we learn about the processes that underpin the behavioral, cognitive, and motor differences that we can measure in the premorbid phase of schizophrenia, we may become able to identify those who are vulnerable with enough precision to be able to do something useful for them.

DEVELOPMENTAL PRECURSORS OF ADOLESCENT-ONSET SCHIZOPHRENIA

There are precursors of schizophrenia prior to the first onset of psychosis in many, but not all, adolescents who develop schizophrenia. As will be seen below, the precursors of schizophrenia can be subtle changes in basic brain functions like motor functions, attention and memory, certain behavior problems, or attenuated schizophrenic symptoms. Identifying the developmental precursors of adolescent-onset schizophrenia has important implications both for enhancing our understanding of the underlying neurobiology of schizophrenia, and for the development of preventive interventions for schizophrenia.

Neurobiological factors present in individuals at high risk for developing a schizophrenic disorder, prior to the onset of frank psychotic symptoms, may represent potential etiological factors for schizophrenia. A number of brain systems known to be disturbed in schizophrenia, including prefrontal and medial temporal lobes (Selemon & Goldman-Rakic, 1999; Weinberger, 1986), may underlie certain neurocognitive impairments in children at risk for schizophrenia (R. Asarnow, 1983; Cannon et al., 1993). Determining how these neurobiological factors evolve when a schizophrenic disorder develops could provide important clues about how the diathesis for schizophrenia is potentiated into the overt disorder. A combination of disease-related progressions and maturational changes is hypothesized to exacerbate these dysfunctions when individuals at risk for the disorder convert to having the disorder.

Two broad classes of methods have been used to identify developmental precursors of schizophrenia. The first class of methods is *prospective* studies of children. A common feature of prospective methods is identifying, then characterizing, a group of children and following them up to determine which children subsequently develop a schizophrenic disorder. One important prospective method is to study children who are at increased statistical risk of developing a schizophrenic disorder. The lifetime risk for schizophrenia in the general population is less than 1%, so very large samples are required to prospectively identify the precursors of schizophrenia by following up children drawn from the general population. Given the population base rate of schizophrenia (<1%), you would need to start off with at least 2,500 children (without accounting for subjects being lost to follow-up) to identify the developmental precursors of schizophrenia in 25 individuals. High-risk studies ascertain individuals with an increased lifetime risk for schizophrenia for inclusion in prospective, longitudinal studies. This is typically accomplished by studying the children of parents with schizophrenia. The lifetime risk for schizophrenia for children of one parent with schizophrenia is approximately 10% to 12%, an approximately 10-fold increase in the risk for the disorder. High-risk studies frequently measure putative etiological factors for schizophrenia prior to the onset of the disorder. In this way, studies of children at risk for schizophrenia provide a vehicle for testing hypotheses about etiological factors in schizophrenia.

Most (85%–90%) patients with schizophrenia do not have parents with a schizophrenic disorder. This has raised the concern that findings from "genetic high-risk" samples may not accurately describe the developmental precursors of schizophrenia in the much larger number of individuals who develop schizophrenia but do not have a schizophrenic parent. Recognition of this problem has led to an interest in complementary strategies for identifying developmental precursors of schizophrenia. *Birth cohort studies* are prospective studies that can provide information on precursors of schizophrenia that do not have some of the ascertainment biases inherent in high-risk studies. In contrast to studies of children at risk for schizophrenia, birth cohort studies follow up large, representative samples of entire birth cohorts. Birth cohort studies are designed to provide information about a wide range of medical, psychiatric, and social conditions, so they use very large samples, literally thousands of subjects. For example, the 1946 British birth cohort study that provided important data on developmental precursors of schizophrenia studied almost 5,400 children born in the week of March 9, 1946, then systematically followed them up to determine that 30 children developed schizophrenia, as well as a broad range of other psychiatric and medical outcomes. A great strength of birth cohort studies is the large, representative sample size. However, a limitation of birth cohort studies is that since they are not typically designed to test hypotheses about any particular disorder, they use a rather broad range of measures, which are not specifically tailored to measure potential precursors of schizophrenia.

By studying children prior to the onset of the disorder, it becomes possible to identify the precursors or antecedents of the disorder, as opposed to the consequences of the disorder—for example, the initiation of antipsychotic drug treatment. We will review some of the key findings that have emerged from three decades of studies of children at risk for schizophrenia and birth cohort studies.

A second class of methods involves the collection of information on the premorbid development of individuals, usually adults, who have been diagnosed with schizophrenia. Some of the earliest studies of this type relied on *retrospective* reports from informants who knew the patient as a child. This approach has obvious limitations, among them being the fact that recollections of the past may be subject to bias. The *follow-back* method features the ascertainment of individuals with schizophrenia and then, using different types of archival material, characterizing them prior to the onset of psychosis. Since the focus of this section is on adolescent-onset schizophrenia, we will emphasize those few studies that ascertained adolescent-onset schizophrenics.

Follow-back studies vary in the type of archival material used to describe the premorbid characteristics of individuals who develop schizophrenia. There is wide agreement (see Watt et al., 1982) about the advantages of using contemporaneous childhood records over retrospective interviews to reconstruct the premorbid histories of individuals who develop schizophrenia. The major limitation of follow-back studies is that the childhood evaluations were not guided by specific hypotheses about the age-specific manifestations of schizophrenia; as a consequence, the most informative measures may not have been collected. They also have ascertainment biases, the nature of which varies depending on how the sample of schizophrenia patients was identified.

Birth cohort and follow-back studies can show associations between childhood characteristics and the development of schizophrenia because in both types of studies individuals with schizophrenia have been identified. These associations are prospective in birth cohort studies and retrospective in follow-back studies. Because the data used to describe childhood risk factors in birth cohort and follow-back studies were not collected with the intent of testing hypotheses about schizophrenia, the measures may not be sensitive to some of the more subtle manifestations of liability to schizophrenia. In contrast, the measures included in studies of children at risk for schizophrenia were specifically designed to tap liability to schizophrenia. On the other hand, most studies of children at risk for schizophrenia, while intended to be longitudinal, were not able to follow up subjects through the age of risk to determine which high-risk subjects developed a schizophrenic disorder. Consequently, while there are extensive cross-sectional comparisons of children at risk for schizophrenia to controls, there is much less information on the long-term predictive validity of childhood risk factors identified in high-risk studies.

If the results of follow-back studies of adolescent-onset schizophrenia patients yield converging results to those of children at risk for schizophrenia and birth cohort studies, this would provide reassurance about the generalizability and validity of the results.

A DEVELOPMENTAL PERSPECTIVE ON RISK FACTORS

There are relatively age-specific manifestations of liability to schizophrenia (see J. Asarnow, 1988; R. Asarnow, 1983; Erlenmeyer-Kimling et al., 2000; Walker, 1991, for reviews), and the manifestations to liability to schizophrenia are somewhat different at different ages. For example, one of the interesting findings that emerges from a review of developmental precursors of schizophrenia is that some deficits observed during infancy frequently found in high-risk, birth cohort, and follow-back studies are not found in later stages of development. Another important reason to attend to the developmental progression of risk factors is that from the point of view of targeting individuals for prevention, risk factors more proximal to the period of time when schizophrenia develops may have better diagnostic accuracy than, for example, infancy predictors.

Table 7.1 summarizes some of the major findings concerning precursors of schizophrenia at three different developmental periods: infancy, early childhood, and middle childhood/early adolescence. Table 7.1 is not an exhaustive summary of the results of high-risk, birth cohort, and follow-back studies; rather, it presents the characteristics that best differentiate high-risk children from controls or predict later development of schizophrenia that have thus far been identified in the literature. Cited below are comprehensive reviews of the results of high-risk, birth cohort, and follow-back studies.

The format of Table 7.1 was modeled after a review by J. Asarnow (1988). The entries in Table 7.1 for studies on high-risk children come from reviews by J. Asarnow (1988), Erlenmeyer-Kimling (2000, 2001), R. Asarnow (1983), and Cornblatt and Obuchowski (1997). The entries for birth cohort studies are based on reviews by Jones, Rogers, Murray, and Marmot (1994) and Jones and Tarrant (1999). The data for entries of follow-back studies of adolescent-onset schizophrenia come from Watkins, Asarnow, and Tanguay (1988), and Walker, Savoie, and Davis (1994). Watt and Saiz (1991) provided a broad review of follow-back studies of adult-onset schizophrenia.

Two types of risk characteristics are differentiated into separate columns in Table 7.1: "endophenotypes" versus clinical and behavioral features. Endophenotypes are putative reflections of the underlying schizophrenic genetic diathesis. Most of the putative endophenotypes employed in high-risk studies are neuromotor or neurocognitive functions (e.g., language, attention, and memory) believed to tap central nervous system disturbances that reflect liability to schizophrenia. In contrast, clinical and behavioral features are either non-schizophrenia psychiatric symptoms or behavior problems that, while they may reflect the underlying genetic diathesis, are much more proximal to the overt symptoms of schizophrenia. The reason for making this distinction is that these two different classes of risk characteristics have somewhat different implications as targets for prevention.

High-Risk Studies

The results of high-risk studies have to be considered in the context of a major limitation: there are limited data on how well the cross-sectional differences between children at risk for schizophrenia and matched controls predict the later onset of schizophrenia. Only six studies of children at risk for schizophrenia have obtained diagnostic evaluations in adulthood or late adolescence:

1. The New York High-Risk study (Fish, 1984)
2. The Copenhagen High-Risk project (Cannon et al., 1993; Mednick & Schulsinger, 1968)
3. The Israeli High-Risk study (Ingraham et al., 1995)
4. The New York High-Risk project (Erlenmeyer-Kimling et al., 2000)
5. The Swedish High-Risk study (McNeil et al., 1993)
6. The Jerusalem Infant Development study (Hans et al., 1999).

The New York High-Risk project studied the largest number of subjects for the longest period of time, and therefore provides the most extensive data on the diagnostic accuracy of childhood and adolescent predictors of schizophrenia-related psychoses. None of these studies focused on the prediction of adolescent-onset schizophrenia. Indeed, there are very few cases of adolescent-onset schizophrenia in the entire high-risk literature. As a consequence, we are making the assumption that the factors that predict adult-onset schizophrenia are germane to the prediction of adolescent-onset schizophrenia.

Infancy

During infancy in most, but not all, studies (see Walker & Emory, 1985, for review), neurological signs or neuromotor dysfunctions are found more frequently in children at risk

Table 7.1 Developmental Precursors of Schizophrenia Identified by Means of Three Different Research Strategies

	Retrospective Studies		*Birth Cohort Studies*		*Follow-Back Studies*	
Life Stage	*CNS Functioning*	*Symptoms and Behaviors*	*CNS Functioning*	*Symptoms and Behaviors*	*CNS Functioning*	*Symptoms and Behaviors*
Infancy (0–2 years)	Impaired motor and sensory functioning High or variable sensitivity to sensory stimulation Abnormal growth patterns Short attention span Low IQ	Difficult temperament Passive, low energy, quiet, inhibited Absence of fear of strangers Low communicative competence in mother–child interaction, less social contact with mothers	Delays in motor milestones Speech problems or delays Delayed potty training		Abnormal motor functioning Impaired language	
Early childhood (2–4 years)	Low reactivity Poor gross and fine motor coordination Inconsistent, variable performance on cognitive tests	Depression and anxiety Angry and hostile disposition Schizoid behavior (i.e., emotionally flat, withdrawn, distractible, passive, irritable, negativistic) Low reactivity More likely to receive a diagnosis of developmental disorder	Speech problems Motor problems	Solitary play	Impaired language Neuromotor impairments	
Middle childhood/ early adolescence years (4–14 years)	Neurological Passive impairment (poor fine motor coordination, Socially balance, sensory perceptual isolated signs, delayed motor development) Poor social adjustment Attentional impairment under ADD overload conditions Anxious/Variance-scatter on depressed intellectual tests	Poor affective control (emotional instability, aggressive, disruptive, hyperactive, impulsive) Poor interpersonal relationships, withdrawn Cognitive slippage disturbance Mixed internalizing-externalizing symptoms, fearful ADD-like syndrome	Twitches, grimaces Poor academic achievement Poor balance, clumsiness	Solitary play Less socially confident "Schizoid" social development	Reduced general intelligence Poor academic achievement Poor attention Neuromotor impairments	Passive Especially isolated Poor social adjustment ADD

ADD, attention-deficit disorder; CNS, central nervous system.

for schizophrenia than controls. In these studies neuromotor anomalies were assessed by observation during a pediatric neurological examination or by performance on standardized tests of infant development (e.g., the Bayley). Neurological signs and neuromotor dysfunctions are not specific to infants at risk for schizophrenia and are not rare events in the general pediatric population. Neurological abnormalities in neonates typically tend to improve. In contrast, it appears that these abnormalities in children at risk for schizophrenia persist, and may worsen over time. Infants with neurological or neuromotor abnormalities are the high-risk infants most likely to develop schizophrenic disorders in adolescence and early adulthood (Fish, 1987; Marcus et al., 1987; Parnas et al., 1982). Neurological dysregulation in infancy predicts the development of schizophrenia spectrum disorders (Fish, 1984). Impaired performance on tasks with extensive motor demands during middle childhood also predicts the presence of schizophrenia spectrum disorders during adolescence (Hans et al., 1999).

Disturbances in early social development are found more frequently in children at risk for schizophrenia than controls. Depending on the study, these disturbances are manifested in difficult temperaments, apathy or withdrawal, being inhibited, less spontaneous and imitative, reduced social contact with mothers, and the absence of fear of strangers. The absence of fear of strangers during infancy could be an indication that the child does not differentiate between familiar adults with whom the child is attached (e.g., their parents) versus others. This absence of the fear of strangers may reflect inadequately developed attachment. These disturbances are not specific to children at risk for schizophrenia; they are also associated with broad risk factors such as socioeconomic status, general maternal distress, early trauma or neglect, and poor quality of parenting. There are scant data on how well these disturbances in infant social development predict the development of schizophrenia. However, many of these findings are related to the development of social competencies (Watt & Saiz, 1991).

Early Childhood

During early childhood (2–4 years of age) children at risk for schizophrenia are more likely to show poor fine and gross motor coordination, and low reactivity than controls. While poor fine and gross motor coordination was found in a different sample of children than the samples of infants at risk for schizophrenia who showed a variety of neurological signs and neuromotor dysfunction, these data suggest that the dysfunctions observed in infancy are persistent.

In early childhood there is an increased occurrence of internalizing symptoms (depression and anxiety), angry and hostile dispositions, and schizoid behavior (emotionally flat, socially withdrawn, passive and distractible) in children at risk for schizophrenia. Again, these characteristics are not specific to children at risk for schizophrenia, and there is no evidence that these characteristics are strongly predictive of the later development of schizophrenia.

Middle Childhood/Early Adolescence

Neuromotor impairments, including gross motor skills (Marcus et al., 1993), are found more frequently in children at risk for schizophrenia than in controls during middle childhood/early adolescence (4–14 years of age). One of the most robust cross-sectional findings during middle childhood and early adolescence is the presence of neurocognitive impairments, especially on measures with high attention demands. A subgroup of children at risk for schizophrenia show impairments on some of the same tasks for which patients with schizophrenia show impairments. The neurocognitive tasks for which children at risk for schizophrenia show impairments include measures of sustained attention (various continuous performance tests) and secondary memory (e.g., memory for stories). For example, children at risk for schizophrenia, as well as acutely disturbed and partially remitted schizophrenia patients, perform poorly on a partial report span of apprehension task (R. Asarnow, 1983) in the high attention/processing demand condition. The span of apprehension measures the rate of early visual information processing (Fig. 7.6).

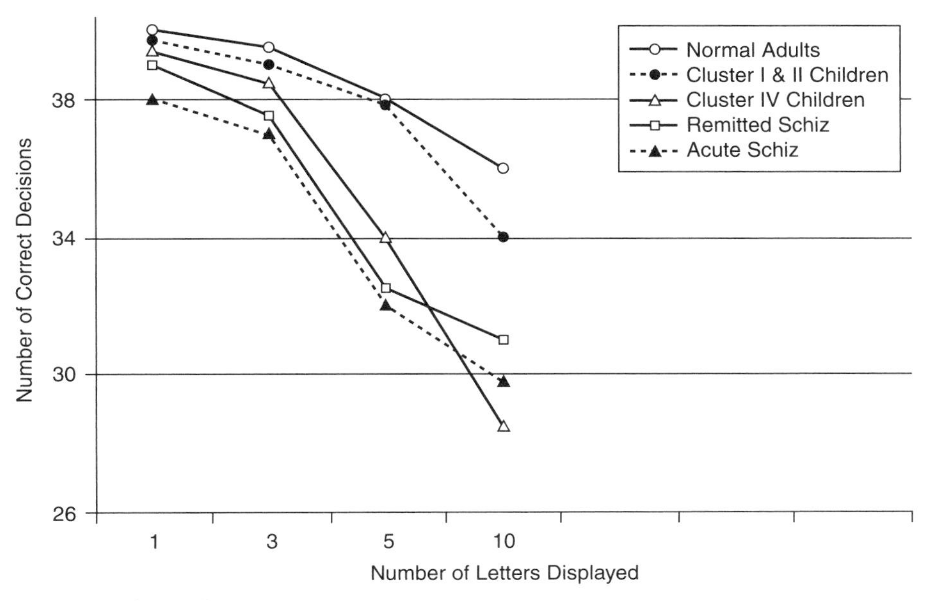

Figure 7.6 Span of Apprehension Data.

There are some data on the predictive validity of the neurocognitive impairments identified during middle childhood and early adolescence. In the New York High-Risk project the presence of impairments on a number of attentional tasks (an "Attentional Deviance Index") given in middle childhood predicted 58% of the subjects who developed schizophrenia-related psychoses by mid-adulthood (Erlenmeyer-Kimling et al., 2000). Attentional impairments in middle childhood were also associated with anhedonia (Freedman et al., 1998) in adolescents prior to the onset of schizophrenia and social deficits during early adulthood (Cornblatt et al., 1992; Freedman et al., 1998). Neuromotor dysfunction during childhood (assessed by the Lincoln-Oseretsky Motor Development Scale) identified 75% of the high-risk children who developed schizophrenia-related psychoses during adulthood (Erlenmeyer-Kimling et al., 2000). A verbal short-term memory factor that included a childhood Digit Span task and a complex attention task predicted 83% of the New York High-Risk project children who developed schizophrenia-related psychoses during adulthood, and showed high specificity to those psychoses (Erlenmeyer-Kimling et al., 2000). If replicated, these findings would suggest that the combination of genetic risk (being the child of a parent who has schizophrenia) and neurocognitive impairments during middle childhood might identify individuals with a greatly increased risk for developing schizophrenia. The sensitivity (correctly predicting the onset of schizophrenia-related psychoses) was higher for the verbal memory (83%) and motor skills (75%) factors than for the attentional factor (58%). Conversely, the false-positive rate (incorrectly predicting that a child would develop schizophrenia) was lower for the Attentional Deviance Index (18%) than for the memory factor (28%) and motor factor (27%).

The short-term follow-up in the Jerusalem High-Risk study provides an important link between the attentional impairments frequently observed in children at risk for developing schizophrenia during adolescence and the motor impairments found during infancy and early childhood. The children who showed impaired neuromotor performance during childhood were the subjects most likely to show impairments on a variety of measures of attention and information processing during early adolescence (Hans et al., 1999).

During middle childhood, children at risk for developing schizophrenia receive an increased frequency of a variety of psychiatric diagnoses, including an AHDH-like syndrome. Poor affective control, including emotional instability and impulsivity, as well as aggression and disruptive behaviors are found more frequently in children at risk for developing schizophrenia than controls. Early precursors of thought disorder may be reflected in the presence of cognitive slippage. Poor peer relations are one of the most frequently found behavioral characteristics during middle childhood and early adolescence. None of these symptoms is specific to children at risk for schizophrenia; for example, poor affective control is found in children who subsequently develop an affective disorder.

Birth Cohort Studies

A British birth cohort study of almost 5,400 people born in the week of March 9, 1946, complements the studies of individuals at risk for developing schizophrenia by virtue of being representative of the general population. Thirty cases of schizophrenia were identified among individuals between the ages of 16 and 43 in this cohort, which reflects the population base rate of the disorder. A 1956 birth cohort study in northern Finland (Isohanni et al., 2001) yielded 100 cases of DSM-III schizophrenia.

Across the major birth cohort studies, a number of developmental precursors of schizophrenia have been identified. These include the British birth cohorts of 1946 (Jones, Rodgers, Murray, & Marmot, 1994) and 1958 (Done, Crow, Johnson, & Sacker, 1994; Jones & Done, 1997) and the northern Finland 1956 birth cohort (Isohanni et al., 2001). Neurological signs, reflected in various forms of motoric dysfunction ranging from tics and twitches, poor balance and coordination, and clumsiness to poor hand skill, are consistently identified as developmental precursors of individuals who later develop schizophrenia (Done et al., 1994; Jones et al., 1994). There was an increased frequency of speech problems up to age 15 in persons who subsequently developed schizophrenia. Low educational test scores at ages 8 and 11 were also risk factors (Jones et al., 1994).

During early and late middle childhood, individuals who subsequently developed a schizophrenic disorder could be differentiated from their peers by their preference for solitary play, poor social confidence, and in general a "schizoid" social development.

In general, birth cohort studies suggest that there appears to be "consistent dose-response relationships between the presence of developmental deviance and subsequent risk" (Jones & Tarrant, 1999). The more deviant an individual is toward the "abnormal" end of a population distribution, the greater the risk of the disorder.

There is considerable overlap between the developmental precursors of affective disorders and schizophrenia (Van Os et al., 1997). For example, lower educational achievement is associated with affective disorders in general, while delayed motor and language milestones are associated with childhood onset of an affective disorder. As in schizophrenia, there is evidence of persistence of motor difficulties, with an excess of twitches and grimaces noted in adolescents.

Follow-Back Studies

In regard to endophenotypic characteristics, during infancy children who subsequently developed schizophrenia as adolescents are characterized by the presence of abnormal motor functioning and impaired language. Neuromotor and language impairments, and decreases in positive facial emotion, are also present in early childhood (Walker et al., 1993). During middle childhood the language impairments fade; however, the neuromotor impairments persist. In addition, during middle childhood children who subsequently develop a schizophrenic disorder are characterized by poor academic achievement, poor attention, and reduced general intelligence.

During middle childhood children who subsequently develop a schizophrenic disorder are characterized as being passive and socially isolated, with poor social adjustment. They frequently present with symptoms of attention-deficit/hyperactivity disorder (ADHD) and/or anxiety and depression.

A novel approach to using archival data to characterize the premorbid histories of individuals who develop schizophrenia is the use of home movies to identify infant and childhood neuromotor dysfunctions (Walker, Savoie, & Davis, 1994). Ratings were made of neuromotor functioning in children who subsequently developed schizophrenia, their healthy siblings, pre–affective disorder participants, and their healthy siblings. The pre-schizophrenia subjects showed poorer motor skills, particularly during infancy, than their healthy siblings and pre–affective disorder participants and their siblings. The abnormalities included choreoathetoid movements and posturing of the upper limbs, primarily on the left side of the body.

Consistency of Findings Across Methods

Endophenotypes

Inspection of Table 7.1 reveals a consistency across studies of children at risk for schizophrenia, birth cohort studies, and retrospective studies in the presence of motor and language problems during infancy. This consistency is particularly impressive given the considerable variation across studies in how motor functioning and language were assessed.

During early childhood (2–4 years of age) neuromotor problems are observed in all three types of studies. In birth cohort studies and retrospective studies, impaired language is noted. In high-risk studies children at risk for schizophrenia are noted as being depressed, anxious, angry, and schizoid, while in birth cohort studies they are noted as preferring solitary play.

During middle childhood (4–14 years of age) there is a persistence of neurological impairments reflected in poor motor functioning in high-risk, birth cohort, and follow-back studies. High-risk studies, unlike birth cohort studies and retrospective studies, included laboratory measures of attention information processing. On these tasks, children at risk for schizophrenia showed attentional impairment under conditions of high processing demands. This may be related to the poor academic achievement that is observed in birth cohort studies and retrospective studies during middle childhood as well as the frequent diagnosis of ADHD. In contrast to the persistence of neuromotor problems, language problems tend to diminish over time so by middle childhood they are rarely noted across the three classes of studies. In adolescents who develop a schizophrenic disorder, language functions are relatively preserved compared to visual-spatial and motor functioning (Asarnow, Tanguay, Bott, & Freeman, 1987).

The results of this brief review suggest a developmental pathway from precursors first identified in infancy to the development of schizophrenia-related psychoses in late adolescence and early adulthood. Neurological signs or neuromotor dysfunctions are present in infancy and persist through early and middle childhood and early adolescence. Neuromotor dysfunction in early childhood predicts the presence of attentional impairments under high processing demands during early adolescence. Neuromotor dysfunctions and attentional impairments during adolescence predict the development of schizophrenia-related psychoses. Since the characterization of key points in this developmental sequence is based on only one or two studies, clearly this model needs to be tested in future research.

The developmental pathway sketched here has potentially interesting implications for our understanding of the neurobiology of schizophrenia. What brain systems are involved in the control of simple motor functions and attention? The developmental link between early neuromotor dysfunction and later attentional impairments may implicate cortical-striatal pathways that support both motor functions and attentional control mechanisms. Striatal dysfunction results in impaired sequential motor performance and chunking of action sequences. Impairments in a variety of attentional functions, including set shifting and self-monitoring, are also associated with striatal dysfunction (Saint-Cyr, 2003).

Clinical/Behavioral Characteristics

In high-risk studies the precursors of later difficulties in developing social relations can first be detected in infancy. In some studies, children at risk for schizophrenia have less social contact with their mothers and less fear of strangers, as well as having a difficult temperament.

Poor peer relations are one of the most frequently found behavioral characteristics during middle childhood and early adolescence. A preference for solitary play, poor social confidence, and in general a "schizoid" social development are frequent precursors of schizophrenia.

Studies of children at risk for schizophrenia, birth cohort studies, and retrospective studies all find an increased frequency of nonpsychotic symptoms, particularly internalizing symptoms and poor affective control (including emotional instability and impulsivity) during middle childhood and early adolescence. However, none of these symptoms are specific to children at risk for schizophrenia; many of these symptoms and behavioral characteristics are found in children who subsequently develop an affective disorder.

LIMITATIONS: WHAT WE DON'T KNOW

Neuromotor and attentional dysfunctions appear to be putative developmental precursors to schizophrenia. They consistently appear with increased frequency in high-risk, birth cohort, and follow-back studies. In a number of high-risk studies, infancy and childhood neuromotor impairments predicted the later onset of schizophrenia-related psychosis. Attentional impairments during middle childhood and early adolescence in the New York High-Risk project predicted the development of schizophrenia-related psychosis.

The endophenotypic indices that appear to have the greatest predictive validity are neuromotor dysfunction and impaired performance on measures that tap processing under high attention demands, or measures of secondary memory. It remains unclear whether these measures tap schizophrenic-related processes specifically. A number of the measures (including continuous performance tests, partial report span of apprehension tasks, and secondary verbal memory tests) that are sensitive to subtle neurocognitive impairments in children at risk for schizophrenia in middle childhood/adolescence also detect neurocognitive impairments in children with ADHD and learning disabilities. It is unlikely that these impairments have cross-sectional diagnostic specificity.

While the ability of childhood/adolescent measures of attention to predict schizophrenia-related psychosis in the New York High-Risk project is promising, those results need to be replicated in an independent sample. Future studies will need to determine the extent to which childhood/adolescent neurocognitive measures predict schizophrenia-related psychosis conditioned on the presence of a second risk factor, having a parent who is schizophrenic. In effect, the analyses reported by the New York High-Risk project contained two risk factors that predicted schizophrenia-related psychosis—being the child of a schizophrenic parent and having attentional, verbal, short-term memory, or neuromotor impairments. These factors did not predict the onset of schizophrenia in the children of parents with an affective disorder nearly as well as they did in the children of parents with schizophrenia. As noted above, children with other, more common psychiatric diagnoses show deficits on these types of tasks. More research is needed on the diagnostic accuracy of these measures when they are used in the general pediatric population before they can be used to screen children for precursors for schizophrenia. At present, all that we know is that these measures have some promise in predicting which children who have a parent with schizophrenia are likely to develop a schizophrenic disorder themselves.

What is needed in the next generation of studies is not merely the demonstration of group mean differences between high-risk and control groups. If endophenotypic measures are to be used as candidates for preventive intervention programs, what is required are diagnostic accuracy analyses that specify the sensitivity and specificity of tasks using various cutting scores. Cutting scores can be created, depending on the purpose, that optimize sensitivity (detecting true positives) or specificity (false negatives). For example, if the intervention can produce significant adverse events, it might be desirable to set a cutting score to minimize false positives.

Poor peer relations, a preference for solitary play, a "schizoid" social development, various nonpsychotic symptoms (particularly internalizing symptoms), and poor affective control occur frequently during middle childhood and early adolescence in high-risk, birth cohort, and follow-back studies. While these behavior problems and symptoms are precursors of schizophrenia, they are not diagnostically specific; many of these symptoms are associated with other psychiatric disorders. For example, poor affective control is both a symptom of and a precursor to affective disorders. Poor peer relationships are associated with the presence of both externalizing and internalizing disorders. There are relatively few data on the diagnostic accuracy (i.e., specificity and sensitivity) of symptoms and behavior problems detected in middle childhood and early adolescence as predictors of schizophrenia-related psychoses.

The behavior problems and symptoms that are putative precursors of schizophrenia are associated with psychiatric disorders (e.g., depression and ADHD) that are much more common than schizophrenia in the general population. This suggests that they will produce high false-positive rates if they are used in the general pediatric population in an attempt to identify individuals likely to develop schizophrenia.

IMPLICATIONS FOR PREVENTIVE INTERVENTION

There is great interest in developing preventive interventions for schizophrenia, in part because of the belief that once the disorder emerges, a neurodegenerative process is initiated that can only be partially forestalled by currently available treatments. The neurocognitive impairments, non-schizophrenia symptoms, and behavior problems that are putative developmental precursors of schizophrenia may have important implications for the development of preventive interventions for this disorder. These precursors could be used to identify children who might benefit from preventive intervention and serve as targets of interventions.

The neurocognitive impairments that are putative developmental precursors of schizophrenia have potential utility in identifying candidates for preventive interventions. Depending on the risk profile of the intervention, cutting scores on neurocognitive indices could be constructed to either maximize sensitivity or minimize false positives. However, as noted above, before the cutting scores for putative neurocognitive precursors of schizophrenia can be applied to the general pediatric population, additional research is required to evaluate the diagnostic efficiency of these measures in populations without a genetic risk. The neurocognitive precursors of schizophrenia seem to be unlikely targets for preventive interventions. There is no evidence that mitigating attentional, memory, and neuromotor impairments forestalls the development of schizophrenia-related psychoses. Identifying neurocognitive precursors of schizophrenia does advance attempts to develop new somatic treatments for schizophrenia by helping to elucidate the dysfunctional neural networks that underlie this complex disorder.

The diagnostic accuracy of the behavior problems and symptoms that are putative precursors of schizophrenia thus far identified in high-risk, birth cohort, and follow-back studies have not been carefully examined. Given the nonspecificity of these behavior problems and symptoms, it seems likely that they would yield high rates of false positives if used to identify candidates for preventive interventions for schizophrenia. It may be that clinical features more proximal to the onset of schizophrenia-related psychoses, such as prodromal signs and symptoms, have greater diagnostic accuracy in predicting which children will develop schizophrenia. A number of research groups are currently addressing this question.

The behavior problems and symptoms that are putative precursors of schizophrenia are potentially interesting targets for interventions. To the extent that poor peer relations, the presence of internalizing symptoms, and poor affective control pose difficulties for the child and parent, they become worthy targets of therapeutic interventions. Behavioral (e.g., social skills training) and pharmacological (mood-stabilizing drugs) interventions for these problems are based on symptomatic presentations. The nonspecificity of these problems is not particularly problematic in this case. While there is no reason to believe that enhancing social skills and controlling affective symptoms will forestall the development of schizophrenia, there is good reason to believe that they will enhance the patient's current quality of life, and may also improve his or her adaptation after a psychotic episode. The best predictor of post-psychotic psychosocial functioning is the level of premorbid social competencies.

WHAT ARE THE PRECURSORS OF SCHIZOPHRENIA?

One of the best ways to develop early intervention efforts for schizophrenia is to start by identifying key features of those individuals who are or will become schizophrenic and determine how these features differ from those seen in individuals who are not ill and are not likely to ever become afflicted with the illness. Several research designs can accomplish this goal. For example, cross-sectional studies of patients and control subjects can be used to characterize each group on as many potentially meaningful variables as possible, including behavior, personality, social activity, neuropsychological abilities, brain structure and function, and genetics. One problem with this method, however, is that any differences observed between the two groups cannot necessarily be attributed a causal role in the development of disease. For example, if total brain volume were lower among a group of schizophrenic patients than it was among a group of well-matched controls, this might indicate that low brain volume is a precursor or predictor of the development of schizophrenia. However, from such a cross-sectional design, it is unclear if the brain volume deficit in the patient group actually preceded the onset of schizophrenic illness. In fact, it is possible that it did, but it is also possible that the onset of schizophrenia caused a decline in brain volume due to some degenerative process. Alternatively, other factors, such as treatment with antipsychotic medication, may have precipitated the decline in brain volume. It is further possible that the brain volumetric decline in the patient group was concurrent with the onset of illness but causally unrelated to it.

Numerous cross-sectional studies have unearthed a wealth of information regarding the ways in which schizophrenic patients are different from patients with other psychiatric illnesses and from normal control subjects. However, because of the limitations on causal inference that exist in these types of studies, their results can only guide further research; they are not powerful enough to dictate a specific pattern of behavioral, neuropsychological, or biological characteristics that would be useful for identifying individuals for targeted prevention efforts. As already mentioned, studies of individuals with prodromal signs of schizophrenia and individuals with schizotaxia provide more insight into those traits that precede the disorder than cross-sectional studies. Thus, great efforts have been made to enable identification of individuals in the earliest stages of the illness or even in the premorbid period so that they may be targeted for intervention.

By characterizing the prodromal phase of schizophrenia, subtle changes in behavior have been noted in those who are beginning to deteriorate into the early stages of the disease, and these changes are now being used to identify other clinically at-risk individuals for inclusion in early intervention programs. Some of the more pronounced changes observed during the prodrome occur in domains of thought, mood, behavior, and social functioning (Phillips et al., 2002). Specifically, difficulties in concentration and memory may emerge, as well as preoccupations with odd ideas and increased levels of suspiciousness. Mood changes may include a lack of emotionality, rapid mood changes, and inappropriate moods. Beyond simply odd or unusual behavior, the prodrome may also be characterized by changes in sleep patterns and energy levels. Social changes can be quite marked, with withdrawal and isolation as the most predominant features. These characteristics may be particularly informative of the disease process in schizophrenia, because they are by definition not related to the effects of medication or the degenerative effects of being ill for a prolonged period.

Perhaps the most powerful window into the premorbid changes in pre-schizophrenia individuals comes from the longitudinal study of children and adolescents who are genetically at high risk for the illness. By studying the biological children of schizophrenic parents, the clinical, behavioral, and biological features of schizotaxia can be revealed. Longitudinal studies of individuals such as these, who harbor the latent genetic liability toward schizophrenia, can be extremely informative for early intervention and prevention efforts because they can track the emergence of schizophrenia precursors before any signs of illness are apparent. Thus, any differences observed between children of schizophrenic patients and children of control subjects can be definitively attributed to factors other than the effects of antipsychotic medication, the degenerative effects of the illness, or any other factors that are subsequent to disease onset. The observed differences can be viewed as antecedents to the illness, which is as close to a causal relationship as can be ascribed in human research studies in which group membership cannot be experimentally assigned.

Studies of children of patients with schizophrenia have yielded a variety of findings of altered behavioral, neuropsychological, and biological processes. The richness and diversity of measures taken on these subjects can make profiling the premorbid genetic susceptibility to schizophrenia difficult. On the other hand, such studies have also produced some surprisingly uniform findings, which simplify our understanding of what may be the most central or universal deficits among those who are at the highest risk for schizophrenia.

Certain personality characteristics seem to reliably differentiate children of schizophrenic parents from children of control subjects (Miller et al., 2002). For example, schizotypal personality features, including social withdrawal, psychotic symptoms, socioemotional dysfunction, and odd behavior, have been shown to precede the onset of psychosis among genetically high-risk children. Deficits of social functioning are also commonly observed in this group (Dworkin et al., 1993). Specifically, children of schizophrenic patients are more likely than children of controls to have more restricted interests, significantly poorer social competence (especially in peer relationships and hobbies/interests), and greater affective flattening. Some neuropsychological deficits have also been reliably observed in these high-risk individuals (Asarnow & Goldstein, 1986; Cosway et al., 2000; Erlenmeyer-Kimling & Cornblatt, 1992; Schreiber et al., 1992). For example, several studies have replicated a pattern of impaired discrimination, sustained attention, and information processing on the visual continuous performance test among children of schizophrenic patients. These high-risk individuals also exhibit marked impairments on memory for verbal stimuli and in executive functioning, as well as neuromotor deficits such as soft neurological signs, gross and fine motor impairments, and perceptual-motor delays.

Perhaps underlying these personality, social, and neuropsychological deficits, children of schizophrenic patients have also been shown to have altered brain structure and function compared to children of control subjects (Cannon et al., 1993; Berman et al., 1992; Liddle, Spence, & Sharma, 1995; Mednick, Parnas, & Schulsinger, 1987; Reveley, Reveley, & Clifford, 1982; Seidman et al., 1997; Weinberger et al., 1981). The most commonly observed structural brain abnormality among children of schizophrenic patients is a reduced volume of the hippocampus and amygdala region. Loss of volume in the thalamus has also been observed in these children, and there has been some support for enlarged third ventricular volume and smaller overall brain volume in this group. Children of schizophrenic patients also have been found to exhibit linear increases in cortical and ventricular cerebrospinal fluid to brain ratios with increasing genetic load—that is, children with the greatest number of affected biological relatives showed the highest ratios.

Ultimately, these clinical, behavioral, social, and biological profiles of risk for emergent schizophrenia will be augmented by information on specific genes that increase susceptibility. Genes coding for neuregulin 1 (NRG1; Stefansson et al., 2002), nitric oxide synthase (NOS1; Shinkai et al., 2002), and dystrobrevin-binding protein 1 (DTNBP1; Straub et al., 2002) have been reported to have an association with schizophrenia, but these findings will require verification. Many other polymorphisms have shown a positive association with the disorder, but attempts to replicate these findings have often failed. For several of these widely studied polymorphisms, meta-analysis has been used to clarify the presence or absence of a true allelic association with the disorder in the presence of ambiguity. In fact, using this approach, some candidate genes, including those that code for the serotonin 2A receptor (HTR2A) and the dopamine D2 (DRD2) and D3 (DRD3) receptors, have already been shown to have a small, but reliable, association with the disorder (Dubertret et al., 1998; Glatt, Faraone, & Tsuang, 2003; Williams et al., 1997). Eventually, other gene variants, including perhaps NRG1, NOS1, and DTNBP1, will be found to be reliably associated with schizophrenia. This may make it possible to create a genetic risk profile that will be predictive of future onsets of schizophrenia, especially in combination with other known risk indicators.

Together, the various abnormal features of children of schizophrenic patients provide a "composite sketch" of the underlying premorbid susceptibility toward schizophrenia. Because the probability of developing schizophrenia among children of one or two affected individuals (12% and 46%, respectively) is far greater than that probability among children of control subjects (1%), these abnormalities signal the subsequent development of schizophrenia with a relatively high degree of sensitivity and reliability. However, it is also clear that these trends are not absolute, and many children of schizophrenic patients will not exhibit these signs, nor will they ever develop schizophrenia.

DO EARLY INTERVENTION AND PREVENTION EFFORTS WORK?

It has been recognized for some time that the duration of untreated illness in schizophrenia is correlated with the prognosis for the disease, such that those with the longest period of untreated psychosis experience the least favorable outcomes (Browne et al., 2000). It has also been discovered that outcome correlates with the duration of illness as measured from the onset of the prodrome rather than only from the onset of frank psychosis. From this line of evidence, the rationale for early intervention efforts was born. It was reasoned that if early treatment of the illness led to a more favorable outcome, early intervention even before the onset of the illness might further inhibit the progression of the illness, either delaying its onset, decreasing its severity, or both.

A fundamental question in designing early intervention protocols is, "What will be the target of the intervention?" There is no single best answer to this question, which may be why various targets are being used in current early intervention efforts. The earliest interventions might realize the greatest opportunities to divert high-risk individuals from the subsequent development of schizophrenia, but the ability to predict schizophrenia accurately might be greatest in the period closest to disease onset. For example, targeting attention problems in young children of schizophrenic parents might allow the identification of the children who are at highest risk of transitioning to psychosis and afford ample time to intervene in that process, yet because of the restricted sensitivity and specificity of this deficit, targeting attention problems may also cause some high-risk children to be excluded from the protocol while, inevitably, some of the children who were included in the protocol would not go on to develop the illness. On the other hand, targeting the changes of the prodrome, such as the emergence of odd behaviors or increased suspiciousness, might lower false-positive and false-negative classification errors, but the ability of the intervention protocol to influence the course of the illness might be relatively restricted compared to earlier interventions. Thus, a balance must be maintained between the potential effectiveness of the intervention and the specificity of the intervention to the target population.

Another key question in developing early intervention protocols is, "At what level should the intervention be administered?" Again, this is a question without a simple answer. Universal and selected interventions will have the greatest likelihood of reaching those individuals most in need of intervention—that is, they will have the greatest sensitivity. However, these may also be too expensive to implement successfully. Indicated interventions will be more feasible due simply to their more restricted nature, but this will prevent such protocols from reaching some individuals who may benefit from them. In fact, interventions administered at multiple levels may work better than protocols designed to intervene only at a single level.

Perhaps the least consensus in the design of early intervention trials is on the form of the intervention. The effectiveness of various early intervention programs is currently an active area of research and, fortunately, multiple types of interventions have shown promise for keeping at least some high-risk individuals from developing schizophrenia. In fact, educational programs, as well as psychosocial and psychotherapeutic interventions, have all shown some degree of promise in either reducing the duration of untreated psychosis or postponing the onset of schizophrenia, suggesting that these methods may also be useful in decreasing the likelihood of schizophrenic illness altogether. In Norway, for example, the establishment of a comprehensive, multilevel, multitarget psychosis education and early detection network reduced the average duration of untreated psychosis in the catchment area by approximately 75% over a 5-year period (Johannessen et al., 2001).

The preventive effects of various psychotherapeutic techniques, such as individual cognitive-behavioral therapy or family-based cognitive remediation, have yet to be evaluated with great rigor, but pharmacological intervention has received a fair amount of empirical support for efficacy in preventing or delaying the transition from prodrome to psychosis. A variety of psychopharmacological compounds may have efficacy in suppressing schizophrenia, including second-generation antipsychotic drugs like risperidone, antidepressants such as the selective serotonin reuptake inhibitors, mood stabilizers such as lithium and valproate, and antianxiolytics such as benzodiazepines, but few of these have so far been tested for such a role. Of these, the novel antipsychotic risperidone has shown tremendous promise in preventing the descent into schizophrenia among prodromal individuals when compared with needs-based therapy alone, even up to 6 months after discontinuation of treatment (McGorry & Killackey, 2002). Of note, risperidone has also been shown to improve neuropsychological functioning among the nonpsychotic, nonprodromal schizotaxic relatives of schizophrenic patients (Tsuang et al., 2002).

In light of these successes, it is not so troubling that consensus is difficult to reach on which form of intervention is the most appropriate; it seems that the method of intervention is not quite as important as the fact that any intervention is better than none. There are, however, a number of problems with current early intervention efforts. For example, because our screening criteria cannot definitively identify individuals who are at risk for developing psychosis, early intervention efforts are sometimes administered to individuals who do not need them or cannot benefit from them. Alternatively, because the warning signs of psychotic decompensation sometimes go unrecognized, some individuals who should have received intervention do not. Furthermore, little is known about the potential harm that may be caused by informing individuals that they are at risk for schizophrenia; presumably there may be some negative consequences of receiving this knowledge. In addition, the benefits of some of our most promising early intervention and prevention protocols (pharmacotherapies) may be offset by the potential side effects of individual compounds.

A careful analysis of the benefits and the risks of early intervention has led to the general consensus that intervention in the prodrome of schizophrenia is warranted. There is less agreement about the feasibility of selective and indicated intervention in the premorbid phase of schizotaxic individuals, who may or may not ultimately develop a schizophrenia-spectrum illness. Studies have shown that pharmacological intervention can improve the subclinical deficits experienced by some non-schizophrenia genetically at-risk individuals; however, at such an early stage of research and with a limited understanding of schizotaxia, it is not yet clear if these benefits outweigh their associated risks when the selection of proper candidates for intervention may still be suboptimal. As the phenomenology and time course of schizotaxia become better understood, criteria for inclusion in preventive and early intervention efforts will improve, along with the efficiency of such protocols in treating only those individuals who will receive maximal benefit while sustaining little harm. A comprehensive summary on the early intervention literature is provided by Srihari and Shan (2012).

Research Agenda for Schizophrenia

Raquel E. Gur
Ruben C. Gur
Matcheri S. Keshavan
Christian Kohler
Judith Rapoport
Elaine Walker

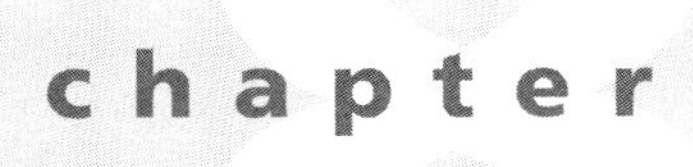

8

We have learned a great deal about the early course of schizophrenia during the past two decades, with increased focus on the prodromal phase of illness. Complex brain disorders such as schizophrenia spectrum disorders pose special challenges, including the heterogeneous clinical presentation, impact on multiple cognitive and functional domains, the chronic course that requires a lifespan perspective, and the lack of validated biomarkers. While these are major obstacles to aligning clinical neurosciences with a precision medicine approach, there has been a paradigm shift in research that is currently helping elucidate the underlying neurobiology of psychosis and building bridges essential for implementation of precision medicine (Insel & Cuthbert, 2015).

Recognizing that schizophrenia spectrum disorders are neurodevelopmental, a key focus has been on early signs of the emergence of psychosis and integration of clinical phenotypic measures with quantitative dimensional neurocognitive and neuroimaging parameters. Such efforts evaluate the presence of abnormalities before the emergence of psychosis that meets current diagnostic criteria. Early identification with reliable measures can lead to early intervention that can help bend the developmental trajectory of youths at risk for psychosis and, it is hoped, bring it closer to that of typically developing young people. This early identification may provide vulnerable individuals with yardsticks to measure and tools to achieve milestones that are critical in the transition to adulthood and independent functioning. This paradigm shift requires complementary studies of populations at an early age before symptoms reach diagnostic criteria, and it is therefore important to study individuals who are at high clinical or genetic risk for psychosis in order to maximize the potential clinical relevance of findings.

Several key areas of research continue to be a priority:

1. In the clinical domain, we need to identify specific clinical characteristics in the premorbid and prodromal phases that can help us predict the individuals at a high risk for developing psychosis.
2. We need to better understand the pathways to care for these individuals. Educating the public and healthcare providers in early signs and symptoms can reduce the delay in care.
3. We need to further clarify the phenotypic features in the first psychotic episode that can help us predict subsequent illness course.
4. We need to better understand the neurodevelopmental and neurodeteriorative processes that may underlie both the emergence and the subsequent course of the first psychotic episode.

An important research need regarding the early course of psychosis is more studies on brain development in relation to behavior during adolescence and early adulthood. While schizophrenia is among the most widely studied psychiatric disorders that emerges in late adolescence and early adulthood, adolescence seems to be a pivotal time for the emergence of a variety of behavioral symptoms that require further study. Such work will be facilitated by the Research Domain Criteria (RDoC) approach, since dimensional measures can be obtained during childhood and adolescence and these can be predictive of future diagnostic features. It is necessary to conduct such studies, as early-onset forms may not just reflect an enrichment of risk factors for schizophrenia or greater severity of the illness but may in fact have their own distinct etiologies and separate ranges of severity. To determine the degree of continuity and etiological similarity between adolescent- and adult-onset schizophrenia, twin, adoption, and longitudinal studies of the early-onset form of the disease should be considered a priority.

With the growing interest of characterization of the early stages of psychosis, the study of brain and behavior in schizophrenia has moved from investigation of chronically ill individuals to those with shorter illness duration, first episode (Andreasen et al., 2011; Gur et al., 2000a, 2000b), and prodromal (Fusar-Poli et al., 2012a;

Giuliano et al., 2012). The focus on early subthreshold signs of psychosis provides a unique opportunity to address potential confounding effects of multiple factors in neurobiological research. Such factors, including psychoactive medications, limited functioning, and social isolation, which are common in patients with long duration of illness, are less likely to be present or as prominent at the time when the psychotic process emerges. Furthermore, symptoms emerge during a dynamic period of brain maturation, resulting in a fluid clinical presentation requiring longitudinal studies. Advances in and the availability of tools to examine brain and behavior have stimulated the integration of such measures into the study of clinical risk.

The rapidly growing literature on individuals at risk for psychosis (Dickson et al., 2012), while different in terms of sample sizes, rigor of reporting inclusion and exclusion criteria, and tests administered, affords quantitative meta-analyses that examine neurocognitive domains. In a meta-analysis of 14 studies, 1,214 individuals at risk for psychosis were compared to 851 healthy controls (Giuliano et al., 2012). Small to medium effect sizes of neurocognitive impairment in the psychosis risk group were observed. Significant deficits were noted in general cognitive abilities, attention, working memory, episodic memory, language functions, and visuospatial abilities. The only domain that did not differ between the groups was motor skills. Seven of these studies conducted longitudinal follow-up demonstrating that participants in the psychosis risk group, who transitioned to psychosis at follow-up, had medium to large effect sizes of neurocognitive deficits at baseline compared to healthy participants, supporting the utility of neurocognitive assessment.

Another meta-analysis (Fusar-Poli et al., 2012b) included 19 studies with a sample of 1,188 participants at clinical risk and 1,029 healthy comparison participants. The clinical risk group manifested lower general intelligence, and deficits in several domains were observed: executive functions, attention, working memory, verbal fluency, verbal and spatial memory, and social cognition. Processing speed did not distinguish between the groups. Transition to psychosis was examined in a subset of seven longitudinal studies with mean follow-up duration of 19 months (Becker et al., 2010; Brewer et al., 2005; Koutsouleris et al., 2012; Pukrop et al., 2007; Riecher-Rossler et al., 2009; Seidman et al., 2010; Woodberry et al., 2010). Findings indicated that individuals who transitioned to schizophrenia, compared to those who did not develop psychosis at follow-up, were more impaired at baseline. They had lower general intelligence and poorer performance in verbal fluency, verbal and visual memory, and working memory.

Most studies on clinical risk for psychosis have examined "cold" cognition and relatively few have focused on social cognition. Impaired social functioning has long been evident in people with schizophrenia, including premorbidly. Systematic studies evaluating affective processes have been more limited. The development of measures that relate to the perception, interpretation, and response to display of emotions is a relatively recent addition to the range of neurobehavioral probes available to evaluate this capacity. The first meta-analysis summarized above (Giuliano et al., 2012) included three studies that examined social cognition. Deficits in emotion processing and "theory of mind" tasks were noted in the group at clinical risk (Addington et al., 2008; Chung et al., 2008; Pinkham et al., 2007). In the second meta-analysis (Fusar-Poli et al., 2012b), data from six studies, some overlapping, with measures of social cognition were included (Addington et al., 2008; An et al., 2010; Chung et al., 2008; Green et al., 2012; Szily & Keri, 2009; van Rijn et al., 2011). Significant impairment in clinical risk participants compared to healthy controls was noted. This literature is growing (Kohler et al., 2014), indicating that the domain of social cognition is important in transitioning to schizophrenia and is related to level of functioning.

Neuroimaging has been applied to people at risk for psychosis, enabling examination of brain integrity as psychosis unfolds. Measures obtained include structural parameters such as gray matter and white matter volumes, cortical thickness, and diffusion tensor imaging (DTI) measures of structural connectivity, as well as functional parameters, including functional connectivity and activation in response to neurobehavioral tasks designed to probe a specific circuitry. The neuroimaging literature on clinical risk for psychosis is growing, although it is still relatively limited in size of samples examined and follow-up (Fusar-Poli et al., 2012a). The largest body of studies has evaluated structural magnetic resonance imaging (MRI) focusing on gray matter volume (Brent et al., 2013).

A meta-analysis of 14 voxel-based morphometry studies, most using a 1.5 Tesla scanner, compared psychosis-risk and first-episode schizophrenia patients to healthy controls (Fusar-Poli, et al., 2012c). The clinical risk group had lower gray matter volume in several regions, including the right temporal, limbic, and prefrontal cortex, whereas the first-episode group had lower volumes in the temporal insular cortex and cerebellum. Notably, the onset of psychosis was associated with decreased gray matter volume in temporal, anterior cingulate, cerebellar, and insular regions. These regions are implicated in cognitive and emotional processing functions that are aberrant in schizophrenia, and volume reduction in these regions has likewise been reported in multiple studies of schizophrenia.

Other brain parameters have been evaluated in fewer studies. Thus, white matter abnormalities have been reported in schizophrenia, early in the course of illness, as well as in individuals at risk for psychosis (Carletti et al., 2012; Fusar-Poli et al., 2011a). The resting the blood oxygenation level-dependent (BOLD) signal in functional MRI paradigms provides a measure of connectivity, reflecting "cross-talk" integration among brain regions. It examines the time-series correlations among brain regions, indicating which regions show synchronized activation. Aberrations in schizophrenia in frontotemporal connectivity have been reported and have also been seen in those at clinical risk (Crossley et al., 2009; Satterthwaite et al., 2015).

DTI quantifies restricted water diffusivity in white matter, enabling noninvasive detection of subtle white matter abnormalities and facilitating the understanding of complex large-scale brain networks. Abnormalities in DTI have been reported in schizophrenia, both in chronic patients and in first-episode presentation (Peters & Karlsgodt, 2015; Roalf et al., 2013), with reduced white matter integrity in frontotemporal tracts. The literature on psychosis risk is limited to several cross-sectional studies, with differing findings such as reduced fractional anisotropy in the frontal lobe (Bloemen et al., 2010) and in the superior longitudinal fasciculus (Schmidt et al., 2015). In a longitudinal study (Carletti et al., 2012), individuals at risk for psychosis (n = 32) were compared to healthy controls (n = 32) and first-episode patients with schizophrenia (n = 15), on a 1.5 Tesla scanner. The psychosis-risk and control participants were rescanned after 28 months. At baseline, the first-episode group had decreased fractional anisotropy and increased diffusivity relative to controls, and the psychosis-risk group was intermediate between the other two groups. At follow-up, further reduction in fractional anisotropy was evident in the left frontal region only in those psychosis-risk individuals (n = 8) who transitioned to psychosis. This suggests that progressive changes occur at disease onset, which has been reported before for gray matter (Andreasen et al., 2011; Borgwardt et al., 2007; Gur et al. 2000a,b; Smieskova et al., 2010). These findings encourage large-scale studies.

Functional MRI has been applied to individuals at risk for psychosis, commonly in small samples with neurobehavioral probes that have shown differences between schizophrenia patients and controls. Neurobehavioral domains examined include working memory, typically using the n-back paradigm. Overall, psychosis-risk groups show decreased activation in the BOLD response in dorsolateral and medial prefrontal regions (Fusar-Poli et al., 2012c). The pattern of activity is similar to that seen early in the course of schizophrenia, but less pronounced abnormalities are observed. To evaluate activation changes with disease progression, longitudinal designs are necessary. Such designs have been applied in several functional MRI studies (Smieskova et al., 2010).

This growing literature suggests that individuals who transition to psychosis differ from those who do not, with the latter group showing normalization. Thus, the application of functional MRI holds promise as a tool that may facilitate identifying brain circuitry dysfunction that may underlie the psychotic process.

Another potentially informative avenue for elucidating pathways to psychosis is the study of neurogenetic disorders that increase vulnerability to psychosis. The 22q11.2 deletion syndrome is the most common copy number variation, occurring in approximately 1:2,000 to 1:4,000 live births (Botto et al., 2003). It is typically caused by a sporadic uneven recombination event resulting in hemizygous deletion of approximately 3 Mb on the long arm of chromosome 22. This deletion of approximately 50 genes results in heterogeneous medical and neuropsychiatric manifestations. In addition to craniofacial and cardiovascular abnormalities, there are cognitive delays, with mild to moderate intellectual disability. There is increased risk for several psychiatric disorders, including anxiety, attention-deficit/hyperactivity disorder, and autism spectrum in childhood, with depression and schizophrenia emerging in adolescence and early adulthood (Gothelf et al., 2013; Tang et al., 2014; Yi et al., 2015). Perhaps the most striking effect of the 22q11.2 deletion is about a 25-fold increased risk of schizophrenia relative to the general population (Bassett et al., 2003). Although the frequency of psychiatric disorders in 22q11.2 deletion syndrome is relatively high, the developmental patterns and phenotypes are similar to manifestations of major psychiatric disorders in the general population (Antshel et al., 2006; Green et al., 2009). Therefore, the 22q11.2 genetic variation may provide a unique window for elucidating mechanisms of schizophrenia spectrum disorders.

As efforts at early identification with convergence of endophenotypic measures are under way, larger samples of individuals at clinical risk will become available for genomic studies. Applying to these samples tools established in the large-scale schizophrenia consortium, such as the polygenic risk score (Purcell et al., 2014), will extend the approach to the full spectrum of psychosis. As clinical risk studies are collecting increasingly large samples with multiple endophenotypic measures, the utility of neurocognitive, neuroimaging, and neurophysiological parameters can be examined in efforts to create gene networks explicating the underlying neurobiology of schizophrenia. Many genes implicated (e.g., GRM3, GRIN2A, SRR, GRIA1) are involved in glutamatergic neurotransmission and synaptic plasticity, corroborating a growing literature on underlying aberrations in schizophrenia. Both genome-wide association investigations of common variants and rare genetic variation studies converge in efforts to provide a mechanistic understanding of the etiology of schizophrenia while examining the psychosis continuum (Fromer et al., 2014; Gulsuner et al., 2013; Owen et al., 2010).

The extension of genomic research to earlier phases of the psychotic process can also contribute to investigations of gene–environment interactions. Multiple environmental risk factors contribute to schizophrenia (Iyegbe et al., 2014; van Os et al., 2009; Walker et al., 2013). The study of large samples of youths, in informative and integrated epidemiological, genomic, and endophenotypic paradigms, can advance the field and help clarify the pathophysiology of psychosis. Such advances will facilitate the development of interventions that can affect the developmental trajectory of individuals as psychosis emerges.

The developments in genetics and neurobiology provide investigators with powerful new tools to extend our understanding of the evolution of schizophrenia. Such an understanding will go beyond the current emphasis on symptomatic characterizations and include measures of behavioral and neurobiological endophenotypic vulnerability markers that are currently applied globally. Adolescence is pivotal for brain maturation, and longitudinal data are necessary to establish bridges between the phenotypic manifestations of schizophrenia and the neurobiological substrate. It is likely that multimodal intervention methods will be shaped by such knowledge in a way that will eventually delay, ameliorate, and perhaps even thwart the devastating impact of schizophrenia.

Anxiety Disorders

COMMISSION ON ADOLESCENT ANXIETY DISORDERS

Edna B. Foa, *Commission Chair*

Second Edition

Martin Franklin
Carmen McLean
Richard J. McNally
Daniel Pine

First Edition

E. Jane Costello
Martin Franklin
Jerome Kagan
Philip Kendall
Rachel Klein
Henrietta Leonard
Michael Liebowitz
John March
Richard McNally
Thomas Ollendick
Daniel Pine
Robert Pynoos
Wendy Silverman
Linda Spear

part III

Defining Anxiety Disorders

Edna B. Foa
Martin Franklin
Carmen McLean
Richard J. McNally
Daniel Pine

chapter 9

Before discussing the anxiety disorders, it is important to consider the concept of anxiety and its heterogeneity. Anxiety refers to multiple mental and physiological phenomena, including a person's conscious state of worry over a future unwanted event, or fear of an actual situation. Anxiety and fear are closely related. Some scholars view anxiety as a uniquely human emotion and fear as common to nonhuman species. Another distinction commonly made between fear and anxiety is that fear is an adaptive response to realistic threat, whereas anxiety is a diffuse emotion, sometimes an unreasonable or excessive reaction to current or future perceived threat.

DISTINGUISHING ANXIETY FROM ANXIETY DISORDERS

Defining the boundaries between extremes of normal behavior and psychopathology is a dilemma that pervades all psychiatry. For some extreme conditions, such as Down syndrome, diagnostic decisions are straightforward. Milder forms, by contrast, present problems when one attempts to define the point at which "caseness" begins. A few symptoms escape this definitional conundrum by virtue of their being deviant, regardless of their severity. This applies to symptoms such as delusional beliefs or hallucinations. In the case of anxiety, however, it is especially problematic to distinguish between normal behavior and pathology. Anxiety plays an adaptive role in human development, signaling that self-protective action is required to ensure safety. Because anxiety can be rated on a continuum, some investigators suggest that extreme anxiety represents only a severe expression of the trait, rather than a distinct or pathological state. Distributions may consist of distinct entities, however. For example, some cases of mental retardation, as caused by neurological injury, represent a qualitative departure from factors influencing normal variations in intelligence. By analogy, the fact that anxiety falls on a continuum of severity does not preclude the presence of qualitatively distinct disorders at any point in the distribution (Klein & Pine, 2001).

Anxiety may become symptomatic at any age when it prevents or limits developmentally appropriate adaptive behavior (Klein & Pine, 2001). However, anxiety about certain circumstances may arise at different developmental stages, based on the typical age-related experiences that occur during a stage. For example, anxiety about separation is a normal aspect of development experienced by many young children. Similarly, in adolescence, questions arise concerning anxiety about social situations, given changes in the social milieu that many adolescents find stressful. A useful rule of thumb for determining the diagnostic threshold is the person's ability to recover from anxiety and to remain anxiety-free when the provoking situation is absent. For example, it is not necessarily deviant for adolescents to respond with acute shyness when meeting an attractive peer. Such reactions reach clinical levels, however, when adolescents are unable to recover from the anxiety (as manifested by recurrent doubts or ruminations about how they behave) or when they avoid such encounters on a consistent basis. Similarly, clinical anxiety could manifest as persistent worry about future meetings with unfamiliar peers or even avoidance of activities that might require peer interactions. Therefore, an adolescent's lack of flexibility in affective adaptation is an important pathological indicator. In addition, the degree of distress and impairment influences diagnostic decisions; these vary with developmental stage as well as with cultural and familial standards. When anxiety symptoms are developmentally inappropriate, subjective distress is relatively more informative. For example, separation anxiety is developmentally more congruent with early childhood than with adolescence. In brief, three clinical features figure in the definition of pathological anxiety. Two features (distress and impairment) vary in importance as a function of developmental stage, whereas the third (symptomatic inflexibility) is diagnostically relevant regardless of age.

The ability to draw firm conclusions regarding the ideal criteria for disorders will remain limited so long as signs and symptoms are the exclusive basis for establishing the presence of psychiatric disorders. Longitudinal research can provide some answers by identifying specific symptom patterns and thresholds that have long-term significance. In practice, however, such evidence has proved to be informative but rarely conclusive.

The past three decades have witnessed a great expansion in the study of anxiety disorders. An earlier emphasis on rating scales or interviews assessing multitudes of unrelated fears and worries has yielded to an emphasis on the study of diagnostic groups characterized by explicit clinical criteria. Scale ratings can be grouped to generate overall scores of anxiety, or what have come to be called "internalizing" symptoms, such as in the widely used Child Behavior Checklist (Achenbach, 1991), but as the evidence shows, scale ratings correspond poorly to clinical entities.

Difficulties separating "normal" from "pathological" anxiety are especially apparent in results from epidemiologic studies, in which the prevalence of anxiety disorders changes markedly with relatively minor changes in the definition of impairment (reviewed by Klein & Pine, 2001). However, adolescents with anxiety disorders who seek treatment typically suffer from markedly impairing anxiety, and there is little ambiguity about determining whether they have "normal" or abnormal levels of anxiety.

This challenge poses both practical and conceptual problems. The practical problem concerns the timing of treatment. Two mistakes are possible: an adolescent who needs treatment may fail to receive it if the threshold for diagnosing the disorder is set too high ("a false negative"), and an adolescent whose anxiety reflects a reasonable response to adverse circumstances may receive unnecessary treatment ("a false positive"). The decision to treat versus not treat is linked to costs and benefits that inform decisions about each adolescent.

The conceptual problem concerns the need to provide a principled basis for distinguishing disorder from nondisorder beyond the current imperfect clinically based principles. Ideally, these principles would be based on understandings of pathophysiology. Consistent with this perspective, some philosophers of medicine have attempted to provide objective, biological criteria for demarcating disorder (e.g., major depression) from distressing states that fall within the bounds of normal unhappiness (e.g., grief). Others have claimed that all ascriptions of disorder reflect nothing more than socially determined value judgments about undesirable states and behavior.

Merging these polarized views, Wakefield (1992) proposed a harmful dysfunction account of disorder, holding that disorder is a hybrid concept comprising a factual component and an evaluative component. The factual component specifies what is dysfunctional (a derangement in a psychobiological function) and the value component specifies the resultant harm (usually emotional suffering, social maladjustment, or both). Therefore, ascription of disorder requires that two interrelated criteria be met: a psychobiological mechanism is malfunctioning, and this underlying dysfunction results in suffering, maladaptation, or both.

Wakefield's criteria imply that a person may be characterized by internal dysfunction but not qualify as having a disorder because no resultant harm occurs. For example, some youngsters characterized by extreme shyness or behavioral inhibition may find niches for themselves that enable them to flourish without marked distress. Even though the dysfunction requirement is met, these children would not be considered disordered because their dysfunction does not result in suffering or maladaptation. Conversely, some youngsters who are bullied by larger children may experience chronic anxiety at school, but because their suffering does not arise from dysfunction in the psychobiological mechanisms for estimating threat, Wakefield's criteria would prohibit their diagnosis as disordered. Mechanisms for detecting threat work precisely as they are "designed" to work: the bullied youngsters experience chronic anxiety because they are continually under threat, not because they have a mental disorder. It is important to note that this is only one definition of *mental disorder*.

Wakefield's (1992) framework is not without its limitations (McNally, 2011, pp. 69–96).

Attempts to elucidate a value-free perspective on function—especially when cast within an evolutionary framework—raise yet another set of thorny problems. Nevertheless, the harmful dysfunction provides a useful model for posing questions regarding the distinction between normal psychological distress and its pathological variants.

DESCRIPTIONS OF THE ANXIETY DISORDERS

In the following sections, we describe each of the anxiety disorders listed in the fifth edition of the *Diagnostic and Statistical Manual of Mental Disorders* (DSM-5; American Psychiatric Association, 2013). DSM-5 no longer classifies posttraumatic stress disorder (PTSD) and obsessive-compulsive disorder (OCD) as anxiety disorders. Conversely, separation anxiety disorder, selective mutism, substance/medication-induced anxiety disorder, and anxiety disorder due to another medical condition have been included among the anxiety disorders in DSM-5. As these latter two conditions are attributable to other causes rather than truly counting as independent syndromes, we do not discuss them here. Finally, reverting to the DSM-III scheme, DSM-5 conceptualizes agoraphobia as a disorder in its own right rather than as a complication of panic disorder.

For each anxiety disorder, DSM-5 stipulates that fear or anxiety must persist for at least 6 months, must be out of proportion to any genuine threat or danger, must produce significant distress or impairment in social, occupational, or other areas of functioning (e.g., school), and must not be attributable to another medical condition or explainable by another mental disorder. For an accompanying list of signs and symptoms, see Table 9.1.

Specific Phobia

A specific phobia is an intense fear or anxiety about a specific object or situation (e.g., animals, heights, flying in airplanes, receiving injections, seeing blood) that far exceeds any genuine danger. Phobic individuals usually experience anxiety when they anticipate encountering the dreaded object or situation, and they experience sudden, intense fear when they encounter it. They avoid their feared situations or endure them with intense distress. A diagnosis of specific phobia requires that the person experience extreme distress and impairment in normal functioning for at least 6 months. Although phobic disorders can begin at an early age, they often occur in childhood. Most children fear the same limited range of objects or events. Encounters with feared objects incite increases in physiological arousal (e.g., heart rate), with one notable exception: people who fear viewing blood (or receiving injections) exhibit a distinct biphasic cardiac response. After a brief, minor increase in heart rate, their blood pressure and heart rate plummet, often resulting in a faint.

Separation Anxiety Disorder

The onset of separation anxiety disorder, defined by unrealistic worry accompanying separation from home or caretaker that interferes with appropriate behavior, usually occurs in late childhood but before adolescence. Because separation anxiety disorder is accompanied by a reluctance to engage in activities that require separation from a caretaker, it can take the form of fear of school attendance. Although some adolescents develop separation anxiety disorder, school refusal among adolescents can occur because of social anxiety rather than anxiety over separation.

Social Anxiety Disorder (Social Phobia)

People with social anxiety disorder have intense fear or anxiety about situations where they might encounter scrutiny by others. They worry that they will exhibit anxiety symptoms or otherwise act in ways that provoke ridicule or rejection by those observing them. Their dread of embarrassment, humiliation, and negative evaluation leads to them to avoid social situations or to endure them with marked distress. Although socially anxious children avoid these situations, some are unable to articulate their concerns and simply feel uncomfortable in unfamiliar social

Table 9.1 Signs and Symptoms of Adolescent Anxiety Disorders

Disorder	*Key Diagnostic Feature*	*Other Criteria for the Disorder*	*Other Relevant Clinical Signs & Symptoms*
Panic Disorder	The occurrence of spontaneous panic attacks; these are paroxysms of fear or anxiety associated with somatic symptoms, such as palpitations or shortness of breath	Panic attacks must be recurrent and must be associated with either concern about additional attacks, worry about the implication of the attacks, or changes in behavior. Panic disorder is frequently associated with agoraphobia, anxiety about being in places where escape might be difficult.	Spontaneous panic attacks are very rare before puberty. Typical developmental course for progressive forms of the disorder involves initial development of isolated spontaneous panic attacks around puberty, followed by recurrent panic attacks, and then agoraphobia in adulthood. This process can take years to unfold across maturation from adolescence to adulthood.
Social Anxiety Disorder	The occurrence of marked or intense fear in social situations where an individual may be scrutinized by others	Exposure to social situations provokes anxiety associated with severe distress or impairment; avoidance is common. The individual must show the capacity for age-appropriate social relationships.	This condition typically develops in late childhood or early adolescence. The disorder is associated with shyness or other subclinical behavioral features, such as certain temperamental types such as behavioral inhibition.
Separation Anxiety Disorder	Developmentally inappropriate or excessive anxiety about being separated from home or from an individual to whom a child is attached	Anxiety is associated with either distress upon separation, worry about harm to an attachment figure, avoidance of situations requiring separation, or physical complaints when separation is anticipated.	This condition is among the most prevalent mental disorders in children. The condition typically develops in early childhood, showing high rates of remission between childhood and adolescence. Some data suggest a familial or longitudinal association with panic disorder in adults.
Obsessive-Compulsive Disorder (OCD)	Recurrent, persistent, intrusive, anxiety-provoking thoughts (obsessions) and associated repetitive acts (compulsions) that a person feels driven to perform	This pattern of intrusive thoughts and compulsions is time-consuming and causes functional impairment or distress. There is a range of insight among OCD patients, although younger children may be less likely to recognize the senselessness of their obsessions and compulsions.	This condition typically presents with stereotyped thoughts or acts. These might include concerns that the individual is in some way dirty or that s/he has sinned. The disorder is frequently associated with tics and attention-deficit disorder during childhood.

(*continued*)

Table 9.1 Continued

Disorder	*Key Diagnostic Feature*	*Other Criteria for the Disorder*	*Other Relevant Clinical Signs & Symptoms*
Posttraumatic Stress Disorder (PTSD)	Following exposure to trauma, which includes actual or threatened death, serious injury, or sexual violence, an individual develops recurrent re-experiencing of the event, attempts to avoid associated symptoms, negative alterations in cognition and mood associated with the event, and increased arousal symptoms.	Re-experiencing can involve flashbacks, nightmares, or images. Avoidance can involve changes in behavior, changes in cognition, or new-onset feelings of detachment. Increased arousal can involve insomnia, exaggerated startle, or irritability.	PTSD is associated with many comorbid disorders, including major depression, other anxiety disorders, and behavior disorders. Different types of traumas may involve different symptomatic manifestations. For example, symptoms may differ in acute vs. chronic trauma.
Generalized Anxiety Disorder (GAD)	A pattern of excessive worry on most days for a period of six months. This worry is difficult to control.	Worry is characterized as apprehension when anticipating an upcoming feared event. Worry is associated with restlessness, fatigue, reduced concentration, or difficulty falling asleep. The individual finds it difficult to control the worry.	GAD shows very high rates of comorbidity with a range of conditions, particularly anxiety disorders. In clinical settings, GAD virtually never presents as an isolated condition but is complicated by another comorbid disorder. Beyond the relationship with other anxiety disorders, GAD shows an unusually strong association with major depression.
Specific Phobia	Marked and excessive fear of a specific object, such that exposure to the object precipitates extreme anxiety	The fear either causes avoidance that interferes with functioning or produces marked distress in the individual.	Specific phobia generally produces lower levels of impairment than other anxiety disorders. Phobias can be divided based on the nature of the feared object into various types, including animal type, natural environment type, blood injury type, or situational type.

settings. To receive the diagnosis, children must be anxious among their peers, not merely in the presence of adults. Some people with this disorder experience anxiety only while performing in front of others (e.g., speaking in public, taking tests), whereas others experience distress in diverse social settings (e.g., attending parties, meeting new people, eating in public).

Selective Mutism

Selective mutism refers to a persistent failure to speak in certain social situations, such as school, despite doing so in other situations, such as at home. The failure to speak persists for at least 1 month (not limited to the first month of school), and it interferes with educational achievement. The problem does not arise from a communication disorder, another mental disorder (e.g., autism), or unfamiliarity with the spoken language.

Generalized Anxiety Disorder

A diagnosis of generalized anxiety disorder (GAD) is given to adolescents who worry about a variety of events or life circumstances—usually schoolwork, appearance, money, or their future. The age of onset of GAD is usually later than for most other disorders, although many patients report having been anxious for many years. Further, GAD is likely to be comorbid with other symptoms, but the primary symptom is a chronic state of worry rather than chronically avoidant behavior.

Panic Disorder

People with panic disorder experience sudden, unexpected surges of terror that peak within minutes and can occur without any obvious precipitants. Panic attacks are characterized by at least four of 13 symptoms, such as racing heart, sweating, trembling, smothering sensations, and fears of dying, losing control, or "going crazy." The diagnosis requires a period of least 1 month of worry about further attacks or maladaptive behavior designed to prevent them (e.g., avoidance).

Panic disorder usually begins in late adolescence or early adulthood. Many young people develop the full-blown disorder only after experiencing occasional, sporadic attacks that culminate into persistent worry and maladaptive behavior to forestall their occurrence (Pine, Cohen, Gurlet, Brook, & Ma, 1998). Although young, prepubertal children can have occasional intense distress reactions, it is unclear whether these attacks are accompanied by thoughts of impending danger. Moreover, it is extremely rare for children to experience such episodes in the absence of a trigger. The apparent absence of spontaneous, unexpected panic attacks renders the diagnosis controversial in preadolescent children. If this disorder does occur in children, it is relatively infrequent. Some investigators believe that the essential missing component in early childhood is the unprovoked change in bodily sensations, whereas others believe that it is the inability to impose a catastrophic interpretation on these sensations.

Agoraphobia

Agoraphobia is intense fear and avoidance of a wide range of situations such as shopping malls, bridges, theaters, crowds, enclosed spaces, public transportation, or being away from home alone. The motivation for avoidance rests on fears that panic attacks or panic-like episodes (e.g., dizziness) may occur in places where escape or assistance from others would be difficult. Agoraphobia is not a fear of open or public places per se; rather, it constitutes fear of sudden, alarming bodily dysregulation in settings where such episodes would be problematic. A minimum of two situations is necessary for the diagnosis, and the fear must persist for at least 6 months and be out of proportion to any real danger. For example, fear of walking alone in a crime-ridden neighborhood would not qualify, whereas fear of walking alone for fear of having a sudden panic attack would.

Beginning with DSM-III-R, agoraphobia was classified not as a separate syndrome, but as a subtype of panic disorder. Indeed, dread of panic attacks or subsyndromal panic episodes falling short of the minimum of four symptoms required for a panic attack, motivates the hallmark avoidance behavior of people with agoraphobia. Agoraphobia's reappearance as a distinct syndrome in DSM-5 does not signify a major discovery in psychopathology; it merely denotes the realization that some people can develop agoraphobia after experiencing insufficiently frequent panic attacks to qualify for panic *disorder*, attacks with fewer than four panic symptoms, and other, sudden physical problems (e.g., loss of bowel control, migraine headaches).

PREVALENCE OF THE ANXIETY DISORDERS

Accurate estimates of the prevalence of DSM anxiety disorders are only available for children older than 8 years of age. Studies on younger children have lacked population-based samples, explicit diagnostic criteria, or both. The best estimates of the prevalence of anxiety disorders in preschool children, based on a primary care clinic sample (Lavigne et al., 1996, 1998, 2001), were very low. The following sections summarize prevalence data based on samples from the general population and studies published over the past decade (Costello, Egger, & Angold, 2004). The prevalence of any anxiety disorder increases with the duration of time over which the symptom's presence is counted. Thus, 3-month estimates range from 2.2% to 8.6%, 6-month estimates from 5.5% to 17.7%, 12-month estimates from 8.6% to 20.9%, and lifetime estimates from 8.3% to 27% (for more information see Kessler, Chiu, Demler, & Walters, 2005).

Anxiety and Disability

The relation between the diagnosis and everyday functioning remains a focus of controversy. Health maintenance organizations, insurance companies, and governmental agencies question whether children diagnosed with anxiety disorders require treatment (Costello, Burns, Angold, & Leaf, 1993). One perspective requires that impairment or disability attributable to the problem be apparent before a child receives a diagnosis. Clinicians could rate a child's psychological functioning but fail to make a clinical diagnosis (Hodges, Doucette-Gates, & Liao, 1999; Shaffer et al., 1983).

The prevalence of anxiety disorders varies according to whether disability is a diagnostic requirement. If a child must meet the criteria for a diagnostically relevant symptom as well as impairment in everyday functioning, the prevalence of a diagnosis drops by 67%. Further, requiring both specific impairment and severe scores on the Children's Global Assessment Scale (Shaffer, Fisher, Dulcan, & Davies, 1996), reduced the prevalence of disorder by almost 90%. This occurred most dramatically for specific phobia: requiring impairment in daily functioning lowered the prevalence from 21.6% to only 0.7%. Thus, all estimates of the frequency of the anxiety disorders depend in a serious way on the source of evidence and the criteria adopted. There is no "correct" prevalence in the sense that there is a correct height, in meters, for the Empire State Building.

Gender and Age Differences in Prevalence

Most investigators report that girls are more likely than boys are to have an anxiety disorder. For example, more girls than boys between ages 9 and 16 years had an anxiety disorder in the Great Smoky Mountains Study (12.1% vs. 7.7%; Costello et al., 2004). Three studies revealed more phobias in girls, two reported more panic disorder and agoraphobia in girls, and only one study found more separation anxiety disorder and overanxious disorder (OAD) in girls than in boys. In one of the few studies that examined the potential confounding factors linked to gender, the excess of anxiety disorder in girls remained even after the researchers controlled for 15 possible confounding variables (Lewinsohn, Gotlib, Lewinsohn, Seeley, & Allen, 1998). One confound was the frequent correlation between a child's age and the timeframe for assessing symptoms. Investigators who used 3-month prevalence rates reported the lowest prevalence but studied the youngest subjects. By contrast, investigators using 12-month estimates had the highest prevalence but worked with the oldest children. In the Great Smoky Mountains Study, the prevalence of separation anxiety decreased with age, whereas social phobia, agoraphobia, and panic disorder increased with age. It is difficult to draw conclusions about gender differences in the fears, worries, and anxieties of clinic-referred samples given the modest amount of extant research. Further research in this area is of critical importance (see Silverman & Carter, in press).

Summary

On any day, between 3% and 5% of children and adolescents suffer from an anxiety disorder. Rates of GAD and specific phobia remain constant across childhood and adolescence. Although girls are more likely than boys are to have an anxiety disorder, the gender difference is less prominent in the general population than it is in the clinical population, perhaps because boys are less likely to receive referral for treatment than girls are. Numerous studies have demonstrated that girls who mature earlier than their peers exhibit higher rates of anxiety symptoms and disorders (e.g., Caspi & Moffitt, 1991); such findings have not been obtained with boys.

COMORBIDITY

Marked comorbidity among the anxiety disorders has been a problem for nosology, epidemiology, diagnosis, and treatment. It occurs in the community as well as in the clinic (Brady & Kendall, 1992; Kendall & Clarkin, 1992; Kendall, Kortlander, Chansky, & Brady, 1992; Table 9.2). A review by Costello et al. (2004) yielded equivocal results because not all diagnoses were present in every study, there was a lack of consensus regarding controls for comorbidity, and concurrent comorbidity and sequential comorbidity were not always distinguished.

GAD

Beginning with DSM-IV, children who once received a diagnosis of OAD now receive one of GAD. Permissively conceptualized, the latter diagnosis was assignable if the child had only one of six symptoms (restlessness, fatigue, difficulty concentrating, irritability, muscle tension, or sleep disturbance), and these criteria

Table 9.2 Summary of Comorbidity from Pediatric Samples

Anxiety Disorder	*Community Samples*	*Clinical Samples*
Social Anxiety Disorder / Selective Mutism	Specific phobias, separation anxiety disorder	Other anxiety disorders, major depression, substance abuse
Generalized Anxiety Disorder (formerly OAD)	Depression, possibly alcohol & other substance abuse	Separation anxiety disorder, specific phobia, social anxiety disorder
Separation Anxiety Disorder	GAD, specific phobia, social anxiety disorder, possibly *subsequent* panic disorder	GAD, specific phobia, social anxiety disorder
Specific Phobias	Separation anxiety disorder, social anxiety disorder	Separation anxiety disorder, social anxiety disorder
Panic Disorder	Possibly social anxiety disorder, specific phobia	GAD
Obsessive-Compulsive Disorder	Other anxiety disorders, depression, tic disorders	Depression, other anxiety disorders, tic disorders
Posttraumatic Stress Disorder	Depression, other anxiety disorders, externalizing disorders	Depression, panic disorder, social anxiety disorder, GAD, externalizing disorders

differ from defining OAD (worry about the past or future, concern about one's competence, need for reassurance, somatic symptoms, excessive self-consciousness, and muscle tension). Further, the newer criteria for GAD resemble those used to diagnose major depressive episodes; examination of the overlap between OAD and GAD should take into account the possibility of a correlation with depression.

The Great Smoky Mountains Study, involving 1,420 children, which examined comorbidity among OAD, GAD, and depression (Costello, Mustillo, Erklani, Keeler, & Angold, 2003), found that among children who were comorbid (5.4% of the entire sample, or 47% of those with any of the three diagnoses), more than half had all three disorders. Only 12 children (16% of those with GAD or OAD) had both disorders but no signs of depression.

Comorbidity Between Panic Disorder and Separation Anxiety Disorder

There is no significant concurrent comorbidity between panic disorder and separation anxiety, but this does not preclude possible sequential comorbidity. Early appearance of separation anxiety appears to predict panic disorder (Black, 1994; Klein, 1995; Silove, Manicavasagar, Curtis, & Blaszczynski, 1996), but no community studies have tested this hypothesis adequately. A meta-analysis of 25 studies (prospective, retrospective, and case-control) revealed that a childhood diagnosis of separation anxiety disorder significantly increased the risk for subsequent anxiety disorders (Kossowsky et al., 2013). Although the effect size was largest for panic disorder with or without agoraphobia, it was not significantly greater than that for anxiety disorders in general. After correcting for publication bias, the authors found that separation anxiety did not increase the risk for depression or substance use disorders.

Comorbidity with Other Disorders

Comorbidity between any one anxiety disorder on the one hand, and attention-deficit/hyperactivity disorder (ADHD), conduct disorder, depression, or substance abuse disorder on the other, reveals the highest level of comorbidity with depression. The median odds ratio is 8.2 (95% confidence interval [CI], 5.8–12; Costello, Egger, et al., 2004).

There is also a sequential link between early anxiety and later depression (Costello et al., 2003; Orvaschel, Lewinsohn, & Seeley, 1995). It is unclear whether depression or anxiety increases the subsequent risk for the complementary disorder or whether the natural sequence is from an initial anxiety disorder to subsequent depression.

The odds ratio for the comorbidity of anxiety with risk for conduct disorder/oppositional disorder is 3.1 (95% CI, 2.2–4.6), and with ADHD it is 3.0 (95% CI, 2.1–4.3). These CIs imply a significant degree of comorbidity. Although the bivariate odds ratios that involve substance use or abuse were significant in some studies, an association between anxiety and substance abuse disappeared when comorbidity between anxiety and other psychiatric disorders was controlled for (Costello et al., 2004).

Although there is little concurrent comorbidity for anxiety and substance abuse (Weissman et al., 1999), childhood onset of an anxiety disorder might predict either lower or higher rates of substance abuse in adolescence. Kaplow, Curran, Angold, and Costello (2001) reported that children with separation anxiety were less likely than others were to begin drinking alcohol, and if they did, they began at a later age than that of most youth. But children with GAD were more likely to begin drinking and abuse alcohol earlier in adolescence.

Using a large British twin registry, behavior geneticists found more support for environmental than genetic sources of comorbidity among specific phobia and both social phobia and separation anxiety in school-age children (Eley, Rijsdijk, Perrin, O'Connor, & Bolton, 2008). In contrast to such studies on adults, shared environment accounted for significant variance, implying anxiogenic parental childrearing practices for all children within families or other sources of similarity among siblings (e.g., exposed to the same bullies at school).

ONSET AND COURSE

The evidence does not permit a confident reply to the question of whether anxiety disorders in preschool children are precursors of similar disorders in adolescents. Invariably fallible retrospective data indicate that adolescents with anxiety disorders recalled their first onset at about 7 years of age (Costello, Erkanli, Federman, & Angold, 1999; Orvaschel et al., 1995). The Great Smoky Mountains Study revealed that specific phobias, GAD, separation anxiety, and social phobia all appeared around the time the child began school, whereas agoraphobia and OAD appeared several years later, usually at 9 to 11 years of age (Costello et al., 2003).

Although early anxiety disorder forecasts later depression (Alloy, Kelly, Mineka, & Clements, 1990; Breslau, Schultz, & Peterson, 1995; Kendler, Neale, Kessler, Heath, & Eaves, 1992; Lewinsohn, Zinbarg, Seeley, Lewinsohn, & Sack, 1997; Silberg, Rutter, & Eaves, 2001a, 2001b; Silberg, Rutter, Neale, & Eaves, 2001), we do not know the influence of anxiety on the timing or occurrence of other psychiatric disorders, with one exception: early separation anxiety and GAD have different predictive consequences for the later abuse of alcohol (Kaplow, Curran, Angold, & Costello, 2001).

Separation anxiety and phobic disorders occur in early childhood but are rare in adolescence. Panic disorder and agoraphobia have the opposite developmental profile: they are rare in childhood and increase in adolescence. We do not yet know whether some adolescent disorders are later manifestations of a syndrome that appeared earlier or whether they represent new forms of psychiatric illness. An answer to this question requires longitudinal research.

THEORIES OF ETIOLOGY AND MAINTENANCE

Learning Theories

Early behavioral models for the treatment of anxiety rested on two primary suppositions. First, fears and phobias are acquired through classical conditioning—that is, through the formation of an association between a neutral stimulus and an aversive stimulus such that the former acquires the aversive properties of the latter. The aversive unconditioned stimulus (US) converts the formerly neutral one into a conditioned stimulus (CS) possessing the capacity to evoke the conditioned response (CR) of fear. Second, the acquired fears can be unlearned through extinction—that is, through presentation of the CS in the absence of the US. This conceptualization gave rise to exposure therapy, in which patients are taught systematically to confront their feared situations, objects, responses (e.g., tachycardia), or memories under safe circumstances with the goal of extinguishing their phobic fear.

However, merely because exposure therapy can reduce fears does not mean that they originated in classical conditioning. Indeed, many phobias of animals, heights, and so forth emerge in childhood without any apparent conditioning events involving a painful US (e.g., dog bites, falls from high places) whatsoever. Such findings motivated the nonassociative theory of phobias, which holds that the key question is explaining why many apparently innate fears fail to extinguish, not to explain why these fears emerge in the first place (Poulton & Menzies, 2002).

Although the original classical conditioning theory of fear acquisition that inspired exposure therapy encountered difficulties explaining the etiology of phobias (e.g., Rachman, 1977), 21st-century conditioning theory has evolved markedly in ways promising to provide a nuanced account of the etiology of anxiety disorders (e.g., Field, 2006). Rather than viewing conditioning as solely the acquisition of associations between physically realizable CSs and biologically significant USs, contemporary views conceptualize it as a form of predictive, causal learning embodied in cognitive representations of events occurring in context. Likewise, in contrast to early views that viewed verbal transmission of threat information and vicarious acquisition of fear as pathways to phobia distinct from conditioning (cf. Rachman, 1977), contemporary views emphasize the procedural similarities among the three pathways as exemplifying causal learning about the world (Field, 2006). The upshot is that developments in human associative learning may prove more theoretically fruitful in accounting for etiology than was the original classical conditioning model. Debates about the mechanisms mediating exposure therapy notwithstanding, considerable research documents its therapeutic benefits (cf., Barlow, 2001; Ollendick & March, 2004).

Discontent with the original, noncognitive accounts of the acquisition and extinction of pathological anxiety led to the development of theories that posited a pivotal role for cognitive factors in anxiety (e.g., Beck, Emery, & Greenberg, 1985). The assumption here is that it is not the events themselves but rather their threat "meaning" that is responsible for the evocation of anxiety. Meaning is represented in language. Accordingly, in cognitive therapy for anxiety disorders, verbal discourse provides the basis for challenging the patient's threat interpretations of events in order to help replace them with more realistic ones, especially so with adolescents. The focus on the meaning of events paralleled the reconceptualization of conditioning in learning theories. For example, as Rescorla observed, "conditioning depends not on the contiguity between the CS and US but rather in the information that the CS provides about the US" (Rescorla, 1988, p. 153). Hence, the "organism is better seen as an information seeker using logical and perceptual relations among events along with its own preconception to form a sophisticated representation of its world" (Rescorla, 1988, p. 154). In the same vein, when discussing the phenomenon of extinction, Bouton (1994, 2000) stated that "in the Pavlovian conditioning situation, the signal winds up with two available 'meanings'" (Bouton, 2000, p. 58).

Advances in information-processing theories of conditioning and of pathological anxiety (e.g., Lang, 1977) inspired similar views of anxiety disorders and their treatment. For example, in their emotional processing theory, Foa and Kozak (1986) conceptualized fear as a cognitive structure in memory that serves as a blueprint for escaping or avoiding danger that contains information about the feared stimuli, fear responses, and the meaning of these stimuli and responses. When a person is faced with a realistically threatening situation (e.g., an accelerating car in one's path, or the approach of a fierce dog), the fear structure supports adaptive behavior (e.g., swerving away, running away). A fear structure becomes pathological when the associations among stimulus, response, and meaning representations do not accurately reflect reality; in this instance, harmless stimuli or responses assume threat meaning. In emotional processing theory, meaning is embedded in associations among stimuli, responses, and consequences (as in Rescorla, 1988), as well as in language, especially in the form of thoughts, beliefs, and evaluations (as in Beck, 1976).

According to emotional processing theory, anxiety disorders reflect the operation of specific pathological fear structures (Foa & Kozak, 1985). For example, the fear structure of individuals with panic disorder is characterized by erroneous interpretations of physiological responses associated with their panic symptoms (e.g., tachycardia, difficulty breathing) as dangerous (e.g., leading to a heart attack). Such misinterpretations motivate avoidance of situations and bodily sensations where these individuals anticipate panic attacks. Accordingly, the core pathology in panic disorder lies in the erroneous meaning of physiological responses. The supposition that inaccurate negative cognitions underlie the anxiety disorders has also been at the heart of theories posed by cognitive therapists (e.g., Clark, 1986; Rapee & Heimberg, 1997; Salkovskis, 1985).

If fear reflects the activation of an underlying cognitive fear structure, then changes in the fear structure should result in corresponding changes in emotions and behavior. Indeed, Foa and Kozak (1986) proposed that psychological interventions known to reduce fear, such as exposure therapy, achieve their effects through modifying the fear structure. According to emotional processing theory, two conditions are necessary for therapeutic fear reduction to occur. First, the fear structure must activate; second, information incompatible with the pathological aspects of the fear structure must be available and incorporated into the structure. Thus, within this framework, exposure therapy corrects the erroneous cognitions that underlie the specific disorder (e.g., tachycardia = heart attack). This is also the presumptive mechanism mediating the anxiolytic effects of cognitive therapy. Accordingly, exposure therapy and cognitive therapy work through overlapping mechanisms. Moreover, some cognitive therapists explicitly posit that fear activation is necessary to refute the patient's false interpretations, and cognitive therapy programs routinely include an exposure component in the form of "behavioral experiments." The evidence for cognitive change as the central mechanism in fear reduction remains incomplete. Accordingly, we need additional work on the mediators or mechanisms of change in both the cognitive and behavior therapies, especially in children and adolescents, for whom the role of cognition remains understudied (Prins & Ollendick, 2003).

COGNITIVE CORRELATES OF ANXIETY DISORDERS

The cognitive approach to anxiety disorders comprises two research traditions (McNally, 2001). In one tradition, researchers assume that introspective self-reports of anxious individuals can reveal aberrant cognition mediating symptom expression. These scholars administer questionnaires and conduct interviews to ascertain, for example, the intensity, frequency, and content of the worries and fears of children and adolescents. One such study revealed that school-age children worry most about school, health, and personal harm, especially the latter (Silverman, La Greca, & Wasserstein, 1995). Another indicated that children and adolescents with anxiety disorders report the same kinds of worries as those of their healthy counterparts, but that the intensity (not the number) of worries distinguished youngsters with anxiety disorders from those without anxiety disorders (Weems, Silverman, & La Greca, 2000). Researchers in this tradition have also studied the fear of anxiety symptoms (i.e., anxiety sensitivity; Reiss & McNally, 1985). Silverman and colleagues have developed the Childhood Anxiety Sensitivity Index (CASI; Silverman, Fleisig, Rabian, & Peterson, 1991; Silverman & Weems, 1999) to investigate this phenomenon.

In the second tradition, researchers eschew self-report as insufficiently sensitive to measure abnormalities in cognitive mechanisms that often operate rapidly, outside of awareness. These scientists apply the methods of experimental cognitive psychology to elucidate biases favoring processing of threat-related information in patients with anxiety disorders (McNally, 1996; Williams, Watts, MacLeod, & Mathews, 1997). In this section, we review experiments on information-processing biases in anxious children and adolescents (see also Vasey, Dalgleish, & Silverman, 2003; Vasey & MacLeod, 2001).

Attentional Bias for Threat

Because attentional capacity is limited, people can attend only to certain stimuli at a given time, and any bias for selectively attending to threat-related stimuli should increase a person's likelihood of experiencing anxiety. Two experimental tasks have indicated that adults with anxiety disorders often exhibit an attentional bias for processing information about threat. In the emotional Stroop task (Williams, Mathews, & MacLeod, 1996), subjects view words of varying emotional significance, quickly naming the colors in which they appear while ignoring the meanings of the words. Delays in color naming ("Stroop Interference") occur when the meaning of the word captures the subject's attention despite the subject's effort to attend to the color in which the word is printed. Most studies have shown that patients with anxiety disorders take longer to name the colors of words related to their threat-related concerns than to name the colors of other emotional or neutral words, and take longer to name the colors of threat words than do healthy subjects. It is debatable whether this task provides a pure measure of attentional bias; for example, an emotional response to threatening words might delay color naming.

Studies on the emotional Stroop in children have yielded mixed results. Relative to control subjects, spider-fearful children take longer to name the colors of spider words (Martin, Horder, & Jones, 1992) and colors of line drawings of spiders (Martin & Jones, 1995). However, not all Stroop studies have confirmed an anxiety-linked attentional bias for threat cues in youngsters. For example, nonanxious as well as anxious children have exhibited delayed color naming of threat words (Kindt, Bierman, & Brosschot, 1997; Kindt, Brosschot, & Everaerd, 1997). A pictorial version of the spider Stroop (naming colors of background against which spider pictures appeared) did not reveal a fear-related effect in children (ages 8–11; Kindt, van den Hout, de Jong, & Hoekzema, 2000).

A second paradigm provides a less controversial measure of attentional bias. In the dot probe attentional deployment task (MacLeod, Mathews, & Tata, 1986), subjects view two words on a computer screen, one appearing above the other. On some trials, one word is threat related, whereas the other is not. After the words disappear, a small dot appears in the location of one of the words. Subjects press a button as soon as they detect the dot. Relative to healthy control subjects, patients with anxiety disorders are faster to respond when the dot replaces a threat word than when it replaces a neutral word. Because threat cues capture attention in anxious patients, these individuals are especially quick to respond to the neutral dot that follows a threat cue.

Using this task, Vasey, Daleiden, Williams, and Brown (1995) found that children (ages 9–14 years) with anxiety disorders exhibited an attentional bias for threat, whereas control children did not. The attentional bias increased with age and with reading ability. Relative to their nonanxious counterparts, test-anxious schoolchildren (ages 11–14 years) exhibited an attentional bias for threat words (both socially and physically threatening; Vasey, El-Hag, & Daleiden, 1996). Patients with GAD (ages 9–18 years) exhibited an attentional bias for threat words, whereas patients with mixed anxiety and depression or healthy control subjects did not (Taghavi, Neshat-Doost, Moradi, Yule, & Dalgleish, 1999). The GAD patients did not show an attentional bias for depression-related words, and the attentional bias for threat words was unrelated to the age of the subject.

Interpretive Bias for Threat

Anxious children tend to interpret ambiguous information in a threatening fashion. In one study, children (ages 7–9 years) heard homophones (e.g., whipping) that could be interpreted in either a threatening or a nonthreatening fashion (Hadwin, Frost, French, & Richards, 1997). The higher a child's trait anxiety, the more likely the child selected threatening pictures (e.g., rope) over nonthreatening pictures (e.g., cream) that made the homophones (e.g., whipping) unambiguous. In another study, GAD patients (ages 8–17 years) and healthy control children were shown homographs (e.g., hang), each possessing a threatening and a nonthreatening meaning (Taghavi, Moradi, Neshat-Doost, Yule, & Dalgleish, 2000). They were asked to construct a sentence including the homograph. Relative to the sentences constructed by control children, the anxious children more often constructed sentences incorporating the threatening interpretation of the homograph, implying that they had interpreted the ambiguous word in terms of its threatening meaning. This interpretive bias was unrelated to the age of the subjects.

Bell-Dolan (1995) asked anxious and nonanxious children to provide interpretations of ambiguous scenarios. Anxious fourth- and fifth-graders were more likely than were their nonanxious peers to interpret nonhostile scenarios in a threatening fashion, whereas both groups interpreted ambiguous scenarios in a hostile fashion. Patients with anxiety disorders (ages 9–13 years) exhibited a bias for interpreting ambiguous scenarios in a threatening manner, and this effect was strongly predicted by level of trait-anxiety (Chorpita, Albano, & Barlow, 1996). Relative to healthy control children, patients ranging in age from 7 to 14 years who had OAD, separation anxiety, social phobia, or specific phobia exhibited a bias for interpreting ambiguous scenarios in a threatening fashion

(Barrett, Rapee, Dadds, & Ryan, 1996). This bias was even more pronounced in patients with oppositional-defiant disorder.

Conclusion

Anxious children and adolescents exhibit threat-related attentional and interpretive biases that resemble those exhibited by anxious adults. Moreover, within most studies, the extent of bias did not vary as a function of the child's age. Yet questions remain. In one study, the responses of anxious children to two measures of attentional bias (dot probe and emotional Stroop) were uncorrelated, indicating that these tasks tap distinct processes (Dalgleish et al., 2003). Further, researchers have yet to test whether these biases disappear following successful psychological or pharmacological treatment. A more detailed critique of information processing in adolescent psychopathology is available elsewhere (Vasey et al., 2003).

BIOLOGIC FEATURES OF ADOLESCENCE AND ANXIETY STATES

Human adolescence is both a biological and a social construction, defined as the period in life between puberty (a biological event) and achievement of independence (a socially determined event). Although the exact timing of puberty is not easy to specify, at its core puberty involves changes in the hormonal milieu, albeit ones shaped by the cultural setting. The end of adolescence, when independence is achieved, is more heavily shaped by culture. Some cultures, like our own, delay the assumption of adult roles; others require a clear transition, with or without a rite-of-passage ceremony (Schlegel & Barry, 1991). Nonetheless, across cultures, a period does exist between the ages of 12 and 18 years that is seen as unique. This period involves changes in hormones, brain structure, and behavior. These properties may have been conserved over evolution to promote autonomy and to foster dispersal of some individuals from the natal territory to another in order to avoid inbreeding (Schlegel & Barry, 1991; Spear, 2000). This is the period of adolescence.

Adolescence is marked by a reactivation of the hypothalamic–pituitary–gonadal axis, development of secondary sexual characteristics, and the onset of reproductive capacity, even though the increased circulation of sex hormones does not account for much of the variance in the behavior of adolescents (Brooks-Gunn, Graber, & Paikoff, 1994). The timing of pubertal signs is influenced by gender and environment; onset of puberty may be influenced more strongly by environmental stressors in girls than in boys (Moffitt, Caspi, Belsky, & Silva, 1992).

The brain undergoes changes throughout life (Eriksson et al., 1998), with intervals of modest change punctuated by periods of more rapid transformation (Spear, 2000). Periods of more dramatic change include not only prenatal and early postnatal eras but also adolescence (Spear, 2000). Rakic, Bourgeois, and Goldman-Rakic (1994) estimate that up to 30,000 cortical synapses are lost every second during portions of the pubertal period in nonhuman primates, resulting in a decline of nearly 50% in the average number of synaptic contacts per neuron, compared with the number prior to puberty. There is a similar loss of synapses in the human brain between 7 and 16 years of age (Huttenlocher, 1979), but the scarcity of human postmortem tissue prevents a more detailed description of this phenomenon. Although the functions of pruning are not fully understood, scientists do agree that pruning reflects an aspect of normal brain maturation. Pruning may lead to changes in functional capacities, facilitated by appropriately arranged neurons, given that some forms of mental retardation are associated with an unusually high density of synapses (Goldman-Rakic, Isseroff, Schwartz, & Bugbee, 1983).

The elimination of synapses that are presumed to be excitatory, accompanied by a reduction in brain energy utilization, is thought to transform the adolescent brain into one that is more efficient and less energy consuming (Chugani, 1996; Rakic et al., 1994). These changes could permit more selective reactions to stimuli that in younger children activate broader cortical regions (Casey, Geidd, & Thomas, 2000).

Considerable research has accumulated on changes in the structures of the brain from childhood through adolescence. This research used refinements in magnetic resonance imaging (MRI), which has allowed for longitudinal studies. Despite inconsistencies across studies, a few areas of consensus have emerged. First, the immature state of the adolescent brain has been repeatedly demonstrated. That is, adolescence involves marked changes in the relative volumes, levels of activity, and connections among brain regions. For example, there is an increase in cortical white matter density, which is thought to reflect changes in the brain's myelination and connections among regions, as well as a corresponding decrease in gray matter (Giedd et al., 1999; Sowell et al., 1999a, 1999b). Complex changes also occur in subcortical structures, including the hippocampus and the amygdala (Giedd et al., 1997; Yurgelun-Todd, Killgrove, & Cintron, 2003). Second, consensus has emerged on the broad pattern of changes in these regions. That is, phylogenically older regions, such as primary sensory and motor cortices, mature earlier than the older regions of association cortex. Finally, consensus has emerged on a few areas of brain development during adolescence as involving relative changes in the brain's circuitry, as reflected in connections among regions.

Conversely, areas of disagreement persist. One area of disagreement concerns the precise nature of changes among the various regions. Thus, some models suggest that adolescence involves a relative imbalance between late-maturing prefrontal regions and earlier-maturing subcortical structures, such as the amygdala and striatum (Casey, Duhoux, et al., 2010; Casey, Jones, et al., 2010; Ernst, Pine, et al., 2006). Other models suggest that adolescence involves more complex, nonlinear changes (Crone & Dahl, 2012). Another area of disagreement concerns the precise timing of maturity for individual brain regions. This reflects differences in the methods among studies reporting different findings. Whereas older studies relied largely on cross-sectional data, newer studies use longitudinal methods and increasingly sophisticated data collection techniques (Giedd, Raznahan, et al., 2012; Raznahan, Lee, et al., 2010; Raznahan, Lerch, et al., 2011; Raznahan, Shaw, et al., 2014).

Studies in rodents and nonhuman primates use more invasive methods than can be employed in humans. Such invasive studies provide more fine-grained analysis of particular connections among brain regions. This research finds developmental shifts in patterns of innervation, including the circuits involved in the recognition and expression of fear, anxiety, and other emotions (Charney & Deutsch, 1996). This work also shows that the responsiveness of the cortical gamma-amino butyric acid (GABA)–benzodiazepine receptor complex to challenge increases as animals approach puberty (Kellogg, 1998); it also delineates changing function in the hippocampus involving GABA transmission (Benes, 1989; Wolfer & Lipp, 1995; Nurse & Lacaille, 1999) and changes in neurogenesis. Further, pubescent animals show lower utilization rates of serotonin in the nucleus accumbens than younger or older animals (Teicher & Andersen, 1999).

Studies in laboratory animals specifically demonstrate developmental increases in amygdala–prefrontal cortex (PFC) connectivity (Cunningham, Bhattacharyya, & Benes, 2002), along with alterations in amygdala activation (Terasawa & Timiras, 1968). This may explain the unique effects of amygdala lesions in immature and mature primates (Prather et al., 2001). Findings from functional MRI research in human adolescents provide some parallels with these data in laboratory animals. However, findings on aspects of normal adolescent development in functional MRI remain less consistent than in structural MRI (Casey, Jones, et al., 2008, 2010; Casey, Pattwell, et al., 2013; Crone & Dahl, 2012).

Maturational changes in the cerebellum, and the circuitry connecting the cerebellum to the prefrontal cortex, continue through adolescence. Lesions of the adult cerebellum disrupt the regulation of emotion and interfere with performance on tasks requiring executive functions (Schmahmann & Sherman, 1998), although this is less apparent in those younger than 16 years (Levisohn, Cronin-Golomb, & Schmahmann, 2000).

One consequence of this restructuring of the brain during adolescence is that early developmental compromises might be exposed. That is, brain regions vulnerable to dysfunction, due either to genetics or to adverse early experience, might be unmasked by the combination of brain restructuring and stressful life experiences (Goldman-Rakic et al., 1983; Hughes & Sparber, 1978).

BIOLOGY AND ANXIETY DISORDERS

There is great interest in detecting the biological variables that might distinguish anxious from nonanxious patients. Many, but not all, of these biological measures are influenced directly or indirectly by a brain circuit that connects a series of regions. This includes inferior aspects of the frontal cortex, the hippocampus, the amygdala, bed nucleus, and their projections to the brain stem, autonomic nervous system, endocrine targets, cortex, and central gray matter (Blackford & Pine, 2012; Pine, 1999, 2001, 2002; Pine, Cohen, & Brook, 2001; Pine, Fyer, et al., 2001; Pine, Grun, et al., 2001). It is relevant that connectivity between the amygdala and prefrontal cortex, along with level of amygdalar activation, increases during adolescence (Cunningham, Bhattacharyya, & Benes, 2002; Terasawa & Timiras, 1968).

How Does One Define a Circuit That Responds to Threats?

As neuroscience research over the past decade repeatedly demonstrates the complexity of the human brain, questions have arisen regarding the degree to which one or another neural circuit mediates a relatively specific series of functions. Thus, as noted above, considerable research does implicate a collection of brain regions in the response to threats. This circuit encompasses ventral PFC, amygdala, hippocampus, and interconnected structures (Davis, Walker, et al., 2010; Davis & Whalen, 2001; LeDoux, 2012, 2013). However, neural circuits are now understood to serve many different functions (Bilder, Howe, et al., 2013). As a result, this circuit is engaged in many scenarios besides those involving threat. Moreover, fear is now understood to be a heterogeneous construct, with different forms of fear varying based on the contexts of the situation, the nature of the particular threat, and the types of cognitive processes engaged (Davis, Walker, et al., 2010; LeDoux, 2012, 2014). This complicates attempts to define a particular set of brain structures that regulates humans' response to threat. Of course, because these same structures continue to evolve with adolescent maturation, it is even more difficult to define a particular circuit that relates to aspects of fear or threat responding in adolescence.

This broader debate concerning the nature of a so-called fear circuit encompasses a number of related issues. For example, some questions persist regarding the functions of particular structures. Hence, there is debate over whether the amygdala is activated primarily by events that are potentially harmful or events that are unexpected or discrepant (Davis 1992, 1998; LeDoux 1996, 1998, 2000). Clearly, because the amygdala responds to discrepant and unexpected events that are harmless as well as to positive events, the amygdala is not merely a fear-related structure. Select neurons in the amygdala, as well as in the bed nucleus, hippocampus, and brain stem sites, reliably respond to unexpected or discrepant events, regardless of whether they are threatening or harmful (Wilson & Rolls, 1993). And the reactivity of amygdalar neurons to unexpected or discrepant events habituates, often rapidly, as the event becomes expected and loses its surprise value (La Bar, Gatenby, Gore, Le Doux, & Phelps, 1998).

Other questions relate specifically to development. Some aspects of fear responding reflect the developmental experiences of the organism. The behavioral reactions of monkeys, chimpanzees, and human infants to a snake are no different from their reactions to discrepant events that are harmless (e.g., a tortoise or seaweed). Only 30% of monkeys born and reared in the laboratory showed more prolonged withdrawal to a live snake than to blue masking tape (Nelson, Shelton, & Kalin, 2003). If snakes were a biologically potent incentive for fear, a majority of monkeys should have shown an immediate withdrawal reaction.

A final set of questions relates to individual differences in fear- and anxiety-related behaviors. Do these relate to differences in particular brain structures or interactions among a series of regions? Moreover, do individual differences in fear-related behaviors reflect ontogeny, as appears to be the case for other aspects of individual differences (Giedd, Raznahan, et al., 2012)? This final set of questions has been addressed most completely through research on anxiety disorders in adolescence.

Biological Correlates of Adolescent Anxiety Disorders

Advances in genetics, imaging, and cognitive neuroscience provide the opportunity to combine discoveries in neuroscience with insights from clinical psychobiology. Current views of adolescent anxiety disorders are influenced by two limiting facts. The first is that the research on adolescents has been modeled on investigations of adults; the second is that all current anxiety disorders are heterogeneous in their origin. This second fact means that investigators would profit from using biological variables to distinguish between patients with transient symptoms and those with more persistent disorders (Merikangas, Avenevoli, Dierker, & Grillon, 1999; Pine, Wasserman, & Workman, 1999).

Autonomic Nervous System

Many, but not all, adults with anxiety disorders show abnormalities of autonomic regulation, especially lability of the cardiovascular system. This feature is most common among adults with panic disorder, social anxiety, and GAD (Gorman & Sloan, 2000). These abnormalities occur in both the sympathetic and parasympathetic systems and probably contribute to the association between anxiety disorder and cardiovascular mortality (Gorman & Sloan, 2000). Although children at risk for one or more anxiety disorders, because of a temperamental bias, show high sympathetic tone in the cardiovascular system (Kagan, Snidman, McManis, & Woodward, 2001), this relation is not robust, and children with different disorders often display similar autonomic profiles (Pine et al., 1998). One mechanism that ties autonomic regulation to psychology is the result of peripheral feedback from the cardiovascular system to the brain. If this somatic activity pierces consciousness, the person might conclude that a threat is imminent (Moss & Damasio, 2001).

Despite a consistent interest in autonomic correlates of anxiety over three decades, findings in this area remain relatively inconsistent. Such inconsistency manifests across particular autonomic measures, such as heart rate, skin conductance, and fear-potentiated startle (Craske, Waters, et al., 2008; Craske et al., 2012; Grillon, Dierker, et al., 1998). Such inconsistencies manifest based on the degree to which state- or trait-related anxiety is assessed (Craske, Waters, et al., 2008; Grillon, Dierker, et al., 1998). Finally, such inconsistencies vary with the nature of the paradigm employed (Britton, Grillon, et al., 2013; Britton, Lissek, et al., 2011; Davis, Walker, et al., 2010; Waters, Craske, et al., 2008).

Assessment of respiratory function represents one area where findings have appeared relatively consistent. Thus, perturbations in respiratory function are characteristic of panic disorder (Pine, 1999) and lead panic patients to experience a heightened feeling of anxiety (Coryell, Fyer, Pine, Martinez, & Arndt, 2001; Pine et al., 2000). Such perturbations are thought to occur in a relatively select set of anxiety patients, including patients with either panic disorder or separation anxiety disorder but not social anxiety disorder. The specificity of such findings generally has been replicated across studies performed over the past decade (Battaglia, Pesenti-Gritti, et al., 2009; Roberson-Nay, Klein, et al., 2010).

Hypothalamic–Pituitary–Adrenal Axis

Patients with an anxiety disorder often show perturbations in the hypothalamic–pituitary–adrenal (HPA) axis. Further, both rodents and nonhuman primates show changes in the HPA axis during acute stress, as well as after a stress experienced early in life (Essex, Klein, Cho, & Kalin, 2002; Kaufman, Plotsky, Nemeroff, & Charney, 2000; Meaney, 2001; Monk, Pine, & Charney, 2002). The strongest association between activation in the HPA axis and anxiety disorder is seen in PTSD (Bremner, 1999; Bremner et al., 1999; Yehuda, 2002). Although enhanced feedback sensitivity in the HPA axis is often associated with an anxiety disorder, some children with an anxiety disorder exhibit the opposite pattern of reduced feedback sensitivity (Coplan et al., 2002; De Bellis, 2001; Heim & Nemeroff, 2002).

Neurochemistry

Brain chemistry can affect the excitability of a particular brain region in diverse ways. Neurochemical regulation in adult anxiety disorders is studied most often with pharmacological challenges, positron emission tomography, or measurement of peripheral neurochemical metabolites. Because the first two techniques are invasive, data on adolescents are restricted primarily to peripheral measures.

Adults with anxiety often show enhanced activity in the neurons of the locus ceruleus (Coplan et al., 1997; Sullivan, Coplan, & Gorman, 1998; Sullivan, Coplan, Kent, & Gorman, 1999). For example, adults with panic disorder and children with separation anxiety disorder show an abnormal response to the administration of yohimbine (Sallee, Sethuraman, Sine, & Liu, 2000). However, children and adults with a diagnosis of OCD show an abnormal, neurohormonal response to clonidine (Sallee et al., 1998). There is also an association between environmental stress and a prolactin response to serotonergic probes (Heim & Nemeroff, 2002), and adults with anxiety disorders show abnormalities in serotonergic regulation.

Immunology

A dramatic indication of a relation between immunology and anxiety disorder comes from studies of children with OCD. Earlier work had found a specific association between OCD and neurological conditions affecting the basal ganglia, including pediatric Sydenham's chorea. This discovery led to the recognition of a specific form of OCD called pediatric autoimmune neuropsychiatric disorder associated with streptococcus (PANDAS; Swedo, 2002), marked by anxiety, OCD, and motor tics that emerge following infection with group A ß-hemolytic streptococcus. This syndrome is thought to occur when an immunological reaction disrupts fronto-striatal-thalamo-cortical-circuitry. It may be relevant that the offspring of adults with panic disorder show selected allergic disorders reflecting anomalies in the immune system (Kagan et al., 2001; Slattery et al., 2002). Of note, controversy has continued to surround research in this area over the past two decades. This controversy relates primarily to the range of conditions that have been tied to similar immunological perturbations. Thus, OCD may in fact relate to streptococcal infection, but this finding may reflect a broader association between a range of immunological insults and a range of emotional disorders that occur in adolescence (Leckman, King, et al., 2011). Work by Storch et al. (2006, 2011) highlights the importance of proper identification of the "sawtooth pattern" of infection, symptom increase, treatment of infection, and symptom alleviation, followed by at least one additional symptom increase associated with re-infection; moreover, biological treatments such as high-dose antibiotics may be brought to bear to treat the infection itself, but cognitive-behavioral therapy and selective serotonin reuptake inhibitors also play an important role in reducing symptoms both acutely and in the long term. More recently, Swedo et al. (2015) and Murphy et al. (2014) have described clinical presentation of pediatric acute-onset neuropsychiatric syndrome (PANS), which implicates more than just the streptococcal virus in the development of acute-onset OCD and related symptoms.

Brain Imaging

A variety of techniques have been used to study anxiety disorders. These include MRI, functional MRI, and electrophysiology. Findings from brain imaging studies in adolescent anxiety disorders using these varied methods generally conform to findings in adults. Moreover, at both ages, the data generally suggest that anxiety disorders can be divided into three large groups, comprising OCD and related disorders, PTSD and related disorders, and the remaining anxiety disorders, including social anxiety disorder and GAD. This broad grouping also is reflected in DSM-5 and conforms to the pattern of findings from longitudinal research.

Morphometric MRI evidence, which provides information on brain structure, reveals that OCD adults have abnormalities in the circuit involving the PFC, basal ganglia, and thalamus (Rauch, Savage, Alpert, Fischman, & Jenicke, 1997). Some of these abnormalities have been observed in children and adolescents with OCD (Blackford & Pine 2012; Rosenberg & Hanna, 2000; Rosenberg, MacMillan, & Moore, 2001). Adults with PTSD have reduced volume in the hippocampus, but children with PTSD do not show these specific reductions, even though they have a smaller brain volume (De Bellis et al., 1999; De Bellis, Spratt, et al., 2011). Children with GAD show increased volume of the amygdala and superior temporal gyrus of the right hemisphere (De Bellis et al., 2002).

Functional MRI quantifies brain activity. Despite its advantages, it relies on measures of blood flow and therefore is an indirect index of neuronal events. Moreover, it measures not the absolute amount of blood flow but rather differences in changes in blood flow during an experimental task compared with a control task.

Despite these caveats, available functional MRI studies do generally differentiate patterns of responding in anxious and non-anxious individuals. Thus, adolescents and adults with a range of anxiety disorders show enhanced amygdalar activation (Blackford & Pine, 2012; Rauch et al., 2000; Thomas et al., 2001a, 2001b). Other research suggests that patterns of responding might differ among OCD, PTSD, and other anxiety disorders when activation is examined in various regions outside of the amygdala, including the striatum and PFC (Blackford & Pine, 2012; Carrion, Garrett, et al., 2008; De Bellis, Spratt, et al., 2011). However, these conclusions remain tentative, since most available studies are small, and few individual studies directly contrast activation across groups of adolescents with anxiety disorders. Rather, conclusions on specificity arise by comparing patterns across different studies targeting different groups of anxiety disorder patients.

Electroencephalogram Activity

The electroencephalogram (EEG) represents the synchronized activity of large numbers of cortical pyramidal neurons that, at any moment, have a dominant frequency of oscillation at particular sites. A state of mental and physical relaxation is usually but not always associated with more power in the alpha frequency band (8–13 Hz) in frontal areas. A state of psychological arousal is associated with greater power in the higher-frequency beta band (14–30 Hz). The change to higher frequencies could be the result of more intense volleys from the amygdala to the cortex.

In addition, there are usually small hemispheric differences in the amount of alpha power on the right, compared with the left, at frontal and parietal sites. Because alpha frequencies are associated with a relaxed psychological state, the less alpha power at a particular site, the more likely that site is neuronally active. The technical term for loss of alpha power is *desynchronized*, and investigators assume that desynchronization of alpha frequencies is a sign that the individual has moved to a more aroused state.

Subjects reporting higher anxiety tend to have greater activation in the right frontal area than the left, whereas normal controls show more activation in the left frontal area. A preference for display of right versus left frontal activation could reflect either a stable trait or a transient state. It appears that a stable preference for right or left frontal activation can be influenced by an individual's temperament and, therefore, could reflect a stable property (Fox, Henderson, Rabin, Caikins, & Schmidt, 2001). McManis, Kagan, Snidman, and Woodward (2002) have found that 11-year-old children who had been highly reactive infants and fearful toddlers were likely to show right frontal activation under resting conditions. However, an asymmetry of activation can also reflect a transient state. Infants watching the approach of a stranger showed greater right frontal activation during that brief period of time (Fox & Bell, 1990). Hagemann et al., who gathered EEG data on four separate occasions on a sample of 59 adults, concluded that 60% of the variance in asymmetry of activation reflected a stable trait while 40% was attributable to the specific occasion of testing (Hagemann, Naumann, Thayer, & Bartussek, 2002).

The event-related potential is a time-locked, postsynaptic potential generated by large numbers of cortical pyramidal neurons to a specific stimulus. The first waveform that represents the detection of a discrepancy is called N2 because it usually peaks at about 200 msec to an unexpected event. The two most frequently studied waveforms, P3 and N4, appear a bit later, with peak voltages at about 400 msec, and are prominent at frontal sites when the subject is passive and has no task to perform. Kagan et al. have unpublished data indicating that 11-year-old children who had been highly reactive infants and fearful toddlers showed a larger negative waveform at 400 msec to nonthreatening discrepant scenes. Interest also has focused on an earlier-appearing potential, the error-related negativity (ERN), which typically manifests in the first 100 msec after a research participant makes an errant motor response. Various forms of anxiety disorder have been linked to an enhancement of the ERN (Hajcak, MacNamara, et al., 2010; McDermott, Perez-Edgar, et al., 2009).

Genetics

Years of work have affirmed that genetic factors influence the risk for anxiety disorders. One study of adults found modest heritability for GAD for both men (15%) and women (20%) and no effect of shared environment (Hettema, Prescott, & Kendler, 2001; Table 9.3). Other research affirms the heritability of panic disorder (Crowe, 1985; Gorwood, Feingold, et al., 1999; Marks, 1986; Skre, Onstad, Torgersen, Lygren, & Kringlen, 1993). Merikangas and Risch (2003) suggested heritability estimates of 50% to 60% for adult panic disorder, with risk ratios ranging from 3 to 8 for first-degree relatives of adult probands with panic disorder. A meta-analysis by Hettema, Neale, and Kendler (2001) uncovered a modest genetic contribution to four anxiety categories and little or no effect of shared environment. One of the most extensive explorations of the contribution of genes to anxiety disorders is the Virginia Twin Study of Adolescent Behavioral Development (Eaves et al., 1997). This corpus, which relies primarily on self-report data, discovered strong additive genetic effects for OAD in both boys and girls (37%), with little effect of shared environment (Topolski et al., 1997). Silberg, Rutter, Neale, and Eaves (2001) reported that 12% to 14% of the variance in OAD in girls was attributable to genes, and most of the remaining variance was due to nonshared environment.

The Virginia Study indicated a smaller genetic contribution to separation anxiety (only 4%) but large nonshared environmental effects (40% and 56%). The data for girls revealed minimal genetic effects on separation anxiety and a greater contribution of shared environment

Table 9.3 Genetics of Anxiety Disorders: Result of Meta-analysis of Studies of Adults

Disorder	*Odds Ratio**	*Heritability*	*Shared Environment*	*Nonshared Environment*
Panic Disorder	5	.37–.43		.57–.63
GAD	6	.22–.37	0–.25	.51–.78
Phobias	4	0–.39	0–.32	.61–.80
OCD	4			

*Relative prevalence in relatives of probands compared with relatives of comparison subjects

From Hettema et al., 2001.

(11% for children 8–12 years old, 23% for children 14–17 years old; Silberg, Rutter, Neale, et al., 2001). However, parent-report checklists from an Australian national twin registry found a higher genetic loading for separation anxiety symptoms in girls (50%) and a much lower one for boys (14%) (Feigon, Waldman, Irwin, Levy, & Hay, 2001).

The Virginia Study indicated that about 9% to 10% of the variance in phobic symptoms was genetic in girls; the remainder was attributable to nonshared environment (Topolski et al., 1997). However, a Swedish study found that shared environmental factors explained considerably more of the variance for fears of animals, unfamiliar situations, and mutilations than nonshared environment (Lichtenstein & Annas, 2000). Thus, it is important to appreciate that conclusions based on twin studies can vary markedly as a function of the site of the laboratory, as well as the informant supplying the relevant information. When mothers reported on separation anxiety disorder in a population-based sample of female twins living in Missouri, heritability estimates were high (62%) and there was only a modest effect of shared environment.

Weissman (1988) argued that high rates of separation anxiety in children of parents who were comorbid for panic and depression disorder implied an association between separation anxiety disorder in childhood and the later development of panic disorder. There was a fairly specific association between separation anxiety in children who had been brought to clinics and separation anxiety in the parents when they were children years earlier (Manicavasagar, Silove, Rapee, Waters, & Momartin, 2001).

In addition, there is evidence for genetic contributions to personality traits such as neuroticism and introversion (Eaves, Eysenck, & Martin, 1989), shyness (Daniels & Plomin, 1985), and behavioral inhibition (DiLalla, Kagan, & Reznick, 1994; Kagan, 1994). A group of very shy 7-year-old Israeli children were more likely than others to inherit the long form of the allele for the serotonin transporter promoter region polymorphism (Arbelle et al., 2003); however, not all studies have found this association.

Some research has focused on aspects of genetics that might vary in anxiety disorders, expressed at particular ages. Thus, twin studies on depression suggest that different genetic factors might shape risk before and after puberty (Silberg, Rutter, et al., 2001). Data suggest that similar developmental variation may occur for anxiety (Kendler, Gardner, et al., 2008). Relatively few studies focus on differences among the particular forms of pathological anxiety. In fact, limited research targets any specific disorder, tending to focus more on patterns for symptom ratings or temperament. Sufficient research does exist on separation anxiety disorder, where 18 cohorts provide data to demonstrate high heritability (Scaini, Ogliari, et al., 2012). However, insufficient research exists to draw similar conclusions regarding any other adolescent anxiety disorder.

Despite these findings, many studies fail to meet the highest research standards, which include the following:

1. Clearly operationalized diagnostic criteria
2. Systematic ascertainment of probands and relatives
3. Direct interviews with a majority of subjects
4. Diagnostic assessment of relatives by investigators blind to the proband's status
5. Family studies with inclusion of comparison groups (Hettema, Neale, & Kendler, 2001)

These standards are occasionally met in studies with adults, but rarely in studies with children and adolescents.

Genes are only expressed within a certain envelope of environments, and individuals both shape and select their environments (Rutter, Silberg, O'Connor, & Siminoff, 1999a, 1999b). Finally, it should be appreciated that the attribution of a genetic risk to an individual should not invite fatalism (Rutter et al., 1990). Some heritable conditions can be treated, and a few can be controlled. The classic example is phenylketonuria, for which the cognitive impairment is caused by an inherited metabolic defect that can be controlled by restricting the child's diet.

By developing personalized treatment plans, the revolution in molecular genetics promises to transform the identification and treatment of anxiety disorders across the lifespan. Two complementary approaches are described. Pharmacogenomic studies use genomic technologies to identify chromosomal areas of interest and, hence, potential drug targets (see, e.g., Arbelle et al., 2003; Smoller et al., 2003). Pharmacogenetic studies identify candidate genes that moderate drug response (see, e.g., Basile, Masellis, Potkin, & Kennedy, 2002) or adverse event profile (see, e.g., Murphy, Kremer, Rodrigues, & Schatzberg, 2003). Identified difference may interact with age, gender, race, and ethnicity (Lin, 2001).

In the adult literature on genetic factors, the most robust findings involve polymorphisms in the serotonin transporter (Weizman & Weizman, 2000). In comparison to progress in ADHD (Rohde, Roman, & Hutz, 2003), however, little is known about pharmacogenetic or pharmacogenomic approaches to anxiety disorders in the pediatric population. Shyness (Arbelle et al., 2003) and behavioral inhibition (Smoller et al., 2003) but not internalizing symptoms (Young, Smolen, Stallings, Corley, & Hewitt, 2003) all have been linked to candidate gene variation, illustrating how lack of consistency in phenotypic identification, among other factors, limits progress despite clear evidence from statistical genetic methods regarding the importance of genetic factors (Stein, Chavira, & Jang, 2001).

Future progress will depend on an improved understanding of the nature and identification of disease states and their natural course, which in turn will allow the development of more specific treatments, better risk prediction, and the implementation of preventive strategies based in pharmacogenomic and pharmacogenetic approaches (Gottesman & Gould, 2003; Pickar, 2003).

SUMMARY

The research of the past few decades has expanded our understanding of the phenomena linked to the concepts of anxiety and anxiety disorder. A comparison of contemporary reports with those of the last half-century provides reason for optimism, for we have learned several important facts.

First, the state we call anxiety in humans is not unitary in origin or consequence and can be the result of living with realistic threat, past history, conditioning, or a temperamental bias for unexpected somatic sensations that are interpreted as meaning one is anxious. Second, epidemiological and genetic data imply distinct biological profiles for the varied anxiety disorders, many of which implicate neurochemical processes. Finally, clinicians and investigators now have an initial set of cognitive and biological procedures that promise to aid differential diagnosis of individuals who report anxiety. Major advances will occur when investigators and clinicians add these procedures to their interview data. The results of this work will permit the parsing of individuals who have a particular diagnosis into subgroups with more homogeneous biological and psychological features. This knowledge should lead to a more fruitful set of psychiatric classifications.

Treatment of Anxiety Disorders

Edna B. Foa
Martin Franklin
Carmen McLean
Richard J. McNally
Daniel Pine

chapter 10

OVERVIEW

Concurrent with the emergence of a growing psychopathology literature, child and adolescent clinical psychology and psychiatry have moved away from nonspecific interventions toward problem-focused treatments keyed to specific diagnoses and, within diagnoses, targets (Holmbeck & Kendall, 2002; Kazdin, 1997). The past several decades have seen the emergence of diverse, sophisticated, empirically supported, cognitive-behavioral and pharmacological therapies that cover the range of childhood-onset anxiety disorders (Ollendick & March, 2004; Rapee, 2011), with the development and empirical evaluation in the past decade of a few adolescent-specific protocols designed to take developmental factors into account (e.g., Foa et al., 2013; Pincus et al., 2010). Before reviewing what is known about the treatment of anxiety disorders in adolescence, however, we first provide a brief overview of the history and rationale for cognitive-behavioral therapy (CBT), pharmacotherapy, and their combination in the treatment of youth with anxiety disorders. Because of increasing emphasis in the field on evidence-based approaches, interventions without empirical support from randomized controlled trials (RCTs), such as psychodynamic approaches, "play therapy," and other approaches, are not reviewed.

COGNITIVE-BEHAVIORAL THERAPY

Current cognitive-behavioral theories regarding the etiology and maintenance of anxiety disorders posit that internal mental phenomena play an important role in mediating pathological anxiety. Foa and Kozak (1985, 1986) proposed that specific "fear structures" that contain erroneous information about the fear stimuli, fear responses, and their meaning underlie the anxiety disorders. Kendall (2000) also referred to "cognitive structures" as important in anxiety disorders in childhood. Accordingly, the goal of CBT is to provide information that is incompatible with the erroneous elements of the fear structure and thus correct the erroneous information.

Most mental health clinicians are familiar with treatments that assume that psychological distress stems from historical relationship problems that must be uncovered in therapy. In contrast to this approach, the CBT clinician addresses the anxiety symptoms directly by confronting the patient with the feared stimuli in a therapeutic environment and/or by teaching the patient a set of adaptive coping skills for specific symptoms that are associated with distress and impairment (O'Neil et al., 2012). Thus, unlike some other psychotherapeutic approaches, CBT fits into a problem-management framework in which the symptoms of the disorder and associated functional impairments are targeted for treatment.

The cognitive-behavioral approach is not a single monolithic approach; quite the contrary. The generic approach labeled cognitive-behavioral involves working with parents, enhancing emotional processing, changing social and peer influences, and using behavioral contingencies and cognitive processing. Similarly, CBT is not one treatment. Rather, treatments of childhood anxiety disorders, though held together by common components and guiding theory, have emerged from different clinics, in different countries, and with variations in the length and specifics of treatment. Nevertheless, there are numerous common themes, strategies, and guiding principles.

One CBT program has received research attention, and though not exactly prototypic, serves as an illustrative example of this approach and will be described here. (For greater detail, the reader is referred to the several programs that are described in detail within each of the sections on the several disorders.) This program, known as the Coping Cat (O'Neil et al., 2012), is manual-based and time-limited; it integrates elements of cognitive information processing associated with anxiety with behavioral techniques (e.g., relaxation, imaginal and in vivo exposure, role playing) known to be useful in reducing anxiety. In this program, children with anxiety typically participate in a structured 16- to 20-week treatment program that is divided into two phases: education and practice.

The first phase includes training, education, and skill building, during which the therapist works with the child to recognize signs of anxiety, to acquire relaxation skills, and to identify anxious cognitive processing. Through self-monitoring homework assignments and in-session role playing, the child learns about anxiety and, more importantly, the cognitive, somatic, emotional, and behavioral aspects of his or her own personal anxious experience. These sessions also allow the child to begin to think about various ways to overcome his or her anxiety.

Education and Skill Building

During initial sessions, the anxious child learns to distinguish between various bodily reactions to emotions as well as the somatic reactions that are specific to his or her anxiety. It is helpful to do this by reviewing the various physical symptoms that occur most frequently in anxious youth (e.g., Crawley et al., 2014). Coupled with this awareness, the child is taught exercises designed to help develop further awareness of, and control over, physiological and muscular reactions to anxiety (see King et al., 1998). This segment may be especially beneficial for children whose worry is accompanied by more severe somatic symptoms (see also Eisen & Silverman, 1998). In this way, anxious children may develop an awareness of their physiological responses to anxiety and use this as an "early warning signal" to remind themselves that what they are experiencing in their bodies is a "false alarm," and to refrain from responding to false alarms as if they were true alarms (e.g., Piacentini et al., 2007).

Next, children are taught how to identify and modify anxious cognition (their internal dialog). Therapist and child then discuss such thoughts, and the child is encouraged to ask himself or herself the various possibilities that may occur in a given situation. It is believed that helping a child to challenge his or her distorted or unrealistic cognition will promote more constructive ways of thinking and less dysfunctional emotional and behavioral responses. For example, the "perfectionistic" nature of many anxious children can be challenged as these children become better able to examine, test out, and reduce their negative self-talk, modify unrealistic expectations, generate more realistic and less negative self-statements, and create a plan to cope with their concerns. Importantly, the idea here is not necessarily to fill the child with positive self-talk. Rather, the ameliorative power rests in the reduction of negative self-talk, or the "power of non-negative thinking" (Kendall & Treadwell, 2007). This phenomenon is supported by evidence indicating that changing children's anxiety-ridden and negative self-talk—but not positive self-talk—mediates changes in anxiety associated with treatment-produced gains (Kendall & Treadwell, 2007; Treadwell & Kendall, 1996). Children learn problem-solving skills that help them to devise a behavioral plan to cope with their anxiety. This includes learning to recognize the problem, brainstorming and generating alternatives to manage their anxiety, weighing the consequences of each alternative, and then choosing and following through with their plan (see D'Zurilla & Goldfried, 1971; D'Zurilla & Nezu, 2001). The therapist serves as a model during each phase of problem solving by, for example, reminding the child that problems and challenges are part of life or by brainstorming ideas without judgment. With the acquisition of problem-solving skills, children develop confidence in their ability to handle anxiety-provoking situations as well as everyday challenges that arise. They learn to judge the effectiveness of their efforts and reward themselves for these efforts. They also learn to identify those things they liked about how they handled a situation and those things that they may want to do differently. Here, children are encouraged to reward both complete and partial successes. Children with anxiety may place exceedingly high standards for achievement on themselves and be unforgiving and critical of themselves if they fail to meet these standards. Therefore, it is important for the therapist to emphasize and encourage self-reward for effort and partial success.

Exposure Exercises

The second phase of treatment focuses on exposure exercises in which children practice the newly acquired skills. In these sessions, participants are prepared for and exposed to various situations that induce pathological, unrealistic anxiety. They first confront low-anxiety situations and gradually proceed to confront moderate- and then high-anxiety ones. Through exposures, the therapist assists the patient in preparing for the exposure by, for example, discussing aspects of the situation that are likely to be troubling, working through the plan, and rehearsing these situations. The exposures are extremely important, as they disconfirm the patient's unrealistic expectations of negative outcomes associated with these situations.

The therapist also facilitates children's processing of the exposures after the experience, helping them to evaluate their performance and modify their unrealistic negative expectations. In so doing, the therapist helps to frame the current exposure experience in terms of a pattern for future coping. When designing the graduated hierarchy of exposures, it is important for the therapist to establish a collaboration with the patient to create the list of exposures and ensure that they are meaningful to the patient.

Homework assignments are an important feature of this program. Throughout the treatment, patients complete tasks in a personal notebook. This allows them to practice their steps and to use their skills outside of session.

As the end of the time-limited treatment approaches (starting with 3 weeks left), the therapist and patient begin to discuss the patient's experiences in the program in an effort to help the patient retain knowledge and consolidate gains. Children are encouraged to use their imagination to chronicle their experiences with strategies for coping with anxiety. This effort is designed not only to help children organize their own experiences but also to afford them the opportunity to "go public" with their newly acquired skills and to recognize their accomplishments.

Developmental Considerations

Treatment manuals evaluated in research trials (e.g., Kendall et al., 2008; Walkup et al, 2008) have typically been designed for children between the ages of 8 and 13 years. Although some manual-based treatments are thought to be somewhat rigid, the therapist working with such cognitive-behavioral programs is allowed flexibility, as life can be "breathed" into the manual to better fit the needs and functioning of the child (Kendall, Chu, Gifford, Hayes, & Nauta, 1998). Adaptations can be made when working with older children and adolescents, but very young children may not have yet developed the cognitive skills necessary to participate fully in, or benefit maximally from, this intervention; children with an IQ below 80 may also not have the prerequisite skills. CBT protocols that take the relevant developmental factors in young childhood into account have been developed (see Cartwright-Hatton, 2013; Freeman et al., 2007), and evidence of their efficacy is now available (e.g., Freeman et al., 2014; Hirshfeld-Becker et al., 2010). It is important to be cognizant of developmental considerations pertaining to adolescents in treatment, including age-related changes in physiological functioning, emotional vulnerability, social and peer pressures, and comorbid conditions.

PHARMACOTHERAPY

Progress in the neurobiology of anxiety has focused on (1) identifying the central nervous system substrates of anxiety and (2) the effects of rearing and environment in the progression of anxiety states with reference to their somatic substrates (Pine & Grun, 1999) in an evolutionary context (Leckman & Mayes, 1998). Convergent evidence from both child studies of stress and trauma and primate rearing and deprivation studies suggests that the effects of stress in the genesis of anxiety disorder can be profound (Perry & Pollard, 1998). Important substrates for this "stress response system" include the following:

- Brain stem arousal centers, particularly the locus coeruleus, which provides noradrenergic input to brain stem and more rostral arousal mechanisms (McCracken, Walkup, & Koplewicz, 2002)
- The amygdala located in the anterior temporal lobe, which processes threat cues and safety signals, with particular

emphasis on social threat (Bremner, Krystal, Charney, & Southwick, 1996)
- The septal-hippocampal system that mediates glucocorticoid-sensitive context conditioning within the framework of learned experience (Takahashi & Goh, 1996)
- Striatal and neostriatal structures, such as the caudate nucleus, which with their cortical targets represent the circuitry that mediates habitual automatic behaviors, such as those seen in obsessive-compulsive disorder (OCD; Rosenberg & Hanna, 2000)
- The orbital-frontal cortex, which assigns complex negative affective valence to cognitive attributions (Amenori et al., 2015)
- Paralimbic structures, such as the anterior cingulate gyrus, which play an important role in directed and selective attention to threatening stimuli (Davidson, Abercrombie, Nitschke, & Putnam, 1999)
- The dorsolateral and ventromedial prefrontal cortex, which respond to and modulate subcortical input and output, generating adaptive responses or, in the case of disease states, maladaptive anxiety-maintaining behaviors (Davidson et al., 1999)

From an integrationist point of view, extensive afferent and efferent connections between these brain regions process a wide variety of internal and external threat cues and safety signals, integrate current experience with previous experience, and generate affective and cognitively mediated approach and avoidance behaviors that are either appropriate or inappropriate to the individual's current context.

The understanding of the neurobiology of anxiety has been propelled by pharmacological agents that impact central nervous system receptors within the "stress-response system" (Heim, Owens, Plotsky, & Nemeroff, 1997). For example, the serotonin system is involved in generating and maintaining normal and pathological fear (Stein, Westenberg, & Liebowitz, 2002). Modulation of this system with a serotonin reuptake inhibitor provides an effective treatment for OCD (e.g., March et al., 1998; POTS Team, 2004) and for separation anxiety, panic, and social phobia (e.g., Walkup et al., 2008). Other major neurotransmitter systems that appear to be involved in pathological anxiety include the GABA-ergic/glutamergic, noradrenergic, and dopaminergic systems, with evidence also suggesting important roles for the neuropeptides cholecystokinin, neuropeptide Y, and corticotrophin-releasing hormone (Sallee & March, 2001). These neurotransmitter systems appear to work in concert to provide homeostasis with respect to the phasic management of threat, and dysregulation in the information processes linked to these substrates may be linked to anxiety states in children and adolescents. They also appear to interface with Kagan's notion of "behavioral inhibition," which as a stable temperamental characteristic appears to be an index of biological vulnerability that under certain circumstances (e.g., separation-stress exposure) can contribute to the generation of an anxiety disorder (Biederman, Rosenbaum, Chaloff, & Kagan, 1995).

Brain mechanisms of response to threat are highly conserved in evolutionary terms. They are exquisitely sensitive to learned experience provide the central nervous system substrate for the information processes that, when dysregulated, produce pathological anxiety as well as for normal fears and worry. For example, McLure et al. (2007) demonstrated fear circuit hyperactivation on functional magnetic resonance imaging (fMRI) measures in a sample of adolescents with generalized anxiety disorder (GAD) attending to their own subjective levels of fear during a face-emotion recognition task. Pharmacotherapy presumably biases these processes directly by influencing the neurotransmitter milieu within which these hierarchically distributed neural networks operate.

Ryan et al. (2011) presented a comprehensive review of novel pathways and neurotransmitters potentially implicated in child and adolescent anxiety. The study showed evidence for a potential role of glutamergic, GABA-ergic, and adrenergic pathways as well; medications that affect these compounds are being developed and tested. The authors noted that thus far there is only evidence to support the potentially beneficial role of the glutamate modulating compound D-cycloserine (DCS) in anxious youth, and that these effects are modest at best thus far. As explicated below, however, the selective serotonin reuptake inhibitors (SSRIs) have typically yielded a partial response at best for pediatric anxiety disorders, so the search for efficacious novel compounds remains of importance to the field.

COMBINED TREATMENT

In a perfectly evidence-based world, selecting an appropriate treatment for the anxious child or adolescent from among the many possible options would be reasonably straightforward. In the complex world of research and clinical practice, however, choices are rarely clear-cut. In this regard, the treatment of the anxious child can be thought of as partially analogous to the treatment of juvenile-onset diabetes, with the caveat that the target organ, the brain in the case of mental disorders, requires psychosocial interventions of much greater complexity. The treatment of diabetes and anxiety disorder can both involve medication, insulin in diabetes and typically a serotonin reuptake inhibitor in anxiety disorders. Each also involves an evidence-based psychosocial intervention. In diabetes, the psychosocial treatment of choice is diet and exercise; in anxiety, it is exposure-based CBT. Depending on the presence of risk and protective factors, not every participant has the same outcome. Bright youngsters from well-adjusted, two-parent families typically do better with either diabetes or anxiety than those with psychosocial adversity and family hardship. Also, not everybody recovers completely even with the best of available treatment, so some interventions need to target coping with residual symptoms, such as diabetic foot care in diabetes and helping patients and their families cope with residual symptoms in anxiety disorders.

Psychosocial treatments may be combined with a medication for one of several reasons:

1. In the acute treatment of the severely anxious child, two treatments may provide a greater "dose" and thus may promise a better and perhaps speedier outcome. Patient preference also plays a role in the selection of acute treatments: for example, patients with OCD may opt for a combined treatment even though CBT alone may offer equal benefit (March & Leonard, 1998).
2. Comorbidity may require two treatments, since different targets may require varied treatments. For example, treating an 8-year-old who has attention-deficit/hyperactivity disorder (ADHD) and separation anxiety disorder with a psychostimulant and CBT is a reasonable treatment strategy.
3. In the face of partial response, an augmenting treatment can be added to the initial treatment to improve the outcome. An SSRI can be added to CBT, or CBT can be added to an SSRI. In an adjunctive treatment strategy, a second treatment can be added to a first one to have a positive impact on one or more additional outcome domains. For example, an SSRI can be added to CBT to address comorbid depression.

As our understanding of both mental disorders in youth and adolescent development increases, treatment innovations inevitably will accrue, including knowledge about when and how to combine treatments. The good news is that large-scale, National Institute of Mental Health–funded comparative treatment trials that include a combination cell as well as CBT and medication monotherapy conditions have been completed. These trials, as well as other treatment outcome studies that have examined either specific anxiety disorders or permitted recruitment of several anxiety disorders into the same trial, will be reviewed below. The largest of these trials, the Child & Adolescent Anxiety Management Study (CAMS; Walkup et al., 2008), will be reviewed in a separate section below, since its recruitment included very large numbers of children and adolescents (N = 488) with either social anxiety disorder, separation anxiety disorder, or GAD. Its findings are complex and warrant close consideration.

Because the state of knowledge varies by disorder, our review will consider each of the anxiety disorders separately: social anxiety disorder, GAD, separation anxiety disorder, specific phobia, panic disorder, OCD, and posttraumatic stress disorder (PTSD). The information will be provided within the categories of (a) acute treatment, (b) maintenance treatment, and (c) management of partial response and nonresponse. In each category we summarize what is known about the treatment of adults and then provide a more detailed coverage of treatments for youth. As noted above, there are few studies of combined treatments of any kind in child/adolescent samples. Moreover, with few exceptions (e.g., Barlow et al., 2000; Davidson et al., 2004), most of the combined treatment studies in adults have not included a CBT-plus-pill-placebo condition, which leaves an important mechanism question essentially unanswered by the extant literature.

ACUTE TREATMENT

Advances in the field over the past decade have resulted in a fairly large number of new RCTs to review. Accordingly, and in the interest of focusing on the most important scientific findings, we have attempted to reduce discussion in the text of open trials or other studies with significant methodological limitations. The fact that we were able to replace discussions of small open studies with data from RCTs is a sign of the progress that has been made since the previous edition.

Table 10.1 provides some tentative recommendations regarding acute treatment strategies for use with adolescents with anxiety disorders. The outcome literature remains underdeveloped, and thus our suggestions should be viewed as just that, rather than as specific recommendations that have been rigorously tested with large samples.

Social Anxiety Disorder

Treatment of Social Anxiety Disorder in Adults

CBT is the most studied psychotherapy for social anxiety disorder, and it is considered the treatment of choice for adults. CBT, which includes cognitive therapy, exposure therapy, and their combination, has been found efficacious for social anxiety disorder when delivered either

Table 10.1 Recommendations for Acute Treatment Strategies

Anxiety Disorder	*Psychosocial Treatments*	*Pharmacotherapy*
Social Anxiety Disorder / Selective Mutism	CBT involving some form of exposure; needs to be adjusted to address specific fears in selective mutism (e.g., hearing own voice)	SRIs
Generalized Anxiety Disorder	CBT; development of problem-focused coping strategies to handle frequently changing themes	SRIs; possibly also TCAs, benzodiazepines, buspirone
Separation Anxiety Disorder	CBT; graded exposure rather than flooding	SRIs
Specific Phobias	Exposure for most fears, possibly 3-hr sessions	If CBT is not available & problem is severe, possibly SRIs
Panic Disorder	CBT, exposure to interoceptive cues	SRIs, possibly imipramine or benzodiazepines
Obsessive-Compulsive Disorder	CBT involving both exposure and response prevention	SRIs
Posttraumatic Stress Disorder	CBT involving exposure to traumatic memories and to objectively safe yet fear-evoking trauma-related situations	SRIs

in groups or individually. Other CBT interventions such as applied relaxation and social skills training have demonstrated greater efficacy than waitlist but have not been studied as extensively. Several meta-analyses now indicate that CBT is superior to waitlist, psychological placebo, and pill placebo at posttreatment, and that these effects are maintained at 6-month and 1-year follow-up assessments (for a review, see Jørstad-Stein & Heimberg, 2009). One RCT found that CBT was superior to psychodynamic therapy for remission and equivalent for response (Leichsenring et al., 2013). Direct comparisons of different forms of CBT have yielded mixed results. Thus, while it is clear that CBT is efficacious for social anxiety disorder, it remains unclear whether there is a strong advantage for one component over the other.

There are now a number of trials supporting the efficacy of Internet-delivered CBT for social anxiety disorder. These studies indicate that Internet-delivered CBT is superior to minimal contact control and waitlist, with large effect sizes comparable to face-to-face CBT. One study found that Internet-delivered CBT was as effective as group CBT for SAD (Hedman et al., 2011). Overall, preliminary evidence supports the utility of delivering CBT for social anxiety disorder over the Internet.

In addition to CBT, interpersonal therapy and mindfulness therapies have shown superiority over waitlist in a small number of trials. Direct comparisons of these treatments with CBT have been mixed (e.g., Koszycki et al., 2007; Stangier et al., 2011), and there are too few studies to draw conclusions about the relative efficacy of these therapies compared to CBT.

In terms of pharmacotherapy, SSRIs and serotonin-norepinephrine reuptake inhibitors are considered the treatments of choice and have been found efficacious in the acute treatment of social anxiety disorder (for a review, see Blanco, Bragdon, Scheier, & Liebowitz, 2013). Research comparing medication with CBT (either alone or combined with medication) has not provided clear evidence in favor of one approach over the other; some studies, but not all, have found medication to be superior to CBT during the acute phase of treatment. However, there is some evidence that patients who receive CBT have a lower risk of relapse after treatment is withdrawn.

In summary, evidence-based treatments for social anxiety disorder in adults include various forms of CBT (e.g., cognitive therapy, exposure therapy) and medication (e.g., SSRIs). These treatments are superior to waitlist and credible placebo conditions but there is no clear advantage for one over the other. More research on treatments that combine CBT with medication that include long-term follow-ups may clarify the relative utility of these interventions. Importantly, the typical response rates in these trials are around 50% (defined as a 1 or 2 on the Clinical Global Impression Improvement [CGI-I] scale), leaving plenty of room for improvement. Also, most RCTs for social anxiety disorder exclude patients with comorbid major depressive disorder or alcohol or substance use disorders, which limits the generalizability of the results.

Social Anxiety Disorder in Children and Adolescents

Increased self-consciousness and preoccupation with social matters are extremely common during late childhood and early adolescence, a developmental stage in which the importance of peers is typically heightened. Differentiating normative adolescent social concerns from the clinical social anxiety disorder poses difficulties for clinicians, parents, teachers, and adolescents alike, and perhaps the best way to parse the two is to examine functional impairment and concomitant symptoms. Compared to their nonanxious counterparts, youth with social anxiety disorder more often report depressed mood, high trait anxiety, and perceived social incompetence (Albano, Chorpita, & Barlow, 2003), higher levels of loneliness and fewer friends (Beidel et al., 1999; Bernstein et al., 2008), a wide range of social avoidances (Hofmann et al., 1999), and learning problems (Bernstein et al., 2008); in at least some cases, social anxiety is associated with school refusal (Kearney & Drake, 2002). Given the potentially serious consequences of social anxiety disorder and its sequelae for the life trajectory of adolescents, detection and treatment are especially important.

Psychosocial Treatment

There is now a robust body of evidence demonstrating the efficacy of CBT approaches for children and adolescents with anxiety disorders. A number of controlled trials targeting anxious children have included those diagnosed with social phobia (Barrett et al., 1996, 1998; Beidel et al., 2000, 2007; Cobham et al., 1998; Dadds et al., 1997, 1999; Flannery-Schroeder & Kendall, 2000; Ginsburg et al., 2002; Herbert et al., 2009; Ingul et al., 2014; Kendall, 1994, 1997, 2008; Last et al., 1998; Lumpkin et al., 2002; Masia-Warner et al., 2005, 2007; Silverman et al., 1999a, 1999b; Walkup et al., 2008). In the context of these mixed anxiety disorder studies, it appears that the diagnosis of social phobia is a predictor of less robust treatment response (e.g., Compton et al., 2014). Perhaps specific aspects of social phobia psychopathology, such as compromised social skills, necessitate the use of different therapeutic approaches.

Six type 1 randomized controlled studies examining the efficacy of CBTs specifically for children and adolescents with social phobia have reported positive clinical response. Hayward et al. (2000) randomly assigned 35 female adolescents with social phobia to cognitive-behavioral group therapy or no treatment. After 16 weeks of treatment, significantly fewer treated patients met the criteria for social phobia. However, at 1-year follow-up, there was no difference between the two groups, suggesting that cognitive-behavioral group therapy may result in a moderate short-term effect. Spence et al. (2000) randomly assigned 50 children with social phobia, ages 7 to 14 years, to either child-focused CBT, CBT plus parent involvement, or a waitlist control. The integrated CBT program involved intensive social skills training with graded exposure and cognitive challenging. After treatment, children in both CBT groups had a greater decrease in social and general anxiety, and a greater increase in parental ratings of child social skills, than those in the waitlist group. At 12-month follow-up, both CBT groups had retained their improvement. Beidel, Turner, and Morris (2000) demonstrated the efficacy of Social Effectiveness Therapy for Children (SET-C) in comparison to an active but nonspecific intervention (Testbusters): children ages 8 to 12 treated with SET-C had enhanced social skills, reduced social anxiety, decreased associated psychopathology, and increased social interaction both at posttreatment and at 6-month follow-up. Beidel et al. (2007) demonstrated the efficacy of SET in a larger randomized comparison (N = 122) to fluoxetine and pill placebo; both active treatments were superior to placebo, but SET was better than fluoxetine in improving social skills, in decreasing anxiety in specific social interactions, and in improving patients' ratings of social competence at 12 weeks.

Two studies have examined CBT protocols developed specifically for adolescents. In the first, Herbert et al. (2009) examined the outcome of group and individual CBT relative to a psychoeducation/supportive counseling condition in 73 adolescents with social anxiety disorder, and found significant and clinically meaningful reductions of social anxiety in all three conditions, but greater improvements on behavioral outcomes for the two conditions that included behavior therapy. There were no differences between individual and group CBT immediately posttreatment, although in a completer analysis at follow-up there was an advantage for those who received group treatment compared to the other two groups. More recently, Ingul et al. (2014) tested treatments based on the cognitive model of social anxiety developed by Clark and Wells (1995), which was developed for use in adults. They conducted a comparison of 128 entrants randomized to individual CBT, group CBT, or an attention control, and found that individual CBT was superior to group CBT and to the attention control group on most outcome measures. These findings diverge from Herbert et al.'s outcomes that favored group treatment, and thus the literature does not provide a clear answer with respect to the benefit of individual versus group therapy for social anxiety disorder in youth.

Researchers have also examined whether CBT can be delivered in the school context, which presumably would help with patient access issues that plague the field at present. Masia et al. (2001) piloted a school-based behavioral treatment for adolescents and concluded that their initial open trial supported the notion that the school setting is a logical place to deliver the treatment since it is where the individuals with social anxiety endure the most distress. Randomized trials now support the effectiveness of this approach as well (Masia-Warner et al., 2005, 2007), which may foster the further development of efforts to disseminate CBT for social anxiety into the school context.

Pharmacological Treatment

In 2001, fluvoxamine, an SSRI, was studied in children and adolescents 6 to 17 years of age with either social phobia, separation anxiety disorder, or GAD (Walkup et al., 2001). Youth (n = 153) were evaluated and enrolled in a 3-week open treatment trial with supportive psychoeducational therapy. Only five children improved with brief psychoeducation and did not go on to medication therapy. One hundred twenty-eight children were assigned to either fluvoxamine or placebo for 8 weeks. The medication was generally well tolerated; five children in the fluvoxamine group and one in the placebo group discontinued because of adverse effects. Adverse effects were more common in the medication group; abdominal discomfort was significantly greater in the fluvoxamine group than in the placebo group, and there was a trend toward a greater frequency of increased motor activity in the fluvoxamine group. The youth in the fluvoxamine group had significantly greater reductions in symptoms of anxiety and higher rates of clinical response than the children in the placebo group. The study led to the conclusion that fluvoxamine is an effective treatment for children and adolescents with social phobia, separation anxiety disorder, or GAD.

In follow-up analyses, Walkup et al. (RUPP, 2003) examined the data for moderators and mediators of pharmacological response. Interestingly, no significant moderators of efficacy were identified, except that lower baseline depression scores, based on parent (but not child) report, were associated with greater improvement. Patients with social phobia and greater severity of illness, irrespective of medical assignment, were less likely to improve. Further study will be needed to determine why the diagnosis of social phobia predicted a less favorable outcome in this specific study.

In the past decade, several social phobia–specific pharmacotherapy trials have been conducted and have yielded convergent findings. The efficacy of venlafaxine (March et al., 2007) and paroxetine (Wagner et al., 2004) has been demonstrated in large RCTs, as has the efficacy of fluoxetine in Beidel et al.'s study reviewed above that also examined the efficacy of SET. Side effects have generally been greater in the medication conditions than with placebo, but the medications have also for the most part been well tolerated. As discussed above, however, the diagnosis of social anxiety disorder has proven to be a negative predictor of outcome in studies that have included multiple anxiety disorders, and there have been no published studies of social anxiety–specific CBT and pharmacotherapy in combination.

Selective Mutism

Consensus places selective mutism among the anxiety disorders, and, although some debate remains (e.g., Anstendig, 1999), it is thought to represent a childhood form of social phobia (for a review see Bögels et al., 2010; Viana et al, 2009). It tends to be a problem that almost exclusively affects younger children so will not be discussed extensively here.

Psychosocial Treatment

Behavioral treatment of selective mutism has generally been the initial and the primary intervention in clinical practice, but until recently has been supported only by case reports and small, uncontrolled trials. Using cognitive-behavioral procedures developed to treat social anxiety disorder, Bergman et al. (2010) conducted a small randomized trial in which the behavioral treatment was found superior to a waitlist control in terms of response rate as well as improved functional speaking as rated by both parents and teachers.

Pharmacological Treatment

Despite the paucity of controlled trials on the efficacy of medications for the treatment of selective mutism, pharmacotherapy is often used in clinical practice. In the only RCT reported, Black and Uhde (1994) treated 16 children with selective mutism with single-blind placebo for 2 weeks. The 15 placebo nonresponders were then randomly assigned to double-blind treatment with fluoxetine (N = 6) or placebo (N = 9) for 12 weeks. Patients on fluoxetine were significantly better than those on placebo based on parental rating of mutism change and global change, but clinician and teacher ratings did not show any significant differences between those receiving medication and those on placebo. The authors suggested that this could in part be due to the small number of patients or the more severe baseline symptoms of the medication group. Nevertheless, the authors cautioned that despite improvement for some, patients in both groups remained very symptomatic at the end of the study. There are no combined treatment studies as yet, which might be a useful direction to pursue given the severity of the condition and its implications for normal development.

GAD

Treatment of GAD in Adults

Psychosocial Treatment

Several CBT programs have been developed and empirically evaluated for GAD. Meta-analyses of traditional CBT and cognitive therapy (CT) programs for GAD have found large within-subjects effect sizes and medium to large effect sizes in comparison to active therapeutic controls (Cuijpers et al., 2014; Hanrahan, Field, Jones, & Davey, 2013; Hunot, Churchill, & Silva de Lima Teixeira, 2007; Mitte, 2005). Although the efficacy of several CBT programs has been established, outcome studies also suggest that there is significant room for improvement; only about 50% of treatment completers achieve high end-state functioning (Hunot et al., 2007) or recovery (Fisher, 2006) following treatment. This observation has prompted scrutiny and refinement of GAD theories and treatments.

Treatment developments for GAD include metacognitive therapy, which was associated with large effect sizes and a high proportion (91%) of loss-of-diagnosis (van der Heiden, Muris, & van der Molen, 2012) as well as CBT focusing on intolerance-of-uncertainty, which has been found superior to waitlist (Dugas et al., 2003; Ladouceur et al., 2000) but not superior to applied relaxation (Dugas et al., 2010). The addition of interpersonal and emotional processing elements into the existing CBT programs was not found to augment CBT alone (Newman et al., 2011). Mindfulness and acceptance-based strategies have been integrated with behavioral approaches (acceptance-based behavioral therapy; ABBT, Roemer & Orsillo, 2009). ABBT has been found superior to waitlist control (Roemer, Orsillo, & Salters-Pedneault, 2008) and applied relaxation (Hayes-Skelton, Roemer, & Orsillo, 2013). In the first RCT of mindfulness-based stress reduction (MBSR) for GAD, it was found to be equivalent to stress management education on the primary outcome but was superior to education on most secondary outcomes, including stress reactivity during a stress challenge test (Hoge et al., 2013).

Internet-based CBT programs for GAD have been developed with the hope of increasing access to treatment. One such program has demonstrated large effect sizes compared to waitlist, with results either improved or maintained at 1 and 3 years posttreatment (Paxling et al., 2011). Moreover, Internet-delivered CBT, with and without clinician assistance, was associated with large effect sizes comparable to those associated with face-to-face treatment (Robinson et al., 2010).

Pharmacological Treatment

Several medications have been found effective for acute treatment of GAD. Benzodiazepines, such as alprazolam, have demonstrated short-term efficacy for reducing GAD symptoms, but antidepressant medications have shown the highest efficacy for GAD in controlled trials (see Baldwin et al., 2011, and National Institute for Health and Clinical Excellence, 2011). A meta-analysis of drug treatments for GAD (Baldwin, Woods, Lawson, & Taylor, 2011) found that fluoxetine was associated with the highest rate (63%) of response (≥50% reduction in symptoms from baseline) and sertraline was associated with the highest rate (50%) of tolerability (proportion withdrawing from trial because of adverse events).

GAD in Children and Adolescents

GAD is, primarily, excessive worry in one or more areas of one's life. Youth with GAD are often viewed by others as "little adults" because their worries may focus on keeping schedules, family finances, the environment, health issues, relationships, and perfectionism—themes that are more typically concerns for adults. Youth with GAD may not be disruptive or acting out in their behavior, so their difficulties may go unnoticed by parents, family, and teachers. Nevertheless, their internal distress interferes with their overall functioning, and they may go on to develop substantially more impairment over time.

Psychosocial Treatment

Historically, a wide range of treatments has been used to treat youth with GAD, including various psychological approaches (e.g., behavioral, cognitive-behavioral, psychodynamic, family, play) as well as medications. Only a very small number of treatments have met the criteria for and have been assigned the label of "empirically supported." And, with regard to GAD, much of this research has been with children, not with adolescents. Our descriptions of the treatment of GAD in youth will place an emphasis on the treatments that have received empirical support.

The results of several type 1 RCTs using CBT conducted by different research groups support the application of this approach in studies that have included GAD patients (Barrett et al., 1996; Flannery-Schroeder & Kendall, 2000; Kendall, 1994, 1997; Mendlowitz et al, 1999). Evidence suggests that CBT for children and adolescents is effective compared to no-treatment control conditions (e.g., Barrett, Dadds, Rapee, & Ryan, 1996; Kendall, 1994, 1997) and that CBT for youth with GAD is a "probably efficacious" treatment (American Psychological Association Task Force on Promotion and Dissemination of Psychological Procedures, 1995; Chambless & Hollon, 1998).

An initial type 1 RCT evaluated a CBT protocol with 8- to 13-year-old children (Kendall, 1994). The manual-based CBT intervention (called the "Coping Cat") targets one or more of the following disorders: social anxiety disorder, social phobia, and GAD. A large percentage of the cases in the report were highly comorbid, and many had GAD as the primary disorder. CBT addresses the cognitive biases associated with anxiety through psychoeducation, cognitive restructuring, changing self-talk, relaxation training, guided imagery, problem solving, and numerous graded-exposure tasks. In this RCT, 47 children ages 8 to 13 years were randomized to either CBT or a waitlist condition. Children in the CBT condition demonstrated significant improvement from pretreatment to posttreatment on self-reported distress, on parent-reported distress of child, and, importantly, on diagnostic status: specifically, 66% of treated children no longer met the criteria for their principal anxiety diagnosis following treatment.

In a second type 1 RCT (Kendall, Flannery-Schroeder, Panichelli-Mindel, Southam-Gerow, Henin, & Warman, 1997), 94 children ages 9 to 13 years were randomized to the CBT protocol or a waitlist condition. Over 50% of treated youth were free of their principal diagnosis at posttreatment, with significant reductions in disorder severity even for the youth remaining symptomatic. Other controlled trials (e.g., Barrett,

1998) support the efficacy of CBT in childhood anxiety (for review see Kazdin & Weisz, 1998; Ollendick & King, 2000), and multiple CBT protocols have also been adapted to the group format (Flannery-Schroeder & Kendall, 2000; Manassis et al., 2002; Silverman et al., 1999a).

Kendall et al. (2008) examined another pressing issue in the field, the role of parent involvement, in an RCT of youth with anxiety disorders, including GAD. Participants were randomized to receive either individual CBT (Coping Cat), family-based CBT, or a family-based education/support/attention condition. Patients in each condition improved from pretreatment to posttreatment, yet individual CBT and family-based CBT were superior to the family-based education/support/attention condition in reducing symptoms of the primary disorder. Of note, family psychopathology was a moderator of outcome: family-based treatment was superior to individual treatment only when both parents had an anxiety disorder diagnosis.

When considering the treatment of adolescents with GAD, one must take into account that the literature on the treatment of "child and adolescent" anxiety is primarily based on studies that have evaluated treatments for youth ages 7 to 14. Moreover, in one of these studies (Barrett et al., 1996), the treatment effects were not the same across age ranges, showing that a combined CBT and family intervention was significantly more effective than CBT alone for 7- to 10-year-old children but not for 11- to 14-year-old children, suggesting that older children might respond differently than younger children to the same treatment. Such findings have not been replicated in subsequent studies involving youth with GAD, however. To date, no controlled studies have investigated CBT for adolescent GAD specifically, and it is important for such studies to be conducted because GAD is prevalent in adolescents (see Merikangas & Avenevoli, 2002).

Pharmacological Treatment

Medication options for the clinical treatment of GAD in children and adolescents include the benzodiazepines, the non-benzodiazepine anxiolytic buspirone, the SSRIs, and tricyclic antidepressants (TCAs). However, due to inconsistency in results, the lack of evidence from randomized trials, reports of potentially serious side effects (Rickels et al., 1990), and the risk of dependency and withdrawal, the benzodiazepines cannot be considered a frontline treatment.

The majority of clinical trials performed using TCAs did not have children and adolescents with GAD only but rather the much more complicated comorbid group of "school refusing" children. The several type 1 placebo-controlled studies of TCAs for children with anxiety-based school refusal provide conflicting results (Berney et al., 1991; Bernstein, Garfinkel, & Borchardt, 1990; Gittelman-Klein & Klein, 1973; Klein et al., 1992). None of these studies were designed to examine children with the primary diagnosis of GAD, so no conclusions can be drawn as to the efficacy of TCAs for this anxiety disorder. Another issue of concern is that TCA use in children is associated with a growing recognition of cardiac risk (Popper et al., 1995; Riddle et al., 1991, 1993; Varley & McClellan, 1997). Given the uncertain clinical efficacy of TCAs for children with anxiety disorders (including GAD) plus the significant side effects, this class of medication is also not a first choice.

The SSRI antidepressants are the best potential pharmacotherapy candidates for the treatment of GAD in youth. The safety of the SSRIs recommends them, as does their effectiveness in treating depression, which is commonly comorbid with childhood GAD. Fluoxetine has shown some preliminary benefit for overanxious disorder (GAD), social anxiety disorder, and social phobia (Birmaher et al., 1994; Fairbanks et al., 1997; Manassis & Bradley, 1994).

Rynn, Siqueland, and Rickels (2001) randomized 22 children meeting the criteria for a GAD diagnosis to receive either placebo or 50 mg (maximum dose) of sertraline for 9 weeks, with positive results. The main side effects reported by the sertraline-treated children compared to the placebo-treated children were dry mouth, drowsiness, leg spasms, and restlessness. The RUPP Study, mentioned earlier, also provides supportive evidence. Rynn et al. (2007) went on to examine the efficacy of extended-release venlafaxine versus pill placebo in a randomized trial and found an advantage for the active medication condition (69% vs. 48% response rate at posttreatment) despite a robust placebo response. However, the side-effect profile for venlafaxine was not especially favorable (e.g., increased anorexia, differences between active medication and placebo in height, weight, heart rate, blood pressure, and cholesterol level), which serves as a reason for trying other medication options first.

There have been reports of activation or agitation with the SSRIs, and this side effect appears to be dose-related (Apter et al., 1994; Riddle et al., 1990, 1991). With these positive studies, it appears that SSRIs are the first-line medication treatment for childhood anxiety disorders. Due to withdrawal symptoms reported upon the discontinuation of SSRIs, including nausea, headache, dizziness, and agitation (Labellarte et al., 1998), these medications should not be abruptly discontinued.

Separation Anxiety Disorder

Distress upon separation from home or caretakers is a normal developmental feature, but such distress can become intense enough to interfere with ordinary functioning. In the extreme, children or adolescents with separation anxiety become so limited in their independent activities that they cannot venture out alone and may resist going to school. In young children, fear of going to school (school phobia) is almost invariably due to separation anxiety, whereas in adolescence, social anxiety or depression may be involved. Childhood school refusal is often due to separation anxiety disorder, whereas school refusal behavior in adolescents may be more strongly linked to social anxiety disorder (Kearney, 2007). Separation anxiety disorder is more common in young children than in adolescents, although some work has suggested that it can be seen in adolescents leaving for college for the first time.

Psychosocial Treatment

Type 1 studies of CBT for children with school refusal behavior, many if not most of whom had separation anxiety, have been conducted (King et al., 1998; Last et al., 1998). King et al. (1998) found that 4 weeks of CBT was superior to a waitlist control. School attendance was higher in the treated than untreated children (89% vs. 60%), and ratings of anxiety also showed meaningful differences. In contrast, Last et al. (1998) found no significant difference in improvement rate between CBT and standardized educational support treatment: mean percentages of school attendance were 67% and 60%, respectively. The more stringent criterion of 95% school attendance was met by 22% of the CBT group and 21% of those receiving educational support. In both treatments, a high rate of children judged themselves to be improved, as did parents and clinicians (90% to 100%), but considerably fewer were considered well by independent raters.

Other studies of CBT have not focused solely on separation anxiety but have included youth with this disorder in addition to other anxiety disorders. These studies have reported efficacy in treating separation anxiety (e.g., Kendall, 1994, 1997). Another type 1 study (Silverman et al., 1999) focused mostly on specific fears; the majority (67%) consisted of anxiety at bedtime requiring the presence of a parent, a cardinal symptom of separation anxiety. Following 10 weeks, children showed similar patterns of improvement with CBT, behavior therapy focusing on training parents in contingency management, or educational support.

Some investigators have examined whether parental involvement in treatment contributes to children's improvement. Of all the childhood anxiety disorders, separation anxiety disorder can be said to have the most direct impact on the family, so there is a strong rationale for parental involvement in treatment. A study of anxious school refusers reported significant superiority for the condition that involved parents and teachers in the children's treatment compared to treatment without this component (Heyne et al., 2002), but the advantage was not sustained over a 5-month follow-up. In a study conducted in Australia, group CBT was compared to a group family anxiety management program and a waitlist control for youth with mixed anxiety disorders, 43% separation anxiety (Barrett, 1998). The treatments were superior to the waitlist but did not differ from each other on most outcome measures.

Schneider et al. extended the CBT literature in separation anxiety disorder by conducting two RCTs. In the first (Schneider et al., 2011), 43 youths ages 5 through 7 were randomized to a family-based CBT condition developed specifically for use with separation anxiety or to a waitlist control condition. Findings indicated a clear advantage for CBT over waitlist in terms of loss-of-diagnosis at posttreatment (76% vs. 13%, respectively) as well as on independent evaluator–rated measures of distress and functional impairment. The second RCT conducted by this group (Schneider et al., 2013) extended the age range (8–13) and examined the relative efficacy of a family-based CBT that included parent training versus a generic child anxiety protocol (Coping Cat). Acute and long-term (12 month) outcomes failed to find a strong advantage for the more specific protocol versus the generic one, likely because the latter yielded substantial and durable reductions in symptoms and associated impairments.

No studies have examined the outcome of separation anxiety treatment in adolescence specifically, although the relatively low base rate of this condition may make conducting a study of this kind impractical.

Pharmacological Treatment

The first use of a pharmacological agent, imipramine, in separation anxiety disorder derived from a postulated relationship between this childhood condition and adult panic disorder (Klein, 1964; Klein & Fink, 1962). A marked clinical benefit for imipramine (mean 125 mg/day) versus a placebo was reported in a type 1 study of 45 children with school phobia and separation anxiety (Gittelman-Klein & Klein, 1971). A smaller study (N = 20) failed to replicate earlier positive findings (Klein et al., 1992). These two treatment studies targeted separation anxiety disorder specifically. Another study failed to observe a significant advantage in school phobic children treated with relatively low doses of clomipramine (75 mg/day; Berney et al., 1981). A type 1 controlled trial in adolescent school refusers reported efficacy for imipramine (Bernstein et al., 2000), but interpretation is complicated by the comorbidity of major depression. The well-documented cardiotoxic effects of high doses of TCAs have limited their usefulness, especially since SSRIs do not present such a risk.

Clinical reports have claimed benefit from high-potency benzodiazepines (i.e., clonazepam) in mixed anxiety, but the only type 1 controlled trial did not confirm these clinical observations (Graae et al., 1994). Benzodiazepines can induce behavioral disinhibition in children, which limits their application.

As noted earlier, a type 1 multisite placebo-controlled study (n = 128) of fluvoxamine (up to 300 mg/day) in children with separation anxiety disorder, social anxiety disorder, and GAD reported marked advantage for the medication (RUPP, 2001) with an overall improvement rate of 78% for fluvoxamine versus 29% for placebo. There were no interactions for diagnosis and treatment outcome, except for the lesser response rate among patients with social phobia compared to other diagnoses (RUPP, 2003). The CAMS trial, discussed below, also shows that the diagnosis of separation anxiety disorder did not predict or modify treatment response to conditions involving medication treatment (Compton et al., 2014). Therefore, it can be surmised that separation anxiety disorder responds to fluvoxamine.

At this time, SSRIs may be the first-line pharmacological treatment for childhood separation anxiety disorder, but we need information specifically regarding adolescents. On the whole, they are well tolerated, have a favorable side-effect profile, and show some efficacy.

Specific Phobia

Treatment of Specific Phobia in Adults

Although few adults seek treatment for specific phobias, collectively the phobias constitute the most common and treatable of the anxiety disorders. The primary treatment for specific phobias is CBT. Several controlled studies have found that significant symptom reduction can be achieved with a single (~2 hour) therapy session (Koch, Spates, & Himle, 2004; Öst, 1989; Ost, Ferbee, & Furmark, 1997; Öst, Salkovskis, & Hellstroem, 1991). The outcome of a single session of longer-duration CBT for specific phobias was found equivalent to a longer, five-session course of CBT (Vika, Skaret, Raadal, Ost, & Kvale, 2009), and treatment gains appear well maintained at follow-ups of up to 1 year (Koch et al., 2004; Tortella-Feliu et al., 2011; Vika et al., 2009). Exposure is considered the key ingredient in CBT for specific phobias (e.g., Schneider, Matai-Cols, Marks, & Bachofen, 2005), although studies have found evidence supporting cognitive therapy (e.g., Jerremalm, Jaansson, & Ost, 1986) and multicomponent nonexposure treatment (Bornas, Tortella-Feliu, & Llabérs, 2006).

Researchers have examined the effectiveness of benzodiazepines, beta-blockers, and SSRIs in treating specific phobias. Some controlled studies have found benzodiazepines to be helpful for patients who are averse to initial exposures to feared stimuli (e.g., Schmidt, Koselka, & Woolaway-Bickel, 2001). However, other research indicated that medications either do not facilitate (Coldwell et al., 2007) or interfere with the treatment efficacy of exposure (e.g., Marks et al., 1993; Wilhelm & Roth, 1997).

Specific Phobia in Children and Adolescents

Fear is a normal response to active or imagined threat that is characterized by affective, behavioral, and cognitive components. As discussed elsewhere (Hagopian & Ollendick, 1997; King et al., 1998; Ollendick, King, & Muris, 2002), nearly all children and adolescents experience some degree of fear. For the most part, these fears are adaptive—they appear to emanate from day-to-day experiences of children and they reflect their emerging cognitive and representational capabilities. Moreover, most of these fears do not involve intense or persistent reactions, and they are short-lived. Not so with specific phobias.

Psychosocial Treatment

Using criteria established for empirically supported treatments (see Chambless & Hollon, 1998; Chambless & Ollendick, 2001), Ollendick and King (1998, 2000) have indicated that two psychosocial treatments have attained "well-established" status (participant modeling, reinforced practice) and five treatments have achieved "probably efficacious" status (imaginal desensitization, in vivo desensitization, live modeling, filmed modeling, and verbal self-instruction) in the treatment of phobic disorders in children. The well-established treatments have been shown to be more effective than credible placebo controls in at least two RCTs, whereas the probably efficacious treatments have been shown to be more effective than waitlist control conditions in at least two RCTs or to be more effective than a credible placebo control in at least one RCT. Support for these interventions to date has come solely from intervention studies with children 12 or 13 years of age and younger. None of the studies treated specific phobia in adolescents. More research is needed with adolescents to determine the efficacy of behavioral treatments for them. However, several studies have now examined cognitive-behavioral interventions in samples that included adolescents.

In the first type 1 study examining the treatment of both children and adolescents, Silverman et al. (1999) examined the relative benefits of an operant-based contingency management treatment and a cognitive-based self-control treatment in comparison to an education support control group. Graduated in vivo exposure was used in both the self-control and the contingency management conditions but not in the education/support condition. Phobic children (n = 81) between 6 and 16 years of age and their parents were evaluated using child, parent, and clinician measures. The children were assigned randomly to one of the three 10-week manualized treatment conditions (self-control, contingency management, or education support). Although all three conditions were found to impart improvement in the child's functioning as measured by the reports of children, parents, and clinicians, clinically significant improvements were noted only in the two CBT conditions. Specifically, on a measure of clinical distress at posttreatment, 80% of the participants in the self-control condition and 80% of the participants in the contingency management condition reported very little or no distress compared to only 25% in the education/support condition. Notably, 88% of the participants in the self-control condition no longer met diagnostic criteria at posttreatment compared to 55% in the contingency management condition and 56% in the education/support condition.

In the second type 1 study, Öst, Svensson, Hellström, and Lindwall (2001) evaluated the effects of a cognitive-behavioral procedure referred to as "one-session treatment" with phobic children and adolescents ages 7 to 17 years old. The hallmark of this "one-session treatment" is a graduated, systematic, prolonged exposure to the phobic stimulus combined with the active dissuading and repair of faulty cognition. As such, it involves a combination of strategies including cognitive restructuring, in vivo graduated exposure, participant modeling, and social reinforcement. Notably, this treatment has been designed to be maximally effective in one session, and therefore lasts 3 or more hours. Results indicated that the treatment was superior to waitlist and produced significant gains both immediately posttreatment and at 1-year follow-up (Öst et al., 2001). Also, in a type 3 study, one-session treatment was found to be comparable to other, longer treatments with more sessions, and perhaps superior to some (see Muris, Merckelbach, Holdrinet, & Sijsenaar, 1998).

In a large international collaborative (United States and Sweden) study of pediatric anxiety disorders, Ollendick et al. (2009) randomized 196 phobic youth ages 7 to 16 who were randomized to receive either one-session treatment, education/support, or waitlist. Findings indicated a clear and durable advantage for the one-session treatment over the other two conditions; education/support was superior to waitlist. In a subsequent randomized study, Ollendick et al. (2015) examined the efficacy of one-session treatment with and without parent involvement in 97 youth ages 6 to 15. Contrary to expectations, there were no differences between the two conditions, with each yielding response rates (loss-of-diagnosis) of approximately 50%. Of particular relevance to the current chapter, age was found to be a predictor of outcome: older participants tended to do better irrespective of which treatment they received.

Pharmacological Treatment

At present, no randomized pharmacological treatment studies of specific phobia in children and adolescents have been completed. The lack of such studies appears to be related to the common misconception that specific fears are a part of normal experience and not a condition associated with impairment. This could also be attributable to the fact that the functional impairment associated with specific phobia may not be as evident if the object of the fear is not omnipresent in the environment of the child (e.g., snake phobias for suburban residents), so it may not rise to the level of impairment that would warrant pharmacotherapy. Pharmacotherapy might be more appropriate for patients with significant psychiatric comorbidity, and judging from Ollendick et al. (2009) it appears that the majority of treatment-seeking phobic youth have a second disorder. However, no research has examined whether targeting these comorbid disorders with pharmacotherapy has any augmentative effects on the specific phobia. To date, no RCTs have examined the joint efficacy of psychosocial and pharmacological treatments with children or adolescents.

Panic Disorder

Treatment of Panic Disorder in Adults

CBT programs are well established for panic disorder. The panic control treatment developed by Barlow and colleagues (PCT; Barlow & Craske, 1989; Craske & Barlow, 2007) and cognitive therapy by Clark and colleagues (Clark,

1997) are two of the most well-established CBT programs for panic disorder. Furthermore, CBT has been found effective at 2 years (Marchand, Roberge, Primiano, & Germain, 2009) and 6 to 8 years posttreatment (Kenardy, Robinson, & Dob, 2005). CBT for panic disorder has been found efficacious when delivered individually or in a group format (Sharp, Power, & Swanson, 2004) and when delivered over the Internet with minimal therapist contact via email (Carlbring, Ekselius, & Anderson, 2003; Calbring et al., 2006; Klein, Richards, & Austin, 2006) or telephone (Wims, Titov, Andrews, & Chol, 2010). CBT has also been found superior to treatment as usual when delivered in combination with pharmacotherapy by CBT-naïve behavioral health specialists in primary care settings (Roy-Byrne et al., 2005).

Other psychological treatments such as Eye Movement Desensitization and Reprocessing (EMDR; Feske & Goldstein, 1997; Goldstein et al., 2000), emotion regulation therapy (Shear, Houck, Greeno, & Masters, 2001), interpersonal psychotherapy (Vos, Huibers Diels, & Arntz, 2012), and Gestalt therapy (Chambless, Goldstein, Gallagher, & Bright, 1986) have not provided such clear benefits in reducing panic and agoraphobia symptoms.

Pharmacological agents with established efficacy for the treatment of panic disorder include benzodiazepines (e.g., Marks et al., 1993) and antidepressants such as SSRIs and TCAs (Bakker, Van Balkom, & Spinhoven, 2001; Barlow et al., 2000), with SSRIs as the first-line pharmacological treatment because they have fewer side effects than TCAs.

Several meta-analyses that have examined the differential efficacy of psychological and/or pharmacological treatment for panic disorder have shown good results for both cognitive-behavioral and pharmacological interventions, alone or in combination (e.g., Chambless & Gillis, 1993, Gould et al., 1995, Mitte, 2005, Van Balkom et al., 1997, Westen & Morrison, 2001). These studies have consistently demonstrated the efficacy of cognitive therapy, exposure therapy, and their combination, although there is some evidence that exposure is the key treatment component (effect size d = 0.78–1.34 in terms of the standardized mean difference). In fact, intensive interoceptive exposure (exposure to internal sensations) was found more efficacious than "low-dose" interoceptive exposure as prescribed in PCT (Deacon et al., 2013). Notably, although PCT typically includes breathing retraining, a procedure designed to increase CO_2 and thereby minimize panic sensations, a controlled study indicated that the inclusion of breathing retraining did not provide incremental benefit above and beyond CBT alone, and on some outcome measures actually yielded a less favorable outcome (Schmidt et al., 2000). Moreover, given that slow breathing and rapid breathing were found equally efficacious in reducing the panic disorder severity, it seems that the efficacy of breathing retraining is not related to the alteration of CO_2 levels.

Panic Disorder in Children and Adolescents

Panic disorder can be a disabling condition accompanied by psychosocial, family, peer, and academic difficulties (Birmaher & Ollendick, 2004; Moreau & Weissman, 1992; Ollendick et al., 1994). In addition, it is associated with increased risk for other anxiety disorders, major depressive disorder, and substance abuse (Birmaher & Ollendick, 2004; Moreau & Weissman, 1992). Moreover, such adverse outcomes are more prevalent in adults whose panic disorder starts early in life (before 17 years of age; see Weissman et al., 1997). Despite this, it takes on average 12.7 years from the onset of reported symptoms for adults to initiate and seek treatment (Moreau & Follet, 1993); unfortunately, it appears that very few youngsters with panic disorder seek help at all (Essau et al., 1999).

Psychosocial Treatment

Psychosocial treatments for panic disorder have been based largely on cognitive and cognitive-behavioral theories (Chambless & Ollendick, 2001), and the few studies of CBT for panic disorder in children and adolescents have used a protocol based largely on PCT (Barlow, 1988).

This treatment comprises three primary strategies: (1) relaxation training and breathing retraining to address neurobiological sensitivities to stress, (2) interoceptive exposure to address heightened somatic symptoms, and (3) cognitive restructuring to address faulty misinterpretations associated with the somatic symptoms. Nelles and Barlow (1988) raised questions about whether young children would be able to develop the kinds of cognitive misperceptions that characterize panic disorder (e.g., catastrophic misinterpretation of physical cues vs. attributing those physical cues to the external environment). These developmental issues may be at the heart of why panic is rarely diagnosed until adolescence. An examination of panic disorder in 35 adolescents seeking treatment in a mental health clinic affiliated with an academic site found that more than half met criteria for agoraphobia, the vast majority had a comorbid internalizing or externalizing disorder, and none had received prior treatment at a specialty clinic for panic disorder (Doerfler et al., 2007).

Pincus et al. (2010) conducted the first RCT of any treatment for panic disorder in adolescents, randomizing 26 adolescents to either 11 weeks of PCT for Adolescents (PCT-A) or a self-monitoring control condition. PCT-A was superior to self-monitoring on independent evaluator–rated panic symptoms as well as self-rated anxiety, depression, and anxiety sensitivity. Posttreatment discussions with participants led the investigative team to develop a more intensive protocol in light of feedback that the treatment took too long. A second RCT initiated by this research group supported the efficacy of an 8-day intensive version of PCT-A that was found superior to a waitlist control condition (Gallo et al., 2012).

Pharmacological Treatment

No RCTs for the pharmacological treatment of panic disorder in children and adolescents have yet been completed (Birmaher & Ollendick, 2003). In children and adolescents, anecdotal case reports suggest that benzodiazepines and the SSRIs (Birmaher & Ollendick, 2003) may be efficacious for panic disorder. For example, in a prospective type 3 open trial, Renaud, Birmaher, Wassick, and Bridge (1999) treated 12 children and adolescents with panic disorder with SSRIs for a period of 6 to 8 weeks. Nearly 75% of the youth showed much to very much improvement with SSRIs without experiencing significant side effects. At the end of the trial, eight (67%) no longer fulfilled the criteria for panic disorder, whereas four (33%) continued to have significant and lasting effects.

Panic disorder is accompanied frequently by a variety of other mental health disorders (Biederman et al., 2001; Mattis & Ollendick, 2002). Treatment of these comorbid conditions may be needed to improve the youngster's overall functioning. Fortunately, two of the common comorbid disorders, depression and other anxiety disorders, also respond to CBT and/or SSRIs (e.g., Walkup et al., 2009).

To date, no RCTs have examined the joint efficacy of psychosocial and pharmacological treatments with children or adolescents with panic disorder. Given the independent promise of both treatments, however, there is reason to believe that synergistic effects could occur. Nevertheless, research into their separate and combined effects, like that pursued in adult populations (e.g., Barlow et al., 2000), is still needed.

OCD

Treatment of OCD in Adults

Effective treatments for OCD include medication and CBT. In terms of pharmacotherapy, serotonin reuptake inhibitors are the only medications approved by the U.S. Food and Drug Administration for OCD. The serotonin reuptake inhibitors include both clomipramine, a TCA with strong serotonin reuptake inhibition, and the SSRIs (fluoxetine, fluvoxamine, paroxetine, sertraline, citalopram, escitalopram). Serotonin reuptake inhibitors have demonstrated efficacy in treating OCD and are recommended as a first-line treatment (March et al., 1997, National Institute for Health and Clinical Excellence [www.nice.org.uk/]). Depending on the study and the definition of response, 14% to 65% of patients respond to an adequate trial of serotonin reuptake inhibitors. However, most responders continue to have clinically significant symptoms, which affect their functioning and quality of life.

Two types of CBT for OCD have been studied in RCTs most frequently: Exposure and Ritual Prevention (EX/RP) and cognitive therapy. Studies suggest that both treatments are effective in reducing OCD symptoms (e.g., Cottraux et al., 2001; Whittal et al., 2005), although results from a meta-analytic review indicate that cognitive therapies that included exposure were superior to those that did not (Abramowitz et al., 2005). American Psychiatric Association practice guidelines for OCD recommend EX/RP as a first-line treatment for OCD, with cognitive therapy a secondary option (Koran et al., 2007). EX/RP teaches patients new strategies to cope with obsessions and compulsions (Foa, Yadin & Lichner, 2012). Specifically, patients are taught to confront situations that elicit obsessional distress (e.g., sitting on the floor, where they feel contaminated by germs) and to refrain from performing compulsions (e.g., excessive washing and cleaning).

EX/RP has been found superior to a variety of control treatments, including placebo medication, relaxation, and anxiety management (for a review see Franklin & Foa, 2002). Foa and Kozak's (1996) review of 12 treatment studies involving a total of 330 patients found that 83% of patients who completed EX/RP therapy were classified as responding favorably to treatment. In 12 studies reporting long-term follow-up of a total of 376 patients, 76% were considered to have maintained their gains. CBT programs comprising cognitive and exposure techniques have been found efficacious for OCD when delivered individually or in group formats (Anderson & Reese et al., 2007; Jaurrieta et al, 2008; Jónsson, Hougaard, & Bennedsen, 2011).

Only one RCT to date has examined the efficacy of EMDR for OCD. This study found that 12 weeks of EMDR was superior to citalopram at posttreatment (Nazari, Momeni, Jariani, & Tarrahi, 2011). The study used a dose (20 mg) of citalopram that is lower than the recommended dose for OCD and did not include a follow-up assessment. Thus, additional research is needed to evaluate the efficacy of EMDR for OCD.

RCTs examining the efficacy of combined treatment in OCD (e.g., Cottreaux et al., 1990; Hohagen et al., 1998; Marks et al., 1988; van Balkom et al., 1998) suggest that combined treatment is not superior to EX/RP alone. For example, in a trial comparing 12 weeks of intensive EX/RP with and without clomipramine or placebo, EX/RP was superior to placebo, not significantly different from clomipramine plus EX/RP, and superior to clomipramine alone at reducing OCD symptoms (Foa et al., 2005). Similarly, cognitive coping therapy plus pharmacotherapy was found superior to pharmacotherapy alone for OCD (Ma et al., 2013). A recent meta-analysis of 468 patients with OCD found that pharmacotherapy combined with CBT was superior to pharmacotherapy alone, but that combined therapy was not superior to CBT alone (Huang, Li, Han, Xiong, & Ma, 2013).

Studies examining novel delivery systems for psychotherapy have found promising results. EX/RP was also found effective when delivered by telephone or face to face, with similar levels of patient-reported satisfaction (Lovell et al., 2006). A small open trial of Internet-delivered CBT (N = 23) found that at posttreatment, 61% of participants had a clinically significant improvement and 43% no longer fulfilled the diagnostic criteria for OCD.

OCD in Children and Adolescents

Children and adolescents with OCD typically present with both obsessions and compulsions, although the youngest sufferers may have difficulty articulating their obsessions. As is the case with adults, the cardinal feature of OCD in youth is neutralizing: when a patient describes anxiety-inducing thoughts and/or images and attempts to relieve this anxiety and/or reduce the chances that feared consequences would occur by performing some overt or covert neutralizing behavior, an OCD diagnosis should be considered. Functional impairment is required for diagnosis as well, as subclinical obsessions and compulsions are probably ubiquitous. Insight into the senselessness of obsessional concerns is not required for diagnosis in children and adolescents and, as with adults, probably exists along a continuum from complete awareness of their senselessness to no insight (Foa et al., 1995).

In general, pediatric OCD is formally similar to OCD in adults, yet the content of obsessions and compulsions is likely to be influenced by developmental factors. For example, younger children are generally more "magical" in their thinking and thus may have more superstitious OCD symptoms (e.g., "If I don't retrace my steps then something really bad will happen to my little sister"). As with adults, some pediatric OCD patients are able to identify feared consequences of not ritualizing (e.g., books will be stolen if locker is not checked), whereas others experience anxiety and distress in the absence of articulated consequences. Further, although the logic of some patients' feared consequences is shared by many in their culture (e.g., contracting disease via direct contact with a public toilet seat), other patients' fears are extremely unusual (e.g., losing their essence by discarding trash that has touched them). Bizarre content does not necessarily preclude a diagnosis of OCD, and patients with such unusual fears may also be responsive to CBT (Franklin et al., 2001).

A subgroup of children with pediatric onset of either OCD or a tic disorder has been described by the term PANDAS (pediatric autoimmune neuropsychiatric disorders associated with streptococcal infection). These children have an abrupt onset of symptoms after a group A β-hemolytic streptococcal infection (GABHS), and their course of illness is characterized by dramatic acute worsening of symptoms with periods of remission (Swedo, 1994; Swedo et al., 1998). The PANDAS subgroup is defined by five clinical characteristics: (1) presence of OCD and/or a tic disorder; (2) prepubertal symptom onset; (3) dramatic onset and acute exacerbations with an episodic course of symptom severity; (4) temporal association between symptom exacerbations and GABHS infections; and (5) associated neurological abnormalities (e.g., choreiform movements) (Swedo et al., 1998). Identifying this subtype is important because these patients may require a different assessment and treatment. In a child who has an acute onset of OCD and/or tics or has had a dramatic deterioration, medical illnesses (including seemingly benign upper respiratory infections) in the prior months should be carefully considered. Obtaining a throat culture, antistreptolysin O (ASO) titer, and anti-DNaseB streptococcal titer may help to diagnose such an infection, even in the absence of clinical symptoms of pharyngitis (Murphy et al., 2002; Swedo et al. 1998). Notably, an examination of treatment and treatment response in youth with PANDAS indicated that disorder-specific CBT and SSRIs play an important role in treatment, in addition to antibiotic treatments (Storch et al., 2006).

Psychosocial Treatments

Expert Consensus Guidelines (March et al., 1997) and AACAP Practice Parameters for OCD (AACAP, 2012) consider CBT, specifically the features of exposure and response prevention, an important intervention, and recommend starting with CBT or CBT plus an SSRI, depending on the severity and comorbidity. EX/RP involves therapist-assisted in vivo exposure to feared situations, imaginal exposure to feared "disasters," and instructions to refrain from rituals and avoidance behaviors. In the treatment of OCD, cognitive therapy procedures are sometimes used to identify faulty cognition, engage in cognitive restructuring and, with behavioral experiments, expose the patient to situations designed to "disconfirm" the faulty cognition. Notably, exposure exercises provide patients with the information that is needed to "correct" their distorted thinking without formal cognitive therapy.

There are now a fairly large number of trials that support the practice parameter conclusions about the efficacy of CBT. Barrett et al. (2004) compared individual cognitive-behavioral family-based therapy (CBFT), group CBFT, and a truncated waitlist control in 77 OCD youngsters ages 7 to 17 years. Both active treatments consisted of a 14-week manualized protocol that included both parent and sibling components; what differentiated the two active conditions was the use of a group format for group CBFT. Both active treatments were associated with significant improvement compared to the truncated waitlist group: at posttreatment, 88% of CBFT, 76% of group CBFT, and 0% of waitlist youngsters no longer met the criteria for OCD according to parental report on structured interviews. CBFT was associated with a 65% reduction in OCD symptoms according to child-only reports, compared to 61% for group CBFT and no change for the waitlist group. The two active treatments did not differ significantly from each other.

Piacentini et al. (2011) directly compared individual CBT (exposure and response prevention plus cognitive therapy) supplemented with a weekly manualized family intervention (FCBT) to a psychosocial comparison condition (relaxation training/psychoeducation) in 71 participants ages 8 to 17 years. Both treatment conditions consisted of 12 manualized sessions delivered over 14 weeks. Findings indicated that FCBT was superior to the comparison condition in terms of clinician-rated response rate (CGI-I score of much or very much improved; 57% vs. 27% in intention-to-treat analysis) and remission rate (Children's Yale-Brown Obsessive Compulsive Scale [CY-BOCS] score < 11; 43% for FCBT vs. 18% for the comparison condition). In addition, parents reported significantly less involvement in OCD symptoms at posttreatment, and changes in accommodation preceded child improvements, which shed light on a potential mechanism by which the treatment effects were realized.

Storch et al. (2011) conducted a trial designed to address the limited availability of CBT for youth by adapting an evidence-based treatment protocol for real-time delivery via webcam. Thirty-one youth with OCD (ages 7–16) were randomly assigned to 14 sessions of web-CBT or a 4-week truncated waitlist control. Participants received 14 60- to 90-minute sessions of family-based CBT over 12 weeks, with adaptations made so that sessions could be conducted via webcam (e.g., handouts emailed before sessions, completed homework assignments read aloud to therapist, parents instructed on coaching child through within-session exposures conducted out of therapist's view). When controlling for baseline group differences, web-CBT was superior to waitlist control on all primary outcome measures with large effect sizes and pre–post change scores on the CY-BOCS of approximately 25 to 11 for web-CBT and 21 to 19 for the waitlist condition. Thirteen of the 16 youth (81%) in the web-CBT arm were treatment responders (defined as at least 30% reduction in CY-BOCS score and a 1 or 2 on CGI-I) versus only two of the 15 youth (13%) in the waitlist group. Despite its limitations (e.g., small sample size, brief waitlist control), this study suggests that web-based delivery is a promising strategy for improving the reach of CBT to select patients whose access to in-person CBT is limited geographically or for other practical reasons (e.g., family scheduling difficulties).

Bolton and Perrin (2008) examined the effects of a behaviorally oriented protocol that excluded formal discussions of feared consequences and other cognitive conceptualizations of OCD and its treatment. Twenty participants ages 8 to 17 were randomized to a waitlist control group or 7 weeks of exposure and response prevention (mean 35.2 days, range 14–47 days) delivered once to three times per week. Findings indicated statistically and clinically significant reduction in OCD symptoms for the exposure group at the end of treatment that were superior to those found in the waitlist group (42% reduction in mean scores for exposure group vs. no reduction for the waitlist group). The potential advantages of exposure and response prevention, as the authors state, are that it is relatively brief, easily manualized, and not overly complicated. Collectively these advantages could prove to be of particular relevance for youngsters, who for developmental reasons may not be especially adept yet at describing the content of their thoughts. The absence of a direct comparison to a blended protocol or a more cognitively oriented one leaves the relative efficacy question unanswered by this trial.

In examining the efficacy of a more cognitively oriented protocol, Williams et al. (2010) randomized 21 youth with OCD (ages 9–18) to either 10 1-hour sessions of CBT or a 12-week waitlist. At posttreatment, the CBT group demonstrated significantly more improvement on the CY-BOCS than the waitlist group (48% vs. 7% reduction). The waitlist group then was treated using the same protocol and made similar gains, with no significant differences between the groups noted at 6-month follow-up (60% symptom reduction from baseline to 6-month follow-up in CBT group vs. 52% reduction in the waitlist-plus-CBT group). Another important aspect of the study involved its setting: patients were treated in an outpatient clinical setting as opposed to an academic clinic, which suggests that the treatment can be disseminated despite the more complex rationale for treatment as compared to the relatively straightforward theoretical model and rationale typically used for exposure and response prevention.

Bolton et al. (2011) further examined the efficacy of a more cognitively oriented treatment for OCD in a substantially larger study (N = 96) of youth ages 10–18 in which they compared the full CBT protocol (12 sessions on average) to a brief CBT (five sessions on average, plus bibliotherapy augmentation) and a waitlist control condition. The study's design permitted an extension of the Williams et al. (2010) study with respect to examining the efficacy of a cognitively oriented protocol and also addressed a question related to dissemination of treatment in that limited resources in many community clinical settings necessitate maximizing a given treatment's efficiency. Both active treatments were superior to waitlist but were not significantly different from one another (e.g., 61% remission rate in full CBT, 49% remission in brief CBT, 8% remission in waitlist control). These findings provided further support for the efficacy of a cognitively oriented program and also indicated that treatment could be delivered efficiently when augmented with bibliotherapy materials.

Pharmacological Treatment

The systematic efficacy studies of the serotonin reuptake inhibitors for the treatment of pediatric OCD form the largest body of work in the pharmacotherapy of the childhood psychiatric disorders, other than that of ADHD. An extensive literature now supports the acute efficacy of clomipramine and the SSRIs in the treatment of children and adolescents with OCD, and there is now evidence for the relative and combined efficacy of CBT, pharmacotherapy, and their combination.

The TCA clomipramine (a serotonin reuptake inhibitor) was the first medication systematically studied in children and adolescents with OCD. Three studies supported its efficacy for pediatric OCD (DeVeaugh-Geiss et al., 1992; Flament et al., 1985; Leonard et al., 1989). The largest of these studies (DeVeaugh-Geiss et al., 1992) led to U.S. Food and Drug Administration approval for a serotonin reuptake inhibitor in pediatric OCD (children 10 years and older). The studies reported that clomipramine was generally well tolerated and has an anticholinergic adverse-effects profile. Periodic electrocardiograms are obtained during ongoing clinical care because of concerns about tachycardia and prolongation of the QTc interval.

The SSRIs have emerged as the first-line pharmacotherapeutic agent for OCD. They have the advantage over clomipramine of having a generally more tolerable side-effect profile with few anticholinergic effects, they have a safer profile in overdoses, and they do not require heart monitoring. Large multicenter type 1 efficacy studies have shown that fluoxetine, fluvoxamine, and sertraline were each superior to placebo for children and adolescents with OCD (Geller et al., 2001; March et al., 1998; Riddle et al., 2001).

March et al. (1998) reported on 187 children and adolescents (ages 6–17) with OCD in a randomized double-blind placebo-controlled 8-week trial of sertraline (forced titration to 200 mg/day) versus placebo. Patients on sertraline versus those on placebo showed significantly greater improvement on several scales. Significant differences (with intent-to-treat analyses) between the two groups were seen as early as week 3 and continued for the entire study.

Riddle et al. (2001) reported the safety and efficacy of fluvoxamine for 120 youth (ages

8–17) with OCD in a randomized controlled study where they received either fluvoxamine (50–200 mg/day) or placebo for 10 weeks. Patients in the fluvoxamine group had a significant improvement (as measured on the CY-BOCS) compared to the placebo group, and a difference could be measured as early as week 1. In the fluvoxamine group, 42% were responders (defined as a 25% decrease in measure of OCD symptom severity, CY-BOCS) in comparison to 26% in the placebo group; the difference was significant.

Geller et al. (2001) randomized 103 youth with OCD to either fluoxetine (starting at 10 mg/day) or placebo (in a 2:1 ratio) for 8 weeks. Intent-to-treat analyses reported that those in the fluoxetine group had significantly better improvement on CY-BOCs than did the placebo group. They concluded that fluoxetine at 20 to 60 mg/day was effective and well tolerated in the pediatric group. In contrast, Liebowitz et al. (2002) randomized 43 patients to either fluoxetine or placebo for 8 weeks. Responders then went into an 8-week maintenance phase. The fluoxetine dose was fixed at 60 mg/day for 6 weeks and then could be increased to 80 mg/day. At week 8, fluoxetine was not significantly better than placebo on the CY-BOCs or CGI-I scale; the authors attributed this to either low power or short duration of treatment. The fluoxetine group continued to improve during the maintenance phase such that at week 16, 57% of the fluoxetine patients versus 27% of the placebo patients (using data at week 8) were much or very much improved. The authors concluded that fluoxetine's effect took more than 8 weeks to develop.

Review of adverse effects of the SSRIs suggests that dropouts from blinded active medication assignment are usually less than 13%, and in many studies there are no significant differences between the dropouts receiving medication or placebo (March, 1999). Generally, the most common side effects seen with the SSRIs include sedation, nausea, diarrhea, insomnia, anorexia, tremor, sexual dysfunction, and hyperstimulation (March et al., 1998; Riddle et al., 2001). Children and adolescents may be more vulnerable to agitation or activation while on SSRIs than are adults, but this is not well studied. Rare adverse reactions include apathy syndrome, serotonin syndrome, and extrapyramidal symptoms. Pharmacokinetic studies of sertraline (Alderman et al., 1998) and of paroxetine (Findling et al., 1999) reported wide intra- and between-individual pharmacokinetic variability but generally similar results as those reported in adults.

How large is the treatment response on an SSRI? The pediatric treatment response is similar to that reported in adults. In general, a 30% to 40% reduction in OCD symptoms, which corresponds to an average six- to eight-point decrease on the CY-BOCS (Scahill et al., 1997), is reported in the medication treatment group in the SSRI controlled studies (March, 1999). Unlike some of the other disorders, there is little or no placebo effect reported. Clinical benefits may begin as early as 3 weeks and typically plateau at about 10 weeks (March, 1999).

The first direct comparison of CBT and pharmacotherapy for pediatric OCD indicated that while CBT and clomipramine both appeared to reduce OCD symptoms, CBT delivered twice weekly was superior to clomipramine. Building upon these findings and on the multisite, randomized, placebo-controlled trial establishing the efficacy of sertraline for pediatric OCD (March, Biederman, et al. 1998), the Pediatric OCD Treatment Study I (POTS I, 2004) directly compared the efficacy of an established medication (sertraline), CBT, and their combination to a control condition, pill placebo (Franklin, Foa, et al. 2003), in a volunteer sample of 112 participants ages 7 to 17. Findings from the intent-to-treat analyses of this three-site study indicated a significant advantage for all three active treatments—CBT, sertraline, and the combination—over placebo; the two monotherapies did not differ from one another. When examining excellent response, a somewhat different picture emerged: approximately 54% of the combination-treatment patients and 39% of the CBT-alone group achieved this designation, in comparison to 21% who received sertraline alone and only 3% who received placebo. A significant site effect was also detected, which indicated that CBT alone at Penn was clearly superior to CBT at Duke (the Brown site did not contribute enough subjects to the trial for its potential site effects to be examined), whereas the reverse was true for the patients treated with sertraline alone, although not as robustly so. Notably, no site-by-treatment effects were found for the combination group or for placebo, suggesting that the effects of combined treatment are less vulnerable to site-specific influences.

Storch et al. (2010) evaluated CBT with DCS, a partial agonist at the NMDA receptor. This work initially was based on animal research showing that the N-methyl-D-aspartate (NMDA) receptor is critically involved in fear extinction, and that DCS enhances extinction of learned fear. Although preliminary results partially supported the use of DCS to augment exposure therapy in adult anxiety disorders, this was the first study to examine its role in augmenting treatment of pediatric anxiety. All 30 participants (ages 8–17) received 10 60-minute CBT sessions based on the POTS I and POTS II protocol. Using a double-blind design, participants also were randomized to either receive either DCS (25 or 50 mg., depending on participant's weight) or a placebo 1 hour before sessions 4 through 10, which all focused on exposure. These sessions were held a minimum of 5 days apart based on prior research that a DCS-free period between administrations maintains the positive effects of DCS on learning and fear extinction. Although no statistically significant differences were found, compared to the CBT-plus-placebo group, youth in the CBT-plus-DCS arm showed small to moderate treatment effects (72% vs. 58% symptom reduction on CY-BOCS; 57% vs. 41% on clinical severity ratings). Further research on the utility of DCS augmentation is ongoing.

Investigational Treatments

Hypotheses concerning whether Sydenham's chorea and PANDAS might share similarities in their pathophysiology led to the question of whether penicillin prophylaxis would reduce neuropsychiatric symptom exacerbation in children with PANDAS by preventing streptococcal infection. An 8-month type 1 double-blind placebo-controlled crossover trial of oral penicillin V (250 mg b.i.d.) and placebo was conducted in 37 children (Garvey et al., 1999). There was no significant between-phase difference in either the OCD or tic symptom severity; however, penicillin administration failed to provide adequate prophylaxis against GABHS (as evidenced by the fact that 14 of 35 GABHS infections occurred during the penicillin phase). A number of children received antibiotic treatment multiple times during the placebo phase. The authors concluded that because of the failure to achieve an acceptable level of streptococcal prophylaxis, no conclusions could be drawn regarding the efficacy of penicillin prophylaxis in preventing tic or OCD symptom exacerbation. Further studies are needed that employ a more effective prophylactic agent and include a larger sample size. Clinical work would recommend workup for GABHS infection in children with an abrupt and sudden onset of OCD or tics and dramatic exacerbations (Murphy et al., 2002; Swedo et al., 1997).

If post-streptococcal autoimmunity is the cause of the exacerbations in this subgroup, then children with PANDAS might benefit from immunomodulatory therapies that have been shown in preliminary findings to treat symptoms of Sydenham's chorea. In a type 1 study, children with severe, infection-triggered exacerbations of OCD or tic disorders were randomly assigned to plasma exchange (five single-volume exchanges over 2 weeks), intravenous immunoglobulin (IVIG) (1 g/kg daily on two consecutive days), or placebo (saline solution given in the same manner as IVIG). Plasma exchange and IVIG were both effective in lessening symptom severity for this group of children. Ratings were completed at 1 month, and symptom gains were maintained at 1 year (Perlmutter et al., 1999). These children were more much significantly impaired than the average child with OCD or tics, which is why these invasive interventions were considered. These interventions are investigational and should only be considered in the context of research approved by a Human Investigations

Committee and not in the context of routine clinical care (Leonard & Swedo, 2001).

PTSD

Treatment of PTSD in Adults

The treatments that have been examined the most for PTSD in adults are psychotherapies derived from behavioral and cognitive theoretical models. CBT has been deemed the treatment approach of choice in clinical practice guidelines for PTSD (American Psychiatric Association, 2004; Foa, Keane, & Friedman, 2000; National Collaborating Centre for Mental Health, 2005; Veterans Affairs and Defense, 2004). Several specific CBTs for PTSD have received empirical support, including prolonged exposure (e.g., Foa et al., 1993), cognitive processing therapy (e.g., Resick et al., 2008), cognitive therapy (e.g., Duffy, Gillespie, & Clark, 2007), stress-inoculation therapy (e.g., Foa et al., 1999), and narrative exposure therapy (e.g., Stenmark, Catani, Neuner, Elbert, & Holen, 2013). EMDR has also been found efficacious for PTSD (e.g., Rothbaum, Astin, & Marsteller, 2005). Prolonged exposure and cognitive processing therapy have been studied in a large number of RCTs and have been found efficacious in a wide range of civilian trauma survivors, including rape survivors (e.g., Foa et al., 1999, 2005; Resick et al., 2002) and veterans (e.g., Forbes et al., 2012; Schnurr et al., 2007).

There is some evidence that implementing an evidence-based treatment within the first few months following a traumatic event can be effective in reducing PTSD (Ehlers et al., 2003; Neuner, Schauer, Klaschik, Karunakara, & Elbert, 2004; Sijbrandij et al., 2007). We have also seen promising results in studies that have integrated prolonged exposure with treatments for PTSD and comorbid alcohol dependence or substance dependence (Mills et al., 2012; Sannibale et al., 2013) or provided these treatments concurrently (Foa et al., 2012). A small number of RCTs have also demonstrated the efficacy of CBT delivered over the Internet relative to waitlist (Spence et al., 2011) and Internet-delivered supportive counseling (Litz, Engle, Bryant, & Papa, 2007).

There is preliminary evidence supporting several other treatment programs for PTSD, including written exposure therapy (Sloan, Marx, Bovin, Feinstein, & Gallagher, 2012), affect regulation–based CBT (Ford, Steinberg, & Zhang, 2011), CBT for couples in which one partner has PTSD (Monson et al., 2011), and intensive cognitive therapy (Ehlers et al., 2014). Group CBT has been found effective but was not more beneficial than a present-centered group comparison treatment (Schnurr et al., 2003).

In terms of pharmacotherapy, multiple medications and classes of medications have been found to be effective in treating PTSD, but there are relatively few placebo-controlled trials of medications outside the class of SSRIs (Watts et al., 2013). The SSRIs (e.g., paroxetine, sertraline, and fluoxetine) are considered the first-line pharmacotherapy for PTSD (Mooney, Oakley, Ferriter, & Travers, 2004). Little is known about combined treatment for PTSD, save for one study that found that the SSRI paroxetine plus prolonged exposure was more effective than placebo plus prolonged exposure in the treatment of PTSD related to the 9/11 attack (Schneier et al., 2012).

PTSD in Children and Adolescents

Adolescence represents a developmental transition in the maturation of self-efficacy in the face of danger. There is increasing reliance on the peer group for appraisal of danger and estimation of needed protective actions, along with greater engagement of the peer group in dangerous and protective behavior. Developmental epidemiology suggests that adolescence carries a high risk of exposure to a spectrum of traumatic situations, subsequent PTSD, comorbid psychopathology, and age-related impairments. There are differential rates of exposure, with boys more likely to experience criminal assault and girls more likely to experience dating violence and rape. A national survey of adolescents found that 23% reported having been both a victim of assault and a witness to violence, and that over 20% met lifetime criteria for PTSD (Kilpatrick, Saunders, Resnick, & Smith, 1997).

In addition to general rates of exposure to war and disasters, international studies indicate that adolescents in these situations are often engaged in resistance and rescue efforts (Nader et. al., 1989) that expose them to many stressful experiences. Studies among adolescents suggest that there may be multiple forms of exposure, with comorbid admixtures of PTSD, depression, and separation anxiety disorder (Warner & Weist, 1996). Finally, adolescent exposures may be superimposed on prior trauma histories and untreated chronic posttraumatic stress symptoms.

Considerable evidence indicates that traumatized adolescents are at increased risk for a spectrum of adverse psychosocial difficulties and functional impairments. These include reduced academic achievement; aggressive, delinquent, or high-risk sexual behavior and substance abuse and dependence (Cavaiola & Schiff, 1988; Farrell & Bruce, 1997; Saigh, Mroueh, & Bremner, 1997 Kilpatrick et al., 2000; Saltzman, Pynoos, Layne, Steinberg & Aisenberg, 2001); and nonadherence to prescribed posttraumatic medical treatment (Shemesh et al., 2000). Further, trauma in adolescence has been linked with long-term developmental disturbances, including disrupted moral development, missed developmental opportunities, delayed preparation for professional and family life, and disruptions in close relationships (Goenjian et al., 1999; Layne, Pynoos, & Cardenas, 2001; Pynoos, Steinberg, & Piacentini, 1999). Ongoing reactive behavior to trauma reminders in adolescence carries the bimodal risk of reckless behavior or extreme avoidant behavior that can derail the adolescent's life.

Psychosocial Treatment

Beginning in the early 1980s, school-age children and adolescents were found to be able to describe their posttraumatic stress symptoms and to engage in the work needed to address their acute traumatic experiences. Pilot studies suggested clinical improvement in posttraumatic stress symptoms after (1) exploring the complexity of the experience; (2) selecting the most traumatic moments; (3) paying repeated attention to the subjective and objective features of these moments, especially experiences of helplessness, fear, and ineffectiveness; (4) clarifying distortions, misattributions, and confusions; and (5) identifying current trauma reminders and increasing cognitive, emotional, physiological, and behavioral management. At the same time, features of traumatic bereavement were distinguished from primary PTSD (Pynoos, 1992). Similar to the treatment of adults, the researchers found that school-age youth were capable of being helped to contend with their anticipatory anxieties about addressing their traumatic experience and also capable of mustering the courage needed to participate in treatment.

Given the high rates of trauma and serious adverse consequences, the treatment of PTSD in adolescence is emerging as an important area for the identification of evidence-based interventions. In the past two decades, there have been continuous advances. Approaches have included individual, group, and family therapy modalities and psychopharmacology. Studies among school-aged children, adolescents, and young adults have provided preliminary evidence about the effectiveness of different interventions for adolescent PTSD. Significant advances include the development of Prolonged Exposure for Adolescents (PE-A; Foa, Chrestman, & Gilboa-Schechtman, 2009), which is based on the adult work by Foa et al. with adults reviewed earlier. The efficacy and effectiveness of PE-A has been evaluated in the United States and Israel, and these trials are described below.

Key type 1 randomized studies among school-age children have primarily examined CBT approaches for sexually abused children, using both symptoms and sexually inappropriate behavior as outcome measures. Deblinger et al. (1996, 1999a, 1999b), in a study of 100 sexually abused children, provided evidence for the effectiveness of a 12-week CBT treatment that emphasizes gradual confrontation of traumatic thoughts, feelings, and memories, using response to even subtle trauma reminders to more fully explore their traumatogenic origins and ongoing cognitive, emotional, and physiological reactions. The CBT treatment included exposure components and cognitive therapy. Children treated alone or with their parents were significantly improved in terms of PTSD, depression, and externalizing behavior compared with treatment for the mothers only and with treatment as usual in community-based clinics. Pertinent to adolescent treatment strategies, when the age range of subjects extended from school-age through late adolescence, an RCT treating child sexual abuse found no effect of parent involvement in treatment (King et al., 2000). Cohen and Mannarino (1996, 1998) provided evidence for the effectiveness of CBT in comparison to supportive therapy for preschool and early adolescent subjects. Their CBT emphasizes developmental skills in emotional labeling and regulation. Of interest, the effect size among adolescents was considerably greater than that for younger children. Each of these three treatment protocols includes a section devoted to promoting safety behaviors both currently and in the future.

Using a staggered-start comparison group, March et al. (1998) reported a robust beneficial effect of an 18-week CBT for school-age children and adolescents who experienced a single traumatic experience. In this small study (14 of 17 completers), there was significant improvement in PTSD, depression, anxiety, and anger. The treatment was modeled on prolonged exposure (Rothbaum, Kozack, Foa, & Whitaker, 2001) and included the following:

1. Anxiety management techniques
2. A preparatory individual breakout session to establish a trauma hierarchy and initial trauma narrative
3. Group exposure work
4. A focus on "worst moments"
5. Homework that addresses avoidant behavior and anger management skills
6. Restructuring of future expectations
7. Relapse prevention

The study confirmed that adolescents can engage in this extended, demanding treatment with acceptance, safety, and effectiveness.

Two comparison studies reported the effectiveness of delayed, intermediate school-based trauma-focused interventions for school-age children and adolescents after large-scale disasters. Goenjian et al. (1997), 1.5 years after the catastrophic 1988 earthquake in Armenia, employed a five-foci approach (trauma reminders, traumatic experience(s), traumatic bereavement, secondary adversities, developmental progression) over six 90-minute combined classroom and individual sessions for adolescents with severe chronic PTSD. Three years after the earthquake, treatment was associated with significant improvement in PTSD and stable depressive symptoms, whereas untreated adolescents suffered a worsening of PTSD and exacerbation of depressive symptoms that reached clinical diagnostic levels. In this extremely traumatized population with persistent and pervasive post-earthquake adversities, treatment gains were maintained for 1.5 years posttreatment. Even without specific strategies to ameliorate depression, this intervention appeared to have protected adolescents against depression.

In a lagged-group design, Chemtob et al. (2002), 3.5 years after Hurricane Iniki, treated a group of school-age children who continued to experience moderate levels of PTSD after being unresponsive to an earlier psychoeducational intervention. Using a form of EMDR, this intermediate intervention sequentially addressed in four sessions positive cognition, worst memories, worst reminders, and fears about future hurricanes. Both groups demonstrated pretreatment-to-posttreatment reductions in PTSD symptoms and moderate reductions in anxiety and depression. These gains were maintained at 6-month follow-up.

These studies demonstrated the potential usefulness of school-based interventions across disasters of different magnitudes and ranges of PTSD outcomes, even if delayed by postdisaster circumstances.

Manualized school-based trauma-focused adolescent group therapy has been studied among adolescents exposed to multiple traumatic experiences during war or urban community violence using the same five foci of treatment as in the Goenjian et al. study (1997). Specific adolescent measures were employed to evaluate the targeted outcome improvement for each module. Layne et al. (2001) reported on the treatment of 55 war-traumatized students from schools in Bosnia-Herzegovina 3 years after the Dayton Accords ended the war. The treatment resulted in significant reduction in PTSD, depression, and traumatic grief reactions. Saltzman et al. (2002) reported on the treatment of chronic PTSD and academic impairment among urban adolescents living in a high-crime area. Similar results were achieved as in the Layne et al. study, with additional evidence for significant improvement in grade-point average, especially reflected in a reduced number of failed classes. As the study authors pointed out, the improvement of grade-point average to a "C" range carries significant developmental importance, as these adolescents could then once again participate in many school interpersonal and enrichment activities that promote adolescent developmental progression. The group intervention was preceded by an individual session in which the adolescent formed a hierarchy of prior traumatic experiences, identified salient features and developmental impact, and selected one to focus on in treatment. As a prelude to core trauma-specific group and homework exposure exercises, these clinical researchers found that the use of beginning strategies to inventory and enhance management of current trauma and loss reminders serves as a useful introduction for adolescents to make the work immediately relevant, understandable, and acceptable. Since many adolescent exposures entail traumatic deaths, a specific module directed at traumatic bereavement was included. Beyond a focus on PTSD-related avoidant behavior, the last module focuses on resumption of adolescent activities in response to missed developmental opportunities, restoration of investment in the social contract, and engagement in prosocial activities. These programs indicate the advantage of school-based interventions, with each study reporting nearly 100% completion rates. They also suggest that group formats may be powerful among adolescents, providing the opportunity to engage the peer group in reexamination of appraisal of danger and protective action. School-based group interventions also provide a potentially cost-efficient method of delivering mental health services to the underserved population of youth with unaddressed PTSD.

Cohen et al. (2004) conducted a large study (N = 209) of the trauma-focused CBT protocol in victims of child sexual abuse ages 8 to 14. Trauma-focused CBT was found superior to client-centered therapy on measures of PTSD, depression, behavior problems, and shame. Parent improvements were seen as well in the trauma-focused CBT group, which further underscores the effects of PTSD symptoms on family members.

PE-A was first evaluated in an efficacy study conducted in Israel, in which 38 adolescents with PTSD from a variety of traumatic experiences (e.g., terror attacks, rape, motor vehicle accidents) were randomized to receive either PE-A or a time-limited psychodynamic therapy. Although both groups evidenced significant reductions in PTSD and related symptoms, participants in the PE-A condition made significantly more progress in reduction of PTSD and depressive symptoms as well as improvements in functioning. Approximately 68% of PE-A participants lost the PTSD diagnosis at post-treatment, and 74% achieved good end-state functioning; this stands in contrast to 37% and 32%, respectively, for the comparison group. PE-A was well tolerated as well, which is especially relevant given concerns about how difficult the treatment might be since it involves confronting traumatic memories directly.

The empirical evaluation of PE-A was extended to an effectiveness context, wherein Foa et al. (2013) compared the protocol to a client-centered therapy condition in a community mental health clinic devoted to delivery of trauma-related services but not expert in the delivery of PE-A. The study's masters-level clinicians were supervised by PE-A experts. Sixty-one participants were randomized to PE-A or client-centered therapy; findings indicated clear advantages for PE-A over client-centered therapy in reducing PTSD symptoms, functioning, depression, and loss of PTSD diagnosis. The fact that PE-A was more effective than client-centered therapy in the hands of clinicians naïve to PE-A prior to the study and accustomed to delivering counseling is notable. Next-stage studies to examine PE-A should include large-scale dissemination work in rape crisis centers, where many sexual survivors seek services after the trauma.

Pharmacological Treatment

Research on pharmacotherapy for PTSD in children and adolescents remains limited, with multiple open trial reports and one study comparing trauma-focused CBT plus either sertraline or placebo (Cohen et al., 2007). In this study, 24 youths with PTSD associated with confirmed sexual abuse were randomized to one of the two active conditions. Both groups experienced significant improvement in their PTSD symptoms as well as on secondary outcome measures, with few differences between the group that received concomitant pharmacotherapy and the one that did not. The authors concluded that their data, in concert with the robust evidence base for trauma-focused CBT programs, suggested that youth who have PTSD should be given a trial of one of these psychological treatments before a medication monotherapy or combined-treatment trial is considered.

Pharmacotherapy could be used either to target PTSD symptoms directly or to address other aspects of PTSD such as sleep disturbance, which carries significant functional consequences. With evidence for the efficacy of SSRIs in the treatment of adult PTSD discussed above, there is interest in conducting large-scale RCTs with children and adolescents, perhaps in comparison to or in combination with the CBT protocols of established efficacy.

CHILD/ADOLESCENT ANXIETY MULTIMODAL STUDY (CAMS)

The largest RCT ever conducted in child or adolescent anxiety disorders is CAMS, a multicenter trial that was conceived as a means of testing the relative and combined efficacy of manualized CBT (Coping Cat), sertraline, and their combination against a credible control (placebo) for youth with a primary diagnosis of separation anxiety disorder, GAD, or social phobia. The rationale, design, and methods for CAMS are explained in detail elsewhere (Compton et al., 2010). Baseline data (Kendall et al., 2010) from the CAMS sample (N = 488) indicated that the sample had moderate to severe anxiety and was highly comorbid (55% had at least one other DSM-IV disorder other than one of the three targeted anxiety disorders). The racial composition of the sample was Caucasian (78%), African American (9%), Hispanic (12%), and Asian (2.5%). Many participants had more than one anxiety disorder: 36% of the sample met the criteria for all three conditions. Anxiety symptom severity and comorbidity patterns did not differ by race or gender. Major depressive disorder was an exclusion in CAMS, which limits the degree to which conclusions can be drawn about this population.

Acute treatment outcomes indicated that all three of the active conditions were superior to placebo on both continuous outcome measures and dichotomous CGI-I responder rates, which were 81% for combination treatment, 60% for CBT, 55% for sertraline, and 24% for placebo (Walkup et al., 2008). Adverse events between the sertraline and placebo groups did not differ, which indicates that the side-effect profile does not contraindicate the use of sertraline as one of the first-line options for pediatric anxiety. At the same time, adverse events in the CBT group were lower than those in the sertraline group, which thus offers a potential reason to start with CBT if available. Accordingly, all three of these treatments can be offered to families of anxious youth, which allows clinicians to take into consideration family preferences and burdens, treatment availability, and associated costs. The search for moderators, baseline characteristics that associated with differential response to conditions, or nonspecific predictors, yielded a few key findings: low anxiety severity and caregiver strain predicted, but did not moderate, anxiety severity at posttreatment (Compton et al., 2014). With respect to moderators, having a principal diagnosis of social phobia was associated with a less favorable response to CBT or placebo, but not to the conditions that included medication (combination or sertraline). Accordingly, the authors recommend that medication may be more helpful, or even necessary, for those with a principal diagnosis of social phobia. Importantly, African-American participants did not differ from Caucasians with respect to treatment response, remission, or relapse (Gordon-Hollingsworth et al., 2015). Follow-up analyses are presented below in the section on maintenance of gains.

MAINTENANCE OF GAINS AFTER ACUTE TREATMENT

There is a paucity of knowledge about what happens after the acute phase of treatment with adults, children, and adolescents. CBT studies have commonly reported uncontrolled follow-up data but did not control the treatments that patients received during the naturalistic follow-up period. These data suggest that on the average, there is a meaningful degree of maintenance of the gains that accrue from CBT, with few studies reporting only mild overall relapse. Traditionally, the vast majority of psychopharmacological trials focused entirely on efficacy during acute, short-term treatment; more recently, more studies have been examining the effects of treatment during longer maintenance phases and after medication discontinuation. Even less is known about children and adolescents. Here we discuss what we know about maintenance and discontinuation in each disorder, collapsing adults, children, and adolescents.

Social Anxiety Disorder

Maintenance trials with phenelzine, paroxetine, and sertraline in adults suggest that responders maintain their gains with continued medication use (Liebowitz et al., 1992; Stein et al., 1996; Walker et al., 2000). However, discontinuation trials with phenelzine (after 9 months of treatment), sertraline (after 20 weeks of treatment), and paroxetine (after 13 weeks of treatment) suggest that relapse rates are high when medication is discontinued. CBT showed good maintenance of gains during maintenance and after discontinuation in a comparative trial with phenelzine, and in another study in comparison with a psychoeducational condition. Knowledge about optimal lengths of treatment to minimize relapse, as well as predictors of which patients can discontinue medication without relapsing, are lacking, as are studies of maintenance of gains and discontinuation in treated children and adolescents.

Separation Anxiety Disorder and Selective Mutism

No adult studies have examined these conditions, which almost invariably occur exclusively during childhood and adolescence. CBT studies that have included children with separation anxiety in the samples have generally shown maintenance of gains following treatment discontinuation (e.g., Barrett et al., 1996; Ginsburg et al., 2014; Kendall, 1994; Kendall et al., 1997; 2004; Kerns et al., 2013). A diagnosis of separation anxiety disorder has not been a predictor of poor outcome in those studies, and the follow-up data reported in the separation anxiety–specific trials by Schneider et al. (2011, 2013) also indicated maintenance of gains in the CBT conditions. Thus, it can be surmised that CBT provides lasting benefits for these children. As mentioned above, separation anxiety disorder may be more common in young children, and its treatment and maintenance of gains have not been studied extensively in adolescent samples.

The treatment of selective mutism has also received little attention in the acute treatment literature, and thus even less is known about maintenance of gains, especially in adolescents. Bergman et al. (2013) reported maintenance of gains in both anxiety reduction and functional speech up to 3 months posttreatment, but there is little else available to guide our expectations regarding the long-term effects of disorder-specific treatment.

GAD

Relapse rates following discontinuation of acute benzodiazepine treatment in adults are as high as 80%, indicating the absence of the maintenance of medication-produced gains (Rickels, Case, & Diamond, 1980; Rickels, Case, Downing, & Fridman, 1986). A few studies demonstrate lasting benefit for GAD patients treated for 6 months or more with benzodiazepines and buspirone. However, concerns over physiological dependence and the potential for abuse make long-term treatment with benzodiazepines controversial. A placebo-controlled trial of venlaflaxine XR showed that the benefits from this medication continued following 6 months of treatment and that it was well tolerated over the long term (Rynn et al., 2007). Several CBT studies involving GAD in youth have indicated maintenance of gains to 12 months after CBT discontinuation. In addition, there are supportive data for 3.5-year (Kendall & Southam-Gerow, 1996), 6-year (Barrett et al, 2006; Ginsburg et al., 2014), and 7.4-year (Kendall, Safford, Flannery-Schroeder & Webb, 2004) follow-ups. Although not all of these treated cases had GAD as the principal diagnosis, and not all evidenced complete initial benefit from CBT, those who do benefit seem to be able to maintain their gains for several years, even without continued treatment.

Specific Phobia

The adult literature on maintenance of gains following treatment of specific phobias generally suggests that the benefits associated with CBT are lasting even when the treatment is delivered in a single 3-hour-long session (Öst, 1989; Öst et al., 1991, 1997). Studies in children and adolescents have indicated that CBT produces significant gains immediately after treatment up to and at 1-year follow-up (Ollendick et al., 2009; Öst et al., 2001; Silverman et al., 1999). The pharmacotherapy literature on this topic is underdeveloped, and thus no conclusions can be drawn about maintenance of gains over time using this approach.

Panic Disorder

A naturalistic study involving 78 adult patients who achieved remission in an 8-week acute phase (with benzodiazepine alone, antidepressant alone, or both) and then received maintenance pharmacotherapy for 2 years found that 46% of these patients relapsed over the maintenance phase and that combination therapy did not confer any added advantage.

As briefly noted earlier, a multicenter trial studied the efficacy of medication therapy and CBT and explored whether combined therapy (medication plus CBT) is more effective than either therapy alone in a randomized, double-blind placebo study (Barlow et al., 2000). In terms of acute response, combined treatment did not differ from medication or CBT alone, but it was better than placebo. The 6-month maintenance response rate of the combination therapy was high (approximately 57% for the Panic Disorder Symptom Scale and 60% for the CGI) and significantly different from medication alone or CBT alone but not significantly different from CBT plus placebo. After the 6-month maintenance phase, patients had treatment discontinued and were followed for 6 months. Improvement in CGI was 41% for CBT plus placebo, 32% for CBT alone, 20% for imipramine alone, and 26% for combined treatment. This study and another large-scale RCT using diazepam (Marks et al., 1993) indicate that combined treatment for panic disorder may be advantageous at posttreatment and during maintenance but may attenuate the benefits of CBT following medication discontinuation (for a review see Foa, Franklin, & Moser, 2002). Pincus et al. (2010) reported stability of gains 6 months after their examination of an 11-week disorder-specific CBT protocol designed for adolescents.

OCD

Pharmacotherapy is frequently prescribed clinically for OCD, yet little is known about how long SRI medication should be continued in OCD. In practice, many adult patients continue taking their medication for at least 1 year; some seem to require indefinite treatment. There are only three published double-blind SRI discontinuation studies in adults with OCD. Each used a different SRI (clomipramine, fluoxetine, sertraline) and reached a different conclusion regarding the effects of discontinuing the SRI: for clomipramine, there was a substantial

(89%) rate of recurrence over 12 weeks; for fluoxetine, there was a moderate rate of relapse (32%) after 1 year and not different from staying on SRI (21%); and for sertraline, there was a low rate of recurrence (24%) after 28 weeks but significantly more than staying on SRI (9%). Given the paucity of blind studies and the methodological differences between them (e.g., relapse definition, length of follow-up, procedure for placebo substitution), the posttreatment effects of SRIs in OCD remain unclear.

A comparative trial of clomipramine and EX/RP in adults suggested that the relapse rate with clomipramine may not be as high (i.e., 45%) as heretofore thought. However, even with this lower relapse rate, EX/RP showed superior maintenance of gains 12 weeks after treatment discontinuation (Simpson et al., 2004). Optimal lengths of SRI treatment to minimize relapse, as well as predictors of which patients can discontinue medication without relapsing, are unknown. Moreover, there is no agreement on the criteria to define relapse. The open studies and randomized trials of CBT in pediatric OCD that have included follow-up data suggest good maintenance of gains following treatment discontinuation (Barrett et al., 2005; Bolton & Perrin, 2008; Bolton et al., 2011; deHaan et al., 1998; Franklin et al., 1998; March et al., 1994; Piacentini et al., 2011; Storch et al., 2007, 2011; Wever & Rey, 1997; Williams et al., 2010), and the one published study of pharmacotherapy discontinuation in pediatric OCD suggests that relapse is common (e.g., Leonard et al., 1991). Relapse rates following medication trials have generally found less stability of gains over time than seen with CBT (Abramowitz, Whiteside, & Deacon, 2005), which also has to be taken into consideration when selecting initial treatment strategies. Although not every patient had attempted discontinuation of medication, this study of patients treated with an SRI suggests that they may require long-term maintenance therapy.

PTSD

Maintenance trials of sertraline at a mean dose of 137 mg/day over 24 to 28 weeks yielded sustained improvement across re-experiencing, avoidance, and hyperarousal PTSD symptom clusters, with an additional 20% improvement in quality of life and functioning measures, and with good tolerance (Rapoport et al., 2002). Additionally, after 64 weeks of treatment, sertraline was found to lower PTSD relapse rates compared to placebo (5% vs. 26%). Double-blind discontinuation of sertraline resulted in recurrence of PTSD symptoms and a worsening of quality of life and functional measures, although degree of exacerbation in symptoms and psychosocial impairment was significantly less than at the time of study entry. Despite the relative paucity of maintenance-phase data, some have recommended that positive responders be maintained on medication for 6 months after remission of acute PTSD and at least 12 months after remission of chronic PTSD (Rapoport et al., 2002). Deblinger and Cohen's (Cohen, Deblinger, Mannarino, & Steer, 2004; Cohen & Mannarino, 1996, 1999) work with sexually abused children provided evidence for the long-term effectiveness of a 12-week CBT treatment. March et al. (1998) reported a robust beneficial effect and maintenance of gains up to 6 months in a small study of CBT for school-age children and adolescents who experienced a single traumatic experience. Follow-up data reported in the PE-A studies (Foa et al., 2013; Gilboa-Schectman et al., 2010) also provide evidence for the durability of treatment gains up to 17 months. Use of medications with adolescents needs to take into account the two adult randomized studies of SSRIs in the treatment of PTSD that indicate relapse with discontinuation of medication (Martenyi et al., 2002). These adult studies raise a similar question as in the treatment of other anxiety disorders—that is, whether the combination of medication and trauma-focused CBT would provide greater resistance against relapse.

Relapse Prevention in Children and Adolescents

No research to date has specifically addressed maintenance treatment and relapse prevention for youth and adolescents with anxiety disorders. However, in general, the ultimate goal of most psychosocial treatment programs for anxiety disorders is to equip the child with skills that will help him or her manage anxious distress after treatment discontinues; a "cure" for anxiety is not the goal (see Kendall, 1989). Because some degree of anxious arousal is likely to persist after treatment, modifying dysfunctional expectations and distorted processing styles can enable more adaptive functioning. The use of in vivo exposure tasks in treatment provides performance-based experiences of coping that bolster confidence for future situations. Therapeutic intervention may be only a first step, but it is a step that helps to alter the maladaptive developmental trajectories of these children so that they are better able to address the inevitable challenges emerging in their lives. Upon completion of a treatment program, the guiding principle (and hope) is for the child to continue to practice the skills learned.

There are several clinical strategies to help guide youth toward consolidation of treatment-produced gains. First, the therapist should shape and encourage "effort" attributions regarding the management of anxiety. Youth are encouraged to reward their hard work and coping efforts, even if the successes are only partial. A second principle for continued post-treatment functioning includes introducing children to the concept of "lapses in efforts" rather than "relapses" (see also Brownell, Marlatt, Lichtenstein, & Wilson, 1986; Marlatt & Gordon, 1985). Mistakes and partial successes are not viewed as incompetence or inability; rather, they can be constructively framed as vital to and inextricably linked to the learning process. Within this framework, children can label and accept inevitable setbacks as temporary and then proceed to work on forward-looking problem solving. Mistakes are viewed as an acceptable part of the learning process and not as excuses for giving up or confirming anxious cognition.

Maintenance treatment may require combinations of CBT and medications, booster sessions, or a return and re-experience of the initial therapy. Alternate approaches or even as-yet-undeveloped treatments may be needed, especially for cases that are refractory to the otherwise reasonably successful programs. To date, the field is lacking information about how best to maintain treatments, prevent relapses, and integrate psychological and pharmacological approaches to maximize long-term gains. Findings from CAMS (Ginsburg et al., 2014), which revealed maintenance of gains in about half of the sample over a 6-year naturalistic follow-up period, clearly suggest that more work needs to be done in this area to help adolescents benefit from treatment and stay well.

MANAGEMENT OF PARTIAL RESPONSE AND NONRESPONSE

Social Anxiety Disorder

There are no controlled studies in any age group on how to address partial response and nonresponse in patients with social anxiety disorder. CBT is a logical candidate to augment partial drug response, given that partial response appears to be the norm. Clinically, gabapentin and clonazepam are also considered possible augmenting agents for partial responders to SSRIs. Complicating this research is the fact that there is no accepted definition of partial response.

GAD

Most adult GAD patients who do improve with acute treatment do not reach full remission of symptoms. In early trials, full remission occurred in as few as one third of GAD patients. There are no systematic studies of treatment options for GAD patients with partial response to medication. Partial response and a significant nonresponse rate also characterize CBT outcomes for GAD. There are no systematic trials assessing nonresponders to initial treatment.

Specific Phobia

There are no controlled data on how to address/augment partial responders, nor are there controlled data on how to treat nonresponders to an initial drug or CBT trial.

Panic Disorder

A double-blind placebo-controlled trial with adults found that pindolol had a beneficial augmentation effect on fluoxetine-treated patients with panic disorder (Hirschmann et al., 2000). Twenty-five patients with panic disorder who had not responded to 8 weeks of fluoxetine (and, prior to that, two other trials of antidepressants) were randomly assigned to pindolol or placebo for 4 weeks. The pindolol group achieved significant improvement on ratings compared to the placebo group. However, since the augmentation period studied was so brief, it is difficult to determine if these effects are sustained and whether they actually lead to remission.

Three studies have examined the effects of benzodiazepine treatment combined with antidepressant treatment. Imipramine plus alprazolam was compared to imipramine plus placebo. The combination group responded with therapeutic effect more quickly. Clonazepam augmentation of paroxetine was shown to be superior to paroxetine alone (Mathew et al., 2001). Goddard et al. (2002) studied 50 panic disorder patients and randomized them to either 0.5 mg of clonazepam t.i.d. plus sertraline or placebo clonazepam plus sertraline for the first 4 weeks. At week 1, 41% of the combination group evidenced improvement compared to 4% of the placebo group. At 3 weeks, the combination group showed a significantly higher (63%) response rate compared to the placebo group (32%), but this difference did not emerge at any other point in the trial. This study suggests that benzodiazepine augmentation of SSRIs at the beginning of treatment can lead to earlier improvement. Kampman et al. (2002) found that paroxetine augmentation of 43 nonresponders to an acute phase of CBT significantly reduced overall anxiety and agoraphobic behaviors.

Nonresponders pose a special challenge, yet there is a paucity of systematic investigation in this area. As far as the clinical management of partial response and nonresponse in adolescents with panic disorder is concerned, the literature does not provide clear guidance about this issue.

OCD

Initial adult studies supported a trial of neuroleptic augmentation in patients with no response or only a partial response to SRI treatment (McDougle et al., 1994), yet a larger study complicated the picture considerably. In a type 1 controlled study of risperidone versus placebo SRI augmentation, risperidone addition was superior in reducing OCD symptoms (McDougle et al. 2000). However, no such effect was found for adults with OCD in a randomized augmentation study comparing CBT (exposure and response prevention), risperidone, and placebo (Simpson et al., 2013). Findings indicated that exposure and response prevention, which had already been found efficacious in augmenting partial response in an earlier RCT (Simpson et al., 2008), was superior to both risperidone and placebo, which did not differ at all from one another.

Neuroleptic augmentation has not been systematically studied in children. In a case series, children who were refractory to SRI therapy improved significantly after risperidone was added (Fitzgerald et al., 1999). Owley et al. (2002) reported four cases of 8- to 25-year-olds who were partial responders to an SSRI and subsequently responded after mixed salts of dextroamphetamine (Adderall) was added. The authors speculated that the "delicate" balance of serotonergic and dopaminergic systems may be be affected by both neuroleptic and Adderall augmentation, resulting in increased serotonergic transmission.

In the only RCT of augmentation strategies conducted with pediatric OCD (Franklin et al., 2011), the relative efficacy of three conditions was examined: (1) medication management provided by a study psychiatrist; (2) medication management plus OCD-specific CBT delivered by a study psychologist; and (3) medication management plus instructions in CBT (I-CBT) delivered by the study psychiatrist assigned to provide medication management. The acute treatment phase lasted 12 weeks; notably, CBT followed the 14-session, hour-long session protocol used in POTS I, whereas I-CBT involved seven brief sessions and did not include in-session exposure. A total of 124 children and adolescents ages 7 to 17 were recruited at three sites (Penn, Duke, and Brown). Inclusion criteria required that patients already were taking an adequate dose of a serotonergic medication (either an SSRI or clomipramine) for OCD and yet still were experiencing clinically significant OCD symptoms. Results indicated that medication management plus CBT was superior to medication management alone and to medication management plus I-CBT, which, contrary to study hypotheses, failed to separate statistically from one another (69% response for medication management plus CBT vs. 34% for medication management plus I-CBT and 30% for medication management alone, where response was defined as a 30% reduction in baseline CY-BOCS score). POTS II thus provided further evidence for the efficacy of combined treatment, in this case administered sequentially rather than simultaneously, and also highlighted the potential need for using the "full dose" of CBT in order to achieve optimal outcomes.

There is no accepted definition of a nonresponder. Sometimes the term is used to describe a patient who has had a suboptimal response to one therapy, but such a definition would include both partial responders and nonresponders. If a nonresponder is defined as someone who has had absolutely no improvement from an initial treatment, there are no published controlled data on how to treat such patients.

PTSD

There is only one placebo-controlled study on augmentation for partial responders. Combat veterans with PTSD who were minimally responsive on an SSRI (sertraline) were given augmentation using the atypical antipsychotic medication olanzapine (Stein et al., 2002). Olanzapine augmentation was associated with statistically significantly greater reduction than placebo in specific measures of posttraumatic stress, depressive, and sleep disorder symptoms (Petty et al., 2001).

There are no controlled data on how to treat nonresponders to pharmacological or CBT treatment for PTSD in adults. Given the high rates of comorbidity with PTSD, it is recommended that the patient be given evidence-based treatments for his or her comorbid conditions; thereafter, the patient's PTSD should be reassessed (Stein et al., 2002).

Management of Partial Response and Nonresponse in Children and Adolescents

There is little research regarding the management of partial response and nonresponse in the treatment of adolescent anxiety disorders, and this area is one that sorely needs to be addressed in future research. Several issues warrant our consideration.

The evidence accrued to date informs us about the choice of an initial treatment to be undertaken for anxious children and, at least to some extent, anxious adolescents. There is a noted absence of studies specifically regarding adolescents and about what to do for them at the various other stages of treatment. Studies reviewed above have evaluated the efficacy of various treatments for children identified with anxiety disorders, and these data guide our treatment choices. However, it is likely that some of the patients treated in these studies had prior experience with one or another treatment, and may or may not have been partially refractory to those earlier treatments. More detailed analyses of initial treatment response may reveal useful information about the moderating role of prior treatment experiences in the efficacy of the treatment being evaluated.

The field has made meaningful progress in identifying at least a few initial treatments for anxious youth that are quite promising, but we know little about what to do when the youthful patient is among those whose response to treatment is not favorable. Even when approximately two thirds of cases respond favorably to CBT, for example, there are still one third who did not respond well and may need something additional. One might speculate that, within the CBT approach, a combination of more practice, increased exposure tasks, and help with the use of the new skills in the new challenging situations would be worthwhile. One might also speculate that a combination of approaches may be valuable. The matter of the nonresponsive client is complicated by the fact that a nonresponder to one treatment approach (psychosocial, medication) may then seek the other as a way to rectify the less-than-preferred previous outcomes. Again, more information is needed about prior treatment history and its effect on the evaluation of a current intervention, and there is a dramatic need for studies of the preferred treatment for patients whose response to treatment is less than satisfactory.

Insufficient research in adults and almost none in youth regarding the continuation and maintenance treatment phases for specific phobia has been carried out. In adults with anxiety disorders, it has been recommended to continue the medications for at least 12 to 18 months; thereafter, if the patient's condition is judged to be stable, the medications can be reduced very slowly to avoid withdrawal side effects. Although it is unknown at this time, it is conceivable that at least some children and adolescents will require treatment for years, consistent with findings from the adult literature. Similar to other psychiatric and medical illnesses, after achieving a therapeutic response it is important to continue the same treatment (CBT and/or medications) to prevent relapses. During these phases, depending on the youngster's clinical status, she or he may need to be seen less frequently.

It is important that an adequate trial be conducted (dose and duration of a SSRI; expertise and number of sessions of CBT) before concluding that a patient is a partial responder. For example, Expert Consensus Guidelines for OCD recommend clomipramine after two or three failed SSRI trials (March et al., 1997). CBT would be a first choice for an augmentation strategy after partial response or nonresponse to adequate pharmacotherapy with an agent of known efficacy, although the availability of trained therapists is sometimes limited, and some children are not motivated to participate. Systematic study of CBT dissemination strategies is sorely needed, as is the development of CBT techniques designed to enhance motivation to engage fully in treatment. Such study is well under way in adult anxiety disorders and clearly needs to be addressed next in children and adolescents.

In considering medication augmentation for anxious youth, a benzodiazepine, such as clonazepam, is occasionally added, but disinhibition, dependence, and tolerance to the medication have limited the enthusiasm for this choice in the long run (Leonard et al., 1994). In a controlled study of risperidone versus placebo SRI augmentation for adults with OCD, risperidone addition was superior in reducing OCD symptoms (McDougle et al. 2000); these findings were not, however, replicated in a large subsequent adult study (Simpson et al., 2013). Neuroleptic augmentation has not been systematically studied in children. Owley et al. (2002) reported four cases of 8- to 25-year-olds who were partial responders to an SSRI and subsequently responded after Adderall was added. Much more needs to be done to establish the efficacy and safety of medication augmentation for adolescents with anxiety disorders. Clinically we know that many are treated with this strategy, but the literature supporting this approach has yet to be developed.

Prevention of Anxiety Disorders

Edna B. Foa
Martin Franklin
Richard J. McNally
Carmen McLean
Daniel Pine

chapter 11

THEORETICAL AND CONCEPTUAL MODELS OF PREVENTION AND CHANGE

The rationale for preventing anxiety disorders in youth has been presented elsewhere (e.g., Fisak et al., 2011; Weissberg, Kumpfer, & Seligman, 2003), but warrants brief reiteration here:

1. Anxiety disorders are common (e.g., Baumeister & Harter, 2007; Kessler et al., 2005).
2. Pediatric onset is common (March, 1995; Snyder et al., 2009).
3. Anxiety disorders are associated with significant comorbidity that often extends into adulthood (Costello & Angold, 1995).
4. The economic burden of anxiety disorders in the United States is enormous.
5. Most pediatric sufferers do not receive adequate care (Kendall & Southam-Gerow, 1995; Teubert & Pinquart, 2011).

Prevention efforts should aim to reduce risk factors and foster protective ones associated with the etiology and maintenance of these syndromes. Some risk and protective factors cannot be modified (e.g., familial history, biomarkers), and thus the interventions need to target variables that mediate the relationship between risk factors and disorder. Timing is also important to consider because certain risk and protective factors may be more likely to exert their influence during certain developmental periods than during others. For example, behavioral inhibition may especially heighten risk for anxiety disorders as adolescents transition from middle to high school, when increased social independence is the norm (see Chapter 9 and below). Consequently, the development of effective prevention of anxiety disorders requires the following:

1. Comprehensive knowledge of the risk and protective factors as well as their complex interrelations during different periods in development
2. Advances in methods to detect the presence of these factors
3. Interventions that increase protective factors, reduce risk factors, or both
4. A societal investment in the importance of doing so

The goal of such programs is to reduce the enormous individual and societal burdens imposed by anxiety disorders.

Recognition of the relationship between investment in prevention science and reducing healthcare costs and burdens is not specific to psychiatry and psychology by any means. Referring to medicine more broadly, Yach and Calitz (2014) suggested that "low levels of investment in prevention research and development represent a missed opportunity to further scientific knowledge and improve population health," and that "investing in prevention should be a strategic national priority to improve the lagging population health of the United States compared with peer countries." As we review what is known thus far about the prevention of anxiety disorders, it is important to consider the state of our knowledge through the lens of lagging commitment to prevention in the United States in particular. The review here highlights that what we do not know continues to far outweigh what we do know, which makes it difficult to mount prevention efforts that will reduce the costs and burdens of anxiety disorders.

In our review of intervention studies aimed at the prevention of anxiety disorders in children and adolescents, we continue to follow the system advocated initially by the Institute of Medicine's Committee on Prevention of Mental Disorders (Mrazek & Haggerty, 1994; Munoz, Mrazek, & Haggerty, 1996) and subsequently adopted by prevention experts (e.g., Craske & Zucker, 2001; Donovan & Spence, 2000; Fisak et al., 2011). This system classifies prevention programs as follows:

1. *Indicated* prevention programs, which target at-risk individuals who already have symptoms, a biomarker, or both, but do not meet full diagnostic criteria for a disorder
2. *Selective* prevention programs, which target individuals presumed to be at high

risk for the development of a disorder (e.g., witnesses of violence)
3. *Universal* prevention programs, in which entire populations are targeted regardless of risk factors (e.g., third-graders)

Before considering the intervention studies themselves, it is important to consider briefly what is known about risk and protective factors at the individual, familial, and societal level, because it is knowledge of these factors and their interrelations that should inform the development of intervention strategies. Unfortunately, knowledge of such factors remains limited, and perhaps the paucity of prevention studies in anxiety disorders across the board is a direct result of this limited knowledge. It is also clear that societal factors influence the feasibility of conducting prevention studies with the information that we already have, since investigators from Australia in particular have managed to conduct the lion's share of anxiety disorders prevention research over the past two decades, despite acknowledged gaps regarding the link between risk and protective factors with intervention strategies. This may be an issue of national priorities and how research funds are allocated nation by nation.

What remains of particular concern is the absence of evidence about protective factors that are specific to anxiety disorders. That is, although the youth resilience literature has generally underscored the importance of factors such as high IQ, self-esteem, social support, and positive coping in serving to protect young people from the development of psychopathology in general, there is a paucity of literature regarding whether any protective factor(s) may serve to protect against anxiety disorders in particular. Development of effective prevention programs will continue to be hampered until evidence-based knowledge has accumulated in this area; significant progress has not been made in the last decade in addressing these concerns sufficiently. It is also the case that only recently did investigators of risk factors begin to examine the complex interplay of these factors and examine their unique and shared contribution to predicting anxiety symptoms down the road—there may not actually be a single risk factor that captures the majority of the variance, but perhaps looking at these factors in concert may help us better understand how they exert their influence on the development of anxiety disorders.

INDIVIDUAL RISK AND PROTECTIVE FACTORS

Individual Psychological Characteristics

Elevated but Subsyndromal Anxiety Symptoms

Many children exhibit symptoms of anxiety at some point, and two questions are of particular interest here:

1. Do children with elevated but subsyndromal levels of anxiety show greater-than-normal levels of impaired functioning at home, at school, or with peers?
2. Does subsyndromal anxiety predict later psychiatric disorder, whether an anxiety disorder or some other diagnosis?

To answer both questions it is necessary to control for comorbidity with other symptoms and disorders; that is, impaired functioning or future anxiety disorder must be linked directly to the anxiety symptoms, not to other symptoms or disorders that may co-occur (e.g., depression with generalized anxiety disorder [GAD]).

To address the question of whether adolescents with elevated but subsyndromal levels of anxiety show greater-than-normal levels of impaired functioning at home, at school, or with peers, it is helpful to consider data from the Great Smoky Mountains Study of youth aged 9 to 16 (Copeland, Angold, Shanahan, & Costello, 2014; Copeland, Shanahan, Costello, & Angold, 2009; Costello, Mustillo, Erkanli, Keeler, & Angold, 2004). In this study, in which 1,420 children and adolescents and their parents were interviewed annually, children and adolescents with an anxiety disorder, but no other psychiatric diagnoses, were twice as likely to exhibit impairment relative to those with no disorder. Even among youths with no diagnoses, those with symptoms of anxiety were twice as likely to have impaired functioning compared to those with no symptoms. This was true of both prepubertal and postpubertal youngsters. Thus, in this population-based sample, subsyndromal anxiety symptoms were associated with youths' impaired ability to function well at home, at school, and with peers. Findings at follow-up that spanned up to two decades indicated that more than one in five participants met the criteria for an anxiety disorder by early adulthood, and that these disorders were associated with adverse functioning in at least one domain by that time. Prior history of symptoms was associated with the development of a disorder later on, but having a disorder at time one was more strongly associated with having a disorder at the last follow-up.

Among children and adolescents without a history of anxiety disorders, those who developed one disorder in any given year of the study had three times as many subsyndromal anxiety symptoms in the year before they developed a disorder compared to those who did not develop an anxiety disorder (2.0 vs. 0.7 symptoms). Almost half of the youths who developed a new anxiety disorder the following year had at least two clinically significant symptoms the previous year, compared with one in five youths who would not develop a disorder. This finding suggests that it should be possible to identify high-risk children and adolescents for prevention programs with a high degree of accuracy, although the interview measures used in this particular study to do so are costly since they require highly trained interviewers, close supervision, and expensive quality assurance methods to do properly.

Autonomic Reactivity

Although research findings are consistent in showing that children and adolescents with anxiety exhibit alterations in autonomic reactivity, Sweeny and Pine (2004) have noted limits in studies that have relied on cardiovascular measures as indices of autonomic activity. Cardiovascular measures are regulated by a wide variety of neural structures and thus provide relatively indirect information about the state of brain systems that might be implicated in anxiety disorders. In addition, abnormalities in cardiovascular control appear to occur in other conditions, and thus are not specific to anxiety disorders. The context in which cardiovascular measures are obtained can also influence reactivity, thereby raising a concern about whether such findings are actually epiphenomena (Sweeny & Pine, 2004). A Dutch prospective cohort study with 965 nonselected adolescent participants indicated that, rather than elevated autonomic reactivity per se, reduced autonomic flexibility in the form of limited heart rate variability predicted self-reported anxiety levels in girls 2 years later (Greaves-Lord et al., 2010); this small yet significant effect suggests that limited heart rate variability should be considered within a larger group of risk factors for the development of anxiety.

Respiratory indices, in contrast, are relatively free of the limits that affect cardiovascular measures (Sweeny & Pine, 2004). These include minute ventilation (the amount of air breathed every minute), tidal volume (size of each breath), and respiratory rate. Guided by Klein's (1993) suffocation false alarm theory of panic, most studies involving these measures have concerned patients with panic disorder, other anxiety disorders, and healthy controls who inhale air enriched with carbon dioxide.

Although most studies show that patients with panic disorder experience panic attacks and exhibit changes in respiratory measures more often than do patients with other anxiety disorders or healthy subjects (e.g., Papp et al., 1993; Papp, Martinez, Klein, Coplan, & Gorman, 1995), the data are not uniformly consistent (Rapee, Brown, Antony, & Barlow, 1992; Woods & Charney, 1998).

Pine, Cohen, Gurley, Brook, and Ma (1998) extended this work to young people (ages 7–17; mixed sample of anxiety disorders), but separate analyses were not conducted for the preadolescent versus adolescent subsamples. Pine et al.'s findings with these youths paralleled those with adults. However, considerably more research is needed before firm conclusions can be drawn about the relationships between adolescents' autonomic reactivity and the development of subsequent anxiety disorders per se.

Behavioral Inhibition

A detailed review of the temperamental vulnerability for behavioral inhibition appeared earlier. Two independent laboratories have shown that children who were highly reactive to novel stimuli as infants were more likely than others to display extreme shyness, timidity, and restraint to unfamiliar people, situations, and objects when they were 2, 4, 7, and 11 years of age, and biological differences were found that implicated the amygdala (Fox, Henderson, Rabin, Caikins, & Schmidt, 2001; Kagan, 2002). Labs using less painstaking methods of measuring behavioral inhibition (e.g., parent report measures) have also found an association between behavioral inhibition and the subsequent development of anxiety disorders (e.g., Gar, Hudson, & Rapee, 2005; Hirshfeld-Becker et al., 2008). Notably, although these children appear to be at a threefold to fourfold increased risk for development of an anxiety disorder compared to those without elevated behavioral inhibition, most actually do not go on to develop one; this raises again the issue of the potential and yet clearly understudied role of protective factors in vulnerable children.

Chronis-Tuscano et al. (2009) conducted a prospective longitudinal study of 126 boys and girls enrolled at 4 months of age and repeatedly assessed for behavioral inhibition until age 7. The investigators conducted semistructured interviews with the subjects, then aged between 14 and 17 years. The results revealed that children who had *repeatedly* scored high on maternal ratings of behavioral inhibition across multiple assessment points during their first 7 years were 3.8 times more likely to meet lifetime criteria for social anxiety disorder by the time of the adolescent interview assessment than were other children. However, repeated ratings of behavioral inhibition did not predict a heightened risk for other anxiety disorders, nor did it predict current social anxiety disorder, thus implying that many behaviorally inhibited children lose the diagnosis before leaving adolescence.

All in all, it appears that behavioral inhibition is not an especially strong predictor of later anxiety disorder in and of itself. This finding points to the importance of identifying protective factors that limit the rate of later anxiety disorders in otherwise vulnerable individuals. It also indicates the potential advantage of studying multiple risk factors together and examining their separate and shared contributions to predicting anxiety later on, such as has been done with behavioral inhibition and attachment style (e.g., Muris et al., 2011; Shamir-Essakow et al., 2005).

Cognitive Factors

There are individual difference variables linked to anxiety and its disorders in children and adolescents. In Chapter 9, we mentioned information-processing biases and anxiety sensitivity. In this section, we discuss coping skills and perceived control. Individuals' coping skills—methods they use to manage negative or aversive situations—can be (1) problem-focused, (2) avoidant, or (3) emotion-focused. Problem-focused coping directly addresses or minimizes the effect of the problem. Avoidant coping denotes the avoiding the problem or escaping from it. Emotion-focused coping concerns attempts to attenuate the distress caused by the problem. Research suggests that problem-focused methods, such as actively seeking information, positive self-talk, diversion of attention, relaxation, and thought stopping reduce anxiety and emotional distress in 8- to 18-year-olds (Brown, O'Keefe, Sanders, & Baker, 1986). Generally, children's and adolescents' use of problem-focused coping predicts positive psychological adjustment more than does use of emotion-focused coping. Interestingly, adolescents' use of avoidant coping is associated with high levels of depression in adolescence (Ebata & Moos, 1991). There has been little systematic research on the association between specific types of coping strategies and the development and maintenance of anxiety disorders in adolescence. There also has been little systematic research on which specific coping skills should be taught to adolescents across diverse anxiety-provoking situations. Research in this area is clearly of importance given that training in coping skills remains a feature of cognitive-behavioral treatments (see Chapter 10).

Perceived control is another important individual difference variable. Specifically, Barlow (2001) has suggested that children who experience uncontrollable events early in life may develop a propensity to perceive or process events as not being under their control, which for some youngsters may serve as a risk for the development of anxiety and its disorders. Chorpita, Brown, and Barlow (1998) found that perceived control may serve as a mediator of family environment among youths with anxiety disorders. Clearly, further research on the role of perceived control as a protective and risk factor in anxiety disorders is needed, especially regarding its specificity for anxiety.

Genetics

As discussed in greater detail in Chapter 9, genetic factors influence the risk for anxiety disorders and, taken together, the epidemiologic and genetic data imply distinct biological profiles for the varied anxiety disorders, many implicating neurochemical processes. A meta-analysis found only a modest genetic contribution to four anxiety categories, and no evidence for a significant effect of shared environment (Hettema, Neale, & Kendler, 2001). When the individual studies themselves are reviewed, however, inconsistencies emerge with respect to the degree to which genetics were implicated in transmission of anxiety disorders; rates appear to vary as a function of the site of the laboratory, as well as the informant supplying the relevant information. There is evidence for genetic contributions to personality traits, such as neuroticism, introversion (Eaves, Eysenck, & Martin, 1989), shyness (Daniels & Plomin, 1985), and behavioral inhibition (DiLalla, Kagan, & Reznick, 1994; Kagan, 1994), each of which may increase risk for the subsequent development of anxiety disorder. There is some recent evidence from a large twin study indicating that separation anxiety disorder and adult-onset panic attacks share a common genetic diathesis not shared with childhood anxiety disorder (Roberson-Nay et al., 2012), which implies specificity of effects only between certain phenotypes. At the same time, it is also evident that even with early-onset obsessive-compulsive disorder (OCD), which is thought to be more closely associated with family history of OCD, the majority of families do not actually have a positive family history of OCD (e.g., Chabane et al., 2005), which means that factors other than genetics contribute to the likelihood of developing full-blown OCD. In general, many studies of the genetics of anxiety disorders involving children and adolescents have substantive methodological limitations, so there remains a great deal to discover in this area.

The presence of a genetic influence for anxiety disorders does not imply that the course of illness is immutable. From the perspective of prevention, it may be that studying other risk factors in youth at genetic risk for anxiety disorders may prove especially fruitful and may suggest roads to interventions that reduce the genetic risk, perhaps by improving our understanding of some of the nonbiological mediators by which that risk may be transmitted (e.g., modeling of fearful behavior, parenting styles).

ENVIRONMENTAL FACTORS

Familial Factors

Parent–Child Interactions/Attachment

All four of the attachment styles in children according to the classification by Ainsworth, Blehar, Waters, and Wall, (1978) and Main and Solomon (1990)—secure, insecure-avoidant, insecure-ambivalent, and insecure-disorganized—have been found to be represented in children with anxiety disorders. However, the highest risks for developing an anxiety disorder are associated with disorganized attachment, which is associated with unresolved trauma or loss, and ambivalent attachment (Cassidy, 1995; Manassis, Bradley,

Goldberg, Hood, & Swinson, 1994; Warren, Huston, Egeland, & Sroufe, 1997). The specificity of an association between disorganized attachment in terms of its link with a specific type of anxiety disorder, such as separation anxiety disorder, has not been established.

Retrospective Studies

Lutz and Hock (1995) examined whether adult mental representations of attachment relationships and memories of childhood experiences with parents contributed to a mother's anxiety about separation from her own infant. Mothers with insecure attachment representations, when asked to remember details of their own childhood, reported more negative recollections of early parental caregiving, particularly rejection and discouragement of independence. Cassidy (1995) found that adolescents and adults with GAD reported more caregiver unresponsiveness, role reversal/enmeshment, and feelings of anger/vulnerability toward their mothers than controls. Systematic and formal assessments of the adolescent and adult attachment styles were not conducted in this sample, however. The biggest problem with this entire line of research, however, is that anxious people's current clinical state may influence their retrospective recall of attachment as they search for viable explanations for why they suffer from these symptoms. Accordingly, prospective and even cross-sectional studies allow for a less biased view of these interrelationships and their potential contribution to the development of anxiety disorders.

Prospective Studies

Manassis et al. (1994) examined adult attachment and mother–child attachment in 20 mother–child dyads (children ages 18–59 months) in which the mothers had anxiety disorders. The mothers all had insecure adult attachments, and 80% also had insecure attachments with their children. Among the insecurely attached children, three of 16 met diagnostic criteria for anxiety disorders; none of the secure children did. Two had separation anxiety disorder (one with disorganized attachment, one with avoidant attachment) and one had avoidant disorder (with disorganized attachment). Insecure children also had higher internalizing scores on the Child Behavior Checklist (Achenbach & Edelbrock, 1984) than secure children. When the dyads who had been classified as disorganized and mothers who had been classified as unresolved were assigned their "best" alternate category, and combined with the remaining three attachment categories, a higher-than-expected rate of ambivalent/resistant attachment and a lower-than-expected rate of secure attachment were found.

Warren et al. (1997) studied 172 adolescents aged 17.5 years who had participated in assessments of mother–child attachment at 12 months of age. Of these 172 adolescents, 26 (15%) met diagnostic criteria for anxiety disorders. More of the adolescents with anxiety disorders were classified as anxious/resistant in infancy than the adolescents without anxiety disorders. More adolescents diagnosed with other disorders (not anxiety) were, as infants, classified as avoidant. Furthermore, being classified as anxious/resistant attachment doubled the risk of subsequently developing an anxiety disorder, and better predicted adolescent anxiety disorders than either maternal anxiety or child temperament. The interaction between anxious/resistant attachment and one aspect of temperament (slow habituation to stimuli) further increased the risk of a subsequent anxiety disorder. However, secure, insecure-avoidant, and insecure-resistant attachment were *all* represented among the adolescents with anxiety disorders (data on the insecure-disorganized classification were unavailable).

Linkages also have been found between attachment and subclinical levels of anxiety. Female undergraduates who were insecurely attached were perceived by their friends as being more anxious than their counterparts who were securely attached (Barnas, Pollina, & Cummings 1991). Crowell, O'Connor, Wollmers, and Sprafkin (1991) found that children with behavioral disturbances whose mothers were classified as secure on the Adult Attachment Interview rated themselves as less anxious and depressed than children with behavioral disturbances whose mothers were insecure-dismissing. Cassidy and Berlin (1994) reported increased fearfulness across several studies of insecure-ambivalent/resistant children.

Belsky and Rovine (1987) have suggested a potential linkage between attachment and anxiety when attachment is placed on a spectrum from the style associated with the most overt distress (ambivalent/resistant) to that associated with the least overt distress (avoidant). Secures are in the middle of the spectrum, with some exhibiting relatively high distress and some exhibiting relatively low distress (Belsky & Rovine, 1987). Consistent with Belsky and Rovine (1987), 2.5-year-old children who were either insecure-ambivalent/resistant or secure with relatively high distress showed higher indices of fear and separation distress than children in the other attachment classifications (Stevenson-Hinde & Shouldice, 1990).

A large study (644 adolescents) conducted in the Netherlands (Muris et al., 2002) examined behavioral inhibition, attachment, parental rearing behavior, and self-reported anxiety symptoms, and identified small to moderate correlations among these risk factors but also a modest but significant positive relationship between each of these variables and child anxiety scores, though little was found in the way of interactive effects. The absence of parent- or observer-reported data on adolescents' anxiety levels is a weakness of the study, especially since the overall levels of anxiety reported were not particularly high.

Costa, Weems, and Pina (2009) examined the predictive value of attachment beliefs and parenting behaviors in a sample of 74 youth exposed to Hurricane Katrina. The advantage of this study was the fact that the investigators had assessments of attachment, anxiety symptoms, and parenting behaviors prior to the storm. Upon reassessment after the storm, it was found that youths' perceptions of trust and communication with their mothers as well as acceptance and firm control moderated the association between youths' pre- and post-Katrina anxiety: those with higher levels of anxiety and lower perceptions of trust, communication, or acceptance as well as higher perceptions of firm control before the hurricane were most likely to show increases in anxiety afterward. These data point to several potential intervention points, such as focusing on improving the parent–child relationship and the child's perception of that relationship, in the context of trauma exposure.

In summary, attachment, in particular insecure attachment, has been linked with both clinical and subclinical anxiety in children of different age ranges. The link may be stronger when the child also has a temperamental vulnerability to anxiety, though the evidence there is not as clear. Limitations of this research include the paucity of prospective studies, the varying definitions of "anxiety" (e.g., anxiety symptoms, anxiety disorders) used across studies, and small sample sizes.

Parenting

The research conducted on "parenting" has primarily focused on parental rearing styles, with the latter conceptualized along two orthogonal dimensions: warmth versus hostility, and control versus autonomy (Boer, 1998; Cassidy, 1995; Dadds, Barrett, Rapee, & Ryan, 1996; Festa & Ginsburg, 2011; Lutz & Hock, 1995; Manassis et al., 1994; Rapee 1997; Siqueland, Kendall, & Steinberg, 1996; Warren et al., 1997).

Retrospective Reports

In a meta-analysis of five studies, with a total of 463 patients in the experimental groups, Gerlsma, Emmelkamp, and Arrindell (1990) found that adults with phobias reported a parental rearing style characterized by less affection and more control. Studies of adults meeting diagnostic criteria for panic disorder or social phobia/avoidant personality disorder have demonstrated a similar recollection of childrearing patterns, in that these adults view their parents, and their relationship with them, as low in affection and overcontrolling (Rapee, 1997). Parental overcontrol was also found to be predictive of social anxiety symptoms in a recent study examining the predictive value of parental and social factors (Festa & Ginsburg, 2011).

Empirical research has documented an influence of parental rearing styles on the development of anxiety (see Rapee, 1997, for review). Interestingly, adults with insecure-preoccupied attachments frequently report parental rejection and control (Main & Goldwyn, 1991), suggesting that parenting style may be related to adult attachment status. Here again, the possibility of biased recall cannot be discounted as a source of variance in any retrospective examination of parenting styles in anxious adults or youth.

Prospective Reports and Behavioral Observations

In an early study, Zabin and Melamed (1980), using a self-report measure of parental rearing patterns, found parental reported use of positive reinforcement, modeling, and persuasion was associated with lower levels of child anxiety when the child had to undergo a fearful medical procedure; parental use of punishment, physical force, and reinforcement of dependency was associated with higher levels during the procedure. Siqueland et al. (1996) found that parents of children with anxiety disorders were rated by observers as less granting of psychological autonomy than were the parents of "normal" controls. In addition, children with anxiety disorders rated their mothers and fathers as less accepting and less granting of psychological autonomy than control children rated their parents. The potential for a bidirectional relationship with respect to child anxiety and parental granting of psychological autonomy renders the meaning of these findings unclear, however, especially as they may relate to potential points of intervention. Parental anxiety in and of itself does seem to play a role in the development and maintenance of anxiety in children (e.g., Bögels & Phares, 2008; Kendall et al., 2009), although here again the way in which this risk is transmitted has yet to be clarified and is likely complex. What did emerge from Kendall et al.'s clinical trial, as discussed in Chapter 10, is that the presence of parental anxiety disorders was a moderator of outcome, such that if *both* parents had an anxiety disorder, then the child's outcomes were substantially better in the condition that involved cognitive-behavioral therapy (CBT) including a strong family component, than in the one that was delivered individually. This implicates, but does not isolate, a potential effect of modeling for both anxious behavior and for approach behavior once the family has been familiarized with the CBT model.

Direct observations of parent–child interactions have provided further evidence of family processes that may be specific to families of children with anxiety disorders, and these processes may serve to either bring out and/or maintain these disorders in children (e.g., Chorpita, Albano, & Barlow, 1996; Dadds et al., 1996 see Ginsburg, Silverman, & Kurtines, 1995). For example, Dadds et al. (1996) studied specific sequences of communication exchanged between parents and children (ages 7–14) in a discussion of ambiguous hypothetical situations. Parents of children with anxiety disorders (n = 66) were less likely to grant and reward autonomy of thought and action than controls (n = 18). Dadds et al. also found that these parents fostered cautiousness and avoidance taking a social risk by modeling caution, providing information about risk, expressing doubt about the child's competency, and rewarding the child for avoidance by expressing agreement and nurturance when the child decides he or she would not join in with the other children. Dadds et al. referred to this finding as the FEAR effect (Family Enhancement of Avoidant and Aggressive Responses).

Hudson and Rapee (2002) studied 57 children and adolescents (37 children with anxiety disorders and 20 non-clinic-referred children; ages 7–16 years) and found that mothers and fathers were overly involved not only with their child with an anxiety disorder but also with the child's sibling (without an anxiety disorder). The authors concluded that because parents' overinvolvement does not occur exclusively in youths with anxiety disorders, it probably is not simply a response to difficulties with anxiety and coping that they have observed with the diagnosed youth. It also suggests that parental overinvolvement does not in and of itself cause anxiety disorders.

Anxious parents could increase the risk of anxiety disorders in their offspring by doing the following:

1. Having difficulty modeling appropriate coping strategies
2. Reacting to their children's fears negatively because they represent an aspect of themselves they would rather deny
3. Becoming overly concerned about their children's anxiety, resulting in overprotection and thus reducing opportunities for desensitization.

The latter two reactions are consistent with dismissive and preoccupied adult attachment types, respectively. Anxious parents who are securely attached, on the other hand, may be able to empathize with their children's fears, which may then be perceived as supportive. Thus, the transmission of parental anxiety may depend on the interaction between attachment and parental psychopathology (Radke-Yarrow, DeMulder, & Belmont, 1995).

Peers, School, and Community

The ecology of adolescent development and culture includes an expanded network of peer, school, and community affiliations. The transition to middle school and high school constitutes a period of high developmental risk, in which there is an increased incidence of school truancy, failure and dropout, engagement in high-risk sexual and self-injurious behaviors, smoking and drug use, initiation into gangs, and contact with the juvenile justice system. It is also a time period of increased exposure to interpersonal violence. For example, among high school students who dated, 21% of females and 10% of males experienced physical and/or sexual violence (Vagi et al., 2015). This prevalence rate has remained unchanged in the last decade (Black et al., 2011) despite increased efforts to publicize this problem as an important public health issue. With respect to traumatic experiences more broadly speaking, the majority of 6,483 adolescents (61.8%) who participated in the National Comorbidity Survey Replication Adolescent Supplement study (McLaughlin et al., 2013) reported a potentially traumatic experience, with 4.7% already meeting full criteria for DSM-IV posttraumatic stress disorder (PTSD). In the sections below, particular high-risk activities engaged in by adolescents and their associated risk with the development of anxiety and anxiety disorders are discussed.

Smoking

Initiation into cigarette smoking in adolescence is recognized as a major public health problem. Approximately 3,200 adolescents start smoking each day (U.S. Department of Health and Human Services, 2012, 2014), resulting in about 23% of high-school seniors smoking or using other tobacco products daily. Smoking prevention and early treatment are important components of universal and selective public health prevention strategies, especially given that the American Health Association estimates that addiction to tobacco during adolescence accounts for 80% of adult smokers. As Upadhyaya et al. (2002) discuss, there is continuing interest in the interaction between the onset of adolescent psychiatric conditions and smoking behavior, including experimental smoking and cessation difficulty. Among the disorders studied, Johnson, Cohen, Pine, Kline, Kasen, and Book (2000) report that heavy cigarette smoking (defined as over 20 cigarettes per day) is associated with higher rates of agoraphobia and anxiety and panic disorders in adolescents. Zvolensky and Bernstein (2005) have identified a more specific link between cigarette smoking and the onset of panic-spectrum psychopathology in particular. Other studies have reported an even stronger association of adolescent smoking with attention-deficit/hyperactivity disorder (Johnson et. al., 2000) and major depressive disorder (Dierker et al., 2001). Most of these studies note the importance of the relationship between peer smoking influences and individual psychiatric vulnerabilities. The general conclusion is two-pronged:

1. Smoking prevention and cessation programs need to incorporate screening for adolescent psychiatric disorders, including anxiety disorders.
2. Attention to adolescent anxiety and comorbid disorders need to include strategies to address risks of tobacco addiction.

Drug Use

Adolescence is a developmental period in which experimentation with alcohol and drugs is common. It also a time of risk for early onset of alcohol and substance abuse/dependence. Nelson and Wittchen (1998) found that among youth and young adults, the peak incidence of alcohol disorders occurred at 16 or 17 years of age. Alcohol and drug use problems in adolescence represent a strong predictive factor for adult alcohol and drug dependence (Swadi, 1999). Studies of substance abuse and alcohol motivation in adolescents suggest a multifactorial explanatory framework. Among the many factors, Comeau, Stuart, and Loba (2001) found that high anxiety sensitivity predicts conformity motives for alcohol and marijuana use, while anxiety traits are associated with coping motives for alcohol and cigarette use. Zucker et al. (2002) reported that among young adults with panic disorder, up to one in five patients had an onset related to an adolescent experience with a psychoactive drug. In a review of studies of adolescent use of the recreational drug Ecstasy, Montoya et al. (2002) found a strong association between repeated drug use and anxiety disturbances, with potential neurobiological consequences that are of concern within this critical developmental stage.

Initiation and use of alcohol and drugs among adolescents is also related to life stresses, including traumatic events (Wills, Vaccaro, & McNammar, 1992). In one study, substance-abusing adolescents were found to be five times more likely to have a history of trauma and concurrent PTSD compared to a community sample (Deykin & Buka, 1997). In a large study of adolescents enrolled in four drug treatment programs, a high positive correlation was found between severity of posttraumatic stress symptoms and higher levels of substance use and HIV risk behavior (Stevens, Murphy, & McNight, 2003). Further support for the link between trauma and substance abuse was found in a large study of cannabis dependence and abuse, wherein PTSD diagnosis was directly associated with both the presence of a cannabis use disorder and with peer deviance which, in turn, exposes adolescents to more potentially traumatic experiences (Cornelius et al., 2010).

As with cigarette addiction, prevention strategies in regard to adolescent substance abuse need to include early intervention for anxiety-vulnerable and traumatized youth and, at the same time, recognize that prevention or early intervention for adolescent substance abuse may also constitute an anxiety disorder prevention strategy.

Gang Affiliation and Other Criminal Behavior

Gang affiliation is a serious cultural problem in adolescence. There are an estimated 33,000 gangs, with over 1.4 million members, active across the United States (U.S. Department of Justice, 2011). There is a complexity to youth involvement in gangs. Many studies have examined the confluence of risk factors that predict gang membership, including neighborhood, family, school, peer group, and individual variables (Hill, Levermore, Twaite, & Jones, 1996). There is an emerging literature about the extent of trauma and loss exposure associated with gang membership and delinquent behavior more generally (Wood, Foy, Layne, Pynoos, & James, 2002). Despite high rates of trauma exposure prior to gang membership, commonly youth report their worst traumatic experiences are gang -related and the source of current PTSD symptoms (Wood et al., 2002). Ages 11 to 13 are primary years for solicitation and inculcation into gang affiliation and activities, contributing to years of increased trauma and loss exposure during adolescence. Consequently, intervention programs to prevent youth from becoming involved in gangs should be considered an adjunct prevention strategy for adolescent PTSD.

Attention has turned to the high prevalence of adolescent psychiatric disorder present among juvenile justice detainees. Studies that have assessed PTSD in this setting have found it to be among the highest rates found (Wasserman, McReynolds, Lucal, Fisher, & Santos, 2002). Interestingly, separation anxiety disorder among adolescents (an age range where it is less expected) is surprisingly high among African-American and Hispanic/Latino detained youth (Teplin, Abram, McClelland, Dulkan, & Mericle, 2002). Further, among incarcerated boys with callous-unemotional traits, the rates of negative life events and PTSD were significantly elevated (Sharf et al., 2014). Such effects are also found in female adolescent criminal offenders: a review of the literature revealed high rates of trauma exposure, PTSD, and substance abuse disorders (Foy et al., 2012). The juvenile justice contact thus provides a key opportunity for mental health intervention that can play a significant role in an overall public mental health approach to adolescent anxiety disorders and delinquency prevention programs. Notably, there is evidence from a randomized controlled trial that providing substance abuse and mental health treatment in prison settings significantly reduces recidivism 1 year after release in adult male offenders (Sacks et al., 2012). This offers encouragement to researchers to develop prevention programs centered around treatment of mental health problems in adjudicated teens, which may reduce the risk of re-offending.

Adolescence and Trauma Exposure

Adolescence represents a development transition in the maturation of self-efficacy in the face of danger. There is increasing reliance on the peer group for appraisal of danger and estimation of needed protective actions along with greater engagement of the peer group in dangerous and protective behavior. Developmental epidemiology suggests that adolescence carries a high risk of exposure to a spectrum of traumatic situations, subsequent PTSD, comorbid psychopathology, and age-related impairments. Included among the salient types of exposure are adolescent physical and sexual abuse (Kaplan et al., 1998; Pelcovitz et al., 2000); interpersonal and community violence (Kilpatrick et al., 1997; Wolfe et al., 2001); serious accidental injury, especially traffic accidents (de Vries et al., 1999); traumatic losses, including those by homicide, suicide, and fatal automobile accidents (Minino, 2010); and life-threatening medical illness accompanied by life-endangering medical procedures (e.g., kidney and liver transplant; Shemesh et al., 2000; Meeske et al., 2001).

There also has been a lack of societal recognition that adolescence is the age range with the highest rates of criminal victimization (Menard, 2002). For example, adolescents are two times more likely than adults to be victims of serious violent crime and three times more likely to be victims of simple assault (Sickmund, Snyder, & Poe-Yamagata, 1997; Snyder, 1998). A national survey of adolescents found 23% reported having been both a victim of assault and a witness to violence, and over 20% met the lifetime criteria for PTSD (Kilpatrick et al., 1997). Boys are more likely to experience criminal assault, and girls are more likely to experience dating violence and rape. Despite a lower rate of filing criminal complaints, adolescence is the period in which, by self-report, sexual assault occurs most, with a rate during ages 13 to 17 years of 14.8% among girls and 3.7% among boys (Kilpatrick et al., 2003). In addition to general rates of exposure to war and disasters, international studies indicate that adolescents in these situations often are engaged in resistance and rescue efforts, and can become victims of torture (Nader et al., 1989; Pynoos et al., 2001). Bouwer and Stein (1997) reported that a significant subpopulation of adults with panic disorder had a history of traumatic suffocation experience, including political torture by suffocation in adolescence. Fear and symptom profiles included respiratory phenomena and nocturnal panic. Studies among adolescents indicate that there may be multiple forms of exposure, with comorbid admixtures of PTSD, depression, and separation anxiety disorder (Pelcovitz et al., 2000; Warner & Weist, 1996). Finally, adolescent trauma exposures often are superimposed on prior trauma histories and untreated chronic posttraumatic stress symptoms.

Considerable evidence indicates that traumatized adolescents are at increased risk for a spectrum of adverse psychosocial difficulties and functional impairments. These include reduced academic achievement; aggressive, delinquent, or high-risk sexual behaviors; substance abuse and dependence (Cavaiola & Schiff, 1988; Farrell & Bruce, 1997; Kilpatrick, Acierno, Saundres, Resnick & Best, 2000; Saigh, Mroueh, & Bremner, 1997; Saltzman, Pynoos, Layne, Steinberg & Aisenberg, 2001); and nonadherence to prescribed posttransplant medical treatment (Shemesh et al., 2000). Further, trauma in adolescence has been linked with long-term developmental disturbances, including disrupted moral development, missed developmental opportunities, delayed preparation for professional and family life, and disruptions in close relationships (Goenjian et al., 1999; Layne, Pynoos, & Cardenas, 2000; Malinkosky-Rummell & Hansen, 1993; Pynoos, Steinberg, & Piacentini, 1999). Ongoing reactive behavior to trauma reminders in adolescence carries the bimodal risk of reckless behavior or extreme avoidant behavior that can derail an adolescent's life. Programs to help reduce adolescents' risk of exposure to trauma would thereby seem to play an important role in preserving adolescent development.

Social Support

The adult literature is replete with studies that suggest the possible beneficial effects of social support following exposure to traumatic events, but less is known about its role in mitigating anxiety disorder symptoms outside the context of trauma, and even less about the influence of social support in adolescent anxiety disorders. Studies of veterans from the Vietnam, Gulf, and Lebanon wars have found that veterans' perceptions of poor social support are associated with worse PTSD symptoms; the relationship remains when veterans report retrospectively about the support they received immediately after their return from duty (Barrett & Mizes, 1988; Fontana, Schwartz, & Rosenheck, 1997; Foy, Resnick, Sipprelle, & Carroll, 1987; Solomon et al., 1988; Stretch, 1985; Sutker et al., 1995a, 1995b) and even when controlling for level of combat exposure, another robust predictor of PTSD symptoms among veterans (Boscarino, 1995; King et al., 1998). Among civilian victims of violence, poor social support also has been linked to PTSD symptoms in victims of violent nonsexual assault (Bisson & Shepherd, 1995), domestic violence (Astin et al., 1993; Kemp et al., 1995), and rape (Resick, 1993; Steketee & Foa, 1987; Zoellner et al., 1999). Moreover, Fontana and Rosenheck (1998) found that good postdischarge social support was strongly predictive of less PTSD in female veterans who were victims of sexual harassment, rape, or attempted rape. Social support is also associated with recovery among victims of "noninterpersonal" traumas, such as natural disasters (e.g., Madakasira & O'Brien (1987), motor vehicle accidents (Buckley et al., 1996), and chronic, life-threatening illness, including patients treated for breast cancer (Andrykowski & Cordova, 1998), African-American women with HIV/AIDS (Myers & Durvasula, 1999), and survivors of childhood leukemia and their mothers and fathers (Kazak et al., 1997).

There are a number of shortcomings to the extant adult literature on social support in the wake of trauma. First, although a large body of research supports the conclusion that social support is associated with decreased PTSD symptomology (e.g., Greene et al. 2006; Keane et al., 1985), most of these studies have relied on retrospective reports (some as many as 30 years after the fact) of social support. Second, the studies typically have aggregated and equally weighted the influence of friends, coworkers, and neighbors with that of immediate family, which may obscure the more influential effects for the latter (Griffith, 1985). Third, and perhaps most importantly for the purpose of considering prevention efforts, no studies have attempted to delineate the mechanism responsible for the apparent positive impact of social support on posttrauma recovery. Pennebaker and Seagal (1999) suggest that painful events that have not been structured in a narrative format may contribute to the continued experience of negative feelings and are more likely to remain in consciousness as unwanted thoughts (Wegner, 1989). Foa and Riggs (1993) suggest that trauma disclosure within naturally occurring social support systems provides three potential benefits:

1. Disclosure allows the trauma survivor to confront frightening memories in a relatively safe environment, allowing habituation of fear reactions much as is accomplished in exposure-based treatment of PTSD (Foa et al., 1991, 1997; Keane et al., 1989; Richards et al., 1994).
2. Given the observation that traumatic memories often are often disjointed and confused, disclosure, particularly repeated disclosure, provides the survivor with an opportunity to create a more coherent memory.
3. Disclosure is thought to provide an opportunity for the survivor to evaluate potentially mistaken cognitions regarding the impact on himself or herself (e.g., "I am incompetent or worthless") or the world (e.g., "the world is unpredictably dangerous").

Herman (1992) suggests disclosure may also serve to "reconnect" the trauma survivor to others within the social arena. That is, the act of disclosing the trauma to another person may provide an opportunity for the survivor to redevelop a sense of trust and attachment to others. Thus, disclosing the trauma to a supportive person may function in multiple ways to facilitate recovery.

There also is evidence that social support may mitigate the impact of negative life events in children and adolescents whose parents are divorcing (Cowen et al., 1990) and in those who have been exposed to community violence (Berman, Kurtines, Silverman, & Serafini, 1996; Hill, Levermore, Twaite, & Jones, 1996; White, Bruce, Farrell, & Kliewer, 1998) and hurricanes (e.g., La Greca, Silverman, Vernberg, & Prinstein, 1996; Vernberg, La Greca, Silverman, & Prinstein, 1996). For example, White, Bruce, Farrell, and Kliewer (1998) found a strong negative relation between anxiety level and family social support in a longitudinal study investigating the effects of family social support on anxiety in 11- to 14-year-olds exposed to community violence. In children exposed to the devastation of Hurricane Andrew in south Florida, higher anxiety, less social support, more intervening life events, and greater use of poor emotion coping strategies each predicted chronic distress at follow-up (LaGreca et al., 2010, 2013), which again underscores the importance of social support as a potential protective factor. Perhaps acceptance into a supportive social network attenuates the effects of the putative anxiety disorder risk factors described earlier. Thus, social support serves as one possible explanation for why so many children and adolescents elevated on these risk factors (e.g., behavioral inhibition, parental anxiety disorders) do not go on to develop full-blown disorders (e.g., Derivois et al., 2014; Festa & Ginsburg, 2011). The importance of the adolescent's peer group suggests that social support may be particularly relevant during this period. (See Table 11.1 for a summary of putative risk factors.)

EARLY DETECTION AND SCREENING

The success of prevention intervention programs for anxiety disorders in adolescents depends a great deal on having early detection and screening strategies in place at key access points where youths might be identified. The types of early detection and screening strategies are likely to vary with the type of preventive intervention program being implemented (universal, selective, indicated). In this section, key access points are identified and specific types of screens that might be administered, depending on the type of preventive intervention strategy, are summarized.

Before proceeding with this discussion, a general point is first worth noting. Namely, for the majority of access points or settings where early detection and screening strategies might be conducted, some type of rating scale is recommended for initial use. Because of their objective scoring procedure, rating scales minimize

Table 11.1 Who May Be at Risk?

Individual Factors	
Elevated but Subsyndromal Anxiety Symptoms	Increased risk of developing full-blown disorder in next two years if elevated symptoms are already present
Behavioral Inhibition (Temperament)	Tendency to avoid novel stimuli and experiences; excessive shyness in response to new people
Anxiety Sensitivity	Tendency to interpret physiological sensations of anxiety as threatening and of themselves
Cognitive Factors	Avoidant coping style, low perceived control
Family Factors	
Parenting	Insecure attachment, possibly interacting w/ behaviorally inhibited temperament
Parent–Child Interactions	Parental tendency to suggest avoidant problem-solving strategies; overinvolvement & overprotection in response to child's fears; poor modeling of coping responses
Peer, School, & Community Factors	
Smoking	Association with panic disorder in particular
Alcohol & Other Drug Use	Elevates other risk factors (e.g., motor vehicle accidents), may also elevate risk in and of itself
Gang Affiliation/Criminal Behavior	Exposure to traumatic events, commission of interpersonal violence
Trauma Exposure	Experiencing a Criterion A trauma increases the risk for PTSD and other anxiety symptoms, perhaps especially in those who are already vulnerable or in response to certain traumas regardless (e.g., sexual assault)
Poor Social Support	Associated with more symptoms and poorer outcomes in adults, possibly a mediating factor

the role of clinical inference and interpretation. As a result, there is no need to use highly trained staff for administration and scoring. In addition, most rating scales contain questions that would be of clear concern to non–mental health professionals, such as school board institutional review board members, because the scales contain items that are face valid. Finally, a wide range of rating scales are available for administration to various informants, including children and adolescents, as well as parents, teachers, and clinicians. Consequently, information can be obtained from either a single source (e.g., adolescent only) or multiple sources (e.g., adolescent, parent) depending on available resources. If resources are limited, the consensus in the field is that information from youths themselves should be obtained for screening/assessing for internalizing problems, including anxiety (Loeber, Green, & Lahey, 1990).

Despite the advantages of using rating scales for early detection and screening, two caveats are worth noting. First, although the measures that are mentioned in this section all possess adequate psychometric properties in terms of reliability and validity, their actual utility for screening purposes awaits further empirical evaluation. For example, data on the measures' sensitivity (the percentage of individuals who receive the diagnosis who were positively identified by the rating scale; true positives) and specificity (the percentage of individuals who do not receive the diagnosis and who are not identified by the rating scale as anxious; true negatives) (Vecchio, 1996) are scarce when it comes to child and adolescent samples, particularly nonwhite samples. Second, currently available rating scales are likely to select more false positives than true positives (Costello & Angold, 1988). That is, youths identified as anxious at an initial screen are likely not to be anxious or depressed at the second stage of an investigation. Consequently, a useful/cost-efficient approach for early detection and screening for indicated intervention programs would employ a multistage sampling design (e.g., Ialongo, Edelsohn, Werthamer-Larsson, Crockett, & Kellam, 1993; Kendall, Cantwell & Kazdin, 1989; Roberts, Lewinsohn, & Seeley, 1991). At the first stage, a rating scale would be administered to informants to identify youths who score 1 or 2 standard deviations from the sample mean or who deviate from normative data. These identified cases would then undergo more precise and comprehensive assessments (e.g., structured diagnostic interviews) at the second or third stage of the research.

Potential Access Points for Early Detection and Screening

School

The school setting is an obvious access point for early detection and screening of anxiety and its disorders because this is where the children and adolescents are! If a preventive interventionist were interested in developing and implementing an indicated prevention program, there are several rating scales that could be administered to target high-risk children and adolescents who may demonstrate minimal but detectable symptoms of anxiety and/or anxiety disorders. In general, most of the research studies that have used rating scales for screening anxiety symptoms/disorders have largely used preadolescent samples of children (e.g., McDermott et al., 2013). There is a paucity of work in which the study's samples involved adolescents specifically.

For anxiety symptoms, the most widely used child and adolescent self-rating scale measure is the Revised Children's Manifest Anxiety Scale (RCMAS; Reynolds & Richmond, 1978), which was used as an initial screen in the Queensland Early Intervention and Prevention of Anxiety Project (Dadds, Holland, Laurens, Mullins, Barrett, & Spence, 1999; Dadds, Spence, Holland, Barrett, & Laurens, 1997), described below. The RCMAS is a 37-item scale: 28 items are summed to yield a Total Anxiety score and the other nine items are summed to yield a Lie score. Youths respond either Yes or No to all 37 items. Factor analytic studies also have provided support for the RCMAS's three-factor subscale structure (Physiological, Worry/Oversensitivity, and Concentration) as well as the Lie scale (e.g., Paget & Reynolds, 1984; Reynolds & Richmond, 1979; Scholwinski & Reynolds, 1985). Positive scale convergence between the RCMAS and other widely used child self-rating scales of anxiety and related constructs (trait anxiety, fear, depression) in community samples have been found as well (e.g., Muris, Merckelbach, Ollendick, King, & Bogie, 2002). A 15-item version of this scale has since been developed, and it performed well psychometrically (Ebesutani et al., 2012); this may increase the likelihood of use as a mass screening tool.

For anxiety symptoms linked more directly to DSM-IV anxiety disorders, the Multidimensional Anxiety Scale for Children (MASC; March, Parker, Sullivan, Stallings, & Connor, 1997), the Screen for Child Anxiety Related Emotional Disorders (Birmaher, Khetarpal, Brent, Cully, Balach, Kaufman, et al., 1997), and the Spence Children's Anxiety Scale may be useful. The MASC, for example, is a 45-item scale that yields a Total Anxiety Disorder Index and four main factor scores: Social Anxiety (with performance anxiety and humiliation as subfactors), Physical Symptoms, (with tension-restlessness and somatic-autonomic arousal as subfactors), Harm/Avoidance (with perfectionism and anxious coping as subfactors), and Separation/Panic. In addition, six items yield an Inconsistency Index to identify careless or contradictory responses. Youths may be identified based on either specific subscale scores on these measures or the total score.

For social anxiety, the Social Anxiety Scale for Children—Revised (La Greca & Stone, 1993) and the adolescent version (La Greca & Lopez, 1998) as well as the Social Phobia and Anxiety Inventory for Children (Beidel, Turner, & Morris, 1995) have been found to be helpful in identifying highly social anxious children (Epkins, 2002; Morris & Masia, 1998), though variations in the two measures' classification correspondence indicated variation with sample, age, and sex. In light of this variation, coupled with the fact that both Epkins (2002) and Morris and Masia (1998) did not sample adolescents (Epkins's sample was 8–12 years; Morris and Masia's was 9–12 years), additional research on the utility of these measures for screening among adolescents is needed. A study that examined several screening measures for social anxiety in pediatric primary care found that a single item from the Screen for Child Related Anxiety Disorders (SCARED), which was "my child is shy," was moderately accurate for detecting generalized social phobia in primary care (Bailey et al., 2006). Moreover, research on all of these scales' utility in the context of prevention remains lacking.

The Childhood Anxiety Sensitivity Index (CASI; Silverman, Fleisig, Rabian, & Peterson, 1991) has been used in a number of studies and appears useful as a screen for adolescents who may be at risk for displaying panic attacks and panic disorder (Hayward, Killen, Wilson, & Hammer, 1997; Weems, Hayward, Killen, & Taylor, 2002). The CASI consists of 18 items that assess the extent to which children and adolescents believe the experience of anxiety will result in negative consequences. Sample items include: "It scares me when I feel like I am going to throw up" and "It scares me when my heart beats fast." Youths respond to each item using a 3-point scale: none (1), some (2), or a lot (3). The CASI yields a total score by summing the ratings across all items. CASI scores can range from 18 to 54, with higher scores reflecting higher levels of anxiety sensitivity.

In addition, evidence indicates that a large proportion of children and adolescents who display school refusal behavior are likely suffering from some type of anxiety disorder, particularly separation anxiety disorder in young children and social anxiety, panic, or GAD in older children and adolescents (Kearney & Silverman, 1997). This renders it critical that school counselors and psychologists be informed and educated about the nature of school refusal behavior so that they can help detect such cases and refer them for appropriate therapeutic, rather than disciplinary, action.

If a preventive interventionist were interested in developing and implementing a selective prevention program in a school setting, specific groups or individuals considered to be at risk for developing anxiety and its disorders need to be identified. At the preschool level, Rapee (2002) used a mother-completed rating scale of child's temperament, followed by a laboratory observation of behavioral inhibition, as a screen for selecting youngsters in the Macquarie University Preschool Intervention Program (described subsequently).

In light of the high rates of traumatic exposure among young people, particularly adolescents, youths who have been exposed to traumatic events are another group that should be considered for early detection and screening in the school setting, focusing particularly on posttraumatic stress and anxiety reactions. Successful efforts in such screening, using most frequently the Reaction Index (Frederick, Pynoos, & Nader, 1992), have appeared in the area of community violence (e.g., adolescent sample: Berman, Kurtines, Silverman, & Serafini, 1996), natural disasters (e.g., child sample; La Greca, Silverman, Vernberg, & Prinstein, 1996; Vernberg, La Greca, Silverman, & Prinstein, 1996); and sniper shootings (e.g., child sample; Pynoos, Frederick, Nader, & Arroyo, 1987). March et al. (1997) and Foa et al. (2001) have developed and conducted psychometric evaluation of the Child and Adolescent Trama Survey (CATS) and the Child PTSD Symptom Scale (CPSS), respectively; both have been found to be psychometrically sound.

The CPSS, for example, assesses traumatic stress symptoms in children and adolescents, 8 to 18 years of age. CPSS items assess all 17

DSM-IV symptom criteria for PTSD and yield a Total Severity Score (17 items) and three empirically derived factor scale scores representing DSM-IV clusters B (Re-experiencing), C (Avoidance), and D (Arousal). The CPSS also includes a seven-item impairment rating scale to assess functioning in such domains as family, peers, and school. Evidence has indicated moderate to excellent internal consistency, retest reliability, and concurrent validity as well as excellent sensitivity and specificity (Foa, Johnson, Feeny, & Treadwell, 2001; Gillihan, Aderka, Conklin, Capaldi, & Foa 2013). In a South African sample, Suliman et al. (2005) found that the CATS can be used effectively as a screening tool for PTSD in school settings provided that appropriate cutoff scores are used. Together, these PTSD scales have the potential for use in early detection and screening of youths at high risk in developing posttraumatic stress and anxiety reactions due to their exposure to traumatic events, though further evaluative research regarding their utility for such purposes is needed. In addition, given that many adolescent-onset problems, such as cigarette smoking, frequently co-occur with anxiety and its disorders, as noted earlier, screening for anxiety using one of the anxiety symptoms scales may be worthwhile to include whenever beginning to work with adolescents on such problems.

Finally, Beidel and colleagues (Beidel & Turner, 1988; Beidel, Turner, & Trager, 1994) conducted a series of studies showing that the Test Anxiety Scale for Children (Saranson, Davidson, Lighthall, & Waite, 1958) could serve as a useful screen in identifying children who may show detectable symptoms of anxiety disorders, including social anxiety disorder, specific phobia, and GAD. Clearly, given that "high stakes" testing (e.g., SATs, ACTs) becomes more of a stressor with adolescence, the potential utility of test anxiety as a marker, and the Test Anxiety Scale as a screen among adolescent samples, deserves scrutiny.

Healthcare Settings

There are multiple access points for early detection and screening in healthcare settings, particularly in pediatrics, obstetrics-gynecology, and psychiatry. The pediatric setting, for example, is the natural site for early detection and screening of young children with pediatric onset of either OCD or a tic disorder following an abrupt onset of symptoms after a group A hemolytic streptococcal infection (PANDAS). Indeed, for a large proportion of families, the pediatrician's office is the "first gate" they enter when their child or adolescent begins to show disturbances associated with anxiety and its disorders, such as somatic complaints and panic attack symptoms. A recent study provided preliminary supportive evidence for use of another disorder-specific screening tool in primary care, the Autonomic Nervous System Questionnaire, which is a relatively short adolescent panic disorder screening instrument (Queen, Ehrenreich-May, & Hershorin, 2012). Similarly, Achiam-Montal, Tibi, and Lipsitz (2103) found that 20% of adolescents presenting with noncardiac chest pain screened positive for panic disorder in general outpatient medical settings. In general, it would thus seem to be critical for primary care physicians to have understanding of and knowledge about anxiety disorders so they could inquire about the presence/absence of key symptoms of the various disorders and refer the patient as necessary to a mental health professional for further evaluation based on the results of these initial queries.

Given the preponderance of female cases of anxiety disorders relative to male cases, particularly from adolescence and beyond, obstetrics-gynecology settings represent yet another potentially useful and critically important access point for early detection and screening. Studies have demonstrated that pubertal maturation in adolescent girls, particularly early onset, may constitute a risk factor for developing anxiety symptoms and disorders (e.g., Caspi & Moffit, 1991; Graber, Brooks-Gunn, Paikoff, & Warren, 1994), particularly panic attacks (Hayward, Killen, Kraemer, Blair-Greiner, Strachowski, & Cunning, 1997). Such findings suggest the potential utility of educating OB/GYNs about the risks of anxiety problems in their young adolescent patients. The manner in which such young patients may become overly sensitive to the physical changes that occur during the menstrual cycle (i.e., high anxiety sensitivity) might be carefully considered and even assessed using the CASI (Silverman et al., 1991). Relatedly, research findings, albeit sparse, suggest that hormonal fluctuations during the female reproductive cycle may serve to either exacerbate or reduce anxiety symptoms/disorders. For example, among some women, the postpartum period may be a risk for the onset and exacerbation of anxiety symptoms/disorders (March & Yonkers, 2001). Also among some women, pregnancy may be a period in which panic disorder improves (Shear & Oommen, 1995). In light of such findings, it seems critical for OB/GYNs to carefully consider their female patients' emotional states during regularly scheduled appointments. Adult anxiety rating scales, such as the Hamilton Scales, may be worth administering as a potential screen for the presence of anxiety symptoms in these patients.

Finally, psychiatry departments housed in medical settings, in community mental health settings, or in private practice represent yet another important, though again largely untapped, access point by which to conduct early detection and screening. In light of the strong evidence for familial transmission of anxiety disorders, adult patients who present with anxiety disorders, depressive disorders, or both (Weissman, 1988) should be carefully queried about the functioning of their children and adolescents. For such purposes, parent rating scales such as the Child Behavior Checklist (CBCL; Achenbach, 1991) and the Connors Rating Scales (Conners, 1997) could be administered. Although parents with anxiety problems are likely to endorse high levels of internalizing problems in their offspring using the CBCL (e.g., Silverman, Cerny, Nelles, & Burke, 1988), some of which might be due to the parent's own pathology, as noted earlier, this initial step is a screen. Further follow-up would then be conducted with the children themselves using structured interview schedules, such as the Anxiety Disorders Interview Schedule for Children: DSM-IV (Silverman & Albano, 1996). This interview schedule is the one most widely used in the child and adolescent anxiety disorders area and includes a child and a parent version.

MODEL PROGRAMS

The development of interventions designed to prevent anxiety disorders in adolescents has been hampered by insufficient and sometimes inconsistent information about the longitudinal course of disorders, the efficacy of procedures designed to reduce modifiable risk factors (e.g., anxiety sensitivity), the poorly understood influence of protective factors, and the possible additive if not multiplicative effects of multiple risk factors. Further, immersion in adolescent culture represents a time of increased risk for a variety of negative life experiences, and as such adolescents are at increased risk for the development of at least certain anxiety disorders during this time, such as PTSD and panic disorder. On the whole, the research literature remains underdeveloped, and addressing critical gaps will be important in developing adolescent-specific prevention programs.

The FRIENDS program, developed by Australian researchers led by Paula Barrett and colleagues and described below, has been evaluated extensively and is associated with the strongest effect sizes in the field. The FRIENDS acronym stands for Feeling worried; Relax and feel good; Inner thoughts; Explore plans of action; Nice work, reward yourself; Don't forget to practice; and Stay cool. The program is cognitive-behavioral in orientation, can be delivered by teachers or psychologists, is conducted weekly for 10 weeks, and includes two booster sessions. The program has been used across the full spectrum from childhood to adolescence, but a clear effect for age has yet to emerge (Teubert & Pinquart, 2012); perhaps as a result of this, no adolescent-specific version of the FRIENDS program has been developed as yet. The FRIENDS program has been used in both selective and universal prevention studies. Developed and tested initially in Australia, the FRIENDS program has now been translated and adapted for use in other nations as well.

Types of Intervention

Our review of the extant intervention literature follows the organizational structure recommended by the Institute of Medicine's Committee on Prevention of Mental Disorders: (1) indicated, (2) selective, and (3) universal prevention programs. Notably, some prevention intervention programs have been developed to target general psychopathology risk factors (e.g., children whose parents recently divorced; Pedro-Carroll & Cowen, 1985). However, because the link between these broader risk factors and the development of anxiety disorders is even more tenuous than the link between anxiety disorders and the specific anxiety disorder risk factors described above, we continue to limit our discussion to studies that focused specifically on prevention of anxiety symptoms and anxiety disorders. A comprehensive review of these broad risk factor studies is available elsewhere (Hudson, Flannery-Schroeder, & Kendall, 2004; Neil & Christensen, 2009).

Indicated Prevention Programs

These programs are most similar to the treatments for fully syndromal individuals with which the field is most familiar, in that patients are already experiencing anxiety symptoms that place them at higher risk for the development of the full-blown syndrome. Although prevention work with adults is relatively uncommon given that most who develop significant problems with anxiety or full-blown anxiety disorders do so during childhood or adolescence, traumatic experiences during adulthood can greatly increase the risk for PTSD across the developmental spectrum. Several indicated prevention studies from the adult trauma literature are relevant to discuss briefly here. Foa et al. (1995) conducted the first PTSD prevention study. Women who were recent victims of sexual and nonsexual assault and who met symptom criteria for PTSD except for the duration criteria (3 months posttrauma), received either a brief CBT program consisting of four weekly 1.5-hour sessions or four weekly assessments of their PTSD-related symptoms. At 2 months after the intervention assessment the CBT group had a recovery rate of 70% for PTSD versus 10% in the assessment control group. Using five sessions of Foa et al.'s prevention program (adding one additional session), Bryant, Harvey, Sackville, Dang, and Basten (1998) compared it to supportive counseling in male and female victims of motor vehicle and industrial accidents who met formal diagnostic criteria for acute stress disorder. At posttreatment, only 8% of CBT participants met the criteria for PTSD, compared to 83% of the supportive counseling patients. Although rates of PTSD increased over the course of a 6-month follow-up, CBT remained superior (17% PTSD incidence) to supportive counseling (67% PTSD incidence). In a subsequent study, Bryant, Sackville, Dangh, Moulds, and Guthrie (1999) modified the brief CBT by limiting it to psychoeducation and exposure, eliminating anxiety management (e.g., relaxation training) and cognitive restructuring, and compared this modified protocol to the full protocol and to supportive counseling. At posttreatment, 20% of participants in the full treatment program and 14% of participants in the brief CBT group met the criteria for PTSD, in comparison to 56% of participants receiving supportive counseling. At 6 months, the incidence of PTSD was 23%, 15%, and 67% for the full treatment program, exposure, and supportive counseling respectively.

Another group presumably at risk for the development of an anxiety disorder are individuals who present to emergency rooms with panic attack symptoms. Swinson et al. (1992) conducted an intervention study with such adults, 40% of whom met full symptom criteria for panic disorder, thus rendering this study an indicated prevention/treatment hybrid. Nevertheless, at 6-months follow-up, participants randomized to a 1-hour exposure-based condition were improved on panic and anxiety measures whereas those assigned to a 1-hour reassurance control intervention were no better than at baseline. Subgroup analyses examining outcome for those with full syndromal panic disorder and those who were subthreshold were not reported, however. Gardenschwartz and

Craske (2001) also targeted the prevention of panic disorder, but recruited college students who had experienced a panic attack within the last year, evidenced elevated anxiety sensitivity, and did not meet the DSM criteria for panic disorder. Participants were randomly assigned to either a waitlist or a day-long CBT workshop that included psychoeducation about agoraphobia and panic, behavioral and cognitive strategies, and interoceptive exposure. At 6-months follow-up, 14% of the waitlist group had gone on to develop fully syndromal panic disorder, compared with only 2% of the workshop participants; significant effects also were seen on other relevant indices (e.g., panic attack frequency × intensity index). As the authors noted, a longer follow-up period may not have yielded a similar outcome.

The number of randomized indicated prevention studies remains few. LaFreniere and Capuano (1997) examined the effects of a program directed at mothers of preschool children (N = 43) already exhibiting anxious/withdrawn behavior, comparing it to no treatment. The intervention lasted for 6 months and consisted of four phases: (1) assessment; (2) educating the parents about their child's developmental needs; (3) determining specific objectives for the family; and (4) implementing the intervention during 11 home visits with child-directed interaction, modification of behavior problems, training in parenting skills, and enhancing the effectiveness of social support systems. Given the age of the children, outcome variables included teacher ratings in social competence within the preschool setting and cooperation and enthusiasm during a problem-solving task rather than symptoms of a specific anxiety disorder. Results indicated that maternal stress was reduced and anxious-withdrawn behavior of the child was significantly lower at posttreatment in both conditions, although the social competence of children whose mothers received the intervention was greater prior to intervention than children whose mothers received no treatment. The relatively brief follow-up period and the lack of information about anxiety disorder symptoms limit the utility of the findings. Nevertheless, the study offered some preliminary findings about the potential benefit of such programs for behaviorally inhibited young children.

Chemtob et al. (2002) conducted a school-based, randomized study for youth in grades two through six with elevated PTSD symptoms (but not necessarily full-blown PTSD) 2 years after Hurricane Iniki and found that children assigned to a brief (4-week) CBT-oriented treatment program fared better both immediately posttreatment and at 1-year follow-up than those assigned to a waitlist comparison group. This study followed the recommendations of experts described above in first conducting a large-scale screening of potentially affected youth followed by identifying and then treating those found to have elevated symptoms of the disorder of relevance.

The Queensland Early Intervention and Prevention of Anxiety Project constitutes the most comprehensive effort made thus far in evaluating the efficacy of an indicated prevention program for children and adolescents (Dadds et al., 1997, 1999). As in the Swinson et al. (1992) adult panic disorder prevention study described above, Dadds et al.'s study can be better characterized as a hybrid indicated prevention/early intervention study because 55% of the selected children met diagnostic criteria for at least one anxiety disorder. A total of 1,786 children (ages 7–14 years) were screened for anxiety problems using teacher nominations and children's self-ratings. After initial diagnostic interviews, 128 children were selected and randomly assigned to either a 10-week school-based psychosocial intervention based on Kendall's Coping Cat protocol (1990) or to a monitoring group. The intervention was conducted over 10 weekly 1- to 2-hour sessions at each intervention school. Group sizes ranged from five to 12 children. Parental sessions were conducted at the intervention schools in weeks 3, 6, and 9. Anxiety disorder diagnostic status was assessed at posttreatment, 6-month, 12-month, and 24-month follow-up and yielded interesting results: the CBT and control groups differed significantly with respect to anxiety disorder diagnostic status at 6 months (27% vs. 57%) and at 24 months (20% vs. 39%) but not at 12 months (37% vs. 42%). Notably, treatment benefits were most evident for those children who initially had moderate to severe clinician ratings of severity, with approximately 50% of these children retaining a clinical diagnosis at the 2-year-follow-up, if they did not receive the intervention. For those children who initially showed symptoms of anxiety but did not have a clinically significant anxiety disorder, there was minimal difference between the preventive intervention and the monitoring-only condition at 24-months follow-up, with 11% in the intervention group showing an anxiety disorder and 16% in the monitoring condition. In other words, children with subclinical anxiety problems did not appear to be at a high risk of developing a more severe anxiety disorder if left untreated; they benefited only minimally from the intervention.

In an effort to test an indicated early prevention program in a school setting, Hunt et al. (2009) cluster randomized 260 high school freshmen from Australia with elevated self-reported anxiety symptoms to take part in the 10-week FRIENDS program led by school staff or a monitoring-only condition. Notably, although there was some evidence of improvement over time for the sample on the whole, there were no differences between the groups in terms of self-reported anxiety, depression, or anxiety diagnosis at the 2-year and 4-year follow-up points. Hunt et al. point to the methodological difference of using school personnel to deliver the FRIENDS program rather than CBT experts, as was done in the Queensland Early Intervention and Prevention Project (Dadds et al., 1997) upon which this was based. They also note that while close supervision by experts might have overcome this problem, such a procedure would have countered the aim of testing the FRIENDS program in routine school-based practice.

Selective Prevention Programs

Selective prevention intervention programs are delivered to individuals or groups who are considered to be high on risk factors for anxiety disorders but are not evidencing significant anxiety disorder symptoms yet. To date, most selective prevention intervention programs have targeted individuals or groups exposed to stressful life events such as parental divorce (e.g., Alpert-Gillis, Pedro-Carroll, & Cowen, 1989; Hightower & Braden, 1991; Hodges, 1991; Short, 1998; Zubernis, Cassidy, Gillham, Reivich, & Jaycox, 1999); transition between primary and secondary school, which can be associated with a number of psychological difficulties (e.g., peer relationships, school refusal behavior, substance use) (Felner & Adan, 1988); medical and dental procedures (Peterson & Shigetomi, 1981); and having a chronically ill sibling (e.g., Bendor, 1990). Although the findings from these studies generally yield positive effects, their direct relevance to preventing anxiety disorders in adolescents is unclear.

In a program designed specifically for anxiety disorder prevention, Rapee et al. (2005, 2010, 2013) launched the Macquarie University Preschool Intervention Program. Young children (ages 3.5–4.5 years) were recruited mainly via questionnaires distributed to preschools. Inclusion in the study was based on mother-completed ratings on the Australian version of the Childhood Temperament Scale (Sanson, Pedlow, Cann, Prior, & Oberklaid, 1996), followed by laboratory evaluation confirming behavioral inhibition. One hundred forty-six behaviorally inhibited children were randomly assigned to either an intervention or a monitoring condition. The intervention was conducted with parents only and focused on education about the nature of withdrawal and anxiety, parental anxiety management strategies, information about the importance of modeling competence and promoting independence, development of exposure hierarchies for the children and practice of graded exposure, as well as discussion of future development. The intervention was conducted in groups of six families and lasted for six sessions. Results at 12 months revealed that mothers in the intervention condition had self-ratings that indicated significantly greater decreases in their child's inhibited temperament as well as in the number of child anxiety diagnoses compared to mothers in the control condition. However, laboratory observations at that same point indicated that children in both groups had reduced behavioral inhibition with no significant differences between the two groups. Rapee (2013) more recently reported long-term follow-up on this same cohort (approximately age 15) and found that girls whose parents had received intervention had fewer internalizing disorders and lower maternally reported anxiety symptoms and self-reported functional interference than those whose parents did not; no such lasting effects were evident for boys. The findings are encouraging with respect to the potential utility of selective interventions that can be delivered at relatively low cost. Rapee et al. also argue that young childhood may be the most appropriate time to conduct intervention trials aimed at prevention given what is known about the developmental trajectory of these symptoms and disorders.

Cooley-Strickland et al. (2011) tested a modified version of the FRIENDS program with U.S. urban children exposed to community violence. Ninety-three children ages 7 to 12 were randomized to the FRIENDS program (13 biweekly 60-minute sessions) or to a waitlist control; the active intervention was delivered by trained school personnel supervised by a licensed psychologist. Results indicated reductions in both groups' total exposure to community violence and overall anxiety (RCMAS scores) from baseline to postintervention assessment, but no group-by-time interaction. The absence of a long-term follow-up may have obscured any delayed effects for the intervention, and even participants in the control condition reported that they liked being "members of the FRIENDS Team," which might have influenced the changes observed in that group from pretreatment to posttreatment.

Ginsburg (2009) examined the efficacy of a cognitive-behavioral prevention program in a sample of offspring of adults with anxiety disorders; notably, children were excluded from the sample if they already had an anxiety disorder themselves. The Child Anxiety Prevention Study (CAPS) protocol involved parents and the identified youth and comprised six to eight weekly 60-minute sessions followed by three monthly booster sessions; the CAPS intervention was compared to a waitlist control. Forty families were randomized (20 per cell), and there were no between-group differences in dropout rate. Unlike the FRIENDS program, the CAPS intervention was based on Ginsburg and Silverman's transfer of control model (Ginsburg, Silverman, & Kurtines, 1995; Silverman & Kurtines, 1996), which strongly emphasizes the importance of using parents in the delivery of treatment. Findings indicated that 30% of children in the waitlist condition had developed an anxiety disorder at the 1-year follow-up assessment, compared to none of the children randomized to CAPS. Moreover, anxiety symptoms as measured on the SCARED were significantly reduced at the 1-year follow-up in the CAPS children but not in those assigned to waitlist. Sample size limits strong conclusions and the use of a waitlist control leaves open the possibility that nonspecific treatment effects accounted for the results, yet these data provide an encouraging route for potential next steps in selective prevention research.

Universal Prevention Programs

In a large-scale examination of the FRIENDS program as a universal prevention intervention, Lowry-Webster et al. (2001) randomly assigned 594 children (10–13 years) within different schools to receive either the FRIENDS program or assessment only. The intervention was implemented by trained classroom teachers, and three separate sessions for parents also were conducted. Pretreatment to posttreatment intervention changes were examined universally and for children who scored above the clinical cutoff for anxiety at pretest. Children in the FRIENDS intervention condition reported fewer anxiety symptoms regardless of their risk status relative to the comparison condition. The 12-month follow-up data indicated that prevention effects were maintained for those who participated in the FRIENDS intervention. Notably, those who were already in the clinically anxious range on the Spence Children's Anxiety Scale fared better in the FRIENDS program than the waitlist condition, as was found by Dadds et al. (1997). This suggests again that the FRIENDS program may be a useful intervention for children who are already experiencing significant problems with anxiety.

Lock and Barrett (2003) conducted another large trial (N = 733) that is of particular relevance here since they examined effects of the FRIENDS program in younger (sixth-graders) and older (ninth-graders) children; their schools were randomized to receive either FRIENDS or a standard curriculum, which served as a control. Results indicated overall reductions in anxiety over time, but also a group-by-time interaction at 6- and 12-month follow-up indicating greater reductions in the FRIENDS group than in the comparison condition. The children in the younger age range fared better than those in the older group, which may suggest that the optimal time for anxiety prevention efforts is before rather than during adolescence. In a longer-term follow-up study examining this same sample, Barrett et al. (2006) found significantly fewer high-risk students at the 36-month follow-up in the FRIENDS condition than in the control group. Gender effects indicating that girls had a larger reduction of anxiety at 12- and 24-month follow-ups were no longer evident at the 36-month follow-up, which may mean that either more booster sessions or more intensive forms of intervention are needed to help girls maintain their gains from universal prevention programs.

Stallard et al. (2008) also adopted a universal prevention approach when they tested the FRIENDS program in British schools in an open trial designed to examine its transportability beyond the centers in which it was developed. As was the case in several prevention intervention programs discussed above, school personnel (trained school nurses) conducted the FRIENDS intervention rather than clinical psychologists from outside the school system. One hundred six youth ages 9 and 10 participated in the FRIENDS program, 63 of whom were available at 12-month follow-up. Improvements in total self-reported anxiety (Spence Children's Anxiety Scale) and self-esteem were evident at the follow-up assessment, as were improvements in panic, separation anxiety, and OCD subscales of the Spence scale. Despite the limitations inherent in any open trial, findings support the implementation of the FRIENDS Program with non–mental health professionals, which has important implications for service delivery and, perhaps more importantly, sustainability. Such findings are not consistent across the literature, however, which raises questions about the ideal training protocol, optimal school-based personnel to run the FRIENDS program, provision of ongoing supervision, and cost-effectiveness of using school personnel to implement the program rather than hiring outside experts to do so.

Farrell and Barrett (2007), who each played critical roles in the development and evaluation of the FRIENDS program, describe the following advantages of a universal prevention approach when it comes specifically to anxiety:

1. It eliminates the need for multiple-gate, presumably expensive screening procedures.
2. It allows for a broader reach for symptoms that may be virtually ubiquitous at least at lower levels of severity.
3. It reduces stigma by not targeting specific youth for participation.
4. It increases peer support by exposing all to the problems associated with anxiety.
5. It promotes a healthy learning environment for all.

In initial evaluations of its effects, children who received the intervention had lower self-rated anxiety levels than did controls at posttreatment; moreover, no statistical differences were found between the FRIENDS program delivered by either teachers or psychologists (Barrett & Turner, 2001), and this intervention when tested by its developers.

What Are the Active Ingredients?

The prevention intervention studies conducted thus far have not shed sufficient light on the mechanisms involved in producing the observed effects, since most of the designs used have compared active treatment packages to repeated assessment only (e.g., waitlist, standard curriculum). The superiority of the CBT packages examined thus far could therefore be attributable to a wide variety of nonspecific factors, such as treatment credibility and therapist contact. Dismantling studies typically follow the establishment of efficacy (e.g., Schmidt et al., 2000), and thus the field may still be a long time from discovering the impact of specific treatment interventions and their underlying mechanisms. Dismantling studies of this sort also requires interest in psychological rather than biological mechanisms of change, which may well be at issue at present in the United States with respect to the priorities of federal agencies that fund clinical research.

What Outcomes Are Targeted?

As noted above, in the studies conducted to date, the outcomes targeted have primarily focused on anxiety symptoms and disorders. As also noted, it might be worthwhile for future research to move beyond symptoms and diagnosis and pay increased attention to whether functional impairment has improved. For example, are there improvements in the adolescent's grades or in his or her peer relationships? These are the outcomes that would seem to matter most and should be seriously considered in the design and evaluation of future prevention studies. As of yet there has not been a significant movement toward emphasizing these functional outcomes.

In addition, the potential of "positive psychology" has yet to be seriously considered in the context of preventing anxiety disorders in adolescents and targeting outcomes. Positive psychology is devoted to creating a science of human strengths that act as buffers against mental illness, including anxiety (Seligman, 2002). Dick-Niederhauser and Silverman (2003) have adapted positive psychology principles and have suggested their utility in serving as outcome targets for anxiety prevention studies. Thus, potential outcome targets might include instilling hope and the active pursuit of goals in young people, which in turn have been linked to the development of courage. Courage in turn has been linked with increased optimistic cognitive processing, a sense of self-efficacy, and skillful coping. Although measures exist to assess some positive psychological concepts, further instrument development and evaluation will be needed for positive psychology principles to be fully implemented and studied in the context of anxiety prevention research. Research on resilience (e.g., Zeller et al., 2015) and grit (e.g., Duckworth et al., 2007), psychological constructs that may well overlap, could potentially serve as points of emphasis in prevention intervention research as society aims to reduce the effects of anxious psychopathology on youth.

CONCEPTUAL, METHODOLOGICAL, AND PRACTICAL ISSUES

Methodological and conceptual issues vary across types of prevention programs. That is, the methodological concerns that arise in universal prevention (targeting the broad population of adolescents) are different from those in selected/indicated prevention intervention trials. The former require more streamlined assessments to increase participation and compliance (thus ensuring sample representativeness) and reduce cost (thus ensuring feasibility). Accordingly, a major issue in universal prevention program research involves identifying the best ways to encourage adolescents to participate in a study that addresses a problem that they probably do not have. Universal prevention programs are especially likely to be conducted with involvement from school administrators, and thus capitalizing on the schools' past successes in encouraging student participation will be important. As noted earlier, a brief survey conducted via a website might capture the interest of teens in particular, and thus computer technologies may prove essential in this kind of work. The costs of universal programs ultimately require a serious political commitment on the level of state or federal government, which exists in Australia in particular. For the selective/indicated programs, the primary methodological concern is how to encourage participation while at the same time protecting student confidentiality—this is all the more a concern in an era characterized by concerns about Health Insurance Portability and Accountability Act (HIPAA) violations. This may be especially important if the intervention itself is conducted at school and during school hours, when absence from regular classes might be conspicuous and thus negative social costs both real and imagined may impact participation. Moreover, if the intervention is conducted in groups, confidentiality among group members needs to be considered. Students who have been identified for intervention participation because of having experienced a trauma or for being excessively shy might be reluctant to share their experiences if they do not have assurance that what is discussed in session will not be discussed outside with nonmembers. Providing sufficient time to foster group cohesion to alleviate this concern would therefore be important in any selective/indicated prevention effort that involves discussion of personal material in a group setting.

Another issue that warrants consideration is when to intervene. As discussed above in relation to trauma exposure, immediate intervention provided to all individuals exposed to the trauma has not been found especially helpful with adults and thus should probably be avoided when conducting interventions with youth who have been exposed to a traumatic event such as shootings at the school.

Yet another issue is the match between the type of intervention and the developmental stage of the individuals being targeted. Perhaps group interventions can be particularly successful in adolescence when the value of the peer group is quite powerful and, if properly harnessed, may enhance the efficacy of the intervention. On the other hand, interventions in the managed-care context must take into account the limited amount of time available in a given medical visit to discuss seemingly peripheral issues such as anxiety symptoms; accordingly, the development of brochures, self-help programs, or interventions that can be delivered by support staff should be considered.

Prevention research by its nature requires longitudinal follow-up, and thus one major issue is how best to retain participation in the study, and how to guard against attrition over time. Here again informed consent from the student/family and active collaboration with the school will be helpful, but it is important to keep in mind that the most valuable assessment points for prevention programs take place years after the intervention is delivered. Thus, it is imperative to fund studies in a manner that will ensure the collection of data well into the future; inadequate participation in follow-up for these kinds of studies imperils the entire enterprise, as detection of sampling bias (e.g., better follow-up with less impaired participants or vice versa) threatens to compromise conclusions that could be drawn about the efficacy of intervention. Treatment studies have had to address this problem and have requested that the family provide the names of family and friends who will know how to contact them in the future if they move, social security numbers, and other such information to facilitate participation in long-term follow-ups (see Marchand et al., 2011).

A final issue that affects all prevention programs involves the ongoing assessment of risk, and responsibility for risk. Those at risk for anxiety also may be at increased risk for other psychiatric comorbidity, and thus procedures must be enacted within prevention intervention programs to manage clinical emergencies. Moreover, the role of the parent in these programs must be considered: if the child or adolescent is found to be at increased risk for anxiety disorders upon screening and is then eligible to participate in the program, how much or how little the parent should be involved or have access to the information discussed in assessment and/or treatment needs to be specified up front, as it will certainly impact both entry and active participation.

Problem of Sustainability (Boosters, Ongoing Programs, Training)

The prevention studies that have included follow-up have generally suggested maintenance of the intervention effects in those trials that found positive initial benefits, but here again these studies have typically focused on young or very young children and thus cannot inform the field about retention of benefits into and through adolescence and adulthood. A related question is whether booster sessions are needed to retain the gains from prevention programs, since the fairly predictable stressful life events that face young children growing into adolescence might compromise long-term maintenance. For example, studies discussed earlier suggest that young children with elevated but subclinical anxiety levels may benefit most from prevention programs; transition from middle school to high school may threaten these gains, and thus it may be reasonable to reinstitute the intervention during this transition. It is unknown whether this is the case, but the relation between loss of gains and stressful life events constitutes an especially important area for future study.

Problem of Contagion

There is no evidence of such undesirable effects from the studies of group treatment of youth that have been conducted thus far (e.g., Kendall, Flannery-Schroeder, Panichelli-Mindel, & Southam-Gerow, 1997), but the possibility for such effects remains. Although it is possible that discussion of anxiety themes may activate new fears in those who are already vulnerable, especially if the interventions involve group discussions, there is no evidence of such undesirable effects from group treatment studies (e.g., Kendall et al., 1997; Silverman, Kurtines, Ginsburg, Weems, Lumpkin, & Carmichael, 1999), including in groups in which the patients involved were very heterogeneous with respect to age (i.e., child and adolescent patients) as well as primary anxiety diagnosis (e.g., OCD, specific phobia) and other clinical features (e.g., presence/absence of school refusal behavior; Lumpkin, Silverman, Weems, Markham, & Kurtines, 2000). However, the example of Critical Incident Stress Debriefing (CISD) suggests that the long-term recovery of certain adults who have experienced a trauma and have attended group meetings may be impeded by participating, and possibly the mechanism by which this effect is realized involves exposure to other participants' narratives of the traumatic event (e.g., Mayou et al., 2001). Provided that secondary gains (e.g., missing trigonometry class) for attending prevention intervention sessions are minimized, there is little reason for concern that students without anxious symptoms or risk factors would feign such problems.

Age-Appropriate Interventions (Developmental Approach)

The prevention intervention programs that have been evaluated thus far in research (e.g., Lowry-Webster et al., 2001) were designed for children rather than for adolescents; when these programs have been applied specifically with adolescents, an attenuation of benefit relative to that observed with younger children has been observed (e.g., Barrett et al., 2006). Accordingly, adaptations to accommodate the developmental needs of adolescents should be made, with specific attention to possible age-related increases in physiological functioning, emotional vulnerability, social and peer pressures, and comorbid conditions, as well as any other changes that these youngsters may be experiencing. In particular, prevention programs must consider the importance of the peer group within the intervention program itself, but also with an eye toward the social implications of participating in the program among nonparticipating students, especially if the program is either a selective or indicated one. Insufficient attention to these factors may reduce the number of teens willing to enter the program altogether, and can limit active participation within the program itself if a group format is implemented. One way to address this potentially important concern is to incorporate program graduates, who may serve as role models for new participants, as a way to alleviate concerns that program participants may not be perceived as "cool" among the larger student population. Another way to make participation more palatable is to present information about adult role models who have struggled with anxiety and have openly discussed their difficulties, such as actresses Emma Stone and Lena Dunham, who have openly acknowledged having been treated for anxiety-related difficulties in the past. However this is accomplished within a protocol, the culture of adolescence and the importance of the peer group must be taken into consideration when developing appropriate interventions for teens.

ETHICAL ISSUES

A Note of Caution from Adult Early Intervention Research

Longitudinal studies of trauma survivors (e.g., Mayou, Ehlers, & Bryant, 2002; Riggs et al., 1995; Rothbaum et al., 1992; Silver, Holman, McIntosh, Poulin, & Gil-Rivas, 2002) indicate that most individuals experience elevated levels of PTSD symptoms shortly after the traumatic event. In addition, elevated levels of depression and general anxiety often accompany PTSD symptoms. However, epidemiological studies indicate that for most trauma survivors these symptoms decline significantly over time without any professional intervention (Kessler, Sonnega, Bromet, Hughes, & Nelson, 1995). That said, a significant minority of trauma survivors continues to experience high levels of posttrauma distress that, without professional treatment, may persist for months or years (Kessler et al., 2005).

As discussed above, it is now well established that various forms of CBT are effective in reducing PTSD symptom severity as well as associated anxiety and depression (e.g., Nayak, Powers, & Foa, 2011). Although there are effective treatments for individuals who have chronic PTSD, many sufferers either do not seek treatment for their trauma-related symptoms or do not have access to treatment. As a consequence, individuals' suffering and their inability to function can be prolonged. They also are vulnerable to associated comorbidity such as substance abuse (McLean & Foa, 2014). Such considerations have prompted trauma therapists to develop brief interventions applied shortly after the traumatic event in order to facilitate recovery and thereby prevent the development of chronic PTSD.

Two approaches to facilitating recovery following a traumatic event have been researched. Abbreviated CBT packages such as those developed by Foa et al. (1995) and adopted by Bryant and colleagues (e.g. Bryant, Sackville, Dang, Moulds, & Guthrie, 1999; Bryant, Moulds, Guthrie, & Nixon, 2005; Bryant et al., 2008) have been found to be efficacious in accelerating recovery and reducing the likelihood of chronic PTSD. The other approach involves psychological debriefing. Debriefing programs typically last only one session and are applied shortly after a traumatic event (frequently within 48–72 hours). In this session (which can be conducted in groups or individually), participants are encouraged to describe the traumatic event, including their thoughts, impressions, and emotional reactions. The session also includes normalization of the trauma survivors' reactions and planning for coping with the trauma and its sequelae. Results of randomized controlled trials for debriefing are somewhat mixed, but a set of recommendations from early intervention experts (Bisson et al., 2009, p. 101) may provide some guidance as to how best to proceed:

1. Pragmatic psychological support and psychoeducation about common reactions should be provided in the immediate wake of trauma.
2. No formal intervention should be mandated for all exposed to trauma.
3. Culturally and developmentally sensitive interventions should be provided that are related to the local formulation of problems and ways of coping.
4. Lack of distress and/or rapid recovery may not necessarily be desirable.
5. The absence of strong evidence supporting early interventions necessitates careful monitoring of outcomes in individual patients provided with these treatments.

Stigmatization

As noted earlier, unlike universal prevention programs, selective and indicated prevention programs specifically select participants based on elevations of anxious symptoms or on putative anxiety disorder risk factors. In the school context where most prevention interventions are likely to take place, the latter program types require identification of a subgroup of participants from among the broader population, who will be either encouraged or required to participate. The potential negative implications of this strategy have already been considered in the academic context with respect to educational issues, and have led to the gradual reduction of labeling for academic tracking systems (e.g., honors, regents, and basic classes) and to increased mainstreaming of special education students. Similar problems may be encountered in identifying already anxious or anxiety-vulnerable students for special attention or services. As discussed above, adolescence is a stage in life when similarity with the relevant peer group is valued, and intervention efforts that do not deal sensitively with this issue may be poorly attended or, worse yet, yield unintended negative consequences. Little has been written about this issue in the context of anxiety prevention programs implemented thus far, but methods to prevent such unintended consequences should be carefully considered.

POSTINTERVENTION FOLLOW-UP AND DISSEMINATION

The studies conducted thus far have involved acute treatment and, at least in some studies, follow-up assessment only. It is unknown how to encourage ongoing use of skills learned in the prevention programs, nor is it known how best to encourage participation in follow-up assessments. Because the primary dependent variable of interest in prevention programs must be measured years later than the intervention was conducted, it is imperative to develop methods that encourage cooperation with long-term follow-up. Given that most prevention interventions will likely be conducted in the school context, active collaboration with the school administration will be critical to promote collection of these data. Families also may be able to facilitate participation, and thus direct contact with families may be advisable. However, this raises issues with respect to confidentiality and the need to discuss up front with the young participant what will and will not be shared with parents and/or guardians.

The preliminary success of the FRIENDS program in the hands of teachers and school nurses in some but not all trials bodes well for transportability of this program to treatment providers other than mental health professionals with expertise in CBT. Clearly, the implementation of CBT-oriented prevention programs cannot realistically be limited to PhD-level psychologists, and a multidisciplinary approach may be the best way to proceed. This raises interesting questions about how best to disseminate CBT prevention programs and how much expert supervision will be needed in the short and long run to optimize treatment delivery; these questions touch on the cost-effectiveness of prevention programs. A similar line of research needs to be pursued in adolescent anxiety disorder prevention in particular, since the broad application of such interventions appears to be dependent on successful training of school personnel to implement these programs in the school context.

IMPEDIMENTS TO PREVENTION

The first set of impediments to developing successful prevention intervention is the lack of knowledge about the complex interrelations among the various risk and protective factors for the development of anxiety disorders. Much is known about some specific factors but little is known about how they interact, which leaves the field bereft of a strong theoretical foundation upon which to build prevention programs. This may be why prevention research has continued to languish relative to treatment and now more basic neurobiological research on psychiatric disorders: the factors associated with etiology may not be same as those associated with maintenance, and thus comprehensive knowledge about the latter will allow for the development of treatment interventions even in the relative absence of the former.

Practical considerations have stunted the development of prevention programs as well.

Prevention efforts are costly, as they necessarily involve collection of data from large samples over a long period of time. Large samples are needed because of the relatively low base rates of anxiety disorder in the population of interest, and because there is insufficient information about who will actually go on to develop an anxiety disorder. Consequently, it is important to conduct broad screens to obtain sufficient numbers of vulnerable children and adolescents for inclusion in indicated and selected prevention studies. For example, most behaviorally inhibited infants do not develop an anxiety disorder later in life, and thus a large sample of inhibited children would be needed to detect the efficacy of a prevention program targeting behavioral inhibition. Further, because the relevant outcome is the future development of anxiety disorders and perhaps of subsequent comorbid conditions (e.g., depression, substance abuse), prevention studies require data collection for years after the intervention to determine its ultimate impact. The need to conduct longitudinal follow-ups of these large numbers for long periods of time renders the study of prevention programs impractical, especially when the primary funding sources for anxiety disorders research (e.g., National Institute of Mental Health) typically have favored shorter studies with more tangible impact, and now appear to be much more strongly emphasizing biological research above intervention science. Thus, new sources of funding must be identified to generate knowledge that will inform the development of anxiety disorder prevention programs. Given the potential of anxiety disorders to derail adolescent development and thereby result in a substantial personal and economic impact, this should be a major priority for a society that alleges to leave no child behind.

Research Agenda for Anxiety Disorders

Edna B. Foa
Martin Franklin
Richard J. McNally
Carmen McLean
Daniel Pine

12

chapter

THE ANXIETY DISORDERS THEMSELVES

What We Know

Much of the research conducted in the last 10 years has explicated in greater detail the complexity of anxiety, which appears more clearly now not to be a unitary construct. Indeed, anxiety is a complex interplay of realistic threat, prior history, conditioning experiences, and anxiety sensitivity. The central role of the amygdala across anxiety disorders has now been clarified, although it also appears that the various anxiety disorders do have distinct biological profiles as well. The field has seen significant advances in terms of the development of a set of cognitive and biological procedures that can be used to aid differential diagnosis; greater methodological consistency across studies will provide increased clarity about the biological and cognitive underpinnings of these conditions. We have also learned that there are genetic contributions to anxiety disorders, although these appear to be modest; here again, methodological consistency across studies will improve our understanding of these contributions across and within the disorders themselves.

What We Do Not Know

The genetic findings that indicate modest effects thus far raise interesting questions about what we do not know, which is how shared and non-shared environmental factors exert their influence over the development and maintenance of pathological anxiety. There is also a great deal to learn about pharmacogenetics and pharmacogenomics, which may elucidate new drug targets based on improved understanding of chromosomal areas of interest. It is widely accepted that extremely large sample sizes are needed to identify a signal and test rather than explore genetic hypotheses, which in turn raises questions about the robustness of such effects. Continuing lack of clarity about the disease states themselves (i.e., the nature and underpinnings of anxiety) continues to hamper our ability to establish anxious phenotypes that will lead to research to improve risk prediction, predict longitudinal course of the various phenotypes, and inform prevention strategies.

Research Priorities

The development of large-scale, multicenter collaborations using shared interview, cognitive, and biological procedures will be necessary to move the research agenda forward, as the complex interactions of interest pose serious challenges when data are derived from smaller, underpowered studies. Such advances will require improvements in data-sharing techniques as well as identification of funding to support the substantial infrastructures needed to support studies on this scale. Team science approaches must also be developed that allow investigators and institutions to work together toward completion of next-stage research studies that have a better chance of addressing the issues that have yet to be explored.

In a recent paper, LeDoux and Pine (2016) suggested that the field will advance further when the distinction is more fully drawn in anxiety between circuits underlying two classes of responses elicited by threat. This conceptualization, which they refer to as the two-system framework, poses two distinct circuits: (1) behavioral responses and accompanying physiological changes in brain and body and (2) conscious feeling states reflected in self-reported fear and anxiety. Accordingly, one would not expect high convergence among the variables across these circuits. Instead, research could focus instead on improving our understanding of how these circuits interact at the behavioral and biological levels of analysis. The hope is that basic knowledge of this sort will inform the development of empirically informed targets for intervention, which could foster improvements in the efficacy of our interventions as well as improved understanding of which forms of intervention are likely to be effective for which patients under which conditions.

TREATMENT

What We Know

In the last decade what we know about cognitive-behavioral therapy (CBT) and pharmacotherapy has increased substantially. Practicing clinicians, parents, and other professionals who encounter adolescents in their own work now have a solid evidence base that broadly supports the efficacy of these procedures across the anxiety disorders in adolescents. The methodological quality, large sample sizes, and encouraging results of multiple randomized controlled trials support the efficacy of CBT protocols for multiple anxiety disorders, and promote confidence that most patients who complete treatment will likely experience a substantial reduction in anxiety and related symptoms at post-treatment. Moreover, these studies have included, if not focused exclusively on, adolescents, so there is greater certainty that protocols and procedures initially developed for adults are comparably efficacious in adolescents, if not even more so. There is much reason for optimism that CBT protocols that involve some form of exposure to feared stimuli will be helpful in reducing anxiety; multiple studies that tested relaxation or other anxiety management strategies in the last decade also converge in indicating that these procedures, while not entirely inert, are less efficacious than those that encourage "leaning into" fears rather than away from them. As far as medications are concerned, research over the last decade has expanded our knowledge and our confidence that the selective serotonin reuptake inhibitors (SSRIs) are efficacious relative to placebo, but their average response rates often leave patients with clinically relevant residual symptoms. Some research has examined the augmentative effects of CBT and pharmacotherapy in patients already taking SSRIs, but there is still much to be learned about those effects in disorders other than obsessive-compulsive disorder (OCD), where we have the most evidence for the augmentative efficacy of CBT.

We also know that the long-term outcomes for both CBT and pharmacotherapy have been less robust than those observed at posttreatment, and we are now beginning to better understand the patient and therapeutic factors associated with partial response to initial treatment. Immediate and long-term responses to both monotherapies are neither universal nor complete, and these outcomes have spawned efforts at treatment development in order to increase the number of adolescents whose anxiety disorders can be treated effectively and durably.

The last decade also brought important developments in the examination of combined treatments in which CBT and SSRI pharmacotherapy were administered concurrently. Those trials, most notably the Child/Adolescent Anxiety Multimodal Study (CAMS; social anxiety disorder, generalized anxiety disorder, and separation anxiety disorder) and the Pediatric OCD Treatment Study I (POTS I), supported the relative and combined efficacy of CBT and sertraline, but the findings for combined treatment versus the monotherapies were mixed. In CAMS there was a clear combined treatment effect at posttreatment with no caveats; in POTS I the combined treatment effect was moderated by a site effect, whereby combined treatment was more efficacious than CBT alone at one site but both were highly effective and equivalent at the other. Exploration of these effects continues, but suffice it to say now that the evidence base supports starting an anxious adolescent with CBT alone or combined treatment; in the absence of clear moderators of outcome for the most part, clinical judgment at this point can be used to determine which of those regimens would be best as an initial treatment. In the absence of CBT availability, SSRIs are also an efficacious and safe option, as informed by the last decade of large-scale studies that have included adolescents in the sample. The black-box warning for the SSRIs must be taken into consideration, but the data from these large-scale studies in the last decade speak to the safety and tolerability of these medications for anxious teens.

What We Do Not Know

We still need more relative and combined treatment trials across the anxiety disorders, especially those in which comorbid depression is common, such as posttraumatic stress disorder (PTSD). Synergistic effects for combined treatments may be more likely realized in such a context; it is also the case that we have insufficient information to inform treatment sequencing when both CBT and pharmacotherapy options are available. What continues to haunt the treatment field, however, is the search for the "Holy Grail" of moderators of treatment outcome: which treatments, for which patients, under which conditions? Efficacy studies are typically underpowered to detect such effects, though there are a handful of studies now that have at least explored whether patient characteristics (e.g., comorbidity, anxiety disorder diagnosis) influence the likelihood of a positive or negative outcome to specific treatments.

Another major issue that needs to be addressed is the dissemination of empirically supported protocols and methods into the clinical settings where most patients receive care. The last decade's focus on efficacy studies that emphasize internal validity was certainly necessary given the paucity of information about this crucial topic just 10 years ago. These trees have borne fruit, but trial design decisions that favor internal validity pose threats to external validity. Now that we know much more about the efficacy of CBT and pharmacotherapy for anxious adolescents, the next critical steps must now be taken to examine the effectiveness of empirically supported therapies in clinical settings. An entire subfield known now as implementation science has developed in the last decade, and clinical scientists involved in these endeavors seek to examine the role of therapist, training, clinic variables, and patient variables and their interactions to see whether the treatments developed in the efficacy context can be delivered effectively in settings that are more generalizable to "real-life" clinical practice. This work has begun in earnest already, and we await the outcomes of large-scale studies to inform treatment development and an improved understanding of the complex interactions among all of these factors that can and likely will influence our capacity to deliver effective treatments to all adolescents suffering from anxiety disorders who wish to receive help.

Research Priorities

In keeping with the critical areas in need of further study described above, we advocate for the following:

1. More efficacy studies of individual anxiety disorders as well as transdiagnostic approaches that cut across our current DSM entities
2. Increased focus on the relative and combined efficacy of CBT and pharmacotherapies, as well as trials examining varying treatment sequences to determine if there is an optimal way to initiate treatment and to optimize outcomes with augmentative strategies. SMART trials that explore the implications of various decision rules (e.g., whether to switch to an SSRI vs. provide more CBT) would be especially beneficial for treatment providers who currently need to make such complex clinical decisions in the absence of sufficient guiding evidence.
3. More research connecting the putative biological and behavioral underpinnings of anxiety disorders in youth; engagement of these theoretical targets with methods designed specifically to do so (e.g., response inhibition deficits targeted with training methods) and accompanying symptom reduction would provide crucial information about causality, which at present the field continues to lack.
4. Identification of new funding sources to support treatment development, examination of efficacy, empirically driven treatment modifications, and dissemination/implementation. Many of the suggested avenues of pursuit listed above are expensive, and shifting priorities within government agencies that have supported the last decade of treatment research make the search for such resources perhaps the most important pursuit of all, since none of the issues identified as still needing exploration can be examined productively without external funding.

PREVENTION OF ANXIETY DISORDERS IN ADOLESCENTS

What We Know

We know that the ecology of adolescent development and culture involves an expanded network of peer, school, and community affiliations and that this expanded network increases adolescents' risk for exposure to events and circumstances that have been empirically linked with the development of anxiety disorders. The events and circumstances associated with the development of anxiety disorders include possible high-risk sexual and self-injurious behaviors, smoking and drug use, and exposure to traumatic events (e.g., interpersonal and community violence). Identifying which young people are most at risk to develop anxiety disorders after experiencing negative life events is an important next step toward developing selective treatment and prevention intervention programs.

Specifically, we already know that there are distinct temperamental vulnerabilities to anxiety disorders and anxiety symptoms in some individuals. Moreover, anxiety disorders tend to aggregate in families, and such familial aggregation is due to genetic contributions as well as family environment. A family environment that limits youth independence may particularly put young people at risk. Furthermore, the interactions of children and parents, in which either the child or parent has an anxiety disorder, maintain anxiety and its disorders in young people. Accordingly, one intervention program can involve working directly with the parents to reduce the negative effects of the parent–child interaction. Another individual characteristic, anxiety sensitivity, also serves as a potential risk factor for anxiety disorders, especially panic disorder and PTSD. A third factor, the presence of anxiety symptoms, at a subthreshold level, may also place young people at risk for developing full-blown DSM-5 anxiety disorders.

We know that not all vulnerable children develop anxiety disorders—in fact, relatively few do. Thus, there are factors that protect young people (i.e., children *and* adolescents) from developing anxiety disorders. Similar to why it is important to know about risk factors, knowledge about protective factors constitutes the building block for developing selective preventive intervention programs that will foster protection from pathological anxiety. In fact, the study of resilience factors has gained traction in recent years.

Specifically, individual characteristics such as child perceived competence, child coping skills and behavior, level of intelligence, and general "resourcefulness" (e.g., knowing how to solve problems and whom to seek out to help solve problems) serve a protective function. Certain environmental resources, such as adequate social support systems (and knowing how to reach out to these systems), and parents who are relatively free of psychopathology and who serve as models of coping also may serve a protective function.

Another fact that is known after decades of clinical trials is that even the best, most well-researched, evidence-based treatments leave at least some youth unresponsive and many still symptomatic. Accordingly, support for research on the anxiety disorders and their treatment must continue to be prioritized.

What We Do Not Know

Although research has informed us some about potential risk and protective factors, we do not know enough about which factors are linked *specifically* to anxiety disorders rather than being *general* risk and protective factors that play a role in the development of either internalizing or externalizing disorders in general. Moreover, we do not know how the risk and protective factors differentially affect specific anxiety disorders. This is because the research conducted to date was based on categorical entities rather than continuous measures of psychopathology across a broader range of symptom manifestation. Further, we know much less about protective and risk factors of anxiety disorders in ethnically/racially diverse groups and in socially/economically disadvantaged groups.

Studies of risk and protective factors conducted thus far have primarily used "main effects" models rather than "interactive models." Consequently, we do not know how risk and protective factors interact with one another and whether they serve to mediate or moderate (or both) anxiety or other psychopathology. We also do not know when in the developmental trajectory of the child potential risk and protective factors have particular influence. Most of the research on risk factors has included either mixed samples of younger and older children (including adolescents), or younger children only. Studies using samples of adolescents only are still rare. We should not presume that potential risk and protective factors operate in similar fashion across developmental stages.

From a selective preventive intervention perspective, we do not know whether targeting of identified risk factors, protective factors, or some combination (or "packages") of risk and protective factors in certain subsamples of adolescents would in fact lead to a prevention of anxiety disorders. Relatedly, we still do not know enough about whether targeting either particular risk factor(s) (i.e., reducing risk factors), protective factors (i.e., enhancing protective factors), or some combination thereof (i.e., reducing *and* enhancing risk and protective factors, respectively) would lead to "resilience building" in adolescence. Indeed, no prevention or resilience-building research in the context of anxiety and its disorders has been conducted in adolescents.

We also do not know whether prevention programs aimed at a universal level (in that they target particular facets of the ecology of adolescent development and culture) reduce anxiety disorders in adolescents. For example, does participation in smoking cessation programs reduce or prevent anxiety disorders in teens? If yes, what might be the mediational processes that are operating, and might they be moderated by certain adolescent characteristics? We are not even close to knowing the answers to such questions.

Research Priorities

It is critical that more research be conducted on obtaining basic knowledge about *specific* risk and protective factors of pathological anxiety in adolescents. This research must carefully consider the context of adolescent development and culture in trying to discern the particular factors and the manner in which these factors *interact*. Future research should focus on continuous variables related to psychological anxiety rather than on homogeneous samples to evaluate the specificity of these factors to abnormal anxiety. In addition, research needs to focus exclusively on the specificity of protective factors in adolescents. This research needs to consider carefully the role of these factors not only using the "mainstream" population, but using diverse samples that represent the adolescent population.

As with the development of treatment interventions, recognition of the social, biological, cognitive, and emotional changes that emerge during adolescent development should be used to design prevention programs specific for adolescents; thus far this important work has not been done. Given pubertal development and the critical role of the social network for teenagers, programs developed for adolescents should carefully consider how best to provide such interventions in the school setting, and at the same time should take into account the possible issues that arise by implementing interventions in schools (e.g., problems with confidentiality).

Eating Disorders

COMMISSION ON ADOLESCENT EATING DISORDERS

B. Timothy Walsh, *Commission Chair*

Second Edition

Evelyn Attia
Anne E. Becker
Cynthia M. Bulik
Alison E. Field
Neville H. Golden
Richard E. Kreipe
Daniel Le Grange
James E. Mitchell
Kathleen M. Pike
Robyn Sysko
C. Barr Taylor

We acknowledge the assistance of

Patricia E. Dunne

First Edition

Cynthia M. Bulik
Christopher G. Fairburn
Neville H. Golden
Katherine A. Halmi
David B. Herzog
Allan S. Kaplan
Richard E. Kreipe
James E. Mitchell
Kathleen M. Pike

First Edition cont.

Eric Stice
Ruth H. Striegel-Moore
C. Barr Taylor
Thomas A. Wadden
G. Terence Wilson

We acknowledge the assistance of

Meghan L. Butryn
Eric B. Chesley
Michael P. Levine
Marion P. Russell
Robyn Sysko

part IV

Defining Eating Disorders

Evelyn Attia
Anne E. Becker
Cynthia M. Bulik
Alison E. Field
Neville H. Golden
Richard E. Kreipe
Daniel Le Grange
James E. Mitchell
Kathleen M. Pike
Robyn Sysko
C. Barr Taylor
B. Timothy Walsh

OVERVIEW

The wide range of human food preferences and of human practices surrounding food preparation and consumption make the definition of an "eating disorder" challenging. This challenge is amplified during adolescence by the dramatic changes in energy requirements required to support normal growth and development. For example, between ages 9 and 19, the estimated caloric requirements for girls increases by almost 50% and, for boys, by 80% (Wadsworth, 2003). Adolescence therefore provides a fertile environment for the development of disordered eating; however, surprisingly little attention has been devoted to precisely how to define an eating disorder. The most widely used definitions are those provided by the fifth edition of the American Psychiatric Association's *Diagnostic and Statistical Manual of Mental Disorders* (DSM-5; APA, 2013), which are described in detail below. In this and previous versions of the DSM, the presence of excess body fat alone (i.e., being overweight or obese) is classified as a general medical problem, not a mental disorder (Marcus & Wildes, 2009).

Further, although most eating disorders begin in adolescence, a limited amount of research has focused on this age range. This part of the volume will review what is known and unknown about defining eating disorders, their treatment, and their prevention. This chapter includes a discussion of the etiology of eating disorders; the DSM-5 diagnostic criteria for feeding and eating disorders, and how well the criteria apply to adolescents; the demographics and prevalence of eating disorders among adolescents; issues of comorbidity, outcome, and diagnostic migration for adolescents with eating disorders; and the medical complications of eating disorders. Chapter 14 describes psychological and pharmacological treatments for adolescents with eating disorders, and studies of relapse prevention using psychological or pharmacological interventions. Chapter 15 addresses the risk factors for the development of eating disorders, culture and eating disorders, and prevention. Chapter 16 suggests promising directions for future study.

ETIOLOGY OF EATING DISORDERS

A variety of biological, environmental, and psychosocial factors are associated with the development of an eating disorder, suggesting that such factors may play a causative role in their evolution. However, as is discussed in detail in Chapter 15, there is no conclusive evidence that any characteristic or event is specifically associated with the development of anorexia nervosa (AN), bulimia nervosa (BN), or binge-eating disorder (BED). AN and BN primarily affect women and usually begin around the time of, or soon after, puberty, suggesting that developmental factors during adolescence play a crucial role in their onset. However, it is not clear whether the biological changes that accompany adolescence, psychological changes, and/or an interaction between the two types of phenomena account for the occurrence of eating disorders. BED is less common in adolescence, but aberrant behaviors (e.g., loss of control over eating) may be observed prior to the onset of a full threshold diagnosis, and can be influenced by risk factors occurring during this developmental period. As discussed more extensively in Chapter 15, there is growing evidence of genetic and cultural influences playing an important role in eating disorders, but precisely how genetic or cultural factors may contribute to an individual's vulnerability to develop an eating disorder is poorly understood. There is little question that psychological distress is common within the families of adolescents with serious eating disorders, but it is not clear to what degree such disturbances precede rather than follow the development of the eating disorder. In short, despite extensive information about the clinical characteristics of eating disorders and much theoretical discussion, solid knowledge of the etiology of eating disorders is elusive.

In addition, it is likely that different factors contribute to the onset and to the maintenance of eating disorders. If risk and maintenance factors are distinct, prevention efforts and treatment interventions need to be directed at different targets and, potentially, separate populations. However, there is currently insufficient evidence to differentiate with confidence those factors that increase the risk of developing an eating disorder from those that perpetuate a disorder once it has begun. The lack of knowledge about such issues clearly limits the development of more effective prevention and treatment interventions.

DIAGNOSTIC CRITERIA FOR FEEDING AND EATING DISORDERS

The most widely used diagnostic classification system for feeding and eating disorders is presented in the DSM-5 (APA, 2013). This manual describes individuals with feeding and eating disorders as exhibiting persistent disturbances in behavior leading to changes in the consumption or absorption of food that produce significant impairments in health or psychosocial functioning. The DSM-5 diagnoses for feeding and eating disorders were revised and expanded and include pica, rumination disorder, avoidant/restrictive food intake disorder, AN, BN, and BED. The DSM-5 categories are intended to be mutually exclusive, allowing an individual to receive only one diagnosis in a given episode, with the exception of pica, which can be assigned in the presence of any other feeding or eating disorder.

Anorexia Nervosa

The DSM-5 criteria for AN are listed in Box 13.1.

The first criterion (A) is a significantly low body weight for the individual (e.g., not within normal limits or expectations) brought about by a restriction of calorie intake relative to factors such as age, sex, development, physical activity, and overall health. Low weight can result from acute weight loss, but with younger patients, longitudinal information about height and weight may be the best metric to identify whether the individual has failed to follow his or her expected growth trajectory. Although a specific cutoff is not provided for this criterion in the DSM, clinicians are directed to BMI-for-age percentile calculators (e.g., Center for Disease Control and Prevention; http://apps.nccd.cdc.gov/dn-pabmi/) with the guidance that a body weight associated with a BMI-for-age below the fifth percentile suggests a low body weight.

The B criterion (fear of weight gain/becoming fat, behavior interfering with weight gain) for AN can be assigned if the clinician notes behaviors that suggest an intense fear of gaining weight or becoming fat, as this diagnostic feature may not be acknowledged, especially among younger patients (Becker, Thomas, & Pike, 2009).

Body shape and weight distortions are the focus of Criterion C, and a variety of manifestations of this disturbance are possible among patients with AN. Adolescents may not have developed the complex reasoning skills required for endorsing some of the cognitive aspects of this criterion (e.g., expressing the role of body shape and weight in influencing self-worth; Bravender et al., 2010); however, the clinician may consider behaviors suggesting a failure to recognize the seriousness of low weight (e.g., lack of interest in receiving treatment because the adolescent does not believe he or she has a problem).

DSM-5 suggests that individuals with AN be further described as belonging to one of two mutually exclusive subtypes, the restricting type (AN-R) and the binge-eating/purging type (AN-B/P). Subtype is determined by the presence or absence of persistent binge eating and/or purging behavior over the 3 months prior to assigning a diagnosis, as crossover between categories during the longitudinal course of AN occurs frequently (Peat, Mitchell, Hoek, & Wonderlich, 2009). New provisions for partial remission, the absence of low body weight while continuing to meet criteria B and C, full remission, and current severity (mild, moderate, severe, extreme) on the basis of BMI are also provided in DSM-5.

Bulimia Nervosa

The DSM-5 diagnostic criteria for BN are listed in Box 13.2.

Criterion A provides a definition of a binge eating episode in terms of amount ("definitely larger than most people would eat"), time-frame ("in a discrete period of time"), and

Box 13.1 DSM-5 Diagnostic Criteria for Anorexia Nervosa

A. Restriction of energy intake relative to requirements, leading to a significantly low body weight in the context of age, sex, developmental trajectory, and physical health. *Significantly low weight* is defined as a weight that is less than minimally normal, or, for children and adolescents, less than that minimally expected.
B. Intense fear of gaining weight or becoming fat, or persistent behavior that interferes with weight gain, even though at a significantly low weight.
C. Disturbance in the way in which one's body weight or shape is experienced, undue influence of body weight or shape on self-evaluation, or persistent lack of recognition of the seriousness of the current low body weight.

Specify whether:

Restricting type: During the last 3 months, the individual has not engaged in recurrent episodes of binge eating or purging behavior (i.e., self-induced vomiting or the misuse of laxatives, diuretics, or enemas). This subtype describes presentations in which weight loss is accomplished primarily through dieting, fasting, and/or excessive exercise.

Binge-eating/purging type: During the last 3 months, the individual has engaged in recurrent episodes of binge eating or purging behavior (i.e., self-induced vomiting or the misuse of laxatives, diuretics, or enemas).

Specify if:

In partial remission: After full criteria for anorexia nervosa were previously met, Criterion A (low body weight) has not been met for a sustained period, but either Criterion B (intense fear of gaining weight or becoming fat or behavior that interferes with weight gain) or Criterion C (disturbances in self-perception of weight and shape) is still met.

In full remission: After full criteria for anorexia nervosa were previously met, none of the criteria have been met for a sustained period of time.

Specify current severity:

The minimum level of severity is based, for adults, on current body mass index (BMI) (see below) or, for children and adolescents, on BMI percentile. The ranges below are derived from World Health Organization categories for thinness in adults; for children and adolescents, corresponding BMI percentiles should be used. The level of severity may be increased to reflect clinical symptoms, the degree of functional disability, and the need for supervision.

Mild: BMI ≥ 17 kg/m^2

Moderate: BMI 16–16.99 kg/m^2

Severe: BMI 15–15.99 kg/m^2

Extreme: BMI < 15 kg/m^2

psychological state ("a sense of a lack of control"). Clinical judgment is required to determine whether an eating episode meets the definition of a binge episode.

Criterion B describes recurrent and inappropriate behaviors, including some easily characterized (self-induced vomiting) and others that are less straightforward, like the "misuse" of laxatives and diuretics or what constitutes excessive exercise.

The frequency criterion (Criterion C) for BN was decreased for DSM-5 and requires that episodes of binge eating and inappropriate compensatory behaviors occur on average at least once weekly for 3 months.

Criterion D attempts to capture an important psychopathological parameter (self-evaluation based on body shape and weight), which is also required for a diagnosis of AN. Younger patients

Box 13.2 DSM-5 Diagnostic Criteria for Bulimia Nervosa

A. Recurrent episodes of binge eating. An episode of binge eating is characterized by both of the following:
   1. Eating, in a discrete period of time (e.g., within any 2-hour period), an amount of food that is definitely larger than what most individuals would eat in a similar period of time under similar circumstances.
   2. A sense of lack of control over eating during the episode (e.g., a feeling that one cannot stop eating or control what or how much one is eating).
B. Recurrent inappropriate compensatory behaviors in order to prevent weight gain, such as self-induced vomiting; misuse of laxatives, diuretics, or other medications; fasting; or excessive exercise.
C. The binge eating and inappropriate compensatory behaviors both occur, on average, at least once a week for 3 months.
D. Self-evaluation is unduly influenced by body shape and weight.
E. The disturbance does not occur exclusively during episodes of anorexia nervosa.

Specify if:

In partial remission: After full criteria for bulimia nervosa were previously met, some, but not all, of the criteria have been met for a sustained period of time.

In full remission: After full criteria for bulimia nervosa were previously met, none of the criteria have been met for a sustained period of time.

Specify current severity:

The minimum level of severity is based on the frequency of inappropriate compensatory behaviors (see below). The level of severity may be increased to reflect other symptoms and the degree of functional disability.

Mild: An average of 1–3 episodes of inappropriate compensatory behaviors per week.

Moderate: An average of 4–7 episodes of inappropriate compensatory behaviors per week.

Severe: An average of 8–13 episodes of inappropriate compensatory behaviors per week.

Extreme: An average of 14 or more episodes of inappropriate compensatory behaviors per week.

may deny this symptom and clinicians may have difficulty distinguishing between "undue influence" and the normative overconcern with shape and weight among female adolescents.

Specifiers for partial remission of BN and current severity, determined on the basis of the frequency of inappropriate compensatory behaviors and functional impairment, are also provided.

Binge-Eating Disorder

Criteria for the diagnosis of BED are provided in Box 13.3. Binge-eating disorder was officially recognized in DSM-5 on the basis of data accumulated after the inclusion of this category as a provisional diagnosis in the prior version of the DSM.

The definition of binge eating for individuals with BED (Criterion A) is identical to that used for BN, with the requirement that at least three additional features associated with these episodes (Criterion B; e.g., eating until uncomfortably full, eating alone because of embarrassment) be endorsed. Further, the individual must report "marked distress" related to binge-eating episodes (Criterion C) that occur at least once weekly over a 3-month period (Criterion D). To receive a diagnosis of BED, the recurrent use of inappropriate compensatory behavior must be denied (Criterion E). Definitions for partial remission, full remission, and current severity (mild, moderate, severe, extreme) derived from binge-eating frequency are also provided in DSM-5.

Box 13.3 DSM-5 Diagnostic Criteria for Binge-Eating Disorder

A. Recurrent episodes of binge eating. An episode of binge eating is characterized by both of the following:
   1. Eating, in a discrete period of time (e.g., within any 2-hour period), an amount of food that is definitely larger than what most people would eat in a similar period of time under similar circumstances.
   2. A sense of lack of control over eating during the episode (e.g., a feeling that one cannot stop eating or control what or how much one is eating).

B. The binge-eating episodes are associated with three (or more) of the following:
   1. Eating much more rapidly than normal.
   2. Eating until feeling uncomfortably full.
   3. Eating large amounts of food when not feeling physically hungry.
   4. Eating alone because of feeling embarrassed by how much one is eating.
   5. Feeling disgusted with oneself, depressed, or very guilty afterward.

C. Marked distress regarding binge eating is present.

D. The binge eating occurs, on average, at least once per week for 3 months.

E. The binge eating is not associated with the recurrent use of inappropriate compensatory behavior as in bulimia nervosa and does not occur exclusively during the course of bulimia nervosa or anorexia nervosa.

Specify if:

In partial remission: After full criteria for binge-eating disorder were previously met, binge eating occurs at an average frequency of less than one episode per week for a sustained period of time.

In full remission: After full criteria for binge-eating disorder were previously met, none of the criteria have been met for a sustained period of time.

Specify current severity:

The minimum level of severity is based on the frequency of episodes of binge eating (see below). The level of severity may be increased to reflect other symptoms and the degree of functional disability.

Mild: 1–3 binge-eating episodes per week.

Moderate: 4–7 binge-eating episodes per week.

Severe: 8–13 binge-eating episodes per week.

Extreme: 14 or more binge-eating episodes per week.

Although the onset of BED typically occurs in late adolescence or young adulthood (Hudson, Hiripi, Pope, & Kessler, 2007), little is known about the presentation of BED in this age group. However, loss of control over eating (with and without the consumption of an objectively large amount of food) is known to be an important clinical characteristic among youth (e.g., Decaluwé, Braet, & Fairburn, 2003; Tanofsky-Kraff et al., 2009). Relationships have been noted between broadly defined forms of binge eating, weight gain, increased body fat, depressive and anxiety symptoms, low self-esteem, and other eating pathology (Decaluwé & Braet, 2003; Isnard et al., 2003; Sonneville et al., 2013; Wildes et al., 2010). It is possible that episodes of loss-of-control eating may develop into full-syndrome BED (Tanofsky-Kraff et al., 2011), but additional studies are needed to better characterize the course of patients with this diagnosis.

Pica

Pica is characterized by the developmentally inappropriate, persistent consumption of substances that are nonnutritive and nonfood (e.g., paper, clay) over at least a 1-month period, and to a degree that merits clinical intervention. Such eating cannot be culturally sanctioned or developmentally normal. If the individual has another diagnosis, such as intellectual developmental disorder, pica should only be assigned if it is severe enough to warrant clinical attention independent of the other co-occurring condition.

Rumination Disorder

Rumination disorder is diagnosed when an individual frequently and repeatedly over a period of at least 1 month regurgitates food following eating. The regurgitation must not simply be due to a gastrointestinal/medical illness, and as with pica, rumination disorder should be assigned as a co-occurring diagnosis for an individual with another mental disorder only if the feeding disturbance is severe enough to require additional intervention. Preliminary data suggest that rumination disorder occurs infrequently among older children and adolescents presenting for an evaluation to an adolescent medicine physician (Ornstein et al., 2013).

Avoidant/Restrictive Food Intake Disorder

Unlike pica and rumination disorder, which were not substantially changed between DSM-IV and DSM-5, the DSM-IV diagnosis "feeding disorder of infancy or early childhood" was rearticulated and renamed "avoidant/restrictive food intake disorder." Individuals with avoidant/restrictive food intake disorder consistently fail to achieve nutritional or energy needs and display at least one clinically significant symptom, such as notable weight loss/failure to gain weight, a nutritional deficiency, a need for food supplementation, or impaired psychosocial functioning. The feeding disturbance is not attributable to cultural or religious practices or problems obtaining food, is not associated with the shape or weight concerns characteristic of AN and BN, and is not merely a symptom of another co-occurring mental or physical disorder. Among the presentations subsumed within the avoidant/restrictive food intake disorder category are (1) food avoidance emotional disorder, or emotional distress leading to insufficient calorie consumption; (2) an aversion or avoidance of foods because of their appearance, smell, taste, or texture; and (3) food avoidance due to a specific fear, or functional dysphagia or fear of swallowing (Bryant-Waugh et al., 2010). Differentiating avoidant/restrictive food intake disorder from AN requires a careful assessment of the rationale for food restriction to determine the most appropriate diagnosis, which may be especially challenging among adolescents, whose level of insight may be limited.

Emerging evidence since the publication of DSM-5 suggests that avoidant/restrictive food intake disorder has significant clinical utility. Five percent to 20% of youngsters presenting to adolescent medicine physicians with eating problems may meet the criteria for avoidant/restrictive food intake disorder (Norris & Katzman, 2015; Ornstein et al., 2013). Individuals with avoidant/restrictive food intake disorder appear to be younger than those presenting with AN, have been ill longer, and are more likely to be male. Body weights are intermediate between those with AN and those with BN (Fisher et al., 2014).

Other Specified Feeding and Eating Disorder, Unspecified Feeding or Eating Disorder

The DSM-5 categories of other specified and unspecified feeding or eating disorder are provided to permit identification of subsyndromal feeding or eating symptoms that nonetheless lead to notable distress or impairment in functioning (e.g., social, occupational, other important areas of functioning; APA, 2013). The other specified feeding or eating disorder category is distinguished from the unspecified feeding or eating disorder category by the provision of five descriptions: for atypical AN, subthreshold BN and BED (of low frequency and/or limited duration), purging disorder, and night eating syndrome. The final category, unspecified feeding or eating disorder, is assigned to individuals with an eating disorder that does not meet the criteria for any of the officially recognized disorders and does not match one of these descriptions. Adolescents assigned an "other" eating disorder may not have a less severe illness, as exemplified by serious medical conditions or comorbidities (e.g., a prolonged QTc interval) observed in this heterogeneous diagnostic group (Peebles et al., 2010).

Summary

The DSM-5 criteria for feeding and eating disorders were published in 2013. Although relatively limited information is available at this time to evaluate the utility of these new categories, emerging data from adults and adolescents (Norris & Katzman, 2015; Ornstein et al., 2013; Stice, Marti, & Rohde, 2013; Sysko et al., 2012; Thomas et al., 2015) suggest that the revised categories improve on the DSM-IV scheme, which failed to capture many adolescents and adults with clinically significant eating problems. Although pica, rumination disorder, and avoidant/restrictive food intake disorder are likely particularly relevant to adolescents, limited information is available about these disorders. Thus, these conditions are not further considered in the sections that follow.

DEMOGRAPHICS AND PREVALENCE OF EATING DISORDERS

Relatively few large population-based studies conducted during the past two decades are available to provide estimates of the prevalence of eating disorders. Since only a minority of individuals with a mental illness, including eating disorders, seek treatment (Demyttenaere et al., 2004; Merikangas et al., 2011; Preti et al., 2009; Swanson, Crow, Le Grange, Swendsen, & Merikangas, 2011), prevalence estimates from clinical samples are likely biased. Healthcare system databases also provide estimates of the age-specific prevalence and incidence of eating disorders (Currin, Schmidt, Treasure, & Jick, 2005; Nicholls, Lynn, & Viner, 2011; Pinhas, Morris, Crosby, & Katzman, 2011; van Son, van Hoeken, Bartelds, van Furth, & Hoek, 2006a, 2006b). Although many of these studies are large and carefully conducted and make important contributions to the literature on eating disorders, it is unclear whether the results are generalizable since many cases of eating disorders are not detected by the healthcare system (Keski-Rahkonen et al., 2007). Therefore, the literature cited in the sections that follow focuses on population-based samples, including nationally or locally representative ones (e.g., Hudson et al., 2007; Kessler et al., 2013; Swanson et al., 2011), cross-sectional convenience samples (e.g., Preti et al., 2009), and birth or population-based cohort studies (e.g., Field et al., 2012; Machado, Goncalves, & Hoek, 2013).

The typical onset of eating disorders is during preadolescence or adolescence, but most epidemiological samples are too small to study eating disorders meeting full diagnostic criteria. Thus, the majority of studies of children and adolescents instead focus on weight concerns, unhealthy weight-control behaviors, and/or bulimic behaviors. However, age of onset of AN, BN, and BED is primarily derived from studies asking adults to recall retrospective information about symptoms at younger ages and symptoms in the past year, data that are subsequently used to generate age-specific or lifetime prevalence. The accuracy of such information is unknown, and the results should therefore be interpreted cautiously.

Anorexia Nervosa

In DSM-IV, the nosological system used for eating disorders until very recently, only AN and BN were specifically recognized as eating disorders, and the diagnostic criteria were very stringent. Thus, extremely large samples were needed to accurately assess current prevalence. For example, Machado et al. (2013) reported a point prevalence of 0.6% among adolescent and young adult females, and estimates from other large population-based samples of female youth report an even lower prevalence of 0%

to 0.3% (see Box 13.1), suggesting that samples of at least 300 to 500 adolescent females are needed to identify one current case of AN among adolescents, and even larger samples to assess the prevalence among males or adults. Therefore, studies with more than 1,000 females and as many or more males are desirable. Unfortunately, a relatively small number of studies with samples of approximately 500 or more females is available (Table 13.1).

Most large epidemiological studies have used rigorous assessment tools, such as the Composite International Diagnostic Interview, the Eating Disorder Examination, or the Structured Clinical Interview for DSM-IV. With these measures, the point prevalence of AN ranges between 0.04% and 0.6% among adolescent females (Ackard, Fulkerson, & Neumark-Sztainer, 2007; Machado et al., 2013; Swanson et al., 2011; Wittchen, Nelson, & Lachner, 1998), between 0% and 0.1% among adolescent males (Ackard et al., 2007; Swanson et al., 2011; Wittchen et al., 1998), and between 0% and 0.1% among adults (Bulik et al., 2007; Hudson et al., 2007; Preti et al., 2009; see Table 13.1).

In the National Survey Replication Survey sample of 9,282 adults, median age of recalled onset of AN was 18 years, with an interquartile range of 16 to 22 years (Hudson et al., 2007). Among the 21,425 adults in the European Study of the Epidemiology of Mental Disorders project, all cases of anorexia developed before 20 years of age (Preti et al., 2009). Lifetime rates appear to decrease as age increases among adults, which has been interpreted as a cohort effect with eating disorders becoming more prevalent in recent decades. However, this may also reflect greater awareness of eating disorders among younger individuals.

The low incidence of AN has made it challenging to conduct prospective studies of individuals with subthreshold variants who may be at risk for the development of full-syndrome AN (see also Chapter 15). The dearth of empirical data evaluating subthreshold versions of AN is particularly important in adolescence, as most cases of AN develop during this period. The identification of clinically significant cases of subthreshold AN prior to meeting full criteria is complicated by the weight trajectories of children and adolescents, as they may have lost weight, or failed to make adequate gains, but are not yet at a low weight. Unlike cancers, which are staged into in situ (completely local and not entirely cancerous) and stages I through IV depending on the size and spread of the tumor, the diagnostic criteria for AN identify an already severe eating disorder. Numerous investigators have attempted to study less severe AN (atypical, broad AN, etc.) but without employing standard definitions, making comparisons across studies very difficult.

Finally, in DSM-5, amenorrhea is not required for a diagnosis of AN, and in combination with a more flexible weight standard, prevalence estimates may increase (Keski-Rahkonen et al., 2007; Wade, Bergin, Tiggemann, Bulik, & Fairburn, 2006).

Bulimia Nervosa

In the DSM-IV and DSM-5 diagnostic schemes, a hierarchy prevents the concurrent diagnosis of BN if an individual meets the criteria for AN. The following sections therefore focus on studies employing DSM-IV or DSM-5 criteria so estimates of BN can be compared across studies. Using data from 24,124 adults in the World Health Organization World Mental Health Surveys, the highest prevalence of BN was noted in Brazil (0.9%) and the lowest in Romania (0%; Kessler et al., 2013). Similar studies have not been conducted with adolescents, but it is reasonable to assume that the same patterns exist among younger individuals.

Studies have consistently found that BN is more common among females than males (see Table 13.1). Among 10,123 adolescents in the National Comorbidity Survey Replication Adolescent Supplement, a nationally representative sample, current BN prevalence was higher (0.3% of males and 0.9% of females) but lifetime rates were similar (0.5% males and 1.3% of females; Swanson et al., 2011) to the adults in the National Comorbidity Survey Replication, which suggests that there is either a secular trend in rising rates or poor recall of past history of BN. There is some evidence to suggest that

Table 13.1 Prevalence Estimates from Population-Based Epidemiological Studies

Authors	*Sample Size*	*Sampling*	*Age*	*Country*	*Assessment*
Ackard et al.	4,746	Cohort study	Adolescents	USA	Self-report questionnaire
Swanson et al.	10,123	Nationally representative	Adolescents	USA	Composite International Diagnostic Interview (CIDI)
McKnight Investigators	1,103 females	Prospective cohort study	Preadolescents	USA	McKnight Eating Disorder Examination (EDE)
Machado et al.	3,048 females	Convenience sample	Adolescents and young adults	Portugal	2-stage design: Eating Disorder Examination Questionnaire (EDE-Q) followed by EDE
Stice et al.	496 females	Prospective cohort study	Adolescents and young adults	USA	EDD Interview
Wittchen et al.	3,021	Convenience sample?	Adolescents and young adults	Germany	M-CIDI
Keski-Rahkonen et al.	2,881	Cohort study of twins	Adolescents and young adults	Finland	2-stage design: Structured Clinical Interview for DSM-IV (SCID)
Hudson et al.	9,282	Nationally representative	Adults	USA	CIDI
Preti et al.	21,425	Probability sample	Adults	6 European countries	CIDI
Micali et al.	5,256 females	Birth cohort study	Adults	Netherlands	
Kessler et al.	24,124	Nationally representative	Adults	14 countries around the world	CIDI
Bulik et al.	31,406	Twin registry	Adults	Sweden	SCID Screen Patient Questionnaire
Trace et al.	13,295 females	Twin study	Adults	Sweden	SCID Screen Patient Questionnaire
Wade et al.	1,002 females	Cohort study of twins	Adults	Australia	EDE
Swanson et al.	10,123	Nationally representative	Adolescents	USA	CIDI
Machado et al.	3,048 females	Convenience sample	Adolescents and young adults	Portugal	2-stage design: EDEQ followed by EDE
Field et al.	8,594 females	Prospective cohort study	Adolescents and young adults	USA	Self-report questionnaire
Stice et al.	496 females	Prospective cohort study	Adolescents and young adults	USA	EDD Interview
Trace et al.	13,295 females	Twin study	Adults	Sweden	SCID Screen Patient Questionnaire
Bulik et al.	41,157 females	Birth cohort study	Adults	Norway	Self-report questionnaire

DSM	AN		BN		BED	
	Point	Lifetime	Point	Lifetime	Point	Lifetime
DSM-IV	0.0% M, 0.04% F		0.2% M, 0.3% F		0.3% M 1.9% F	
DSM-IV	0.2% (0.1% M, 0.2% F)	0.3% (0.3% M, 0.3% F)	0.6% (0.3% M, 0.9% F)	0.9% (0.5% M, 1.3% F)	0.9% (0.4% M 1.4% F)	1.6% (0.8% M, 2.3% F)
DSM-IV	0.0% F		0.4% F			
DSM-IV	0.6% F		0.5% F			
DSM-IV		0.6% F		1.6% F		1.0% F
DSM-IV	0.0% M, 0.3% F	0.1% M, 1.0% F	0.0% M, 0.7% F	0.0% M, 1.7% F		
DSM-IV		2.2% F		2.3%		
DSM-IV	00 0	0.6% (0.3% M, 0.9% F)	0.3% (0.1% M, 0.5% F)	1.0% (0.5% M, 1.5% F)	1.2% (0.8% M, 1.6% F)	2.8% (2.0% M, 3.5% F)
DSM-IV	0% (0.0% M, 0.0% F)	0.5% (0.0% M, 0.9% F)	0.2% (0.0% M, 0.3% F)	0.5% (0.1% M, 0.9% F)	0.3% (0.1% M, 0.6% F)	1.1% (0.3% M, 1.9% F)
DSM-IV	0.3% F	2.1% F				
DSM-IV			0.4%	1.0%	0.8%	1.9%
DSM-IV		1.2% F 0.3% M				
DSM-IV				1.2% F		0.2% F
DSM-IV		1.9% F		2.9%		2.9%
DSM-5	0.2% (0.1% M, 0.2% F)	1.1% (0.4% M, 1.8% F)			2.0% (1.4% M, 2.6% F)	4.1% (3.4% M, 4.6% F)
DSM-5	0.7% F		0.6% F		0.6% F	
DSM-5			0.8% F		1.8% F	
DSM-5		0.8% F		2.6% F		3.0% F
DSM-5				1.6% F		0.4% F
DSM-5	0.1% F		0.7%		3.5%	

past recall of binge eating and purging results in underestimation (Field, Colditz, Herzog, & Heatherton, 1996), but it is difficult to draw conclusions about secular trends since there are not large-scale studies that have been done repeatedly over time. However, Hudson et al. (2007) did note a cohort effect in the National Comorbidity Replication Sample.

Another methodological concern is the challenge of assessing criteria for BN among adolescent males. The definition of binge eating requires the consumption of an abnormally large amount of food, larger than others would eat in a similar circumstance, and a sense of loss of control during the episode of eating. Adolescent males, especially if physically active, require prodigious caloric consumption to support normal growth and development (Shomaker et al., 2010), making the assessment of an "unusually large" amount of food difficult. In addition, adolescent males may be reluctant to admit that their eating sometimes feels out of control.

Binge-Eating Disorder

Although BED was not formally recognized until the publication of DSM-5, numerous studies have investigated the prevalence and correlates of this disorder using the DSM-IV definition in both adolescent and adult samples. The prevalence of BED is higher than AN and BN combined, with a range in population-based samples from 0.6% to 4.6% among adolescent and young adult females (Ackard et al., 2007; Field et al., 2012; Machado et al., 2013; Stice et al., 2013; Swanson et al., 2011). Since DSM-5 BED includes a lower binge-eating frequency cutoff than the provisional criteria for BED in DSM-IV and reduces the required timeframe (>3 months) for diagnosis, rates of BED will be higher in studies using the most recent criteria, although it is not clear by how much (Hudson, Coit, Lalonde, & Pope, 2012; Trace et al., 2012).

Apart from Brazil, studies in U.S. populations report higher prevalence rates (Ackard et al., 2007; Field et al., 2012; Hudson et al., 2007; Swanson et al., 2011) than other countries (Kessler et al., 2013; Machado et al., 2013; Preti et al., 2009). Few differences in prevalence estimates are noted in studies using clinical interviews (Hudson et al., 2007; Swanson et al., 2011) and self-report questionnaires (Ackard et al., 2007; Field et al., 2012). As with other eating disorders, a cohort effect appears to occur with BED such that samples with large numbers of older adults report lower prevalence rates. For example, Hudson et al. (2007) found a lifetime rate for BED of 4.2% among 18- to 29-year-old women but a much lower (2.4%) rate among women older than 60 years.

Other Specified Eating Disorders

In both clinical samples and research studies, the majority of adolescents with an eating disorder do not have either AN or BN and were classified as (1) not having an eating disorder, (2) having an eating disorder not otherwise specified, or (3) having BED, a specific variant of eating disorder not otherwise specified, the residual category of DSM-IV. In DSM-IV, eating disorder not otherwise specified captured a wide range of eating pathology, making comparisons across studies difficult. Moreover, although the boundary between full-criteria disorders and an eating disorder not otherwise specified is clear, there has been no discussion about the lower bound for inclusion in the eating disorder not otherwise specified category, further complicating an understanding of the prevalence of clinically significant eating pathology.

Although not recognized by the DSM-IV, and only listed as a specific example of other specified feeding and eating disorder in DSM-5, a nontrivial number of youths engage in frequent purging but do not binge eat. Whether they have a "purging disorder" or are a non-binge-eating variant of BN is not yet completely understood. Purging disorder has not been as thoroughly studied as other eating disorders; however, a growing number of large population-based epidemiological samples are beginning to include this category. Among the 9,000 girls in the Growing Up Today Study, 4.1% developed purging disorder during adolescence or young adulthood (Field et al., 2012). A slightly lower rate (3.4%) was observed by Stice et al. (2013) in a smaller sample followed for 8 years.

Population-Based Studies of Eating Disorder Symptoms and Behaviors

All of the recognized eating disorders require frequently engaging in bulimic behaviors and/or a low weight resulting from use of extreme weight-control behaviors over an extended period of time. Many researchers, particularly epidemiologists and others interested in prevention, have examined less frequent or extreme weight-control behaviors and binge eating, which might be particularly relevant for adolescents if these symptoms represent an early stage of an eating disorder or are associated with harmful outcomes regardless of whether they progress to a full-threshold eating disorder.

Cross-sectional studies of disordered eating among adolescents and young adults and a growing number of prospective investigations have provided information about other forms of eating disorder psychopathology. Neumark-Sztainer et al. (2012) reported that among 2,793 adolescents in Project Eating Among Teens, 9.6% of females and 6.3% of males had engaged in binge eating at least once during the past year. Lower rates of binge eating were observed among 10,334 young adults in the Longitudinal Study of Adolescent Health. In a nationally representative sample, Striegel-Moore et al. (2011) found that among Caucasians, 1.3% of females and 0.4% of males reported binge eating, but rates were much higher among American Indians and Native Americans (3.8% and 0.8%, respectively). Large ethnic differences in purging were also observed among the more than 10,900 adolescents assessed in the Youth Risk Behavior Surveillance System, with Chao et al. (2008) reporting purging in the past 30 days among 6.7% of whites and 6.8% of Hispanics, but in only 4% of blacks. For boys, rates were highest among Hispanics (3.9%) and lowest among whites (2.3%). Even larger disparities were observed among 16,978 children from 47 Massachusetts middle schools participating in the Healthy Choices overweight prevention study (Austin et al., 2011). In females, the prevalence of use of vomiting, laxatives, or diet pills to control weight was lower among whites (2.7%) than blacks (6.7%), Hispanics (6.6%), Pacific Islanders (24.2%), or American Indians (23.3%), and a similar pattern was observed among boys. Fewer studies have assessed the incidence of bulimic behaviors, but among 12,534 adolescents in the Growing Up Today Study, during 7 years of follow-up, 4.3% of females and 2.3% of males started to binge eat at least weekly and 5.3% of females and 0.8% of males started to purge at least weekly, but few adolescents engaged in weekly binge eating and purging (Field et al., 2008).

Summary

A growing number of studies have been published on eating disorders and disordered eating among adolescents and young adults. Comparisons between studies can be challenging because of sample characteristics (i.e., size and sampling methodology) and lack of standard definitions for the most common behaviors and disorders (e.g., eating disorder not otherwise specified) among adolescents. For example, some studies include only presentations that miss the duration criterion for BN or BED, while others include all disordered eating not captured by a full-threshold eating disorder diagnosis (Box 13.4). Comparisons between studies of disordered eating are equally

Box 13.4 Red Flags for Eating Disorders

- An abnormally low weight or significant fluctuations in weight not due to medical illness
- Purging behaviors intended to induce weight loss
- Persistent intense concerns with weight or shape
- Persistent attempts to diet or lose weight despite being at a normal or low weight
- Social withdrawal and avoidance of activities involving food and/or eating
- Unexplained amenorrhea

challenging. Some studies focus only on frequent binge eating and purging; others examine any use of a large variety of weight-control behaviors (diet pills, laxatives, vomiting, etc.), or include dieting in the same category as vomiting and laxatives. Despite these methodological challenges, more females than males try to control their weight, engage in weight-control behaviors including purging, and binge eat. Eating disorders are also more common among females, but the gender difference in rates of BED may appear to be much smaller in future studies using DSM-5 criteria.

COMORBIDITY, OUTCOME, AND DIAGNOSTIC MIGRATION

In addition to examining the diagnostic categories and data on the prevalence of eating disorders, it is important to know what other forms of psychopathology individuals with eating disorders are prone to develop, and to describe what is likely to occur over time to individuals with eating disorders in terms of stability of diagnoses and outcome. Knowledge of comorbidity, outcome, and migration among diagnostic categories is important to match patients to interventions and to assessing the overall effectiveness of treatments. A number of studies have addressed comorbidity, course, and outcome of adult patients with eating disorders, but studies of adolescents are limited. The available literature suggests that the comorbidities commonly seen in adults with eating disorders are also seen in adolescents with such problems, with elevated rates of affective disorders, anxiety disorders, and substance abuse compared to control groups (Castro-Fornieles et al., 2010; Herpertz-Dahlmann, 2009; Kirkcaldy, Siefen, Kandel, & Merrick, 2007; Swanson et al., 2011; Touchette et al., 2011).

Comorbidity

Comorbidity of Anorexia Nervosa

Overall, the lifetime rates of psychiatric comorbidity among patients with eating disorders are substantial (Halmi et al., 1991, Spindler & Milos, 2007; Villarejo et al., 2012; von Lojewski, Boyd, Abraham, & Russell, 2012). Affective disorders, anxiety disorders, substance use disorders, and personality disorders are all commonly associated with AN. The affective disorder that most commonly co-occurs with AN is major depressive disorder, with a lifetime comorbidity of 50% to 70% (Herzog, Nussbaum, & Marmor, 1996; von Lojewski et al., 2012). Lifetime rates of anxiety disorders are seen in between 50% and 70% of these patients (Dellava, Kendler, & Neale, 2011; Godart, Flament, Perdereau, & Jeammet, 2002; Swinbourne & Touyz, 2007; Strober, Freeman, Lampert, & Diamond, 2007); common comorbid anxiety diagnoses are social phobia (40%–55%) and obsessive-compulsive disorder (OCD; 5%–69%; Godart et al., 2002; Halmi et al., 1991). Of particular note, AN seems to commonly develop following childhood anxiety disorders (Bulik et al., 1997; Raney et al., 2008; Swinbourne et al., 2012). Also of note, there is a clear association between OCD and AN, and similarities between the two conditions have often been cited (Altman & Shankman, 2009). Lifetime prevalence of substance use disorders ranges between 12% and 21% (Bulik, Sullivan, McKee, Weltzin & Kaye, 1994; Herzog, Keller, Sacks, Yeh, & Lavori, 1992; Root, Pisetsky, et al., 2010; Stock, Goldberg, Corbett & Katzman, 2002), and patients with the binge/purge subtype are more likely than those with restrictor subtype to manifest such problems (Herzog, Keller, Sacks, Yeh & Lavori, 1992; Root, Pinheiro, et al., 2010). Current prevalence rates are also notable, with over 70% meeting criteria for a current psychiatric disorder when presenting for treatment (Braun, Sunday & Halmi, 1994; Herpertz-Dahlmann, Müller, Herpertz, Heussen, Hebebrand & Remschmidt, 2001; Herzog et al., 1992; Wonderlich & Mitchell, 1997).

The developmental sequence of AN in relation to other comorbid conditions varies significantly. Affective disorders may begin before or after the onset of AN, or the disorders can begin concurrently (Braun et al., 1994). Anxiety disorders, in particular social phobia and OCD, frequently predate the onset of AN (Anderluh, Tchanturia, Rabe-Hesketh & Treasure, 2003; Braun et al., 1994; Bulik, Sullivan & Joyce, 1997;

Swinbourne & Touyz, 2007), whereas substance use disorders often develop after the onset of AN (Braun et al., 1994).

Comorbidity of Bulimia Nervosa

Approximately 70% to 85% of patients with BN report a lifetime history of another psychiatric disorder, and the rates of current disorders at time of presentation are also elevated (Fichter & Quadflieg, 1997; Halmi et al., 2002; Herzog et al., 1992; Mitchell, Specker, & de Zwaan, 1991; Wonderlich & Mitchell, 1997). Affective disorders, anxiety disorders, substance use disorders, and personality disorders are commonly associated with BN, with major depressive disorder the most common mood disorder among patients with BN. In community samples, approximately one third meet lifetime criteria, a rate that increases to 65% in inpatient and outpatient samples. In clinical samples, the lifetime rates of comorbidity with at least one anxiety disorder range from 3% to 65% (Herzog et al., 1992; Swinbourne & Touyz, 2007), with social phobia, OCD, panic disorder, and posttraumatic stress disorder (PTSD) commonly observed (Brewerton et al., 1995; Mitchell, Mazzeo, Schlesinger, Brewerton & Smith, 2012; von Ranson, Kaye, Weltzin, Rao & Matsunaga, 1999). Some literature also suggests that eating disorders, in particular BN, may also be associated with attention-deficit/hyperactivity disorder (ADHD; Nazar et al., 2008; Yates, Lund, Johnson, Mitchell, & McKee, 2009).

The lifetime prevalence of substance use disorders is approximately 25% (Bulik et al., 1994); alcohol is most frequently cited, followed by cocaine and marijuana. A meta-analysis suggested that substance abuse problems primarily cluster among those with binge-eating behaviors, such as those with BN, BED, and the binge/purge subtype of AN (Gadalla & Piran, 2007). Patients with BN and substance use disorders commonly exhibit impulsivity in multiple domains, including suicide attempts, self-injurious acts, and stealing. Some reports describe an increased prevalence of bipolar affective disorders among those with eating disorders, particularly those with BN (Brietzke, Moreira, Toniolo & Lafer, 2011; Fornaro et al., 2010, Lunde, Fasmer, Akiskal, Akiskal & Oedegaard, 2009; McElroy et al., 2011).

As in AN, the sequence of development of BN and comorbid conditions varies, as onset of the comorbid disorder can occur prior to, at the same time as, or following the development of BN (Braun et al., 1994). As with AN, anxiety disorders commonly predate the onset of BN, whereas substance use disorders more often develop after the onset of BN (Braun et al., 1994; Bulik et al., 1997; Swinbourne & Touyz, 2007).

Comorbidity of Binge-Eating Disorder

Although the literature on BED and comorbidity remains limited, there again appears to be an increased rate of various forms of other psychopathology, although this issue has yet to be adequately addressed in adolescent populations (Grilo, White, Barnes & Masheb, 2012; Grilo, White, & Masheb, 2009).

Outcomes

Outcome of Anorexia Nervosa

One of the problems in examining the outcome of eating disorders is that widely varying criteria for recovery have been employed (Noordenbos, 2011; Williams, Watts, & Wade, 2012). However, the available data suggest that approximately 40% to 70% of adolescents with AN recover, 20% to 30% are improved but continue to have residual symptoms, and 10% to 20% develop a chronic form of illness (Herpertz-Dahlmann et al., 2001; Morgan, Purgold, & Welbourne, 1983; Steinhausen, 1997, 2002, 2009). Most adolescents with AN continue to recover over time; for example, Strober, Freeman, and Morrell (1997) reported a 1% probability of adolescents reaching full recovery at 3 years, which increased to 72% after 10 years. Patients experiencing persistent symptoms typically display abnormalities in weight, eating behaviors, menstrual function, comorbid psychopathology, and difficulties with psychosocial functioning (Herpertz-Dahlmann et al., 2001; Steinhausen, 2009; Strober et al.,

1997; Wentz, Gillberg, Gillberg, & Rastam, 2001). Relapse is common after weight gain in hospitalized patients, with up to one third of adolescent AN patients relapsing soon after discharge (see also Chapter 14; Herzog, Nussbaum, & Marmor, 1996; Strober et al., 1997).

AN has one of the highest mortality rates among psychiatric disorders. Approximately 5.6% of patients diagnosed with AN die per decade of illness, and long-term follow-up studies consistently find increased rates of death from both medical complications and suicide (Crow et al., 2009; Franko et al., 2013; Keel & Brown, 2010; Papadopoulos, Ekborn, Brandt, & Ekselius, 2009; Sullivan, 1995). Although the combined mortality rate for AN among adolescents and adults is over 5% (Steinhausen, 2002), the mortality rate during adolescence is believed to be low.

Some studies have found lower weight at presentation, longer duration of illness, and severe comorbid alcohol use to be associated with higher risk of mortality. Few variables are consistently associated with outcome in adolescents with AN, but the most positive outcomes are seen in patients between the ages of 12 and 18 with a short duration of illness. Poor outcome in adolescent patients is associated with extremely low weight at presentation and, in some studies, with vomiting.

Outcome of Bulimia Nervosa

Most adolescents and adults with BN improve over time, with recovery rates ranging from 35% to 75% at 5 or more years of follow-up (Fairburn, Cooper, Doll, Norman, & O'Connor, 2000; Fichter & Quadflieg, 1997; Keel & Brown, 2010; Steinhausen & Weber, 2009). However, approximately one third of individuals with BN relapse (Keel & Brown, 2010; Keel & Mitchell, 1997; Keel, Mitchell, Miller, David, & Crow, 1999), often within 1 to 2 years of recovery. Although approximately 40% to 60% of patients with BN eventually recover, the remaining individuals continue to be symptomatic, often with substantial impact on physical and psychosocial functioning (Steinhausen & Weber, 2009). While there have been some hints of an elevated mortality associated with BN (e.g., Crow et al., 2009), recent data indicate that BN without a history of AN is not associated with a significant increased risk of premature death (Franko et al., 2013). Few prognostic factors have been consistently reported across studies, but low self-esteem, longer duration of illness prior to presentation, higher frequency or severity of binge eating, substance abuse history, and a history of obesity have been associated with poorer outcome (Bulik, Sullivan, Joyce, Carter & McIntosh, 1998; Keel et al., 1999; Keel & Brown, 2010; Steinhausen & Weber, 2009).

Diagnostic Migration

Few studies address diagnostic migration, or the movement from one eating disorder subtype or eating disorder to another within the adolescent eating disorder population. While some patients migrate from BN to AN (Kassett, Gwirtsman, Kay, Brandt, & Jimerson, 1988), the most frequent change is from the restrictor subtype to the binge/purge subtype, reflecting the development of bulimic symptoms, and this migration may herald an increase in various other problems, such as suicidal ideation (Foulon et al., 2007). Some individuals gain weight in association with the binge eating, leading to a change in diagnostic status from either subtype to BN (Peat et al., 2009). In one study, more than 50% of restrictor AN patients, both adolescents and adults, developed BN symptomatology (Eddy et al., 2002), and only a small fraction of patients with the restrictor subtype remained in that diagnostic subtype. The remaining patients with the restrictive subtype who did not develop binge eating or purging were partially or fully recovered. It is unknown what factors lead to the development of binge/purge symptoms among patients with the restrictor subtype, and the precise time course of this development; however, overall diagnostic crossover should be regarded as a common phenomenon (Castellini et al., 2011).

Summary

The occurrence of other psychiatric disorders is very common in association with AN, BN, and

BED, and this comorbidity complicates both diagnosis and treatment. Many treatment studies of eating disorders exclude patients with serious comorbid disorders, such as substance use disorders, resulting in few available data regarding the appropriate treatments for such high-comorbidity patients. Although information about the course and outcome of eating disorders in adolescents is limited, adolescents with AN appear to have a better prognosis when they receive treatment early in the course of the illness. Diagnostic migration appears to be common from the restrictor subtype to the binge/purge subtype to BN. Little is known about the course and outcome of BN among adolescents; among adults, full recovery is common, but BN can be a chronic condition. Excess mortality has been clearly demonstrated for those with AN.

MEDICAL COMPLICATIONS OF EATING DISORDERS

Eating disorders are associated with significant medical morbidity and significant mortality. Most complications result from physiological adaptations to the effects of malnutrition, or occur as a result of unhealthy weight-control behaviors. Many, but not all, of the complications are reversible with nutritional rehabilitation and symptomatic improvement. However, in an adolescent whose growth and development are not yet complete, the medical consequences of eating disorders can be long-lasting and potentially irreversible. Particularly worrisome complications for adolescents include growth retardation, pubertal delay or arrest, impaired acquisition of peak bone mass, and structural brain changes. During normal pubertal development, body weight doubles and maturation of various organs occurs, with increases in the size of the heart, brain, lungs, liver, and kidneys. Approximately 17% to 18% of final adult height is achieved (Abbassi, 1998), and between 40% and 60% of peak bone mass is accrued (Golden & Shenker, 1992; Katzman, Bachrach, Carter, & Marcus, 1991).

The medical complications of AN and BN are listed in Table 13.2. Individuals with symptoms of both disorders (e.g., patients with AN and episodes of binge eating and/or purging) are at risk for complications of both AN and BN. Adolescents with symptoms of eating disorders that do not meet the full criteria for AN or BN are also at risk for medical complications (Peebles, Hardy, Wilson & Lock, 2010). Most complications occur with equal frequency in adults and adolescents, but in contrast to adults, a young adolescent with incompletely formed stores of body fat and other substrates can suffer significant medical compromise after a relatively small degree of weight loss.

Medical Complications of Anorexia Nervosa

The most notable medical complications of AN result from malnutrition. Subcutaneous tissue and muscle mass are lost, and patients display sunken cheeks and prominence of bony protuberances. Body temperature is usually low and patients often wear multiple layers of clothing to keep warm. The hands and feet may be cold and blue (acrocyanosis); the skin may be pale, dry, and yellow. Fine downy hair (lanugo) may be present over the arms, back, and abdomen. Scalp hair is dry, listless, and brittle, and there may be evidence of hair loss. Resting pulse and blood pressure are both low, and dizziness and fainting may occur upon standing as a result of orthostatic changes in pulse and blood pressure. There may be generalized muscle weakness.

Life-threatening complications of AN include electrolyte disturbances and cardiac arrhythmias. Patients may present with dehydration and abnormal serum levels of sodium, potassium, chloride, phosphorus, magnesium, carbon dioxide, and blood urea nitrogen. Electrolyte disturbances are more likely in those who are vomiting or abusing laxatives or diuretics. Hyponatremia (low sodium levels) can occur in those who drink excessive amounts of water either to satisfy hunger urges or to falsely elevate body weight prior to a medical visit. Water intoxication with hyponatremia can cause seizures, coma, and death. Serum phosphorus levels may be normal on presentation but may drop upon refeeding, and hypophosphatemia may play a role in the development

Table 13.2 Signs and Symptoms of Eating Disorders in Adolescence[1]

Factor	*AN*[2]	*BN*
Weight	Markedly decreased	Usually normal
Menstruation	Absent	Usually normal
Skin/Extremities	Growth of fine downy hair (lanugo)	Calluses on back of hand
	Cold blue hands and feet (acrocyanosis)	
	Swelling of feet (edema)	
Cardiovascular	Low heart rate (bradycardia)	
	Hypotension	
	Orthostasis	
Gastrointestinal	Elevated liver enzymes	Parotid and salivary gland enlargement
	Delayed gastric emptying	
	Constipation	Dental erosion
		Esophagitis
		Barrett's esophagus
Hematopoietic	Normochromic, normocyctic anemia	
	Leukopenia	
	Thrombocytopenia	
	Low erythrocyte sedimentation rate	
Fluid/Electrolytes	Increased blood urea nitrogen	Hypokalemia
	Increased creatinine	Hypochloremia
	Hyponatremia	Alkalosis
	Hypophosphatemia	
	Hypomagnesemia	
Endocrine	Hypoglycemia	
	Low estrogen or testosterone	
	Low luteinizing hormone	
	Low follicle-stimulating hormone	
	Low-normal thyroxine, low T3	
	Normal thyroid-stimulating hormone	
	Increased cortisol	
	Delayed puberty	
	Growth retardation	
Skeletal	Reduced bone mineral density	
	Increased bone fragility	

[1]Partially adapted from Walsh, B. T., & Attia, E. (2011). Eating disorders. In: D. L. Longo, A. S. Fauci, D. L. Kasper, S. L. Hauser, J. L. Jameson, & J. Loscalzo (Eds.), *Harrison's principles of internal medicine* (18th ed.). New York: McGraw Hill.

[2]Individuals with AN who engage in binge eating and/or purging may also develop signs and symptoms of BN.

of cardiac arrhythmias and sudden unexpected death seen in the "refeeding syndrome" (Kohn, Golden, & Shenker, 1998). Hypomagnesemia is more likely to occur in those who are purging (Raj, Keane-Miller, & Golden, 2012).

Resting pulse rates among patients with AN may be as low as 30 to 40 beats per minute (Palla & Litt, 1988), and systolic and diastolic blood pressures are low. Within the first 4 days of hospitalization, 60% to 85% of patients demonstrate orthostatic pulse changes on standing (Shamim, Golden, Arden, Filiberto, & Shenker, 2003). Both cardiac structure and function are affected (Casiero & Frishman, 2006), left ventricular mass and cardiac output are reduced (Mont et al., 2003; Moodie & Salcedo, 1983), heart rate variability is increased (Kosche et al., 2010; Mont et al., 2003), and exercise capacity is diminished (Nudel, Gootman, Nussbaum & Shenker, 1984). Electrocardiographic abnormalities have been noted in up to 75% of hospitalized adolescent patients (Galetta et al., 2002; Palla & Litt, 1988). A prolonged QTc interval, one type of electrocardiographic abnormality, is particularly concerning because it appears to precede ventricular arrhythmias and sudden death in patients hospitalized with AN (Isner, Roberts, Heymsfield, & Yager, 1985). A mild to moderate pericardial effusion (fluid around the heart) that is clinically silent, has been reported in 60% to 70% of patients with AN (Ramacciotti, Coli, Biadi, & Dell'Osso, 2003; Silverman & Krongrad, 1983; Silvetti et al., 1998). Congestive heart failure does not usually occur in the starvation phase and is more likely to occur during refeeding (Powers, 1982).

Bloating and constipation are frequent complaints of patients with AN and reflect delayed gastric emptying and decreased intestinal motility. Liver enzyme levels are elevated in 4% to 38% of patients (Mickley, Greenfeld, Quinlan, Roloff, & Zwas, 1996; Palla & Litt, 1988; Sherman, Leslie, Goldberg, Rybczynski, & St. Louis, 1994). Liver enzyme elevations are usually mild, most frequently are present before refeeding has been initiated, and usually respond to nutritional rehabilitation (Narayanan, Gaudiani, Harris, & Mehler, 2010; Rautou et al., 2008). On occasion, they can be aggravated by refeeding. Acute liver failure can occur but is rare (De Caprio et al., 2006; Furuta et al., 1999). Cholesterol levels may be high but most frequently are normal (Arden, Weiselberg, Nussbaum, Shenker, & Jacobson, 1990; Boland, Beguin, Zech, Desager, & Lambert, 2001; Mehler, Lezotte, & Eckel, 1998). Serum carotene levels may be elevated in 13% to 62% of cases and may lead to a yellowish discoloration of the skin (Boland et al., 2001; Sherman et al., 1994). The cause of the high serum carotene levels is not clear but is thought to be a combination of increased dietary intake of pigmented vegetables such as carrots and derangements of hepatic conversion of beta-carotene to vitamin A. In contrast to other forms of malnutrition, serum albumin levels are usually normal. Rapid weight loss is associated with gallstone formation. With malnutrition, metabolic rate slows as an adaptive response to starvation. In AN, measured resting energy expenditure may be 65% to 70% of predicted values (Schebendach et al., 1995), and consequently, caloric requirements are lower in the malnourished state. With nutritional rehabilitation, metabolic recovery occurs over a 4- to 6-week period and caloric requirements increase dramatically (Schebendach, Golden, Jacobson, Hertz, & Shenker, 1997).

Suppression of the bone marrow occurs frequently in AN, resulting in low white blood cell, red blood cell, and platelet counts (Misra et al., 2004). Leukopenia (low white blood cell count) has been reported in one third to two thirds of patients with AN and is thought to be secondary to bone marrow suppression (Palla & Litt, 1988; Sharp & Freeman, 1993). Despite the low white blood cell count, there does not appear to be an increased risk of infection. Once a bacterial infection is present, however, low complement levels may prolong the course of the infection. All hematological abnormalities are reversed with nutritional rehabilitation.

The major neurological complications of eating disorders are seizures and structural brain changes, found on computed tomography and magnetic resonance imaging scans (Enzmann & Lane, 1977; Golden et al., 1996; Katzman et al., 1996; Nussbaum, Shenker, Marc, & Klein, 1980). Muscle weakness and a peripheral neuropathy can also occur. Neuropsychological testing notes impairments of attention, concentration, and memory, with deficits in visuospatial ability (Kingston, Szmukler, Andrewes, Tress, & Desmond, 1996). While the ventricular enlargement and white matter changes revert to normal after weight restoration (Golden et al., 1996; Katzman, Zipursky, Lambe, & Mikulis, 1997), the gray matter volume deficits and regional blood flow disturbances may persist, suggesting that these changes may predate the illness (Golden et al., 1996; Gordon, Lask, Bryant-Waugh, Christie, & Timimi, 1997; Katzman et al., 1997). Similarly, some, but not all, of the cognitive deficits improve with weight restoration (Kingston et al., 1996).

Adolescents who develop AN prior to the completion of growth can exhibit growth retardation and short stature. Patients are shorter than expected (Nussbaum, Baird, Sonnenblick, Cowan, & Shenker, 1985), and growth stunting may even be the presenting feature (Modan-Moses et al., 2003; Root & Powers, 1983). Growth retardation is more likely to occur in adolescent boys because boys grow, on average, for 2 years longer than girls. In girls, growth is almost complete by menarche, which occurs at an average age of 12.4 years in the United States (Chumlea et al., 2003). Catch-up growth can occur with nutritional rehabilitation; even with intervention, however, these adolescents may not reach their genetic height potential (Lantzouni, Frank, Golden, & Shenker, 2002).

Hypothalamic dysfunction is evidenced by amenorrhea (loss of menses) as well as disturbances in satiety, difficulties with temperature regulation, and ability to concentrate urine (Mecklenberg et al., 1976). There is activation of the hypothalamic–pituitary–adrenal axis with elevated levels of serum cortisol. Clinically, patients with AN have symptoms that look very much like those seen in hypothyroidism (dry yellow skin, low heart rate, low metabolic rate, amenorrhea, and constipation). Disturbances in thyroid function tests resolve with improved nutrition and should not be treated with thyroid hormone replacement.

Pubertal delay is frequently found among patients who develop AN prior to the completion of puberty (Palla & Litt, 1988; Russell, 1985). Amenorrhea occurs as a result of suppression of the hypothalamic–pituitary–ovarian axis secondary to an energy deficit associated with poor nutritional intake and excessive exercise. Levels of pituitary and ovarian hormones controlling menstruation are all low, and the uterus and ovaries shrink (Golden & Shenker, 1992). In most instances, amenorrhea is associated with weight loss, but in approximately 20% of cases, loss of menses may precede significant weight loss (Golden et al., 1997). Weight gain is usually accompanied by restoration of normal hypothalamic–pituitary–ovarian function and resumption of spontaneous menses, but in many cases, amenorrhea may be prolonged.

Provided weight is restored and menses are regular, the ability to conceive should be normal. Persistence of low body weight and weight-control behaviors, however, may be associated with infertility (Bates, Bates, & Whitworth, 1982). Women with a past history of AN have similar pregnancy rates and are no more likely to have received treatment for infertility than healthy controls, but they are more likely to have a miscarriage, presumably because of continuation of inappropriate weight-control behaviors during pregnancy (Bulik et al., 1999). Although the majority of women with eating disorders have positive pregnancy outcomes, some studies have demonstrated an increased risk of birth by cesarean section (Bulik et al., 2009; Franko et al., 2001) and higher rates of preterm delivery and low birth weight (Micali, Simonoff & Treasure, 2007; Sollid, Wisborg, Hjort, Secher, 2004).

Osteoporosis is a serious long-term medical complication of AN (Golden, 2010). Bone formation is impaired and bone resorption is increased, resulting in net reduction in bone mineral density (BMD) and increased fracture risk. Compared to controls, fracture risk is estimated to be increased twofold to threefold in women who have previously had AN (Lucas, Melton, Crowson & O'Fallon, 1999; Vestergaard et al., 2002). BMD reduction may occur after a relatively short duration of illness, and those who develop AN prior to menarche have lower BMD than those who develop it after menarche

(Bachrach, Guido, Katzman, Litt, & Marcus, 1990; Golden et al., 2002; Grinspoon et al., 2000). Contributing factors include poor nutrition, low body weight, estrogen deficiency, excessive exercise, and high levels of cortisol in the bloodstream. In women, the degree of BMD reduction in AN is more severe than that seen in women with other conditions associated with amenorrhea and a low estrogen state, suggesting that, in addition to estrogen deficiency, nutritional factors play an important role (Grinspoon et al., 1999). Low BMD is also found in males with AN and is associated with low testosterone levels (Andersen, Watson, & Schlechte, 2000; Mehler, Sabel, Watson, & Anderson, 2008; Misra, Katzman, et al., 2008).

Adolescence is a critical time for bone mass acquisition: approximately 60% of peak bone mass is accrued during the adolescent years, and there is very little net gain in bone mass after 2 years following menarche (Bonjour, Theintz, Buchs, Slosman, & Rizzoli, 1991; Golden & Shenker, 1992; Katzman et al., 1991; Theintz et al., 1992). Whether or not a young woman will develop osteoporosis in later life depends not only on the rate of bone loss in adulthood, but also on the amount of bone present at skeletal maturity, often referred to as "peak bone mass." Multiple studies have shown that peak bone mass is achieved toward the end of the second decade of life (Bonjour et al., 1991; Faulkner et al., 1996; Katzman et al., 1991; Southard et al., 1991). A woman who develops AN during adolescence will not reach peak bone mass, placing her at increased risk of developing fractures, and since she has a lower peak bone mass, the increased fracture risk may persist for years after recovery from AN. More than 90% of adolescents and young adults with AN have reduced BMD at one or more skeletal sites (Grinspoon et al., 2000). Both intermediate (Bachrach, Katzman, Litt, Guido, & Marcus, 1991; Golden et al., 2002; Rigotti, Neer, Skates, Herzog, & Nussbaum, 1991; Soyka et al., 2002) and long-term studies (Hartman et al., 2000; Herzog, Minne, et al., 1993; Ward, Brown & Treasure, 1997) have demonstrated that BMD reduction is persistent and may be irreversible despite full recovery from the eating disorder. In women recovered from AN for an average of 21 years, hip BMD remained lower than in controls, and a relatively high percentage of patients reported a history of pathological bone fractures (Hartman et al., 2000). Weight gain is associated with some BMD improvement, but levels do not return to normal (Bachrach et al., 1991; Golden et al., 2005; Misra, Prabhakaran, et al., 2008).

Medical Complications of Bulimia Nervosa

Patients with BN can have large fluctuations in body weight, reflecting cycles of dehydration, electrolyte disturbances, and water retention associated with vomiting and abuse of laxatives and diuretics. Massive swelling of the hands and feet can occur among those who abruptly discontinue the use of laxatives or diuretics. Examination of the hands may reveal calluses or scars over the knuckles or skin of the dominant hand (Russell's sign), caused by abrasions by the teeth during self-induced vomiting.

Hypokalemia, a reduced level of potassium in the blood, is the most frequently found significant electrolyte disturbance in patients who vomit or use laxatives or diuretics. Hypokalemia can be associated with life-threatening cardiac arrhythmias, and a low serum potassium level should be carefully corrected. Periods of caloric restriction result in episodes of bradycardia and vital sign instability, though not to the same degree as that seen in patients with AN.

Ipecac, a medication used to induce vomiting after accidental poisoning, is abused by some patients with BN. Ipecac contains the alkaloid emetine, which is toxic to both skeletal and cardiac muscle; excessive intake may cause muscle weakness, congestive heart failure, and cardiac arrest. Ipecac use is cumulative, and ipecac abuse can be a cause of sudden death among adolescents with BN (Schiff et al., 1986).

Enlargement of the parotid and salivary glands occurs in 10% to 30% of patients with BN and is thought to be secondary to binge eating and vomiting (Ogren, Huerter, Pearson, Antonson, & Moore, 1987). Erosion of the dental enamel is most evident on the lingual aspects of the anterior teeth and is caused by exposure to gastric acid while vomiting. Recurrent vomiting may also lead to gastroesophageal reflux, esophagitis, tears of the esophagus, and, less frequently, esophageal rupture. Small tears may be evidenced by bloodstained vomitus. Esophageal rupture is a catastrophic event and is usually fatal. Esophagitis is associated with epigastric or retrosternal chest pain and warrants treatment. Chronic exposure of the distal esophagus to acidic stomach contents can lead to precancerous changes in the mucosal lining of the esophagus, known as Barrett's esophagus.

Patients with BN with a prior history of AN or amenorrhea may have reduced BMD, though not to the same degree as those with active AN (Naessen, Carlstrom, Glant, Jacobsson, & Hirschberg, 2006).

TREATMENT OF MEDICAL COMPLICATIONS

The goals of medical management of patients with eating disorders are threefold: acute medical stabilization, normalization of eating, and reversal of medical complications. In AN, weight restoration is an important early goal of treatment and is usually associated with improvements in mood and eating disorder symptoms.

Refeeding in Anorexia Nervosa

The greatest risk of cardiac decompensation and electrolyte disturbances occurs during the refeeding phase, in particular during the first 7 to 10 days of refeeding. It is during this time when the "refeeding syndrome," a constellation of cardiac, neurological, and hematological complications, is most likely to occur. The refeeding syndrome can occur after intravenous, nasogastric, or oral refeeding. Hypophosphatemia is a hallmark of this syndrome and occurs in over one quarter of adolescents hospitalized with AN (Ornstein, Golden, Jacobson, & Shenker, 2003). Hypophosphatemia is more likely to occur in those who are severely malnourished (<70% of expected body weight) and may predispose patients to ventricular arrhythmias and sudden death.

The refeeding syndrome can be prevented by monitoring heart rate and serum electrolytes (especially phosphorus) during the first 7 to 10 days of treatment. Some authorities (American Dietetic Association, 2006; American Psychiatric Association, 2006; National Institute for Clinical Excellence, 2006) have recommended slow advancement in caloric intake as a measure to prevent the refeeding syndrome, but there is limited evidence to support this recommendation. Hypocaloric diets are associated with initial weight loss (Garber, Michihata, Hetnal, Shafer, & Moscicki, 2012; Solanto, Jacobson, Heller, Golden & Hertz, 1994) and prolonged hospitalization (Garber et al., 2012). Recent studies have demonstrated that more aggressive regimens, starting patients on 1,400 to 2,000 kcals/day, are safe on units where cardiac monitoring is performed to detect cardiac arrhythmias and electrolytes are frequently checked (Gentile, Pastorelli, Ciceri, Manna, & Collimedaglia, 2010; Golden, Keane-Miller, Sainani, & Kapphahn, 2013; Whitelaw, Gilbertson, Lam, & Sawyer, 2010). Because of the metabolic effects of carbohydrates on insulin secretion and cellular phosphorus uptake, the macronutrient composition of the diet, specifically the carbohydrate content, may be more important in the genesis of the refeeding syndrome than total number of calories prescribed (Kohn, Madden & Clarke, 2011).

The caloric requirements of children and adolescents with AN are usually higher than for adults, and may reach 3,000 to 4,500 kcals/day. The rate of weight gain should be 2 to 3 pounds per week for inpatient programs, 1 to 2 pounds per week for partial hospitalization programs (when such programs are stepdown programs from inpatient units), and 0.5 to 1 pound per week for outpatient management (Yager, Anderson, & Devlin, 2000).

Treatment of Osteoporosis in Anorexia Nervosa

Few controlled trials have evaluated the treatment of reduced bone mass in AN, fewer specifically focused on adolescents, and most studies enrolled only a modest number of subjects.

Therefore, the preferred treatment of AN-related osteoporosis is unknown.

Calcium supplementation is known to improve bone mass in healthy adolescents (Cadogan, Eastell, Jones, & Barker, 1997; Johnston et al., 1992; Lloyd et al., 1993) and in postmenopausal women with osteoporosis (Reid, Ames, Evans, Gamble, & Sharpe, 1995), but no randomized controlled trials have documented the impact of calcium supplementation on BMD in AN. The Institute of Medicine (2011) recommends a dietary intake of 1,300 mg/day of calcium for healthy girls ages 9 to 18 years, and most authorities recommend calcium supplementation (1,000–1,200 mg/day of elemental calcium) for those patients with AN whose dietary intake contains less than the recommended amount.

Vitamin D, a fat-soluble vitamin that is often deficient in the diets of those with eating disorders, is necessary for absorption and utilization of calcium. Vitamin D supplementation increases bone mineral accretion in a dose-dependent manner in adolescent girls (Viljakainen et al., 2006). The American Academy of Pediatrics (2014) now recommends a daily intake of 600 IU vitamin D for adolescents to optimize bone health. Once again, no randomized controlled trials have studied the efficacy of vitamin D supplementation to increase BMD for adolescents with AN. Most authorities recommend supplementation with at least 600 IU vitamin D per day. Patients found to be deficient in vitamin D should be treated with vitamin D2 or D3, 50,000 IU weekly for 6 to 8 weeks, followed by a maintenance dose of 600 to 1,000 IU daily (American Academy of Pediatrics, 2014).

A number of studies have shown that body weight, and in particular lean body mass, is a significant determinant of BMD in healthy subjects (Glastre et al., 1990; Henderson, Price, Cole, Gutteridge, & Bhagat, 1995; Southard et al., 1991) and in those with AN (Bachrach et al., 1990; Goebel, Schweiger, Kruger, & Fichter, 1999; Golden et al., 2002; Gordon et al., 2002; Grinspoon et al., 1999; Soyka et al., 2002). While BMD increases with weight gain, even with weight restoration, reduced bone mass is not entirely reversible (Bachrach et al., 1991; Golden et al., 2002; Hartman et al., 2000; Rigotti et al., 1991). One study of adolescent girls with AN found that weight gain and resumption of menses was associated with arrest of the BMD decline, but lack of weight gain was associated with continued BMD decline. Girls who gained weight but did not resume menses had similar BMD to those who did not gain weight (Misra, Prabhakaran, et al., 2008).

Both weight-bearing and resistance exercise programs increase the spine BMD in children and young women (McKay et al., 2000; Snow-Harter, Bouxsein, Lewis, Carter, & Marcus, 1992), and, in AN, even 5 days of bed rest is accompanied by a reduction in markers of bone formation (DiVasta, Feldman, Quach, Balestrino, & Gordon, 2009). Exercise programs for patients with AN have not been studied. Excessive exercise, commonly used by patients with AN to control weight, could interfere with weight gain and produce amenorrhea. Therefore, any exercise should be undertaken cautiously.

Hormone replacement therapy is frequently prescribed to treat reduced BMD in adolescents with AN (Robinson, Bachrach, & Katzman, 2000) on the assumption that estrogen deficiency contributes to the bone loss. There is no evidence that oral contraceptives increase BMD in either adult (Klibanski, Biller, Schoenfeld, Herzog, & Saxe, 1995) or adolescent (Golden et al., 2002; Strokosch, Friedman, Wu, Kamin, 2006) females with AN, and oral contraceptives should not be prescribed for this purpose. Furthermore, oral contraceptives cause exogenously induced monthly menstrual bleeding even at a low weight, which may incorrectly be interpreted as indicative of adequate weight restoration. Studies investigating the use of IGF-1 (Grinspoon et al., 1996; Grinspoon, Thomas, Miller, Herzog, & Klibanski, 2002), DHEA (Gordon et al., 1999; Gordon, Grace, et al., 2002), and the bisphosphonates (Golden et al., 2005; Miller et al., 2004, 2011) have proved disappointing.

Current treatment recommendations focus on weight restoration with resumption of spontaneous menses, calcium supplementation

(1,000–1200 mg elemental calcium /day), vitamin D supplementation (600 IU/day), and carefully monitored weight-bearing exercise (Golden, 2010).

Treatment to Goal Weight for Adolescents with Anorexia Nervosa

Treatment goal weight should be individualized, taking into account pubertal stage, prior growth percentiles, height, and age. For adolescents, the treatment goal weight is a "moving target," and normal growth and development necessitates a recalculation of this number every 3 to 6 months. Height and weight tables used for adults are inappropriate for adolescents. The Centers for Disease Control and Prevention growth charts (available at cdc.gov/growthcharts) provide a useful resource of normative height and weight data for children and adolescents in the United States; however, the tables provide only normative weight and BMI data, not specific guidance for what is an "ideal body weight." Absolute BMI values should not be used in children and adolescents. For example, a BMI of 17.5 would be on the third percentile for a 19-year-old but on the 50th percentile for an 11-year-old.

Treatment goal weight should be the weight at which normal physical and sexual development occurs, and for girls, the weight at which menstruation and ovulation are restored. In postmenarcheal adolescent girls, 86% of patients resumed menses within 6 months of achieving a weight at or above 90% of median weight for age and height (Golden et al, 1997). However, there was wide variability, with some subjects resuming menses at a lower weight and others doing so at a higher weight. When using the CDC growth charts to calculate expected body weight (expected body weight in kilograms = median BMI times height in meters squared), 90% of median weight for age and height corresponds to a weight approximately 95% of expected body weight (Golden, Yang, Jacobson, Robinson, & Shaw, 2012). For those who were previously overweight, treatment goal weight may need to be higher. In a premenarcheal girl or an adolescent boy whose growth and development are not yet complete, treatment goal weight should be 100% of expected body weight in order to maximize growth potential. It is preferable to provide a weight range for treatment goal weight, with a clear message that this range will change with growth and development. This is done in order to avoid focusing on a single weight and to acknowledge that there are daily fluctuations in weight as well as expectations that both height and weight will change as puberty progresses.

Once an individualized treatment goal weight range is reached, serial estradiol levels or pelvic ultrasonography can be used to assess restoration of normal hypothalamic–pituitary–ovarian function and readiness for spontaneous resumption of menses. A serum estradiol level above 30 pg/mL is predictive of resumption of menses within 3 to 6 months (relative risk 4.6, confidence interval 1.9–11.2) (Golden et al., 1997). One clinical approach is to aim for weight maintenance in the treatment goal weight range for 3 months. If after 3 months the patient remains amenorrheic, a serum estradiol level can be measured. If the level is above 30 pg/mL, the patient can wait a further 3 months at that weight in anticipation of resumption of menses. An estradiol level below 30 pg/mL indicates that the treatment goal weight needs to be higher and the patient needs to gain further weight. Another approach is to use serial pelvic ultrasound scans to assess ovarian and uterine maturity to provide an individualized weight when reproductive maturity has been achieved or restored (Allan et al., 2010; Key, Mason, Allan, & Lask, 2001; Lai, De Bruyn, Lask, Bryant-Waugh, & Hankins, 1994; Sobanski, Hiltmann, Blanz, Klein, & Schmidt, 1997; Treasure, Wheeler, King, Gordon, & Russell, 1988).

Summary

Most of the medical consequences of eating disorders are secondary to malnutrition and/or purging and are reversible with nutritional rehabilitation and interruption of binge/purge activity (Table 13.2 provides a summary). Heart rate returns to normal after approximately 12 days, vital sign instability resolves after approximately 2 to 3 weeks, and resting energy expenditure increases slowly and normalizes after approximately 6 weeks (Schebendach et al., 1997; Shamim et al., 2003). The amount of time needed for weight gain varies, and resumption of menses usually occurs within 3 to 6 months after achieving treatment goal weight. Difficulties with body image distortion and preoccupation with weight and shape, however, may take longer to resolve. While most of the medical complications are reversible with weight restoration, growth retardation, reduced BMD, and, possibly, structural brain changes may not be entirely reversible.

Treatment of Eating Disorders

Evelyn Attia
Anne E. Becker
Cynthia M. Bulik
Alison E. Field
Neville H. Golden
Richard E. Kreipe
Daniel Le Grange
James E. Mitchell
Kathleen M. Pike
Robyn Sysko
C. Barr Taylor
B. Timothy Walsh

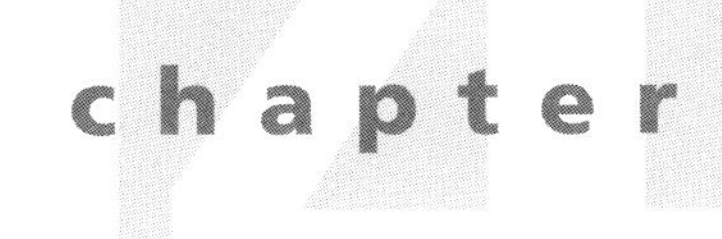

14

OVERVIEW

Treatment efficacy is most definitively established using randomized controlled trials (RCTs); unfortunately, only a handful of relatively small RCTs focusing on adolescents with eating disorders have been conducted. Although some additional studies have been published since the first edition of this book, much is still unknown about the utility of different treatment modalities for adolescents. The evaluation and the recommendations described in this chapter are derived from the following sources: (1) RCTs conducted with adolescent samples and (2) extrapolation from evidence-based treatments for eating disorders in adults.

PSYCHOLOGICAL TREATMENTS

Adolescents with Anorexia Nervosa

Although the peak onset of anorexia nervosa (AN) occurs during adolescence (Hoek & van Hoeken, 2003), to date only seven RCTs focused on this population have been published. As described below, most of these studies have examined the utility of familial involvement in the treatment of adolescents with AN. Given the morbidity and mortality associated with AN (e.g., Bulik, Berkman, Brownley, Sedway & Lohr, 2007), there is a clear need for additional empirical examination of treatment efficacy in this age group. This section first presents a description of the content of family and individual treatment modalities and subsequently details the methods and results of the seven RCTs for adolescents with AN.

Family and Individual Treatments

Family therapy for adolescents with AN, sometimes referred to as the "Maudsley Approach," was first developed in the 1980s at the Maudsley Hospital in London. Following this work, behavioral family systems therapy, a close relative of family therapy for adolescent AN (Robin & Le Grange, 2010), was used in an RCT by Robin et al. (1999). More recently, this treatment modality was formally manualized, given the name "family-based treatment," and articulated in a guide for clinicians (Lock et al., 2001; Lock & Le Grange, 2013). The main focus of family-based treatment is putting the parents in charge of their child's weight restoration, before eventually returning control over eating back to the adolescent. Adolescent development is promoted, but only once the prominence of the eating disorder has receded. Family-based treatment proceeds through three clearly defined stages:

1. The parents are guided by the therapist to support their child's nutritional rehabilitation.
2. Once the adolescent approaches a healthier weight (~90% expected body weight), and the impact of the eating disorder begins to recede, the therapist supports the parents to carefully return control over eating to the adolescent.
3. With the eating disorder largely in the background, the therapist engages the family in discussions about adolescent development. The tenor of this discussion is based on the adolescent's age and the extent to which the eating disorder has interrupted his or her adolescent developmental process.

Adolescent-focused therapy (Fitzpatrick, Moye, Hoste, Lock, & Le Grange, 2010; initially called ego-oriented individual therapy; Robin et al., 1999) is a primarily individual treatment for adolescents with AN, although the parents also have a role in their child's treatment. As described in its manualized form, this therapy is conducted in 32 treatment sessions over 12 months, with each session lasting about 45 minutes. During this course of treatment, the therapist conducts about eight to 10 collateral sessions with the parents (without the adolescent), typically on a bimonthly basis, to update them on the progress in treatment, provide psychoeducation, and encourage parents to be supportive, nonjudgmental, and empathic of their teen's struggles. In the individual sessions with the adolescent, the therapist focuses mainly on supporting the patient's ego strength, self-efficacy, coping skills, and individuation from the family. In addition, the therapist also reviews more general issues regarding social, physical, and emotional development and helps the adolescent consider how these relate to eating, weight expectations, and body image. The therapist's stance is nurturing but also authoritative: the therapist shows respect toward the adolescent's autonomy, but at the same time expresses understanding that the adolescent's attempts at establishing autonomy are at the center of his or her struggle with the eating disorder. The therapist supports the adolescent to identify common daily life issues that present as obstacles in the adolescent's path to lead a healthy life and encourages the adolescent to find solutions other than dieting to address these issues. Adolescent-focused treatment progresses through three phases:

1. The first phase focuses on developing rapport and identifying the adolescent's psychological issues and how the eating disorder serves as a coping strategy to manage these issues.
2. The second phase provides the platform for exploring the various issues identified in the first phase of the treatment.
3. The third phase serves to prepare the patient with coping strategies for typical adolescent issues and to encourage age-appropriate behaviors and strategies toward independence.

The pediatrician or adolescent medicine physician plays a key role in the treatment of adolescents with eating disorders, regardless of treatment modality. In family-based treatment, for instance, the pediatrician serves as a consultant to the parents and the primary therapist. In this role, the pediatrician provides a regular medical assessment and treatment as indicated, and provides guidance and support to the parents and adolescent in a way that supports this treatment. For a detailed description of the role of the pediatrician, see Katzman, Peebles, Sawyer, Lock, and Le Grange (2013).

Clinical Trials

The first RCT for AN (Russell, Szmukler, Dare, & Eisler, 1987) included 80 patients discharged from the inpatient service after an average of 10 weeks of nutritional rehabilitation. During the inpatient stay, participants reached an average of 89.5% of expected body weight and were randomized to either outpatient family therapy or individual supportive therapy. The main findings of interest pertain to a subgroup of adolescents with AN with an age of onset less than 18 years of age who were ill less than 3 years (n = 21), where family therapy significantly outperformed individual supportive therapy after 1 year of outpatient treatment in terms of weight maintenance, nutritional status, menstrual function, psychosexual adjustment, and socioeconomic status. Although the sample size was modest, a strength of this study was the 5-year follow-up of all 80 patients (Eisler, Dare, Russel, Szmukler, Le Grange, & Dodge, 1997). The benefits of family therapy at the end of 12 months of outpatient treatment were maintained at 5-year follow-up for 90% of patients in the subgroup characterized by an earlier age of onset and shorter duration of illness. In contrast, 50% of patients in the subgroup who received individual supportive therapy still presented with significant eating disorder symptoms 5 years later.

Following this initial work, the Maudsley team conducted a pilot study (n = 18) comparing two forms of family therapy: conjoint (family seen together) or separated (adolescent and parents seen separately) family therapy (Le Grange, Eisler, Dare, & Russell, 1992a). Unlike the first study (Eisler et al., 1997; Russell et al., 1987), all patients were treated on an outpatient basis. After approximately 6 months of treatment, both therapies produced positive outcomes and appeared to be effective for short-term reductions in AN symptoms. This study identified an important effect of parental criticism of the ill adolescent as measured by Expressed Emotion (Vaughn & Leff, 1976). While no differences in overall levels of this characteristic were noted between the two treatment groups, families with high Expressed Emotion at the beginning of treatment were more likely to drop out, or, if they stayed in treatment, to do more poorly than families with low baseline levels of Expressed Emotion (Le Grange, Eisler, Dare, & Hodes, 1992b).

This study was extended by comparing the same two forms of family therapy in a larger outpatient sample of adolescents with AN (n = 40; Eisler, Dare, Hodes, Russell, Dodge, & Le Grange, 2000). Treatment assignment for this study was stratified by the number of critical comments made by the parents toward the patient. At the end of treatment, patients in both forms of family therapy made significant gains across nutritional and psychological domains, with no differences between the treatment groups. However, there was a significant difference between treatments when baseline Expressed Emotion was considered. Adolescents from high Expressed Emotion families fared better with separated, versus conjoined, family therapy, whereas the outcomes of those from families with low Expressed Emotion were comparable. Similarly, adolescents from families with high Expressed Emotion treated with separated family therapy demonstrated additional weight gain over a 5-year follow-up, while those treated with conjoined treatment did not (Eisler, Simic, Russell, & Dare, 2007).

Taken together, these studies suggest that family therapy is effective for adolescent AN, and that most patients remain well long after they have received this intervention.

Subsequently, Robin et al. (1999) randomized 37 participants to behavioral family systems therapy, a treatment similar to the intervention in the aforementioned studies, or ego-orientated individual therapy (later referred to as adolescent-focused therapy), which is perhaps more psychodynamically informed than the individual supportive therapy used in other research. Findings were mixed. In comparison to individual therapy, behavioral family systems therapy produced significantly greater changes in BMI percentile, and significantly more patients resumed menstruating (89% vs. 60%). However, on secondary outcome measures (eating-related and general psychopathology, family functioning), both treatments produced comparable improvements. The authors concluded that both treatments were effective for adolescents with AN, although family therapy was perhaps more efficient in terms of weight gain.

The publication of a manual of family therapy for adolescent AN (Lock & Le Grange, 2001) facilitated use of this treatment by providing a detailed description of this approach (Lock & Le Grange, 2013; Lock, Le Grange, Agras, & Dare, 2001). The first study using the manual compared two doses of family-based treatment (Lock, Agras, Bryson, & Kraemer, 2005). A total of 86 adolescents with AN were randomized to either short-term (10 sessions over 6 months) or long-term family-based treatment (20 sessions over 12 months). At the end of treatment, no differences were found between forms of family-based treatment, with weight gain averaging in excess of 6 pounds. Longer-term treatment did, however, produce better outcomes on one measure of eating disorder symptoms. Two preliminary treatment moderators were identified, suggesting that most adolescents with AN could be treated with the short version of family-based treatment, while those with more severe and persistent eating-related obsessive-compulsive thinking or from single-parent families benefited more from a longer version of family-based treatment. A 4-year follow-up assessment confirmed that the short course of family-based treatment is as effective as the longer course (Lock, Courturier, & Agras, 2006).

The largest RCT for adolescents, and the first to test the efficacy of treatment intensity, randomized 167 adolescents to inpatient treatment, specialist outpatient individual treatment (cognitive-behavioral therapy [CBT]), and treatment as usual (Gowers et al., 2007). Weight gain and improvements in self-reported psychopathology were evident across all three treatment groups, and about 25% of patients had a good outcome using the Morgan-Russell Assessment Schedule. Outcome improved at the 2-year follow-up, with one third of patients, regardless of treatment group, categorized with a good outcome. Still, close to 30% had a poor outcome and still met criteria for AN, suggesting that inpatient management did not provide any advantage over outpatient treatment.

In another large published controlled trial (n = 121), adolescents were randomized to family-based treatment or adolescent-focused therapy (ego-orientated individual therapy; Lock, Le Grange, Agras, Moye, Bryson, & Jo, 2010). Unlike other trials, the definition of recovery required a weight of more than 95% expected body weight plus a score on a global measure of eating disorder psychopathology within 1 standard deviation of published normative means. While no differences between the treatments were noted in terms of full remission at the end of treatment, significantly more patients were remitted in family-based treatment at both 6-month follow-up (40% vs. 18%) and 12-month follow-up (49% vs. 23%). Family-based treatment showed significantly greater improvement at the end of treatment (89%) compared to adolescent-focused therapy (67%) using the criteria for partial remission by the Morgan-Russell categories (weight >85% expected body weight plus menses) but failed to reach significance at the two follow-up time points. These results provide strong evidence for the efficacy of family-based treatment as a first-line outpatient treatment for medically stable adolescents with AN.

A recent Australian study compared parent-focused treatment and family-based treatment for adolescents aged 12 to 18 years with DSM-IV or partial AN (N = 107) (Le Grange et al., 2016). Parent-focused treatment does not require the involvement of the whole family, the family meal is omitted, and the clinician focuses on the parents for the full 50-minute session. In this study, the primary outcome was remission, or more than 95% of median BMI and Eating Disorder Examination Global Score within 1 standard deviation of community norms. At the end of treatment, a higher rate of remission was observed with parent-focused treatment (43%) in comparison to family-based treatment (22%), but statistically significant differences were not noted between the interventions at the two follow-up assessments (6 or 12 months posttreatment). Given the reduced therapist burden and efficacy data, parent-focused therapy may be a more "user friendly" version of family therapy for adolescents with broadly defined AN, thereby facilitating access to this treatment and dissemination.

Secondary analyses of the previously described trials suggest mechanisms for family-based treatment. Using data from 121 patients receiving family-based treatment or adolescent-focused therapy (Lock et al., 2010), two moderators of outcome at the end of treatment were identified: eating-related obsessionality (Yale-Brown-Cornell Eating Disorder Total Scale) and eating disorder–specific psychopathology (EDE-Global; Le Grange, Lock, Agras, Moye, Bryson, Jo, & Kreamer, 2012). Participants with higher baseline scores on these measures benefited more from family-based treatment than adolescent-focused therapy. While the binge-eating/purging type of AN was also found to respond less well than the restricting type, this moderator was much less robust given the relatively small number of binge-eating/purging type patients with AN in this sample. Taken together, these findings highlight that better outcomes are achieved for patients with more severe eating-related psychopathology with family-based treatment, which allows the parents to target the behavioral symptoms in comparison to adolescent-focused therapy, an individual approach.

Evaluation of Research

Some progress has been made in the past 25 years in testing psychological treatments for adolescents with AN, although the work has focused on extending studies from the original trials at the Maudsley Hospital. Taken together, the following conclusions can be offered on the basis of empirical evidence from controlled trials and clinical experience:

1. Family-based treatment is effective for medically stable adolescents with AN, especially for those with a short duration of illness.
2. Benefits of family-based treatment appear to be well maintained at long-term follow-up.

3. Adolescent-focused therapy may be a credible alternative if the family is unable or unwilling to participate in family-based interventions.
4. Inpatient treatment is critical for medical stabilization but may not be needed for complete weight restoration in younger patients.

The available studies are informative, but controlled studies are few, and many are hampered by significant methodological limitations (e.g., modest sample size; Le Grange & Lock, 2005). Thus, there is a need for replication with larger sample sizes for greater confidence in the findings of the trials. We do not yet know what to do when families are unable to implement or do not respond to family-based treatment; more definitive studies of moderators and mediators of treatment outcome are needed; and the benefit of other treatments, such as enhanced CBT (CBT-E), is unknown (cf. Dalle Grave, Calugi, Doll, & Fairburn, 2013). The need for larger, better controlled, systematic studies in adolescents is clear; without them, clinical guidance for best care practice remains hampered (Agras et al., 2004).

Several larger studies have begun to examine varying forms of family involvement. The Maudsley group completed a large study comparing multiple-family versus single-family therapy (Eisler, 2010). In New York, family-based therapy has been adapted for subsyndromal AN and tested in a small RCT (Loeb et al., 2012). Six sites in the United States and Canada completed an RCT of family-based versus systemic family treatment (Agras et al., 2013). The results of these studies consistently underscore the importance of family involvement in the treatment of adolescents with AN, although it is not clear there is a single "best" method for doing so.

Summary

Parental involvement appears crucial in outpatient treatment of adolescents with AN. Additional studies are needed and are more completely considered in the final chapter of this section.

Adolescents with Bulimia Nervosa

There are even fewer data evaluating the efficacy of psychological treatments among adolescents with BN, with three published controlled studies, all of which include family-based treatment interventions. In light of the positive effects observed for adolescents with AN (see above), the first trial adapted and evaluated the aforementioned manualized form of family therapy (Le Grange & Lock, 2007). A total of 80 outpatients ages 12 to 19 with a DSM-IV diagnosis of BN or a subthreshold variant received 20 sessions of either family-based treatment (n = 41) or supportive psychotherapy (n = 39) over a 6-month period (Le Grange, Crosby, Rathouz, & Leventhal, 2007). At the end of active treatment, a significantly larger proportion of those receiving family-based treatment were abstinent from binge eating and purging (39%) in comparison to supportive psychotherapy (18%), a directional difference that persisted at the 6-month posttreatment follow-up. Benefits of family-based treatment were also observed on secondary variables (e.g., eating-disordered behaviors and cognitions).

The second trial (Schmidt et al., 2007) also examined family therapy for adolescents with BN and subthreshold BN, and included a group receiving a guided self-help form of CBT, an evidence-based treatment for adults (Wilson & Zandberg, 2012). A total of 85 adolescents participated (n = 41 family-based treatment, 44 = guided self-help). Binge-eating episodes were significantly reduced in the guided self-help group in comparison to family-based treatment, but this difference was not sustained at the 12-month follow-up. Differences between groups were not found for other measures of eating disorder symptoms.

The third study (Le Grange et al., 2015) compared family-based treatment and CBT, adapted for adolescents, among 130 youth ages 12 to 18. At the end of treatment, a significantly higher rate of abstinence from binge eating and purging in the 4 weeks prior to the assessment was observed for family-based therapy (39.4%) in comparison to CBT (19.7%). This difference in favor of family treatment persisted at the

6-month follow-up but was no longer significant at the 12-month follow-up assessment. Family pathology was found to be a significant moderator of treatment: adolescents with lower conflict scores on the Family Environment Scale demonstrated a better response to family-based therapy than CBT, but patients from families with higher levels of conflict showed no difference between the treatments. Thus, as described above with studies of adolescent AN, adolescents with BN from high-conflict families may not be the best match for family-based therapy.

To summarize, based on the available trials, for adolescents with BN, both family-based treatment and guided self-help based on CBT are empirically supported interventions. Additional data are needed to evaluate the utility of other forms of treatment for this population.

Adolescents with Binge-Eating Disorder

At this time, there are no RCTs for the treatment of adolescents with binge-eating disorder (BED). In adults, manual-based CBT and interpersonal psychotherapy are efficacious for the treatment of patients with BED (Wilson, Grilo, & Vitousek, 2007; Wilson, Wilfley, Agras, & Bryson, 2010). Other treatments, including dialectical behavior therapy and guided self-help, may also be useful interventions (Iacovino et al., 2012; Wilson et al., 2010). At this time, it is not known whether any of the data regarding the treatment of adults with BED are applicable to adolescents.

PHARMACOLOGICAL TREATMENTS

With rare exceptions (e.g., Biederman et al., 1985), there are few published RCTs of the efficacy of pharmacological treatment for adolescents with eating disorders. Therefore, information about pharmacological interventions must be adapted from the literature for adults.

Adolescents with Anorexia Nervosa

Significant challenges in conducting medication trials for both adults and adolescents with AN have been described (Halmi et al., 2005; Lock et al., 2012; Norris et al., 2007), and there are currently no empirically supported pharmacological treatments for the acute symptoms of AN in either group. Conceivably, however, as adolescents with AN appear to be more responsive to psychological interventions, pharmacological interventions might be more effective as well.

Antidepressant Medications

Four placebo-controlled trials of antidepressants for underweight individuals with AN have been published (Attia, Haiman, Walsh, & Flater, 1998; Biederman et al., 1985; Halmi, Eckert, LaDu, & Cohen, 1986; Lacey & Crisp, 1980). None of the trials documented more than a slight therapeutic effect. Similarly, a small retrospective study of adolescents found few benefits of adjunctive selective serotonin reuptake inhibitors (SSRIs; fluoxetine, fluvoxamine, or sertraline) during inpatient treatment or at 3 and 6 months following discharge (Holtkamp et al., 2005). Given the evidence of utility of antidepressant medication for conditions with substantial symptomatic overlap with AN, such as major depression and BN, the lack of any significant effect is surprising and raises the theoretical possibility that malnutrition or other physiological disturbances (e.g., alterations in serotonin pathways; Kaye, Fudge, & Paulus, 2009) inherent in AN interfere with the therapeutic action of antidepressant medication.

Atypical Antipsychotic Medications

Two early small placebo-controlled trials of antipsychotic medication found little evidence of efficacy (Vandereycken, 1984; Vandereycken & Pierloot, 1982), but more recently, the atypical antipsychotics have prompted reconsideration of this class of medication as a treatment for acute AN, as many of these drugs are associated with notable weight gain. Several open and a few controlled studies have described improvements associated with adjunctive olanzapine (Barbarich et al., 2004; Boachie, Goldfield, & Spettigue, 2003; Dennis, Le Grange, & Bremer,

2006; Hansen, 1999; Jensen & Mejlhede, 2000; La Via, Gray, & Kaye, 2000; Leggero et al., 2010; Mehler et al., 2001; Mondraty et al., 2005; Powers, Santana, & Bannon, 2002), aripiprazole (Frank, 2016; Trunko, Schwartz, Duvvuri, & Kaye, 2011), quetiapine (alone: Bosanac et al., 2007; Powers, Bannon, Eubanks, & McCormick, 2007; adjunctive: Mehler-Wex, Romanos, Kirchheiner, & Schulze, 2008), or risperidone (Fisman, Steele, Short, Byrne, & Lavallee, 1996; Newman-Toker, 2000) for the treatment of children, adolescents, and adults with AN. Three placebo-controlled RCTs published since the first edition of this book have also suggested the utility of olanzapine for the treatment of adults with AN. Three studies found improvements in obsessionality among patients receiving olanzapine as an adjunctive treatment (Bissada et al., 2008; Brambilla et al., 2007; Marzola et al., 2015), two studies also noted a greater rate of increase in weight with olanzapine (Attia et al., 2011; Bissada et al., 2008), and one trial found that patients receiving olanzapine had an earlier achievement of target BMI (Bissada et al., 2008). A meta-analysis of double-blind RCTs studying individuals less than 19 years of age found positive results for mean weight gain with olanzapine, risperidone, and aripiprazole (Almandil et al., 2013). On the other hand, one pilot placebo-controlled trial of adjunctive olanzapine for adolescents did not find a medication benefit above the improvements noted with standard eating disorder treatment (Kafantaris et al., 2011); similarly, Hagman et al. (2011) found no significant benefit from risperidone versus placebo.

At this time, although these medications have some promise for enhancing weight gain and reducing co-occurring anxiety and depressive symptoms, additional research is needed to evaluate their use among "representative patients" in "high quality randomized-controlled trials" (McKnight & Park, 2010, p. 18).

Other Medications

Zinc deficiency is associated with weight loss, a decrease in appetite, changes in taste perception, amenorrhea, and depression, all symptoms described by patients with AN. This observation, coupled with reports of zinc deficiency associated with AN, prompted several trials of zinc supplementation. While one controlled study in adults found zinc to be associated with an increased rate of weight gain (Birmingham, Goldner, & Bakan, 1994), two other studies of adolescents found no effect (Katz et al., 1987; Lask, Fosson, Rolfe, & Thomas, 1993).

The benefits of lithium for the treatment of bipolar disorder among adults are well established, and, like many antipsychotic medications, the use of lithium is often associated with weight gain. These considerations prompted a single controlled trial of lithium among inpatients with AN, but it provided little support for the utility of this agent (Gross, Ebert, Faden, Goldberg, Nee, & Kaye, 1981).

Adolescents with Bulimia Nervosa

Antidepressant Medications

Virtually every class of antidepressant medication has been studied in placebo-controlled double-blind trials for adult patients with BN. Antidepressant medications, including both tricyclic antidepressants and SSRIs, appear to have approximately equal efficacy in the acute treatment of BN; however, because SSRIs are generally better tolerated and have fewer side effects (Golden & Attia, 2011), they are the pharmacological treatment of choice for adults with BN. The SSRI fluoxetine is the only drug approved by the U.S. Food and Drug Administration for the treatment of BN. It is most effective at a dose of 60 mg/day, significantly higher than the 20 mg/day typically used to treat major depression. No pretreatment characteristics predict response to pharmacotherapy among patients with BN, but by the third week of treatment, eventual nonresponders to fluoxetine can be reliably identified, making early response one of the only indicators available to guide clinical management (Sysko et al., 2010). One open trial suggests that fluoxetine at this dose is well tolerated and may be useful for adolescents with BN (Kotler, Devlin, Davies, & Walsh, 2003). Limited controlled data on SSRIs other than fluoxetine in the treatment of BN are available for adults, and some of the existing studies note benefits (fluvoxamine: Milano, Siano, Putrella, & Capasso, 2005; sertraline: Milano, Petrella, Sabatino, & Capasso, 2004) while others have failed to identify significant reductions in binge eating and vomiting (fluvoxamine: Schmidt et al., 2004; citalopram: Sundblad, Landén, Eriksson, Bergman, & Eriksson, 2005).

Although wide variability exists across studies, a comprehensive review of RCTs found a reduction in binge eating and vomiting of about 70% and complete abstinence in less than 20% of subjects (Bacaltchuk & Hay, 2003). The mechanism of action of antidepressant medications in BN may be different than in depression, as response to antidepressant drugs in BN is independent of mood state; nondepressed patients with BN respond equally as well as depressed BN patients to these drugs (Hughes, Wells, & Cunningham 1986; Walsh, Hadigan, Devlin, Gladis, & Roose, 1991).

Attrition rates are notable in most studies of medications for BN (Hay & Claudino, 2012), and in clinical practice many patients with eating disorders are reluctant to use medication and a significant number of patients who initiate medication terminate treatment prematurely.

Several studies have examined the effectiveness of a combination of antidepressant pharmacotherapy and psychotherapy (usually CBT) for adults with BN. Two meta-analyses of combined treatments for BN (Bacaltchuk et al., 2001; Nakash-Eisikovits et al., 2002) demonstrated an advantage for combined treatments, but the number of studies available for analysis may not be sufficient to determine whether combination therapy or psychotherapy alone is superior to treatment with antidepressants (Bacaltchuk, Hay, & Trefiglio, 2001).

Other Medications

Other pharmacological agents may also be useful in the treatment of BN. The anticonvulsant topiramate was superior to placebo in two placebo-controlled studies (Hoopes et al., 2003; Nickel et al., 2005). Although these trials were conducted in adults, this medication is approved for the treatment of seizure disorders in patients as young as 2 years. The serotonin antagonist ondansetron, which is used for the treatment of chemotherapy-induced nausea and vomiting, has been found to be of use in the treatment of adults with refractory BN (Faris et al., 2000), and the GABA-b agonist baclofen has been shown to decrease binge-eating episodes in an open trial (Broft et al., 2007). Additional work is required to confirm these preliminary findings and extend them to adolescents.

Adolescents with Binge-Eating Disorder

A number of medications have been studied among adults with BED, including antidepressants (fluoxetine, fluvoxamine, escitalopram, citalopram, sertraline), the serotonin-norepinephrine inhibitor duloxetine, the selective norepinephrine reuptake inhibitor atomoxetine, the anticonvulsant topiramate, the anti-obesity medication orlistat, and the psychostimulant lisdexamfetamine (Flament, Bissada, & Spettique, 2012; Golden & Attia, 2011; McElroy et al., 2016). In 2015, lisdexamfetamine was approved by the U.S. Food and Drug Administration for the treatment of moderate to severe BED in adults. Most of these agents were associated with greater decreases in binge eating than was placebo, but weight loss tended to be modest or nonexistent. A notable exception was lisdexamfetamine, which led to significant short-term weight loss; longer-term outcome data regarding binge eating and weight have not yet been published. None of these trials included adolescents.

Issues to Consider in Treating Adolescents with Pharmacotherapy

The pharmacokinetics and pharmacodynamics of psychotropic drugs in children and adolescents are not well studied. Some biological factors inherent in adolescents may affect the metabolism and efficacy of psychiatric medications, such as immature neurotransmitter systems, rapid hepatic metabolism, and shifting hormonal levels (Hazell, O'Connell, Heathcote, Robertson, & Henry, 1995). As a result, there may be differences in the metabolism and/or the effects of medications in adolescents with eating disorders, which could necessitate adjustments in dosage and medication response.

The safety of psychotropic medications should be considered when prescribing medications for eating disorder patients, especially medically unstable ones. Tricyclic antidepressants and mood stabilizers, which tend to be less frequently used today than in the past, have the potential for serious side effects. In particular, although no clear causal link has been documented, tricyclic antidepressants have been associated with sudden death among adolescents without eating disorders (Geller, Reising, Leonard, Riddle, & Walsh, 1999), and the cardiac abnormalities associated with AN, in theory, should increase the risks of tricyclic use in this population. Careful medical and psychiatric monitoring is required when prescribing psychotropic drugs to adolescents with eating disorders. As with adults, adolescents with eating disorders are prone to develop other behavioral problems, such as substance abuse, which may increase the risk of side effects. In addition, in sexually active adolescents, ensuring adequate birth control is important to prevent potentially harmful effects of medications during pregnancy (Kotler & Walsh, 2000).

In 2004, the U.S. Food and Drug Administration issued a black-box warning disclosing the potential for some SSRIs to increase suicidal ideation among adolescents and suggesting a need for close monitoring for suicidal ideation when such treatment is initiated. The warning was subsequently expanded to include individuals ages 18 to 24 on the basis of data indicating "increasing benefit and decreasing risk across the age span" (Leon, 2007, p. 1787). Although the warning highlights the hazards of untreated depression and was intended to increase monitoring of patients initiating antidepressant medications, not to discourage the prescription of antidepressants (Leon, 2007), the number of children and teenagers prescribed antidepressants has decreased significantly since the implementation of the warning (e.g., Nemeroff et al., 2007; Olfson et al., 2008).

Finally, as noted in the discussion of psychotherapeutic approaches, the motivation of adolescents regarding treatment is quite variable, and a lack of motivation may compromise patients' adherence to treatment recommendations, including taking psychotropic drugs as prescribed. For adolescents, compliance may be increased by family psychoeducation and parental involvement with treatment.

Summary

Despite the widespread use of psychotropic medications for adolescents with eating disorders, there is little empirical information about their utility and safety. Reports that atypical antipsychotic medications may be useful for adolescents with AN are encouraging but need to be examined further in controlled trials. Antidepressant medications have been shown to be useful in the treatment of adults with BN, but additional studies are needed to document their utility and safety for adolescents with BN.

Combined Pharmacological Treatments for Anorexia Nervosa and Bulimia Nervosa

Virtually all of the studies of acute pharmacological treatment for AN have been conducted in settings such as hospitals, where patients receive psychological treatment in addition to medication. Brambilla et al. (2014) conducted a three-part study relating biochemical markers to outcomes of combined CBT with olanzapine or placebo in patients with AN but found no correlation between biochemical and psychological effects. There have been no controlled trials examining the combination of psychological and pharmacological treatment for underweight patients with AN. Given the dearth of evidence that medication is useful in the treatment of AN, it is not possible to draw any conclusions about the potential utility of combined treatments.

For adults with BN, studies suggest that the addition of antidepressant medication to psychotherapy leads to a small but detectable increase in improvement of bulimic symptoms (Walsh et al., 1997). There have been no controlled studies of combined treatments in adolescents with BN.

RELAPSE PREVENTION USING PSYCHOLOGICAL TREATMENTS

Relapse prevention, as initially formulated by Marlatt et al., was conceptualized as a maintenance therapy for individuals who had completed initial treatment and had achieved a certain measure of symptomatic recovery (Brownell, Marlatt, Lichtenstein, & Wilson, 1986; Marlatt & Gordon, 1985). In the case of eating disorders, relapse is a major issue, and attention to the prevention of relapse is viewed as an essential goal and an integral step in the course of recovery. Some of the challenges that the field continues to face are the lack of standardized definitions of relapse and inconsistency of goals in terms of relapse prevention interventions. By definition, relapse occurs when there is a resurgence of symptoms or deterioration of condition subsequent to attaining a clinically significant degree of improvement. Thus, central to advancing the study of relapse prevention is the establishment of consistent, operationalized definitions of initial treatment response. Such standardized definitions would also reduce the risk of conflating reports of chronicity and relapse in follow-up studies.

With AN, the definition of relapse usually involves weight loss associated with clinical deterioration in terms of more restrictive eating and increased purging efforts or increased energy expenditure in the form of excessive exercise. Attitudinal variables are also a core feature of AN, and an increase in concerns about weight and shape is a prominent feature of relapse. Relapse prevention interventions for AN have primarily focused on the need for continuing care following initial response to inpatient treatment and have focused on weight maintenance, healthy regulation of energy expenditure, prevention of purging, and continuing improvements in attitudes about weight and shape.

For BN, binge eating and purging are the core behavioral components that define treatment response and relapse, and for BED, binge eating is the primary behavioral target. In addition, for both BN and BED, treatment response and recovery include changes in a range of attitudinal and psychological variables. As with AN, the field does not have accepted standards for defining "response" and "relapse" for BN or BED, and reports of response and relapse vary considerably across studies. An illustration of this phenomenon is a posttreatment study of 54 women with BN that compared relapse rates based on differing definitions of "remission" and "relapse"; depending on the definitions employed, relapse rates at 19 months ranged from 21% to 55% (Olmsted, Kaplan, & Rockert, 2005).

In light of these limitations and variations in terminology across studies, the COST Action B6 group, representing 19 European countries, adapted the principles set forth by Frank et al. (1991) for depression and reached a consensus on operational definitions for partial remission, full remission, relapse, recovery, and recurrence for eating disorders (Kordy et al., 2002). They tested the empirical validity of these operationalized terms against data collected over 2.5 years as part of a longitudinal study of 233 and 422 patients with AN and BN, respectively (German Project TR-EAT), concluding that the operationalized terms had substantial validity. Bardone-Cone et al. (2010) have also contributed to operationalizing these terms, and adoption by the field of such standardized definitions would greatly facilitate understanding of the frequency and prevention of relapse.

In addition to standardizing terminology, another priority for the eating disorders field is expanding information regarding treatment outcomes for adolescents. With some notable exceptions, much of the eating disorders outcome research has been conducted with adults, and the results may not fully apply to adolescents. Providing support for the notion that adolescents and adults may respond differently to treatment and experience different rates of relapse following treatment, a study that assessed 30-month outcomes after treatment noted that no differences were seen between diagnostic eating disorder groups among adolescent participants, whereas adult patients with anorexia-like diagnoses of eating disorder not otherwise specified showed significantly poorer clinical outcome compared to others (Helverskov et al., 2010).

Relapse Rates and Relapse Prevention for Anorexia Nervosa

Outpatient Treatment

Data from outpatient trials of psychological treatments for AN report that an overwhelming percentage of older adolescents and adults, between 60% and 70%, fail to achieve full recovery or even a good response to treatment (Dare, Eisler, Russell, Treasure, & Dodge, 2001; McIntosh et al., 2005). In some studies, attrition rates among outpatients are so high that it is impossible to analyze treatment response (Serfaty, Trukington, Heap, Ledsham, & Jolley, 1999). Family-based therapy, as described in previous sections, currently has the largest evidence base for adolescents with AN (Couturier, Kimber, & Szatmari, 2013; Lock et al., 2010), with a significant percentage of adolescents achieving full recovery at the end of treatment (Lock et al., 2006). While a recent meta-analysis found no differences between family-based therapy and individual therapy at the end of treatment, at 6- to 12-month follow-up, family-based therapy demonstrated an overall better outcome (Couturier et al., 2013). These data suggest that although family-based therapy is not uniquely focused on relapse prevention, it may nonetheless be the most effective treatment as judged by long-term outcome. However, the data available to evaluate relapse prevention after family-based therapy are limited, and significant numbers of adolescents continue to be at least partially symptomatic regardless of the initial therapy. Thus, continuing treatment aimed at full recovery, and ultimately relapse prevention, is still warranted.

Inpatient Treatment

The data indicate that, across the lifespan, the majority of hospitalized patients with AN respond to treatment (Anderson, Bowers, & Evans, 1997; Attia et al., 1998; Baran, Weltzin, & Kaye, 1995), despite their greater severity of illness. However, follow-up studies also indicate that the post-hospital period is fraught with difficulty, with a significant resurgence of symptoms and relapse rates generally ranging from 30% to 50% (Carter, Blackmore, Sutandar-Pinnock, & Woodside, 2004; Pike, Walsh, Vitousek, Wilson, & Bauer, 2003). Some studies report post-hospital relapse rates as high as 70% (Lay, Jennen-Steinmetz, Reinhard, & Schmidt, 2002). In a study of AN and BN, Richard, Bauer, and Kordy (2005) reported rates of relapse within 2.5 years of successful inpatient treatment completion of 32.6% for patients with AN and 37.4% for patients with BN, with the highest risk of relapse being within the first 6 or 7 months after achieving partial remission.

Post-hospital relapse rates are significant for both adolescent and adult patients. In a study of 95 patients between the ages of 12 and 18, Strober et al. (1997) reported that nearly 30% of those who successfully completed their inpatient program relapsed following discharge, with a mean time to relapse of 15 months and a median of 11 months. In an older sample (mean age = 20 ± 5.4 years), Eckert et al. reported that 42% of women who achieved weight normalization in the hospital relapsed within 1 year of discharge; however, if weight normalization was maintained for 1 year, the risk of subsequent weight loss declined dramatically (Eckert, Halmi, Marchi, Grove, & Crosby, 1995). Taken together, these data indicate that relapse prevention strategies are critically important, particularly during the first year after effective hospital-based treatment due to the high rate of relapse during that period, even among those who achieve remission during the acute treatment phase.

Psychological Treatments for Anorexia Nervosa Aimed at Post-Hospital Relapse Prevention

Family Therapy

As discussed above, the Maudsley Approach to family therapy for AN was originally designed as a post-hospital treatment, delivered over the course of 1 year following inpatient treatment. The findings from the initial study of this treatment (Russell et al., 1987) and 5-year follow-up assessment (Eisler et al., 1997) indicated that changes effected by family therapy serve to prevent relapse and enhance long-term efficacy for this group of patients with AN. The most recent studies of family-based therapy have not been relapse prevention studies but rather outpatient studies conducted during the acute phase of treatment that focus on weight gain and normalization of eating. As noted above, these studies indicate that family-based therapy is associated with significant remission rates (Lock et al., 2010); however, insufficient evidence exists to establish definitively that family-based therapy is superior to other psychological interventions with regard to relapse prevention (Ball & Mitchell, 2004; Couturier et al., 2013; Fisher, Hetrick, & Rushford, 2010).

Cognitive-Behavioral Treatment

A version of CBT has been designed to treat patients with AN in the year following the successful completion of inpatient treatment. Consistent with the fundamental components of CBT for eating disorders (Fairburn, Marcus, & Wilson, 1993; Garner, Vitousek, & Pike, 1997; Pike, Devlin, & Loeb, 2003), this intervention focuses on the cognitive and behavioral processes involved in the overvaluation of weight and shape, dysregulation of eating behavior, and deficits in self-esteem and self-schemata thought to be at the core of maintenance of the eating disorder (Pike, Carter, & Olmsted, 2009). Initially, treatment focuses on specific cognitive distortions and behavioral dysfunction pertaining to eating and weight that increase the risk of relapse. As treatment progresses, schema-based approaches are used to address a range of issues that extend beyond the specific domains of eating and weight but remain fundamental to the individual's self-schema, self-esteem, and eating disorder. Based on a sample of 33 patients, a survival analysis demonstrated a statistically significant advantage of CBT over the comparison treatment of nutritional counseling. Using adapted Morgan Russell outcome criteria, 44.4% of the CBT group met criteria for a good outcome, compared to 6.7% of the nutrition counseling group, and an additional 16.7% of the CBT group met criteria for a full recovery compared to none in the nutritional counseling group (Pike, Walsh, et al., 2003). A recent uncontrolled trial also suggests the utility of an enhanced form of CBT to prevent relapse among adolescents (Dalle Grave et al., 2014).

Further support for the efficacy of CBT in maintaining treatment gains following hospital discharge is provided by a 2009 study that compared CBT versus maintenance treatment as usual in 88 patients with AN (mean age = 24.1; Carter et al., 2009). At 1-year follow-up, 65% of the CBT group compared to only 34% of the treatment-as-usual group had not relapsed. Furthermore, based on a definition of "relapse" as BMI less than or equal to 17.5 kg/m^2 for 3 months or the resumption of binge-eating/purging behaviors for 3 months, the time to relapse among CBT participants was significantly longer than in the treatment-as-usual group (Carter et al., 2009). Both these studies included adults and older adolescents. Larger studies and studies that focus specifically on relapse prevention for younger adolescents are still needed to draw more definitive conclusions about relapse prevention for adolescents (Bodell & Keel, 2010).

Risk Factors for Relapse for Anorexia Nervosa

In recent years, a number of studies have explored predictors of relapse among individuals with AN. A study of 58 women who had either fully or partially remitted from their eating disorder following intensive day hospital treatment found that more severe pretreatment caloric restriction, higher residual symptoms at time of discharge, slower response to treatment, and higher weight-related self-evaluation were significant predictors of relapse (McFarlane, Olmsted, & Trottier, 2008). Associations between energy density and diet variety and clinical outcome have also been found in the 12 months following inpatient hospitalization. A lower diet energy-density score (eating fewer energy-dense foods) prior to hospital discharge was associated with poor clinical outcome in the first year following hospitalization (Schebendach et al., 2008; Schebendach, Mayer, Devlin, Attia, & Walsh, 2012). Diet variety score (the number of foods consumed) was found to predict relapse in one study (Schebendach et al., 2008) but not another (Schebendach et al., 2012). A relationship between body composition and clinical outcome has also been observed among patients with AN over the year following discharge from inpatient treatment, with a lower percentage of adipose tissue after short-term weight normalization identified as a risk factor for relapse (Bodell & Mayer, 2011). Conversely, higher BMI at the conclusion of inpatient treatment for AN is associated with a lower risk of relapse (Kaplan et al., 2009). The best predictors of weight maintenance at 6-month and 12-month follow-up from inpatient treatment for AN were level of weight restoration at the end of acute treatment and the avoidance of weight loss immediately following the end of intensive treatment (Kaplan et al., 2009). Finally, a retrospective study of 680 women found that likelihood of recovery was significantly predicted by vomiting, impulsivity, and trait anxiety. Self-induced vomiting and greater trait anxiety were negative prognostic factors and predicted a lower likelihood of recovery (Zerwas et al., 2013).

Relapse Rates and Relapse Prevention for Bulimia Nervosa

A significant percentage of individuals with BN achieve partial recovery following initial treatment (Steinhausen & Weber, 2009), and studies generally estimate a relapse rate of approximately 30% (Herzog et al., 1999; Keel & Mitchell, 1997; Richard et al., 2005). A study of eating disorder outcomes found that a bulimia-like variant of eating disorder not otherwise specified was the most frequent relapse diagnosis over 30 months, while more severe binge-eating and purging behaviors predicted a worse clinical outcome for participants with BN (Helverskov et al., 2010). None of the published clinical trials evaluating psychological treatments for BN specifically focus on relapse prevention for this disorder; instead, relapse prevention is typically an integrated component of the initial intervention. Given the likely relationship between partial recovery and relapse in BN, it may be beneficial to develop relapse prevention treatments specifically targeting those who achieve partial recovery at the end of acute care.

Follow-up data on CBT and interpersonal psychotherapy, two evidence-based treatments for BN, indicate that they do not differ in rates of relapse at 1-year follow-up. Therapeutic changes appear to be well maintained for the majority of individuals who respond well to initial CBT or interpersonal psychotherapy, with the most enduring recovery being reported by individuals who achieve complete remission of binge eating and purging by end of treatment (Agras, Walsh, Fairburn, Wilson, & Kraemer, 2000; Fairburn et al., 1995). However, as many as 30% of individuals who are abstinent from binge eating and purging at the end of CBT report some resurgence of symptoms during a 1-year follow-up (Halmi et al., 2002). A similar rate of 30% relapse has been reported among individuals who had responded to an eating disorders day program (Olmsted, Kaplan, & Rockert, 1994). Given that a significant percentage of individuals who respond to CBT or interpersonal psychotherapy fail to achieve full remission, developing interventions that target not only those individuals who fail to respond to initial treatment but also those who have a significant but incomplete response to treatment could enhance treatment outcome in the long term.

Relapse Rates and Relapse Prevention for Binge-Eating Disorder

Numerous studies examining the efficacy of psychotherapies for BED have been reported over the past 10 years. However, with few exceptions, study participants have been adults, and in all cases, the treatments were not uniquely focused on relapse prevention (Hay, 2013). Interpersonal psychotherapy, CBT, and various forms of guided self-help have been shown to be effective in the short-term treatment of BED and related forms of eating disorder not otherwise specified; however, a significant percentage of individuals remain at least partially symptomatic, and follow-up data report significant symptomatology. Although it is not always clear whether this impairment represents enduring symptomatology or relapse, it does indicate that follow-up treatments aimed at more lasting recovery are needed.

Risk Factors for Relapse for Bulimia Nervosa and Binge-Eating Disorder

Studies of BN and BED have aimed to identify potential predictors of relapse. Olmsted et al. (1994) identified a relapse rate of 31% over a 2-year follow-up period for individuals with BN, with most relapses in the first 6 months after treatment. The strongest predictors of relapse were younger age, higher vomiting frequency, a higher pretreatment score on the bulimia subscale of the EAT-26, and posttreatment higher frequencies of purging and higher scores on the interpersonal distrust subscale of the Eating Disorder Inventory (Olmsted et al., 1994). A naturalistic study including 35 individuals with BN and 82 individuals with BED/an eating disorder not otherwise specified reported a relapse probability of 43%, with no significant differences in time to relapse in either diagnostic group. Stressful life events (e.g., elevated work and social stressors) significantly predicted relapse, while psychiatric comorbidity, duration of illness, and personality disorder status did not (Grilo, Pagano, et al., 2012). A 9-year prospective study in 136 women with AN and 110 with BN reported relapse rates of 36% and 35%, respectively (Keel, Dorer, Franko, Jackson, & Herzog, 2005). Greater body image disturbance significantly predicted risk of relapse in both groups, while worse psychosocial functioning increased relapse risk among women with BN. A significant minority of women with the AN restricting subtype at intake risked developing bulimic symptoms during relapse, whereas women with the binge-purge subtype of AN or BN at intake evidenced bulimic symptomatology during relapse (Keel et al., 2005). Another study (Halmi et al., 2002) observed a relapse rate of 44% among young adults with BN who were abstinent from binge eating and purging following CBT. Greater preoccupation with and ritualization surrounding eating, less motivation to change, and a shorter period of abstinence during the treatment phase significantly predicted relapse. Among patients with BN who responded well to CBT, interpersonal psychotherapy, or behavior therapy, shape and weight overvaluation has also been shown to predict relapse (Fairburn, Peveler, Jones, Hope, & Doll, 1993).

Internet-Based Relapse Prevention for Eating Disorders

In the last few years, interest in the feasibility and efficacy of Internet-based relapse prevention programs has grown steadily. In many ways, the emergence of these interventions represents a logical next step following the development and assessment of acute treatments for BN or BED. In the case of Internet-based interventions, most programs are designed for use across the full range of eating disorders rather than one specific diagnostic category. As with guided self-help interventions, virtually all of the Internet programs are based on CBT manuals (Fichter et al., 2012). Advantages of these interventions include the ease of accessibility, cost-effectiveness, and the possibility of reaching individuals who otherwise would not seek out treatment (Fichter et al., 2012). Internet-based interventions have shown promise in the reduction of symptoms in a range of other psychiatric disorders, including depression and anxiety disorders such as panic disorder, specific phobias, and posttraumatic stress disorder. The use of therapist-guided Internet chat groups reduced the rate of relapse following inpatient treatment for a range of disorders (e.g., mood disorders, somatoform disorders, personality disorders) while also increasing the length of survival time until relapse (Bauer, Wolf, Haug, & Kordy, 2011).

Most Internet-based programs have focused on BN- and BED-like symptoms (Carrard et al., 2011; Fernandez-Aranda et al., 2008; Marrone,

Mitchell, Crosby, Wonderlich, & Jollie-Trottier, 2009; Sanchez-Ortiz et al., 2011; Schmidt et al., 2008; Shapiro et al., 2007). However, Fichter et al. (2012) conducted a multisite study of 258 women (aged 16 or above) with AN. This Internet-based relapse prevention program was more effective than treatment as usual in the 9 months following inpatient treatment. Other studies that make use of Internet technologies such as Internet chat groups following inpatient psychotherapy (Bauer et al., 2011) or self-guided Internet programs (Gulec et al., 2011) show promise with adults and should be evaluated for their utility with adolescents.

Summary

Post-hospital relapse rates for patients with AN are high, and the achievement of enduring recovery may often follow periods of relapse. Early intervention for AN (i.e., among those with short duration of illness at time of presentation for treatment) is likely to be associated with a better long-term prognosis, especially for younger patients receiving family-based therapy. CBT has support for relapse prevention among adults with AN, but there are no data regarding the efficacy of this treatment for adolescents. Clinical trials have not specifically targeted adolescents with BN and BED, and the limited data on relapse among younger patients are not sufficient to analyze separately. Family-based therapy is effective in treating adolescents with BN, but the efficacy of maintenance and relapse prevention is limited (Le Grange, Crosby, Rathouz, & Leventhal, 2007). More data regarding the clinical efficacy of treatments for adolescents with BN and BED, both in the short term and in preventing relapse in the longer term, are needed to help inform evidence-based clinical practice.

RELAPSE PREVENTION USING PHARMACOLOGICAL TREATMENTS

Anorexia Nervosa

As described above, trials evaluating antidepressant medications for underweight patients with AN have failed to show a difference between active medication and placebo for the treatment of eating-disordered or mood symptoms. As antidepressant medications might be hypothesized to lack efficacy in this population due to neurochemical disturbances associated with low body weight (e.g., Attia et al., 1998), these medications have also been evaluated for the prevention of relapse after weight gain.

Two placebo-controlled studies addressed this issue (Kaye et al., 2001; Walsh et al., 2006). In the study by Kaye et al., a small number of patients who did not binge eat ($n = 35$), half of whom had reached a near-normal weight, were randomized to receive either fluoxetine or placebo in double-blind fashion following an inpatient hospitalization. Some patients also received unstandardized psychological treatment. Fluoxetine-treated patients were more likely to complete the trial (63% completed) in comparison to patients receiving placebo (16% completed, $p = .0001$). Patients who completed the trial tended to experience more weight gain and psychological improvement than patients who did not complete the trial. The average age of the patient sample was 22.5 years old, and it is not clear whether any adolescent patients were included. In the largest controlled medication trial for individuals with AN, Walsh et al. (2006) randomized 93 weight-restored women to receive either fluoxetine or placebo. All of the patients were also provided with a CBT intervention, which consisted of 50 individual treatment sessions. The authors found no evidence for any significant benefit of fluoxetine compared to placebo on most measures; in contrast to the findings of Kaye et al., fluoxetine did not affect time to relapse regardless of how dropouts from the study were classified. A minority (5.4%) of patients with AN included in this study were younger than 18, and a larger subgroup (37.6%) were less than 21 years of age.

Bulimia Nervosa

Although pharmacological interventions reduce bulimic symptoms in the short term, as previously described, the role of continued pharmacological treatment in sustaining clinical improvement over time is unclear. Several controlled trials have examined the efficacy of antidepressant medications in preventing relapse among BN patients.

Some studies have evaluated continuing treatment with pharmacotherapy to prevent relapse after an initial positive response to medication (Pyle et al., 1990; Romano, Halmi, Sarkar, Koke & Lee, 2002; Walsh et al., 1991) and an additional study randomized patients to receive either medication or placebo for relapse prevention after receiving a course of inpatient treatment (Fichter, Kruger, Rief, Holland & Dohne, 1996). A consistent finding across studies has been a significant rate of symptomatic relapse despite continued pharmacological treatment. There is also an indication that tricyclic antidepressants, specifically imipramine and desipramine, and the SSRI fluoxetine may diminish the rate of relapse for patients maintained on antidepressant medications, in comparison to patients maintained on placebo. Combined, these studies suggest that although there is a significant rate of relapse in patients on antidepressant medications, the rate of relapse is greater when medication is discontinued after a few months (Romano et al., 2002). Although the studies evaluating pharmacotherapy as a means to prevent relapse have generated similar results, there have been relatively few studies in this area, with modest sample sizes and large dropout rates across trials. Further, at this time, all of the trials of medication treatment for relapse prevention for BN are more than 10 years old, and there have been no additional studies of adults or adolescents since the publication of the first edition of this book.

All four controlled trials evaluating pharmacotherapy to prevent relapse enrolled only adult BN patients. Therefore, it is unclear whether the results of these studies are applicable to an adolescent population, or if there are special considerations for using antidepressant medications with younger patients for the prevention of relapse.

Binge-Eating Disorder

To date, there are no published studies examining pharmacological interventions specifically for preventing relapse among individuals with BED (adults or adolescents).

Summary

On the basis of evidence described in this chapter, Crow et al. (2009, p. 1) concluded, "at present, there is no convincing evidence of efficacy for any drug treatment for [AN] in either the acute or chronic phase of the illness." For some adult patients with BN who initially respond to medication, symptomatic relapse occurs despite continued pharmacotherapy. Therefore, continued treatment with medication after an initial positive response cannot guarantee against relapse. On the other hand, data from placebo-controlled studies suggest that, when BN patients respond to a medication, and are maintained on that medication, they experience lower rates of relapse than patients who are switched to placebo (Pyle et al., 1990; Romano et al., 2002; Walsh et al., 1991). Therefore, continuing to administer an effective pharmacological intervention likely reduces the rate of relapse, but does not ensure against the return of bulimic symptoms. The question remains as to the optimal length of time to maintain a patient on medication to prevent symptomatic relapse. Additionally, given the absence of data in adolescent samples, it is not known if the pattern of results from the controlled studies of pharmacotherapy for relapse prevention apply to a younger population.

EVALUATION OF THE EFFICACY AND EFFECTIVENESS OF TREATMENTS FOR EATING DISORDERS IN ADOLESCENTS

The previous sections focused on the specific efficacy of psychological and pharmacological treatments. A number of other questions should also be considered in evaluating the treatment of eating disorders in adolescents, such as the following:

1. When is the best time to begin treatment?
2. What is the optimal treatment setting?
3. Do adolescents with eating disorders need specialized services?
4. Who should provide the treatment?

When Should Treatment Begin?

Ideally, patients would be identified at the earliest possible point in the course of the disorder, and treatment would begin as soon as the adolescent, the parent(s), or other professional(s) recognize a clinically significant eating problem. Changes in the DSM-5 diagnostic criteria for AN (elimination of any specific number with respect to percent body weight and of the requirement for amenorrhea) and for BN (reduction in the minimum average frequency of binge/purge behavior to once a week over 3 months) will lower the threshold to make a clinical diagnosis, potentially aiding earlier identification and treatment. Among the factors to be considered in initiating treatment are the intensity, severity, and duration of symptoms, their trajectory, and the motivation of the adolescent and his or her family for treatment.

Where Should Adolescents Be Treated?

A fundamental and uncontroversial tenet is that treatment should occur in the least restrictive setting in which effective treatment can be provided, and it should be directed toward the adolescent eventually maintaining healthy weight-control habits in home, school, and work settings. A primary real-world consideration is the availability of treatment settings to which the adolescent has access. Larger cities are more likely to have university-based programs, with a full spectrum of treatment options such as outpatient clinics, intensive outpatient and partial hospitalization programs, and inpatient hospitalization. Even if available, more intensive treatment settings, such as residential facilities or inpatient units, may be less useful for the treatment of some adolescents (e.g., Gowers et al., 2007; Morton et al., under review) and can be resisted by adolescents and/or their parents due to distance from home, disruption of family life or schooling, or financial burden. However, these options may be necessary if other types of treatment are not effective. Treatment options in smaller towns or rural areas are often limited to clinicians with varying degrees of interest and expertise in treating adolescents with eating disorders. The skills and interests of the adolescent's treatment providers help to determine where an adolescent will be treated, as some primary care physicians may not feel comfortable monitoring the physical health of adolescents with eating disorders, and some therapists may limit their practices to adults. In these situations, adolescents who might otherwise be treated in their home community may need to be referred to a specialty program. If an appropriate treatment team or program is available locally, allowing an adolescent to live at home and engage in outpatient therapy, while also remaining in school and continuing to develop important peer relationships, is optimal. The challenge for the provider is to determine the balance between what treatment is ideal and what is available.

Another "setting" that holds promise but has not been adequately studied in the treatment of eating disorders is cyberspace, detailed in the previous section as a venue for relapse prevention. The delivery of reminders or responses from professionals treating adolescents with eating disorders to patients or their parents via smartphone or email (possibly automated) could enhance the messages and skills being focused on in treatment.

Even when services are available, there are very few data to guide the determination of the most appropriate type and duration of clinical services for adolescents with AN. One study suggests that providing more expensive, intensive inpatient treatment early in the course of AN is associated with reduced relapse rates and long-term personal, social, and financial costs (Striegel-Moore, Leslie, Petrill, Garvin, & Rosenheck, 2000). On the other hand, combining less intensive and more intensive and specialized care, particularly family-based treatment, may be efficacious and cost-effective (Garner & Needleman, 1997; Gowers et al., 2007; Wilson, Vitousek, & Loeb, 2000).

Currently, there are no agreed-upon specific treatment protocols for adolescents with eating disorders to guide how the treatment setting and intensity are best matched to the patient's clinical status. Instead, adolescents tend to begin in outpatient treatment settings, having visits for medical and mental health services, then progress to more intensive treatment approaches if they do not have a positive response.

Are There Special Considerations in Treating Adolescents with Eating Disorders?

One aspect of treatment that is unique to adolescents is the involvement and authority of the family in the treatment process. As previously described, parental criticism (Eisler et al., 2007; Le Grange et al., 1992b) can significantly affect treatment outcome. Thus, the development of a therapeutic relationship between care providers and parents can be critical to success, but it can also be challenging if parents deny the existence of a problem, or blame the adolescent. Conversely, if the care providers attribute blame or fault to the parents, it will be difficult to foster a collaborative relationship with the parents. It is crucial to empower parents to effectively address at home the challenging behaviors exhibited on a daily basis.

Who Should Provide the Treatment?

Especially for AN, treatment often begins with an adolescent medicine specialist because of physical symptoms associated with weight loss (e.g., amenorrhea, fatigue, cold intolerance, weakness, fainting). A general medical evaluation is helpful in ruling out the potential contribution of other conditions known to affect eating and weight (e.g., Crohn's disease, central nervous system tumors, gastric outlet obstruction) and assessing potential physical complications related to the eating disorder (see also Chapter 13). Adolescents with AN tend to be more willing to be evaluated for these "medical problems" than for associated psychological symptoms. In addition to addressing the presenting medical symptoms, primary care providers can suggest the need for additional mental health services. By focusing on the signs and symptoms that precipitated a medical evaluation, and emphasizing healthy meal planning and completion, the primary care provider can shift the focus away from the presence of an eating disorder and toward the behaviors needed to improve health, and thereby enhance motivation for treatment. In the case of continuing medical instability or significant eating problems, adolescent patients can be referred for additional specialist services. Appropriately trained healthcare professionals may be able to treat BN on an outpatient basis, but some BN patients need to be monitored for potential medical complications.

Summary

There are no rigorous studies to guide the optimal treatment for adolescents, in terms of when treatment should begin, where that treatment should be delivered, or who should provide the treatment. The consensus view is that therapy should begin as soon as possible after a clinically significant eating problem has been identified, with the treatment provider, parents, and patient working to individualize treatment. The setting for the treatment is partially determined by availability, but the severity and duration of illness, especially with regard to medical complications, must also be considered. The optimal professional to treat an adolescent with an eating disorder is again determined, in part, by availability. Eating disorders can be effectively managed by a variety of different professionals, including physicians (psychiatrists, primary care providers, and adolescent medicine specialists), psychologists, social workers, and nutritionists who are familiar with efficacious eating disorder treatments.

Prevention of Eating Disorders

Evelyn Attia
Anne E. Becker
Cynthia M. Bulik
Alison E. Field
Neville H. Golden
Richard E. Kreipe
Daniel Le Grange
James E. Mitchell
Kathleen M. Pike
Robyn Sysko
C. Barr Taylor
B. Timothy Walsh

chapter 15

OVERVIEW

For any disorder, understanding risk factors, or variables that predict the development of the disorder, is vital to prevention efforts and informative for treatment development. The accurate prediction of risk for eating disorders requires not only that a factor or constellation of factors predicts the onset of a disorder, but also that there is some degree of specificity to the prediction. The eating disorders field has evolved over the past several decades to reach consensus that both biological and psychological factors need to be incorporated into any risk models for anorexia nervosa (AN), bulimia nervosa (BN), and binge-eating disorder (BED). Models that include only sociocultural factors, such as the influence of societal emphasis on thinness, ultimately fail, given the ubiquity of exposure to that risk factor. Refinement of the concept, for example, to capture the extent to which the cultural ideal of thinness is internalized by an individual, or to account for temperamental or behavioral factors that increase the likelihood of extreme weight-control behaviors, or to include biological vulnerabilities to negative energy balance, all hone prediction of risk. Furthermore, refinement of our predictive models should also encompass protective or buffering factors, although traditionally these are more difficult to identify and verify.

To review the state of the science of risk factors for eating disorders, we will first discuss what is known about biological risk factors for AN, BN, and BED and then cover behavioral and environmental risk factors. Ultimately, our understanding will be enhanced by delineating ways in which biological and environmental risk factors interact to influence ultimate risk.

A *risk factor* can be defined as an agent or exposure that increases the probability of an adverse outcome—in this case, an eating disorder. In order to be demonstrated conclusively to be a risk factor, the agent in question should be assessed prospectively (prior to the development of the eating disorder), show temporal precedence to the onset of the eating disorder, and show some degree of specificity with the eating disorder (i.e., not merely a general risk factor for psychopathology). This discussion will include a range of potential risk factors that have been associated with eating disorders via a variety of research designs. Excellent previous reviews are available (Jacobi, Hayward, de Zwaan, Kraemer, & Agras, 2004; Striegel-Moore & Bulik, 2007). In all cases it is important to consider whether temporal precedence was established ("Did the event occur prior to the onset of AN?") and time of reporting ("Was the temporal precedence determined prospectively or retrospectively?").

RISK FACTORS FOR ANOREXIA NERVOSA

Biological Risk Factors

Genetics

The familiality and heritability of AN are well established. First-degree relatives of individuals with AN are about 11 times more likely also to have AN over the course of their lifetime than relatives of individuals without AN (Strober, Freeman, Lampert, Diamond, & Kaye, 2000). Population-based twin studies support this finding and implicate genetic factors in the observed familial patterns. Heritability estimates using different definitions of AN range from 28% to 74%, with the remaining variance largely due to unique environmental factors (Bulik, Slof-Op't Landt, van Furth, & Sullivan, 2007). Genome-wide linkage studies were largely unsuccessful at identifying specific genetic markers of risk for developing AN and carrying findings through to true biological targets (Bacanu et al., 2005; Devlin et al., 2002; Grice et al., 2002). As with genetic risk for many other diseases, many initial findings from candidate gene studies of AN have not been replicated (Bulik et al., 2007; Hinney, Scherag, & Hebebrand, 2010; Slof-Op't Landt et al., 2005). Three association studies using genome-wide approaches have been conducted in AN. First, a Japanese study using microsatellite markers with follow-up genotyping suggested an association with rs2048332 on chromosome 1, but this finding was not significant at the genome-wide level and has not been replicated (Nakabayashi et al., 2009). Two small genome-wide association studies using AN cases from around the world failed to detect genome-wide significant findings (Boraska et al., 2012; Wang et al., 2011). Given what is now known about the sample sizes necessary for detection of significant loci in such genome-wide investigations in complex traits, this is not surprising. However, encouragingly, sign tests in the second study (which determine whether the direction of effect was the same in discovery and replication analyses) strongly suggest that increasing sample size would yield significant findings. Indeed, amassing larger sample sizes is an immediate priority for the field, and efforts are under way globally in order to allow AN to experience advances in genomic science similar to those that have been witnessed for other psychiatric disorders, especially schizophrenia (Collins & Sullivan, 2013; Schizophrenia Working Group of the Psychiatric Genomics Consortium, 2014). Genetic risk factors clearly meet the requirement for temporal precedence, and further advances in gene expression and epigenetics may refine temporality even further to enable the uncoupling of biomarkers of starvation from biomarkers of disease.

Neurocognitive and Social Cognitive Functioning

The most robustly documented neurocognitive deficit in AN is in the domain of set-shifting: the ability to flexibly shift a cognitive response set. This neurocognitive feature may be permissive of *rigid* self-focus, as individuals with AN inflexibly stick to a cognitive domain (Roberts, Tchanturia, Stahl, Southgate, & Treasure, 2007; Tchanturia et al., 2004). Impaired set-shifting is evident in individuals who are acutely ill with AN and following weight restoration (Tchanturia et al., 2012), and in long-term recovery, and similar deficits are seen in family members who are unaffected by AN (Holliday, Tchanturia, Landau, Collier, & Treasure, 2005; Nakazato et al., 2010; Roberts, Tchanturia, & Treasure, 2010; Tchanturia et al., 2004; Tenconi et al., 2010). Altogether, these findings suggest that set-shifting deficits may represent a trait rather than a state characteristic of AN. Additional research has shown that individuals with AN exhibit impairment in some facets of interpersonal functioning (Zucker et al., 2007), as well as deficits in social reward and attention dysfunction (Watson, Werling, Zucker, & Platt, 2010).

Neurobiology

Numerous behavioral traits associated with AN, including premorbid anxiety, obsessive behaviors, negative emotionality, impaired cognitive flexibility, increased harm avoidance and perfectionism, and altered interoceptive awareness, may be related to underlying abnormalities or alterations in brain structure and function (for a review of these behavioral traits, see Kaye, Wierenga, Bailer, Simmons, & Bischoff-Grethe, 2013).

Individuals with AN display alterations in both the dopamine and serotonin neurotransmitter systems (Kaye, 2008; Kaye, Fudge, & Paulus, 2009). Dopamine plays a role in reward, motivation, and executive functioning (Kaye, 2008), while serotonin is generally implicated in mood, satiety, and impulse control (Kaye, 2008; Kaye et al., 2013).

Neuroimaging investigations have revealed that abnormalities in neurocircuits in at least two brain regions, including the temporal lobe and anterior insula (Kaye et al., 2009) and the cortico-striatal-thalamo-cortical pathways (Foerde et al., 2015; Stahl, 2008; Steinglass & Walsh, 2006), are associated characteristics frequently observed in AN (DeSocio, 2013). In a review, DeSocio (2013) hypothesized that research and clinical evidence are converging on an observable phenotype, with identifiable underlying abnormal neurocircuitry, which may be useful in evaluating risk for AN and designing preemptive interventions that may avert symptom onset or decrease severity.

Studies using genetic, pharmacological, and physiological methods suggest that individuals with AN have abnormal dopamine function in the striatum, one of many areas of the brain linked to reward processing, which persists even in recovery from AN (Bergen et al., 2005; Delgado, Nystrom, Fissell, Noll, & Fiez, 2000; Friederich et al., 2006; Kaye, 2008; Lawrence et al., 2003; Montague, Hyman, & Cohen, 2004; Schultz,

2004). Such disturbances may contribute to vulnerability to disordered eating behaviors, and to the ability of individuals with AN to inhibit appetite and demonstrate high levels of self-control (Kaye, Wagner, Fudge, & Paulus, 2011).

Sex

Being female is perhaps the most obvious and established risk factor for AN. The female-to-male ratio for AN has been consistently estimated to be approximately 10:1 in both clinical and epidemiological samples (American Psychiatric Association, 2013). The uneven gender distribution cannot yet be explained, although theories ranging from sociocultural to biological exist. Sociocultural theories explain the sex imbalance by suggesting that "Western" culture's female beauty ideal of extreme thinness leads to body dissatisfaction and subsequent dieting. Additional factors may interact with exposure to this thin ideal to increase risk, including social pressure to be thin, perfectionism, social anxiety, overweight or obesity, and high impulsivity. Differences in an individual's biological response to starvation, including effects on reward pathways, may also play a role (Striegel-Moore & Bulik, 2007).

Perinatal Events

A number of studies have suggested that prenatal and perinatal events may increase the risk for developing AN. Possible risk factors include prematurity, birth complications, multiple birth, and maternal health, including the mother's history of AN (Cnattingius, Hultman, Dahl, & Sparen, 1999; Favaro et al., 2006; Goodman et al., 2014; Micali et al., 2012; Shoebridge & Gowers, 2000). Some studies suggest that perinatal complications may be independent risk factors that may interact with, but are not caused by, genetic risk factors (e.g., Favaro et al., 2011).

Puberty/Reproductive Milestones

The onset of AN typically occurs during the peripubertal or postpubertal period (Lucas, Beard, O'Fallon, & Kurland, 1988, 1991). Prepubertal AN exists (Cooper, Watkins, Bryant-Waugh, & Lask, 2002; Nicholls, Lynn, & Viner, 2011), and age at onset of AN appears to be decreasing in some studies (Favaro, Caregaro, Tenconi, Bosello, & Santonastaso, 2009). However, disturbances in eating and weight-related behaviors are clearly present in preadolescent girls (Graber, Brooks-Gunn, Paikoff, & Warren, 1994; Killen et al., 1994; Nicholls, et al., 2011; Sands, Tricker, Sherman, Armatas, & Maschette, 1997). The extent to which these disturbances overlap with AN is not entirely known (Kotler, Cohen, Davies, Pine, & Walsh, 2001). Theories for the peripubertal period's association with onset range from sociocultural (during puberty, girls become more vulnerable to social pressures to be thin, especially in the context of their changing bodies; Gowers & Shore, 2001) to biological (hormonal changes during puberty trigger other relevant biological processes; see Young, 2010, for a review). Early menarche has not been associated with risk for AN (Fairburn, Cooper, Doll, & Welch, 1999; Mangweth-Matzek, Rupp, Hausmann, Kemmler, & Biebl, 2007; Ruuska, Kaltiala-Heino, Koivisto, & Rantanen, 2003; Stice, Presnell, & Bearman, 2001).

Body Mass Index

Familial obesity is less frequently associated with risk for AN than for BN (Fairburn et al., 1999). Only one older study explored the opposite phenomenon, whether parents of individuals with AN tend to be thinner than parents of healthy controls (Halmi, Struss, & Goldberg, 1978), and there was no evidence to suggest that either mothers or fathers weighed less than parents of controls.

Personality/Temperament/Negative Affectivity

Psychometric studies have consistently linked AN to a cluster of personality and temperamental traits—specifically, negative self-evaluation, low self-esteem, extreme compliance, obsessionality, perfectionism, neuroticism, negative affect, and harm avoidance (Anderluh et al., 2003; Bulik, Tozzi, et al., 2003; Gual et al., 2002;

Halmi, Tozzi, et al., 2005; Pike et al., 2008). These traits continue to characterize individuals with AN after recovery (Bulik, Sullivan, Fear, & Pickering, 2000). In addition, a twin study suggests that AN may represent the expression of a common underlying familial liability to a temperament style that reflects a striving for perfectionism, a need for order, and a sensitivity to praise and reward (Wade et al., 2008).

Behavioral/Environmental Risk Factors

Dieting/Negative Energy Balance

One of the first factors mentioned in most discussions of risk factors for eating disorders is dieting. However, the term *dieting* is complex, laden with many meanings, and used to refer to a variety of attitudes and behaviors. The National Task Force on the Prevention and Treatment of Obesity (2000) defines dieting as "the intentional and sustained restriction of caloric intake for the purposes of reducing body weight or changing body shape, resulting in a significant negative energy balance." This useful and relatively straightforward definition implies that dieting, because it results in negative energy balance, must be associated with weight loss. Therefore, attempts to restrict caloric intake that do not result in weight loss might properly be termed unsuccessful dieting; such attempts are frequently described by individuals with symptoms of eating disorders. The literature on eating disorders uses dieting to refer to both successful and unsuccessful attempts to restrict caloric intake, making it difficult to determine whether successful and unsuccessful dieting play similar roles in the development of eating disorders.

The operative condition relevant to risk for AN is indeed the state of negative energy balance. The prevalence of dieting has been estimated to be between 14% and 77% and is highest in young women (French, Perry, Leon, & Fulkerson, 1995). In the majority of these studies, dieting was simply defined as whether individuals had ever restricted their intake in order to lose weight, and therefore likely captured both successful and unsuccessful dieters. In a study of 36,320 public school students, dieting frequency was strongly related to poor body image, fears of being unable to control eating, and more prevalent history of binge eating. Dieting was also related in a "dose-response" fashion to a range of psychosocial and health behavior variables (French, Story, Downes, Resnick, & Blum, 1995). The risk of achieving a negative energy balance as a risk for the development of eating disorders appears to differ between adolescents who are initially within a normal weight range versus those who are overweight or obese. Professionally administered weight loss programs for overweight children and adolescents produce significant improvements in psychological status and pose minimal risks of precipitating eating disorders (Butryn & Wadden, 2005).

Walters and Kendler (1995) found dieting status to be associated with AN in a population-based sample of twins; however, dieting was not measured prior to the onset of AN. In contrast, in a series of studies of AN, BN, and BED in which subjects were asked to report on the premorbid presence of potential risk factors, Fairburn et al. (1999) found that although dieting dimensions were relevant to the emergence of both BN and BED, they were not associated with AN. Dieting was not elevated in a study of affected sisters in discordant sister pairs (Karwautz et al., 2001). Thus, the data from clinical and epidemiological studies do not resolve whether dieting should be considered a risk factor for AN.

Internalization of the Thin Ideal

Weight concerns and dieting are normative in developed countries (Rodin, Silberstein, & Streigel-Moore, 1985). The concept of thin ideal internalization refers to the extent to which an individual adopts cultural pressures toward thinness and is thought to be a necessary but not sufficient precondition for the development of eating disorders (Brownell, 1991). Exposure to thin ideals and dieting are nearly universal in industrialized countries, but only a very small number of young women actually develop clinically significant eating disorders.

Individuals may be susceptible to the cultural pressures toward dieting and body dissatisfaction in proportion to their degree of genetic predisposition (Bulik, 2005). Thus, although all individuals are exposed to these forces, those at greater genetic risk may be more adversely affected. In addition, mediating factors could influence how the thin ideal gets internalized. Fitzsimmons-Craft et al. (2013) suggest that social comparison mediates the impact of thin ideal internalization on disordered eating. Peer context has also emerged as a risk factor, as personality factors influence peer selection, and the chosen peer environment has been shown to influence disordered eating. However, peers may also serve as a buffer against development of eating disorders, and peer groups may prove to be an important intervention target (Keel & Forney, 2013).

Body Dissatisfaction

Dissatisfaction with the size or shape of one's body is often thought to be the key psychological motivator for dieting behavior (Stice, 1994) and a key contributor to the gender differential in the prevalence of eating disorders. In puberty, body dissatisfaction begins to increase in young girls, and may be secondary to the increase in body fat percentage associated with female pubertal development (Marino & King, 1980).

Comorbidity

As also described in Chapter 13, other psychiatric disorders, especially major depression and anxiety disorders, commonly co-occur with AN (Fernández-Aranda et al., 2007; Godart, Berthoz, Perdereau, & Jeammet, 2006). Well over half of women with AN report a lifetime presence of an anxiety disorder, most commonly overanxious disorder, obsessive-compulsive disorder, or social phobia. In most cases, onset of the anxiety disorder precedes the onset of AN (Bulik, Sullivan, Fear, & Joyce, 1997). Retrospective accounts of premorbid symptoms among children who later develop AN often emphasize the presence of pervasive anxiety (Bruch, 1973; Lask & Bryant-Waugh, 2000). This pattern of onset may reflect the natural course of the two disorders (i.e., the average age of onset of many anxiety disorders is younger than the average age of onset of AN), but it may also indicate that childhood anxiety is a significant risk factor for the development of AN. In a population-based sample of over 2,000 female twins, odds ratios for generalized anxiety disorder, phobias, and panic disorder were significantly elevated among women with varying definitions of AN (Walters & Kendler, 1995).

In addition, several outcome studies suggest that depression and anxiety commonly persist after recovery from AN (Berkman, Lohr, & Bulik, 2007; Holtkamp, Muller, Heussen, Remschmidt, & Herpertz-Dahlmann, 2005; Löwe et al., 2001; Mischoulon et al., 2011). In addition, high trait anxiety is associated with a lower likelihood of recovery from AN (Zerwas et al., 2013). Significantly elevated relative risks for mood disorders have been reported among relatives of probands with AN (Hudson, Pope, Jonas, & Yurgelun-Todd, 1983; Logue, Crowe, & Bean, 1989; Rivinus et al., 1984), although these rates may be highest among relatives of individuals with AN who are themselves depressed (Strober, Lampert, Morrell, Burroughs, & Jacobs, 1990). Twin studies have shown that the genetic risk factors for AN and depression are correlated (Wade, Bulik, Neale, & Kendler, 2000), and there appears to be a unique genetic factor that influences the emergence of both early eating and early anxiety disorder symptoms (Silberg & Bulik, 2005).

Race and Socioeconomic Status

Traditionally, AN was considered to be a disorder confined to the white upper middle class. However, this perception may result from the failure of many community-based studies to include non-white participants or from sampling highly homogeneous populations. AN occurs across races and cultures (Hoek et al., 1998; Katzman, Nasser, & Gordon, 2001). In terms of socioeconomic status, in a large population-based study of female twins, Walters and Kendler (1995) found that a greater number of years of parental education (a proxy variable for socioeconomic status) was associated with AN. In addition, there is some suggestion that the risk of developing AN is somewhat lower in individuals who are African-American (Taylor, Caldwell, Baser, Faison, & Jackson, 2007). Striegel-Moore et al. (2003) found that 15 white women (1.5%) and no black women in a geographically and economically diverse community sample of young women who previously participated in the 10-year National Heart, Lung, and Blood Institute Growth and Health Study met lifetime criteria for AN. Our understanding of why risk may be lower is incomplete.

Family Environment

Research does not support the existence of a "typical" AN family. Murphy et al. (2000) reported that sisters with AN had higher levels of maternal control and more antagonism toward and jealousy of their sisters than did their unaffected sisters. Walters and Kendler (1995), in a population-based sample of female twins, reported higher maternal overprotectiveness in individuals with AN. Consensus in the field tends to be that many of the behaviors noted in families of individuals with AN reflect the challenges of dealing with the disorder rather than being causal factors.

Trauma

Childhood sexual abuse has been reported in women with AN (Herzog, Staley, Carmody, Robbins, & van der Kolk, 1993; Horesh et al., 1995) and may be more prevalent in women with AN who exhibit purging behavior (Carretero-Garcia et al., 2012; Carter, Bewell, Blackmore, & Woodside, 2006; Waller, Halek, & Crisp, 1993). Given the relative rarity of AN, few population-based estimates of the prevalence of childhood sexual abuse in these women exist. Romans et al. (1994) studied 3,000 women in New Zealand and found that there was a higher frequency of AN and BN in women who reported childhood sexual abuse. However, childhood sexual abuse did not appear to act independently, as poor parenting and growing up away from both parents also contributed independently to the risk of eating disorders.

Life Events

Adolescents with AN report more adverse life events than healthy controls, and more adverse life events relating to family than psychiatric controls (Horesch et al., 1995). A history of events including abuse and death of close relatives increases the risk of AN (Fairburn et al., 1999). Schmidt et al. (1997) found that individuals with AN experienced significantly more adverse events and difficulties with the potential to evoke sexual shame or disgust in the year prior to onset of AN. An increase in such events was also found by Karwautz et al. (2001) using discordant sisters, where sisters with AN reported more teasing about breast development. Whether individuals with eating disorders actually experience more adverse life events, whether they remember adverse life events better than patients without such events, or whether they are more susceptible to the impact of life events is unknown.

Participation in Sports/Activities/Professions with Body Shape/Weight Focus

Activities that place substantial emphasis on weight and appearance (e.g., ballet, gymnastics) have been investigated as independent risk factors for the development of AN. Ballet participation has received substantial attention (Klump, Ringham, Marcus, & Kaye, 2001; Nascimento, Luna, & Fontenelle, 2012; Penniment & Egan, 2012; Thomas, Keel, & Heatherton, 2011; Van Durme, Goossens, & Braet, 2012). Unlike data from other athlete groups (Powers, Schocken, & Boyd, 1998), ballet dancers' scores on measures of eating pathology are similar to those of individuals with diagnosable eating disorders. In addition, disturbed eating attitudes and behaviors appear to persist after retirement in ballet dancers (Khan et al., 1996). Athletic, artistic, and professional environments may attract individuals who are preoccupied with facets central to eating disorder pathology, which then contributes to the emergence of the syndromes.

A greater prevalence of both subthreshold and threshold eating disorders, including AN, has been described among elite athletes compared with controls, especially among female athletes competing in aesthetic and endurance sports (Hulley & Hill, 2001; Sundgot-Borgen & Torstveit, 2004). Some have proposed a distinct variant of AN deemed "anorexia athletica," where reduction in body mass is for the purpose of athletic performance rather than appearance or weight/shape concerns. However, evidence suggests that anorexia athletica can precede or overlap with AN or other eating disorders, so this distinction is not clear-cut (Sudi et al., 2004). Additional risk factors for eating disorders in athletes include dieting, personality factors, pressure to lose weight, frequent weight cycling, overtraining, injuries, and sport-specific training at a young age (Sundgot-Borgen & Torstveit, 2010). Indeed, many of the personality factors that are associated with the development of AN are the same ones that lead individuals to self-select into certain individual sports. Thus, these third variables (i.e., personality features such as determination, perfectionism, perseverance) may contribute both to sport selection and risk for eating disorders.

Summary

Identifying prospective risk factors for AN in the population is challenging due to the relative rarity of the condition. High-risk paradigms (i.e., focusing on offspring of individuals with AN) might identify factors associated in the development of the disorder in multiply afflicted families. Such studies, although potentially highly valuable, would be representative of only a subset of the population with AN. Inclusion of AN in large epidemiological studies and national surveillance is one way to ensure that incident cases are captured. With recent advances in genetics and neurobiology, the field is well positioned to make inroads into understanding the biological substrates of AN. Central to this understanding is the ability to disaggregate biomarkers of starvation from biomarkers of illness. Given the widespread adverse effects of AN on bodily systems and organs, retrospective studies face serious challenges in attempting to distinguish between factors that existed prior to the disorder and psychological and biological scars of the illness.

RISK FACTORS FOR BULIMIA NERVOSA

Biological Risk Factors

Genetics

Controlled family studies suggest that relatives of individuals with either AN or BN have a significantly elevated prevalence of these disorders compared to relatives of unaffected controls (Lilenfeld et al., 1998; Strober et al., 2000). However, no studies have examined the prevalence of only BN in family members of affected individuals. Heritability estimates for BN from twin studies range from 28% to 83% (Bulik, Sullivan, Wade, & Kendler, 2000). A single linkage study has been conducted to date to investigate markers of genetic risk for BN, examining 308 families with eating disorders. This study found significant linkage on chromosome 10, while a region on chromosome 14 met criterion for genome-wide suggestive linkage (Bulik, Devlin, et al., 2003). The majority of molecular genetic investigations in BN are candidate gene association studies exploring genes in the serotonergic and dopaminergic systems and genes related to appetite and weight regulation. No genes have yet emerged with significantly strong and replicated signals to be considered concrete risk factors for BN. There have been no genome-wide association studies of BN.

Neurobiological

Individuals with BN demonstrate abnormalities of the dopamine and serotonin neurotransmitter systems (Kaye, 2008). Individuals recovered from BN show higher-than-normal levels of CSF 5-hydroxyindoleacetic acid (Kaye, 2008) and altered responses to serotonin behavioral challenges (Kaye et al., 2003; Ward, Brown, Lightman, Campbell, & Treasure, 1998). Serotonin abnormalities have also been implicated in binge eating (Akkermann, Nordquist, Oreland, & Harro, 2010) and in the frequency of binge-eating episodes in BN (Jimerson, Lesem, Kaye, & Brewerton, 1992; Monteleone, Brambilla, Bortolotti, Ferraro, & Maj, 1998). Perspectives that view BN as an appetitive or even addictive behavior are using various paradigms to explore how the brains of individuals with BN respond to food reward or nonreward (e.g., Bailer & Kaye, 2011; Frank et al., 2012; Uher et al., 2004).

Sex

As with AN, females with BN outnumber males by a considerable margin. Data from the National Comorbidity Survey Replication, which includes a nationally representative sample of U.S. households, estimate the female-to-male ratio at approximately 3:1, with lifetime prevalence estimates for BN of 1.5% in women and 0.5% in men (Kessler et al., 2004; Kessler, Chiu, Demler, Merikangas, & Walters, 2005). However, although BN is more prevalent in females, recurrent binge-eating behavior is found equally in both sexes. Striegel-Moore and Bulik (2007) hypothesized that this discrepancy may be explained by the fact that men who binge eat are significantly less likely to report extreme weight-control behaviors (e.g., purging) than women (Hay, 1998) and often use different compensatory methods in an attempt to reduce body fat and increase muscularity (Anderson & Bulik, 2004; Striegel-Moore & Bulik, 2007).

Early Menarche

Early menarche is associated with increased adipose tissue, which may result in a perceived deviation from the thin ideal and decreased body dissatisfaction, and could, in turn, lead to dieting, negative affect, and bulimic symptoms. Early sexual development can also lead to increased sexual attention and unwanted comments and teasing. Early menarche has been associated with BN (Fairburn, Welch, Doll, Davies, & O'Connor, 1997) and especially early onset of BN (Day et al., 2011; Favaro et al., 2009).

Body Mass Index

Elevated body mass, or being at a higher weight, has been shown to predict increases in perceived pressure to be thin, body dissatisfaction, attempted dieting, and purging (Field et al., 1999; Stice & Whitenton, 2002). Therefore, individuals at a higher weight may experience pressure to be thin from family or peers, which could result in increased drive for thinness or body dissatisfaction, and increased risk for bulimic symptoms. In addition, weight suppression (i.e., the difference between the highest previous weight and the current weight), and the interaction between weight suppression and body mass index (BMI), predicted binge-eating frequency in a study of women with threshold and subthreshold BN, with participants with low BMI and high weight suppression having the highest frequency of binge eating (Butryn, Juarascio, & Lowe, 2011). However, in a study of college freshmen, weight suppression did not predict future increases in bulimic symptoms (Stice, Durant, Burger, & Schoeller, 2011). Thus, while increased weight is a risk factor for pressure to be thin, body dissatisfaction, and attempted dieting, it may play a more important role in promoting other risk factors for BN than in directly fostering bulimic symptoms.

Personality/Temperament

Perfectionism has been examined as a risk factor for eating pathology because this trait may promote a relentless pursuit of the thin ideal. Several studies have provided support for a model in which high perfectionism, high weight and shape concern, and low self-esteem interact to cause the onset and maintenance of bulimic symptoms (Bardone-Cone, Abramson, Vohs, Heatherton, & Joiner, 2006; Vohs, Bardone, Joiner, Abramson, & Heatherton, 1999). However, attempts to replicate the results from this model have been mixed (Downey & Chang, 2007; Shaw, Stice, & Springer, 2004; Steele, Corsini, & Wade, 2007; Watson, Steele, Bergin, Fursland, & Wade, 2011). Another personality characteristic, a deficit in impulse control, has also been considered as a risk factor for bulimic pathology, as deficits in impulse control might increase the propensity for episodes of uncontrollable binge eating. Several investigators have found associations between symptoms of bulimia and indicators of impulsivity (Kaltiala-Heino, Rissanen, Rimpela, & Rantanen, 2003; Peñas-Lledó, Vaz, Ramos, & Waller, 2002; Rosval et al., 2006).

Behavioral/Environmental Risk Factors

Perinatal and Early Feeding Problems

Several studies have examined the extent to which early problems with feeding constitute risk factors for the later development of broadly defined eating disorder symptoms. In data obtained from a long-term prospective study, Marchi and Cohen (1990) found that symptoms of BN in later adolescence were related to both digestive problems and pica in early childhood and to efforts at weight loss in early adolescence. Early feeding difficulties were endorsed by 21% of individuals with early-onset (childhood) eating disorders in a British national surveillance study (Nicholls et al., 2011), though most met criteria for AN or an eating disorder not otherwise specified rather than BN. Higher infant BMI and birthweight for gestational age predicted the emergence of overeating and BN (Goodman et al., 2014; Stice, Agras, & Hammer, 1999), while Jacobi, Schmitz, and Agras (2008) found that disturbed eating behavior was associated with higher BMI in 8- to 12-year-old German children. However, the relationship of these phenomena to the development of BN is unknown.

Dieting/Negative Energy Balance

Dieting is commonplace in adolescence. Although the intention of dieting is generally to lose weight and control eating, dieting has in fact been associated with weight gain, obesity, and the development of binge eating (Haines, Kleinman, Rifas-Shiman, Field, & Austin, 2010; Neumark-Sztainer et al., 2006; Stice, Cameron, Killen, Hayward, & Taylor, 1999; Stice, Presnell, & Spangler, 2002; Tanofsky-Kraff et al., 2006). Yet very few individuals who diet go on to develop BN, indicating that the relationship between dieting and BN must be complex. Various models propose that binge eating develops in response to "dietary restraint" (Polivy & Herman, 1985) or as a means of alleviating low mood that arises secondary to restraint or dieting (Stice, 2001). Retrospective data suggest that a history of dieting is common among adults with BN (de Zwaan et al., 1994; Kurth, Krahn, Nairn, & Drewnowski, 1995). Prospective studies suggest that low self-esteem, depression, and teasing may increase the likelihood of dieting resulting in binge eating (Goldschmidt, Wall, Loth, Le Grange, & Neumark-Sztainer, 2012; Presnell, Stice, & Tristan, 2008; Stice, 2001).

Internalization of the Thin Ideal

As with AN, the cultural emphasis on thinness has been implicated as a risk factor for the development of BN, and pressure to be thin predicts increases in body dissatisfaction, dieting, negative affect (Cattarin & Thompson, 1994; Field et al., 2001; Stice & Bearman, 2001; Stice & Shaw, 2002), and bulimic symptom onset (Field et al., 1999; Stice et al., 2002). Higher levels of thin ideal internalization are also predictive of greater time to remission of binge eating in women with subthreshold and threshold BN (Bohon, Stice, & Burton, 2009). Experiments have found that acute and long-term exposure to ultra-slender media images and peers produces increased body dissatisfaction, negative affect, dieting, and bulimic symptoms, which are mediated by thin ideal internalization (Bair, Kelly, Serdar, & Mazzeo, 2012; Nouri, Hill, & Orrell-Valente, 2011), but that these effects are stronger for girls with preexisting body image disturbances and social support deficits (Cattarin & Thompson, 1994; Groesz, Levine, & Murnen, 2002). Furthermore, inclusion of a disclaimer or warning about thin ideal media images showed no effect on body dissatisfaction in female college students (Ata, Thompson, & Small, 2013) and may even have unintended harmful effects in some individuals (Tiggemann, Slater, Bury, Hawkins, & Firth, 2013).

Body Dissatisfaction

Body dissatisfaction predicts increases in attempted dieting (Cooley & Toray, 2001; Wertheim, Koerner, & Paxton, 2001), negative affect (Rierdan, Koff, & Stubbs, 1989; Stice & Bearman, 2001), bulimic symptom onset (Field, et al., 1999), and increases in bulimic symptoms (Cooley & Toray, 2001). As mentioned previously, social comparison may be an important mediator of body dissatisfaction (Fitzsimmons-Craft et al., 2013). In a longitudinal investigation in Norway, appearance dissatisfaction (as well as anxiety and depressive symptoms, alcohol consumption, self-concept instability, and loneliness) was particularly associated with purging behavior in a population-based sample (Abebe, Lien, Torgersen, & von Soest, 2012).

Trauma

Childhood sexual abuse is a nonspecific risk factor for BN, especially in the presence of psychiatric comorbidity (Kendler et al., 2000; Wonderlich, Brewerton, Jocic, Dansky, & Abbott, 1997). A history of abuse has been reported by as many as 71% of individuals receiving inpatient treatment for BN (Claes & Vandereycken, 2007), and in the Victorian Adolescent Health Cohort Study, the incidence of BN was 2.5 times higher in females reporting one childhood sexual abuse episode and nearly five times higher among those reporting two or more episodes, even after adjusting for age, background factors, and other potential mediators and confounders (Sanci et al., 2008). Childhood physical or sexual abuse may influence the long-term outcome of BN. In patients who were hospitalized for treatment of BN and interviewed 2 to 9 years later, poor outcome was associated with childhood physical abuse (Fallon, Sadik, Saoud, & Garfinkel, 1994). In addition, adult childhood sexual abuse survivors with a history of AN or BN were significantly more depressed and had lower self-esteem than those without an eating disorder history (Harper, Richter, & Gorey, 2009).

Comorbidity (Impulse Control Disorders/Substance Use/Depression/Anxiety)

The most commonly diagnosed comorbid disorder in individuals with BN is major depressive disorder, with a frequency estimated at 25.3% (Giovanni et al., 2011), and rates may be higher among adolescents (Fischer & le Grange, 2007).

The majority of individuals with BN have at least one comorbid anxiety disorder, most commonly obsessive-compulsive disorder, social phobia, and specific phobia (Godart et al., 2002; Kendler et al., 1995; Walters & Kendler, 1995; Kaye, Bulik, Thornton, Barbarich, & Masters, 2004). Generally, the onset of the anxiety disorder precedes the onset of BN (Bulik et al., 1997; Godart, Flament, Lecrubier, & Jeammet, 2000).

The comorbidity of BN and substance abuse is also common. In a sample of 2,436 females receiving inpatient treatment, 22% had a comorbid substance use disorder, with patients with BN twice as likely to have comorbid alcohol abuse or dependence and three times as likely to have polysubstance abuse/dependence as patients with other eating disorders (Blinder, Cumella, & Sanathara, 2006). Using data from the Swedish Twin Registry, Root, Pisetsky, et al. (2010) found a similar prevalence of comorbid alcohol abuse/dependence among individuals with BN (22%). In the National Women's Study, the prevalence of alcohol abuse was higher in women with BN compared to those without BN or BED, but only after controlling for comorbid major depressive disorder and post-traumatic stress disorder, suggesting that these disorders may influence or mediate the relationship between BN and alcohol use disorders (Dansky, Brewerton, & Kilpatrick, 2000). BN is also associated with drug use disorders, an association mediated by depression, neuroticism, and childhood sexual abuse (in both directions; Baker, Mazzeo, & Kendler, 2007).

The lifetime prevalence of impulse control disorders in a sample of females receiving inpatient treatment for BN was 23.8%, with lifetime compulsive buying (17.6%) and intermittent explosive disorder (13.2%) most commonly reported. Across eating disorders, individuals with BN are characterized by high impulsivity, sensation seeking, novelty seeking, and traits associated with borderline personality disorder (Cassin & von Ranson, 2005).

Summary

A number of factors, including thin ideal internalization (possibly mediated by social comparison), body dissatisfaction, and negative affect have been identified as risk factors for the development of bulimic symptoms. Some studies suggest that attempted dieting and weight suppression can contribute to risk, but it is not clear whether dysfunctional dieting, especially severe caloric restriction, is a risk factor for full-syndrome BN. A history of AN is clearly a risk factor for BN given the high rates of diagnostic crossover. There are some tentative suggestions that early feeding problems may be associated with later BN. The data are mixed on the impact of early menarche, with some indications that it may be related to early-onset BN. More than in AN, child maltreatment and childhood sexual abuse emerge as precursors to BN, although, again, this is not a specific predictor as these histories predispose to a number of psychiatric disorders. Finally, complex comorbid profiles including anxiety disorders, depressive disorders, substance-related disorders, and disorders of impulse control all suggest that several psychological dimensions likely contribute to the development of bulimic pathology.

RISK FACTORS FOR BINGE-EATING DISORDER

Considerably fewer risk factor investigations have been conducted for BED relative to AN and BN. In addition, in the absence of official diagnostic criteria before the publication of DSM-5, studies have had to rely on approximate definitions that have varied depending on the questions that were used to identify symptoms. Dimensions such as the nature of a binge, the presence of loss of control or distress, and the frequency and duration criteria for binge eating have varied widely across studies. To avoid becoming lost in these details, the following review takes the case definitions at face value, but it is important to note that subtle definitional differences may ultimately lead to slightly different conclusions.

Biological Risk Factors

Genetics

With the exception a 1999 family study (Lee et al., 1999), which failed to show a significant familial relationship, the majority of research suggests that BED is familial (Fowler & Bulik, 1997). A large direct-interview family study (Hudson et al., 2006) interviewed overweight or obese individuals with and without BED, along with all available first-degree relatives. BED aggregated strongly in families, independent of obesity. Similarly, Lilenfeld et al. (2008) reported significantly increased rates of BED in first-degree family members of individuals with this diagnosis. Three population-based twin studies have estimated the heritability of the DSM-IV diagnosis of BED or a broader definition of BED to be between 39% and 45%, with the remaining variance due to unique environmental factors (Javaras et al., 2008; Mitchell et al., 2010; Reichborn-Kjennerud, Bulik, Tambs, & Harris, 2004).

Candidate gene association studies of binge eating have examined neurotransmitter systems or genetic variants implicated in appetite and obesity, including the serotonin and dopamine systems, but none of the few reported findings has as yet been replicated (Burnet et al., 1999; Davis et al., 2008). No genome-wide association studies have been performed for BED.

Neurobiological

Individuals with BED have higher meal-induced levels of cholecystokinin and peptide YY than age- and BMI-matched controls, which Munsch et al. (2009) suggest could indicate a physiological response to the release of satiety hormones in order to prevent binge eating. In addition, dopamine has been hypothesized to play a role in the development and perpetuation of BED by modulating reward pathways (Bello & Hajnal, 2010; Mathes, Brownley, Mo, & Bulik, 2009). Results from neuroimaging studies in adolescent and young-adult females by Stice, Spoor, et al. (2008) suggest that the dorsal striatum is less responsive to food reward in obese individuals, which could be due to diminished dopamine (D2) receptor density or altered dopamine signaling, which would explain overeating as compensation for a deficit in reward pathways. However, these studies have not been replicated in individuals with BED.

Body Mass Index

In comparing women with BED to those with other psychiatric disorders, Fairburn et al. (1998) and Striegel-Moore et al. (2005) found that those with BED reported more childhood obesity. Comparing girls with BED and no eating disorder in the National Heart, Lung, and Blood Institute Growth and Health Study, girls with BED were found to have a higher BMI, even in the 2 years prior to the onset of the eating disorder (Striegel-Moore et al., 2004). A modest genetic correlation between obesity and binge eating has also been reported (Bulik, Sullivan, & Kendler, 2003).

Sex

Sex differences are far less pronounced in BED than AN or BN, which both have a higher prevalence in females (Swanson et al., 2011). Differential prevalence across sexes is also less evident when broader definitions of all of the eating disorders are used, including partial syndromes (Hudson et al., 2007; John, Meyer, Rumpf, & Hapke, 2006; Woodside et al., 2001). Recurrent binge eating is equally as common in men as in women (Hay, 1998; Lewinsohn, Seeley, Moerk, & Striegel-Moore, 2002; Reagan & Hersch, 2005; Woodside et al., 2001).

Age and Development

Unlike AN or BN, adolescence does not appear to be a unique period of risk for onset of BED. Onset has been reported to occur well into adulthood (Hudson et al., 2007). Moreover, pregnancy has been identified as a risk period for the onset of BED (Bulik et al., 2007).

Dieting

Several studies have examined differences between BED subtypes delineated by whether binge eating or dieting occurred first. Collectively, they have found that the prevalence of "binge eating first" in patients with BED is approximately 35% to 55%, though there were differences across studies in terms of how "dieting" was defined (Abbott et al., 1998; Grilo & Masheb, 2000; Mussell et al., 1995; Spurrell, Wilfley, Tanofsky, & Brownell, 1997). Across studies, the "binge eating first" group reported (1) starting to binge eat at an earlier age (11–13 years vs. 25 or 26 years for the "dieting first" group); (2) higher frequency of weight-related teasing; (3) earlier onset of overweight and BED diagnosis; and (4) higher number of lifetime psychiatric diagnoses (including substance use disorders; Abbott et al., 1998; Grilo & Masheb, 2000; Spurrell et al., 1997). Using a diverse community-based sample, and a strict definition of dieting, Manwaring et al. (2006) did not find significant differences in risk factors for BED between "binge eating first" and "dieting first" groups, though the "binge eating first" group had an earlier onset of BED, and the "dieting first" group endorsed greater eating disorder psychopathology and lifetime substance use disorder diagnosis. However, a history of childhood weight loss attempts has been associated with a greater risk of BED in adults (Rubinstein, McGinn, Wildman, & Wylie-Rosett, 2010).

Loss-of-Control Eating

The onset of BED typically occurs in adolescence or adulthood, and full-syndrome BED is uncommon in children. However, both retrospective studies in adults and prospective studies in children suggest several childhood risk factors, including loss-of-control eating (i.e., the inability to stop eating or control the amount/

type of food consumed). Children who report loss-of-control eating also endorse greater disordered eating attitudes and depressive symptoms, have increased adiposity, and may be at higher risk for excess weight gain (Tanofsky-Kraff et al., 2006; Sonneville et al., 2012), metabolic syndrome (Tanofsky-Kraff et al., 2012), and BED. One candidate gene (*FTO* rs9939609) is associated with loss-of-control eating in children, even after controlling for body weight (Tanofsky-Kraff et al., 2009). Psychosocial factors, including parental underinvolvement and critical comments, may also increase the risk for loss-of-control eating (Field et al., 2008; Tanofsky-Kraff et al., 2013).

Teasing

Several prospective and retrospective studies have suggested that weight-related teasing and negative comments about shape, weight, and eating are risk factors for BED or binge eating (Fairburn et al., 1998; Field et al., 2008; Haines, Neumark-Sztainer, Eisenberg, & Hannan, 2006; Jacobi et al., 2011; Neumark-Sztainer et al., 2002, 2007; Stormer & Thompson, 1996). Intriguingly, victims, bullies, and bully-victims (i.e., individuals who both bully and are bullied) are at risk for developing eating disorder symptoms (Copeland et al., 2015).

Comorbidity

Comorbidity is the norm in BED. In a large population sample in Sweden, individuals with BED were at significantly elevated risk for major depressive disorder, anxiety disorder, post-traumatic stress disorder, and suicide attempts (Welch, 2016). In a sample of more than 400 patients with BED, Grilo et al. (2009) found that 73.8% met diagnostic criteria for at least one additional lifetime psychiatric disorder, while 43.1% had at least one current comorbid psychiatric disorder. Mood (54.2% lifetime, 26.0% current) and anxiety (37.1% lifetime, 24.5% current) disorders were the most common comorbid diagnoses. Nearly a quarter of the patients also met criteria for a lifetime substance use disorder, with higher rates among males than females. In addition to psychiatric comorbidity, individuals with BED are at increased risk for medical comorbidity across a range of bodily systems (Thornton et al., 2017) and demonstrate high medication utilization (Watson et al., 2016).

Summary

Our understanding of risk factors for BED is currently limited. Different developmental patterns in comparison to AN or BN, sex distribution, and weight and weight history profiles argue against "lumping" BED together with risk factor studies of other eating disorders. Now that DSM-5 has provided a consensus definition for the disorder, studies should be more consistent. A critical issue to address is the extent to which loss-of-control eating in childhood is etiologically similar to binge eating in adults. As many, but not all, individuals with BED are overweight or obese, a major challenge is to extricate risk factors for binge eating from risk factors for weight dysregulation. This is in many ways as complicated as separating biomarkers of illness from biomarkers of starvation in AN and represents one of the most important challenges facing the field.

CULTURAL ISSUES AND EATING DISORDERS

A wide variety of evidence—including historical, epidemiological, ethnographic, and experimental data—indicates that sociocultural factors influence the risk for eating disorders, although their pathogenesis is incompletely understood and undeniably complex. The salience of the impact of culture on eating disorders has been inferred, in part, from robust epidemiological evidence that the prevalence varies across diverse social contexts and populations, including across ethnic groups and national regions. Other studies demonstrate that the prevalence has changed for certain populations over time—for example, concurrently with modernization or following transnational migration. Importantly, putative sociocultural contributions to risk do not preclude biological factors—including genetic and physiological vulnerabilities—as risk factors. Indeed, social and biological factors likely exert complementary impact, as noted above, and are even plausibly synergistic in contributing to risk.

Eating disorders are now recognized to have a broad global distribution, and the World Health Organization (2003) named eating disorders as a priority area for adolescent mental health in 2003. In 2012, the Global Burden of Disease Study published data for the first time on the estimated burden of disease for eating disorders. This global burden (measured as disability-adjusted life-years), while lower than for other major mental disorders such as schizophrenia, depression, and bipolar disorder, was estimated to have increased by 65.7% between 1990 and 2010 (Murray et al., 2012). Because even in well-resourced health systems a substantial number of eating disorders remain undetected or untreated (Hudson et al., 2007), it is likely that the health and social impacts of eating disorders are underestimated in low- and middle-income countries. Moreover, few community-based epidemiological studies have assessed the prevalence of eating disorders in these regions.

Cross-Cultural Studies

Cultural influences on the presentation of eating disorders are elegantly illustrated in series of scientific papers by Lee et al. in Hong Kong, who first described "non-fat-phobic AN" as a common clinical variant in Hong Kong. This variant was distinguished by its absent "fear of fatness," and the expressed alternative rationales for dietary restriction—for example, gastrointestinal discomfort—were notable for their cultural relevance to the local context (Lee, 1991, 1995). Whereas the non-fat-phobic AN phenotype initially represented approximately one third of cases seen in a major psychiatric clinic in Hong Kong, the number of cases declined relative to the fat-phobic phenotype over the past decade, coinciding with greater exposure to global culture among the Hong Kong Chinese (Lee, Ng, Kwok, & Fung, 2010). Other reports from non-Western populations of AN-like presentations in the absence of overt weight concerns support the impact of cultural environment on the local phenomenology of eating disorders (Becker et al., 2009; Keel & Klump, 2003). For example, a latent profile analysis of adolescent girls in Fiji who self-reported purging identified a culture-specific variant distinguished from BN-like presentations by the use of traditional herbal purgatives for weight management. Notably, this culturally particular phenotype was associated with significantly more distress than BN-like presentations even though it does not mesh with the conventional diagnostic criteria for BN (Thomas, Crosby, Wonderlich, Striegel-Moore, & Becker, 2011). Indeed, because the diagnostic criteria for the eating disorders are based on data primarily drawn from Western populations, unique cultural variations in their patterning and presentation may not be readily discerned by conventional diagnostic criteria, and opportunities to appreciate etiologic social factors or pathogenic cultural exposures likely have not been fully exploited. These culturally distinctive phenotypes suggest a complex interplay between biological vulnerabilities and social context.

The variation observed across culturally distinct populations is consistent with major theoretical models of etiology (Stice, 1994; Striegel-Moore & Bulik, 2007; Thompson & Shroff, 2006) positing a link between social pressure to be thin and eating disorders. These models are appealing insofar as they can account for the observed cross-cultural variation in eating disorder prevalence and phenomenology since key risk factors, such as internalization of a thin ideal, appearance-based comparison, body dissatisfaction, and dieting, are underpinned by prevailing—but highly variable—social norms. To the extent that body size ideals are socially constructed, how they are valued, perceived, and pursued varies substantially across cultural contexts.

The plasticity of social norms for body size ideals has also been well documented historically, famously illustrated in the early-20th-century debut of the thin ideal for women in the United States (Brumberg, 1988). This ideal emerged alongside increasing food security, social autonomy for women, expanding opportunities to commercialize beauty, and widespread distribution of both images and ideas through the mass media that associated slenderness with social prestige. During this era, the introduction of standardized clothing sizes by the ready-to-wear clothing industry (Brumberg, 1988) and the ensuing migration of social norms for self-presentation, style, diet, and fitness also set the stage for the deep cultural resonance with concerns about weight. Although cases consistent with AN are reported over a century ago, the historical record supports the emergence of prevalent eating disorders in Western cultural settings only later, during the 20th century.

An increasing prevalence of disordered eating over time has also been reported in non-Western cultural contexts, for example among Japanese adolescents in Japan (Chisuwa & O'Dea, 2010) and among ethnic Fijian teenagers in Fiji (Becker, Burwell, Gilman, Herzog, & Hamburg, 2002). The impact of cultural context on eating disorder risk for adolescents is illustrated by a series of studies conducted in the Western Pacific island nation of Fiji during a period of rapid modernization. Prior to the electrification of rural areas and introduction of broadcast television with largely Western-produced content, the aesthetic ideal for women's bodies in Fiji was robust and strong; this was in contrast to the slender ideal with social currency in Euro-American populations, but similar to the ideal large body size preferred elsewhere among Pacific Islanders. Eating disorders were also reportedly rare in Fiji prior to the 1990s (Becker, 1995). A two-wave cohort study supported the emergence of serious eating disorder behaviors among adolescent ethnic Fijian girls following the introduction of television in the mid-1990s (Becker et al., 2002). Subsequently, a study with a large, representative sample of school-going adolescent Fijian girls also demonstrated a significant association between certain Western-based cultural exposures—overseas travel, a media-exposed peer network, and Western cultural orientation—and eating pathology as measured by the Eating Disorder Examination Questionnaire (Becker et al., 2011).

Elevated eating disorder risk in populations following migration to new social contexts with novel Western cultural values also illustrates the impact of sociocultural exposures (Nasser, Katzman, & Gordon, 2001). For example, despite the low incidence of AN in Curacao, Antilleans living in the Netherlands have a comparable incidence of AN to the native Dutch population there (van Hoeken, Veling, Smink, & Hoek, 2010). Similarly, a large study of Latinos in the United States found the lifetime risk of BN to be significantly higher among those who had spent more than 70% of their lifetime in the United States (Alegria et al., 2007). Likewise, U.S.-born African-American and Caribbean blacks were more than twice as likely to develop an eating disorder as those who were foreign born (Taylor et al., 2013).

These and other studies have also raised the question of whether the process of acculturation (or associated transnational migration) or exposure to specific cultural content is inherently pathogenic. Notwithstanding some reports of increased risk following transnational migration, the scientific literature, in aggregate, has not demonstrated a consistent pattern relating culture change per se to eating disorders. For example, transnational migration may impact risk both by proximal exposures to new social norms that specifically influence aspects of disordered eating and by juxtaposition of norms characterizing the culture of origin and the host culture. Simultaneous or serial exposures to divergent norms may, in turn, engender transgenerational or other conflicts (Bhugra & Bhui, 2003; Pike & Borovoy, 2004) around engagement with host cultural values, or otherwise result in "acculturation stress" (Berry & Annis, 1974), related, for example, to social marginalization (Bhugra & Arya, 2005).

Whereas some studies demonstrate the association between acculturation and disordered eating, others suggest that acculturation is either protective or unrelated to eating disorders. Undoubtedly this observed inconsistency is, in part, attributable to methodologic limitations in operationalizing and measuring processes—migration, assimilation, and acculturation—that are both heterogeneous and multidimensional (Becker et al., 2010b). The relation of ethnicity to eating disorder risk is similarly complex.

Ethnicity and Adolescent Eating Disorders in the United States

Although high socioeconomic status was once identified as a risk factor for AN (Garfinkel & Garner, 1983), numerous studies have upended the previous clinical stereotype that eating disorders are uncommon among women of color or the economically disadvantaged. Indeed, some data support that disordered eating may be even more common among Hispanic and American Indian teens than in their white, non-Hispanic peers (Croll, Neumark-Sztainer, Story, & Ireland, 2002). Bulimic features may be relatively more common in African-American girls than their white counterparts, whereas the latter show comparatively greater body dissatisfaction and dietary restraint (Striegel-Moore et al., 2000). This is consistent with evidence that BN is more common in African-Americans and Latinos than in non-Latino whites among U.S. adults (Marques et al., 2011). That being said, studies have yielded a rather mosaic picture of ethnicity, disordered eating, and risk correlates (Judge, Thomas, & Becker, 2006) with temporal fluidity (Shaw, Ramirez, Trost, Randall, & Stice, 2004). The upshot is that rigorously collected community-based data support that eating disorders occur across the major ethnic groups in the United States (Marques et al., 2011).

In addition, comparative data demonstrate that etiologic pathways for disordered eating may have some common features across diverse social groups. For example, a large-scale study of middle school–age youth showed that dietary weight management behaviors were associated with increased odds of "disordered weight control behaviors" (e.g., purging) for boys and girls across ethnic groups in Massachusetts (Wang et al., 2013). Another large study found weight was associated with body dissatisfaction, independently of ethnicity, among fourth-graders through sixth-graders in urban Philadelphia, although body dissatisfaction was significantly higher among Asian children (Xanthopoulos et al., 2011). In addition, study findings from the National Longitudinal Study of Adolescent Health showed an association between body dissatisfaction and dietary restraint as well as bulimic symptomatology among a large sample of Latina and Latina multi-ethnic female adolescents (Granillo, Jones-Rodriguez, & Carvajal, 2005).

Notwithstanding commonalities across ethnic groups suggesting that etiologic pathways may be similar across diverse social contexts, there are also examples of differences in how these might be culturally mediated or moderated. For instance, although exposure to and internalization of the thin ideal has been associated with body dissatisfaction among Asian-American college students, Asian-American respondents also showed less internalization of the thin ideal compared with their European-American counterparts (Nouri et al., 2011). Similarly, whereas internalization of beauty ideals was associated with disordered eating in a sample of African-American college women, ethnic identity was inversely associated with internalization of beauty ideals (Rogers, Wood, & Petrie, 2010). Other research demonstrates that there may be ethnic-based differences with regard to which body ideals—those of one's own ethnic group or those of the dominant and broad U.S. culture—are salient to body dissatisfaction (Gordon, Sitnikov, Castro, & Holm-Denoma, 2010) or which aesthetic dimensions of self-presentation are most highly valued (Rubin, Fitts, & Becker, 2003). Finally, a large longitudinal study of black and white girls in the United States found that the relation of BMI to body dissatisfaction was moderated significantly by ethnicity; that is, despite no differences in the lowest BMI quintile, white respondents had significantly greater body dissatisfaction than black respondents in the top four BMI quintiles (Striegel-Moore et al., 2000). In this respect, there is evidence that ethnicity affects eating disorder risk.

In summary, some data support variation in patterning of symptoms such as dietary restriction, purging, or binge eating across ethnic groups (e.g., Franko, Becker, Thomas, & Herzog,

2007; Striegel-Moore et al., 2000). However, ethnicity is only one of multiple dimensions of social identity, and individuals may be influenced by multiple kinds of social norms, such as those relating to their occupation as well as geography or cultural heritage. Moreover, the major ethnic groups in the United States are characterized by substantial cultural heterogeneity, partly determined by national origin. Further, adolescents may relate variously to social norms endorsed by peers and/or represented and amplified in the mass media. Such norms, moreover, are fluid and tied to both local and global contexts.

Although "culture" is often treated as a static construct, it is useful to understand culture as dynamic, with many cross-cutting dimensions and micro-pockets. Culture can be operationalized as comprising mutually shared values and conventions, which, in turn, stem from shared history, heritage, language, geography, and experience and inform both perspectives and practices related to quotidian life, the organization of family and community, and broader economic and political domains. Modern platforms for communication and travel facilitate globalized distribution of goods, services, ideas, and news that result in wide circulation of various "local" cultural exposures and also allow community building to transcend geographic locale. Transnational commerce and geopolitical pressures on migration result in unprecedented rapid spread of exposures associated with "local" cultures. To the extent that "youth culture" and contemporary ideas and trends transcend cultures tied to populations with shared history and geography, cultural exposures associated with risk for eating disorders now have global distribution.

It is precisely this broad and rapid distribution of ideas, images, and values that suggests that eating disorders are no longer confined to narrow regional or demographic distribution, if we accept the premise that social context mediates and moderates risk. When culture is operationalized in this way, instead of being associated with "exotic" or remote ideas or traits, it is more straightforward to understand how it exerts influence on social norms for body cultivation, self-agency, self-presentation, dietary patterns, physical activity, and values governing aesthetic ideals and self-discipline.

The observed variation across national regions, ethnicity, and historical periods strongly supports the influence of sociocultural factors on eating disorders. It therefore behooves clinicians to appreciate that behavioral symptoms, their disclosure, and associated care seeking for eating disorders may vary across ethnic groups. This heterogeneity in presentation, moreover, potentially complicates diagnostic assessment (Kelly, Cotter, & Mazzeo, 2012), and standard diagnostic criteria may undermine detection in some groups (Taylor et al., 2013). However, formulaic characterization of prevalence and phenotypes for any particular ethnic or cultural group is unwarranted since it would be misguided to presume temporal stability of socially mediated risk factors for eating disorders. Rather, studies reporting comparative findings should be understood as a snapshot that can inform our understanding of risk and resilience with respect to social norms and cultural values in a specific community at a specific historical moment. For this reason, broad patterns reported in the literature that relate ethnicity to differential risk for either eating disorders or one of their many putative or candidate risk factors, such as body dissatisfaction, overweight, dietary restriction, or acculturative stress, are more informative to etiologic models than to practice.

Social Barriers to Caring for Patients with Eating Disorders

In addition to cultural influences that exert their impact on values, conventions, and practices that shape preferences and motivation, and structure the environment in which eating behaviors and symptoms emerge, social structural factors powerfully influence economic and social opportunities and risks of stigma and discrimination. These, in turn, impact health literacy and access to information that underwrite care-seeking patterns. Ethnic-based disparities in healthcare access are well known, and mental health services utilization is significantly lower among ethnic minority individuals with a lifetime history of an eating disorder than it is for non-Latino whites in the United States (Marques et al., 2011). Social barriers include challenges relating to the affordability of medications, feasibility of obtaining time off from work, and the cost of transportation to the clinic. Additional social barriers to care for eating disorders include both clinician and lay stereotypes about the demographics of eating disorders (Becker, Arrindell, Perloe, Fay, & Striegel-Moore, 2010a). For example, in a voluntary college-based screening program, counselors were less likely to refer Latino and Native American participants than non-Latino, white participants for further care based on a standardized referral protocol, adjusting for clinical severity of symptoms, which suggests possible clinician referral bias (Becker, Franko, Speck, & Herzog, 2003). Understanding and reducing the multiple social barriers to care for mental disorders are pragmatic and essential first steps toward abrogating disparities in care access for treatment.

Culture, Eating Disorders, and Clinical Practice

Although cultural variation in both eating disorder risk factors and presentations has been described across major ethnic groups in the United States, clinicians practicing in multicultural settings will enhance the cultural sensitivity and relevance of their care if they understand that no particular ethnic group is "immune" to eating disorders. Further, it is neither feasible nor useful to characterize fixed, relative differences in risk or presentation across ethnic groups. Ethnic identities, moreover, are potentially fluid and dynamic, especially among teenagers who may engage in multiple social networks through school, work, family, and community, resulting in hybrid cultural identities. Therefore, clinicians would be well advised to engage patients with an interview approach, such as the Cultural Formulation Interview in DSM-5 (APA, 2013) that provides an avenue for eliciting the clinically relevant features and experience of a patient's social identity. Setting aside social and cultural differences that have been observed, the phenomenological heterogeneity of eating disorder presentations is well known, and changes to the diagnostic criteria for eating disorders in the DSM-5 will likely encompass greater heterogeneity of symptom presentations, including those relating to cultural diversity.

Despite some cultural variation in presentation and risk, there is also evidence of certain uniform mechanisms—peer influence and mass media exposure—that impact adolescents across diverse populations (e.g., Becker et al., 2011), possibly because these are chief vectors for diffusing new ideas and establishing social norms relevant to body dissatisfaction and disordered eating. These commonalities can inform both prevention programs and therapeutic approaches, although further research on how other cultural dimensions may moderate their impact will be of great benefit. Patients will be best served when clinicians understand how patients' experience, engagement, and identification with sometimes multiple cultural traditions, practices, and values relate to their body image, weight concerns, and disordered eating. These cultural exposures are, moreover, continually changing, so attunement to their mutability and multifaceted dimensions, as well as their endlessly complex interactions with psychological and biological resilience and vulnerabilities, is warranted in both research and clinical settings.

PREVENTION OF EATING DISORDERS

This section reviews empirical studies of prevention, with a focus on universal and targeted prevention activities. Universal prevention attempts to reduce the incidence of a disease by eliminating or reducing risk factors in a population. Increasing exercise levels and reducing intake of high levels of saturated fat to reduce the prevalence of obesity is a universal prevention intervention. Ideally, the reduction of risk factors would decrease the incidence of eating disorders, such that the benefits of the change outweigh any attendant risks for the population as a whole. Universal prevention could also target cultural norms that affect risk. Targeted (sometimes called selective) preventive interventions focus on reducing risk factors in individuals who are at high risk of developing subthreshold or threshold eating disorder syndromes. Indicated prevention programs focus on reducing symptom progression in individuals who have subclinical or early symptoms.

Since the previous edition of this book, considerable progress has been made in developing and evaluating models for prevention (e.g., Stice, Becker, & Yokum, 2013), although the majority of the work has focused on college and university students. In addition, several large effectiveness trials were published, models have been developed to prevent the onset of AN, eating disorder prevention and weight maintenance/loss programs have been combined, and interventions for both boys and girls are now available.

For both universal and targeted interventions, risk factors must be identified and subsequently tested to determine whether a reduction in the risk factor decreases the incidence of the disorder. Of the many risk factors discussed previously, most preventive programs have focused on reducing the thin body ideal, weight/shape concerns, dieting/restriction, and low-rate binge eating and/or compensatory behaviors. As discussed below, there is some evidence that reduction in these risk factors can reduce the incidence of the disorder at least in older adolescents. Although reducing the incidence of a disorder is the holy grail of prevention efforts, the use of a dichotomous outcome (case or no-case) often requires very large numbers of individuals to show effects because of the low prevalence of full-threshold eating disorders. Demonstrating that a preventive intervention reduces symptom progression/onset requires smaller samples. Given data that eating disorders exist on a continuum with little distinction between "clinical" and subclinical disorders (Wildes & Marcus, 2013), reductions in symptom progression/onset may therefore be a more meaningful outcome. Although some have argued that preventive activities should also focus on "protective" factors, such as building higher levels of self-esteem to reduce the risk of developing an eating disorder, no such protective factors have been identified in prospective risk factor studies.

Theoretical Models

Thus, the overall theory of prevention is that reduction in risk factors reduces the onset of a disorder. Some evidence in college students and other subpopulations has indicated that a decrease in eating disorder risk factors can reduce the onset of eating disorders (Stice, Rohde, Shaw, & Marti, 2013; Taylor et al., 2006), with evidence of long-lasting significant reductions in eating disorder symptoms (Stice et al., 2015), although this has yet to be demonstrated in those under the age of 18. Five general models have guided the nature of eating disorder preventions: psychoeducation, social cognitive learning theory, dissonance theory, feminist theory, and media literacy and advocacy (for a review see Sinton & Taylor, 2013). One meta-analysis found that programs that included body acceptance and dissonance content had larger effects than programs that focus on psychoeducation (Stice, Shaw, & Marti, 2007). Interventions based on these theories will be discussed in greater detail in the sections that follow.

Universal Prevention

A majority of studies evaluating universal prevention efforts use curricula designed to change the knowledge, beliefs, attitudes, intentions, and behaviors of individual students. Most of these programs discourage calorie-restrictive dieting, and address ways in which body image and eating are influenced by developmental, social, and cultural factors, thereby promoting a healthy weight regulation model. Other studies of universal prevention focus on broader issues such as increasing self-esteem, empowerment, confidence, and general skills, or a self-esteem/social competence model, or focus on reducing the onset of eating disorder symptoms, particularly bulimic pathology.

Elementary School

Studies of elementary school universal prevention efforts demonstrate increases in awareness of eating disorders but are less successful in altering attitudes and behaviors. A meta-analysis of

13 studies to improve body image in children ages 8 to 12 found increases in children's post-test and follow-up knowledge, but little effect was noted for preventing body image concerns and/or problem eating (Holt & Ricciardelli, 2008). McVey et al. (2009) used a somewhat different approach, focusing on using a web-based prevention program (Student Body) designed to alert teachers and others to factors that can trigger dieting among children. Seventy-eight elementary school teachers and 89 local public health practitioners providing support to schools were assigned to either the intervention or comparison groups. Student Body teacher and public health recipients were found to have an improved knowledge of facts about dieting and increased efficacy to fight weight bias, respectively. Participants reported an overall improvement in awareness of how weight bias can be presented in their teaching practices, and potential effects of weight bias in triggering body image concerns among students.

Middle School

At least 23 studies have evaluated universal prevention interventions with middle-school children, including several notable publications since the previous edition. McVey et al. (2007) examined the long-term effects of a comprehensive school-based universal prevention program involving male and female students, parents, teachers, school administrators, and local public health professionals. A total of 982 male and female middle-school students in grades six and seven and 91 teachers/school administrators participated. The intervention was associated with a reduction in the internalization of media ideals among male and female students and in disordered eating among female students, with the positive effects most pronounced among high-risk students.

More recently, programs have begun to provide interventions for males and females, as eating disorders occur in both genders. Two studies used programs focused on eating disorder risk factors (self-esteem and body image, eating-related problems), and two papers examined media literacy interventions. In Australia, Richardson et al. (2008) randomized 277 boys and girls in seventh grade to Body Think, a "self-esteem/body image" program, or a control condition. At 3-month follow-up, girls in the intervention group reported higher media literacy and lower internalization of the thin ideal compared to the control group. Boys in the intervention group reported higher media literacy and body satisfaction than the control group. A follow-up study with another cohort of students had similar results, but the effects were small. The effects of a German school-based primary prevention program ("Torera") were assessed by Berger et al. (2014) among seventh graders ages 11 through 13. The coeducational intervention involved nine manual-guided lessons on a wide range of eating-related problems. Results were compared between 10 schools that had agreed to participate and 12 schools that had declined. At follow-up approximately 1 year later, girls and students at risk showed significant improvements with small (0.35) to medium (0.66) effect sizes on eating behavior. Boys only improved with respect to eating attitudes with a small effect size (0.35). A media literacy program was evaluated in Spanish adolescents ages 12 to 14 (254 girls and 189 boys) by randomizing participants to a control group, media literacy program, or media literacy plus nutrition awareness (Espinoza, Penelo, & Raich, 2010). At 30-month follow-up, participants in the two media literacy conditions demonstrated improved body image. Wilksch and Wade (2009) also examined the effects of a media literacy class, called Media Smart, for eighth-graders, with a total of 11 classes in four schools receiving the eight-lesson media literacy program (126 girls and 107 boys) and 13 comparison classes receiving their normal school lessons (147 girls and 160 boys). Significant effects were found for the literacy program in reducing weight and shape concern (effect size = 0.29), dieting (0.26), body dissatisfaction (0.20), ineffectiveness (0.23), and depression (0.26).

Recently, Wilksch et al. (2014) compared three eight-session programs for early adolescents: Media Smart, which targets media internalization; Life Smart, which targets obesity risk factors (Wilksch & Wade, 2013); and Happy Being Me, which targets internalization of social appearance ideals and appearance comparisons (Richardson & Paxton, 2010). The Happy Being Me program was expanded from an original three-session version to eight sessions for comparability with the other two programs and was relabeled HELPP. A total of 1,316 girls and boys in grades seven and eight (mean age = 13.21 years) across three Australian states were randomly allocated by classroom to one of these three interventions or control (usual school class). Risk factors were measured at baseline, after the program (5 weeks later), and at 6- and 12-month follow-ups. At the 6-month follow-up, both Media Smart and control girls scored significantly lower than HELPP girls on eating concerns and perceived pressure. Media Smart girls showed half the rate of onset of clinically significant concerns about shape and weight in comparison to control girls at the 12-month follow-up. In addition, Media Smart and HELPP girls reported significantly lower weight and shape concerns than Life Smart girls at the 12-month follow-up.

Promising interventions for preventing eating disorders in middle schools have come from interventions focused on healthy weight regulation combined with other activities. For example, Austin et al. (2007) randomized sixth- and seventh-grade girls and boys in 13 middle schools (n = 749 and 702, respectively) to "5-2-1Go!," an intervention that combines an obesity prevention curriculum and the CDC's School Health Index for Physical Activity and Healthy Eating: A Self-Assessment and Planning Guide, Middle/High School Version. At follow-up, a significant effect was noted for disordered weight-control behaviors for girls, with 3.6% of girls in control schools and 1.2% of girls in intervention schools engaging in disordered weight-control behaviors ($p = .04$). No intervention effect was observed in boys. Subsequently, the authors evaluated the effects of Planet Health, a program designed to promote healthful nutrition and physical activity and to reduce television time, when disseminated in 45 schools in Massachusetts (n = 16,369; Austin et al., 2012). After 3 years, lower odds of disordered weight-control behaviors were observed among students in schools with (1) a high number of participants with Planet Health lessons on reducing television viewing and (2) active staff teamwork and programs for staff addressing television viewing goals.

In combination, these studies are notable for addressing issues of both effectiveness and dissemination, and by suggesting that healthy weight regulation interventions focusing on middle schools may have a major benefit of reducing eating disorder risk. Effects of other healthy weight interventions/combined healthy weight eating disorder prevention efforts are discussed later. As noted above, the Media Smart program, which does not directly address obesity, was nonetheless the only program of the three studied to show benefit on both disordered eating and obesity risk factors (Wilksch et al., 2015).

High School

In reviewing the effects of eating disorder prevention programs, Stice and Shaw (2004) identified seven universal prevention studies designed for high school–age students. The programs were generally effective in producing changes in knowledge but, with one exception, had little impact on behaviors and attitudes. Neumark-Sztainer, Butler, and Palti (1995) found effects for knowledge and eating pathology at follow-up and observed sustained effects 7 years later.

Targeted Prevention

Two programs (the Body Project and StudentBodies), delivered as targeted or combined universal/targeted interventions, have been studied in both high school–age and college-age populations. Both programs show some promise in reducing risk factors for eating disorders, although the impact on reducing the onset of these diagnoses in adolescence remains uncertain.

The Body Project (Stice, Rohde, & Shaw, 2013) uses a cognitive dissonance approach to reduce thin ideal internalization. In a study of

481 girls (mean age 17) assigned to a cognitive dissonance intervention (three sessions), a control healthy weight regulation condition (three sessions), an expressive writing condition, or an assessment-only control, dissonance participants showed significantly greater reductions in eating disorder risk factors and bulimic symptoms than participants in the other conditions (Stice, Marti, Spoor, Presnell, & Shaw, 2008). Further, participants in the healthy weight regulation condition showed significantly greater reductions in risk factors and symptoms than expressive writing and assessment-only participants from pretest to posttest. Although no differences were observed at 1-year follow-up, at 2 and 3 years of follow-up, the two control conditions (healthy weight and expressive writing) had similar outcomes to the dissonance intervention; all three were better than the assessment-only condition. In a subsequent study, female high school students with body image concerns (n = 306, mean age 15.7 years) were randomized to the dissonance intervention or an educational brochure control condition (Stice, Rohde, Gau, & Shaw, 2009). Dissonance participants showed significantly greater decreases in body dissatisfaction at 2-year follow-up and eating disorder symptoms at 3-year follow-up than controls; effects on other risk factors, risk for eating disorder onset, and other outcomes (e.g., body mass) were marginal or nonsignificant. By 3-year follow-up, nine participants in the educational brochure control condition (5.5%) and five participants in the dissonance condition (4.0%) showed onset of a threshold or subthreshold eating disorder, but the difference was not significant.

The researchers and their colleagues have generated a number of studies related to this program and suggest that this and related programs can be delivered by college health educators (Matusek, Wendt, & Wiseman, 2004) and peer leaders in sororities (Perez, Becker, & Ramirez, 2010). Moderators of the program's effects and issues for widespread dissemination of the program have also been reviewed (see Stice, Becker, & Yokum, 2013), and the program has also been adapted to the Internet (Stice et al., 2014).

The Stanford StudentBodies program has also been widely studied in adolescent and college-age populations. This 8-week structured cognitive-behavioral online program addresses factors presumed to lead to or allay eating pathology (Taylor et al., 2006). The program includes an online self-monitoring journal and an asynchronous online discussion board moderated by a health professional. In a study of 480 college-age women at risk for developing an eating disorder, a significant reduction in the main risk measure, the Weight Concerns Scale, was noted in the first 2 years of the study among the intervention group in comparison to the control group (Taylor et al., 2006). While there was no overall significant difference in the onset of eating disorders between the intervention and control groups, moderator analyses identified two subgroups (about half of the participants) for whom the intervention significantly reduced the onset of eating disorders: (1) participants with an elevated BMI at baseline and (2) at one site, participants with baseline compensatory behaviors (e.g., self-induced vomiting, laxative use, diuretic use, diet pill use, driven exercise). A comparison of six U.S. and four German randomized controlled trials of female high school and college students (total n = 990) found that the intervention was associated with moderate improvements in eating disorder–related attitudes, especially negative body image and the desire to be thin (Beintner, Jacobi, & Taylor, 2012); these effects remained significant at follow-up. No differences between samples were found on any of the outcome measures after the intervention, suggesting the suitability and effectiveness of StudentBodies for American and German students.

These and other targeted prevention programs employ screening to identify at-risk students and, in newer models, to partition populations into groups at low/no risk, high risk, and subclinical/clinical. Screening items are based on evidence from prospective risk factor studies, but less is known about the characteristics of screenings that attempt to separate high-risk from clinical populations. A detailed discussion of this issue is beyond the scope of this chapter (see Jacobi, Abascal, & Taylor, 2004, for a review); however, the screening developed by Stanford/Washington University is unique in providing sensitivity/specificity and measuring psychometric characteristics with nonclinical, high-risk, and clinical populations for both DSM-IV and DSM-5 (Wilfley, Agras, & Taylor, 2013; for psychometrics see: http://bml.stanford.edu/resources/index.html).

Combining Targeted and Universal Prevention

Prevention programs delivered through schools benefit from universal content relevant to all students, but universal programs designed for eating disorder prevention have had limited effect. Targeted programs are effective, but identifying high-risk students through schools can be challenging. Some researchers have begun to combine universal healthy weight-regulation programs with embedded targeted programs for high-risk students, as these skills are relevant to all students and appear to have some benefit in reducing disordered eating and weight behaviors. This type of model allows the content to be appropriate to the risk status of the participant and could be applied to younger populations. Luce, Osborne, Winzelberg, and Taylor (2005) demonstrated that students can be screened for eating disorder risk and participate in interventions appropriate to their needs and interests. Answers to an online risk factor screen and self-reported height and weight were used to offer various online options, including a general nutrition/healthy weight-regulation program or an intensive psychoeducational program focused on body image enhancement and/or weight maintenance. Students completed one program, provided 1 hour a week for 4 weeks, and participated in a monitored discussion group germane to their group. Of the 11 students who reported vomiting and/or laxative abuse before the intervention, 10 reported a decrease after the intervention, and the 11th entered therapy.

The Stanford/Washington group has since developed a universal, targeted, and indicated prevention program for college students (Wilfley et al., 2013), and a similar model has been used in Ireland and Germany (Lindenberg, Moessner, Harney, McLaughlin, & Bauer, 2011). Students are assessed for risk and then assigned to the appropriate intervention, and preliminary data are also positive (Wilfley et al., 2013).

Meta-Analysis of Universal and Targeted Programs

Several meta-analyses of eating disorder programs have been published, and they often include both universal and targeted programs. Stice, Shaw, and Marti (2007) identified 66 published and unpublished studies evaluating 51 different eating disorder prevention programs, and found that 51% of programs reduced eating disorder risk factors and 29% reduced current or future eating pathology, with larger effects for selected (vs. universal) programs. Larger effect sizes were found for interactive versus didactic programs, multiple-session versus single-session programs, programs offered solely to women and participants over 15 years of age, and programs with body acceptance and dissonance induction content. Langmasser and Verscheure (2009) examined four studies and noted strong effect sizes for knowledge, smaller effect sizes for behaviors ($d = 0.17$ to 0.21), and stronger effects in the targeted group, and no evidence for harmful effects from the interventions. A meta-analysis of 51 media literacy interventions (not specific to eating disorders) found positive effects ($d = 0.37$) on outcomes including media knowledge, criticism, perceived realism, influence, behavioral beliefs, attitudes, self-efficacy, and behavior (Jeong, Cho, & Hwang, 2012). Taken together, individual studies and meta-analyses suggest that prevention programs, delivered universally or in targeted fashion, have a positive impact on older, higher-risk individuals.

Combined Eating Disorder and Obesity Prevention

A major shift in thinking has occurred since the previous edition of this book, with a new emphasis in prevention on providing programs in schools that address both eating disorder prevention and weight management. The core messages for healthy weight regulation/positive body image are similar for both eating disorder prevention and weight maintenance (Neumark-Sztainer, 2012; Sanchez-Carracedo, Neumark-Sztainer, & López-Guimerà, 2012). Universally delivered healthy weight-regulation programs have been shown to reduce disordered weight-control behaviors in middle school students (Austin et al., 2007, see above) and high school students (Neumark-Sztainer, 2012). Stice et al. (Stice, Becker, & Yokum, 2013; Stice, Marti, et al., 2008) also found support for the effect of a healthy weight-regulation program. A variation of StudentBodies called StayingFit, designed to teach healthy weight regulation, has been shown to reduce weight and shape concerns in high school students (Taylor et al., 2012). Taken together, these studies suggest that interventions designed to promote healthy weight regulation and/or prevent eating disorders may help with body weight maintenance.

Indicated Prevention

New models include programs designed to provide universal, targeted, *and* indicated prevention. The last generally uses intervention strategies developed for clinical populations and will not be reviewed in detailed here; however, at least two studies have extended a prevention model to populations with early symptoms, and showed promising results in reducing symptom progression (Jacobi, Volker, Trockel & Taylor, 2012; Ohlmer, Jacobi, & Taylor, 2013). Integrated interventions with comprehensive universal, targeted, and indicated prevention programs are currently being evaluated (Wilfley et al., 2013), but it is not known if this intervention would work in younger populations.

Preventing Anorexia Nervosa

Although significant progress has occurred in prevention programs for high-risk individuals, most benefits are noted for reducing bulimic symptoms and binge eating, and reductions in subclinical/subthreshold cases of BN and eating disorder not otherwise specified. No evidence suggests that AN can be prevented, in part because of its low prevalence. However, given the success of family-based interventions for adolescents with AN (e.g., Lock et al., 2005), early prevention of AN might focus on the parents of high-risk students. Jones et al. (2012) developed a 6-week online intervention focused on encouraging parents to address their child's behavior. Overall, only 22% of eligible parents agreed to participate, and of those, only 39% completed the whole program. While 16 of 19 completers had reduced risk for AN at the end of the study, this method was inefficient. Indicated prevention, including early identification of subclinical cases, may be the most feasible approach for preventing AN.

High-Risk Settings/Environmental Interventions

Eating-disordered attitudes and behaviors are difficult to alter because they are strongly reinforced by a variety of family, peer, medical, and other cultural factors. Consequently, some prevention researchers have argued to change the environment of children and adolescents and consider a more public health approach (Austin, 2012; Taylor, Franko, Neumark-Sztainer, Paxton, & Shapiro, 2007), specifically focusing on the school environment (e.g., Neumark-Sztainer, 1996; Piran, 1999). These initiatives assume that defined populations should be considered for targeted outcomes, and environmental, policy, and provider education should be integrated into a comprehensive approach. Examples of this approach include those by Piran (1999), who demonstrated that system-wide changes can reduce eating disorders in the high-risk setting of an elite ballet school, and Neumark-Sztainer et al. (2000), who designed a community-based intervention to prevent disordered eating among preadolescent girls. A total of 226 Girl Scout troop members were randomized to receive six 90-minute sessions focusing on media literacy and advocacy skills, with some training for troop leaders, or a control group. At 3-month follow-up, the program demonstrated a positive influence on media-related attitudes and behaviors, including internalization of sociocultural ideals, self-efficacy to impact weight-related social norms, and print media habits (Neumark-Sztainer, Sherwood, Coller, & Hannan, 2000), suggesting the potential for such efforts.

Aside from a few studies with ballet dancers, preventive interventions for particular at-risk populations or high-risk settings have received little attention. Olmsted, Daneman, Rydall, Lawson, and Rodin (2002) randomly assigned adolescent girls with insulin-dependent diabetes to a psychoeducational program and found significant reductions in body dissatisfaction, drive for thinness, dietary restraint, and eating concerns at 6-month follow-up. Cheerleading coaches were targeted by Whisenhunt et al. (2008) by training them to recognize the symptoms of eating disorders and reduce the pressures for thinness among their squads. Self-reported improvement in coaches' behavior was noted at 8-month follow-up, but there was no sustained knowledge about eating disorders. Similarly, Buchholz et al. (2008) evaluated the effectiveness of a selective prevention program to reduce pressures to be thin and to promote positive body image and eating behaviors in athletes belonging to gymnastic clubs. The intervention focused on competitive female gymnasts (ages 11–18 years), parents, and coaches. Clubs were randomized to receive a 3-month intervention program (n = 4) or a control intervention (n = 3), with a total of 62 female gymnasts completing the self-report posttest. The program resulted in a perceived reduction in pressure from sports clubs to be thin, although no changes were found in eating disorder attitudes. In older students, Becker, McDaniel, et al. (2012) randomized 157 athletes to an athlete-modified dissonance prevention or healthy weight intervention, and reported that both interventions reduced bulimic pathology, shape concern, and negative affect at 1 year. Finally, in adults, an Internet-based cognitive-behavioral intervention was promising for individuals who were at very high risk for developing an eating disorder and had high concerns about body weight (Taylor et al., 2016). The findings from these studies show the promise of preventive interventions targeted at high-risk settings.

Also relevant to the public health model is an interest by advocacy groups to change policies and practices related to eating disorders at a national level. Recommendations include disclosing and avoiding the digital enhancement of images; banning ultra-thin female models, overly muscular male models, or models under the age of 16 to advertise adult clothes; employing a greater diversity of ethnicities and model body sizes; eschewing editorial and advertising content that promotes negative body image through rapid weight loss and cosmetic surgery; and, for retailers, carrying a wider variety of clothing sizes that better reflects the demands of the community (http://www.youth.gov.au/sites/youth/bodyimage/pages/advisorygroup). However, these policies may not always have the intended effects, as students exposed to images they knew were digitally enhanced showed worsened eating disorder attitudes (Tiggemann et al., 2013). Very little research has been done to examine intended or unintended effects of policy change.

In the past 10 years, the personal products corporation Dove has undertaken media campaigns to increase acceptance of various body sizes and to increase self-esteem (for a review, see Sinton & Taylor, 2010). The program includes "viral films" distributed online through sites like YouTube and Facebook. For instance, "Evolution" depicts the transformation of a real woman into a model and promotes awareness of how unrealistic perspectives of beauty are created, and "Onslaught" shows the barrage of beauty images that girls absorb daily. The impact of these programs is not known, but the campaign has been associated with a 13% increase in worldwide sales of Dove skin and hair products, suggesting some positive response to these strategies.

Oswalt and Wyatt (2007) evaluated a campaign with messages displayed on campus buses, billboards, and magnets, including 10 messages related to sabotaging body image and 10 ways to enhance body image. A follow-up evaluation found that the campaign had little impact.

The Tri Delta sorority has sponsored an annual Fat Talk Free Week, an international

5-day body activism campaign designed to draw attention to body image issues and the damaging impact of the "thin ideal" on women in society. This annual public awareness effort was the result of Tri Delta's involvement with the Reflections program. A recent study found that the campaign was associated with significant declines in self–fat talk and peer physical comparison among both those who attended and did not attend Fat Talk Free Week (Garnett et al., in press).

Many prevention programs include activities that attempt to get students to create campaigns, examine policy, and so forth, but the impact of these activities needs to be evaluated. In general, the promise of environmental and public health approaches to eating disorders remains unproven, although the results of Fat Talk Free Week are promising.

Is Prevention Harmful?

Some have argued that prevention programs may inadvertently be harmful, a concern that stems from two early prevention studies that indicated an increase in eating disorder risk factors (Carter, Stewart, Dunn, & Fairburn, 1997; Mann, Nolen-Hoeksema, Huang, Burgard, Wright, & Hanson, 1997). However, substantial subsequent research failed to identify adverse effects from eating disorder prevention programs or eating disorder risk factors (see Sinton & Taylor, 2010, for a review).

SUMMARY

The prevention of disordered eating is an important issue in public health, and much progress has occurred since the previous edition of this book. Universal prevention efforts with elementary school children produce positive changes in terms of relevant knowledge and attitudes. Programs that focus on changing factors with broad application, such as increasing self-esteem, creating a stronger sense of connection to peers and mentors, and transforming critical awareness into cultural change, have proved promising with middle school students, and a number of studies have shown that healthy weight-regulation programs provided to middle school students may reduce disordered weight-control behaviors.

The most impressive progress has occurred in providing targeted prevention programs to older students. Substantial evidence now suggests that at least two approaches, the dissonance-based approach represented by the Body Project and an Internet psychoeducation/cognitive-behavioral approach, Student Bodies, can reduce risk factors and may even reduce the onset of eating disorders, although the evidence for the latter comes mainly from college-age populations.

However, despite the progress in prevention research, the magnitude and duration of intervention effects still need improvement, and it is not yet clear how to disseminate evidence-based prevention programs more broadly to reduce the population incidence of eating disorders (Stice, Becker, & Yokum, 2013). Further, the prevention of AN remains elusive. One family-based model shows promise, but the parents of at-risk students were reluctant to participate. More focus may need to be placed on altering the environments/settings where relatively more students may be at risk for AN, and models are emerging for how to craft these programs. Very early identification of and intervention with students who are showing early clinical features may also be of benefit. While environmental, cultural, policy, and other broader approaches to prevention have been widely advocated, few data are available to determine their impact.

Research Agenda for Eating Disorders

Evelyn Attia
Anne E. Becker
Cynthia M. Bulik
Alison E. Field
Neville H. Golden
Richard E. Kreipe
Daniel Le Grange
James E. Mitchell
Kathleen M. Pike
Robyn Sysko
C. Barr Taylor
B. Timothy Walsh

chapter 16

Research on eating disorders has produced a substantial base of knowledge regarding the definitions of eating disorders, their treatment, and their prevention. However, there are significant gaps in our understanding of eating disorders, especially among adolescents. Most of the research literature on eating disorders has focused on adults, and the findings may not apply to younger individuals. The research agenda regarding eating disorders among adolescents is large. Future studies, such as those outlined below, could take advantage of the increase in available technology (e.g., smartphones) and use of social media, which are of particular relevance to this age group.

DIAGNOSTIC CRITERIA FOR EATING AND FEEDING DISORDERS

In light of the minor alterations to the diagnostic criteria for anorexia nervosa (AN) and bulimia nervosa (BN), the inclusion of binge-eating disorder (BED), and rearticulated diagnoses (e.g., avoidant/restrictive food intake disorder), it will be important to understand whether the changes described in DSM-5 are helpful in reducing the use of residual feeding or eating disorder categories among adolescents without a loss of diagnostic utility. Further, information is needed about adolescents within novel DSM-5 categories, in particular BED and avoidant/restrictive food intake disorder, as little is known about the clinical characteristics of youth with these diagnoses. Finally, the utility of other diagnostic schemes (e.g., Broad Categories for the Diagnosis of Eating Disorders; Walsh & Sysko, 2009) should be considered in younger populations. A broader system of classification could offer an advantage for adolescents, because it may be able to accommodate the range of symptom presentations noted among youth and is more straightforward for assessing individuals with eating disorders who present to primary care settings, where a large proportion of adolescents with eating disorders are initially seen.

In 2010, the National Institute of Mental Health introduced the Research Domain Criteria (RDoC), a novel framework to support research on clinical symptoms and their linkage to underlying neurobiology (Insel et al., 2010). Several problematic issues related to eating disorders illustrate the rationale for RDoC. The eating disorders as defined by DSM-5 are characterized by a high degree of comorbidity and overlapping symptoms; for example, significant depression is extremely common in AN, BN, and BED, and binge eating occurs among individuals in all three categories. In addition, many individuals with clinically significant eating problems fail to meet DSM-5's diagnostic thresholds, such as a minimum average of one episode of binge eating per week over 3 months for both BN and BED, and therefore receive a "residual" diagnosis. The goal of the RDoC approach is to avoid such problems by eschewing DSM-5 categories, by examining symptoms dimensionally and by linking them to underlying neurobiological constructs such as reward processing and impulse control.

Despite its many deficiencies, the DSM system has well-established clinical utility and broad acceptance, and the RDoC system is, as its name suggests, designed to augment research rather than clinical care. However, the fundamental principles underlying the RDoC framework are sound and provide an important foundation for novel probes of the development and persistence of eating disorders.

GENETICS

As sample sizes for genome-wide association studies (GWAS) of individuals with eating disorders grow, all indications are that the discovery trajectory will mirror that observed in schizophrenia. Future genomic work will identify genes and gene sets ripe for functional study using rapidly developing technologies and methodologies available to neuroscientists. Elucidation of the biology of eating disorders via genomics and other "-omics" will open avenues for the development and testing of novel pharmacological agents that directly target the core biology of the illness.

Emerging GWAS results will also permit the development of genetic risk profiles and the exploration of their ability to identify at-risk children and to predict the course and outcome of eating and comorbid disorders. In the longer term, such risk profiles may be applied in the clinic to inform the personalization of treatment. Finally, the common mechanisms underlying comorbidity identified via genomics will translate immediately into the pilot testing of novel pharmacological agents to tailor and improve treatment for eating disorders.

EPIDEMIOLOGY

More large studies are needed to understand the true prevalence of eating disorders among adolescents. As described above, changes to the diagnostic criteria should result in some increase in the prevalence of AN, BN, and BED and a reduction in the frequency of less-specific diagnostic labels, but only large, nationally representative samples will provide information on the impact of these DSM-5 changes on rates of feeding and eating disorders. Future studies should also examine the prevalence of specific types of other specified feeding and eating disorders (e.g., subthreshold AN, purging disorder), which will facilitate comparisons of results across studies. Large prospective studies would provide clarification about the age of onset of DSM-5 disorders. Research is needed to better understand substantial racial/ethnic and gender differences in the prevalence of disordered eating. Alterations to the method of assessment in epidemiological studies may be needed, as a growing number of studies document weight and shape concerns and related behaviors that are more common in males and not measured in existing studies.

COMORBIDITY, OUTCOME, AND DIAGNOSTIC MIGRATION

Psychiatric comorbidities are common among both adolescents and adults with AN and BN and include mood disorders, anxiety disorders, and substance use disorders. The outcome of adolescent patients with AN who receive treatment soon after the onset of illness appears better than that of patients who do not; however, those patients who remain ill have high rates of psychiatric comorbidity and are at risk for premature death (Franko et al., 2013). Data on the course and outcome of adolescent BN are very limited.

Diagnostic migration occurs frequently from AN-restricting subtype to AN-binge purge subtype, and from AN-binge purge subtype to BN, and it is not currently possible to identify those patients likely to migrate. Future studies should include individuals with comorbidities, such as substance use disorders, to aid in developing treatment strategies for these dual-diagnosis conditions.

Studies of the course and outcome of adolescent BN are needed, and early identification and intervention strategies need to be developed.

MEDICAL COMPLICATIONS OF EATING DISORDERS

While the majority of medical complications associated with eating disorders are reversible with nutritional rehabilitation and cessation of the binge–purge cycle, there are indications that growth retardation, reduced bone mass, and, possibly, structural brain changes may not be entirely reversible. Studies probing structural brain changes in AN and their relationship to neuropsychological changes are needed. In addition, there is a pressing need to develop efficacious treatments for reduced bone mass among adolescents with AN.

A better understanding of the pathophysiology of the refeeding syndrome is required to avoid unnecessarily conservative refeeding protocols, which can lead to prolonged and costly inpatient medical hospitalization. Randomized controlled trials are necessary to examine the safety of different rates of refeeding and the effect of macronutrient composition on development of the refeeding syndrome.

TREATMENTS OF ADOLESCENTS WITH EATING DISORDERS

Psychological Treatment

A significant focus of future research should be on effective psychological treatments for adolescents with eating disorders. Family-based therapy appears useful for adolescents with AN and BN, and self-help forms of cognitive-behavioral interventions show promise for adolescents with BN. However, it is imperative to build on these initial efforts. Several future research priorities should be highlighted. It is clear that additional treatment modalities in this population should be explored. Perhaps the most obvious candidate is Enhanced Cognitive Therapy (CBT-E; Fairburn, 2008), which has been studied in other eating disorder groups. Another priority is to design randomized controlled trials to specifically identify moderators and mediators of treatment outcome so that patients can be matched with the appropriate treatment modality.

Pharmacological Treatment

Few controlled studies have evaluated the utility and safety of pharmacological treatments for adolescents with eating disorders, although medications are frequently used in the clinical treatment of these patients. Antidepressant medications reduce binge eating and vomiting behaviors for adults with BN, but additional study will be necessary before firm conclusions can be reached regarding the use of these medications with younger patients. There is currently no evidence for the efficacy of pharmacological treatments in low-weight adults with AN; however, recent reports have suggested that atypical antipsychotic medications, such as olanzapine, may be useful, and future research should evaluate these medications in a controlled manner among younger patients.

RELAPSE PREVENTION

Psychological Treatments

The field has made significant strides in terms of documenting effective treatments across the range of eating disorders. Although more studies focused on adolescents have been published, more can and should be done to develop interventions for this age group. Data across disorders consistently indicate that early intervention has positive effects, and the field would benefit from continuing to gather data that provide an empirical basis for defining treatment response, relapse, and remission. Promising findings related to Internet-based strategies should be pursued, particularly given the reality that adolescents are technology "natives," and it is likely that they will find such strategies familiar. Privacy issues are a particular concern with Internet-based strategies, especially when working with minors in such a context. However, the economic leverage and extensive reach that are feasible with the Internet represent strong advantages.

As relapse-prevention interventions develop further, it will be useful to analyze the components of the interventions to determine what is most salient and significant in preventing relapse. Relatedly, as data emerge from neuroscience, more targeted interventions informed by basic neuroscience may be important in terms of understanding who is at risk and which specific interventions prevent relapse. Studies also need to pay careful attention to distinguishing between enduring impairment and relapse.

Gone are the days when it was thought that individuals could not fully recover from eating disorders; however, we continue to have much work to do to ensure that more individuals achieve full and lasting recovery.

Pharmacological Treatments

Adolescents have not been the focus of medication trials to prevent relapse, and studies that have included adolescent patients are not sufficient to draw conclusions about relapse prevention for these patients. It is important to determine whether response rates to continued medication regimens are similar in adolescents to the extant data for adults.

RISK FACTORS

Our definition of "risk factor" has evolved in several meaningful ways over the past decade. In the early years of research, the focus was primarily on sociocultural factors, family factors, and life events. The current conceptualization of risk is much more fluid and encompasses not only environmental factors but also neurobiological, genetic, and epigenetic factors, as well as interactions and correlations across these domains, and the impact of adolescent development. Although our conceptualization of risk has evolved, our study of risk has not kept pace. Few truly specific risk or protective factors for the development of eating disorders have been definitively established, and developmentally informed risk profiles have yet to be developed, tested, and validated. Knowledge concerning males and BED is particularly limited. It is important to clarify the developmental nature of BED and determine whether childhood presentations of loss-of-control eating are on the same continuum of pathology as BED in adulthood. The use of prospective designs should be encouraged. Such research methods are a potentially powerful means of elucidating the etiological processes that give rise to eating disorders.

PREVENTION

Although a significant amount of evidence has been generated on prevention interventions since the last edition of this book, additional work is needed to extend the extant studies. Future research should investigate whether the risk factors for symptom onset differ from those for symptom escalation and symptom maintenance. This is important because the former are germane to the design of universal and selected prevention programs, but the latter are necessary for the design of optimally effective indicated-prevention programs and treatment interventions, respectively. Further, given the national and global efforts toward obesity prevention, it is also important that none of these efforts in any way encourages behaviors or attitudes that can increase risk not only for BED but for the other eating disorders as well.

Substance Use Disorders

COMMISSION ON ADOLESCENT SUBSTANCE AND ALCOHOL ABUSE

Charles P. O'Brien, *Commission Chair*

Second Edition

James Anthony

Hui Cheng

Brian Fairman

Dan Romer

Claudia Szobot

Gary Wenk

With contributions from

Richard Spoth

First Edition

James C. Anthony

Kathleen Carroll

First Edition cont.

Anna Rose Childress

Charles Dackis

Guy Diamond

Robert Hornik

Lloyd D. Johnston

Reese Jones

George F. Koob

Thomas Korsten

Caryn Lerman

A. Thomas McLellan

Howard Moss

Helen Pettinati

Richard Spoth

part V

The Neurobiology, Characteristics, and Prevalence of Substance Use

Gary Wenk
James Anthony
Hui Cheng
Brian Fairman
Dan Romer

chapter 17

Most adolescents who experiment with drugs do not progress to clinical problems. The neurobiological mechanisms that underlie the vulnerability of some adolescents, and not others, are explored in this chapter. Some of them progress to the level of abuse and a smaller number progress to addiction (dependence). The latter has been the focus of much biological research because the chronic relapsing nature of addiction suggests that changes in the brain underlie its persistent course. We describe what has been learned about the neurobiological processes that underlie this progression. We then describe the characteristic effects of the most prevalent drugs used by adolescents and trends in their use over the past several decades. We also describe what has been learned about important social and personal risk factors for progression in adolescent drug use.

THE NEUROBIOLOGY OF ADDICTION

Over the past several decades, neuroscientists have uncovered compelling evidence that addiction is a disease modification of brain circuitry and chemistry that primarily involves specific brain regions that mediate motivation and reward. With the help of animal models and direct studies on addicted human subjects, scientists are rapidly unraveling neuronal mechanisms that underlie many of the clinical features of addiction, including drug euphoria, tolerance, withdrawal, craving, and hedonic dysregulation. It is now apparent that brain reward circuitry is stimulated by addictive agents during drug-induced euphoria and disrupted over the course of chronic exposure. Interestingly, despite the diverse initial actions of various drugs on neuronal receptors, they produce many similar neurochemical effects, including disrupted homeostasis of the mesolimbic dopamine system, which produces positive reinforcement after drug intake and negative reinforcement during withdrawal. These common effects support the established classification of different substance dependence disorders within the single category of addiction, and can have implications for polydrug use and the so-called gateway theory.

Why are the actions of these drugs in the brain so similar? Why do they all induce craving? Sometimes the effects of some chemicals are present in the brain for so long that the brain slowly adjusts to their presence. Over time, the brain acts as though the drug or nutrient has become a necessary component of normal brain function. The user experiences the brain's adjustment to the eventual absence of this substance as craving. Consider, for example, the very powerful drug sugar. The brain needs sugar (usually in the form of glucose) to function normally. The many billions of neurons in the brain require a constant supply of glucose to maintain their ability to produce energy and communicate with other neurons. The brain consumes the equivalent of about 12 doughnuts worth of glucose every day. Neurons can tolerate a deprivation of glucose for only a few minutes before they begin to die. Therefore, as blood levels of sugar decrease with the passage of time since your last meal, you begin to experience a craving for food, preferably something sweet. The presence of sugar in your brain is considered normal, and its absence leads to the feeling of craving and the initiation of hunting or foraging behaviors, such as seeking out a vending machine for a chocolate bar.

If you wish to experience the truly overwhelming and powerful nature of drug craving, just stop eating for a full day (Wenk, 2015). Now you can easily recognize a parallel with the experience of a heroin addict. Within a few hours the addict will not be able to think of anything but food (heroin) and will do anything, sell anything, or steal from anyone to get food (heroin); as time passes, nothing is more important than the next meal (shot of heroin). The brain behaves as though it cannot tell the difference between a food and a drug; both are just chemicals. The constant consumption of caffeine, nicotine, or almost any chemical can produce similar types of compensatory changes within the brain and lead to craving with their absence from the brain. This response is exactly what the brain evolved to do: to be flexible and learn how to survive, to adapt to a changing environment and to the variety of chemicals that you consume. When this situation of "normalcy" is lost because of the absence of something that your brain has become accustomed to having regularly available (e.g., sugar, amphetamine, heroin, or anything else that you are accustomed to consuming), your brain reacts by creating in you the urge to replenish its supply. You experience this feeling as craving, regardless of the legality, safety, or cost of the substance being craved.

Whether motivated by curiosity, boredom, peer pressure, or thrill seeking, the initial use of a euphoric drug indelibly embeds the experience into memory. Since we organisms are neurologically "wired" to repeat pleasurable experiences, drug euphoria positively reinforces subsequent use. When used repeatedly, addictive drugs produce unpleasant states (craving, withdrawal, impaired hedonic function) that negatively reinforce use and alternate with euphoria to produce a vicious cycle of addiction that becomes increasingly entrenched and uncontrollable, regardless of negative consequences. Although psychological, genetic, and environmental factors play critical roles in the initiation and perpetuation of addiction, brain involvement explains many of its contradictions and provides important clues for the development of more effective and durable treatments.

Biological Research Based on Animal Models

Since the discovery of "pleasure centers" by Olds in the early 1950s, extensive research has been conducted using animal models that address the acute and chronic effects of addictive drugs on reward-related brain regions. These studies have contributed tremendously to our understanding of addiction by delineating relevant neuronal mechanisms and proposing hypotheses to define the disorder. Drug addiction, also known as substance dependence (American Psychiatric Association, 1994), is a chronically relapsing disorder that is characterized by (1) compulsion to seek and take the drug, (2) loss of control in limiting intake, and (3) emergence of a negative emotional state (e.g., dysphoria, anxiety, irritability) when access to the drug is prevented (Koob et al., 2014). Experimental animal studies have shown that the occasional limited use of an addictive agent is distinct from escalated drug use and the emergence of chronic drug dependence. Therefore, an important goal of current research is to understand the neuropharmacological and neuroadaptive mechanisms within reward-related neurocircuits that mediate the transition between occasional, controlled drug use and the loss of behavioral control over drug seeking and drug taking that defines chronic addiction (Koob et al., 2014).

Drug addiction has aspects of both impulse-control disorders and compulsive disorders (Fig. 17.1). Impulse-control disorders are characterized by an increasing sense of tension or arousal before committing an impulsive act; pleasure, gratification, or relief is felt at the time of committing the act, and following the act there may or may not be regret, self-reproach, or guilt (Schreiber et al., 2011). In contrast, compulsive disorders are characterized by anxiety and stress before committing a compulsive repetitive behavior and relief from the stress by performing the compulsive behavior. As an individual moves from an impulsive disorder to a compulsive disorder, there is a shift from the euphoria driving the motivated behavior to the craving and discomfort driving the motivated behavior. These stages have biological, social, and psychological aspects that feed into each other, intensify, and ultimately lead to the pathological state known as addiction (Koob & Le Moal, 1997).

Given these considerations, the modern view of addiction has shifted from a focus on physical withdrawal symptoms to the motivational aspects of addiction. This shift in emphasis is supported by the clinical axiom that mere detoxification (the elimination of drug from the body with pharmacological suppression of physical withdrawal symptoms) is insufficient treatment for addiction. More central to the transition from drug use to addiction is the emergence of negative emotions, including craving, anxiety, and irritability, when access to the drug is prevented (Koob & Le Moal, 2001). Indeed, some have argued that the development of such a negative affective state should define addiction.

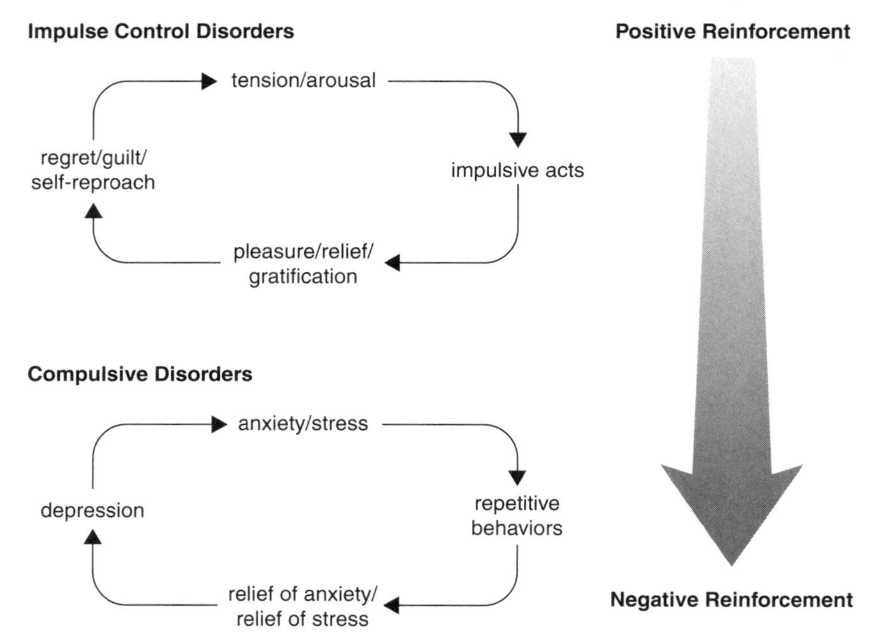

Figure 17.1 Impulse-control disorders and compulsive disorders in drug addiction.

Craving is also associated with another interesting expression of brain function. The removal of a drug or a chemical from the brain is frequently accompanied by biological and behavioral changes that are the opposite of those produced by the drug. For example, the rebound from the euphoria induced by the stimulants cocaine and amphetamine is the depression that follows once the drugs have left the brain. This interesting brain response is apparently only unidirectional. In other words, we often observe depression following stimulant-induced euphoria, but we never see euphoria as part of the rebound experience following use of depressants such as alcohol and barbiturates. No one ever experiences happiness as part of a hangover from a night of binge drinking!

Animal Models of Drug Reward

Through extensive animal research, the neurotransmitters and brain circuits that mediate drug reward have been largely delineated; the biological basis of drug reward is exemplified by the fact that laboratory animals will press levers to receive addictive substances. When provided unlimited access, animals will consistently self-administer cocaine and amphetamine to the point of death, and the power of drug reward should not be underestimated in the clinical setting. Diverse classes of addictive drugs affect different neurotransmitter systems and produce distinct activation patterns within reward circuits. Many addictive substances (including heroin, cocaine, amphetamine, alcohol, nicotine, and marijuana) acutely increase the neurotransmitter dopamine in elements of the ventral striatum, specifically the nucleus accumbens, but this increase is most robust for psychomotor stimulants and much more modest for sedative-hypnotics. Other neurotransmitter systems are also involved, including opioid peptides, GABA, glutamate, and serotonin, and play more critical roles as one moves out of the domain of psychomotor stimulants. Dopamine levels in the nucleus accumbens are also elevated during activities that lead to natural rewards, providing compelling evidence that addictive drugs tap into natural motivational circuits.

A principal focus of research on the neurobiology of the pleasurable effects of drugs of abuse has been the origins and terminal areas of the midbrain dopamine system, and there now is compelling evidence for the importance of this system in drug reward (Koob et al., 2014). The major components of this circuit are the projection of brain cells containing dopamine from the ventral tegmental area (the site of dopaminergic cell bodies) to the basal forebrain, which includes the nucleus accumbens. Other chemical transmitters form the many neural inputs and outputs that interact with the ventral tegmental area and the extended amygdala and include opioid peptides, GABA, glutamate, and serotonin (Koob, 2006). While dopamine is critical for the reward associated with cocaine, methamphetamine, and nicotine, it has a less critical role in the pleasure associated with opiates, phencyclidine (PCP), and alcohol. Endogenous opioid peptides (such as β-endorphin and enkephalin) and their receptors have important roles in opiate and alcohol reward.

Animal Models of Motivational Effects of Withdrawal

Although considerable focus in animal studies has been directed toward neuronal sites and mechanisms that produce drug reward, new animal models have been developed to examine negative emotional states produced by neuroadaptations caused by repeated drug administration. Although drug reward certainly reinforces repeated use, the transition to drug addiction appears to require an additional source of reinforcement, the reduction of negative emotional states that are associated with repeated drug administration. The ability of addictive drugs to produce reward and negative emotional states (which they temporarily alleviate) is a powerful combination that positively and negatively reinforces the compulsive cycle of addiction.

Addictive drugs may produce dysphoric effects during their withdrawal by disrupting the same sites that they activate during drug reward. A part of the forebrain component of the reward system has been termed the extended amygdala (Heimer & Alheid, 1991) and may represent a common anatomic substrate for acute drug pleasure and the dysphoria associated with compulsive drug use. As such, negative emotional states associated with chronic drug exposure may reflect the dysregulation of the extended amygdala and midbrain dopamine systems that are implicated in drug reward. There is considerable evidence that dopamine activity is decreased during drug withdrawal (as opposed to being increased during drug reward), and alterations in the activity of other reward-related neurotransmitter systems, such as glutamate, endogenous opioids, GABA, and serotonin, have also been reported.

Stress-related chemical systems in the extended amygdala may also contribute to the dysphoria associated with dependence. Drugs of abuse not only activate the brain pleasure systems but also activate the "stress" systems within the brain. One major component of the brain stress system is the brain peptide corticotrophin-releasing factor (CRF), which controls the master gland (pituitary) hormonal response to stress, the sympathetic system (fight-or-flight) response to stress, and behavioral (emotional) responses to stress (Koob et al., 2014). Increases in brain and pituitary CRF are associated with the dysphoria of abstinence from many drugs, including alcohol, cocaine, opiates, and marijuana (Koob, 2015). Another component of the brain stress systems is the chemical norepinephrine, which also is associated with the dysphoria of drug withdrawal. Conversely, the acute withdrawal from some drugs such as alcohol is associated with decreases in the levels of the brain "anti-stress" neuropeptide Y (NPY) in the extended amygdala (Koob & Volkow, 2010). It has been hypothesized that decreased NPY activity, combined with increased CRF activity, may contribute significantly to the dysphoric effects of drug withdrawal. This suggests that addictive drugs not only reduce the functional integrity of reward-related neurotransmitter systems but also produce stress by enhancing stress-related chemicals (CRF and norepinephrine) and reducing the NPY anti-stress system. Should even a small part of these changes persist beyond acute withdrawal, a powerful drive for resumption of drug taking would be established.

Animal Models for Conditioned Drug Effects

Through classical conditioning, environmental cues that have been repeatedly paired with drug administration can acquire drug-like (rewarding) and drug-opposite (dysphoria) properties that contribute significantly to drug craving and relapse in the clinical setting. Human studies have shown that the presentation of stimuli previously associated with drug delivery or drug withdrawal produce craving and increase the likelihood of relapse and that these responses are gendered; for example, males were more "cue-reactive" and more successful at establishing control over their reactivity to cocaine stimuli (Rosenberg, 2009; Sterling et al., 2004). A number of animal models are available to characterize the conditioning effects imparted on formerly neutral environmental stimuli that are subsequently paired with drug self-administration. For instance, stimuli that previously signaled drug availability will cause an animal to continue to press the lever even when drug is no longer available. In other situations, animals can be trained to work for a previously neutral stimulus that predicts drug availability. In an extinction procedure, responding with and without drug-related cues provides a measure of the rewarding effects of drugs by assessing the persistence of drug-seeking behavior. Drug-related cues can also reinstate responding by animals long after drug responding has been extinguished. These findings are important because the learning reinforced by drugs persists long after the drug has been eliminated from the body. In humans, these learned or conditioned effects can produce drug craving and possible relapse long after the patient is discharged from a drug-free rehabilitation program.

In summary, brain substrates implicated in conditioned drug effects have been intensely researched, paired both with drug administration and drug withdrawal. The amygdala, and specifically the basolateral amygdala, is an important substrate in reward-related memory and conditioning. This structure has a critical role in the consolidation of emotional memories that have long been recognized as an essential component of the addictive process (Cahill & McGaugh, 1998; Roozendaal et al., 2008). How such drug memories relate to memory circuitry in general and contribute to the dysregulation of already strained reward circuits is a subject for future studies.

Neuroadaptations and Allostasis

While the pleasurable effects of drugs occur immediately in response to the pharmacological activation of reward centers, negative hedonic effects emerge later, persist, and intensify with repeated exposure. Hedonic dysregulation worsens over time because repeated use, while providing temporary relief, merely exacerbates the problem. The concept of "allostasis" has been proposed to explain how physiological brain changes contribute to relapse vulnerability. In contrast to homeostasis, in which a system returns to normal function, allostasis defines a brain reward system that does *not* return to normal but remains in a persistent dysphoric condition because of a shift in the reward set point (Koob, 2013; Koob & Le Moal, 2001). Fueled not only by the dysregulation of reward circuits but also by the activation of brain and hormonal stress systems, this process leads gradually to the loss of control over drug intake. Disruptions in reward-related neurotransmitter systems (dopamine, glutamate, opioids, serotonin, GABA) that contribute to emotional dysfunction in drug addiction persist long into abstinence and are reasonable targets for pharmacological treatments. Restoring normal hedonic function in drug addiction and alcoholism could significantly reduce relapse rates in these treatment-refractory conditions.

Vulnerability of the Developing Nervous System: Focus on Adolescents

Recent brain imaging research with addicted adults suggests that the vulnerability to addiction may lie in the function (and dysfunction) of two critical brain systems: (1) the ancient brain motivational system, which underlies the powerful motivation for natural rewards such as food and sex (as described above), and (2) the brain's inhibitory or executive function systems, responsible for inhibiting behavior and putting on the brakes, for deciding when pursuit of a desired reward would be a danger or a disadvantage in the long term.

Despite great interest and relevance to the ultimate development of drug abuse and dependence, relatively little work has been done on the potentially unique vulnerability of the developing nervous system to drugs of abuse. Researchers have been slow to adapt animal models in the drug abuse field to studies of adolescent animals largely because many of the established models, such as intravenous self-administration, historically have required extensive time and technical expertise to establish, and the window of adolescence in rodent models is quite short (postnatal days 28–42; Spear & Varlinskaya, 2010; Varlinskaya, Spear, & Spear, 2001). However, studies with nicotine and alcohol have begun to characterize a pattern of results in adolescent rats that may provide critical insights into the importance of adolescent exposure for future vulnerability to addiction. When treated with nicotine, amphetamine, and alcohol, for instance, adolescent rodents show smaller responses to the acute effects of the drugs and less of a withdrawal response (Craig et al., 2014; Levin, Rezvani, Montoya, Rose, & Swartzwelder, 2003; Spear, 2002).

Human adolescents commonly experiment with drugs, but relatively few go on to develop entrenched patterns of addiction. It is not known why some individuals are more vulnerable to addiction, although family studies support a contributing hereditary role. Neuroscientists have identified reward-related molecular machinery (circuits, receptors, and enzymes) that could be encoded by specific genetic polymorphisms that significantly affect the rewarding and aversive qualities of addictive drugs (see the genetics summary below). Constitutional factors might thereby enhance addiction vulnerability, affect drug preference, or provide inherent protection.

Based on research with laboratory animals, it is now becoming clear that differences in sensation and novelty seeking are entry points to the drug addiction process (Fig. 17.2). However, although progression toward addiction begins with enhanced interest in the excitement of drug use (Romer & Hennesy, 2007), as use progresses, it is differences in impulsivity that predispose toward continued use and dependency. That is, individuals with elevated levels of impulsive traits, such as impulsive choice (delay discounting) and impulsive action (acting without thinking) (Bickel et al., 2012; Khurana et al., 2015), are less able to discontinue drug use once its adverse effects become evident. This effect was illustrated in a study with rats selected either for high sensation seeking or high impulsivity (Belin et al., 2008). Although the sensation-seeking rats initiated cocaine use at levels equal to or greater than impulsive rats, once they had to endure electric shock to acquire the drug, they desisted to a greater degree than the impulsive rats, who could not withhold the drug acquisition response.

The effects of impulsivity have been conceptually replicated in human adolescents in a longitudinal study in which sensation seeking was predictive of early use of alcohol, cannabis, and tobacco, but impulsive action and choice were predictive of progression in the use of these drugs (Khurana et al., 2015). This early progression was also predictive of substance use disorder for each drug at ages 18 and 19 (Khurana et al., 2017). These findings are also consistent with the observation that sensation-seeking animals do not exhibit deficits in inhibitory control (Jupp & Dalley, 2014) and that sensation-seeking adolescents exhibit greater working memory ability than impulsive youth (Romer et al., 2011). Working memory is an executive function that enables one to make decisions that require active consideration of information relevant to the decision. It is related to other functions, such as inhibitory control, that enable one to resist responding to impulses (Wesleym et al., 2014). Thus, sensation seekers may have greater ability to control their drug use once it becomes aversive.

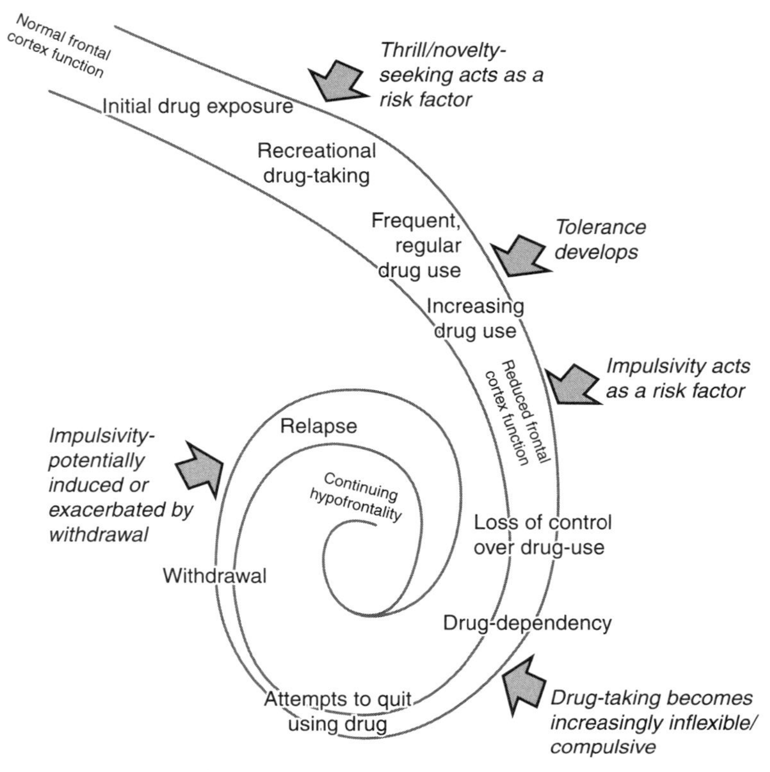

Figure 17.2 Drug use progression from early initiation to later dependence (from Winstanley et al., 2010).

Many questions also exist regarding the effects of addictive drugs on the adolescent brain, which continues to develop and mature well into early adulthood. Existing evidence suggests that heavy use of cannabis and alcohol during adolescence has deleterious effects on brain functions, such as working memory and verbal learning (Squelia & Gray, 2016). However, with some exceptions, the studies have been conducted with small samples that may not be representative of the larger adolescent population, the assessment of drug use has been limited to self-reports, and the use of different drugs makes it difficult to attribute effects to any single one. Although many questions remain unanswered, the current rate of knowledge expansion should shed light on these and other critical issues, enhancing our understanding of addiction and guiding the development of more effective interventions. The National Institutes of Health is about to launch its Adolescent Brain Cognitive Development (ABCD) Study, which will follow a cohort of 10,000 children ages 9 and 10 at baseline into early adulthood using structural and functional brain imaging as well as neuropsychological testing to assess trajectories of brain development in relation to drug use and other experiences.

Differences in Reward Systems of Addicted Individuals

The brain's reward circuitry is composed of an ancient network of interconnected structures whose evolutionary function is to ensure pursuit of the natural rewards necessary for daily survival (food) and for survival of the species (sex). As previously discussed, drugs of abuse activate the brain's circuitry for natural rewards. However, reward center activation by addictive drugs greatly exceeds that of natural rewards, which explains why drugs like cocaine can produce euphoria that is outside the range of normal human experience. The powerful subjective effects (which, in the case of cocaine and heroin, are likened to "orgasm, but much stronger") of drugs result in powerful reactions to drug cues.

Although many chemical messenger systems are involved in the brain circuitry for reward and reward signals, the neurotransmitter dopamine has been the focus of most research in human brain imaging (Takahashi, 2013; Volkow et al., 1990; Volkow, Wang, Fischman, et al., 1997; Volkow, Wang, et al., 1999). This focus is due in part to the large number of animal studies that implicate a role for dopamine in reward function (Di Chiara et al., 2004; Di Chiara, Acquas, Tanda, & Cadoni, 1993; Koob & Nestler, 1997; Miliano et al., 2016; Roberts & Ranaldi, 1995; Schultz, 2002; Wise, 1996). The focus on dopamine is also due to a current research limitation: there are several dopamine-related tracers available for human imaging research, but very few are available for the other transmitter systems. As previously noted, most drugs of abuse acutely increase the level of dopamine in the nucleus accumbens and other reward-related brain regions. This allows more dopamine to bind specialized dopamine receptors, increasing transmission of the dopamine message. Increased dopamine neurotransmission may be associated with an increase in positive mood, energy, arousal, and motor activity, all of which are effects that have been linked to the dopamine system.

Low D2 Dopamine Receptors

In terms of addiction vulnerability, one might expect that individuals with more dopamine receptors would potentially experience a greater (positive) drug effect and might therefore be *more likely* to become addicted. However, brain imaging research suggests the opposite may be true. Cocaine-addicted adults with long histories of addiction had low numbers of dopamine (type D2) receptors in the striatum (a critical way station in the reward circuitry), compared with controls who had no history of any substance abuse (Asensio et al., 2010; Takahashi, 2013; Volkow et al., 1993).

For some years, the finding of low D2 dopamine receptors in cocaine users was regarded as a possible consequence of the cocaine use. This interpretation was based on knowledge (from animal studies) that the increased flood of dopamine caused by cocaine or other drugs of abuse can often trigger adaptive and compensatory responses in the brain. In the case of an excessive dopamine message, as occurs during drug intoxication, reductions in dopamine synthesis, release, or reduction in dopamine receptors could help reduce the transmission of the message and help bring the dopamine system back into homeostatic balance. Dramatic findings from imaging studies suggest that low D2 receptors may also predate drug use and may constitute a vulnerability factor in their own right. In a study of normal controls without addiction, those individuals within the group who "liked" an infusion of the stimulant methylphenidate had D2 receptor levels that were as low as those in cocaine users addicted for many years (Volkow, Wang, et al., 1999; Volkow et al., 2009). In the same study, individuals with a higher level of D2 receptors rated stimulant administration as "too much" and downright unpleasant. The study suggests that a higher level of D2 dopamine receptors may actually be protective against stimulant addiction by reducing the pleasurable effects of the powerful stimulant.

The potential protective effect of higher dopamine D2 receptors and the interaction of environmental experience with this effect was dramatically demonstrated in imaging studies with nonhuman primates given the opportunity to administer cocaine (Morgan et al., 2002; Nader et al., 2012). Individually housed male monkeys were imaged and some were then group housed, allowing dominance hierarchies to be established. Alpha-male monkeys, who had achieved dominance in the group-housing situation, showed a significant increase in dopamine D2 receptors in the striatum and did not find cocaine initially appealing. However, the subordinate monkeys who had low D2 dopamine receptors avidly self-administered cocaine (Czoty et al., 2010; Morgan et al., 2002).

These imaging findings suggest that a genetically determined trait, the initial level of D2 dopamine receptors in the striatal portion of the reward system, may be one vulnerability factor for enjoyment of drugs, drug taking, and eventual addiction. The findings equally demonstrate the critical role of the environment in determining whether a genetic vulnerability is expressed or even is reshaping the trait itself. For example, the human control subjects with low D2 receptors (those who liked drugs in the methylphenidate study) had survived adolescence and early adulthood without developing addiction. The mastery experiences of the alpha-male monkeys apparently reshaped a biological risk factor for addiction into one of protection.

We do not yet know whether human adolescents with low D2 dopamine receptor levels will have more preference for stimulants and experience enhanced vulnerability to future addiction. However, recent animal studies suggest that immature D2 interactions in adolescents underlie their unique responses to drugs of abuse and vulnerability to psychopathology (Dwyer & Leslie, 2016). Research in humans also suggests that impulsive persons as assessed by questionnaire have weaker D2 receptor binding in the ventral striatum, a finding that is consistent with the model of drug use progression presented in Figure 17.2 (Jupp & Dalley, 2014).

For those at risk, an implication of these findings for prevention and treatment might be to reset the D2 receptor numbers to a more protective level. The teaching of social and behavioral coping tools to increase mastery and control over stressors could help turn a vulnerable individual (with low D2 dopamine receptors) into one who is more like the alpha monkey: ready to take on challenges and challengers. Once these monkeys had established dominance, they were much less attracted to cocaine. Another approach might be to train youth with impulsive tendencies to develop greater executive control over drug-related impulses. Working memory training in adults with substance use disorder was found to reduce delay discounting, an effect that could increase control over substance use (Bickel et al., 2011).

Other approaches could include a medication to reset the reward system to a more protective level. Agents that occupy the dopamine D2 receptors but block their action should, over time, lead to a compensatory increase in the D2 receptors. Unfortunately, the chronic administration of dopamine-blocking drugs (e.g., the typical antipsychotic neuroleptic medications such as chlorpromazine and haloperidol) often have prohibitive side effects, including sedation and a Parkinson's-like neurological syndrome, that make these medications undesirable for long-term treatment. Medications that reduce the activity of the dopamine system but do not completely block it are better tolerated. For example, GABA agonists reduce dopamine neurotransmission without producing the side effects associated with neuroleptics and might theoretically produce a gradual (compensatory) increase in D2 dopamine receptors. Consistent with this prediction, the GABA-B agonist baclofen has shown some early promise in the treatment of cocaine (Kampman, 2010; Ling, Shoptaw, & Majewska, 1998), alcohol (Addolorato et al., 2000; Agabio & Colombo, 2014), and opiate (Akhondzadeh et al., 2000) dependence (trials in nicotine dependence are just beginning). Whether GABA-B agonists could also have a prophylactic effect in those *at risk* for addiction has not yet been tested, but this benefit might be predicted by the adult imaging findings with D2 dopamine receptors.

Brain Response to Drugs of Abuse and Drug-Related Cues

As previously described, drugs of abuse increase dopamine in critical parts of the reward circuitry, and this increase is most robust for psychomotor stimulants. Animal research also shows that the learned signals, or "cues," for these drugs (as well as for natural rewards) also increase dopamine release in these same brain regions. In humans, drug cues trigger strong craving and arousal and may precede relapse. The brain's responses to drugs and to cues that signal the availability of drugs thus represent two additional sources of potential addiction vulnerability in the reward system.

Research in animals has shown that under certain circumstances, the brain response to drugs of abuse (as measured by either brain dopamine release or behavioral activation) can "sensitize" or increase with repeated exposures to the drug. This might lead to the prediction that chronic drug use in humans would similarly lead to an increased brain response, compared with those who have not previously used the drug. Contrary to this expectation, imaging studies in chronic cocaine users have shown that the brain dopamine response to administration of a stimulant in chronic users is actually *lower* than the response of non-drug users (Volkow, Wang, et al., 1997; Volkow et al., 2009). Though this lower brain response can be interpreted as evidence for tolerance (a reduced response to drug with repeated administrations), we do not yet know whether the response is indeed an effect of cocaine exposure or (as with lower D2 receptors) possibly a preexisting neurochemical condition that predated chronic cocaine use. How could a lower brain response to rewards be a risk factor in adolescence? One possibility is that a lower brain dopamine response to natural rewards would mean that these rewards are insufficiently engaging, whereas the powerful, supranormal stimulation by drugs of abuse might be experienced as "just right." Some theories of sensation seeking and thrill seeking take this view. For sensation seekers, the arousal produced by natural rewards may be low, and thus high-intensity, high-arousal experiences are pursued and experienced as pleasurable (Zuckerman, 1986; Zuckerman & Kuhlman, 2000). In contrast, for those with a normal response to natural rewards, the high-intensity (often higher-risk) experiences (parachuting, bungee jumping, etc.) could be experienced as overwhelming and unpleasant.

We do not yet know whether adolescents at risk for substance dependence have a blunted brain response to natural rewards or to drugs of abuse. Although imaging studies that probe dopamine tone require small amounts of radioactive tracers and thus would not be permitted in adolescents, other nonradioactive imaging techniques could be used to measure response to the presentation of common rewards (money, food, etc.). Nonradioactive techniques such as functional magnetic resonance imaging (fMRI) use magnetic fields to map the regional change in brain blood flow, an index of increased brain activity. This technique is currently being used with adults to map the normal response of the brain to monetary (Elliott, Newman, Longe, & Deakin, 2003; Pedroni et al., 2011), food (Asmaro et al., 2012; Small, Zatore, Dagher, Evans, & Jones-Gotman, 2001), or sexual stimuli (Karama et al., 2002; Stoleru et al., 2012). These studies demonstrate that research on the reward circuitry could be conducted in adolescents.

As previously described, animal research has shown activation of the brain reward circuitry by both drugs of abuse and the cues signaling these drugs. The drug and the cues for the drug lead to dopamine increases at important nodes in the reward circuitry. In humans, cues regularly associated with drug use (e.g., the sight of a drug-using friend, dealer, location, or drug paraphernalia) can come to trigger profound craving and motivation for their drug of choice, potentially leading to drug use and relapse (Childress, Franklin, Listerud, Acton, & O'Brien, 2002; Wetherill et al., 2014). Brain imaging studies of this conditioned motivational state in addicted adults have shown activation of several way stations in the motivational/reward circuitry, including those linked to attention, affect, autonomic arousal, and the rapid assignment of emotional valence to incoming stimuli (Lam et al., 2013). Studies also demonstrate significant similarity in the brain regions activated by the cues for cocaine (Bonson et al., 2002; Childress, Mozley, et al., Garavan et al., 2000, 1999; Grant et al., 1996; Kilts et al., 2001), heroin (Daglish et al., 2001; Sell et al., 1999), alcohol (Schneider et al., 2001), and cigarettes (Brody et al., 2002; Wetherill et al., 2015). Similar actions by diverse drugs on motivational circuitry provide biological evidence that supports the commonality of substance abuse disorders. This circuitry also normally manages the motivation for natural rewards, as demonstrated by human brain imaging studies using food (chocolate) (Salem & Dhillo, 2015; Small et al.,

2001) or sexual (Karama et al., 2002) stimuli. Addicted adults often report their craving for drugs exceeds their desire for natural rewards. An fMRI study in adolescents with alcohol use disorder indeed found that the brain response (which included regions in the reward circuitry and cue recognition, such as the fusiform gyri, temporal gyri, parahippocampal gyrus) to visual cues of their preferred alcohol beverage was larger than the response to pictures of a nonalcohol beverage (Park et al., 2007; Tapert et al., 2003).

Most substance-dependent individuals find that behavioral techniques are difficult to apply when they are already in the throes of a full-blown craving episode. Therefore, medications that help bring the powerful brain reward system into a more manageable range are much needed. The GABA-B agonist medication baclofen, described above as having the potential to reset dopamine receptors, has also shown promise in blunting the response to cocaine (Brebner, Childress, & Roberts, 2002; Roberts, 2005; Roberts, Andrews, & Vickers, 1996) or heroin and nicotine (Di Ciano & Everitt, 2003; Spano et al., 2007) cues in animals, and it also blunts the craving and brain activation by cocaine cues in humans (Brebner et al., 2002; Childress, McElgin, et al., 1999; Young et al., 2014). Other candidate medications for reducing the brain response to drug cues are discussed in Chapter 18.

Conclusions on Neurobiology

The neuroscience research reviewed in this section supports the notion that addiction involves disruption in brain pleasure, reward, and memory centers, including the extended amygdala and its numerous connections with other reward-related systems. Extended use of addictive drugs also undermines executive control over drug taking, making it even harder for the addicted individual to withdraw from drug use. Neurobiological research has provided an understanding of brain mechanisms that can guide treatment and prevention development and potentially improve outcome. In contrast, we know little about molecular changes within these regions that mediate the transition into addiction, enhance relapse vulnerability, and produce hedonic dysregulation. Although addictive drugs produce pleasure by activating brain reward circuits, their long-term effect is to inhibit these regions, leading to hedonic dysregulation and unpleasant emotional states. The short-term fix of more drug use provides temporary relief but then merely worsens this vicious cycle. Animal models of addiction have identified specific neurochemical alterations in reward-related and stress-related systems that contribute to dysphoric motivational states associated with drug abstinence, and the pharmacological reversal of these neuroadaptations is a promising strategy to improve outcome in clinical practice. Human studies likewise demonstrate functional and structural brain abnormalities associated with addiction, especially in the prefrontal cortex and amygdala, although the issue of causality has not been adequately addressed. Are these abnormalities produced by repeated drug administration, or do they predate and even contribute to addictive vulnerability? Can they be normalized with abstinence or through specific interventions? Will brain abnormalities identified through imaging techniques eventually serve to identify individuals who are most at risk of developing addiction? The issue of vulnerability is particularly important in order to identify adolescents who might benefit from specific interventions, be they preventive or therapeutic. Closing the gaps in our knowledge of the neurobiology of addiction in adolescents represents an important goal for future research.

THE ROLE OF GENETICS

Overview of Genetic Models

Genetic analyses of susceptibility to drug use and progression have identified major pathways of influence between genetic variation and drug use. The biobehavioral model in Figure 17.3 developed by Audrain-McGovern and Tercyak (2011) provides a useful overview of genetic effects on drug dependence that, with minor

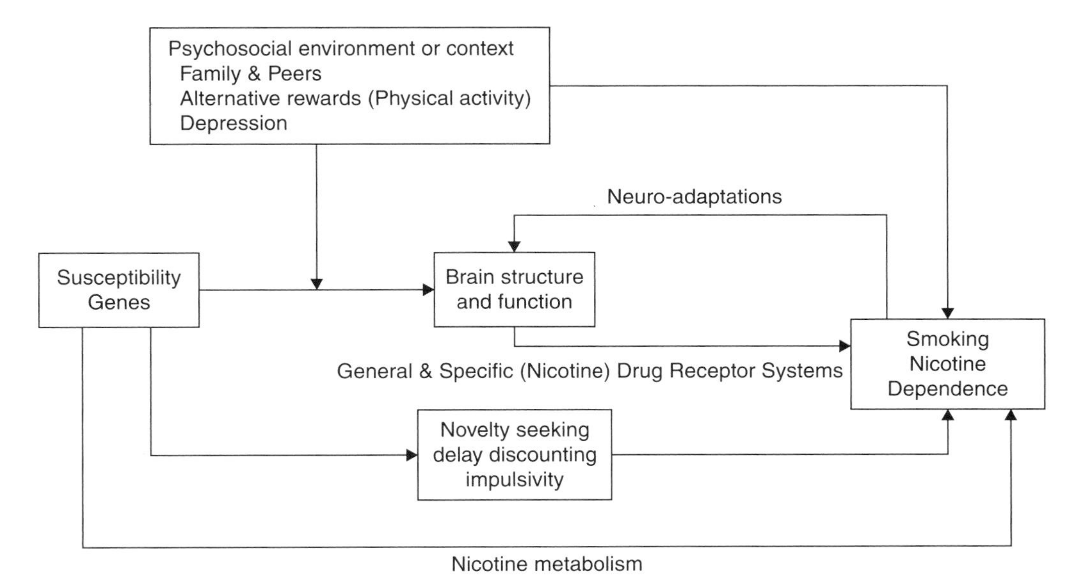

Figure 17.3 Biobehavioral model of genetic effects on drug use and dependence. Developed by J. Audrain-McGovern & K. P. Tercyak. (2011). Genes, environment, and adolescent smoking: Implications for prevention. In K. S. Kendler, S. R. Jaffee, & D. Romer (Eds.), *The dynamic genome and mental health: The role of genes and environments in youth development* (pp. 294–321). New York: Oxford University Press.

modifications for each drug, encompasses the role of genetic variation in drug use. As is evident, genes affect drug use through two mediating processes as well as a direct effect on metabolism. A good example of the effects of metabolic processes involves the uptake and progression of smoking. Slower metabolism of nicotine reduces the reward value of the drug and is protective against smoking and the development of nicotine dependence in adolescents (Audrain-McGovern et al., 2007).

With regard to the mediated pathways, one operates through the expression of personality differences that are important in predisposing youth to try and to progress in the use of drugs. These differences include novelty seeking and two important forms of impulsivity, delay discounting and impulsive action, that influence control over drug seeking and progression. Various dopamine and serotonin genes have been implicated in these personality differences (Bevilacqua & Goldman, 2013). The second pathway is through effects on brain structure and function that are particularly sensitive to the effects of drugs, such as genes that influence the inhibitory system (Zintzaras, 2012) or that influence the receptors that are sensitive to a particular drug. For example, in the case of nicotine, genes that control nicotinic receptors may reduce the reward threshold and aversive effects of nicotine (Morel et al., 2014). One such gene has been consistently associated with heavier smoking and risk for dependence in adolescents (Rodriguez et al., 2011). The effects of both pathways on drug use can also feed back to brain structure, producing changes in brain function that have enduring effects on brain and behavior, such as the development of dependence and the undermining of cognitive control over drug use.

Of great importance to biobehavioral models of genetic influence is the role of psychosocial environments as interacting influences on genetic effects. This influence has been studied under the umbrella concept of gene (G) by environment (E) interplay, which includes G × E interaction (the influence of genes varies with important environmental conditions) as well as forms of gene and environment correlation (rGE: e.g., genetic variation that predisposes the selection of different environments). Some of the environmental factors that play an important role in the relation between genes and behavior are the family and peer group (Dick, 2011). These social influences can moderate effects of genes, such as when families with strong parental monitoring of adolescent behavior reduce the effects of genes that might otherwise strongly predispose to drug use (Dick et al., 2007). Genes also predispose youth to select peer group affiliations, a form of rGE, that can intensify gene effects that might otherwise be muted without the influence of peers (Kendler, 2011). Behaviors that might affect the influence of genes also may moderate their effects. One example is physical activity, such as sports, that might reduce the need to satisfy novelty- and sensation-seeking drives through drug use (Audrain-McGovern et al., 2003). Other mental conditions, such as depression, may be moderated by the effects of genes such that predispositions to use drugs for self-medication are either enhanced or reduced (Shytle et al., 2002).

A final factor that is implicit in the model in Figure 17.3 is the differential role of genes during development. While classical analyses of genetic effects on behavior and personality summarize those relations with a single measure of heritability, it has become increasingly clear that the magnitude of genetic effects varies with age and drug use exposure. For example, twin models have been used to explore the relative contribution of genetic and environmental factors to substance use and dependence. This is accomplished by comparing concordance rates for a particular trait in monozygotic twins, who share all of their genes in common, to those for dizygotic twins, who share roughly 50% of their genes (Kendler, 2001). This methodology has been used to study the role of heritable factors for smoking, alcohol use, and use of illegal drugs. Although these methods tend to find strong heritability in drug use (usually around 50%), these estimates tend to be differentially related to drug use at different developmental stages. For example, heritability for alcohol use is relatively weak for initiation of the drug but grows in strength as the youth ages and alcohol use progresses (Rose et al., 2001). There are also sex differences in the strength of these relations. In early adolescence, genetic influences account for larger variance for alcohol consumption in girls, whereas it is essentially negligible for boys in early adolescence. In contrast, genetic influences appear to be much more pronounced for adult males compared to adult females (Meyers et al., 2014).

Twin studies have uncovered important insights into the genetic underpinnings of drug dependence. It is now clear that the entire spectrum of externalizing behavior, including conduct disorder and dependence on various drugs, is predicted by a common latent trait, characterized as reflecting a variety of disinhibitory predispositions (Iocono et al., 2008; Kreuger et al., 2002). In addition, the strength of these genetic influences appears to grow with age in both males and females, with novel genetic effects appearing in later years (Jacobson et al., 2002). Nevertheless, early signs of these behavior patterns are evident prior to adolescence, as illustrated by the Dunedin birth-cohort study. This study identified children with weak self-control that persisted into adulthood, with dramatic effects on drug use and other dysfunctional behavior (Moffitt et al., 2011).

Once a particular behavioral trait (also referred to as a "phenotype") has been established as heritable, molecular genetic approaches are used to identify the specific genetic variants that may be responsible. One such approach identifies candidate genes based on neurobiological or biochemical pathways (e.g., dopamine or serotonin genes) and uses a case-control study design to compare the frequency of genetic variants (alleles) in these pathways among persons with and without the phenotype (e.g., nicotine-dependent persons vs. nondependent persons) (Sullivan, Jiang, Neale, Kendler, & Straub, 2001). Several studies employing the candidate gene approach to investigate substance abuse genes are described below. The role of specific genetic variants can be also investigated through family-based designs that examine allele sharing or allele transmission for candidate genes within families (Spielman et al., 1996). This latter approach controls for potential bias due to ethnic differences, but it has less statistical power and is more costly to implement.

In contrast to these hypothesis-driven approaches, genetic linkage analysis can be used to search for as yet unidentified genetic variants that may be linked with substance use phenotypes. In this approach, families or relative pairs (e.g., siblings) are studied to look for linkage with anonymous markers across the genome. Because the effect sizes of any individual gene conferring susceptibility to a behavioral trait are expected to be small (Comings et al., 2001), this approach requires a large sample size. Another approach that has gained popularity in recent years is the use of genome-wide association. This method examines the entire genomes in large samples in search of associations with relevant phenotypes. A recent example of the use of this approach is a study of the general disinhibition phenotype underling all externalizing behavior (Vrieze et al., 2014). However, progress in identifying significant associations for complex traits such as externalizing behavior has not always met its initial expectations (Salvatore & Dick, 2016). Effects of individual genes tend to be small, requiring large samples, and the identification of such genes often fails to be replicated in different samples.

The most consistent evidence for genetic effects on drug use comes from studies of drug metabolism. As already mentioned, genes that control the metabolism of nicotine can predict important characteristics of smoking behavior. With regard to alcohol, genetic differences in alcohol metabolism have been strongly implicated in the development of alcohol use disorder. Alcohol is converted to its major metabolite acetaldehyde by the enzyme alcohol dehydrogenase (ADH). Decreased metabolism results in more aversive effects of alcohol consumption, such as flushing and toxicity. A reduced-activity allele of the *ADH2* gene (*ADH2*2*) is found more commonly in Asian populations and has been shown to be protective against alcohol dependence in Chinese (Chen et al., 1999) and European (Borras et al., 2000) populations. There is some evidence that the genetic effect is stronger for males than for females (Whitfield et al., 1998). The reduced-activity allele of *ADH2* is also found more commonly in Ashkenazi Jewish populations and has been associated with reduced alcohol consumption among Jewish college students (Shea, Wall, Carr, & Li, 2001). Nonetheless, a recent study found comparable prevalence of alcohol dependence among males in China compared to those in Western countries (Cheng et al., 2015). Authors speculated that peer pressure and the Chinese drinking culture are major contributors to this observed contradiction to the well-established low metabolism of alcohol in the Han Chinese population. This highlights the complicated interplay between genetic and environmental factors for drinking and the importance of the consideration of social variables in alcohol research.

Key Findings from Research on Genetics of Substance Use

Although heritable factors are clearly important in substance use and dependence as assessed in twin studies, such effects involve a complex interaction between multiple genes in different biological pathways. Some genetic variants may result in a more generalized predisposition to substance use and dependence, while others may influence risk for dependence on specific substances. These genetic effects interact with environmental factors, and any individual genetic variant is likely to account for only a small proportion of the overall variance in a substance use behavior. Indeed, the model in Figure 17.3 suggests that effects of genes are largely mediated by effects on brain structures and functions that actually control drug use. Furthermore, environments can dramatically affect how these processes unfold, making the effects of genes highly conditional on social and personal circumstances.

Findings on the effects of specific genetic variants are not consistent. The use of different study designs and methods of subject ascertainment, the focus on polymorphisms of unknown functional significance, and ethnic admixture have resulted in inconsistent findings in this field. Very large studies using both population-based and family-based designs are needed to validate specific genetic effects and to identify the set(s) of genetic variants that predispose to general addiction potential and dependence on specific substances.

A complete understanding of specific genetic influences on substance dependence will reveal only part of the picture. On average, genetic influences account for roughly half of the variance in specific substance use behaviors. Such effects occur in the context of complex socio-environmental and psychological influences. Even the best panel of genetic tests to identify individuals predisposed to substance abuse will have low sensitivity and specificity unless non-genetic influences are incorporated into the model. Increased understanding of the role of genetic factors in addiction will never diminish the importance of behavioral and social influences.

DRUG EPIDEMICS AFFECTING ADOLESCENTS IN THE UNITED STATES: THE 1960S TO THE PRESENT

Due to public health research largely designed and set up by the early 1970s and maintained over the years, disease surveillance approaches from the field of epidemiology have given the American public a previously unseen view of the nature and extent of adolescent drug use in the United States. In this section we consider whether the experiences of 21st-century adolescents in the United States deserve to be considered an "epidemic." Illustrations are provided in the form of quite recent estimates for the prevalence and incidence for psychoactive drug compounds that include alcoholic beverages, tobacco products, and internationally regulated drugs such as marijuana (cannabis) and prescription pain relievers.

In this update to the previous edition, which presented estimates from the 1970s to 2002, we are mindful that today's 21st-century adolescents do not experience the same agents or environmental conditions that were present during the middle and later years of the 20th century. To illustrate, during the peak years of the cannabis, LSD, and cocaine hydrochloride powder epidemics between 1975 and 1980, fully two thirds (65%–70%) of American adolescents had used one or more of the internationally regulated drugs (generally "to get high") by the time they had finished high school (Johnston, O'Malley, & Bachman, 2002). The available estimates, based on epidemiologic surveillance of the time, represented a dramatic increase over values observed in the 1960s, when the 20th-century "drug epidemic" had its origins (Johnston, 1973; National Commission on Marihuana, 1972).

As for the agents contributing to more recent adolescent drug experiences, cannabis continues to predominate, but the dynamic evolution of drug epidemics in the United States included the emergence of crack cocaine in the 1980s. In addition, the older methamphetamine compounds were reformulated in a "smokeable" form as "ice" and have come into widespread use during the past 20 years, especially in America's rural areas. The stimulant-hallucinogen 3,4-methylenedioxymethamphetamine (MDMA; Ecstasy) of the 1980s and 1990s generally displaced LSD of the 1960s and 1970s. During these years, the pharmaceutical industry also introduced legitimate products with approval from the U.S. Food and Drug Administration (FDA) that are used extra-medically, such as sustained-release opioid prescription pain relievers (e.g., OxyContin; De Andrea, Troost, & Anthony, 2013). Despite efforts to prevent diversion from legitimate supply lines, these compounds have made their way into the black market, sometimes via sales via mass market vendors who started to make use of the Internet once it was "invented" in the early 1990s. Accordingly, concomitant with increased prescribing of prescription pain relievers, there were increases in extra-medical use of these drugs during the 1990s, as well as mounting casualties in the form of overdose deaths and opioid use disorders—a new drug epidemic still in its middle years and not yet in full decline.

As gauged in relation to the retrospectively derived numbers of newly incident adolescents with extra-medical drug-using experience year by year, it can be seen that these epidemic trends turned downward during the late 1970s. Even so, the proportion of young people continuing to use drugs did not decline across the board until later in the 1980s. (This pattern can be seen in epidemiology's "prevalence proportions," which are determined as much by persistence of use, sometimes more than what is determined by occurrence of newly incident use of a drug.) For most of the internationally regulated drugs, the downward trajectory in each year's prevalence proportion persisted into the early 1990s and then stabilized. In some instances (e.g., cannabis and prescription pain relievers), there have been increases from the early 1990s onward into the 21st century.

In our previously published retrospective analysis of the domains of influence that govern youths' appreciation of the hazards of illegal drug use, we were building from a foundation of observations by historian David Musto and others, highlighting (a) media coverage, (b) drug prevention programming, (c) personal experiences, and (d) vicarious experiences (i.e., learning from peers, parents, or other relatives about the drugs' hazards experienced by others). To the extent that society achieves success in dampening the prevalence of adolescent extra-medical drug use (by whatever means), we have come to expect controllable declines in the first two domains: (a) as media coverage falls and (b) as support for prevention programming wanes. Part and parcel with declining prevalence as measured at the population level, there has been a reduction in the diversity of individual-level experience—that is, personal experience with these drug-taking behaviors falls off. Then, there are fewer chances to try the drugs, and fewer young people are experiencing the hurt that often goes along with drug taking. In addition, there is less vicarious experience with the associated hazards as can be gained by personal acquaintance with other young people or adults whose lives have been harmed by their drug use (or by that of others).

It follows that on the downward side of an epidemic curve of such drug use, the same processes that fuel the continuing decline in drug-using behaviors are fueling a decline in adolescents' personal and vicarious knowledge of the associated hazards. In this sense, a "success" in the form of declining prevalence of such drug use sows the seeds for a "failure" and later rebound—to the extent that the knowledge of drug-associated hazards helps to promote resistance when the young person faces the first or subsequent chance to use these drugs to get high or for other extra-medical reasons.

These seeds for a resurgence of extra-medical drug use among American adolescents had been sown in the late 1980s and early 1990s. Thereafter, for most internationally regulated drugs, the epidemic curve turned upward in the early 1990s, with a generally persistent trend of increasing proportions of new users and continuing users into the late 1990s. Cannabis smoking exhibited the sharpest rise during these resurgent epidemic years, but extra-medical use of many drugs in a growing list of alternatives increased during this period as well, most prominently and problematically the prescription pain relievers that had been prescribed for years (e.g., Vicodin) as well as newly introduced products such as sustained-release OxyContin (Johnston et al., 2013, 2014; Substance Abuse and Mental Health Services Agency, 2013, 2014).

With respect to the "environments" contributing to these recent adolescent drug experiences in the United States, there have been some new developments. In the first edition, when we tried to convey an understanding of what might be contributing factors in the succession of drug epidemics during the second half of the 20th century and the earliest years of the 21st century, it was necessary to consider macro-level demographic changes, with concurrent economic, social, and political developments, too complex for in-depth coverage within this chapter. The major contributing environmental factors in the middle to late 20th century included (1) a major demographic change in the form of the post–World War II "baby boom" with rapidly increasing birth rates in the United States, and much-increased numbers of young people entering adolescence between the late 1950s and the 1970s; (2) sustained economic prosperity after the Second World War, giving midcentury adolescents unprecedented "buying power" for products that could be transported from state to state with greater speed, thanks to a new interstate highway system, followed by reduced air transportation costs that promoted travel abroad; and (3) a more cosmopolitan and outward-looking mid- to late-20th-century worldview, in contrast to the more parochial and inward-looking worldview of many Americans in the post-Depression era, prior to the experiences of World War II.

A "youth culture" of the late 1950s and early to mid-1960s emerged from these background conditions, sometimes with deliberate "counter-cultural" facets and loosening of social bonds to conventional social norms and traditional forms of "social adaptation." For many youths, entry into adolescent peer groups required a choice between adaptive bonding to the more transient peer group social norms (including drug use norms) versus the more stable social norms of their families of origin (including antidrug norms).

Additional complexity was introduced by initiation of the military service draft for the Vietnam War, widespread smoking of cannabis by many late adolescents and young adults serving in Southeast Asia, and considerable numbers of veterans returning home to the United States after trying heroin and opium while abroad. These environmental conditions modulated formerly strong antidrug sentiments and cultural values of the parents and grandparents of America's adolescents such that those becoming adolescents in the 21st century are exposed to a much greater diversity of pro-drug and antidrug sentiments among the older generations than was true for adolescents growing up in the mid- to late 20th century.

The sedative-hypnotic drug methaqualone (Quaalude) serves to illustrate a subepidemic that has come and gone, nestled within larger drug epidemic processes within the United States. Ignored by most scholars in drug epidemiology, methaqualone surfaced and then essentially disappeared as an epidemic phenomenon in the United States. As for the "methaqualone epidemic" years, based on epidemiologic surveys conducted in the late 1970s, about 1% of American adolescents ages 12 to 17 years old had tried methaqualone at least once; incidence rates of methaqualone use clearly were greater than expected values based on adolescent experiences in the 1960s and early 1970s, as documented in field survey research at that time. Moreover, corresponding estimates for 18- to 25-year-olds and 26- to 34-year-olds in the late 1970s were 3% and 3.7%, respectively, such that by the time young people in the United States had reached their 30th birthday, almost one in 30 had tried methaqualone, due to major increases in the numbers of newly incident users between 1960 and the late 1970s. However, between 1980 and 1995, there was a major reduction in the incidence of methaqualone use, and very few who started showed persistence. By 2011, comparable epidemiologic values for methaqualone had dropped to below six per 1,000 (0.6%) for all of the age groups just mentioned, including adolescents (data not shown; estimates produced for this report).

We have no definitive explanation for general disappearance of this "methaqualone epidemic" in the United States, although the background includes (1) the marketing of benzodiazepine compounds that promote sleep provided clinicians with less toxic sedative-hypnotics than older compounds such as methaqualone as well as chloral hydrate, and (2) the methaqualone manufacturers in the United States voluntarily put a stop to methaqualone production. (A footnote of interest is that some countries continued to experience methaqualone problems after these problems had ended in the United States—e.g., South Africa.)

Another subepidemic seen for adolescents in the United States has involved smoking of cocaine products, which was an extremely rare behavior for adolescents before the late 1970s. Nasal insufflation of cocaine hydrochloride powder ("snorting") had started to increase in the late 1960s and early 1970s toward peak numbers of newly incident users in roughly 1976, but crack cocaine use was nonexistent until the 1980s. The crack cocaine formulation and its characteristic smoking route of administration became more distributed in the United States toward the late 1980s.

Since that time, as gauged by the estimated numbers of "newly incident" crack cocaine smokers year by year (i.e., those just starting to use crack cocaine), the crack cocaine epidemic has subsided; now we are experiencing what clearly is a "descending limb" of the crack cocaine epidemic curve in the United States (Parker & Anthony, 2014). Incidence rates for snorting cocaine seem to be falling more slowly, but they also have been declining (Substance Abuse and Mental Health Services Agency, 2014).

With these facets of the history of adolescent drug experience in mind, we now focus on newer epidemiologic estimates from this line of surveillance research, including a view of and trends for different forms of drug taking. Some attention is given to clinically defined drug use disorders and associated problems, such as the cannabis dependence syndromes. We stress the plural "problems" as we seek to understand these conditions because when we try to collapse everything into a single "drug problem," we can oversimplify a complex situation to the point of confusion and misunderstanding.

In the case of crack cocaine and other drug use, once drug use starts, it might be persistent and last for many years, with prevalence of recently active use as a reflection of the numbers of past-onset persistent users, and with each year's numbers of newly incident users dwindling toward zero. This seems to be the case in the United States with respect to the crack cocaine epidemic in recent years (Parker & Anthony, 2014).

What about other drugs, such as tobacco? Are we still in the middle of an epidemic of tobacco use? The answer depends upon which set of expected values is chosen. In relation to values observed between 1965 and 1980, the current incidence of tobacco smoking (particularly of cigarettes) now is lower than it was in past decades (since the 1990s). However, as gauged in relation to expected values for adolescent cigarette smoking from the 19th century, the entire 20th century and the early 21st century to date qualify as "epidemic years," notwithstanding important drops in incidence over the past 15 to 20 years (particularly for boys). Throughout most of the 20th century, the United States experienced an epidemic of cigarette smoking, followed by some epidemic years of non-cigarette tobacco product use (e.g., smokeless tobacco). According to recent reports, we now are experiencing a new epidemic in the form of increasing numbers of newly incident adolescent e-cigarette users (Johnston et al., 2016a, 2016b).

Sources of Estimates and Trend Lines

In the United States, our current best estimates for the prevalence and incidence of adolescent drug use are from the National Surveys on Drug Use and Health (NSDUH). However, our longest trend lines for estimated prevalence of adolescent drug use come from the "Monitoring the Future" (MTF) surveys. It may be useful to compare and contrast the NSDUH and MTF survey approaches, starting with the MTF, which began in the 1970s with surveys of 12th-graders in the final semester of secondary school. These school-attending youths have been assessed using self-administered questionnaires, typically in a multiclass group assembly or convocation in a school auditorium or similar room. During more recent years, samples of eighth-graders and 10th-graders have been surveyed as well, with one group of eighth-graders becoming 10th-graders 2 years later and then becoming 12th-graders 2 years after that, but with complications of interpretation that involve dropping out of school and uncertainty about whether the sample each year should be treated as an independent replication. Other details about MTF, including its longitudinal follow-up of the 12th-graders into their postsecondary years, are provided in a series of online reports, books, and other publications (e.g., Johnston et al., 2013, 2014).

The more recently launched NSDUH have involved community fieldwork to draw samples of all noninstitutionalized civilian residents of the United States ages 12 years and older. Most typically assessments are done by audio computer-assisted self-interviews (ACASI) in or near a private location within each participant's dwelling unit. Before the NSDUH, starting in the mid-1970s, there was a National Household Survey on Drug Abuse (NHSDA) with a more restrictive sampling of people living in households but not in other noninstitutional dwelling units or group quarters. Due to methods changes of this type, the trend lines for NHSDA and NSDUH generally cannot be traced from the mid-1970s to recent years, but the NSDUH now has trend lines from 2002 through 2015, and perhaps beyond.

It is the more limited sampling frame of the MTF surveys of young people attending school in the United States that makes the NSDUH estimates for extra-medical use exceptionally valuable. For all intents and purposes, the NSDUH estimates now are based on samples of virtually all adolescents in the United States, including those in all 50 states and the District of Columbia, and excluding only those who are incarcerated or in relatively long-term residence within an institution at the time of the survey. The survey coverage now includes not only households but also dormitories, homeless shelters, and other noninstitutional group quarters, providing a view of adolescents in nontraditional dwelling units, and without being restricted to school-attending adolescents as is the case for school-based surveys.

In addition, the vast majority of sampled dwelling units and almost all adolescents sampled for the NSDUH agree to be assessed via its standardized ACASI or an optional computer-assisted personal interview (CAPI), designed to promote validity and completeness of reporting sometimes illegal and sensitive behaviors (Substance Abuse and Mental Health Services Agency, 2013). In contrast, there is a considerable degree of school-level nonparticipation in the U.S. school surveys such that a large fraction of sampled schools actually do not participate in the survey and must be replaced with schools that have more compliant school administrations (Johnston et al., 2013, 2014).

With respect to accuracy and completeness of assessment about sensitive and sometimes illegal behaviors such as drug use, one might expect the ACASI assessment approach to yield more complete coverage of adolescent drug use. Nonetheless, sometimes it is true that MTF prevalence estimates are larger than corresponding NSDUH prevalence estimates, for reasons not well understood, but possibly due to exaggeration, boasting, or overreporting of drug use by the students in the MTF assemblies, or possibly due to underreporting and nondisclosure of use by young people completing the ACASI assessment at home. The MTF and NSDUH research teams have offered their own perspectives on these variations in prevalence estimates from the two concurrent surveillance approaches in the United States, but at the end of the day, one perhaps should not expect a survey of all youths in the community to yield exactly the same results as a survey restricted to school-attending youths (Johnston et al., 2013; Substance Abuse and Mental Health Services Agency, 2013).

In a final note on methods, it is possible that some of the variation between the MTF and the NSDUH is introduced by variations in the definitions used to explain the survey questions to the participants. Nonetheless, both survey initiatives have produced estimates for alcoholic beverages (hereinafter, alcohol), tobacco cigarettes (hereinafter, tobacco, unless noted otherwise, as in the case of e-cigarettes and smokeless tobacco), inhalant compounds (e.g., volatile glues, gases), and various subtypes of the internationally regulated drug compounds such as (1) LSD and other hallucinogens; (2) cocaine, methamphetamine, and other psychostimulants; (3) heroin and other opioid and nonopioid prescription pain relievers; and (4) sedative-hypnotic-anxiolytic compounds (sometimes called "tranquilizers" or "sedatives" in MTF and NSDUH reports). Coverage of MTF and NSDUH survey items on the internationally regulated drugs does not encompass using medicines exactly as prescribed by a clinician or as taken exactly as described in FDA-approved instructions and indications for use. Rather, the focus is on extra-medical use, such as when a young person has used inhalants or one of these internationally regulated drugs in order to get high or for other feeling states or in ways that are outside the boundaries of indications, frequency of use, and dosing as prescribed by a clinician engaged in the legitimate practice of medicine in the United States.

For shorthand, we will use the abbreviation "extra-medical use" to stand for these forms of extra-medical use of prescription drugs, nonprescription drugs such as opioid-containing cough medicines, and inhalants, as well as internationally regulated drugs such as LSD or heroin, which often will mean using the drug to get high, more than was prescribed, or for feelings or experiences other than a prescribing clinician intended. The distinction between "nonmedical" and "extra-medical" drug use involves the fact that sometimes "extra-medical" use of a drug is outside the boundaries of what a clinician has prescribed but is not strictly speaking "nonmedical." As an example, consider a young person given a small supply of opioid prescription pain relievers after oral surgery, with one tablet left over in the medicine cabinet. Then, the patient experiences a completely independent toothache that wakes her up and disrupts her sleep before an important school examination, and the parent tells her to take the remaining tablet to relieve the pain and get back to sleep. It is clear that this is "extra-medical" and beyond the boundaries of what the oral surgeon prescribed, but it is not so clearly "nonmedical" in this context.

Estimates and Trends in Prevalence of Adolescent Drug Use

Comparison of the just-discussed age-specific NSDUH estimates for recently active users with MTF estimates is not straightforward because MTF results are organized by school grade, and there is heterogeneity of ages within grades. Nonetheless, it might be expected that the NSDUH estimates for 12- and 13-year-olds should be somewhat lower than corresponding MTF values for eighth-graders, in that many eighth-graders have passed or are close to their 14th birthdays; some eighth-graders are 15 (e.g., if they have been held back). Accordingly, it is not surprising that the NSDUH estimate of 6.9% in 2012 is smaller than the MTF estimate for eighth-graders in 2012, which is 13.4% (95% confidence interval [CI] 12.2–14.6).

In contrast, the NSDUH prevalence estimate for 16- and 17-year-olds in 2012 shows 30% to be recently active extra-medical drug users. This value for 16- and 17-year-olds might be larger than the MTF estimate for 10th-graders, most of whom are 15 or 16. However, the estimate for 10th-graders is about the same, at 30.1% (95% CI 28.4–32.0).

A similar NSDUH excess in 2012 might be found when comparing the NSDUH estimate for 18- to 20-year-olds with the MTF estimate for 12th-graders, given that few 12th-graders have reached age 20. However, by age 19 or 20, many young people have entered college, and college-attending students are somewhat less likely than 12th-graders to be active drug users (Johnston et al., 2013, 2014); this fact might bring the estimates into greater balance. As it happens, in 2012, the NSDUH estimate for the prevalence of recently active extra-medical drug use among 18- to 29-year-olds is 40%, as compared to the not-appreciably-different corresponding MTF estimate of 39.7% for 12th-graders (95% CI 37.1–42.3).

The real value of the MTF estimates in research on adolescent drug use can be seen in their capacity to yield a view of very long-term trends. To illustrate, Figure 17.4 depicts an especially important set of trend lines based on what the MTF surveys have learned by asking 12th-graders when they first started to use internationally regulated drugs and/or inhalants extra-medically. These estimates reflect the cumulative incidence of drug use, as estimated retrospectively for each year from 1968 through 2012, with grade in school plotted as a separate line in the figure.

To be clear, each trend line in this figure reflects the reconstructed cumulative experience of students in each grade from grade six to grade 12. The peak values are between 60% and 70%, reflecting the cumulative experience of students who were completing grade 12 during 1976 through 1984. Corresponding MTF estimates for 12th-graders between 2004 and 2012 are lower, at 50% to 55%.

We can gain a sense of dynamic incidence rates by looking at what these 12th-graders reported retrospectively about their drug experiences as of 2006, when they were in sixth grade, and fewer than 5% had engaged in extra-medical drug use by that grade. A corresponding estimate of about 15% is seen 2 years later, in 2008, when these 12th-graders were completing grade eight, and the estimate is 35% to 40% 2 years after that, in 2010, when the 12th-graders were completing grade 10. As was seen in the NSDUH estimates for recently active users, the sequential retrospective MTF estimates for these 12th-graders, and for 12th-graders in prior years, are providing a consistent picture of major increases in risk of starting extra-medical drug use during the years of adolescence.

Was there any single drug subtype contributing to the increasing cumulative occurrence estimates that can be observed to have appeared between 1990 and 2000, after which plateau values are observed? The evidence shows that the answer involves cannabis products, without which there might well have been no tangible increase in the cumulative occurrence estimates across that span of years. This result can be seen in Figure 17.5, which reproduces Figure 17.4's curve for eighth-, 10th-, and 12th-graders in the years from 1975 to 2015 (top panel), and shows the corresponding year-by-year estimates for the same youth when cannabis use is not included in the estimates (bottom panel).

This consideration of drug subtypes leads directly to the topics of the next sections of this chapter. In sequence, these sections consider clinical aspects of adolescent involvement with each in a series of drug subtypes, starting with heroin and other opioid compounds. In these sections, the clinical aspects of primary importance are discussed in relation to DSM-5, which reintroduced concepts of addiction (American Psychiatric Association, 2014). Nonetheless, virtually all epidemiologic evidence on these clinical aspects has been based on the previously specified concept of drug dependence, for reasons articulated by World Health Organization expert committees since 1965; this accounts for the use of the term "dependence" in diagnostic classifications from 1965 until DSM-5 was published in 2014. One might anticipate that it will take 5 to 10 years before epidemiologic studies on a national scale can present estimates for drug addiction as specified in DSM-5. Until then, the drug dependence syndromes of prior DSM editions will prevail, along with epidemiologic research on individual clinical features that are shared across the concepts of drug addiction and drug dependence (e.g., pharmacological tolerance, withdrawal, craving). We present a more detailed description of DSM-5 criteria for addiction in the section on alcohol use disorder.

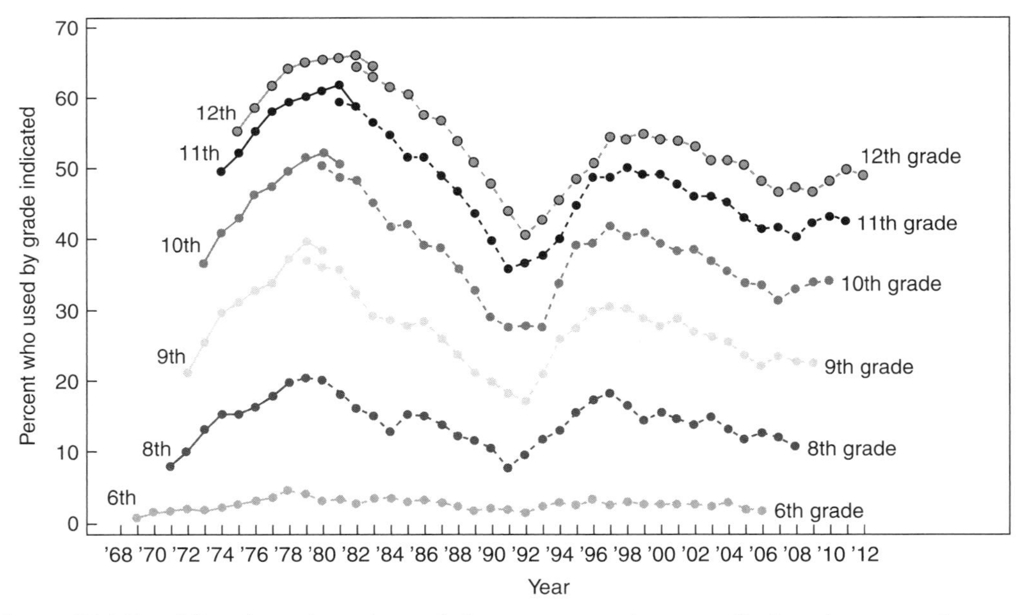

Figure 17.4 Trend lines for estimated cumulative occurrence of extra-medical use (encompassing internationally regulated drugs as well as inhalants). Retrospectively recalled data from the MTF surveys. (From Fig. 6.1 in Johnston et al., 2012.)

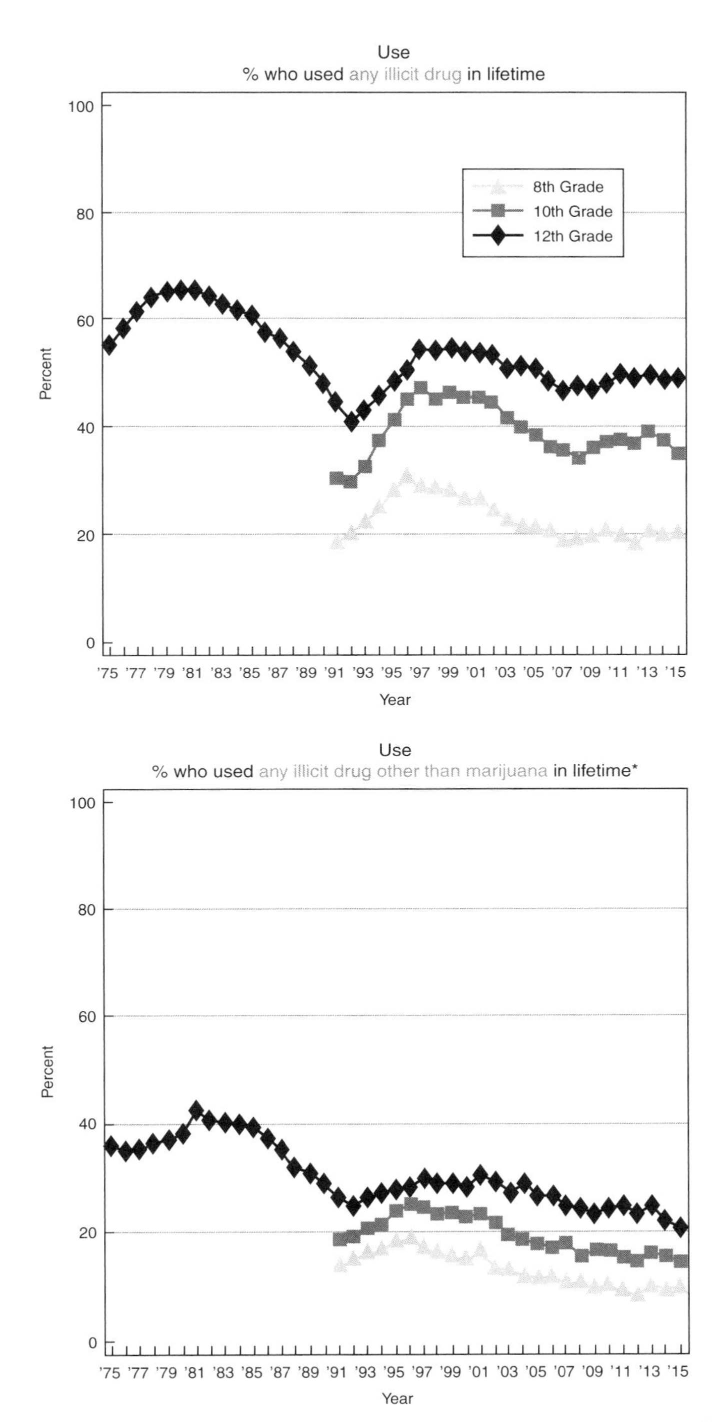

Figure 17.5 Trends in lifetime use of any illicit drug (top panel) vs. illicit drug excluding marijuana. (From Johnston et al., 2016a.)

CLINICAL ASPECTS OF SPECIFIC DRUG USE DISORDERS

Our understanding of adolescent dependence and addiction syndromes, in both pharmacological and behavioral realms, continues to grow but remains somewhat limited. Research advances in this area have been delayed by several considerations. First, the typical pharmacological experiments involving controlled administration of drugs commonly done with adult research volunteers for the most part have not been possible with adolescents. Thus, much of what is known about the pharmacology of drugs in adolescents must be inferred from experience with adults. The logistics, particularly ethical, regulatory, and related informed-consent issues, are such that much of the pharmacological research on drugs that adolescents should not be using must necessarily take place with animal models or with adult volunteers. Of course, useful information can be learned from clinical experience and observations, but even our clinical experience has been limited by adolescents' resistance to treatment, by social stigma, and by an inadequate addiction treatment infrastructure in the United States. Furthermore, anecdotal clinical information is much less reliable than that gleaned from controlled studies, as have been performed on adult patients. Experience from clinical settings, such as emergency rooms and treatment clinics, provides information on the pharmacology of adverse drug consequences but provides less information on the more typical pharmacological effects of extra-medical drug use experienced by the majority of adolescent users who never appear for treatment of adverse consequences.

Another consideration when describing the effects of drugs in adolescents is that it is traditional to present and discuss the pharmacology of each drug or drug class individually. However, adolescents who engage in extra-medical use of drugs, particularly those who use drugs regularly, seldom take only one drug. They might take a combination of drug subtypes during an evening or day of drug use, or they might use different drugs in sequence, on different days. All of the drugs reviewed here often are used more in various combinations rather than individually. For example, until recently, when considering the use of cannabis, there almost always has been prior experience with alcohol and tobacco. More often than not, after becoming a regular user, a person uses all of these three drugs (and often others) in one or several polydrug patterns. This is true to varying degrees for all the drugs sought out by adolescents in the United States. The pharmacology and toxicity of drug combinations can be complex and different from the pharmacology of the drugs used individually (Anthony et al., in press).

HEROIN AND OTHER OPIOID DEPENDENCE IN ADOLESCENCE

Most adolescents, especially those in the middle to late teen years, view heroin use as an extreme form of hazard-laden behavior, too risky to try even one time; few start using with a plan to become dependent or addicted to this drug. They regard the use of the drug to be extremely dangerous; few if any plan to become addicted to this agent when they start to use it. Even so, adolescent heroin use is showing some indication of increases in numbers of newly incident users in recent years. As mentioned in the prior section on drug epidemics, for the 2-year interval from 2010 to 2011, the corresponding estimate for newly incident adolescent heroin users has almost doubled from what it was in prior years of the most recent decade. These increases might be attributable to an increasing adoption of the intranasal route of administration or "heroin smoking" ("chasing the dragon") relative to heroin injection practices. Another explanation involves increases in heroin purity relative to price. During these years, heroin use has diffused beyond the boundaries of densely populated urban neighborhoods and now affects rural drug users as well.

Concurrently, there were increases in the numbers of newly incident extra-medical users of prescription pain relievers, many of which share opioid agonist actions with heroin. As such, the opioid dependence or addiction syndrome after sustained regular use of opioids prescription pain relievers resembles what has been seen for clinical features of heroin dependence. Whereas it seems that the epidemic of prescription pain relievers among adolescents in the United States has stabilized at a relatively high plateau value, unless there are more effective prevention, outreach, and early intervention initiatives, we may expect a growing number of clinical problems due to prescription pain relievers over the next 5 to 10 years.

Some rough projections can be made based on the most recently available estimates for adolescents in the United States, which suggest that the numbers of newly incident adolescent users of heroin might be roughly 140 and 300 new initiates per 100,000 per year. Epidemiologic estimates first published by Anthony et al. in 1994 and updated by Chen et al. in 2009 indicate that roughly 20% to 25% of these newly incident heroin users might eventually qualify as clinically diagnosable cases of heroin dependence (i.e., develop need of treatment services), with possibly somewhat larger transition probabilities for adolescents as compared to newly incident users in adulthood. Even if the transition from first heroin use to onset of heroin dependence occurs no more frequently for adolescents than for adults, as each year passes, the numbers of newly incident adolescent heroin dependence cases in the United States might be increasing by as many as 4,000 new patients in need of heroin intervention services (Anthony et al., 1994; Chen et al., 2009).

By comparison, in recent years, the numbers of newly incident adolescents starting to use prescription pain relievers extra-medically are many-fold greater than these numbers of newly incident heroin users. Estimates obtained from the NSDUH indicate that about 3% of youth between the ages of 12 and 17 have used an extra-medical prescription pain reliever in the past 30 days (www.drugabuse.gov/publications/research-reports/prescription-drugs/trends-in-prescription-drug-abuse/adolescents-young-adults). According to the MTF, heroin use escalated from the early 1990s until 2000, followed by declining values under 1% in the past 12 months (Fig. 17.6). Although it is not shown in the figure, a considerable fraction of heroin users in recent years are taking this drug via smoking or nasal insufflation, with a declining fraction injecting heroin with a syringe. Corresponding MTF trend lines for opioid prescription pain relievers are not shown due to complexities associated with changes in survey questions about specific prescription pain reliever compounds. These changes make it difficult to interpret the trend lines from MTF during the past 10 years. The NSDUH estimates do not have this complexity and are more readily interpreted.

To be sure, there must be many adolescent heroin users who try this drug once or twice and never become dependent, and the same is true for extra-medical users of prescription pain relievers. Otherwise, the estimated transition probabilities would be larger than 1 in 11 to 1 in 4 or 5. For those who progress toward the full clinical syndromes of dependence or addiction, the subjectively felt effects often have been described as a kind of euphoria. Either in conjunction with self-medication of preexisting conditions or in attempts to alleviate the heroin withdrawal syndrome, the experience has been described by heroin-dependent patients as a sense of being wrapped in "God's warmest blanket."

The functional value of heroin as an agent-reinforcer of sustained heroin use can be traced to activation of endogenous opioid receptors that densely populate reward-related brain regions, and this activation also is present for the opioid prescription pain relievers. Opioid receptors that are normally activated by endogenous opioid peptides include β-endorphin, enkephalin, and dynorphin, all of which have been found to play important roles in natural reward and satiety (Dackis & O'Brien, 2003b). As such, for many of the users who have become dependent or addicted, an injection of heroin or other opioid is followed by an immediate "rush" several minutes in duration, followed by a longer interval of sedation and satiety, during which time the user may well "nod off" into a sleep state. Nonetheless, we note that early clinical research by Lasagna et al. suggested that as

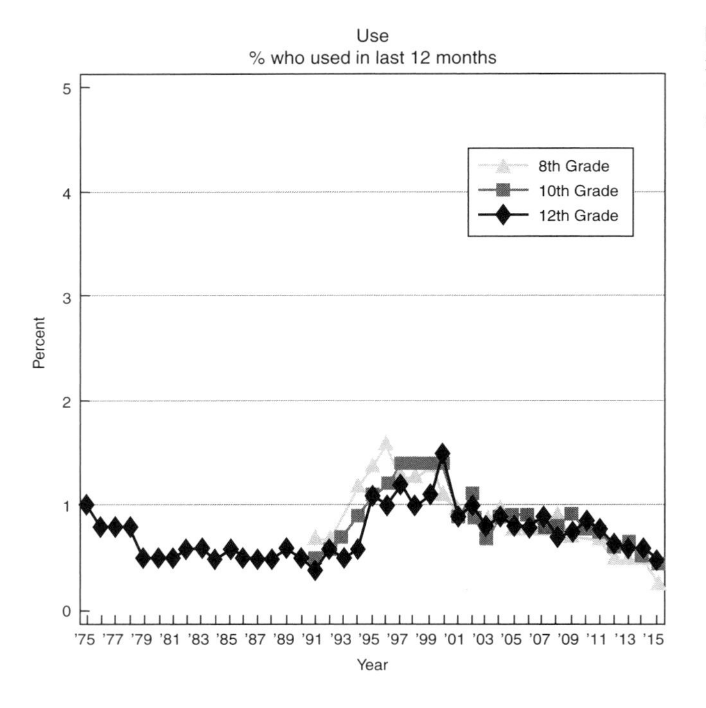

Figure 17.6 Trends in use of heroin in past 12 months for grades eight, 10, and 12 from 1975 to 2015. (From Johnston et al., 2016a.)

many as 50% who take an opioid may describe the experience as somewhat noxious—that is, an experience not to be repeated.

Once heroin is used on several occasions, pharmacological and subjectively felt tolerance to the reinforcing effects of the drug develops more rapidly than is true for the drug's more toxic effects such as respiratory depression. In consequence, there is an increased risk of lethal overdose when users seek the reinforcement that first came at smaller doses, and later requires larger doses, perhaps large enough to induce respiratory depression. In the presence of adequate supply, some heroin users have been known to exhibit progressively increasing daily doses by 100-fold. Enhancing the risk of a lethal outcome, street market heroin varies widely in potency. As a result, when an area's heroin users acquire access to an unusually pure shipment, one result often is a well-traveled trail to the medical examiner's office, fatality by fatality.

Opioid receptor antagonists such as naloxone can be administered to reverse the respiratory depression and cardiorespiratory toxic effects of heroin overdose, but too few users of opioids are using these drugs in close proximity to an effective dose of the antagonist, and timely life-saving medical treatment may be too distant. Additional complications arise when the heroin or other opioids are used in combination with other drugs such as cocaine, alcohol, or benzodiazepines, as occurs in the "speedball" combination of injecting heroin and cocaine simultaneously.

In adolescence as in adulthood, sustained use of heroin or other opioids can be followed by marked functional impairment and failure to fulfill expectations for social role functions at home, in school, at work, or in society at large. These clinical aspects of sustained opioid use with respect to impairment and social maladaptation often are seen together with increasing amounts of time spent procuring the drug, or time required to obtain funds to procure the drug, and with progressive loss of control over the amount used and frequency of use. As such, there can be deterioration in school performance, family relations, and social functioning when heroin becomes the adolescent's first priority. Some adolescents involved with heroin and other opioids resort to illegal activities such as shoplifting, dealing, prostitution, and robbery to pay for their increasing dose requirement. The concomitant risks of arrest, conviction, and incarceration, along with the stigma and disadvantages associated with a criminal record, compound any risks inherent in drug use per se. Users of heroin and other opioids also experience an increased risk of physical trauma associated with contact with the criminals who sell these drugs on the street market. As heroin addiction intensifies, adolescents may be shielded from insight or self-recognition of their growing impairments and socially maladaptive behavior via processes of denial, which may become woven into the fabric of the clinical aspects of addiction. Minimization, rationalization, intellectualization, and other aspects of denial must be addressed by treatment interventions that help adolescents become more aware of these consequences of what might have started as an apparently risk-free first occasion of use.

Once use of heroin and other opioids has started, adolescent users are often surprised by the rapid onset of heroin withdrawal within days or weeks after first use, often within 8 to 12 hours of abstinence and lasting for as many as 3 to 5 days. It is noteworthy that the signs and symptoms of heroin withdrawal are diametrically opposite those of heroin intoxication. This phenomenon results from the fact that compensatory brain responses to chronically administered heroin are unopposed during heroin abstinence, resulting in rebound withdrawal symptoms (O'Brien, 2001). It is fortunate that although the heroin withdrawal syndrome can be extremely unpleasant, it rarely is medically dangerous in and of itself.

Opioid-involved individuals, including adolescents, may experience panic and intense irritability during withdrawal after sustained use, with a subsequent round of sometimes risky drug-seeking behaviors. This tendency may be enhanced by the general impulsivity of adolescence. When possible, opioid users will actively avoid withdrawal symptoms by using these drugs on a regular and daily basis; the binge pattern of use that is more characteristic of cocaine dependence seldom is found among heroin users. Once the syndrome becomes severe, it often is necessary for the user to take the drug several times per day to avoid withdrawal, with resulting oscillation between periods of heroin intoxication and withdrawal. The result is a vicious cycle with positive reinforcement of sustained use (e.g., euphoria) and with negative reinforcement as well (e.g., relief of withdrawal or craving states). This vicious cycle, most often seen in adult patients in treatment services, also may be found among the prominent clinical features seen in adolescent heroin users.

COCAINE AND OTHER STIMULANT DEPENDENCE IN ADOLESCENCE

Among the internationally regulated drugs known for their central nervous system stimulant effects, cocaine is especially noteworthy because there have been a series of cocaine epidemics in the United States, starting with initial epidemic years in the late 19th century and early 20th century, before international regulations were in place, and continuing to the currently waning years of the late-20th-century epidemic. Other drug compounds in this central stimulant drug subtype include methamphetamine, amphetamine, and dextroamphetamine, which also have cocaine-like subjective effects. To a large extent the similarities in subjectively felt effects of the stimulant drugs can be traced back to more-or-less similar neurotransmitter actions in reward-related brain circuits, often involving presynaptic synthesis or blocking of reuptake of dopamine (Dackis & O'Brien, 2001).

Cocaine also deserves special note because the transition probabilities from first use to onset of a cocaine dependence syndrome have been found to be as large as one in five users when cocaine is consumed in its "crack" formulation and is smoked, and as large as one in six users when cocaine is taken intranasally as a powder. (Among first-time adolescent users, these transition probabilities may be larger than these epidemiologic estimates, as was described in relation to heroin users.) Of all the drugs for which these transition probabilities have been estimated on the basis of U.S. population experience, only two other drug subtypes have been found to have larger transition probabilities: heroin (one in four or five users) and cigarettes (one in three users). With cocaine, as with tobacco, a considerable fraction of first-time users develop a cocaine dependence syndrome within 1 to 2 years after first use (Anthony et al., 1994; Chen et al., 2009; Vsevolozhskaya & Anthony, 2016a, 2016b; Wagner & Anthony, 2002a, 2002b).

When only one in five or six first-time cocaine users develops a clinically diagnosable cocaine dependence syndrome, we must ask about sources of variation in this vulnerability such that four of five or five of six do not become dependent, and whether good prediction models have been developed. Environmental conditions and processes surely are at play, including those that govern the availability and price of cocaine during the days and weeks of first use, as well as secondary reinforcement of cocaine use by cocaine-using peers, through which cocaine use may be sustained even in the absence of an effective dose. Nonetheless, host characteristics such as genetic predispositions also deserve attention as we seek to understand these variations in response to the first occasions of cocaine use. Research to isolate these sources of variation in vulnerability only recently has begun to include serious investigations of gene–environment interactions; the resulting prediction models from these studies are not yet optimal, and it is very difficult to predict which adolescents or adults ultimately will become dependent on cocaine.

Prevention of cocaine use and dependence has attracted some public investments, mainly in the domain of supply reduction and law enforcement activities, with much smaller allocations toward prevention via environmental modulations, educational programs, or mass media advertising campaigns (see Chapter 19). As outlined in this section, there also is a need for outreach, early intervention, and treatment resources in order to address clinical aspects of cocaine dependence among adolescents.

The trace of the two separate cocaine epidemics in the 20th century in the United States is of interest because (1) in both epidemics it seems that the possibility of a cocaine dependence syndrome was dismissed and (2) declines from peak incidence values seem to have been accompanied by growing public awareness of hazards attributed to cocaine use. The first epidemic followed chemical isolation of cocaine in the middle of the 19th century, with production of a white cocaine hydrochloride powder that could be efficiently consumed by oral, intranasal, and intravenous routes. Soon thereafter, cocaine became very popular in Europe and the United States and was sold in wine, patent medicine solutions, or soft drinks such as Coca-Cola, with marketing for its presumed but not well-documented medicinal, antidepressant, and energy-enhancing effects. Widespread availability and perceived harmlessness sowed the seeds of the epidemic, and once the risk of tangible medical, psychiatric, and behavioral consequences became known, restrictive laws and eventually international regulations were enacted. Subsequently, the first epidemic came to an end well before the Great Depression.

Another major set of stimulant drug compounds of the amphetamine variety, including methamphetamine, were developed in the mid-20th century and came into widespread use during and right after World War II, not only in the United States but also in countries such as Japan and Sweden, where major epidemics had to be faced during the 1950s. It is said that draconian restrictions helped terminate the amphetamine epidemics in Japan and Sweden, but the available evidence about the causes suggests other factors were active, some of which are now hidden from view.

Other prescription stimulants have been introduced more recently (e.g., Adderall) and have been used extra-medically, not only to get high but also for performance enhancement in academic contexts (e.g., to be able to stay up later to study, or for enhanced attention and concentration during studying and test taking). In the epidemiologic estimates, the amphetamine-type drugs often are combined with the newer stimulant drugs in a subtype known as "stimulants other than cocaine."

After relatively large peak prevalence values for recently active extra-medical use in the early 1980s, the extra-medical use of stimulants other than cocaine in the United States has occurred in waves that might be characterized as relatively small epidemics in comparison to the tobacco, cannabis, and cocaine epidemics. Nonetheless, in recent years, with declining numbers of newly incident cocaine users, especially seen in relation to crack cocaine use, the numbers of extra-medical users of these non-cocaine stimulant-type drugs have been increasing. To illustrate, the most recent NSDUH estimates for stimulants other than cocaine suggest roughly 300,000 to 350,000 recently active extra-medical users, of which slightly more than 50% were newly incident users. By comparison, slightly more than 200,000 recently active cocaine users (including crack cocaine) were observed; slightly more than 50% were newly incident cocaine users (Substance Abuse and Mental Health Services Agency, 2013).

It was during the middle to late 1980s that the increased availability of relatively inexpensive unit dosage forms of crack cocaine increased cocaine access to adolescents. The unit purchase price of as low as $2 was well within the limits of disposable income for American adolescents. In consequence, the second cocaine epidemic of the 20th century in the United States was sustained into the 1990s and the early years of the 21st century; we now are on the descending limb of a crack cocaine epidemic as the numbers of newly incident users each year continue to decline, with concurrent declines in the numbers of newly incident cocaine powder users (Parker & Anthony, 2014).

Trend lines from the MTF surveys show a trace of the cocaine epidemic years from the mid-1970s through 2012, based on MTF assessments of school-attending adolescents each year (Fig. 17.7). As shown, peak values for estimated numbers of recently active cocaine users were seen before the 1980s, with subsequent declines, a wave of increasing prevalence during the 1990s, and then declining values in the 21st century.

In addition to its relatively low price point, the crack cocaine formulation of cocaine provides adolescents with a convenient and highly efficient means of administering cocaine that is particularly acceptable to adolescents who are already smoking tobacco or marijuana. Marketing inexpensive crack, whether by design or chance, has apparently provided the illegal drug industry with adolescent cocaine customers that until recently numbered in the hundreds of thousands.

The observed incidence rates for cocaine and other stimulant drugs, coupled with transition probabilities for becoming cases of the dependence syndrome, imply an accumulation of large numbers of adolescents in need of effective treatment for stimulant dependence. However, specialized adolescent addiction treatment programs are scarce and difficult to access throughout the United States (see Chapter 18). This insalubrious situation is compounded by the fact that cocaine dependence becomes more difficult to treat when it is allowed to progress for months and years without intervention. In addition, as was described in relation to heroin and the opioids, the clinical aspects of stimulant dependence begin to become complicated by secondary impairments in social role functions and by social maladaptation within the family, or at school or work. In fact, effective intervention in adolescence is noteworthy not only because these complications can be prevented, but also because stimulant dependence in adulthood often has secondary complications for the patient's children and other family members. Unfortunately, adolescent-onset cocaine addiction too often persists into adulthood, with predictable medical, psychiatric, behavioral, and societal ramifications. Many of these might be avoided with effective outreach, early intervention, and treatment services in adolescence.

Our understanding of these clinical aspects of cocaine and stimulant use in adolescence has been aided by a series of studies across a range of biomedical disciplines. We already have provided an overview of the

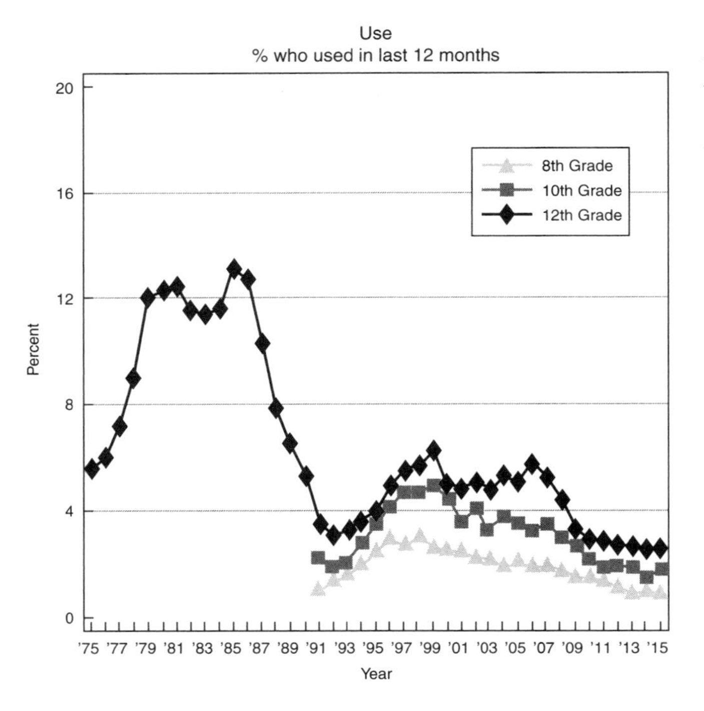

Figure 17.7 Use of cocaine (including crack) in past 12 months for youth in grades eight, 10, and 12 from 1975 to 2015. (From Johnston et al., 2016a.)

epidemiologic evidence, including the importance of the drug's formulation and route of administration on the transition that leads from the first use of cocaine or other stimulants until the onset of a stimulant dependence syndrome (Chen & Anthony, 2004). In other research, various aspects of the environment (Dackis & O'Brien, 2001) and host (constitutional) factors have been found to affect the attractiveness and rewarding qualities of cocaine (Tsuang et al., 1999). Environmental and psychosocial factors strongly influence the likelihood of first-time use. In some communities, drug dealers are viewed as successful role models and are actually emulated by adolescents who have few educational or vocational alternatives. Disenfranchised adolescents might be particularly vulnerable to cocaine or other stimulant use as a means of gaining peer acceptance, and parents are well advised to be cognizant of peer group changes (DuRant, 1995).

Family members, particularly older siblings, are often instrumental in providing adolescents with their first dose of a stimulant or normalizing its use through example and social role modeling. Studies indicate that the vulnerability for stimulant dependence is enhanced when there is a family history of alcoholism or drug dependency. Moreover, the vulnerability to develop dependence upon stimulants is partially inherited: twin studies report significantly higher concordance rates for identical twins than for nonidentical twins (Cadoret, Troughton, O'Gorman, & Heywood, 1986; Tsuang et al., 1996; van den Bree, Johnson, Neale, & Pickens, 1998). Nonetheless, to date, research into candidate genes that encode enzymes involved in cocaine metabolism and receptors that mediate cocaine effects has not identified reliable genetic vulnerability markers.

CANNABIS USE IN ADOLESCENCE

Among the internationally regulated drugs, cannabis is one of the most ancient "plant drugs." Its long history of use in both ceremony and medicine dates back to ancient "materia medica" texts of Central and South Asia, millennia before today's era of evidence-based medicine and governmental mandates for rigorous randomized controlled trials when a medicinal benefit is claimed. Notwithstanding continuing controversies within the United States (and abroad) about the most appropriate cannabis policy regimes for the 21st century, we have many proponents for greater use of "medicinal marijuana" and cannabis-related products (e.g., Sativex) and relaxation of what continue to be draconian criminal justice and other social penalties, such as denial of public benefits, when young people are apprehended by school or law enforcement authorities for simple possession and use of small amounts of this drug.

Notwithstanding the currently restrictive cannabis policy regimes in most U.S. jurisdictions, cannabis smoking is the most prevalent form of extra-medical drug use among adolescents in the United States. Cannabis smoking shares some attributes and possible health consequences with tobacco, another ancient plant drug. Cannabis and tobacco generally are consumed in leaf form or as buds from human cultivation of the commercially grown plant and in this country are most commonly smoked. Both contain hundreds of compounds; there are at least 60 termed cannabinoids that are unique to the cannabis plant.

The pharmacology of most of the cannabinoids is relatively unknown, but the most potent psychoactive agent, δ-9tetrahydrocannabinol (THC), has been isolated, can be synthesized, and has been well researched in adults since the early 1970s. The noncannabinoid materials in the plant and its combustion products when smoked are similar to many of those from tobacco leaf smoking with, of course, the exception of nicotine.

In recent years the technology of growing and distributing cannabis plants, as well as cannabis products, has become sophisticated and much improved. The THC content of plants from different sources and strains varies a great deal. Improved growing techniques, particularly plant breeding, have changed the THC content from a typical 10 mg in a marijuana cigarette in the 1960s to a 1-g marijuana cigarette that contains 150 to 200 mg. One consequence of the increased potency is that much of the human research done in the 1970s and 1980s with relatively low-potency smoked marijuana may be less relevant to the pharmacology of and consequences from marijuana now readily available to adolescents in most parts of the world, unless there is a titration of dose when higher-potency cannabis products are consumed (e.g., by taking fewer puffs on the cannabis "joint" than would be the case with lower-potency material). What is clear from past research is that the biological effects of THC depend on the dose. The availability of potent cannabis has greatly increased so that far higher doses of THC are now available to adolescent cannabis users than was possible 10 or 20 years ago.

Although cannabis is typically smoked in the form of cigarettes or from pipes, THC can also be easily extracted with ethanol and the THC extract or raw plant material can be added to baked goods or to sugar cubes, included within candies, or dispensed via an inhaler or spray or e-cigarette-like delivery device. Because THC and other cannabinoids are not water-soluble, the use of an injection route of administration leads to major toxic effects unless very special preparations and delivery systems are used. Based on clinical case reports, the number of known cases of THC injection is very small, and it seems that no adolescent cases have been reported.

During states of acute cannabis intoxication, it is not difficult to show clear impairments of cognitive and psychomotor performance. Complex and demanding tasks are more affected, and these effects appear in a dose-dependent manner. The spectrum of behavioral effects is similar to the spectrum seen for other central nervous system depressant drugs such as alcohol and can be additive to effects produced by concurrently used depressant drugs.

The magnitude of cannabis-attributable perceptual and psychomotor alterations measurable in research settings is such that it is reasonable to assume that complex tasks such as driving or other tasks that have high demands on attention and information processing and reaction responses might be impaired. Some driving simulator and naturalistic research on cannabis-impaired driving points toward existence of these impairments. Of particular relevance when considering consequences of adolescent marijuana use is that in a laboratory setting, overlearned or well-practiced tasks are relatively less affected by marijuana. Thus, a beginning or relatively inexperienced driver may be more subject to marijuana-induced cognitive, motor, and perceptual impairments than might be true for an adult who has been driving for many years.

Although the evidence for cognitive impairment for some hours after a dose of marijuana is quite consistent and has been repeated in experiments in many laboratories over many years, there is less unanimity about the consequences of long-term regular cannabis use, such as daily or almost-daily use. One consensus based on evidence from accumulating studies is that individuals who have used cannabis over long periods of time can show impaired performance on tests even when not acutely intoxicated, and that there might be long-term decrements in general problem solving (as measured by IQ tests) after sustained cannabis smoking. In these studies, the main cognitive functions found to be impaired in regular cannabis smokers are attention, memory, and processing of complex information. These effects may last for months, perhaps years, after cessation of use. Uncertainty remains as to whether some of the individuals had impaired performance before becoming involved with cannabis, or whether long-term cannabis smoking might disrupt psychometric test performance (e.g., by affecting a motivational component required to perform well on these tests). Nonetheless, there is a pattern of evidence to suggest that the performance of regular cannabis users shows impairments in comparison with nonregular users.

Outside the domain of neurocognitive functions, medical complications experienced by adolescent cannabis users have been more difficult to substantiate in well-controlled studies, in part due to the ethical constraints that preclude deliberate experimentation on adolescents with randomized assignment to varying regimens of dosage and frequency of use. Based on less well-controlled epidemiologic studies of adolescents and adults who have become cannabis users, there may be most concern about pulmonary disease and cardiovascular disease in general, including the possibility of a cannabis-attributable heart attack. On the other hand, in the domain of pulmonary disease, there also is some evidence that symptoms of asthma can be relieved by taking cannabis products. In this context, we note that pulmonary toxins are present in marijuana smoke as they are in tobacco smoke, but the balance of evidence about pulmonary diseases such as lung cancer suggests little tangible excess risk of lung cancer due to cannabis smoking.

One intriguing line of research involves immunomodulation by cannabis smoking and the possibility that active cannabis smokers actually might be less likely to show signs of prediabetes and might be less likely to develop diabetes. Whether this hypothesized protective relationship should be attributed to cannabis smoking or to something else remains an unanswered question, and the relative importance of sustained regular cannabis use versus acute cannabis effects is not yet clear. This line of research still is in its very early stages, and more research is needed, but the global burdens of diabetes are so great that it would be unwise to abandon this work prematurely (Alshaarawy & Anthony, 2015).

Turning to the clinical aspects of cannabis use disorders, the available epidemiologic evidence makes clear that in community populations of cannabis smokers, there is a running together of clinical features attributed to cannabis smoking by cannabis users themselves, similar to the syndromes described in clinical studies of cannabis-smoking patients seeking or referred to treatment. Whether this syndrome should be called a "cannabis dependence syndrome" or a "cannabis addiction syndrome" can be debated; the primary domains of these clinical features fall under both rubrics. These primary domains are (1) disturbances of the mental life such as obsession-like craving for cannabis and cannabis experiences with unbidden and intrusive thoughts about cannabis that disrupt intervals of attempted abstinence; (2) disturbances of behavior such as compulsion-like repetitive rounds of cannabis smoking, which include smoking cannabis even when one has made self-promises not to do so, as well as smoking larger amounts or with greater frequency than was intended; and (3) manifestations of neuroadaptation, such as pharmacological and subjectively felt tolerance with need to increase the dose or frequency of smoking to achieve desired effects previously achieved at lower doses or lower frequency levels.

It seems that tolerance to many of cannabis's subjective and behavioral effects develops rapidly with relatively few exposures, not unlike the pattern of tolerance that develops to nicotine and cocaine effects when smoked. Signs of neuroadaptation in the form of characteristic clinically significant cannabis withdrawal symptoms also have been reported in community samples of smokers, and are well described in both human laboratory studies and clinical settings. With abrupt discontinuation after only a few days of repeated administration of THC or marijuana in a laboratory setting, disturbed sleep, decreased appetite, restlessness, irritability, sweating, chills, nausea, and markedly disturbed sleep rapidly develop within hours of the last dose. Although most symptoms disappear in a day or two, irritability and sleep disturbance can persist for weeks.

Regular cannabis users observed in clinic settings experience similar symptoms when they stop smoking, along with a craving for marijuana, depressed mood, increased anger, wild dreams, and headaches. This pattern of withdrawal symptoms has suggested to some investigators that it may contribute to continued use of marijuana in cannabis-dependent individuals. Nonetheless, the precise links between withdrawal symptoms and continued or relapse to drug use is still a matter of some uncertainty.

In this final subsection on cannabis smoking, we add to epidemiologic estimates concerning the incidence rates of cannabis smoking during adolescence, prevalence proportions for cannabis use, and the transition probabilities for appearance of a cannabis dependence syndrome once cannabis smoking has started. In recent years, the MTF surveys have added questions about adolescent use of synthetic cannabinoids, making it possible to present some epidemiologic estimates on this topic as well. We also consider this epidemiologic evidence in light of current reconsideration of restrictive cannabis policies, at least at the state and local levels, within the United States.

We noted in the section on drug epidemics that the United States has been facing a resurgent epidemic of cannabis product use. Even so, the interval of time from 2002 through 2012 has been one of relatively stable or "endemic" incidence rates for cannabis smoking: based on NSDUH estimates for that span of years, roughly 6% to 7% of adolescents in the United States started to use cannabis each year. It would seem that any increase in the prevalence of recently active cannabis use during these years must be coming from sources other than an increasing number of newly incident users. The most likely alternative source of variation is an increasing persistence or duration of cannabis use—for example, as manifest in a newly incident cannabis user in some year prior to 2012 showing persistence of cannabis use to include at least one day in 2012. Ordinarily, when we see stable incidence rates for cannabis use across a span of 10 years (e.g., a relatively constant number of newly incident users each year) with increasing prevalence proportions, the increase should be interpreted to mean that more newly incident cannabis users are continuing to use this drug from one year to the next.

As more states in the United States have liberalized their "medical marijuana" laws, one might expect that some unknown fraction of the NSDUH's newly incident adolescent users are being supplied with cannabis products from medical marijuana dispensaries and are answering the NSDUH survey items on cannabis smoking so as to acknowledge use that actually might have been accompanied by a prescription. If so, the numbers of newly incident users overall in the United States would not seem to be affected to any material extent by any addition of newly incident users. One might infer that these newly incident adolescent users are now getting cannabis directly or indirectly (e.g., via diversion from an adult patient), whereas in the past the same number of newly incident users would have gotten their first supply of cannabis from some other source. At least one pundit has observed that it is better for these adolescents to be obtaining cannabis directly (perhaps illegally) or indirectly (definitely illegally) from an authorized "medical marijuana" dispensary than to be obtaining it from an unregulated black market, which might expose them to adulterated plant material (e.g., laced with PCP or some other drug) or to misadventures (perhaps assaultive violence or mugging) encountered when buying drugs illegally, as discussed elsewhere in this chapter. If the increasing availability of cannabis via "medical marijuana" sources is having an effect on adolescent cannabis use, this effect is not being seen in the overall U.S. incidence rates. Nonetheless, there is some concern about increasing prevalence of use, and in particular the increasing prevalence of "regular" near-daily or daily cannabis use, which might mean that dispensaries are affecting the persistence of cannabis use but not the numbers of newly incident users. We will return to some implications of the increasing prevalence of "regular" cannabis use later in this section.

Many jurisdictions in the United States are shifting their cannabis policy regimes along lines recommended by the U.S. National Commission on Marijuana and Drug Abuse back in the early 1970s, with discouragement of cannabis use via means other than the traditional threat of law enforcement action and criminal penalties. Some jurisdictions have shifted their policies in the direction of a regulated and taxed "recreational" cannabis marketplace. For example, recently, the state of Colorado enacted a cannabis policy that permits cannabis product sales for extra-medical use (e.g., "to get high" and not only as prescribed by a clinician for an FDA-approved or other legitimate medical indication such as eye disease, seizures, or appetite enhancement in the context of cancer chemotherapy or HIV/AIDS complications). Definitive evidence on the adverse or beneficial effects of this type of change in cannabis policy regime cannot be obtained under naturalistic conditions of this type, except perhaps in the domain of documenting increased tax revenues for a cannabis market that previously generated no tax revenues, along with reductions in the state-level and local law enforcement and criminal justice cost burden of the previous state policies. Too many threats to validity and sources of uncertainty, and too many untestable assumptions, are present when pre-to-post time series designs and nonequivalent control groups are substituted for the experimental research designs that our society requires when manufacturers seek to substantiate claims about the effects, beneficial or harmful, of their newly developed or reformulated medical products, devices, or medicines.

Nevertheless, we already are starting to see published articles with evidence based on nonexperimental evaluations of the changing cannabis policy regimes (e.g., Stolzenberg et al., 2016; Wall et al., 2016). There is good reason to start with skepticism about such evidence, irrespective of whether it claims to show beneficial or harmful effects of new cannabis policies. Leaving aside the threats to validity, sources of uncertainty, and untested assumptions just mentioned, the evidence from any single study of this type is not to be trusted, until and unless there is a consistent trace of replicated convergent evidence from additional studies, preferably conducted by independent research teams. Too much is at stake in this context for our society to base important public policy decisions on any single unreplicated study from any single research team whose starting assumptions might be hidden from view.

Trend lines from the MTF survey depicted in Figure 17.8 show how prevalence estimates for recently active cannabis smoking among students in the United States now are showing some leveling off that remains well below the peak values observed in the late 1970s. In 2015, the estimated prevalence based on use in the year prior to assessment was roughly 35%. Nonetheless, as noted in relation to our discussion of cannabis policy, the stability of NSDUH cannabis smoking *incidence* estimates at 6% to 7% per year in recent years makes it likely that the observed recent increases in these trend lines should be attributed to increasing *persistence* or *duration* of cannabis smoking once it starts, rather than to increasing incidence of cannabis smoking. In light of discussions about how cannabis use might be responsive to increasingly widespread and less restrictive "medical marijuana" laws and cannabis policy liberalization, this distinction between incidence and prevalence is important.

Another interesting feature of Figure 17.8 is the considerable stability of prevalence estimates for students in grade eight, which have been observed at roughly 10% for the past 10 years. If cannabis policy discussions or changes have been affecting adolescent cannabis use, one might expect to see something other than a stable trend line of this type.

We note that study estimates of marijuana use are drawn largely from the present situation in which there continue to be tangible penalties for simple possession and use of small amounts of cannabis, sometimes in the form of fines or community service, sometimes in the form of incarceration, given that few U.S. jurisdictions have adopted the liberalized cannabis policies recently enacted in the states of Colorado and Washington. Some of the authors of this volume express a hope that some jurisdictions might adopt intermediate cannabis policies, perhaps with "public health officers" substituted for "law enforcement officers" in the context of persuasive outreach and early intervention services designed to be more effective and persuasive than is now achieved in the current prevailing cannabis policy regime.

A carefully designed experimental evaluation of intermediate cannabis policies in some jurisdictions, as compared to more draconian and more liberalized policies in other comparable jurisdictions, would provide an evidence base to guide future policy decision making, as well as planning for possibly increasing needs for outreach and early intervention services, if not treatment services for more seriously affected cases. In this comparative context, it would be possible to assemble more definitive evidence on a potentially increasing incidence of problems of "underage cannabis smoking" (e.g., by 12- to 17-year-olds) part and parcel with relaxation of the more draconian criminal justice approach currently in place in most U.S. jurisdictions. Some of the states with currently restrictive cannabis policies are considering liberalization, perhaps encouraged or lured

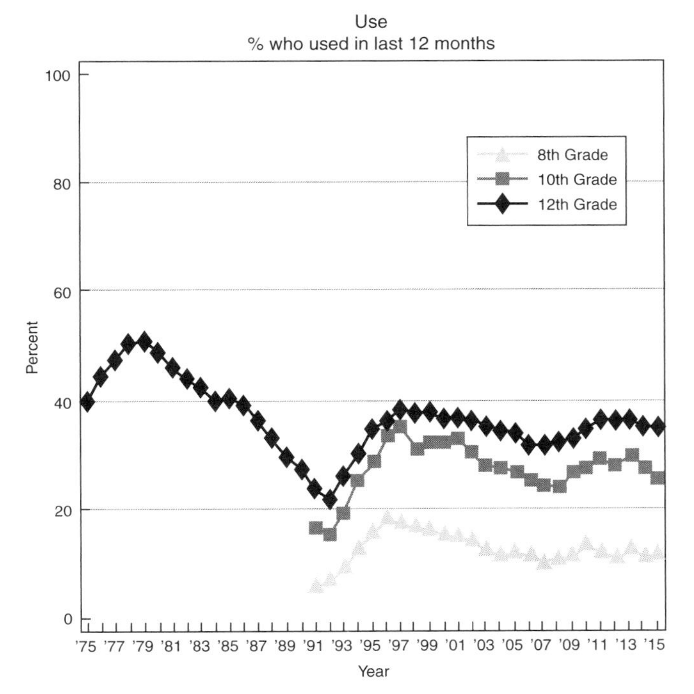

Figure 17.8 Trends in reported use of marijuana in the past 12 months in grades eight, 10, and 12 from 1975 to 2015. (From Johnston et al., 2016a.)

by the prospect of increased cannabis "sin tax" revenues. If several of these states were to participate in a comparative policy experiment of this type, the society would have the benefit of an experiment with systematic replications across the states. We are hopeful that a future revision of this chapter will be able to provide more definitive evidence about the effects of changing cannabis policy regimes on adolescent cannabis use, with the evidence substituted for mere speculation about what might or might not happen to younger adolescents when their older siblings, friends, parents, and acquaintances are granted more liberal access to this ancient plant drug.

ALCOHOL USE AND ABUSE IN ADOLESCENCE

In this section we provide an overview of the phenomenology of alcohol drinking and alcohol use disorders in adolescents ages 11 to 19. Included in this overview is a current description of "drinking youths"; incidence and prevalence rates of adolescent drinking, binge drinking, alcohol use disorders, and drinking-related consequences; pertinent diagnostic issues; and potential etiological factors that may enhance our understanding of alcohol use and the development of problem drinking in adolescents.

Alcohol is a sedative and it is the only drug in this category to be discussed in this chapter; other sedatives such as benzodiazepines, barbiturates, and other sleeping pills are used so uncommonly that they do not merit a full discussion. Notably, a discussion of alcohol leads to some overlap in content with discussions of other substance use disorders in adolescents, discussed elsewhere in this chapter. However, there are some important distinctions to bear in mind. Alcohol use by persons 21 years or older is legal in the United States, making it more readily available to adolescents and exposing them to seductive advertisements. It is noteworthy that although underage drinking is illegal, it is very common in the United States. By the time they reach the legal minimum drinking age of 21, 90% of individuals have already had their first full drink (Cheng et al., 2016a). In addition, low to moderate alcohol use is an integral part of our adult community life. Alcohol is available in many restaurants, it is sold in grocery stores in many states, and it is available in liquor stores throughout the country. It is readily accepted in social settings, frequently accompanying a meal, and incorporated in many religious ceremonies. In recent decades, the health benefits of one or two glasses of wine per day have been widely covered by the media. The alcohol industry has been trying to reach and attract a broader audience. For example, one study found a larger increase in the amount of advertisements targeting girls compared to boys (Jernigan et al., 2004). This can interact with other factors to contribute to a recent discovery of an adolescent female excess in drinking incidence (Cheng et al., 2016b). Finally, parents and other authorities frequently overlook adolescent drinking, relegating it to experimentation or "rites of passage." In contrast, the illegality of many of the other abused substances (e.g., marijuana, cocaine, heroin) makes them taboo in most adult circles and causes much alarm and concern in adult communities when adolescent use is uncovered.

General Description of Adolescent Drinking

Drinking alcohol can be a highly pleasurable experience for many people, regardless of age. It is frequently described as relaxing, euphoric, anxiety reducing, and disinhibiting. Nonetheless, as alcohol is absorbed, metabolized, and eliminated from the body, it can also be associated with poor motor coordination, some confusion, irritability, depression, sleeplessness, nausea, and vomiting, among other adverse effects. Ingesting excessive amounts of alcohol in a relatively brief period of time can cause extreme confusion, unconsciousness, and sometimes death.

Beer is the most commonly consumed alcoholic beverage among adolescents. It has been estimated that youth ages 12 to 20 consume nearly 20% of all alcoholic beverages sold in the

United States (Foster et al., 2003). A more recent analysis found that beer accounted for 42.5% of the alcohol consumed by youth ages 13 to 20 (Siegel et al., 2013). The second most popular category was various kinds of spirits (35.8%), which includes vodka, rum, and bourbon. The third most popular category was flavored beverages (16.1%), which include malt-based drinks with appealing brand names such as Mike's Hard Lemonade. While adolescents will use elaborate means to obtain alcohol (e.g., having fake identification cards made; asking strangers to buy alcohol for them), they more commonly obtain alcohol from their own homes, their friends' homes, their parents, or other adults (Institute of Medicine, 2004).

Adolescents report drinking for many of the same reasons that adults drink; that is, they expect positive effects from drinking. Younger adolescents report that drinking reduces tension, and they like the mild impairment it causes to their cognitive and behavioral functioning. Older adolescents say they drink primarily because of the euphoria they experience and/or the behavioral disinhibition that occurs when they drink. Adolescent males rate the pleasurable effects and sexual enhancement of alcohol more highly than females, who, in contrast, rate the tension-reduction effects more favorably (Institute of Medicine, 2004).

Traditionally, alcohol drinking has been considered a "masculine behavior," with a male excess in the prevalence of alcohol drinking consistently reported among adults around the globe (Erol & Karpyak, 2015). In contrast, smaller and even null male/female differences in recent drinking have been documented for adolescents, especially young adolescents (Patrick & Schulenberg, 2010). Nonetheless, prevalence bears little information about the onset of drinking. Using data from the NSDUH 2002–2009, Seedall and Anthony (2015) found a *female excess* in drinking onset among adolescents, ages 12 to 17, as an aggregate. A more recent study found that this female excess is most prominent among 14- and 15-year-olds, with a 25% higher incidence among 14- and 15-year-old girls compared to boys at the same age (Cheng et al., 2016b).

Problem Drinking in Adolescents

The hallmarks of problem drinking are loss of control over drinking (i.e., drinking more than planned or in inappropriate settings) and the occurrence of negative consequences from drinking (driving under the influence [DUI], high-risk sexual behaviors, fights, medical problems). The development of addiction is associated with repeated, heavy drinking over time, potentially as a continual attempt to recreate the pleasurable state associated with initiating drinking and intoxication. Repeated drinking can also lead to the development of physiological dependence, marked primarily by tolerance to alcohol, and withdrawal symptoms between drinking periods. Tolerance is one of the most commonly reported dependence symptoms in community samples and clinical samples of adolescents (Chung, Martin, Armstrong, & Labouvie, 2002; Martin & Winters, 1998).

Although less frequently reported among adolescents than among adults, heavy drinking can also lead to alcohol withdrawal symptoms between drinking periods (Table 17.1). Severe withdrawal can be life-threatening and may present as delirium tremens (DTs), which include symptoms of confusion, delirium, hallucinations, and psychosis (Dackis & O'Brien, 2003b). Delirium tremens are more likely if patients are malnourished or dehydrated or suffer from an infection or an electrolyte imbalance. A careful history is critical, because withdrawal can produce seizures, especially if they have occurred before.

The psychological, behavioral, and physical effects of alcohol are related to the blood-alcohol level of an individual, which is determined primarily by the quantity, frequency, and potency of alcohol consumed. The blood-alcohol level (the ratio of milligrams of alcohol per 100 mL of blood) can be easily estimated by exhaling into instruments called breathalyzers, which are commonly available to treatment providers and law enforcement agencies. Impaired judgment and impaired coordination due to alcohol are legally determined by a level of 0.08%, and all U.S. states have laws making it illegal to drive with a concentration at this level or

Table 17.1 Signs and Symptoms of Alcohol Intoxication and Withdrawal

Alcohol Intoxication	*Alcohol Withdrawal*
Signs (Observed)	
Decreased heart rate	Increased heart rate
Lower blood pressure	Elevated blood pressure
Lower body temperature	Elevated body temperature
Sedation	Sweating
Decreased respiration	Tremors and muscle spasm
Loss of balance	Vomiting and diarrhea
Restlessness	Seizures
Slurred speech	Confusion
	Delirium
	Psychosis
Symptoms (Reported)	
Relaxation	Craving for alcohol
Sense of well-being	Anxiety
Euphoria	Irritability
Dizziness	Insomnia
Fatigue	Nausea
Nausea	Hallucinations
Blackouts	

higher. Most European countries set the legal limit lower because discernable impairment from alcohol usually begins at about 0.05% or below.

Prevalence and Incidence of Adolescent Use and Abuse of Alcohol

It is generally acknowledged that some use of alcohol is the norm among adolescents (Schulenberg & Maggs, 2002; Windle, 1999). According to national school surveys, alcohol is the most widely used psychoactive substance in adolescents (excluding caffeine) (Grunbaum et al., 2002; Johnston et al., 2016a, 2016b). The most recent MTF survey found that by eighth grade, 26% of students reported some lifetime use of alcohol, a figure that rose to 64% by senior year (Johnston et al., 2016a, 2016b). Using data from the NSDUH, a recent study found sharp increases in the prevalence of recently active drinking during adolescence: the prevalence increases from 6% in 12-year-olds to 56% in 17-year-olds and to 75% in 20-year-olds (see Fig. 2 of Cheng et al., 2016a). Estimated cumulative incidence proportions (so-called lifetime prevalence) follow similar patterns, with slightly larger point estimates.

Although prevalence provides valuable information about the extent of drinking, it bears little information about the risk of becoming a drinker, the epidemiologic parameter that is more relevant to etiology studies. To fill this gap, Cheng et al. (2016a) also estimated the age-specific incidence of drinking, defined as the percentage of new drinkers who had their first full drink during the 12 months prior to the assessment rising from the "at risk" population (i.e., those who had never had a full drink before the 12 months prior to the assessment). They found an interesting pattern: the incidence increases sharply between the ages of 12 and 15; thereafter, a more gradual increase is seen between ages 16 and 18, followed by a clear *drop* in incidence at ages 19 and 20, just before peak incidence at legal drinking age, 21 (Fig. 17.9). Thereafter, the incidence decreases sharply, falling to a quite low value at age 25. This newly discovered nonlinear pattern suggests that most adolescents who are vulnerable to underage drinking encounter their first chance to drink before the age of 19. Furthermore, adolescent girls have surpassed boys in drinking incidence during recent years (Cheng et al., 2016b).

The good news is that alcohol consumption in adolescents has steadily declined since the 1970s. As seen in Figure 17.10, past 30-day use of alcohol in eighth-, 10th-, and 12th-grade students as assessed in the MTF study has dropped from 68.2% in 1975 to 35.4% in 2015 among 12th-graders. The rate of reported drunkenness in the past 30 days has also declined from 31.6% in 1991 to 20.6% in 2015 in 12th-graders (Johnston et al., 2016a, 2016b). Although there are various explanations for these declines (discussed in Chapter 19 on prevention), this is undoubtedly an important trend that has reduced risks to the health of adolescents in the United States.

Binge Drinking

One particular concern is the amount of binge drinking by adolescents. Wechsler, Davenport, Dowdall, Moeykens, and Castillo (1994) are generally credited with first using the term *binge drinking* in referring to excessive alcohol drinking by some adolescent and college-aged drinkers. Excessive or binge drinking has been defined in multiple ways (National Research Council and Institute of Medicine, 2004), but the standard definition is consuming five or more drinks in a single episode (four or more for women) (Wechsler et al., 1994; Windle, 1999). This pattern of drinking in adolescents is associated with a broad range of problems, including date rape, vandalism, and academic failure (Baer, 1993). The 2015 MTF survey (Johnston et al., 2016a) obtained information on binge drinking in the 2 weeks prior to the interview

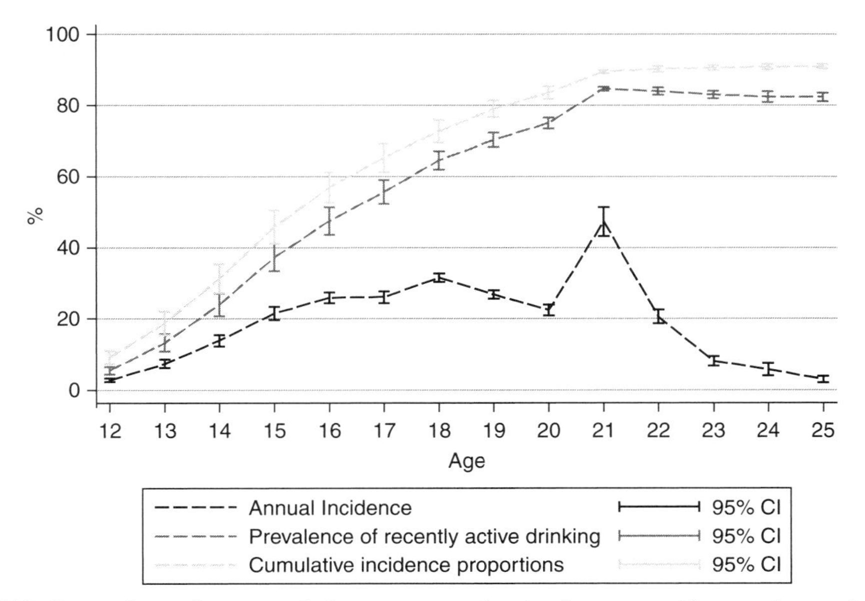

Figure 17.9 Comparison of meta-analytic summary estimates for age-specific prevalence of drinking and estimated age-specific annual incidence. (Data from U.S. NSDUH, 2002–2013; n ~ 420,000 12- to 25-year-olds.)

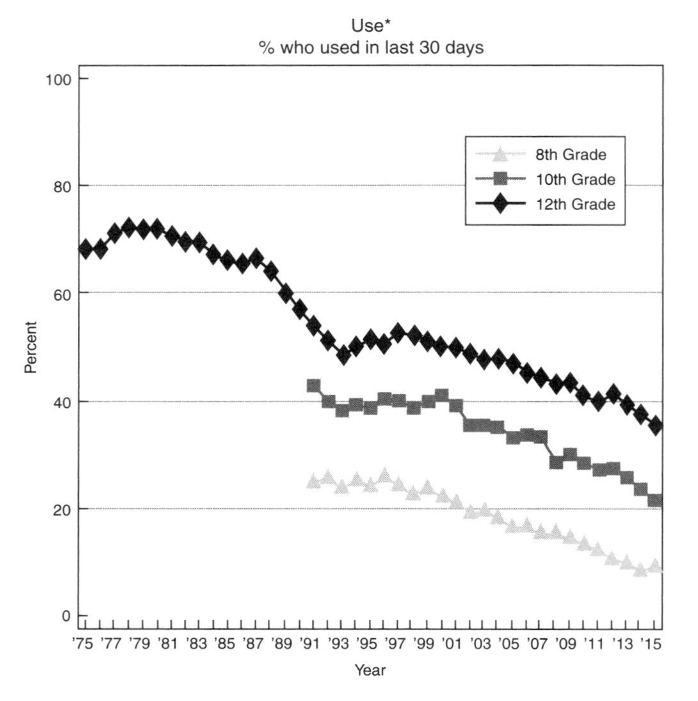

Figure 17.10 Alcohol use in the past 30 days by grade and year. (From Johnston, L. D., Miech, R. A., O'Malley, P. M., Bachman, J. G., & Schulenberg, J. E. [Dec. 16, 2015]. *Use of ecstasy, heroin, synthetic marijuana, alcohol, cigarettes declined among US teens in 2015*. Ann Arbor: University of Michigan News Service. Retrieved from http://www.monitoringthefuture.org.)

and found that 4.6% of eighth-graders, 10.9% of 10th-graders, and 17.2% of 12th-graders had at least one binge-drinking episode. The MTF survey also asked respondents to report if they had been "drunk" in the past month, and found that 3.1% of eighth-graders, 10.3% of 10th-graders, and 20.6% of 12th-graders responded affirmatively.

Perhaps some of the most innovative work to date has combined a developmental perspective in defining more homogeneous adolescent and young adult subgroups with respect to their amount of binge drinking. Schulenberg, O'Malley, Bachman, Wadsworth, and Johnston (1996) identified six different patterns or trajectories of binge drinking on the basis of data from MTF. These trajectories accounted for 90% of the sample. The most common trajectories were "never" (36%) or "rarely" (17%) reported binge drinking; however, the other four trajectories were 12% decreased binge drinking over time, 10% increased binge drinking, 10% increased and then decreased, and 7% sustained chronic binge drinking over time.

Nonetheless, drinking and heavy drinking are two different phenotypes with different etiologies. Therefore, it is not clear whether the observed patterns described above are due to drinking per se or heavy episodic drinking, when the study population includes nondrinkers. In a series of inquiries, Cheng and Anthony (under review) investigated the transition from drinking to heavy episodic drinking among U.S. adolescents. In these studies, heavy episodic drinking is defined as consuming five or more drinks on one occasion. The definition is held constant for both males and females because the focus is on heavy episodic drinking as a behavior instead of physiological effects of alcohol. Additionally, the validity of the five/four drinks thresholds for adolescent boys and girls is unclear, especially among prepuberty adolescents. Moreover, there is an epidemiologic principle that between-group comparisons require the same case definition. Applying this principle, they estimated the age-specific transition from drinking to heavy episodic drinking among newly incident drinkers who had their first drink during the 12 months prior to the assessment. The result was an estimated transition probability at 20% to 30% in girls and 35% to 45% in boys. That is, about one in three new underage drinkers rapidly transition to their first heavy episodic drinking binge each year. In addition, 10% to 20% of new adolescent underage drinkers transition to heavy episodic drinking in the same month they start drinking. Before mid-adolescence, there is no male excess in the risk of heavy episodic drinking.

In another study, Cheng and Anthony (2016) investigated the timing of this transition in four age groups representing four developmental stages using survival analysis methods. They found sex-specific variations across the four developmental stages. In both males and females, 15- to 20-year-olds were at a higher hazard to develop heavy episodic drinking compared to 11- to 14-year-olds. Males who started drinking at 21 years of age were also at a higher hazard to develop heavy episodic drinking compared to 11- to 14-year-old boys, whereas there was no difference in females. The most surprising finding was the *female excess* in the onset of heavy episodic drinking among newly incident drinkers who start drinking during early adolescence (i.e., 11–14 years of age); after 14 years of age, a male excess is observed.

These results indicate that (1) rapid transition to heavy episodic drinking is common in adolescents and (2) there may be sex-specific mechanisms across different developmental stages (i.e., early, middle, and late adolescence) (see also Meyers, et al. 2014).

Drinking-Related Consequences Among Adolescents

According to the National Institute on Alcohol Abuse and Alcoholism (NIAAA, 2003), "underage alcohol use is more likely to kill young people than all illegal drugs combined." As in adult circles, excessive drinking and intoxication have serious consequences in the adolescent population. Most notable are automobile crashes. In 2013, 6.4% of high school students drove after drinking in the past 30 days, and 21.9% rode with a driver who had been drinking (Kann et al., 2014). Not surprisingly, driving skills appear to be more readily impaired by alcohol in adolescent than adult drivers (Voas et al., 2012); nevertheless, the alcohol-involved fatality rate is highest among drivers ages 21 to 24 (National Highway Traffic Administration, 2015).

Other harmful behaviors frequently related to excessive drinking among adolescents are high-risk sexual behaviors (unplanned with no protection); rapes, including date rape; assaults; homicides; and suicides (National Institute on Alcohol Abuse and Alcoholism [NIAAA], 2003; Windle, 1999). Having multiple sexual partners, failing to use condoms, and performing other high-risk sexual behaviors have been associated with alcohol use in adolescents (NIAAA, 2003). Furthermore, alcohol use by the offender, victim, or both has been linked to sexual assault, including date rape. Using the MTF data, Bachman and Peralta (2002) reported that heavy alcohol use increased the likelihood of violence for either gender, even after controlling for home environment, grades, and ethnicity. Alcohol generally is a disinhibiting intoxicant, and it may also potentiate mood and stress states that lead to suicide attempts or other life-threatening behaviors. For example, heavy drinking has been correlated with suicide attempts in eighth-grade girls (Windle, Miller-Tutzauer, & Domenico, 1992).

Alcohol Use Disorders in Adolescents

The national surveys mentioned above are representative of the general population drinking patterns but do not specifically address the prevalence of alcohol use disorders in adolescents. Chung et al. (2002) reviewed the epidemiologic literature on diagnosing alcohol use disorders in adolescents. Although this review summarized both community and clinical groups, the community groups are of specific relevance here. Five community samples were identified from studies in peer-reviewed journals whose sample sizes ranged from 220 to 4,023 adolescents, ages 12 to 19. Two of the studies were representative of the entire U.S. population and the other three were representative of individual states (North Carolina, Oregon, and Pennsylvania). In these surveys, the percentage of adolescents meeting criteria for alcohol abuse ranged from 0.4% to 9.6%; for alcohol dependence, the figures ranged from 0.6% to 4.3%. With the release of DSM-5, definitions have changed for all addictive substances, and we illustrate those changes in the following section on alcohol use disorder in adolescents.

As mentioned above, another important piece of information is the transition from drinking to alcohol dependence. Using nationally representative data from NSDUH, Cheng et al. (2016) investigated the rapid transition from drinking to DSM-IV alcohol dependence among newly incident drinkers across developmental stages. They found that an estimated 3% (95% CI 2–3) of adolescent girls and 2% (95% CI 2–2) of adolescent boys transition to alcohol dependence within the first 12 months of drinking. The transition probability decreases with age among girls, whereas no appreciable variation is observed among boys. Among early adolescents (i.e., 11–14 years of age), there is a *female excess* in the rapid transition from drinking to alcohol dependence.

Issues in Determining Alcohol Use Disorders in Adolescence

In DSM-IV, substance use disorders were defined on the basis of separate criteria for abuse and dependence. Nonetheless, copious empirical evidence suggests that the categorical abuse/dependence approach does not serve well in the general population (Hasin et al., 2013). Therefore, in DSM-5, there is only one alcohol use disorder diagnosis category. The DSM-IV diagnostic criteria for abuse and dependence are combined; the "legal problem" criterion was removed because it is largely determined by the local social environment (e.g., law enforcement); a "craving" criterion was added. In addition, the DSM-5 incorporates a severity dimension in the diagnosis (i.e., mild, moderate, and severe, based on the count of symptoms).

Diagnostic criteria for alcohol use disorder as detailed in the DSM-5 are similar to the criteria for all substance disorders in all populations. To meet a diagnosis of alcohol use disorder, at least two criteria from the following list must be met:

1. Recurrent use causing serious consequences
2. Being physically dangerous
3. Use resulting in persistent social or interpersonal problems
4. Withdrawal
5. Tolerance
6. Larger amounts consumed than intended
7. Unsuccessful attempts to stop
8. Excessive time spent drinking
9. Important activities given up
10. Continued use despite awareness of negative effects of drinking
11. Craving

Meeting two or three criteria indicates a mild disorder, four or five a moderate disorder, and six and above a severe disorder.

While the number and type of symptoms needed to determine an alcohol use disorder diagnosis appear to be valid for adults (e.g., Schuckit et al., 2001), investigators have questioned the validity of these diagnostic criteria in adolescent populations (Winters, 2001). Pollack and Martin (1999) studied 372 adolescent regular drinkers. More than 10% of this sample reported symptoms of alcohol dependence but not enough to have a diagnosis, and they also did not have symptoms of alcohol abuse (termed "diagnostic orphans"). However, these individuals had drinking-related problems similar to those of adolescents who did meet the diagnostic criteria for an alcohol use disorder, and they had significantly more drinking-related problems than did adolescents with no symptoms of alcohol abuse or dependence. In the review by Chung et al. (2002), "diagnostic orphans" represented from 1.9% to 16.7% of adolescent community samples and from 7.5% to 33.7% of adolescent clinical samples.

Finally, the two physiological symptoms (withdrawal and tolerance) that are part of the diagnostic DSM-5 criteria may have limited utility in diagnosing alcohol use disorder in adolescents (Martin, Kaczynski, Maisto, Bukstein, & Moss, 1995). Both tolerance and withdrawal are reported more frequently in young people, and diagnoses of alcohol use disorder are highest in the 18- to 23-year-old age group (Caetano & Babor, 2006), suggesting that young people may use different criteria or attach different meaning to these symptoms. In an earlier study, Dawson et al. (2008) found that those who started drinking before the age of 18 were more likely to experience "withdrawal" and "drinking more than intended" when compared to those who initiated drinking at 18 or older, but they were no more likely to experience impaired control, the hallmark of alcoholism. This finding suggests that alcohol dependence reflects poor decision making rather than loss of control over alcohol among adolescents compared to adults (Dawson et al., 2008). Clearly, additional conceptual and empirical research is needed to adequately diagnose alcohol use disorders in adolescents and young adults.

Etiology: Risk and Protective Factors

The risk for alcohol use disorder increases as the number of risk factors increases (Jaffe & Simkin, 2002; Newcomb, 1997). However, there are protective factors that can counteract risk factors. For example, a strong religious commitment, dedication to constructive activities such as sports, intense anti-alcohol beliefs, and high self-esteem all can serve to neutralize inherent risk factors for developing an alcohol use disorder (Liepman, Calles, Kizilbash, Nazeer, & Sheikh, 2002).

The relevance of some of the risk factors varies with the age, gender, and ethnicity of the adolescent. In addition, other factors have been identified that influence the risk for alcohol use disorder as well as other substance use disorders. Newcomb (1997) classified these risk factors into four generic domains: cultural/societal, interpersonal, psychobehavioral, and biogenetic. The first three factors are summarized here; discussion of genetic factors was given earlier this chapter.

Cultural and Societal Factors

While many factors contribute to the availability and acceptability of alcohol in a community (cultural, economic, legal, etc.), probably the single most influential factor that relates to alcohol consumption in adolescents is the attitude of the adult community in the particular geographic location (see review by Newcomb, 1997). For example, the purchase of alcohol by youth under the age of 21 is prohibited in all 50 states. However, in some places, the laws are not regularly enforced by police, and liquor stores and bars do not consistently require identification from minors (Bonnie & O'Connell, 2004; Windle, 1999). Underage drinking at family gatherings or special celebrations may be acceptable to parents and relatives in some communities. An in-depth examination of the relationship between community attitudes and alcohol availability (economic and legal) is of paramount importance but beyond the scope of this book.

Interpersonal Factors

Interpersonal factors that relate to the risk of alcohol use disorder in adolescents involve parental (referring to other than heredity), sibling, and peer influences. Despite waning parental influence with the passage of time, parents' level of nurturing, monitoring, and communication and their own alcohol use affect the amounts and patterns of alcohol drinking in their adolescents (see reviews by Gilvarry, 2000; Liepman et al., 2002; Schulenberg & Maggs, 2002; Windle, 1999). That is, although adolescents may reject many of their parents' ideas and behaviors, the majority do not seem to reject their parents' drinking behaviors. Higher levels of maternal and paternal alcohol consumption are related to higher levels of alcohol use among adolescents (e.g., Kilpatrick et al., 2000; Webb & Baer, 1995). However, parents can have a positive influence on their adolescents. Higher levels of emotional support and warmth (nurturance), higher levels of appropriate monitoring and limit setting, more time spent together, and higher levels of parent–adolescent communication have been associated with lower levels of adolescent alcohol-related problems (Windle, 1999).

Siblings represent another familial influence. Older siblings typically serve as role models, and there is a greater likelihood that younger siblings will drink alcohol before they are adults if their older siblings drink. This relationship is stronger if the older sibling is closer in age and the same gender (Windle, 1999).

The commonly held notion that peers exert considerable influence on the initiation and maintenance of alcohol use is sustained empirically (Schulenberg & Maggs, 2002), but there is little support for overt peer pressure causing the initiation of alcohol use. Rather, most studies support a more complex, developmental interactional process in which an adolescent selects and unselects peer groups. The individual is influenced by the course of behaviors and attitudes of these groups and in turn influences them (Schulenberg & Maggs, 2002). However, overt peer pressure can play a role in relapse (Brown, 1993).

Early Influences

Newcomb (1997) cites age of onset and comorbid psychopathology as primary psychobehavioral influences in alcohol use. An earlier age of first use of alcohol is frequently associated with increased alcohol-related problems then and later in life. According to adults interviewed as part of the National Longitudinal Alcohol Epidemiological Survey, Grant and Dawson (1997) found that over 40% of adults who had reported using alcohol before age 14 had developed alcohol dependence later in their lives. This compared to a rate of less than 10% of alcohol-dependent adults who said they did not start drinking alcohol until after the age of 18.

Ellickson, Tucker, and Klein (2003) published a 10-year prospective study in which students recruited from 30 Oregon and California schools were assessed at grades seven and 12, and then later at age 23 (N = 6,338, 4,265, and 3,369, respectively). Young drinkers in both middle school and high school, compared to nondrinkers, were more likely to report academic problems, delinquent behaviors, and other substance use. At age 23, compared to nondrinkers, those who had been adolescent drinkers were more likely to report employment problems, continued "other" substance abuse, and criminal and violent behaviors.

As detailed in Chapter 19 on prevention of drug use, a review by Iocono, Malone, and McGue (2008) provides extensive evidence in support of a general liability that predisposes to a wide range of antisocial behavior in children and adolescents, including drug use. They characterize the behavioral expression of this liability as a form of disinhibition that is evident relatively early in development. This predisposition could explain the association between early onset of drug use and heightened risk for later dependence. It also explains comorbidity between drug use and other externalizing behavior. Early identification and intervention efforts for these individuals with childhood antisocial behaviors may ameliorate later alcohol use disorders.

Attention-deficit/hyperactivity disorder (ADHD) has been associated with alcohol use disorder, but its independence from conduct disorder has not been well established (Gilvarry, 2000). In a 4-year longitudinal study of children with ADHD and controls (age 6–15), there was no difference in the prevalence of alcohol use disorder between youths with and without ADHD (Biederman et al., 1997). In contrast, conduct disorder proved to be a significant predictor of alcohol use disorder in the target and control groups. In another study, Moss and Lynch (2001) used structural modeling to illustrate an association between ADHD and alcohol use disorder for adolescent males but not females, yet conduct disorder symptoms had the strongest association with alcohol use disorder in adolescents.

Comorbid Internalizing Disorders

Comorbid psychiatric disorders frequently co-occur with alcohol use disorder (Deas & Thomas, 2002; Gilvarry, 2000), but it is often difficult to distinguish etiological from consequential associations. For example, it is easy to imagine that a psychiatric disorder can result from continual, excessive alcohol consumption, especially in a physiological and psychological developmental period such as adolescence. In this example, the alcohol use disorder would precede the comorbid disorder. Another scenario, however, is drinking alcohol to treat the symptoms of a psychiatric disorder; this is called "self-medication." For example, an individual with a social phobia may desire the relaxing and disinhibitory effects of a few drinks prior to attending a social gathering. In this case, if an alcohol use disorder is identified, it is likely that the comorbid disorder preceded it. Finally, both alcohol use disorder and a psychiatric disorder may have the same etiology (e.g., genetic, neurochemical). Naturally, an understanding of the etiology of both concomitant disorders can guide treatment decisions.

In adults, a person with alcohol dependence is nearly four times more likely to have major depression than a person without alcohol dependence (Petrakis, Gonzalez, Rosenheck, & Krystal, 2002). Gilvarry (2000) reported that up to one third of adolescents in addiction treatment facilities are diagnosed with mood disorders, especially major depression and dysthymia. Deas-Nesmith, Campbell, and Brady (1998) reported that 73% of inpatient adolescents who used substances met diagnostic criteria for depression. Furthermore, in 80% of those cases, the depressive symptoms predated the substance use, suggesting that the mood disorder for these adolescents was an important risk factor for developing a subsequent substance use disorder. In the Biederman et al. (1997) study, bipolar disorder predicted substance use disorders, independent of ADHD. Although not all studies have found that mood disorders predate substance use disorders (e.g., Rohde, Lewinsohn, & Seeley, 1996), these observations suggest that mood disorders may be a risk factor for developing an alcohol use disorder in some adolescents.

A large body of literature has documented associations between stress and alcohol-related problems (Zimmermann et al., 2007). Proposed mechanisms include the anxiolytic effect of alcohol as well as alcohol-induced physiological changes that increase an individual's risk for problematic drinking, especially when drinking starts at a young age. Stress is also a known cause for depression and an array of anxiety disorders. In this context, the role of stress in the relationship between depression and alcohol use disorder merits further exploration. A recent study in China found an inverse association between depression and alcohol drinking (Cheng, Chen, McBride, & Phillips, 2016). The differential distribution of genetic polymorphisms encoding alcohol dehydrogenase and aldehyde dehydrogenase causes low metabolism of alcohol in a large proportion of the Chinese Han population compared to Caucasians. In this context, it is plausible that individuals with low metabolism of alcohol are less likely to use alcohol for tension relief due to the unpleasant "flushing effects." Future investigations on gene–environment interactions will provide more definitive evidence for this interesting observation.

Anxiety disorders, especially social phobia and posttraumatic stress disorder (PTSD), may also be risk factors for alcohol use disorder. Rohde et al. (1996) reported that alcohol use among female high school students was associated with anxiety disorders that preceded the alcohol problems. Deas-Nesmith, Brady, and Campbell (1998) found that 60% of adolescents seeking treatment for addiction met the diagnostic criteria for a social anxiety disorder. The anxiety symptoms generally predated substance dependence by about 2 years.

PTSD has also been implicated as a risk factor for alcohol use disorder. Kilpatrick et al. (2000) explored PTSD as a risk factor for substance use problems in adolescents and found that physical or sexual abuse, assault, or the witnessing of violence (e.g., murder, sexual assault) increased the risk of abuse of several illicit drugs, including alcohol. Clark et al. (1997) found that adolescents with an alcohol use disorder were more likely to have a history of physical and sexual abuse compared to an adolescent control group. The association of PTSD and alcohol dependence was stronger in females than in males.

College Drinking

Thus far, this chapter has focused on alcohol drinking and disorders observed in adolescent youth, with most of this population attending middle school and high school. However, there are significant numbers of adolescents in the age group who have just graduated from high school and may be attending college (average college age ranges from approximately 18 to 24 years). Drinking on college campuses has its own culture, with easy access to alcohol. This clearly distinguishes it from our traditional view of adolescent drinking patterns, prevalence, and disorder development. In addition, access to alcohol on most college campuses, from both attitudinal and economic perspectives, is unparalleled in any other large, established adult community and has been associated with a high frequency of serious and sometimes life-threatening drinking-related negative behaviors. While it is not within the scope of this chapter to detail the phenomenology of college campus drinking, we briefly mention the nature of the problem here and the need for further research.

Basically, the prevalence of drinking and heavy drinking among college students is higher than that of their peers who do not attend college (Johnston et al., 2015). As seen in Figure 17.11, the prevalence of binge drinking in college students (around 40%) has not declined nearly as much as in 12th-graders since 1980. Furthermore, young people not in college ages 19 to 24 report even lower rates of binge drinking than college students. This difference is due to many factors, including the influence of sororities and fraternities, greater amounts of unstructured time, easy access to those who can obtain alcohol legally, differential economic issues (parents or scholarships typically provide some financial support), and special advertising of alcoholic beverages targeted to the college population.

Hingson, Zha, and Weitzman (2009) reported an update on the serious consequences of college drinking in the United States. On an annual basis in 2005, alcohol consumption was associated with 1,825 deaths and an estimated 599,000 injuries, 646,000 assaults, and 97,000 sexual assaults of college students. Approximately 3.4 million college students were estimated to drive while under the influence of alcohol each year, 400,000 report having unprotected sex while drinking, and over 150,000 develop health-related problems due to their drinking (Hingson et al., 2002).

A special issue in the United States is that many college students turn 21, the legal minimum age for autonomous drinking and purchasing of alcohol, during college. Recent studies have found evidence about extreme drinking games as part of the ritual to celebrate the attainment of this adult privilege. For example, a study in a large Midwest university found that 12% of students who drank at a 21st-birthday party consumed at least 21 drinks; it is common even among individuals who had not consumed alcohol before 21 years of age (Rutledge et al., 2008). Another national study found that those who started drinking at 21 years of age were at a much higher risk of experiencing their first heavy episodic drinking during the same month of drinking onset compared to underage drinkers (Cheng & Anthony, 2016). These findings highlight the importance of initiatives targeting these drinking games and call for a more thorough discussion about the role of legislation for alcohol drinking. Perhaps it is not age 21 per se that is crucial; rather, the important experience might be the rite of passage into drinking on one's own, whether at age 21 years or in earlier teen years. Joint efforts from parents, teachers, and clinicians are likely needed to produce the most robust results in order to shape the nature of that ritual experience and to dampen its potentially unhealthy facets.

TOBACCO USE IN ADOLESCENCE

Adolescent tobacco use is widely recognized as a major public health problem (Windle & Windler, 1999). According to recent data, 31% of high school seniors reported ever having smoked cigarettes, 11% reported having smoked on at least 1 day in the past month, and 5.5% reported having smoked cigarettes daily (Miech et al., 2015a). Among 17-year-olds

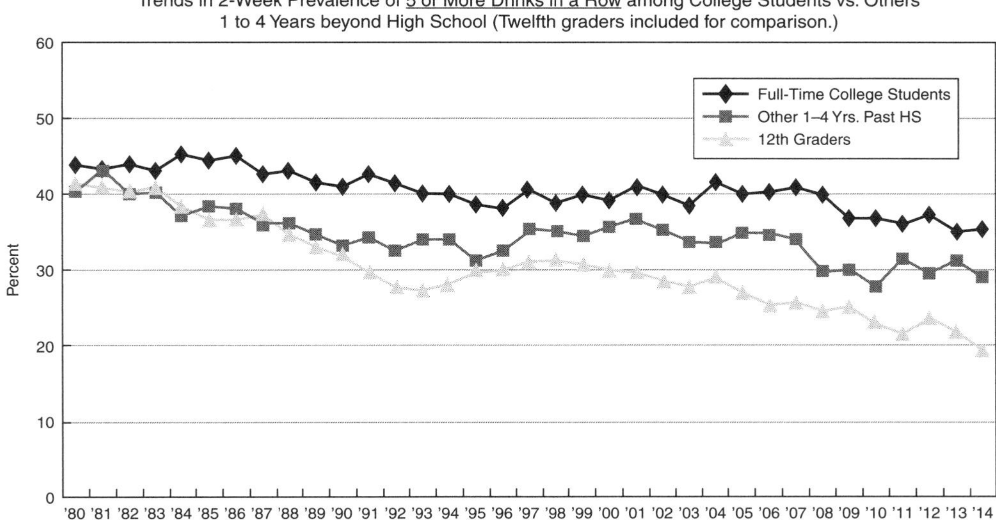

Figure 17.11 Binge drinking in college students, non-college-attending youth, and 12th-graders from 1980 to 2014. (From Johnston, L. D., O'Malley, P. M., Bachman, J. G., Schulenberg, J. E., & Miech, R. A. [2015]. *Monitoring the Future national survey results on drug use, 1975–2014: Volume 2, College students and adults ages 19–55*. Ann Arbor: Institute for Social Research, The University of Michigan.)

who indicated that they currently smoked, 38% reported symptoms that met the criteria for nicotine dependence (U.S. Department of Health and Human Services, 2014). Moreover, over half of adolescents indicated that they experience withdrawal symptoms following a quit attempt and 70% regret ever having started smoking (Centers for Disease Control and Prevention, 1998; Colby, Tiffany, Shiffman, & Niaura, 2000a). Nicotine directly activates the release of dopamine, producing a potent reinforcement effect (Dickson et al., 2011). An earlier study comparatively assessed the transition from use to dependence of an array of psychoactive drugs and found that approximately one in three tobacco users developed tobacco dependence, one of the highest among all drugs assessed (Anthony et al., 1994). This high transition probability is likely a product of various contributing factors, including the strong reinforcement effect of nicotine, high absorption into the brain via smoking, and the wide availability of tobacco products. Thus, early patterns of tobacco use among adolescents may develop into lifelong nicotine addiction.

Nicotine and Nicotine Dependence

One of the more noteworthy developments since the first edition of this volume is the introduction of a novel method of nicotine delivery, the electronic cigarette (e-cigarette). Nicotine, a potent alkaloid in tobacco leaves, is what sustains tobacco smoking, which efficiently delivers nicotine to the brain (Benowitz, 1990). Nicotine, steam distilled from burning tobacco plant material in a cigarette, is inhaled into the lungs on small tar droplets and absorbed rapidly into arterial blood, reaching the brain within 20 seconds after each puff. With the e-cigarette, nicotine can be inhaled without the need to burn tobacco leaves, thereby delivering a potentially potent dose of the drug minus the harmful ingredients contained in the tobacco cigarette.

Nicotine has similarities to the neurotransmitter acetylcholine, binding to a complex family of nicotine cholinergic receptors distributed throughout the brain and elsewhere in the body. During cigarette smoking, with each puff, nicotine levels in brain tissues briefly rise and then decline rapidly, more because of the rapid distribution into tissues than of being broken down by metabolism. Each puff acts like an individual dose of drug.

Blood and brain nicotine levels peak immediately after each cigarette, but gradually nicotine accumulates during 6 to 10 hours of repeated smoking because of nicotine's 2-hour half-life. During sleep, nicotine levels fall, but upon awakening, when the first cigarette of the day is smoked, levels begin to rise. Thus, someone smoking 10 cigarettes a day exposes his or her brain to nicotine 24 hours a day but along with rewarding perturbations in brain levels of nicotine after each of the 100 puffs. Each cigarette in effect delivers about 10 separate doses of nicotine to the brain. With marijuana or cocaine smoking, a similar pattern of drug delivery is involved.

Adolescent smokers quickly learn to regulate, on a puff-by-puff basis, their smoked nicotine dose by maintaining a brain concentration of the drug that just avoids nicotine toxicity but satisfies the increasing need for nicotine as dependence develops. Tobacco smoking is initially aversive for almost everyone. It is unlikely that a young person would begin tobacco or other drug smoking without the support and teaching from peers, the observations of admired or envied adult smokers, and the reinforcement associated with the tobacco industry's multibillion-dollar marketing that promotes the rewards of cigarette smoking.

Nicotine delivered by cigarettes offers a beginning smoker individualized and personal control of psychoactive drug dose unobtainable by any other drug delivery system. Rapid onset of nicotine toxicity, particularly the early symptoms of nausea, weakness, and sweating, gives rapid feedback that the absorbed dose is higher than optimal, exceeding the acquired tolerance level. After repeated exposure to smoking, the difficulty in concentrating and other symptoms of nicotine withdrawal that develop when brain levels are falling offer another set of cues that it is time for a cigarette to be smoked.

If nicotine toxicity is avoided, adult tobacco smokers report enhanced concentration and improved mood. Attention to task performance improves, as does reaction time and problem solving. Adult smokers report enhanced pleasure and reduced anger, tension, depression, and stress after a cigarette. Whether performance and enhanced mood after smoking are due to relief of abstinence symptoms rather than intrinsic effects of nicotine remains unclear. However, enhanced performance of nonsmokers after nicotine suggests some direct nicotine enhancement. Reports from adolescent tobacco users parallel those of adults, which suggests that nicotine has these same pharmacological effects in adolescent smokers (Corrigall, Zack, Eissenberg, Belsito, & Scher, 2001).

Nicotine, by its effects on nicotinic cholinergic receptors in the brain, enhances or modulates release of many neurotransmitters—dopamine, norepinephrine, acetylcholine, serotonin, vasopressin, β-endorphin, glutamate, GABA, and others (Tobacco Advisory Group Royal College of Physicians, 2000). Thus, changes in brain neurochemistry after nicotine exposure are profound. Neurotransmitter release is assumed to mediate nicotine's positive effects on arousal, relaxation, cognitive enhancement, relief of stress, and depression. The mesolimbic dopamine system is important in mediating the pleasurable and other rewards of nicotine, as with other drugs of abuse, and is important for understanding the withdrawal phenomena as well.

When brain nicotine levels decrease, diminished neurotransmitter release contributes to a relative deficiency state. The resulting symptoms of withdrawal—craving, lethargy, irritability, anger, restlessness, inability to concentrate, anxiety, depressed mood, and others—develop rapidly (DiFranza et al., 2002). Regular adolescent smokers report withdrawal symptoms similar to those reported by adults. Whether the withdrawal symptoms experienced by an adolescent nicotine addict are more or less intense after comparable levels of nicotine exposure is not established.

Young smokers who are still experimenting are likely to become regular smokers surprisingly rapidly. The precise numbers who go on to regular smoking and factors that influence the progression from experimentation to regular smoking for any single individual remain uncertain. Measurable symptoms of nicotine dependence occur within weeks of the beginning of occasional nicotine use, probably well before daily smoking has been established. One third to one half of adolescents who experiment with more than a few cigarettes become regular smokers (Colby, Tiffany, Shiffman, & Niaura, 2000b).

The criteria common to all drugs are used to diagnose nicotine dependence as defined in the DSM-5. Nicotine dependence is associated with tolerance, cravings for tobacco, desire to use tobacco, withdrawal symptoms when the nicotine dose is decreased or unavailable, and loss of control over the frequency and duration of use.

Although traditionally it has been assumed that a period of sustained, daily use is required to produce dependence, clinical observations of adolescent smokers and data from animal laboratory experiments suggest that dependence develops rapidly in adolescent smokers and in adolescent laboratory animals (Abreu-Villaca et al., 2003; DiFranza et al., 2000; Slotkin, 2002). Some adolescent smokers demonstrate evidence of nicotine dependence well before becoming daily smokers and possibly after only a few days of intermittent smoking (DiFranza et al., 2000; O'Loughlin, Tarasuk, DiFranza, & Paradis, 2002). This pattern is consistent with a variety of evidence from animal research showing that an adolescent brain is more susceptible to rapid development of nicotine dependence (Abreu-Villaca et al., 2003). Animal researchers have focused on possible brain mechanisms that account for the special susceptibility of adolescent brains (Slotkin, 2002). For example, nicotine exposure in adolescent rats results in greater and more persistent nicotine receptor upregulation and cholinergic activity than in adult animals. The rapidity of change in the animal models is consistent with adolescent smokers who develop evidence of nicotine dependence after only a few days' experience with just a few cigarettes (Di-Franza et al., 2000, 2002). Brief nicotine exposure results in alterations in cholinergic receptor activity lasting at least 1 month after exposure in rats, which suggests that brief exposure to nicotine changes cholinergic tone in a persistent manner. The level of exposure in the animal models was thought to be in the range experienced by adolescents occasionally smoking three to five cigarettes a day. The data suggest the possibility that brain mechanisms that account for nicotine dependence can be activated by nicotine exposure from only occasional smoking. Although nicotine has a variety of systemic effects in a smoker, particularly cardiovascular and neuroendocrine changes, some animal researchers believe they have found evidence of a primary neurotoxicity as well (Slotkin, 2002) with lasting cell injury, particularly cholinergic system cells. There is no evidence of cholinergic toxicity in human studies.

In summary, animal experiments with nicotine suggest rapid and persistent changes in nicotinic receptor and cholinergic function in adolescent rat brains with doses perhaps as little as one tenth of those ingested by regular tobacco smokers.

Recent Trends in Cigarette Smoking and Other Tobacco Products

One of the successes of drug prevention in adolescents is the continued decline in cigarette use among adolescents in the United States. As seen in Figure 17.12, past 30-day cigarette smoking has dropped below 10% of high school students in the most recent year of the survey. Nevertheless, other forms of tobacco use have remained prevalent. For example, the prevalence of past-month use of flavored cigarillos (i.e., small cigar) is now equivalent to cigarette use (11%), and estimates of past-month tobacco use increases by half from 11% to 18% among high school seniors when cigarillo use is included (Miech et al., 2015b). The e-cigarette has emerged as a major tobacco product in recent years, along with greater use of hookahs (i.e., a specialized water pipe) and cigars of various types. The tobacco industry has been introducing new products in order to attract a broader audience; an example is fruit-flavored hookahs to attract females. In a recent national survey, 16% of high school students said they have used an e-cigarette

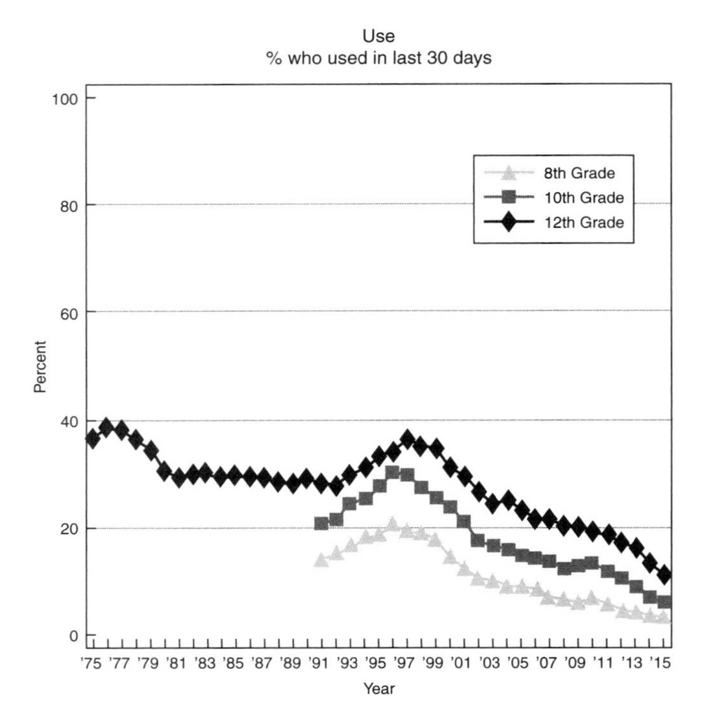

Figure 17.12 Trends in past-30-day use of regular cigarettes among eighth-, 10th-, and 12th-graders. (From http://monitoringthefuture.org/pressreleases/15Ecigfig.pdf.)

at least once in the past month (Miech et al., 2015c), and reported exposure to e-cigarette advertising among adolescents is high (about 69%, Singh et al., 2016). Although students reported curiosity as the primary reason for trying e-cigarettes, few (10%) said their e-cigarette use was to help quit smoking. The annual prevalence of hookah use among these students is about 20%, and estimates for cigarillos (both flavored and unflavored) is about 16%. Nevertheless, these tobacco products may be less harmful to health than cigarettes because they are either used less frequently (i.e., hookahs and cigars) or pose less risk (i.e., e-cigarettes) (Goniewicz et al., 2014).

Determinants of Smoking

Nicotine is essential to maintain tobacco smoking, but the beginning of tobacco addiction, as with other addictions, is influenced mostly by nonpharmacological, learned, or conditioned factors. Peer influence, social setting, personality, and genetics determine who begins and who continues to smoke. In order to develop and implement more effective prevention and treatment programs for adolescent tobacco use, a greater understanding of the determinants of these behaviors is needed. The following summarizes a few of these determinants.

Socioenvironmental Factors

Socioenvironmental factors can have an important influence on youth tobacco use. For example, smoking among peers is a powerful determinant of smoking initiation and progression (Choi, Pierce, Gilpin, Farkas, & Berry, 1997; Conrad, Flay, & Hill, 1992). Tobacco industry promotional activities can also have a significant impact on adolescent smoking behavior (Choi, Gilpin, Farkas, & Pierce, 1998). Of particular relevance to prevention strategies are socioenvironmental factors that protect against youth smoking. For example, adolescents who are involved in interscholastic sports and non-school-related physical activity are less likely to be established smokers (Escobedo, Marcus, Holtzman, & Giovino, 1993; Patton et al., 1998; Thorlindsson & Vihjalmsson,

1991). Religious affiliation appears to be protective against smoking (Heath, Madden, et al., 1999), as are school and home smoking restrictions (Farkas, Gilpin, White, & Pierce, 2000; Wakefield et al., 2000).

Psychological Factors

Relatively less attention has been devoted to the role of psychological factors in youth smoking. Available data suggest that tobacco use and nicotine dependence are more common among adolescents who experience depression symptoms (Escobedo, Kirch, & Anda, 1996; Wang et al., 1999), particularly those with more serious psychiatric conditions (Bresleau, 1995). Adolescents with ADHD are at greater risk for tobacco use (Milberger, Biederman, Faraone, Chen, & Jones, 1997). Weight concerns appear to promote smoking initiation and current smoking in female adolescents (French, Perry, Leon, & Fulkerson, 1994). These findings suggest that multiple causal pathways are involved in tobacco smoking, a common phenotype. The understanding of these pathways is essential to targeted prevention and intervention strategies for subgroups of adolescents.

While some socioenvironmental and psychological factors appear to play an important role in the early stages of smoking uptake, genetic factors may be more influential in the development of nicotine dependence. Differentiation of the precise set of factors that are important in each of these transitions is a critical step toward developing effective strategies to prevent progression to smoking addiction and facilitate quitting.

Individual Variability

There are abundant data supporting the heritability of cigarette smoking (see discussion on genetics earlier in this chapter). This variability influences the subjective effects of nicotine. Nicotine has both positive reinforcing effects (e.g., enhances alertness, arousal, pleasure) and negative reinforcing effects (relieves adverse mood and withdrawal symptoms) (Pomerleau & Pomerleau, 1984). Individual differences in the rewarding effects of the initial dose of nicotine from a cigarette may account for the observation that some young adults become dependent smokers, whereas others can experiment and not progress to nicotine dependence (Eissenberg & Balster, 2000; Flay, d'Avernas, Best, Kersell, & Ryan, 1983). In support of this hypothesis, one cross-sectional analysis found that pleasant emotional and physiological effects of the initial smoking experience discriminated teens who continued to experiment with cigarettes and those who did not (Friedman, Lichtenstein, & Biglan, 1985). Among adults, retrospective reports of the rewarding effects of the initial smoking experience (e.g., pleasurable rush or buzz, relaxation) were associated with current levels of nicotine dependence (Pomerleau, Pomerleau, & Namenek, 1998). On the basis of this knowledge, researchers are testing medications that may reduce the nicotine metabolism rate, thereby increasing aversive effects of initial smoking experiences (Sellers, Tyndale, & Fernandes, 2003).

Personality Traits

Novelty and sensation seeking as a personality trait has been linked to tobacco use during adolescence (Wills, Vaccaro, & McNamara, 1994; Wills, Windle, & Cleary, 1998) and early onset of smoking in adolescent boys (Masse & Tremblay, 1997). Genetic studies have related novelty seeking with genetic variants in the dopamine pathway (Noble et al., 1998; Sabol et al., 1999), suggesting that these genetic effects on smoking behavior may be mediated in part by novelty-seeking personality traits. Research suggests that two forms of impulsivity, acting without thinking (Khurana et al., 2015) and delay discounting (Audrain-McGovern et al., 2009), may be more important for the progression of drug use than novelty seeking per se (Winstanley et al., 2010). Interventions that include messages and formats targeted to adolescents with these predisposing personality traits may be more effective than broad-based appeals (Lerman, Patterson, & Shields, 2003). However, the evidence regarding the use of video messages that target sensation-seeking smokers has not been supportive of this strategy (Langleben et al., 2009).

OTHER SUBSTANCES

MDMA (Ecstasy)

MDMA (3,4-methylenedioxymethamphetamine), also called Ecstasy, Molly, and other names, has similarities to other amphetamines with stimulant and hallucinogen-like properties (Green, Mechan, Elliott, O'Shea, & Colado, 2003). About 4% of high school seniors use Ecstasy annually, with 1% having used it in the past month. Usually taken orally, it can also be injected. MDMA produces feelings of energy along with a pleasurable, altered sense of time and enhanced perception and sensory experiences. MDMA effects last 3 to 6 hours. A typical oral dose is one or two tablets, each containing 60 to 120 mg of MDMA, although recently the average dose may be increasing. As is characteristic of all illicit drugs, the chemical content and potency of the MDMA tablets vary; thus, dose estimates or even unverified assumptions about the actual drug ingested are only estimates (Cole, Bailey, Sumnall, Wagstaff, & King, 2002).

Perhaps MDMA has a special appeal to adolescents because its usual effects include, along with mental stimulation, feelings of relatedness and empathy toward other people and feelings of well-being (Cole & Sumnall, 2003). These mood effects, along with the experience of enhanced sensory perception, make MDMA an appealing drug, particularly as typically used at social gatherings, dances, and concerts. At higher doses or in susceptible individuals, undesirable effects include rapid onset of anxiety, agitation, and feelings of restlessness (Gowing, Henry-Edwards, Irvine, & Ali, 2002). During the period of marked intoxication, memory is impaired, sometimes for days or longer in regular users. Information processing and task performance are disrupted. Regular users and sometimes even occasional users report withdrawal phenomena when MDMA's effects are wearing off. Withdrawal effects include feelings of depression, difficulty concentrating, unusual calmness, fluctuating mood, and feelings of pervasive sadness sometimes lasting a week or more after an evening of moderate MDMA use (Parrott et al., 2002).

As with other amphetamine-like stimulant drugs, high doses of MDMA, particularly if used with other stimulants, can be associated with nausea, chills, sweating, muscle cramps, and blurred vision. Anxiety, paranoid thinking, and, later, depression are common. After higher doses, markedly increased blood pressure, loss of consciousness, and seizures may occur, and under certain conditions of dose or drug combinations and heat, the body's thermoregulation mechanisms fail. The resultant marked increase in body temperature (hyperthermia) under some circumstances is rapidly followed by multiple organ failure and death (Schifano, 2003). MDMA is commonly used with alcohol, increasing MDMA's toxicity.

The nature of MDMA metabolism in the body contributes to toxicity. After a dose of MDMA is rapidly absorbed, it slows its own breakdown, resulting in unexpectedly high MDMA concentrations with repeated doses (Farre et al., 2004; Green, Mechan, et al., 2003). After regular use, tolerance to the desired effects develops (Verheyden, Henry, & Curran, 2003). This tolerance leads regular MDMA users to take larger or more frequent doses, resulting in the accumulation of toxic blood levels because of the drug-induced slowdown in its own metabolism.

As with all psychoactive drugs, the general considerations of gender, dose, frequency of exposure, and concurrent use of other drugs, along with genetic and environmental factors, are probably important determinants of the consequences of MDMA exposure for any specific individual (Daumann et al., 2003; De Win et al., 2004; Obrocki et al., 2002; Roiser & Sahakian, 2003). Certainly many people have used MDMA and appear to have avoided measurable harm, but some have died after taking MDMA. As with nicotine, animal experiments suggest that younger brains may be more susceptible to the neurotoxic effects of MDMA (Williams et al., 2003), although important experiments with adolescent animals have not yet been reported.

Inhalant Abuse

Thousands of chemicals produce vapors or can be delivered as aerosols and inhaled to produce psychoactive effects (Anderson & Loomis, 2003). Inhalants can be organized by their chemical classification (e.g., toluene or nitrous oxide), by their legitimate use (as an anesthetic, solvent, adhesive, fuel, etc.), or by their means of delivery (as a gas, a vapor, or an aerosol) (Balster, 1987). What inhalants have in common is that they are rarely taken by other routes when abused, although some can be swallowed or injected.

Volatile solvents include common household and workplace products: cleaning fluids, felt-tip markers, glues, paint thinners, and gasoline (Anderson & Loomis, 2003). Volatile medical anesthetics, halothane or isoflurane, and other ethers occasionally turn up among adolescent inhalant users. Another category of inhalants, aerosols, is available as the solvents in spray cans that deliver paint, deodorants, hairspray, insecticides, and other products. Inhalant gases include household and commercial gases: butane in cigarette lighters, and nitrous oxide in whipped cream cans or from medical sources. Nitrites are a special class of inhalants occasionally encountered by adolescents. When inhaled, nitrites dilate blood vessels, relax smooth muscles, and, unlike other inhalants, are more stimulating than depressing and are used primarily to enhance sexual activities.

Inhalants have been used as intoxicants for hundreds of years. Inhalants, particularly solvents, are often one of the first psychoactive drugs used by children. An estimated 6% of children had tried inhalants on at least one occasion by the fourth grade. Inhalants stand out among abused drugs by being used more by younger than older children, though on occasion inhalant abuse persists into adulthood (Balster, 1987). Although inhalant abusers generally use whatever is available, preferred agents exist, varying from region to region in an almost fad-like way.

National and state surveys indicate that inhalant use peaks around the seventh to ninth grades, with 2% of eighth-graders reporting use of inhalants within the previous 30 days (compared to only 0.7% by the 12th grade). The prevalence of inhalant use in young adolescents exceeds marijuana use and is more frequent in boys and in adverse socioeconomic conditions. Poverty, childhood abuse, poor grades, and early school dropout are associated with greater inhalant abuse (Beauvais, Wayman, Jumper-Thurman, Plested, & Helm, 2002; Kurtzman, Otsuka, & Wahl, 2001).

When inhaled, the drugs move from the lungs to brain and an onset of effects occurs within seconds. Psychoactive effects dissipate within minutes when inhalation is stopped. The chemicals are distributed to other organs, potentially damaging the liver, kidneys, and peripheral nerves. The experience produced by most inhalants is similar to that of drinking alcohol: an initial feeling of relaxation, anxiety relief, and feelings of disinhibition. As the intoxication increases with repeated doses, speech becomes slurred, fine motor movements and ability to walk are impaired, and, with increasing and repeated doses, loss of consciousness and an anesthetic state or coma occur. The neural mechanisms by which inhalant intoxication occurs are not well understood (Balster, 1998). During the period of intoxication many neural systems become dysfunctional.

As intoxication wears off, a hangover state commonly ensues. The severity of the post-intoxication effect depends on dose, duration of exposure, and the amount used, but typically includes headache or nausea. Inadvertent overdose is possible, particularly when the bag or other inhalant delivery system becomes positioned so that when consciousness or coordination is lost, delivery of the inhalant continues.

A common cause of death during inhalant use is rapid inhalation of large amounts of solvents, followed by strenuous activity. This results in impaired cardiac function and arrhythmias. Injury and death may result from accidents associated with impaired judgment, motor impairment, or falls. Suffocation from inadequate air during the inhalation of concentrated gases or solvents is possible, and because many inhalants are flammable, fires or explosions may lead to injury or death.

When asked, children typically report that they sniff inhalants because it's fun and they like the feeling of intoxication. Initial use is often in a group with considerable peer pressure. Some users report that the intoxicated state is a way to avoid experiencing or dealing with worries and problems. Although most child inhalant use is transient and initially stems from curiosity, with the wrong kind of group pressure, it becomes a repeated behavior.

Gammahydroxybutyrate (GHB)

A potent central nervous system depressant, GHB (Liquid Ecstasy, Georgia Home Boy, and other names) is typically taken to produce euphoria and a relaxed and uninhibited state, similar to that produced by alcohol (Nicholson & Balster, 2001; Teter & Guthrie, 2001). GHB is a clear, odorless, slightly salty-tasting liquid. Because of its steep dose–effect curve, inadvertent overdose is frequent. Nausea, vomiting, slowed heart rate, loss of consciousness, coma, respiratory depression, and seizures can require emergency treatment. Coma, along with vomiting and an obstructed airway, can lead to death. The purity and the strength of individual doses of GHB vary greatly and can contribute to overdoses, particularly by inexperienced users. When GHB is taken with other CNS depressants, lethality increases. Deaths from GHB typically occur after combined use with alcohol. GHB is so rapidly metabolized that postmortem toxicology statistics may underestimate its frequency.

Regular users of GHB report that they must increase the dose to attain euphoric and relaxing effects; thus, tolerance seems likely. A withdrawal state with increased heart rate, restlessness, anxiety, agitation, delirium, and disrupted sleep follows sudden cessation of regular GHB use (Miotto et al., 2001). GHB has been perceived as a safe drug because it was available in health food stores as a dietary supplement. Its potential toxicity may be underestimated by adolescents (Mason & Kerns, 2002). Although now a controlled drug, GHB precursors are readily available through Internet distributors. Because it is odorless and relatively tasteless, GHB has reportedly been added to the drinks of unsuspecting victims. It can sedate or anesthetize an unwary recipient, leading to its use as a date rape drug (Schwartz, Milteer, & LeBeau, 2000).

Flunitrazepam (Rohypnol)

Rohypnol (Roofies, Rophie, Forget Me) is a potent benzodiazepine sedative drug with similarities to Valium or Xanax, except for its increased potency (Simmons & Cupp, 1998). Although a prescribed medication in some countries, Rohypnol is not approved for prescription use in the United States. Taken by mouth in tablet form or when dissolved in beverages, Rohypnol rapidly produces profound sedation or loss of consciousness and marked amnesia for events occurring during the period of intoxication. With no odor, and almost tasteless, it can easily be administered to someone without his or her knowledge. Like GHB, it has been associated with date rape and other sexual assaults (Schwartz et al., 2000; Slaughter, 2000).

Hallucinogens

Hallucinogens are a pharmacologically diverse group of drugs. They have in common the ability to produce profound distortions in sensory perception, but accompanied by a relatively clear level of consciousness (Hollister, 1968). The perceptual distortions are typically termed *hallucinations*, though in fact true hallucinations are relatively uncommon. The sought-after alterations in visual images, perception of sounds, and bodily sensations are sometimes accompanied by intense mood swings and feelings of being out of control that can be disturbing to the uninitiated (Strassman, 1984).

Some humans have valued hallucinogenic drugs for thousands of years. The older hallucinogenic plants (e.g., mescaline, psilocybin, or ibogaine) contain chemicals structurally similar to brain neurotransmitters such as serotonin, dopamine, and norepinephrine. Historically, drug-induced hallucinogenic states were typically part of social and religious rituals rather than entertainment. Plant-based hallucinogens are still available and are even sold over the Internet (e.g., psilocybin mushrooms and peyote cacti), but since the 1960s the prototype hallucinogen has been LSD (lysergic acid diethylamide), an extremely potent, chemically synthesized drug that is readily available through illicit sources and, compared to many drugs, relatively inexpensive (Hofmann, 1994). LSD's physiological effects are relatively few and mild: dilated pupils, increased deep tendon reflexes, increased muscle tension, and mild motor incoordination. Heart rate increases, as does blood pressure and respiration, but not greatly. Nausea, decreased appetite, and increased salivation are common.

In nontolerant users, about 25 μg of LSD is a threshold dose. The psychological and perceptual state produced by LSD is in general similar to that produced by mescaline, psilocybin, and hallucinogenic amphetamine analogs. The major difference is potency: LSD is hundreds to thousands of times more potent. Acquired tolerance to LSD can be profound. After 3 days of successive daily doses, a 4- or 5-day drug-free period is necessary to again experience the full sensory effects. This limits, to some extent, frequency of use.

In recent years, LSD has been distributed as "blotter acid"—that is, on sheets of paper perforated into postage stamp–size squares, with each square containing 30 to 75 μg of LSD, ingested as a chewed dose. The effects of a single dose last from 6 to 12 hours, diminishing gradually.

LSD alters the function of brain serotonin receptors (Aghajanian & Marek, 1999). At higher doses LSD can produce a distressing drug-induced psychosis with similarities to naturally occurring psychotic states, such as acute schizophrenia. The user has difficulty in recognizing reality, thinking rationally, and communicating easily with others (Blaho, Merigan, Winbery, Geraci, & Smartt, 1997; Strassman, 1984).

For reasons not well understood, an LSD-induced experience can be psychologically traumatic, particularly for poorly prepared novices. The symptoms persist long after the pharmacological effects have worn off (Blaho et al., 1997). A persistent psychosis with mood swings ranging from mania to depression, visual disturbances, and hallucinations is relatively uncommon. Individuals who are predisposed, for genetic or other unknown reasons, to developing schizophrenia may be more likely to experience this (Hollister, 1968).

Other hallucinogens such as mescaline, consumed in the form of peyote buttons from cacti, or tryptamine hallucinogens (e.g., dimethyltryptamine [DMT]) are less commonly used, probably because they are less available to adolescents. However, trafficking over the Internet has enhanced their availability (Halpern & Pope, 2001). Psilocybin is occasionally available to adolescents, usually ingested as psilocybin-containing mushrooms. Psilocybin sold illicitly as pills or capsules more likely contains PCP or LSD rather than psilocybin.

PCP and Ketamine

PCP (Angel Dust) and a shorter-acting analog, ketamine (K, Special K, Vitamin K, Kat Valium) were developed as surgical anesthetics (Reich & Silvay, 1989). At lower doses both alter perception and produce feelings of detachment and of being disconnected or dissociated from the environment, leading to use of the term *dissociative anesthetics* to describe this class of drugs and distinguish them from hallucinogens. At anesthetic doses patients are quiet but with eyes open, fixed in a gaze, and in a seeming cataleptic state without experiencing pain during a surgical procedure. Both PCP and ketamine produce similar effects by altering the distribution of an important brain neurotransmitter, glutamate.

PCP anesthesia produced a sometimes distressing delirium as the anesthetic was wearing off, so it was replaced with ketamine, which is shorter-acting and slightly less potent but associated with briefer and less troublesome delirium. Most abusers do not overdose to full anesthetic levels (Freese, Miotto, & Reback, 2002). However, depending on drug dose and tolerance, PCP or ketamine intoxication can progress from feelings of detachment and perceptual changes through confusion, delirium, and psychosis to coma and coma with seizures (Dillon, Copeland, & Jansen, 2003; Jansen & Darracot-Cankovic, 2001). After overdose, the progression to recovery follows the reverse pattern. Treatment of symptoms is primarily supportive. Ketamine produces a shorter period of intoxication; in a surgical setting a single anesthetic dose produces coma for only 10 minutes, as compared to a much longer coma after a single large dose of PCP. When abused, these drugs can be taken by mouth or, for more rapid effects, smoked or sniffed. When used medically they are injected. With frequent use, tolerance and dependence develop (Pal, Berry, Kumar, & Ray, 2002).

Ketamine is odorless and tasteless and can be surreptitiously added to someone's drink to produce a period of impaired awareness and amnesia. Thus, ketamine has been used during sexual assaults and date rape. PCP is inexpensive to produce and distribute so it is often substituted for other illicit drugs—for example, it is misrepresented as MDMA or THC.

Club Drugs

The term *club drugs* refers to a variety of drugs that have in common only that they are typically used at all-night parties or "rave" dances, clubs, and bars (Smith, Larive, & Romanelli, 2002; Weir, 2000). The drugs in this group are varied. Their pharmacology and patterns of use vary in different regions (Gross, Barrett, Shestowsky, & Pihl, 2002). Patterns of use, dose, and popular drug mixes change over time. The most common club drugs, particularly marijuana, cocaine, MDMA (Ecstasy), and methamphetamine, are discussed earlier in this chapter. Club drugs that have come to the attention of adolescents include GHB, flunitrazepam (Rohypnol), and ketamine. Thus the list includes stimulants, depressants, and hallucinogens. MDMA, GHB, and Rohypnol have received the most recent attention as club drugs. The special appeal of club drugs to an adolescent includes their novelty and fad-like qualities. Unfortunately, among users there is a misperception about the relative safety of club drugs (Koesters, Rogers, & Rajasingham, 2002): Their use, particularly by novices, can lead to serious health problems (Tellier, 2002).

Treatment of Substance Use Disorders

Claudia Szobot

chapter 18

OVERVIEW

The high rate of adolescent substance abuse in the United States (Forrester 2012; Jones et al., 2015; Substance Abuse and Mental Health Services Administration, 2014) makes the identification of effective treatment approaches a significant priority. Effective early intervention is crucial. Adolescents who initiate alcohol use by age 14 are significantly more likely to develop alcohol dependence as adults than those who initiate by age 20, with significant reductions in the odds of developing dependence for each year of delayed initiation (Barry et al., 2016; Grant, 1997; Von Diemen et al., 2008). Effective early intervention is also crucial with substance-abusing adolescents because it can play a preventive role in later years (Borduin, 1995; Kazdin, 1991, 1993; Pianca et al., 2016; Santisteban, 2003; Winters, Botzet, & Fahnhorst, 2011).

Alcohol remains the most commonly used age-restricted substance among adolescents in several countries (Brown et al., 2015; Kandel, 1993). However, a marked trend in recent years is the increased use of cannabis among adolescents, which has led to an increased demand for cannabis treatment. According to United Nations Office of Drugs and Crime (UNODC, 2012), North America has one of the highest prevalences of cannabis use (10.8%) worldwide. However, recent surveys indicate small decreases in cannabis use. One study examined time trends in tobacco and cannabis use among 15-year-olds in Europe and North America between 2002 and 2010 (Hublet et al., 2015). The authors included 28 countries, with 142,796 adolescents divided into "non-users," "tobacco and cannabis users," "tobacco-only users," and "cannabis-only users." Tobacco use and concurrent tobacco and cannabis use decreased by 3% and 3.7%, respectively, but prevalence rates varied by region. In the United States, there was an interaction between time and gender for tobacco and cannabis use. This is in agreement with the "Monitoring the Future Study: Trends in Prevalence of Various Drugs for 8th Graders, 10th Graders, and 12th Graders; 2012–2015," where there was a reduction in the prevalence of cannabis use in the past month and daily use among students in 12th grade between 2012 and 2015. In Brazil, in 2012, 4.3% of the adolescents in a national survey reported lifetime use of cannabis, and 3.4% in the last month (Abdalla et al., 2014).

Despite the tendency for a decrease in cannabis prevalence among North American adolescents since the 1970s, there is a significant number of youth in need of marijuana treatment. From 1992 to 1998, the number of adolescents with primary, secondary, or tertiary problems related to cannabis who presented to the U.S. public treatment system grew from 51,081 to 109,875 (a 115% increase) (Dennis, Dawud-Noursi, Muck, & McDermeit, 2002). In 1998, over 80% of these adolescents received treatment in an outpatient setting. The bulk of treatment evaluation studies and clinical trials report that the most prevalent types of substance use in clinical populations are alcohol and marijuana, with some cocaine, heroin, methamphetamine, hallucinogen, and polysubstance use as well, based on setting and sample. The perception of the risks of marijuana use have steadily declined over the past decade among adolescents, possibly related to public debate about legalizing for medicinal and recreational use (Johnston et al., 2014). Medical emergencies possibly related to marijuana use have also increased. The Drug Abuse Warning Network (DAWN) estimated that in 2011, there were 456,000 drug-related emergency department visits in the United States in which marijuana use was mentioned in the medical record (a 21% increase over 2009) (Substance Abuse and Mental Health Services Administration, 2013).

Treatment of substance-abusing adolescents is complicated by a number of factors that appear to be particularly prevalent or problematic among adolescents (although they complicate treatment for adults as well). First, as noted above, adolescents in treatment or community samples use multiple substances, typically alcohol and marijuana, with occasional cocaine use (Kaminer, 2002; Szobot et al., 2007; Winters, 2000) and, increasingly, heroin as well. This reality is also seen among adolescents who use prescription stimulants (McCabe et al., 2014).

Second, as highlighted at several points throughout this volume, substance-using adolescents have very high rates of comorbid psychiatric disorders, which can greatly complicate treatment delivery and outcome. For example, Henggeler (1996) reported that 35% of participants in a clinical trial of family approaches (described in more detail below) met criteria for conduct disorder (CD), 19% for social phobia, 12% for oppositional defiant disorder (ODD), and 9% for major depression. In Waldron's sample (Waldron, 2001), 89.8% had a history of significant delinquent behavior, 29.7% met criteria for anxiety and depressive disorders, and 27.3% had attention problems. Kaminer et al. (Kaminer, 2002) reported that 55% met criteria for an externalizing disorder, 39% for CD, 18% for attention-deficit/hyperactivity disorder (ADHD), 22% for major depression, and 26% for an anxiety disorder. Recently, Pianca et al. (2016) evaluated the comorbidity profile in adolescents hospitalized for crack cocaine use (n = 88) compared to community controls (n = 81). Based on DSM-IV-TR, the authors found a high lifetime prevalence (98.9%) of comorbidity, with 81.8% of CD, 52.3% of ODD, and 44.3% of ADHD; 46.6% had any anxiety disorder. For current comorbidities, the prevalence was also high: 74% for CD, 51.1% for ODD, and 39.8% for ADHD; 15.2% had any current mood disorder and 27.2% had any anxiety disorder. As discussed in more detail below, the presence of a comorbid disorder often indicates the need for evaluation for pharmacotherapy as well and, with it, the need to coordinate treatment to include close monitoring of treatment adherence and response. The presence of CD is particularly significant among substance-abusing adolescents as it is often associated with poor long-term treatment outcome and persistence of antisocial behavior in this population (Myers, 1998). Moreover, in some circumstances (e.g., deviant adolescents assigned to interactional groups), having a high proportion of adolescents with CD in unstructured treatment groups may lead to poor outcomes (Arnold, 1999; Dishion, 1999).

Third, treatment of substance-abusing adolescents is complicated by high rates of substance abuse in their immediate families. Henggeler (1996) reported that a substance abuse problem was present in 18% of birth mothers and 56% of the fathers of youth in his treatment sample. Winters (2000) reported that 66% of participants had at least one parent with substance use disorder. According to the 2009 National Survey on Drug Use and Health (NSDUH), approximately 8.3 million children under the age of 18 years have lived with at least one parent who abused alcohol or illicit drugs during the 12 months prior to the interview (Substance Abuse and Mental Health Services Administration, 2009). This is significant because parental substance use is associated with poor parenting practices and low levels of parent monitoring, which can exacerbate adolescent substance use (Chilcoat, 1995). Furthermore, exposure to drug use and drug-related cues within the household is likely to provoke craving in established adolescent substance abusers.

Fourth, adolescents rarely seek treatment voluntarily but are usually coerced at some level after experiencing school, legal, or medical problems (Brown, 1993). Treatment is also complicated by adolescents' involvement in multiple systems and points of entry, as many have legal problems, school problems, and medical problems that may be identified prior to recognition of the presence of a substance use disorder (Henggeler, 1991). Thus, multiple treatment systems are simultaneously involved with a given individual. In this sense, ethical issues deserve more attention in future studies, as it is often difficult to distinguish between coercion and protection in these systems.

Finally, high attrition in treatment is also a particular problem among adolescents, with treatment completion rates for adolescents in therapeutic communities estimated at less than 20%; completion rates for outpatient programs are generally estimated at 50% (Henggeler, 1996).

Based on all these premises, treatment programs must be designed specifically for adolescents. There has been a lot of progress in recent decades concerning adolescent approaches, and treatment choice should consider, for instance, the severity of drug use and environmental factors, such as family conditions. The American

Society of Addiction Medicine (2001) suggests the following patient placement levels, from least to most intensive:

1. Early intervention services, which commonly consist of educational or brief intervention services
2. Outpatient treatment, in which adolescents typically attend treatment for 6 hours per week or less for a period dependent on progress and the treatment plan
3. Intensive outpatient treatment, in which adolescents attend treatment during the day (up to 20 hours per week) but live at home; the program ranges in length from 2 months to 1 year
4. Residential/inpatient treatment, which includes programs that provide treatment services in a residential setting, lasting from 1 month to 1 year
5. Medically managed intensive inpatient treatment, which is most appropriate for adolescents whose substance use, biomedical, and emotional problems are so severe that they require 24-hour primary medical care for a length dependent on the adolescent's progress

PSYCHOSOCIAL TREATMENTS

Psychosocial approaches are essential when making a treatment plan. The most frequent treatment psychosocial approaches offered in adolescent drug addiction services are family-based therapy (FBT), with several theoretical orientations, and individual and group therapy (Becker & Cury, 2008; Winters, Botzet, & Fahnhorst, 2011). For individual and group therapy, despite the several theoretical available approaches, the most evaluated are cognitive-behavioral therapy (CBT), brief motivational interviewing (MI), and behavioral therapy, where contingency management (CM) reinforcement approaches are included. Some of these studies will be described later in this chapter.

Treatment Evaluation Studies

There are rigorous evaluations of the efficacy and effectiveness of standard treatment approaches for adolescents. As of 2001, two major reviews identified between 32 and 53 published studies (Dennis & White, 2003; Williams et al., 2000). Overall, most of these were program evaluation studies of inpatient services, and only about 15 were randomized clinical trials (RCTs) in outpatient settings. Although the older studies tended to suffer from a range of methodological problems, a number of newer studies have provided more methodologically sound conclusions. These are reviewed by Waldron and Turner (2008) and more recently by Hogue and colleagues (2014). The newer studies are more likely to have high inclusion rates (>80%), experimental designs, manualized protocols, standardized measures, validation sub studies, repeated measures, long-term follow-up (12 or more months), high follow-up rates (80%–90% or more), and an economic analysis of the cost and benefits to society.

Until about 2001, the three more intensive programs (inpatient, residential, and Outward Bound) had received the most attention from investigators. Roughly 30 to 40 studies existed, which primarily involved uncontrolled evaluations of a single treatment program (Williams et al., 2000). In these studies, it was difficult to determine the relative effectiveness of the approaches because few included any type of comparison or control group; however, in some studies, patients who dropped out of treatment served as a quasi-experimental control group (although this is clearly not an ideal comparison because of the possibility of selection bias). The primary outcome measures used in these studies were typically abstinence, drug use reduction, and treatment retention, although different studies tended to define these differently. Outcomes were almost always measured by self-report and often taken from clinical records rather than assessed by an independent evaluator. The use of validated outcome measures or biological indicators of substance use was rare. Thus, the highly positive outcomes typically reported by these studies should be tempered by an understanding of the substantial limitations of their designs. On average about 50% of patients reported significant decreases in substance use, typically measured as number of days with any drug use (Williams et al., 2000). Given that most of these programs emphasized complete abstinence, on average only 38% of those followed reported complete abstinence at 6 months.

A substantial number of studies have been conducted, including two important literature reviews on outpatient treatments for adolescents with substance use disorder. Waldron and Turner (2008), in an empirical review and meta-analysis of 17 RCTs, identified 46 different interventions: 17 with FBT, 13 with group CBT, seven with individual CBT, and nine with minimal treatment controls. Later, Hogue et al. (2014) updated Waldron and Turner´s revision; they included findings from literature reviews and meta-analyses for adolescent substance use disorder treatment from 2009 to 2013. One of the conclusions was the confirmation that protocol-driven interventions were more effective than treatment as usual; also, FBT had the strongest support and several manualized options; CBT (group or individual) and MI interventions also received empirical support. Besides these reviews, the authors selected 19 comparative studies and evaluated them according to sample characteristics, methodological quality, and substance use outcomes (based on *Journal of Clinical and Adolescent Psychology* Levels of Support Evaluation Criteria). One important point is that in this publication, effect size (ES) estimates were noted when available. The studies were evaluated according to the presence/mention of the following: random assignment; blind assessment; clear inclusion and exclusion criteria and sampling process; strong and reliable measures of substance use; sample size; follow-up duration of 6 months or longer; and statistical analysis using intent-to-treat, reporting between-group ESs for substance use disorder. Of the 19 included studies, 11 were considered to have effectiveness (three FBT, five MI, and the remaining integrating treatments such as CBT and MI). The effectiveness for the intervention was based on intra-group comparisons, mostly on ES at follow-up. For instance, in a study comparing Multidimensional Family Therapy (MDFT) versus CBT, an ES of 0.77 for substance frequency favoring MDFT intervention was reported (Liddle et al., 2009). In another study, considered not effective, MDFT was compared to individual CBT; the main outcome variable was self-reported delinquency and the ES was small (Hendriks et al., 2011). This review suggested some topics to improve adolescent substance abuse treatment, since despite the existence of effective interventions, only 7% of the adolescents in the United States meeting the diagnostic criteria for substance abuse receive specific treatment (U.S. Department of Mental Health, 2011). Thus, treatment delivery is an important issue. Some suggestions to make progress in this area are strategies like pursuing partnerships with influential governmental systems in order to achieve great market penetration and to use web-based technology (see Chapter 31 in this volume).

Despite the progress in more recent research, much more evidence is needed, such as longitudinal studies accounting for gene–environment interactions with treatment. For instance, an elegant study by Chung et al. (2014) evaluating 142 adolescents receiving substance use treatment found that the serotonin transporter linked polymorphic region (5-HTTLPR) genotype was associated with externalizing behaviors (S and $L_G > L_AL_A$), and externalizing behaviors predicted alcohol and marijuana problem severity at follow-up. This finding might have treatment implications. Adolescents with substance use disorder and with low-expressing (S and L_G) 5-HTTLPR alleles plus externalizing behavior could benefit from interventions targeting serotonergic functioning and externalizing behaviors, besides drug use–specific treatment. This article points toward integrative goals for further studies.

Also, some outcomes could be added in light of the current knowledge about drug use and its effects on the body. For instance, although most of the abused drugs have a systemic effect on body functions (de Jong et al., 2015; Spring et al., 2014), few studies include clinical data as participant description or as outcome measures, which is especially important for a population, such as adolescents, who are still in a growth period. It would be interesting to have clinical outcomes, like vascular or liver tests, besides infections, in these longitudinal studies, since drug addiction should be understood as a health issue.

Although residential and inpatient treatments warrant more research, focus on improving the effectiveness of outpatient services seems more promising, given that nearly 80% of adolescents with substance abuse at least initially receive outpatient treatment. In addition, outpatient services have many benefits (e.g., ability to characterize or dictate specific treatments, potential use of randomized designs, larger sample size).

Although few well-designed treatment evaluations of outpatient services exist, some of the most important large-scale studies involve primarily cannabis use and are summarized here. These multisite studies of existing practice generally defined minimal or no treatment as less than 90 days (13 weeks) of outpatient service, even though nearly 80% met that criteria. Changes in days of marijuana use were assessed in most of these studies, allowing some cross-study comparison. Among the 111 to 158 youths (under age 21) followed through the Drug Abuse Reporting Program (DARP; Sells & Simpson, 1979; Simpson et al., 1978) in the early 1970s, cannabis use rose from 3% to 10% in the 3 years following their discharge. Among the 87 adolescents receiving outpatient treatment in the Treatment Outcome Prospective Study (TOPS; Hubbard et al., 1985) in the early 1980s, the change in daily cannabis use from the year before to the year after treatment varied from a decrease of 42% (for those with less than 3 months of treatment) to an increase of 13% (for those with 3 or more months of treatment). Among the 156 adolescents receiving treatment (predominantly outpatient) in the Services Research Outcome Study during the late 1980s to early 1990s (SROS; OAS, 2000), cannabis use rose from 2% to 9% between the year before and the 5 years after treatment. Among the 236 adolescents in the National Treatment Improvement Evaluation Study (NTIES; CSAT, 1999; Gerstein, & Johnson, 1999) during the early 1990s, there was a 10% to 18% reduction in use between the year before and year after treatment. Among the 445 adolescents followed up after outpatient treatment in the Drug Abuse Treatment Outcome Study, Adolescents (DATOS-A; Grella et al., 2001; Hser et al., 2001) in the middle to late 1990s, there was a 21% to 25% reduction in cannabis use between the years before and after treatment. These findings are important, since cannabis is the most used illicit drug. However, a significant number of adolescents use more than one drug (polydrug users), usually alcohol, so evaluation in this context is strongly needed.

In recent decades, more outpatient follow-up studies became available, endorsing the idea that development-appropriate approaches are fundamental. One intervention is the Adolescent-Community Reinforcement Approach (A-CRA; Godley et al., 2001). A-CRA takes into account differences in adolescents' patterns of use, addresses life areas that are developmentally appropriate for adolescents, and adds procedures for working with parents/caregivers (Godley et al., 2001). An individually based standalone treatment intervention, A-CRA is generally delivered with 10 individual sessions for adolescents, two with caregivers alone, and two with adolescents and caregivers combined. It has been shown to be among the most effective and cost-effective approaches for the treatment of adolescent substance abuse (Dennis et al., 2004). The treatment also allows polydrug users. Data from 399 adolescents, from one of four RCTs of A-CRA, were used to examine the extent to which exposure to A-CRA procedures mediated the relationship between treatment retention and outcomes. Participants were primarily male (68%), Caucasian (65%), and 15 or 16 years of age (55%). With regard to alcohol and other drug use, 72% reported weekly use of any other drug at intake, with nearly all participants self-reporting DSM-IV criteria for abuse (30%) or dependence (64%) in the year prior to intake. The authors concluded that there was a significant relationship between treatment exposure and reductions in any other drug use and related problems (Bryan et al., 2009). Besides treatment exposure, therapeutic alliance also had an association with cannabis reduction in adolescents. In a longitudinal study

(12 months), patient-rated alliance predicted a reduction in cannabis use at 3 and 6 months and a reduction in substance-related problem behaviors at 6 months (Diamond et al., 2006).

Effectiveness of Specific Approaches: RCTs

RCTs are the gold standard for establishing the efficacy of a given approach, as they are the most rigorous approach that clinical investigators have for evaluating the effectiveness of a given treatment, in comparison with a well-defined control treatment, and while controlling for multiple threats to internal validity. While the number of well-designed controlled clinical trials of well-defined treatment approaches for substance-abusing adolescents is steadily increasing, the knowledge base regarding effective treatments continues to lag well behind that for adult substance use disorders. Drawing firm conclusions about treatment outcome and the relative benefits of different approaches is difficult, as few controlled clinical trials meet the rigorous standards required for determining that a treatment can be called "empirically supported" (Chambless, 1998). Many of the studies reviewed here are characterized by several threats to internal validity, including differential attrition, lack of validated independent outcome measures with objective evaluation of drug use, small sample sizes, lack of specification and evaluation of treatment fidelity and quality, dilution of interventions, and limited follow-up (Cottrell, 2002; Deas, 2001; Kaminer, 2002; Waldron, 1997). Thus, with only a few exceptions, caution must be used in drawing conclusions about the effectiveness of these approaches.

Becker and Curry (2008) conducted a literature review to assess the interventions for adolescent substance abuse. They rated each study (n = 31, published up to 2007) according to methodological issues: objective, sample size, power, outcome measures, sequence, allocation, active comparison, baseline measures, manualized treatment, treatment adherence, collateral report, objective measure, intention-to-treat analysis, treated case analysis, and blind assessment. From the 31 studies, just 16% had blind assessment of the outcome, indicating that this is a point that needs improvement. Eighty-one percent, on the other hand, had manualized interventions. FBT was the most frequently tested approach, with 22 models evaluated across 17 studies. "Brief motivational interventions" was the second most frequently investigated outpatient intervention, and three (out of four) methodologically stronger studies found good results for this modality. CBT was tested by four studies and was the intervention that was supported by the greatest proportion of methodologically stronger studies (100%). CBT models explicitly aimed to modify cognitive processes, beliefs, individual behaviors, or environmental reinforcers associated with the adolescent's substance use.

Since the need for developmentally appropriate approaches became a consensus, much effort has been engaged toward this goal. The release of the Cannabis Youth Treatment (CYT) interventions was a significant advance for better-designed research on adolescent treatment follow-up (Diamond et al., 2002). Briefly, these five manual-guided treatment models were (a) a 6-week intervention consisting of two sessions of individual motivational enhancement therapy (MET) plus three sessions of group CBT (MET/CBT5); (b) a 12-week intervention of two sessions of MET plus 10 sessions of group CBT (MET/CBT12); (c) a 12-week intervention consisting of MET/CBT12 plus the family support network (FSN), a multicomponent intervention that includes parent education, family therapy, and case management; (d) a 12-week intervention based on A-CRA; and (e) MDFT. Dennis et al. (2004) presented the main outcome findings from two interrelated randomized trials conducted at four sites (n = 600 cannabis users, age 15 or 16) to evaluate the effectiveness and cost-effectiveness of five short-term outpatient interventions for adolescents with cannabis use disorders according to CYT. The five CYT interventions demonstrated significant pre–post treatment effects after 12 months in two main outcomes: days of abstinence and the percentage of adolescents in recovery (no use or abuse/dependence problems and living in the community). The outcomes were similar across sites and conditions; however, after controlling for initial severity, the most cost-effective interventions were MET/CBT5 and MET/CBT12 in Trial 1 and A-CRA and MET/CBT5 in Trial 2 (Dennis et al., 2004). The MET/CBT5 (CYT) intervention (n = 174) was tested with community-based outpatient treatment among 323 adolescents with marijuana problems. The outcome measures, over 12 months, were substance use problems, substance use frequency, emotional problems, illegal activities, recovery, and institutionalization. Youth who received MET/CBT5 exhibited greater reductions in substance use frequency, substance use problems, and illegal behaviors 12 months after treatment entry than those who entered community-based outpatient programs (Ramchand et al., 2011).

Another approach, with a manual for outpatient adolescents with substance abuse, thus allowing clinical studies, is Assertive Continuing Care (ACC; Godley et al., 2006). ACC sessions are conducted either with the adolescent individually, the caregiver alone, or the two together. This format is in part dictated by the setting of the intervention: in the adolescent's home or community. ACC led to significantly greater continuing care linkage and retention and longer-term abstinence from marijuana in comparison to usual continuing care. ACC also resulted in better adherence to continuing care (Godley et al., 2007). An RCT including 320 adolescents evaluated the effectiveness and cost-effectiveness of two types of outpatient treatment, with and without ACC. Participants were randomly assigned to one of four conditions: (a) Chestnut's Bloomington Outpatient Treatment without ACC; (b) Chestnut's Bloomington Outpatient Treatment with ACC; (c) MET/CBT, seven-session model (MET/CBT7) without ACC; and (d) MET/CBT7 with ACC. Analysis of the costs of each intervention combined with its outcomes revealed that the most cost-effective condition was MET/CBT7 without ACC (Godley et al., 2010).

An RCT compared the efficacy of individual CBT and MDFT among 224 youth, primarily male (81%), from low-income single-parent homes (58%) with an average age of 15 years. The outcomes were substance use problem severity; 30-day frequency of cannabis use; 30-day frequency of alcohol use; 30-day frequency of other drug use; and 30-day abstinence. Both treatments produced significant decreases in cannabis use and slightly significant reductions in alcohol use, without differences in reducing the frequency of cannabis and alcohol use. Significant treatment effects were found favoring MDFT on substance use problem severity, among other outcomes. MDFT is notable for the sustainability of treatment effects (Liddle et al., 2008).

Another RCT allowed conclusions about treatment predictors. Hendriks et al. (2011) compared MDFT and CBT among 109 adolescents (13–18 years) and found that both approaches were equally effective in reducing cannabis use (ES = 0.14). In a secondary analysis of the trial data, there was an age-specific effect: older adolescents (17 or 18) benefited considerably more from CBT, and younger adolescents benefited considerably more from MDFT ($p < .01$). Similarly, adolescents with a past-year comorbid CD or ODD and those with internalizing problems achieved considerably better results in MDFT, while those without these coexisting psychiatric problems benefited much more from CBT ($p < .01$ and $p = .02$, respectively), again favoring the idea that MDFT is a good approach for more impaired youths (Hendriks et al., 2012).

Family and Multisystem Therapies

A key defining feature of family and multisystem approaches is that they treat adolescents in the context of the family and social systems in which substance use develops and may be maintained. Thus, inclusion of family members in treatment (often with the provision of home visits) is seen as a critical strategy for reducing attrition and addressing multiple issues simultaneously (Henggeler, 1996; Liddle, 2001). Because they are grounded solidly in the knowledge base on adolescence and development and thus are well suited to the specific problems of this population, family-based approaches have been among the most widely studied approaches for adolescents in controlled trials and also have, to date, the highest levels of empirical support (Deas, 2001; Liddle, 1995; Waldron, 1997):

> Reviews of formal clinical trials of family-based treatments have consistently found that more drug-abusing adolescents enter, engage in, and remain in family therapy than in other treatments and that family therapy produces significant reductions in substance use from pre- to post-treatment . . . in seven of eight studies comparing family therapy with a non-family-based intervention, adolescents receiving family therapy showed greater reductions in substance use than did those receiving adolescent group therapy, family education, and individual therapy, individual tracking through schools, or juvenile justice system interventions. (Waldron, 2001)

Moreover, the high level of support for family and multisystem approaches parallels findings from large meta-analyses pointing to the effectiveness of family therapies for adult substance users (Stanton, 1997). Family-based approaches are diverse, and many combine a variety of techniques, including family and individual therapies and skills and communication training, which may broaden the benefits of treatment by allowing greater individualization and enabling clinicians to address multiple factors in treatment (Waldron, 2001). The family-based approaches with the highest level of support with this population include Multisystemic Therapy (MST; Henggeler, 1990), Brief Strategic Family Therapy (BSFT; Szapocznik, 2012), and MDFT (Liddle, 2001).

MST is a manualized approach that addresses the multiple determinants of drug use and antisocial behavior. It is intended to promote fuller family involvement through engaging family members as collaborators in treatment, stressing the strength of the youth and their families, and addressing a broad and comprehensive array of barriers to attaining treatment goals. Therapists must be familiar with several empirically based therapies (including structural family therapy and CBT) and make frequent visits to the home and be available on a full-time basis to families. Henggeler et al. (1996) conducted a controlled trial with 118 substance-abusing or -dependent juvenile offenders (mean age 16) in which participants were randomly assigned to home-based MST and compared with usual community treatment services. The comparison condition involved referral by the youth's probation officer to outpatient adolescent group meetings. Ninety-eight percent of families completed a full course of treatment (an average of 130 days and 40 hours of service provision), compared with very little service access among the youth assigned to the control group (78% of youths received no substance abuse or mental health services, and only 5% received both substance use and mental health services). Other studies showed that MST reduced re-arrest rates by up to 64% and was associated with significantly lower rates of substance-related arrests (Henggeler, 1991, 1997). In a later study, the authors evaluated 80 of the 118 original participants for a 4-year follow-up. A multimethod assessment battery was used to measure the criminal behavior, illicit drug use, and psychiatric symptoms of the participating young adults. In this follow-up, there was a significant long-term treatment effect for aggressive criminal activity, and biological measures indicated higher rates of marijuana abstinence for MST participants (Henggeler et al., 2002).

BSFT (Szapocznik, 2012) is a somewhat less intensive approach (it targets fewer systems and can be delivered in a once-per-week office-based format) that has also achieved an impressive level of empirical support. BSFT targets patterns of interaction in the family system that have been shown to influence adolescent drug abuse and consists of three classes of interventions: engaging all family members in treatment, identifying family strengths as well as roles and relationships linked to adolescent problems, and developing new family interactions (e.g., improved parenting skills and conflict resolution) to protect the adolescent. Home visits and use of specific engagement strategies are encouraged. In a comparison of 126 drug-abusing adolescents and their families that compared BSFT to a group control condition, 75% of those assigned to BSFT showed reliable improvement and 56% could be classified as recovered. In the control condition, only 14% showed reliable improvement, while 43% showed reliable deterioration in marijuana use (Santisteban, 2003). BSFT has also been shown to be associated with improved retention (Santisteban, 1996; Szapocznik, 1988) as well as significant reductions in the frequency of externalizing behaviors (aggression, delinquency) (Szapocznik, 1986).

A multisite randomized trial was designed to evaluate the effectiveness of BSFT compared to treatment as usual as provided in community-based adolescent outpatient drug abuse programs. Family participants were 480 adolescents and their family members. The primary outcome was adolescent drug use, assessed monthly via adolescent self-report and urinalysis for up to 1 year after randomization. BSFT was significantly more effective than treatment as usual in engaging and retaining family members in treatment and in improving parent reports of family functioning (effect size [EF] = 0.4), but differences in adolescent drug use were weak (Robbins et al., 2011).

MDFT is a multicomponent, staged family therapy that targets substance-abusing adolescents, their families, and their interactions. Liddle et al. (2001) assigned 182 substance-abusing adolescents who were referred by the criminal justice system or the schools to either MDFT, group therapy, or multifamily education. Treatment was delivered in weekly sessions over 6 months, with roughly 70% of participants completing treatment across conditions. Superior outcomes for the adolescents assigned to MDFT relative to other approaches were seen at termination and 1-year follow-up. At termination, 42% of those assigned to MDFT, 25% of those in group therapy, and 32% of those in family education had clinically significant reductions in their drug use. Positive outcomes have also been reported for other models of family therapy, including Family System Therapy (Joanning, 1992) and Functional Family Therapy (Friedman, 1989).

Henderson et al. (2010) analyzed two clinical trials on the effectiveness of MDFT with higher-severity substance-abusing adolescents. The first study compared individually focused CBT and MDFT in a sample of 224 ethnic-minority youths (average age 15 years). The second compared a cross-systems version of MDFT with enhanced services as usual for 154 youths (average age 15 years) who were incarcerated. Results favored MDFT, especially in youths with more severe drug use and greater psychiatric comorbidity. It seems, in fact, that this approach is of special interest when dealing with externalizing symptoms among adolescents with drug use (Schaub et al., 2014). Like any other clinical trial, it is always important to evaluate the context in which the intervention is evaluated, especially regarding the comparison intervention (Treatment as usual, or other family therapy approach, or other individual/group technique). In this sense, Hendriks et al. (2011) investigated whether MDFT was more effective than CBT in treatment-seeking adolescents with a DSM-IV cannabis use disorder in the Netherlands. Sample size was 109 adolescents. MDFT was not superior to CBT in terms of cannabis use, delinquent behavior, treatment response, and recovery at 1-year follow-up. Treatment intensity and retention were significantly higher in MDFT than in CBT. Post hoc subgroup analyses suggested that subgroups with high problem severity at baseline may benefit more from MDFT than from CBT, again favoring the idea that the most severely affected adolescents might benefit from MDFT

Behavioral Therapies

A wide range of individual behavioral interventions, including those that seek to provide alternative reinforcers to drugs or reduce reinforcing aspects of abused substances, are based on operant conditioning theory and recognition of the reinforcing properties of abused substances (Aigner, 1978; Bigelow, 1984; Thompson, 1971). For adult substance users, these approaches have among the highest empirical support (Griffith, 2000; NIDA, 2000). Examples include the work of Stitzer et al., which has demonstrated that persons with methadone-maintained opioid addiction will reduce illicit drug use when incentives such as take-home methadone are offered for abstinence (Stitzer, 1978, 1992, 1993), as well as contingency management (CM) incentive systems (Higgins, 1991, 1999; Kirby, 1998; Petry, 2000; Silverman, 1996; Stanger & Budney, 2010), which offer incentives for targeted treatment goals (e.g., retention, drug-free urine samples) on an escalating schedule of reinforcement.

Behavioral approaches have begun to be evaluated among substance-abusing adolescents. Azrin et al. (1994) assigned 26 substance-using adolescents to supportive counseling or behavior therapy, which consisted of therapist modeling and rehearsal, self-monitoring, and written assignments. After 6 months, urine toxicology screens as well as self-reports suggested significantly less substance abuse among the group assigned to behavioral therapy relative to supportive counseling, as well as better school and family functioning.

CM has started to be evaluated in adolescents. In a feasibility study that involved adolescent smokers as a model for drug use, Corby et al. (2000) found that providing cash incentives to adolescents enrolled in a smoking cessation project for not smoking (as assessed by twice-daily carbon monoxide levels) reduced adolescent smoking and also appeared to improve their mood. In a pilot study involving young-adult marijuana users referred by the criminal justice system, Sinha et al. (Sinha, in press) studied the use of vouchers that could be used to purchase items in neighborhood stores. By providing these vouchers as rewards contingent on session attendance, treatment retention improved significantly. Kaminer et al. (2014) investigated the efficacy of a voucher-based reinforcement therapy rewarding drug-free urine samples for adolescents with cannabis use disorder. It was a controlled 10-week study (n = 59; age 14–18 years) in which adolescents were assigned into groups of either integrated CBT and voucher-based reinforcement or CBT with an attendance-based reward program. There was no difference for cannabis use either from sessions 1 to 10 or between end-of-treatment to 3-month follow-up. Good results with CM were achieved when adolescents in the experimental condition (plus CBT, vs. a group without the CM, but just CBT) participated in an abstinence-based CM program based on previous trials for adult marijuana dependence with modification (Stanger, Budney, Kamon, & Thostensen, 2009).

In another study, adolescents received incentives only if they provided a urine specimen and breath specimen that tested negative for *all* substances and parent and self-reports indicated no substance use (including alcohol). For each substance-negative specimen and report during weeks 3 to 14, participants earned vouchers starting at $1.50 and escalating by $1.50 with each consecutive negative specimen. A $10 bonus was earned for each two consecutive negative results. Vouchers were reset back to their initial value if results were positive. Voucher earnings were redeemed for retail goods selected by the teen (e.g., a movie pass). There were two groups, both with Motivational Enhancement and CBT, plus FBT. The experimental group received the above-mentioned intervention and earned a mean of $312 (SD = $237) or $22.28 per week. The control group could earn $5 vouchers twice per week (maximum earnings of $140; average actual earnings = $113). The experimental group had fewer positive urine specimens (ES = 0.48) (Stanger et al., 2009). Another recent study with CM in adolescents and cannabis use demonstrated the effectiveness of this approach (Stanger et al., 2015).

Cognitive-Behavioral Therapies

Cognitive-behavioral approaches, based on social learning theory, are among the approaches with highest levels of empirical support for the treatment of adult substance use disorders. Key defining features of most cognitive-behavioral approaches for substance use disorders are (1) an emphasis on functional analysis of drug use—that is, understanding instances of substance use with respect to their antecedents and consequences, and (2) emphasis on skills training and self-regulation. CBT has been shown to be effective across a wide range of substance use disorders (Carroll, 1996; Irvin, 1999), including alcohol dependence (Morgenstern, 2000; Miller, 2002), marijuana dependence (MTP Research Group, 2001; Stephens, 2000), cocaine dependence (Carroll, 1994, 1998; McKay, 1997; Rohsenow, 2000), and nicotine dependence (Fiore, 1994; Hall, 1998; Patten, 1998). These findings are consistent with evidence supporting the effectiveness of CBT across a number of other psychiatric disorders as well, including depression, ADs, and eating disorders (DeRubeis, 1998).

CBT has also been evaluated as a treatment for adolescent substance use disorders. In an extremely well-done study, Waldron et al. (Waldron, 2001) randomly assigned 120 adolescents who were abusers of illicit drugs (primarily marijuana) to one of four treatment conditions: family therapy alone (Functional Family Therapy), individual CBT alone, a combination of individual and family therapy, and a psychoeducational group. Completion rates were high (70%–80% across groups). In general, while there were meaningful reductions in drug use in all conditions, there were larger and more durable reductions in substance use for the combined and family conditions relative to the individual CBT and group conditions. Treatment effects were strongest immediately after treatment but persisted through a 7-month follow-up.

Kaminer et al. (Kaminer, 2002) compared group CBT to psychoeducational substance abuse treatment for 88 adolescents referred for treatment of a substance abuse problem. Eighty-six percent of the sample completed treatment and 9-month follow-up data were available for 65% of the sample. The presence of a CD was associated with treatment dropout. CBT was significantly more effective than the psychoeducational group only for male subjects; females appeared to improve regardless of treatment condition. Nevertheless, there were no significant differences between the two conditions at the 9-month follow-up. The relatively high rates of relapse in this sample (52% had a urinalysis that was positive for marijuana at the 9-month follow-up evaluation) suggest that an eight-session stand-alone approach may not be adequately intensive or structured for this population.

Since many CBT studies have an RCT design, some of them have already been addressed in this chapter (Dennis et al., 2004; Liddle et al., 2008; Ramchand et al., 2011). Cornelius et al. (2011) compared the long-term (2-year) efficacy of an acute-phase trial of CBT/MET versus naturalistic treatment among adolescents with both major depressive disorder and an alcohol use disorder who had signed consent for a treatment study involving fluoxetine and CBT/MET. Outcomes measures were levels of depressive symptoms and alcohol-related symptoms at a 2-year follow-up evaluation. CBT/MET demonstrated superior outcomes compared to those who had not received protocol CBT/MET therapy. No significant difference was noted between those receiving fluoxetine versus those receiving placebo on any outcome at any time point. Other pharmacological studies also included CBT, and sometimes one of the explanations for the lack of effect, or small pharmacological effect, seen in these adolescents with substance abuse is that receiving CBT reduced the ability to detect the effects of the pharmacological agent (Riggs et al., 2007; Cornelius et al., 2009).

Much attention has been given to meditation and mindfulness interventions, since they may enhance the individual skills of children and adolescents by helping them feel more relaxed, focused, and creative. There are different techniques, and one is closely related to CBT: mindfulness-based cognitive therapy (MBCT) (Simkin & Black, 2014). MBCT aims to relieve negative feelings by targeting negative thoughts or emotions (Gilpin, 2009). Up to now, few studies have evaluated MBCT in adolescents with substance abuse. One of the first studies in this field investigated how to effectively teach mindfulness to 10 incarcerated adolescent substance users in an urban California detention setting (Himelstein et al., 2014). In another study, with 1,051 students, mindfulness-based strategies toward impulsivity and positive and negative urgency were evaluated cross-sectionally. Mindfulness was associated with a lower likelihood of lifetime alcohol or marijuana use. Interactions between urgency and mindfulness were not supported

(Robinson et al., 2014). More studies in this field are recommended, especially because RCTs have demonstrated the effectiveness of diverse psychotherapeutic approaches (CBT, family, behavioral).

Motivational Approaches

Motivational approaches are brief treatment approaches that are designed to produce rapid, internally motivated change in addictive behavior and other problem behaviors. Grounded in principles of motivational psychology and patient-centered counseling, MI (Miller, 1991, 2002) arose out of several theoretical and empirical advances (Miller, 2000). MI has high levels of empirical support in the adult substance abuse treatment literature (Burke, 2003; Dunn, 2001; Miller, 2002; Wilk, 1997). The core principles of MI are as follows: (1) express empathy; (2) develop discrepancy; (3) avoid argumentation; (4) roll with resistance; and (5) support self-efficacy. MI makes the important assumption that ambivalence and fluctuating motivations define substance abuse recovery and need to be thoroughly explored rather than confronted harshly. Ambivalence is considered a normal event, not something that indicates the patient is unsuitable for treatment or needs vigorous confrontation in hopes of forcing a sudden change. The patient's point of view is respected, which in some cases may mean accepting that major change, or even any change, is not what the patient wants, at least at the present time (Carroll, in press). Thus, while the bulk of research on the efficacy of MI is in the adult literature, this nonconfrontational approach appears quite well suited for application to adolescents and young adults, given its flexibility around goals and recognition of abstinence as part of the change process.

Another distinct advantage of using MI with adolescent populations is that it can be implemented in a range of settings, given that adolescents with substance abuse problems rarely seek treatment of their own volition in traditional substance abuse settings. Monti et al. (1999) studied 94 adolescents treated at an emergency room for a problem related to alcohol use (e.g., injuries related to drinking, drunk driving). They were randomly assigned to MI or standard care, with all interventions and assessments conducted in the emergency room. At a 6-month follow-up, there were significantly fewer incidents of drunk driving, traffic violations, and alcohol-related problems in the group assigned to receive MI. Not only does this study suggest the promise of brief motivational approaches for this population, but it also underlines the importance of intervening with adolescents in nontraditional settings.

Kohler and Hofmann (2015), in a systematic review and meta-analysis, investigated the effect of MI delivered in a brief intervention during an emergency care contact on the alcohol consumption of young people who screen positively for risky alcohol consumption. Six trials with 1,433 participants, ages 13 to 25 years, were included. MI was never less efficacious than a control intervention. Two trials found significantly more reduction in one or more measures of alcohol consumption in the MI group. One trial indicated that MI may be used most effectively in young people with high-volume alcohol consumption. MI was effective in reducing the drinking quantity more than control interventions in a meta-analysis of the subset of trials that were implemented in the United States (standardized mean differences [SMD] = -0.12, $p = .04$). The authors concluded that MI is effective and possibly more effective than other brief interventions in emergency care to reduce alcohol consumption in young people. Similar results for alcohol consumption were not confirmed by a Cochrane Review, when studies selected were not limited to emergency department samples (Foxcroft et al., 2014).

MI was tested against brief advice for smoking cessation among adolescent (13–17 years old) smokers hospitalized for psychiatric and substance use disorders. After 12 months, there was no difference between groups regarding quit attempt. Given that MI was associated with greater increases in self-efficacy compared to brief advice, the authors examined whether self-efficacy at discharge was associated with better smoking outcomes when controlling for self-efficacy before treatment. In fact, there was an association between MI, better self-efficacy, and more abstinence (Brown et al., 2003).

Adolescents (n = 48) presenting for treatment intake assessments were randomized to MI (n = 22) or MI plus normative feedback (n = 26) (Smith et al., 2015). Three-month outcomes included the percentage of youth engaged in treatment, the percentage of youth reporting past-month binge drinking, and the percentage of days of abstinence. There were no differences between groups for abstinence rate. MI was also evaluated among adolescents with cannabis use, with positive results when considering, at the 3-month follow-up, number of days of cannabis use and negative consequences of drug use. Reductions in use and problems were sustained at 12 months (Walker et al., 2011).

Overall, MI seems a very interesting approach for adolescents and has been tested in different settings and with different drugs. More studies are recommended, especially to test its efficacy for polydrug use.

Disease Model Approaches

While disease model treatments and other approaches associated with the 12 steps of Alcoholics Anonymous dominate the treatment system for both adults and adolescents, there are no RCTs evaluating the effectiveness of these approaches in adolescents. Reports from RCTs evaluating the efficacy of manualized 12-step approaches have found evidence to suggest their effectiveness with adult substance users (Carroll, 1998; Crits-Christoph, 1999; Project MATCH Research Group, 1997). It is important to note, however, that these manual-guided approaches are highly structured, are delivered as individual (rather than group) therapy, and might be quite different from the nonmanualized group approaches typically delivered in community settings with adolescents. In addition, since individual drug counseling emphasizes and encourages frequent 12-step group attendance, its effectiveness might reflect increased patient involvement in rehabilitative groups. It is important to note that the absence of sufficient research on 12-step treatment should not lead one to conclude that this widespread and popular approach is ineffective; up to now, however, there are no data on those who are younger than 18 years.

Data on the effectiveness of more traditional programs are beginning to emerge, but no data from randomized trials comparing these approaches to alternatives are available. Winters et al. (Winters, 2000) reported on a large nonrandomized evaluation comparing a group of substance-abusing youth who completed the 12-step Minnesota Model Treatment to similar individuals who did not complete treatment and to a group on a waiting list for treatment. The treatment was multimodal, based on the principles of the 12 steps of Alcoholics Anonymous, and included group therapy and individual counseling, family therapy, lectures about the 12 steps, and reading assignments. Better substance-use outcomes and psychosocial outcomes at 6 and 12 months were reported for those who completed treatment compared with those who did not complete or who did not receive treatment. While a high rate of abstinence was reported among treatment completers, it is difficult to interpret these findings, given the self-selection due to lack of randomization and lack of measurement of treatment delivery or process.

Process Research and Mechanisms of Action

As new effective therapies for adolescents are identified, the field must move toward evaluating how these treatments exert their effects by looking at mediators and moderators of outcome. Several investigations have examined these variables. In terms of retention and engagement, Szapocznik's (1983) impressive work on engaging teens and families in treatment has been replicated and further developed (e.g., Coates et al., 2001; Santisteban et al., 1996). Henggeler (1996) demonstrated a 98% treatment completion rate for home-based MST. Henggeler has also demonstrated that adherence to the treatment was significantly associated with better treatment outcome. Liddle has conducted several process studies looking at mechanisms of change, including in-session patterns of change associated with the resolution of parent–adolescent conflict (G. S. Diamond & Liddle, 1996, 1996) and the link between improvement in parenting and better substance use outcome (Schmidt, Liddle, & Dakof, 1996). These kinds of studies will help identify key treatment ingredients hopefully leading to increased treatment potency.

The treatment process in Therapeutic Community (TC) is also a matter of interest. This psychotherapeutic technique emphasizes socioenvironmental and interpersonal influences in the resocialization and rehabilitation of the patient. The setting is usually a hospital unit or ward in which professional and nonprofessional staff interact with the patients. Five points have been considered in this setting: treatment motivation, personal development, problem recognition, family relations, and social network. Stucky et al. (2014) evaluated the validity of the short form of the Dimensions of Change in Therapeutic Communities Treatment Instrument-Adolescent (DCI-A; DCI-A-SF) by examining its associations with demographic and pretreatment characteristics as well as program completion status. The study sample consisted of 442 adolescents in residential treatment at one of seven TC treatment programs in the United States. The majority of participants were referred to treatment by the criminal justice system (62%). Other referral reasons included self/family (18%), social services (9%), transfer (6%), and referral by a medical professional (2%). At the time of the survey administration, 21.7% of respondents had been in treatment for 30 days or less, 19.2% for 31 to 60 days, 14.5% for 61 to 90 days, 29.9% for 91 to 180 days, and 14.7% for more than 180 days. In this study, DCI-A-SF demonstrated correlated with treatment outcomes. It might contribute to further studies on therapeutic process in TC for adolescents.

Assessment

Another area relevant to treatment research that may be influenced by the developmental perspective concerns assessment. While self-report of substance use by adolescents has been confirmed as fairly reliable (Buchan et al., 2002), analysis from the Cannabis Youth Treatment Study suggests that parent reports provide information not given by the adolescent. In terms of substance use symptoms, although adolescents and parents reported about the same number of symptoms, there was a very low concordance in terms of which symptoms were endorsed. Parents tended to report more symptoms related to role failure, tolerance, and substance-induced psychological problems (Dennis et al., 2002). Similar findings were discovered regarding mental health symptoms; specifically, parents tended to endorse more symptoms of depression and attention problems (Diamond et al., in press). This was particularly true for African-American adolescents, suggesting that parent report may have a unique contribution when working with a minority population, a community that has been characterized as suspicious of the research community.

Based on the authors' clinical experience, it seems that parents are good informants for reporting some conduct problems, such as staying out overnight, skipping medications, or school refusal. However, adolescent drug use is usually a hidden behavior, especially at the beginning of the disorder, or when moving toward a new drug (e.g., starts treatment due to alcohol abuse and, under treatment, starts on marijuana). By using the Adolescent Diagnostic Interview (ADI) in 109 adolescents (14–18 years), providers' impressions of adolescents' level of substance use were compared with the resultant diagnostic classifications. Of 50 participants who were classified with a diagnosis of alcohol or drug abuse, providers correctly identified only 10. These data confirm the idea that parents underestimate adolescents' alcohol/drug involvement. According to the Practice Parameter for the Assessment and Treatment of Children and Adolescents with Substance Use Disorders (Bukstein et al., 2005), toxicology tests of bodily fluids should be part of the evaluation and the ongoing assessment of substance use in adolescents. It is important to establish rules regarding the confidentiality of the results before testing, since maintaining the therapeutic alliance is always a matter of concern.

The Challenge of Comorbidity

One area that has received strikingly little research with adolescents is the integration of substance use and other mental health services that can treat adolescents with both kinds of disorders. Historically there has been a divide between treatment systems for substance abuse and mental health disorders, where substance abuse counselors often have little or no training in mental health issues and programs either ignore co-occurring problems or refer patients to other systems during (parallel) or after (sequential) substance abuse treatment. There is emerging consensus that lack of integration leads to poor coordination of services, interagency miscommunication, and funding conflicts that contribute to attrition and poor outcomes for patients (Osher & Drake, 1996; Report to Congress, 2003). This is particularly troubling since co-occurring mental health distress is associated with more severe substance use, greater psychosocial impairment, treatment resistance, and poorer long-term prognosis (Diamond et al., 2005; Drake et al., 1996; Shane et al., 2006). Consequently, the most severe and chronic patients often receive the poorest care, leading to repeated visits to hospital emergency rooms and inpatient and residential facilities (Richardson et al., 1995). The end result is that patients with comorbidities in need of care are consuming a major portion of treatment funding (Ridgely et al.,1990).

The gap between substance abuse and mental health dates back to the 1930s (Rosenthal & Westreich, 1999). At that time, psychodynamic therapists, who dominated the treatment world, believed that persons with substance use disorder had a personality structure that was not amenable to the analytic method, and therefore were not treatable. This attitude may persist today in the mental health community, who tend to view addiction as inhibiting treatment of other "underlying" problems (Blanchard, 2000). Simultaneously, the self-help movement developed independent of the mental health community, and as the self-help philosophies and programs matured, educational and professional licensure pathways emerged that legitimized and strengthened these approaches (Rosenthal et al., 1999). As often happens, then, these ideological differences became institutionalized and perpetuated a division that does not reflect the clinical realities of patients.

Recognition of this schism has inspired many attempts to integrate substance abuse and mental health treatment programs for adult dual-diagnosis populations (Drake et al., 1993; Lehman & Dixon, 1995; Miller, 1994; Minkoff & Drake, 199; Ziedonis & Fisher, 1994). At least 36 studies have evaluated different versions of integrated programs, at all levels of care (e.g., outpatient, day treatment, inpatient, residential). Some studies added a substance abuse group to outpatient mental health services, resulting in reduced dropout, decreased hospitalization, and increased abstinence (e.g., Hellerstein, 1995; Kofoed et al., 1989). Studies that combine substance abuse services with inpatient, day treatment, and residential care have also shown some benefits as long as patients remained in the program. Unfortunately, attrition rates were often high and, once discharged, relapse rates were high as well (e.g., Rahay et al., 1995).

A major contribution to this area was the 1987 funding of 13 dual-diagnosis demonstration projects (National Institute of Mental Health, 1989). These studies demonstrated that integrated programs could be implemented in a number of settings, resulting in increased engagement and services utilization and reduced drug use. Another five studies were conducted on comprehensive integrated systems using more sophisticated treatment programs and quasi- or true experimental designs (e.g., Drake et al., 1997, 1998; Godley,1994; Jerrell & Ridgely, 1995; Ridgely & Jerrell, 1996). These studies showed significant reductions in substance use, program readmission, and hospital admission, and improvement in other functional outcomes (Drake et al., 1998). However, there has been little or no comparable research on the effectiveness of integrated programs for adolescent substance users.

In a multicenter study, 992 adolescents were evaluated considering the presence of some comorbidity (positive in 64% of the sample). The presence of comorbidity was associated with more severe pretreatment condition and poorer outcomes, such as more use of marijuana and hallucinogens and engaging in illegal acts in the 12 months after treatment (Grella et al., 2001).

A review of the literature was conducted to evaluate the effects of comorbid depression on treatment retention and outcomes across 13 adolescent substance use treatment studies. Depression had a mixed relationship with treatment retention and other outcomes, depending on aspects of the study: it could increase or decrease retention (Hersh et al., 2014).

Evaluation of Inpatient/Residential Approaches

As stated by the American Society of Addiction Medicine (2001), intensive inpatient treatment might be appropriate for adolescents whose substance use, biomedical, and emotional problems are so severe that they require 24-hour primary medical care. The length of the intervention should depend on the adolescent's progress. Usually, there are few possibilities, up to now not well studied, ranging from inpatient treatment for detoxification inside general or psychiatric hospitals, to residential programs. Tripodi (2009) reviewed eight studies regarding the effectiveness of residential treatment centers for substance-abusing adolescents, and only three of them used a strong quasi-experimental design. Of the four most rigorous studies reviewed, two found significant differences in substance use reduction between the treatment and comparison groups. In other words, there are important methodological flaws and a small number of studies, limiting more robust conclusions on their long-term effectiveness. However, based on clinical experience, this is an important resource when dealing with risky situations. More studies are needed, since it is a reality in clinical practice.

Summary of Psychosocial Treatment

Clinical research during the past 20 years has identified a number of effective treatments for adolescent substance users. Although the field is still young, this growing body of work has yielded several important findings that support the effectiveness of carefully implemented, structured behavioral approaches for adolescent substance use (Liddle & Rowe, 2001; Stanton & Shaddish, 1997; Williams, 2000). These can be summarized as follows:

- Despite the progress, the field has been inadequately studied.
- Most studies indicate that treatment can be effective for most adolescents. In the bulk of studies, well-defined structured approaches tend to be more effective and durable in reducing adolescent substance use and improving related problems than no treatment, treatment as usual, or other comparison approaches. Treatments that focus on broad aspects of functioning seem to be most promising (Williams et al., 2000). That is, interventions should, in addition to addressing substance use, target domains such as family functioning, school success, delinquency, peer group associations, and other risky behaviors. Confrontational approaches are not recommended.
- Adolescents who complete treatment tend to have the best outcomes, although this may be related to factors such as higher motivation for treatment, better or more intact family/social supports, less severe substance use, better school competency, and less psychopathology, all of which are associated with more treatment success.
- In general, including family members improves retention and outcome among substance-using adolescents. To date, there is no evidence from controlled studies that involvement of family members in treatment has a negative effect on outcome. In the studies of family-based therapy reviewed here, retention rates were generally high (70%–80% range), and retention is often sustained over comparatively long periods. At least two studies have demonstrated that outpatient family therapy was more effective and less

costly than residential placement (Liddle & Dakof, 2000; Schoenwald et al., 1996). Finally, long-term effectiveness of family-based models has also gained some empirical support (Henggler et al., 1998; Stanton & Shadish, 1997). MDFT seems a good choice for more severely impaired adolescents, especially in the presence of externalizing symptoms.

- Behavioral therapies, especially those that target multiple systems, also appear to have some promise. CM approaches have started to be evaluated, with potentially good results. However, CM in adolescents has been, up to now, limited to cannabis users. CM approaches might be used, for example, to target retention, to encourage patients to meet specific treatment goals (e.g., reducing truancy and improving school performance), or to enhance compliance with pharmacotherapies (Carroll, 2003). The literature indicates that adults with antisocial personality disorders respond relatively well to CM approaches (Messina, 2003). In view of the high rates of conduct/externalizing disorders among substance-abusing adolescents, further evaluation of CM approaches with this population is still warranted.
- Cognitive-behavioral approaches are well established and have been often used together with MI. CBT has generally been delivered to adolescents in a group format and for a comparatively brief period. It has also been used as an intervention to be compared against medication in pharmacological studies. Longer or more intensive CBT approaches, or delivery of CBT as an individual treatment, may be necessary with this population. Mindfulness in adolescents with substance abuse needs better evaluation.
- The data suggesting that some deviant, high-risk adolescents may escalate problem behavior in the contexts of interventions delivered in peer groups (Dishion, 1999) have important implications for behavioral treatments of substance-using youth. While poor outcomes for group approaches for adolescents have not uniformly been reported in the studies reviewed here, it is clearly important to be aware of this possibility when group approaches are used, to monitor behavior closely, and to involve adults and parents as well.

PHARMACOLOGICAL TREATMENTS

Pharmacotherapy for substance dependence is a relatively young field of medicine, and the proven treatments for adults have not been adequately researched in adolescents. Therefore, few conclusions regarding this modality can be stated conclusively at this time. However, the actual usage of pharmacotherapy for psychiatric syndromes has been steadily increasing among adolescents and children, despite lack of data. Prescribing for these young patients between 1987 and 1996 rose 300% overall (Magno Zito, 2003). By 1996 stimulants and antidepressants were ranked first and second in terms of total prescriptions. These two medications also had the greatest increase in prescribing (400% each): stimulant prescribing rose from 10 per 1,000 youth to 40 per 1,000 youth, and antidepressants rose from 3 per 1,000 to 13 per 1,000.

Regarding prescription patterns of antipsychotic use among patients aged 1 to 24 in the United States based on calendar years 2006 (n = 765,829), 2008 (n = 858,216), and 2010 (n = 851,874), the percentages of young people using antipsychotics in 2006 and 2010, respectively, were 1.10% and 1.19% for adolescents and 0.69% and 0.84% for young adults. The authors concluded that antipsychotic use increased from 2006 to 2010 for adolescents and young adults, especially among boys (Olfson, King, & Schoenbaum, 2015). Comer, Olfson, and Mojtabai (2010) examined the patterns and trends in multiclass psychotropic treatment among youth visits to office-based physicians in the United States from 1996 to 2007. There was an increase in the percentage of child visits in which psychotropic medications were prescribed that included at least two psychotropic classes. Across the 12-year period, multiclass psychotropic treatment rose from 14.3% of child psychotropic visits (1996–1999) to 20.2% (2004–2007). In the presence of a current mental disorder, the percentage of multiclass psychotropic treatment increased from 22.2% (1996–1999) to 32.2% (2004–2007). Over time, there were significant increases in multiclass psychotropic visits in which ADHD medications, antidepressants, or antipsychotics were prescribed, and a decrease in those visits in which mood stabilizers were prescribed. Specific increases were found for co-prescription of ADHD and antipsychotic medications (adjusted odds ratio [AOR] = 6.22, 95% CI 2.82–13.70, $p < .001$) and for co-prescription of antidepressant and antipsychotic medications (AOR = 5.77, 95% CI 2.88–11.60, $p < .001$).

In a cross-sectional survey in United States, the prevalence of specific classes of psychotropic medications indicated for mental disorders was evaluated between February 2001 and January 2004. Participants were adolescents ages 13 to 18 years who participated in the National Comorbidity Survey Adolescent Supplement (n = 9,244; response rate 74.7%). Among adolescents with substance use disorder based on DSM-IV criteria (n = 854), 9.2% were on antidepressants, 4.1% on stimulants, 1.1% on antipsychotics, 1.0% on mood stabilizers, 2.7% on anxiolytics, and 14.4% on any medication (Merikangas et al., 2013).

This last publication corroborates the association of behavioral problems and substance use disorders in adolescents, since adolescents who abuse drugs and have substance use disorders typically have deviant behavior, skills deficits, academic difficulties, family problems, and mental health problems (Peeters et al., 2014; Rao, 2006; Ridenour et al., 2013; Tarter, 2002; Tims, 2002). While these problems usually reflect more than neurochemical defects that may be reversed with medications, adolescents with substance dependence and comorbid psychiatric disorders can benefit from pharmacotherapy, but pharmacotherapy should be justified by careful evaluations of the diagnoses in these young patients. These medical and psychiatric evaluations can be informed by structured interviews for common comorbid disorders such as depression and bipolar disorders, ADHD, and substance dependence. Medical disorders including infections, endocrine problems, and various developmental disorders also need consideration but are beyond the scope of this review. However, based on Merikangas et al. (2013), comorbidity may not be as treated as it should, perhaps reflecting the lack of studies in this area, or even the lack of positive results, as will be reviewed

Adolescents who enter substance abuse treatment programs are more likely than non-drug-abusing peers to have experienced abuse or neglect, to have significant family problems, and to have developed a psychiatric disorder during childhood such as ADHD and mood disorder. These behavioral, psychosocial, and mental health problems are coupled with the neurohormonal changes of puberty and lead to poor adjustment in the school environment, thereby increasing the risk for school failure (Riggs, 1999; Tarter, 2002). These school experiences also may lead to the early onset of substance abuse (Crowley, 1995; Rutter, 1998). Substance abuse exacerbates preexisting psychiatric disorders such as ADHD, as well as mood disorders and AD (Kruesi, 1990; Markou, 1998; Rutter, 1998).

The multidimensionality of the problems that substance-abusing youth typically bring to treatment underscores their need for multimodal treatment that addresses a broad range of mental health and psychosocial problems integrated with treatment for drug abuse. The role of pharmacotherapy targeted specifically to substance abuse may therefore be relatively limited, and there is no research base to provide guidance on the dosing or duration of treatment for adolescents with dependence on alcohol, nicotine, opiates, or other addictions for which we have pharmacotherapies. Furthermore, the other most commonly abused drug—cannabis—has no specific pharmacotherapy. Pharmacotherapies are also entirely lacking for "club drugs" such as MDMA, GHB, and various hallucinogens.

Specific Pharmacotherapy for Substance Use Disorders in Adolescents

Given the clinical importance of drug euphoria and drug craving, most pharmacological strategies for addiction target these primary reinforcers. Drug-induced reward is attenuated in animal models by a number of agents, depending on the drug in question. These medications act on dopamine, opioid, glutamate, or GABA systems. These reward-blocking medications have been tested in human substance abusers to determine whether they reduce drug euphoria under controlled settings, or promote abstinence in clinical trials. Other means of reducing reward have also been tested, including vaccines that block the entry of an addictive substance into the brain, and agents like disulfiram that produce aversive symptoms when alcohol is consumed. In addition to strategies that reduce drug euphoria, strategies that reduce craving have also been tested and prescribed. Agonist treatment (prescribing a substance that replaces the addictive drug) has been used in opioid (e.g., methadone, buprenorphine) and nicotine (e.g., nicotine gum) dependence with considerable success, providing a means of bypassing dangerous routes of administration or hazards associated with drug procurement. Reversing clinically relevant neuroadaptations associated with chronic exposure to addictive substances has the theoretical ability to reduce craving and other aversive aspects of addiction.

Unfortunately, there has been little research directed toward the pharmacological treatment of substance dependence in adolescents. For a number of reasons, there are not enough controlled trials evaluating the effectiveness of substitution/replacement therapies (e.g., methadone, buprenorphine), antagonists (e.g., naltrexone), aversive therapies (e.g., disulfiram), or anticraving medications (e.g., bupropion, naltrexone) in this subpopulation. Therefore, if such medications are used in adolescents, they must be used with caution, careful monitoring, and consideration of the developmental characteristics that distinguish adult patients from adolescents (e.g., greater impulsivity and polydrug use) (Solhkhah, 1998). More research is clearly needed in this area. In most of the available controlled trials, strength of the therapeutic benefit (number needed to treat) is lacking.

Since the most commonly abused substances by adolescents are nicotine, alcohol, and cannabis, these are the most likely drugs for which pharmacotherapy questions might arise. A few specific relapse-prevention pharmacotherapies are approved by the U.S. Food and Drug Administration (FDA) for nicotine and alcohol dependence in adults, and some of them have started to be evaluated in adolescents in the past decade. For nicotine the medications are nicotine replacement, bupropion, and varenicline, and for alcohol the medications are disulfiram, naltrexone, and acamprosate. We will review these medications briefly, starting with those used in detoxification. Advances in our understanding of the mechanisms of drug craving and drug-induced euphoria should guide future research and shed light on more effective pharmacological treatments for addiction in adolescents.

Detoxification

Medical detoxification is required for alcohol, sedatives, and opiates but not for other abused drugs. In adolescents with alcohol use disorder, withdrawal symptoms occur in only between 5% and 10% of cases (Chung et al., 2002; Langenbucher et al., 2000), and only a small percentage will require pharmacotherapy. Detoxification from alcohol dependence can be effectively attained in adults by using benzodiazepines or barbiturates and anticonvulsants such as valproate and carbamazepine to block or reverse withdrawal symptoms (Kosten, 2003). These medications have not been tested in adolescents with withdrawal symptoms, but detoxification medications should be used in adolescents if withdrawal symptoms are significant, particularly because alcohol withdrawal is potentially life-threatening. Since the combination of alcohol and benzodiazepines is potentially lethal, this approach should only be undertaken in supervised settings (Clarck, 2012).

Detoxification from sedative-hypnotic dependence can be accomplished by prescribing descending doses of benzodiazepines. However, there is currently no approved pharmacotherapy for benzodiazepine use disorder treatment even in adults (Sabioni, Bertram, & Le Foll, 2015).

For opioid dependence, the most common means of detoxification involves prescribing descending doses of methadone for a period of 2 to 4 days while carefully monitoring the patient's response. Methadone is a long-acting opioid agonist that reverses heroin withdrawal by replacing heroin at the opioid receptor. Since methadone has the potential to cause lethal opioid overdose, and opioid withdrawal is not medically dangerous, it is imperative to avoid prescribing an excessive dose of methadone to adolescents. The appropriate dose is best selected by closely monitoring the signs of opioid withdrawal, which should be given more weight than reported symptoms that might be exaggerated or feigned by drug-seeking patients.

A new treatment for detoxification and maintenance was made available in the United States in 2003. This is buprenorphine, a partial μ-opioid receptor agonist. It may be ideally suited to adolescents and is currently in clinical trials in this population. Detoxification with this medication is simple because overdose is almost impossible. The patient can be transferred from the opiate of abuse to buprenorphine, and then the dose is gradually reduced with minimal or absent withdrawal symptoms. Yet another option is the nonopioid clonidine, an antihypertensive medication that blocks many of the opiate withdrawal symptoms (Gold, 1984). Most patients prefer methadone or buprenorphine because of greater comfort. However, up to now, neither methadone nor buprenorphine has been sufficiently evaluated in adolescents.

One of the first studies on adolescent opioid detoxification tested buprenorphine versus clonidine. A significantly greater percentage of adolescents who received buprenorphine stayed in treatment (72%) relative to those who received clonidine (39%) (Marsch et al., 2005). Later, a naturalistic study, conducted in Dublin by Smyth et al. (2012), described the detoxification process safely used in 100 adolescents with opioid dependence (mean age 16.6 years). Induction onto methadone started with a dose of 20 mg, increasing by 10 mg every 2 to 4 days, titrated against withdrawal symptoms, cravings, and ongoing heroin use while also monitoring for evidence of sedation. Stabilization doses were generally between 40 and 70 mg. For buprenorphine, induction usually involved provision of 2 mg during the morning of day 1, with a further 2 to 6 mg later that afternoon. Single daily doses of up to 8 to12 mg were administered from day 2. Stabilization doses were typically in the region of 6 to 12 mg. There were no deaths during treatment among these 100 patients.

Recently, Minozzi et al. (2014a, 2014b) assessed the effectiveness of any opioid detoxification treatment alone or in combination with psychosocial intervention compared with no intervention, other pharmacological intervention, or psychosocial interventions on completion of treatment, reducing the use of substances, and improving health and social status. Two trials involving 190 participants were included in this study. One trial compared buprenorphine with clonidine for detoxification. No difference was found in terms of the dropout rate, and more participants in the buprenorphine group initiated naltrexone treatment. The other trial compared maintenance treatment (buprenorphine/naloxone) versus detoxification (buprenorphine) treatment: in terms of the dropout rate, the results were in favor of buprenorphine/naloxone. In this Cochrane Review, the authors emphasized that it is difficult to draw conclusions on the basis of only two trials and a small sample size. Furthermore, the two studies included did not consider the efficacy of methadone. Thus, there is a need for more studies on adolescent opioid detoxification.

Despite the benefits of pharmacological approaches in the detoxification process, inpatient detoxification treatment should not be restricted merely to the medical management of heroin withdrawal. This intensive intervention provides the physician with an ideal opportunity to establish a therapeutic alliance with adolescent patients by concomitantly addressing the critical treatment issues of honesty, openness, trust, denial, and engagement. Inpatient detoxification also provides an opportunity to fully evaluate patients, assess their readiness for change, and provide critical family therapy. Since families require education, support, and guidance throughout the process, clinicians should be familiar with the psychosocial as well as medical aspects of heroin addiction. It is essential to emphasize that detoxification, in and by itself, is not sufficient treatment for heroin dependence and must therefore be followed by ongoing outpatient drug rehabilitation. The recent fad of very rapid detoxification using general anesthesia has not been shown to produce better outcomes than standard detoxification.

Because detoxification in and by itself is usually insufficient treatment for addiction, medications for relapse prevention are more likely to be useful in promoting abstinence. However, before medicating adolescents, it is imperative to determine that they will be cooperative, that parental consent has been obtained, and that the adolescents and parents have the same understanding of treatment goals and approaches.

Relapse Prevention

The nature of addiction requires that complete abstinence be the treatment goal for addicted adolescents rather than the mere reduction of drug and alcohol use. Indeed, even the use of other addictive agents, such as alcohol by a cocaine-dependent adolescent, often leads to relapse to the drug of choice. Thus, total abstinence from all addicting drugs should be the goal when treating adolescents. Furthermore, since both alcohol purchase and illicit drug use are illegal activities in adolescents, it is hard to argue with a goal of total abstinence. After attaining abstinence, preventing relapse to drug dependence is the primary clinical target in adolescents. The following sections review proven treatments for both initiation of abstinence and relapse prevention for nicotine, alcohol, and opiates.

Smoking Cessation

Despite the prevalence of adolescent tobacco use and nicotine dependence, there have been relatively fewer studies that evaluate adolescent smoking treatment programs. The settings for and approaches to the treatment of adolescent tobacco use are similar to those described for adolescent smoking prevention, with the addition of pharmacological approaches. However, the challenges inherent in adolescent smoking treatment appear to be greater than those for prevention. Another challenge is the role of comorbidity in adolescent nicotine dependence (Goodwin et al., 2014). Recruitment to adolescent smoking treatment programs is difficult, in part because of adolescents' desires to keep their smoking practices confidential. Moreover, among those adolescents who enroll in treatment programs, attrition rates are very high (Mermelstein, 2003).

For the most part, available data on the effectiveness of adolescent smoking treatment have been disappointing. Quit rates for adolescents receiving behavioral smoking cessation treatment are roughly 10% to 15%, compared with 5% to 10% in control conditions (Pomerleau, 1998). The results of pharmacological trials using nicotine replacement therapy (e.g., nicotine patch) have also been disappointing, yielding 6-month quit rates of only 5% (Hurt, 2000; Smith, 1996). While not yet thoroughly investigated, interventions delivered by pediatricians and family physicians may have great promise for assisting youth to quit smoking (Pbert, 2003). E-cigarette use in adolescents is also a matter of interest. It is not clear, up to now, if it might have a protective or a harmful effect, for instance (Rennie, Bazillier-Bruneau, & Rouëssé, 2016; Kinnunen et al., 2015; Schneider & Diehl, 2015; Glasser et al., 2017). Adolescents with comorbid psychiatric conditions are an important target group for treatment, given their greater predisposition to tobacco use (Dune et al., 2014; Moolchan, 2000). The prevalence of anxiety disorders and dysthymia among current smokers appears to have increased from 1990 to 2001. Tobacco cessation interventions should address comorbidities as well, and attention should be paid to this trend in the increase of comorbidity among smokers (Goodwin et al., 2014).

Medications for Smoking Cessation

Nicotine replacement therapy (NRT), varenicline (a partial agonist at the nicotinic receptors) and bupropion (a nicotinic acetylcholine-receptor antagonist that is a dopamine and norepinephrine reuptake inhibitor) are FDA-approved smoking cessation medications for adult smokers. Their role in the adolescent population needs more evidence.

It is unclear if the interventions that are effective for adults can also help adolescents to quit. The forms of NRT include patches, gum, inhalers (oral absorptions), nasal spray, and lozenges (McCance, 1998). NRT might be a reasonable treatment for adolescents who want to quit smoking and are experiencing acute withdrawal symptoms that interfere with abstinence.

A Cochrane Review on tobacco cessation interventions for young people included 28 trials, with 6,000 adolescents (both pharmacological and psychotherapy, together or separately). A small trial testing NRT did not detect a statistically significant effect. Two trials of bupropion, one testing two doses and one testing it as an adjunct to NRT, did not detect significant effects (Stanton & Grimshaw, 2013). Despite the few trials included in this review, there was no evidence for pharmacological interventions (NRT and bupropion) for adolescent smokers.

Scherphof et al. (2014a) conducted a randomized, double-blind, placebo-controlled trial in 257 adolescents (mean age 16.7 years); 136 received NRT and 129 received placebo. The duration was 6 to 9 weeks of treatment. In the NRT group, participants smoking more than 20 cigarettes per day received a higher transdermal nicotine patch dose (3 weeks 21 mg/day, 3 weeks 14 mg/day, and 3 weeks 7 mg/day) to use daily for 9 weeks; those who smoked less than 20 cigarettes per day received a lower dose (3 weeks 14 mg/day and 3 weeks 7 mg/day) to use daily for 6 weeks. Intent-to-treat analyses showed that independent of compliance, NRT was effective in promoting abstinence rates after 2 weeks (OR = 2.02, 95% CI 1.11–3.69) but not end-of-treatment abstinence. However, end-of-treatment abstinence rates were significantly increased in highly compliant participants (OR = 1.09, 95% CI 1.01–1.17) but not in low-compliant ones. The authors tested NRT's long-term effectiveness in the same sample of adolescents, concluding that NRT fails to help patients to quit smoking at 6- and 12-month follow-ups (Scherphof et al., 2014b).

The safety and efficacy of sustained-release bupropion hydrochloride for adolescent smoking cessation was evaluated by and prospective, randomized, double-blind, placebo-controlled, dose-ranging trial. Adolescents (aged from 14–17 years, n = 312), received sustained-release bupropion hydrochloride, 150 mg/d (n = 105) or 300 mg/d (n = 104), or placebo (n = 103) for 6 weeks, plus weekly brief individual counseling for 12 weeks and then 26 weeks. There was a difference, in terms of nicotine abstinence, between placebo and medication at 300 mg (6 weeks: 5.6% vs. 14.5%, p = 0.03; 26 weeks: 10.3% for placebo and 13.9% for bupropion, p = 0.049) (Muramoto et al., 2007). Gray et al. (2011) studied the effects of bupropion for smoking cessation. The study had four arms: bupropion SR alone; bupropion SR + contingency management (CM); Placebo + CM, or just placebo. Combined bupropion SR and CM was efficacious in the short term, and more effective than other study arms (Gray et al., 2011). Varenicline also needs more clinical trials in adolescents. The multiple-dose pharmacokinetics, safety, and tolerability of varenicline in adolescent smokers was tested by Faessel and colleagues (2009). Varenicline was generally well tolerated during the 14-day treatment period. Later, varenicline (n = 15) was compared to bupropion XL (n = 14) in a randomized double-blind study with adolescents (age from 15–20 years). Participants receiving varenicline reduced from 14.1 ± 6.3 to 0.9 ± 2.1 cigarettes/day (CPD), and four participants achieved abstinence, without adverse-event-related discontinuation from the study. In the bupropion XL group, participants reduced from 15.8 ± 4.4 to 3.1 ± 4.0 CPD (two achieved abstinence; two discontinued the study due to adverse events) (Gray et al., 2012).

Discussion has considered vaccines for nicotine dependence (Kosten, 2002; Fahim et al., 2011). These immunotherapies can attenuate the rewarding effects of nicotine and have been considered as a potential prophylactic for preventing nicotine dependence. Immunotherapies might also be used as a secondary prevention for adolescents who have begun to smoke (Kosten, 2002). However, this type of invasive and long-lasting intervention has potential ethical problems, particularly in adolescents who do not want to stop smoking (Feldman, 2013; Lieber & Millum, 2013).

Alcohol Abuse and Alcoholism in Adolescents

One of the actions of alcohol in the body is to release endogenous opioids. Thus, a drug such as naltrexone that blocks opiate receptors will reduce the reward of alcohol and help to prevent relapse. The majority of controlled studies in adults have shown that naltrexone increases abstinence. Although there are case reports in adolescents (Lifrak et al., 1997), we were able to identify only one controlled study of naltrexone in adolescents with alcohol use disorder. Side effects of naltrexone in adults have generally been minimal at usual doses. Naltrexone also has substantial hormonal effects that include raising cortisol and various sex hormone levels (e.g., luteinizing hormone), and these actions could interfere with growth and development in adolescents (Morgan, 1990). Miranda et al. (2014) conducted a randomized, double-blind, placebo-controlled crossover study comparing naltrexone (50 mg/daily) and placebo in 22 adolescents with drinking problems (mean age 18.36 years, SD = 0.95; 12 were women). The primary outcome measures were alcohol use, subjective responses to alcohol consumption, and alcohol-cue-elicited craving. In this study, naltrexone significantly reduced the likelihood of drinking and heavy drinking (p's ≤ .03), reduced craving in the laboratory and in the natural environment (p's ≤ .04), and altered subjective responses to alcohol consumption (p's ≤ .01). The only ES mentioned in this study was related to the naltrexone-reduced likelihood of drinking on a study day (OR = 0.69, 95% CI 0.50–0.97, p = .03, ES d = 0.17 [a small ES]). The medication was well tolerated by the research subjects. The comparison of adverse events between placebo and naltrexone groups became nonsignificant in all analyses, considering neurocognitive, gastrointestinal, and ear, nose, and throat symptoms. These results encourage larger clinical trials with long-term follow-up.

Disulfiram promotes abstinence by blocking the metabolism of alcohol, resulting in the production of acetaldehyde, a noxious compound. It can produce severe reactions when mixed with alcohol, including death, and there is significant risk associated with prescribing this medication to impulsive adolescent alcohol abusers. Thus, disulfiram is rarely used for younger patients. We could identify only one study of disulfiram use in adolescents with alcohol use disorder (Niederhofer & Staffen, 2003a); its efficacy and long-term safety were evaluated in a double-blind, placebo-controlled study (n = 26, ages 16–19 years). Patients were randomly allocated to treatment with disulfiram (200 mg/day) or placebo for 90 days. At the end of treatment, seven disulfiram-treated and two placebo-treated patients had been abstinent continuously (p = .0063). Mean cumulative abstinence duration was significantly greater in the disulfiram group than in the placebo group (68.5 vs. 29.7 days; p = .012). In this pioneering study, the authors concluded that in some cases, disulfiram may be an effective and well-tolerated pharmacological adjunct to psychosocial and behavioral interventions for adolescents with alcohol use disorder.

Other medications such as acamprosate and topiramate are have been found effective in relapse prevention in clinical trials in adult populations but have not yet received FDA approval. There have been few studies of these medications in adolescents. Niederhofer and Staffen (2003b) assessed the efficacy and safety of long-term acamprosate treatment in alcohol dependence of adolescents by a double-blind, placebo-controlled study. Participants were 26 youth, ages 16 to 19 years, with alcohol use disorder. Patients were randomly allocated to treatment with acamprosate (1,332 mg/day) or placebo for 90 days. Thirteen acamprosate-treated and 13 placebo-treated patients completed the treatment phase (50% loss). At the end of treatment, seven acamprosate-treated and two placebo-treated patients had been continuously abstinent (p = .0076). Mean cumulative abstinence duration was significantly greater in the acamprosate group than in the placebo group (79.8 days vs. 32.8 days; p = .012). Despite the limits of the study (small sample size, short follow-up, sampling loss), results indicate that acamprosate was well tolerated and might be an effective pharmacological adjunct to psychosocial treatment programs.

Opioid Dependence

Opioid dependence is relatively uncommon in adolescents, particularly those seeking treatment. However, many regions of the United States have experienced a rise in opioid addiction, particularly with the available of potent, smokeable heroin. Naltrexone, by blocking opiate receptors, can absolutely prevent relapse to opioid dependence as long as it is ingested. Adolescents, however, are not likely to take this medication regularly. Several naltrexone depot preparations are currently in clinical trials. When these become available, a monthly injection will effectively prevent relapse.

Extended-release naltrexone was evaluated on a convenience sample of 16 adolescents and young adults (mean age 18.5 years) treated for opioid dependence by Fishman et al. (2010). The medication was well tolerated over a period of 4 months and its use was feasible in a community-based treatment setting.

Agonist maintenance using methadone or buprenorphine is the most generally effective treatment for adolescent opioid addiction currently available (Gonzalez, 2002).

A recent Cochrane Review that included randomized and controlled clinical trials of any maintenance pharmacological interventions, either alone or associated with psychosocial intervention compared with no intervention, placebo, other pharmacological intervention, pharmacological detoxification, or psychosocial intervention in adolescents (13–18 years), selected two studies involving 189 participants. One study (n = 35) compared methadone with levo-alpha-acetylmethadol (LAAM) for maintenance treatment lasting 16 weeks, after which patients were detoxified. In this trial, the authors concluded that there was no difference in the use of a substance of abuse or social functioning. The other trial (n = 154) compared maintenance treatment with buprenorphine/naloxone and detoxification with buprenorphine. In this second study, maintenance treatment appeared to be more efficacious in retaining patients in treatment but not in reducing the number of patients with a positive urine test at the end of the study. Self-reported opioid use at 1-year follow-up was significantly lower in the maintenance group, even though both groups reported a high level of opioid use (Minozzi et al., 2014a, 2014b).

Cocaine and Stimulants

There has been little research on the treatment of adolescent stimulant dependence, and most regions of the United States do not provide adequate treatment options for the large population of afflicted adolescents. Unfortunately, no pharmacological treatments with proven efficacy have been identified for cocaine dependence in general, and few clinical trials have even included adolescents. Similarly, psychosocial treatments have been minimally researched in stimulant-addicted adolescents. Group-based treatments, following the principles of Alcoholics Anonymous and Narcotics Anonymous, are commonly employed in specialized adolescent treatment programs in the United States. Adolescents will naturally resist treatment approaches that ignore normal developmental issues, including their need for peer acceptance, autonomy, and individualization. In addition, they cannot be treated in a vacuum, and it is important to address maladaptive family patterns with family therapy. Parents should also receive education about cocaine addiction that includes the warning signs of relapse and specific behavioral guidance.

Treatment approaches have limited effectiveness when adolescent patients do not view their use as problematic, or are not sufficiently motivated to quit using cocaine. It is even more difficult to establish a therapeutic alliance when adolescents have been pressured into treatment by their parents, the legal system, or school authorities. Even internally motivated adolescents are often difficult to engage, and treatment facilities should be staffed with practitioners who are familiar with the dynamics of addiction, normal adolescent development, and the nuances of treating adolescent patients.

A large number of medications have been examined, in adults, for reducing cocaine craving and euphoria or helping to promote abstinence, including disulfiram, without promising results, and several agents that enhance GABA activity, such as baclofen, topiramate, and tiagabine, have also been evaluated (Kosten, in press). Some experimental agents include immunotherapies such as a cocaine vaccine (Kosten, 2002) and glutamatergic agents such as modafinil (Dackis, 2003), but these are still waiting for more robust effectiveness evidence. According to a recent Cochrane Review, no current evidence supports the clinical use of anticonvulsant medications in the treatment of patients with cocaine dependence (Minozzi et al., 2015). At present, no medication has been consistently beneficial in preventing relapse to stimulant abuse and dependence in adolescents.

Treatment of Co-occurring Psychiatric Disorders in Adolescents

Current research provides fairly solid support favoring integrated pharmacotherapy of co-occurring psychiatric disorders and substance dependence in adolescents. The first consideration is that comorbid psychiatric disorders in adolescents with substance dependence are associated with poorer treatment outcomes compared to those with single disorders; if the comorbid condition goes untreated, the likelihood of successful engagement, retention, and completion of substance treatment will be reduced (Grella, 2001; Lohman, 2002; Whitmore, 1997; Wise, 2001). Second, pharmacotherapy of comorbid disorders, alone, is not likely to reduce substance use or "treat" substance abuse in the absence of specific substance treatment interventions in adolescents with substance dependence. This has been demonstrated in controlled trials for comorbid ADHD, bipolar disorder, and depression (Deas, 2001; Geller, 1998; Lohman, 2002; Riggs, 2001). Third, treatment of substance dependence (or achievement of abstinence), alone, does not "treat" comorbid psychiatric disorders, such as ADHD, bipolar disorder, or major depression, in the absence of specific pharmacotherapy for the comorbid disorder. Even depression is much less likely to remit with abstinence in adolescents compared to findings in depressed adults with chronic alcohol or drug dependence (Bukstein, 1992; Riggs, 1996). Fourth, controlled trials indicate that some medications commonly used to treat psychiatric disorders in children and adolescents may be safe and effective in treating comorbid disorders in adolescents with substance dependence, even if the adolescent is nonabstinent. Specific studies have examined fluoxetine for depression (Lohman, 2002), lithium for bipolar disorder (Geller, 1998), and bupropion and methylphenidate (MPH) for ADHD (Riggs, 2001).

Taken together, current research supports integrated, concurrent treatment of comorbid psychiatric disorders and substance abuse in adolescents. Sequential treatment models requiring adolescents to first complete substance treatment and achieve abstinence as a prerequisite for medicating comorbidity are much less effective and are probably contraindicated. Although research now supports integrated treatment models, it is understandable why sequential models evolved and have been perpetuated. Some of these reasons include a shortage of child and adolescent psychiatrists with training in addictions; shortages of addiction clinicians with substantial psychiatric training; separate provider networks for mental health and substance treatment services; and poor third-party payer coverage for integrated treatment services. Although coordinated treatment of co-occurring disorders in adolescents provides significant clinical advantages, it is often unavailable due to inadequacies in the health delivery system.

The dearth of research related to pharmacological treatment of addiction in adolescents results, in part, from the traditional exclusion of addicted adolescents from clinical trials evaluating the safety and efficacy of medications, even when prescribed for psychiatric illnesses. Until very recently, virtually nothing was known about the safety and effectiveness of these medications in adolescents with substance dependence or the potential for adverse interactions of medications with drugs of abuse. Clinicians were therefore understandably reluctant to use medications to treat psychiatric disorders in substance-abusing adolescents, often referring such youth for substance treatment before considering treatment of comorbidity. This reluctance to use pharmacotherapy is often cited as one reason for the poorer treatment outcomes in dually diagnosed adolescents, since untreated psychiatric illness significantly diminishes the likelihood of successful substance treatment. The risks of treatment must be balanced with the risks associated with *not* treating psychiatric comorbidity. Some controlled clinical trials have begun to extricate clinicians from this therapeutic conundrum by demonstrating the safety and efficacy of some medications used to treat the most common psychiatric comorbidities, including bipolar disorder, ADHD, and depression (Geller, 1998; Lohman, 2002; Riggs, 2001). When evaluating such studies, it is important to take into account what is considered the outcome measure, which in this case can be complex if we consider, for instance, the self-medication theory for addiction. Usually, studies present multiple outcome variables, including substance use measures (e.g., retention rate, days of abstinence, time to relapse), and comorbidity symptoms (e.g., reduction in depressive symptoms). For the purpose of this section, we will only consider studies specifically treating adolescents.

ADHD

ADHD is highly prevalent among adolescents with addiction (Horner & Scheibe, 1997; Kuperman et al., 2001). The comorbidity is clinically relevant, since ADHD is associated with both earlier and more frequent alcohol relapses (Ercan et al., 2003) and a lower likelihood of cannabis treatment completion (White et al., 2004) in adolescents. Several evidence-based guidelines have suggested that stimulants such as methylphenidate (MPH) should be the first option for treatment of ADHD (see, for instance, Pliszka et al., 2006). However, ADHD treatment studies typically exclude individuals with drug use/misuse or addiction. Given that most abused drugs act on the dopaminergic system (Volkow, Fowler, & Wang, 2004), as does MPH (Volkow, Wang, Fowler, & Ding, 2005), pharmacological studies of subjects with ADHD and addiction are crucial. That is, data from adolescents with ADHD without addiction can not necessarily be generalized to those with comorbid addiction. Pharmacotherapy with psychostimulants is considered the first-line treatment for ADHD in children and adolescents without substance dependence. The stimulants used for ADHD have good efficacy but a relatively high abuse potential and have been grouped with Schedule II psychostimulants (e.g., MPH, dextroamphetamine) (Klein-Schwartz, 2003). This is of special concern for short-action formulations, and some data suggest that long-acting formulations might be safer, such as osmotic-release oral system methylphenidate (OROS-MPH), even despite drug abstinence (Winhusen et al., 2011). Given the lack of evidence-based guidelines for the concurrent treatment of ADHD and substance use disorder, evidence suggests that stimulant medications should not necessarily be avoided for those with both ADHD and substance use disorder; indeed, concurrent treatment may be a successful approach to improve ADHD outcomes without worsening substance use symptoms (Klassen et al., 2012).

Recently, it was described that "medication for ADHD did not protect from, or contribute to, visible risk of substance use or [substance use disorder] by adolescents," based on the multimodal treatment study ADHD (MTA), in an 8-year follow-up. Substance use or substance use disorder rates were greater in the ADHD than in the non-ADHD samples, regardless of sex (Molina et al., 2013). These data do not agree with a previous finding indicating a protective effect of ADHD medication and further substance abuse development. Mannuzza et al. (2008), for instance, found a positive relationship between age at MPH initiation and non-alcohol substance use disorder later on. However, this study excluded children with CD, limiting its external validity. While a protective role for the use of ADHD medication since childhood on adolescent and adult substance use disorder remains an open question, studies have begun on the pharmacological effects of first-line ADHD medications in patients with both ADHD and substance use disorder, specifically in adolescents. An RCT of OROS-MPH, together with CBT, in adolescents with ADHD and substance use disorder showed no group differences in terms of reducing ADHD-RS scores or days of substance use; that is, there were no differences in either ADHD or substance use disorder outcome measures (Riggs et al., 2011). It is interesting to note that in this study, parent ADHD-RS scores was considered a secondary outcome measure, and it favored OROS-MPH at 8 weeks (mean difference = 4.4, 95% CI 0.8–7.9) and 16 weeks (mean difference = 6.9; 95% CI 2.9–10.9). This multicenter study recruited 303 adolescents with ADHD and substance use disorder (ages 13–18 years), and the medication dosage was from 18 to 72 mg/day, or to the highest dose tolerated. Later on, the authors intended to find significant treatment predictors in this sample, which included (1) substance use severity, associated with poorer ADHD and substance use disorder outcomes, (2) ADHD severity, associated with better ADHD and substance use disorder outcomes, (3) comorbid CD, associated with poorer ADHD outcomes, and (4) court-mandated status, associated with better substance use disorder outcomes but poorer treatment completion (Tamm, 2013).

In a less robust study, the authors evaluated the effects of a long-acting formulation of MPH (Spheroidal Oral Drug Absorption System [MPH-SODAS]) on ADHD symptoms in an outpatient sample of adolescents with ADHD and substance use disorder. In this 6-week, single-blind, placebo-controlled crossover study assessing the efficacy of escalated doses of MPH-SODAS, participants were randomly allocated to either group A (weeks 1–3 on MPH-SODAS, weeks 4–6 on placebo) or group B (reverse order). The primary outcome measures were the Swanson, Nolan, and Pelham Scale, version IV (SNAP-IV) and the Clinical Global Impression Scale (CGI). The sample consisted of 16 marijuana users, 7 of whom also used cocaine (43.8%). Subjects had a significantly greater reduction in SNAP-IV and CGI scores ($p < .001$ for all analyses) during MPH-SODAS treatment compared to placebo (Szobot et al., 2008).

Despite a few reports of the use of lisdexamfetamine in adults with ADHD and substance use disorder, we were not able to find studies on adolescent samples.

To date, just one study is available assessing the use of atomoxetine in adolescents with comorbid ADHD and substance use disorder (Thurstone et al., 2010). In this placebo-randomized, controlled trial, change in ADHD scores did not differ between the atomoxetine + MI/CBT and placebo + MI/CBT groups ($F_{4,191} = 1.23$, $p = .2975$). Change in days in which non-nicotine substances were used in the last 28 days did not differ between the groups ($F_{3,100} = 2.06$, $p = .1103$).

Bupropion has a low effect size in children and adolescents with ADHD (0.32 vs. 0.80 for MPH, for instance, and 0.72 for atomoxetine) (Faraone at al., 2006). Thus, it should not be considered as a first option unless there is a contraindication for other medications. Moreover, although several questions remain open, it seems reasonable to state that the use of long-acting formulations of MPH will not worsen substance use disorder. Its effects on ADHD, and in what dosages, need better understanding. It is also interesting to note that the above-mentioned pharmacological protocols did not require drug abstinence for treating ADHD. ADHD diagnoses usually can be made retrospectively, based on the anamnesis (it is difficult to have 12 years as the age of onset for substance use disorder, and it is the upper limit for diagnosing ADHD, based on DSM-5). Thus, we can assume that, in the presence of substance use disorder, ADHD should be investigated, given the high prevalence. No abstinence period is needed to establish an ADHD diagnosis. If present, a long-acting stimulant could be considered, with use closely monitored by the parents, together with a substance use intervention.

Bipolar Disorder

Pharmacotherapy with mood stabilizers (e.g., lithium, valproic acid, carbamazepine) is the first-line treatment for bipolar disorder in adolescents without substance dependence. Only one controlled trial (lithium vs. placebo) has been conducted in adolescents with bipolar disorder and substance dependence (Geller, 1998). In this study, lithium had a relatively good safety profile and was shown to be effective in stabilizing mania or hypomania in adolescents with substance dependence, many of whom were not abstinent during the trial (Geller, 1998). Although there was a somewhat greater decline in substance use in the lithium-treated group compared to those who received placebo, the pharmacological treatment of bipolar disorder did not effectively treat substance dependence in the absence of specific substance treatment. The available data would support treating bipolar disorder only in the context of concurrent treatment for substance dependence in dually diagnosed adolescents. No data are yet available from controlled trials about the safety or efficacy of other mood stabilizers in dually diagnosed adolescents.

Studies have suggested that the second-generation antipsychotics may be more efficacious than the traditional mood stabilizers in the acute phase, and they appear to yield a quicker response (Liu et al., 2011). The FDA has approved several second-generation antipsychotics for the acute treatment of manic/mixed episodes in children and adolescents: risperidone for 10- to 17-year-olds, olanzapine for 13- to 17-year-olds, aripiprazole for 10- to 17-year-olds, and quetiapine for 10- to 17-year-olds. However, up to now, there are no reports on their use in adolescents with a concomitant substance use disorder. Thus, despite the clinical relevance of this comorbidity, there is a lack of studies on this topic.

Depression

In standard practice, adolescents with major (severe) depression would receive both psychotherapy and pharmacotherapy, while those with mild or moderate symptoms might be given a trial of psychotherapy alone before considering medications. When medications are used, selective serotonin reuptake inhibitors (SSRIs) are considered first-line medication choices for adolescent depression without comorbid substance dependence (Emslie, 1997). Fluoxetine is the best studied and has the best evidence of effectiveness. It is approved by the FDA and the European Medicines Agency (EMEA) for those aged 8 years or older. Sertraline, citalopram, and escitalopram have less robust evidence of effectiveness, though they may be effective in patients who did not respond to fluoxetine (Joseph et al., 2015). Escitalopram has been approved by the FDA for adolescents with depression. Paroxetine appears not to be effective in youth and shows more side effects than the other SSRIs. Monoamine oxidase inhibitors and tricyclic antidepressants should be avoided in children and adolescents (Rey, Bella-Awusah, & Liu, 2015).

No adequately powered controlled trials of SSRIs have yet been completed in depressed adolescents with substance dependence. Preliminary data from an ongoing RCT of fluoxetine for depression in 120 depressed and addicted adolescents indicates that it appears to have a very good safety profile even in non-abstinent adolescents with polydrug abuse (Lohman, 2002). A protocol of fluoxetine (20 mg/day) or placebo, both with CBT, for 16 weeks was tested in 126 adolescents (ages 13–19) meeting DSM-5 diagnostic criteria for current major depressive disorder, lifetime CD, and at least one nontobacco substance use disorder. Fluoxetine combined with CBT produced greater changes on the Childhood Depression Rating Scale-Revised (ES = 0.78) but not on the Clinical Global Impression Improvement treatment response (76% and 67%, respectively; relative risk, 1.08). There was an overall decrease in self-reported substance use, without a difference between the groups (Riggs et al., 2007). In a double-blind controlled trial to test the efficacy of fluoxetine over placebo in 50 adolescents with alcohol use disorder and comorbid major depression, concomitant with CBT and MET, there was no significant difference between groups for both depressive symptoms and alcohol use. In this study, alcohol abstinence was not required (Cornelius et al., 2009). Fluoxetine was also evaluated in 70 adolescents and young adults with depression and current cannabis use in a 12-week study, concomitant with CBT and MET. Again, no difference between the fluoxetine (up to 20 mg/day) and the placebo groups was described for either depressive symptoms or cannabis use (Cornelius et al., 2010). This cohort was followed and, after 1 year, 68 of the participants (97%) were retained. Most of the clinical improvements in depressive symptoms and for cannabis-related symptoms persisted at the 1-year follow-up evaluation, despite the study arm (fluoxetine or placebo). The authors suggest that the persistence of the efficacy of the acute-phase treatment might be attributed to the CBT/MET psychotherapy (Cornelius et el., 2012).

It seems that the good results for the SSRIs in nonaddicted youths have not been replicated in adolescents with comorbid substance use disorder. Whether it is a matter of low medication dosage, for instance, or whether there really is no effect in adolescent who are currently using drugs remains to be better understood. Studies demonstrated, however, that fluoxetine was well tolerated. Moreover, there is currently a controversy over whether SSRIs may increase the risk of suicide in adolescents; this issue is thoroughly discussed in Chapter 2 of this volume.

Anxiety Disorders

CBT, often used in combination with SSRIs, are considered standard treatment for a variety of anxiety disorders (including social anxiety disorder, generalized anxiety disorder, and posttraumatic stress disorder) in adolescents without substance dependence. While the use of SSRIs in adolescent anxiety disorders that are comorbid with substance dependence has not yet been well studied, the data support their relatively good safety profile in treating depression in adolescents with substance dependence, as mentioned above. Furthermore, the high rates of co-occurring depression and anxiety disorders suggest that clinicians may wish to consider SSRIs in dually diagnosed adolescents with anxiety disorders. Good target symptoms for SSRIs include the management of sleep problems, depressive symptoms, intrusive memories, and hyperarousal symptoms often associated with posttraumatic stress disorder (Davies, 2001; Lohman, 2002). There is a strong need for studies on this comorbidity.

Benzodiazepines are contraindicated for anxiety disorders in patients with substance dependence because of their well-known abuse potential.

Pharmacotherapy in Adolescents, Special Considerations

In CD, the most common comorbidity in adolescents with substance abuse, the results of pharmacological treatment in adolescents without substance abuse have been poor, but there is some evidence that medications might help, together with an integrative approach. The impulsive/aggressive symptoms of CD seem to be responsive, for instance, to divalproex sodium (Padhy et al., 2011; Saxena et al., 2010; Steiner et al., 2003), aripiprazole (Ercan et al., 2012; Kuperman et al., 2011), and risperidone (Loy et al., 2012). Although most pharmacotherapy studies in adolescent substance abuse enroll adolescents with CD, studies specifically on the pharmacological approach to this common comorbidity are missing.

Eating disorder is another comorbidity that needs more attention. In adolescents with eating disorders, rates of substance use and abuse have also been found to be 20% to 40% greater than that of normal-weight peers (Denoth et al., 2011). Studies evaluating the role of medication in this complex clinical situation, which requires a multidisciplinary team, are needed.

Polypharmacy has become increasingly common in the adolescent population over the past two decades (Jureidini, Tonkin, & Jureidini,

2013). In the United States, among adolescents with mental disorder, polypharmacy increased from 22.2% (1996–1999) to 32.2% (2004–2007), despite the lack of studies on its safety and effectiveness (Comer, Olfson, & Moitabai, 2010). In clinical practice, adolescents with substance abuse usually present with more than one comorbidity (e.g., CD plus ADHD), and there are no studies, up to now, evaluating multiclass drug treatment in adolescents with substance abuse. This is of special interest and concern given the higher rates of psychotropic drug interactions expected when in the presence of a drug of abuse.

Another open question is the best moment to introduce medication in the presence of a comorbidity. Some studies, for instance, did not require abstinence to start comorbidity treatment (like most ADHD studies). If the adolescent has a comorbid disorder for which medication is being considered (e.g., ADHD, major depression), abstinence should be considered before initiating medication for comorbidity. However, abstinence is not a realistic goal for many adolescent patients. Clinicians must therefore weigh the risk of potential interactions between the drug and the medication against the risk that the untreated psychiatric illness will thwart treatment engagement or precipitate early dropout. Once the adolescent is engaged in substance abuse treatment, both urine drug screening and self-report should indicate either abstinence or significant reduction in substance use, although it is often necessary to tolerate some ongoing alcohol or cannabis use. The mental health professional or psychiatrist then should develop a plan for regular drug abuse monitoring (e.g., urine toxicology, breath alcohol) and for information exchange regarding compliance with substance treatment, urine toxicology results, target symptom response, and emergence of adverse side effects. When initiating medications, the patient should be compliant with at least weekly therapy sessions. Our clinical experience suggests benefit from MET coupled with CBT and an empathic, encouraging therapeutic style. Such an approach typically leads to successful medication stabilization for comorbidity during the first month of treatment. Early treatment of a psychiatric disorder can be critically important in facilitating treatment engagement and retention during the initial months of substance abuse treatment.

The following principles also may be helpful when using medications to treat comorbid disorders concurrently with substance dependence:

1. When medication is indicated, consider medications with good safety profiles, low abuse liability, and once-per-day dosing, if possible.
2. Use a single medication if at all possible.
3. Educate the patient and family about the potential for adverse interactions of medications with substances of abuse and the need for abstinence or reduced substance use to ensure safety and efficacy.
4. Establish mechanisms to closely monitor medication compliance (initially weekly), adverse effects, target symptom response, and ongoing substance use (using both self-report and urine drug screening).
5. Monitor compliance with regular substance treatment (generally, individual or family counseling at least weekly) and regular urine drug screening (if not the primary substance abuse treatment provider).
6. Monitor patient treatment motivation and target symptom response as well as behavior changes and psychosocial functioning throughout treatment. If substance abuse or target symptoms of the comorbid disorder do not significantly improve within the first 2 months after initiating treatment, or if there is evidence of escalation in drug abuse or clinical deterioration, consider several options:
   a. Evaluate the medication's efficacy and change the medication.
   b. Reassess the diagnostic formulation (e.g., bipolar vs. unipolar depression).
   c. Increase the treatment intensity (frequency or level of care).

Following these principles should facilitate pharmacotherapy in adolescents who frequently have comorbid psychiatric disorders with their substance dependence. Medications primarily targeted at the substance dependence, such as bupropion or NRT for nicotine dependence, might also be considered, but behavioral treatments should be tried first for most adolescents with primary substance dependence and no other psychopathology.

Approximately one in seven users of prescribed adolescent medication had diverted their controlled medications in their lifetime. Medication must be closely monitored by parents/guardians and physicians, given the high rates of diversion in substance-abusing patients (trading, selling, giving away, or loaning). In a study conducted by McCabe et al. (2011), being approached to divert medications was more prevalent among adolescents who had substance use disorder. Thus, diligent prescribing and monitoring of controlled medications are recommended (McCabe at al., 2011).

Prevention of Substance Use Disorders

Daniel Romer
Claudia Szobot

chapter 19

Extensive epidemiologic research has identified a set of interrelated problem behaviors, typically originating during childhood and adolescence, that are critically important from a public health standpoint. For youth, central among these risk-related health behaviors are alcohol, tobacco, and other drug use (Substance Abuse and Mental Health Services, 2015). Prevalence rates of alcohol, tobacco, and marijuana use among adolescents remain high. For example, recent prevalence of lifetime alcohol use among 12th-graders was 64%; for cigarette use the lifetime rate was 31%, and for marijuana it was 45% (Johnston, O'Malley, Miech, Bachman, & Schulenberg, 2016a, 2016b). Early initiation and progression in the use of addictive substances is associated with a wide range of externalizing behaviors, including conduct disorder (CD), risky sexual practices, and behaviors that result in unintentional and intentional injuries (Iacono, Malone, & McGue, 2008; Taylor et al., 2010). Thus, legal and moral implications aside, adolescent substance abuse must be regarded as a public health issue. The effective prevention and treatment of adolescent substance abuse, like that for any public health problem, requires a clear understanding of causes and the context in which these causes operate.

The review of the epidemiology and neurobiological underpinnings of drug use in Chapter 17 provides important background for the study of prevention. This research has uncovered important determinants of drug use that can guide interventions to prevent the uptake and progression of this behavior. In this chapter, we review the major theories that have guided the development of interventions to reduce drug use in adolescence and examine the evidence that has accumulated regarding the success of these efforts. We then describe major directions for the future development of effective prevention programs.

THEORETICAL AND CONCEPTUAL MODELS OF PREVENTION AND CHANGE

There is no generally agreed-upon theoretical or conceptual model for prevention of substance abuse. What is clear is that the uptake of drugs during adolescence is a product of a wide array of individual, social, and cultural factors that affect adolescent interest in and access to drugs. This is evident in the long-term trends for recent alcohol, cigarette, and marijuana use among adolescents as tracked by the Monitoring the Future study (MTF) and shown below. Since the mid-1970s, recent use of all three drugs has decreased, and quite dramatically for alcohol and cigarettes (Johnston et al., 2016a, 2016b). Although marijuana use has also declined, it is now more prevalent than cigarettes, reflecting a cultural change in the United States of greater acceptance of this drug among adults (see Chapter 17 and Fig. 19.1). Associated with these declines are changes in perceptions of the harmfulness of these drugs, with the correlations between aggregate perceptions of harm and recent use of alcohol (–.83), cigarettes (–.80), and marijuana (–.59) quite high. Over this period, federal education policy has encouraged schools to educate adolescents about drugs, and these programs have proliferated (Kumar, O'Malley, Johnston, & Laetz, 2013; Ringwalt et al., 2011). Media campaigns to discourage the use of tobacco (National Cancer Institute, 2008) and other drugs have also expanded (Ferri, Allara, Gasparrini, & Faggiano, 2013). In addition, the age at which adolescents can purchase alcohol was raised to 21, which researchers believe has reduced the use of and the number of injuries associated with this drug (DeJong & Blanchette, 2014). Although there have been massive efforts over this period to educate adolescents and the public about the harms of alcohol and tobacco, how these perceptions and behavior changed is not well understood.

RISK AND PROTECTIVE FACTORS: THE COMPLEX CAUSES OF ADOLESCENT SUBSTANCE ABUSE

It has been recognized for over 40 years that the risk for becoming a substance abuser is not equally distributed in the population. Originally this observation came from research that followed children into

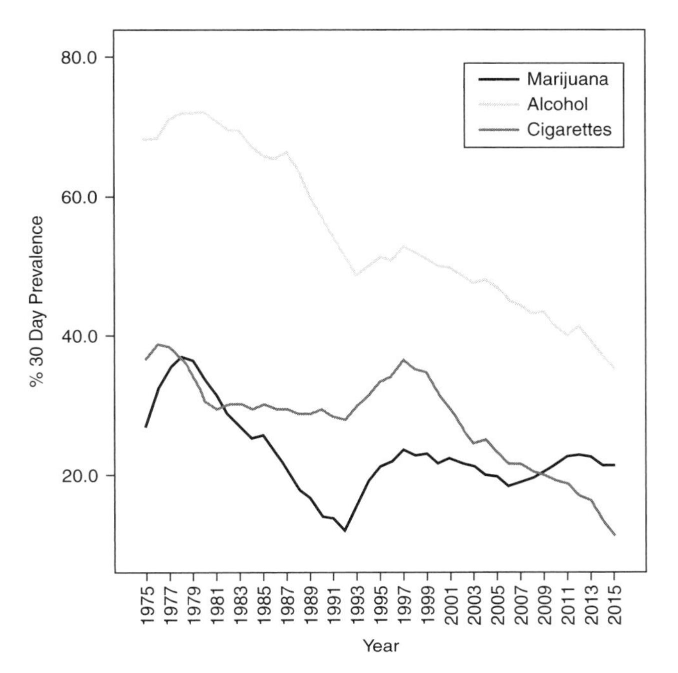

Figure 19.1 Percentages of 12th-grade students reporting past-30-day use of alcohol, cigarettes, and marijuana from the Monitoring the Future study, years 1975–2015. (From Johnston et al., 2016a, 2016b.)

adulthood and used childhood demographic and psychological data to uncover pathways to an adolescent or adult substance abuse disorder. Subsequently, this view was bolstered by epidemiologic surveys in the United States that revealed that only 27% of individuals who have experimentally used drugs six or more times actually progress to become daily drug users, and only about a half of young-adult daily drug users go on to develop a drug abuse or dependence disorder (Robins & Regier 1991). While it is possible that chance plays a role in the acquisition of a substance abuse problem, it is more likely that the complex interplay of risk and protective factors determines who progresses from experimentation to regular use and from regular use to problematic involvement. Furthermore, this interplay of risk and protective factors exists in a maturational context such that at some stages of human development certain biological, psychological, or social factors may be totally benign, while at other stages of development these same factors may confer considerable risk for problematic involvement with drugs of abuse. These risk factors are subject to effects of gender and ethnicity, so risk factors may operate differently in boys and girls, and in different ethnic groups. To further complicate the issue, individual risk and protective factors must be viewed against a backdrop of laws, cultural and social norms, drug availability, economic circumstances, and regional and community factors. For example, a white adolescent male living in the United States who has a variety of individual risk factors for alcohol dependence might develop alcohol problems, but if he were raised in Saudi Arabia (where drinking alcohol is forbidden), it is less likely that he would develop an alcohol problem. However, it is possible that these risk factors might manifest themselves in other forms of problematic behavior (e.g., aggressive behavior). Thus, substance abuse is a multifaceted problem.

Geneticists refer to multidetermined problems like substance abuse as "complex disorders" because a multiplicity of individual biological and behavioral factors interact with environmental factors (e.g., social and societal phenomena) in complicated ways across human development to produce different outcomes. To the best of our knowledge, there is no single cause of adolescent substance abuse, so it is unlikely that there will be a single preventive measure to forestall its development. For this reason, the reader is cautioned to be skeptical of overly simplistic causal explanations for our substance abuse problems and facile and obvious solutions. The likelihood that approaches guided by conventional wisdom will achieve their promised results is diminished by the realities of our current understanding of the complex pathways to a substance use disorder.

INFLUENTIAL THEORIES OF THE DEVELOPMENT OF ADOLESCENT SUBSTANCE ABUSE

Theories develop as an effort to summarize and explain research data generated by observation and experimentation. Theories are used to organize future research studies that ultimately test the validity of the original theory and provide an opportunity for it to evolve and undergo revision. Thus, theories are scientific "works in progress." Several influential theories have guided our understanding of the origins of adolescent substance abuse and provide a framework for ongoing research in this area. These theories also provide a useful structure to guide approaches to the prevention and treatment of adolescent substance abuse problems. The following are among the most influential of these theories. There are many areas of commonality and overlap, yet each has contributed and advanced our understanding of the origins of substance abuse.

The "Gateway" or Stage Theory

This theory comes from epidemiologic research that has examined the patterning of alcohol and other drug use progression among adolescents. However, this theory has become a battleground for those both for and against the decriminalization of marijuana. The theory is based on the delineation of four stages in the sequence of involvement with drugs. The original findings suggested that surveyed adolescents engage in use of either alcohol or cigarettes (as legal and culturally accepted drugs) and then progress to marijuana, and then on to other illicit drugs, such as heroin and cocaine. The legal drugs are necessary intermediates between nonuse and marijuana. Thus, the use of tobacco, alcohol, and marijuana by adolescents was viewed as a crucial step or "gateway" to the use of other illicit drugs (Kandel, 1975; Yamaguchi & Kandel, 1984).

Why would tobacco and/or alcohol trigger marijuana use? It could be a general liability that increases the risk for any drug, with those most prevalent more likely to be initiated first. A secondary analysis of the 2008 MTF 12th-grade data aimed to check which drug (alcohol, tobacco, or marijuana) was the actual "gateway" drug leading to additional substance use among a nationally representative sample of high school seniors. Results indicated that alcohol represented the "gateway" drug leading to the use of tobacco, marijuana, and other illicit substances (Kirby & Barry, 2012). Or, the route of administration could predispose. According to a Dutch study, early-onset tobacco use does not pose a significantly higher risk of initiating cannabis use than early-onset alcohol use. Thus, the route of administration was not a factor. In this same study, early-onset comorbid use of both tobacco and alcohol was associated with a higher likelihood of initiating cannabis use than in adolescents who had tried either tobacco or alcohol. The authors concluded that the gateway hypothesis was not enough to explain their finding, again favoring the general liability model (van Leeuwen et al., 2011). An interesting study that examined East Asian youth with a genetic variation that yields a deficiency in an enzyme that metabolizes ethanol found that they were just as likely to progress to other drugs as those without the deficiency (Irons, McGue, Iacono, & Oetting, 2007). Thus, being unable to tolerate and use alcohol does not appear to influence the progression to other drugs. Furthermore, surveys of American high school students suggest that by 12th grade, 44.7% of students have tried marijuana, while only 0.8% have tried heroin and 4.0% have tried cocaine (Johnston et al., 2016a, 2016b). The discrepancies in these prevalence rates indicate that although illegal drug users may have started with marijuana, it is clear that marijuana use does not invariably progress to adolescent use of other illegal drugs.

Importance of Age of Initiation

Although the gateway theory has remained controversial, a less controversial aspect of this theory deals with age of initiation of experimentation with drugs of abuse (whether alcohol, tobacco, marijuana, or other illegal drugs) and the timing of stages of regular use and problematic involvement. The literature converges around the observation that the earlier the onset of progressive substance use, the greater the likelihood of problematic involvement later in development (Choi et al., 1997, 2001; Kandel & Logan, 1984; Schuckit & Russell, 1983; Yamaguchi & Kandel, 1984). However, this pattern is also consistent with a general liability theory described below. For example, early appearance of any externalizing behavior increases the risk for later antisocial behavior (McGue & Iacono, 2005). Khurana et al. (2015) also showed that impulsive tendencies reflective of poor executive function predict the *progression* rather than *initiation* of drug use in early to middle adolescence. Progression would seem to be the critical factor rather than early initiation, because without progression, there is little chance for addiction or other adverse consequences. Thus, for this reason, substantial effort has been placed on prevention interventions that delay the initiation and progression of substance use during early adolescence.

General Liability for Drug Use and Other Externalizing Behavior

Opponents of the gateway theory suggest that if there were a risk factor that was common to alcohol and other drugs, it could easily account for the relationship between supposed gateway drugs and other drug use. Examples of a theorized "third factor" include the genetic predisposition to drug use, a predisposition toward adolescent risk behavior in general, or shared opportunities to obtain both marijuana and other drugs (Morral, McCaffrey, & Paddock, 2002). The Problem Behavior Theory proposed by Jessor and Jessor (1977) is an early example of a third-factor explanation. They suggested that adolescents differ in a general tendency toward antisocial behavior, perhaps in response to stressors or deviant peers. The theory also posits that substance abuse for some adolescents may be a maladaptive means to cope with the stresses and social pressures that are characteristic of the adolescent stage of development. This theoretical perspective suggests that prevention interventions that offer alternative means of coping and social adaptation might reduce adolescent substance use behavior.

Considerable evidence reviewed by Iocono, Malone, and McGue (2008) suggests that a liability is present for the emergence of a wide range of antisocial behavior in children and adolescents. They characterize this liability as a behavioral disinhibition reflecting lack of control over impulses, which is common in children and adolescents who exhibit such externalizing behavior. Evidence for this pattern is present prior to adolescence, with children showing early signs of disinhibition exhibiting enhanced risk for later drug use (Elkins, McGue, & Iacono, 2007; Moffitt et al., 2011; Wong et al., 2006). More recent research suggests that weakness in executive functions, such as working memory, is an important component of the impulsive tendencies that predict the use of alcohol (Khurana et al., 2013) and other drugs (Khurana et al., 2015).

Consistent with the general liability model of adolescent drug use is evidence for shared genetic risk in twin studies of adolescent drug use (Iocono, Malone, & McGue, 2008). This pattern is further supported by studies showing high heritability of more general externalizing behaviors, including drug use, CD, and other antisocial behavior (Iocono, Malone, & McGue, 2008). Although there are gender differences in the display of these behaviors, the genetic liability appears to be similar for both males and females (Hicks et al., 2007; Kendler, Prescott, Myers, & Neale, 2003). Internalizing tendencies, such as depressed mood and anxiety, are also correlated with externalizing behavior in adolescents and thus are a potential co-occurring liability for drug use (Kreuger & Markon, 2006).

While research clearly reveals that genes are an important determinant of liability for substance abuse, it does not tell us which genes. For other complex traits like high blood pressure, diabetes, or high cholesterol, it is clear that there are multiple genes involved and multiple genetic and biological pathways are involved in producing disease. It is unlikely that there is a single gene for alcohol, cocaine, or nicotine dependence. There may be hundreds or thousands of genes in a given pattern producing risk, and that risk may only be present in a given environmental context. The nature of the genetic risk may be a common factor for abuse across a wide variety of drugs, or a genetic risk for conduct difficulties or problem behaviors, or a set of genes that delay the maturation of the brain so one is less able to control the habituating effects of drugs. The effects of genes may be protective rather than associated with risk, and what we think of as genetic effects producing substance abuse may actually be the *absence* of protective genes. There is good evidence that specific genetic mutations protect against the development of alcohol use disorder in certain ethnic groups, and some evidence that there is a mutation that protects against smoking. There is some evidence that substance use heritability changes across development. It seems that genetics plays a smaller role for substance initiation, but might gain more importance for the progression of drug use (Meyers & Dick, 2010).

In sum, the finding that deficits in inhibitory control and related liabilities are a primary source of risk for drug abuse and other externalizing behavior has been a focus of several interventions that attempt to enhance self-regulatory skills in children and adolescents. A prominent example of this approach is embodied in theories regarding the role of the family in enhancing such skills in at-risk children.

Patterson's Developmental Theory

Patterson's theory was originally proposed to explain the development of juvenile delinquency; consistent with the observation that problem behaviors frequently co-occur in adolescents, it has also been used to understand and address problematic involvement with alcohol and other drugs of abuse. Patterson and colleagues (Dishion et al., 1991; Patterson, DeBaryshe, & Ramsey, 1989) proposed a developmental theory of CD and related externalizing behavior that posits that adolescent problem behavior is a consequence of poor parental family management practices interacting with the child's own aggressive and oppositional temperament. Here, temperament refers to the early and genetically determined behavioral characteristics that over time lead to externalizing behavior. Deficits in parenting skill, such as harsh and inconsistent punishment, increased parent–child conflict, low parental involvement, and poor parental monitoring result in poor behavior and performance in school. The poorly performing and behaving child may be socially rejected by many peers, but he or she may form friendships with other problematic children. This process of forming close peer relationships is augmented by the negative interactions with caregivers in the home. The impact of CD on further drug addiction outcomes is well documented, with CD conferring additional risk for illicit drug use (Hopfer et al., 2013; Sung, Erkanli, & Costello, 2012).

As the child affiliates with more deviant children, he or she adopts deviant behavior as a norm. Other deviant children become powerful social role models, from whom the child learns further deviant and socially unacceptable behavior, including experimentation and progression in the use of drugs of abuse. These children may therefore be viewed as being on a developmental trajectory of deviancy and substance abuse that begins early in development and is compounded by unskilled parenting and the formation of social relationships with other problem children (Vuchinich, Bank, & Patterson, 1992).

The developmental cascade model shown in Figure 19.2 illustrates the influences featured in Patterson's theory. In this model, children who show early signs of externalizing behavior move on to experience school failure and attraction to other antisocial children that is exacerbated by poor family management practices. As the child moves into adolescence, the problems

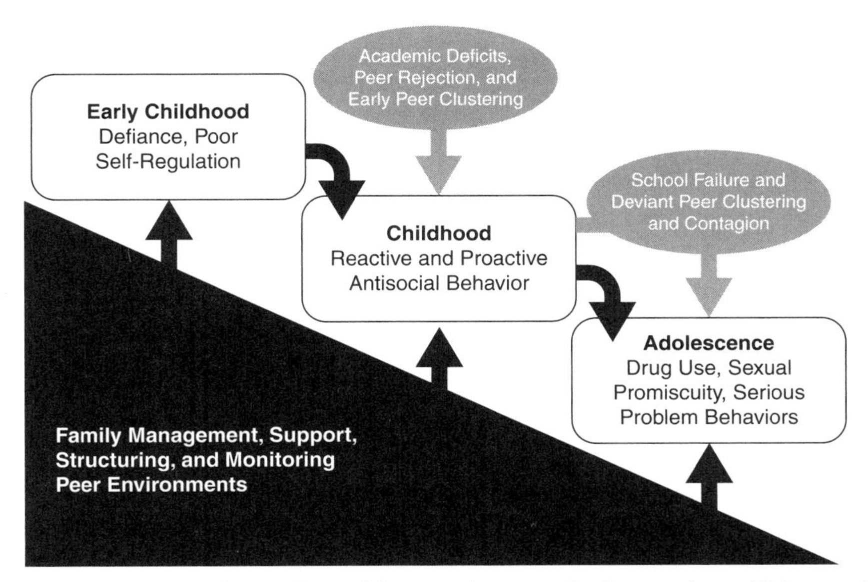

Figure 19.2 A developmental cascade model: parenting contributions and amplifying mechanisms. (From Dishion, Veronneau, Stormshak, & Kavanagh, 2015.)

escalate into various forms of unhealthy behavior such as drug use. Prevention interventions that are based on this theoretical approach offer parenting skill training to teach parents more effective ways to discipline and monitor their children, and to reduce the negative environment of the home. Tutoring and other forms of education support may be provided to reduce academic failure. Social skills training may also be offered the child in order to reduce peer rejection and provide a mechanism to gracefully resist peer pressure to use alcohol and illicit drugs. These interventions are described in greater detail below.

Summary of Factors Influencing Adolescent Drug Use

While adolescents in the United States are widely exposed to a spectrum of drugs of abuse, research suggests that adolescent substance abuse problems are due to multiple factors. Most theories suggest that genetic, psychological, familial, and nonfamilial environmental factors interact in a complex way to determine an adverse or protective outcome. Thus, genes, temperament, attitudes and beliefs, family environment, peer affiliation, and social norms all influence the relationship between the individual and a substance use disorder outcome. The developmental timing of these factors adds an additional level of complexity. The question of "nature or nurture" has been rendered moot, primarily by research conducted over the last 20 years: it is clear that both "nature" and "nurture" are involved, set against the backdrop of child development (Kendler, Jaffee, & Romer, 2011). Thus, there is no single cause of adolescent substance abuse, and any single prevention approach is unlikely to have broad universal success.

The general liability approach does help us to identify high-risk children for prevention interventions. Clearly, offspring of parents with substance abuse problems are themselves at significant risk for becoming substance abusers. Interventions that improve parenting practices may be important, not only in instilling appropriate disciplinary practices in the parents of high-risk children, but also by enhancing parental involvement and monitoring. Social skills training may keep high-risk children from being rejected by less deviant peers and thereby avoid being attracted to more deviant peer groups. A wide range of personality characteristics that have been linked to drug use progression may also provide guidance for more targeted prevention (Audrain-McGovern & Tercyak, 2011). For example, an intervention designed to reduce drug use was found to reduce the risk that a gene conferred to substance use (Brody, Yu, & Beach, 2015).

Other important liabilities include two facets of impulsivity, acting without thinking and delay discounting (Audrain-McGovern et al., 2009; Khurana et al., 2013; Winstanley et al., 2010). Acting without thinking is a phenotypic expression of impulsivity linked to early involvement in a wide range of externalizing behavior, including drug use, gambling, and fighting (Romer et al., 2009). Delay discounting is a related but separate expression of impulsivity characterized by preference for small immediate rewards over larger but delayed rewards (Shamosh et al., 2008). It has been linked to progression in use of various drugs in adolescents, including alcohol (Khurana et al., 2013) and cigarettes (Audrain-McGovern et al., 2009). Prevention programs that target these specific liabilities have yet to be developed, although universal programs described below have components that can help to constrain these liabilities by enhancing decision making and self-regulation skills.

TYPES OF PREVENTION INTERVENTIONS AND MODEL PROGRAMS

Prevention programs are often categorized according to the following definitions based on the audience they are designed to reach (Haggerty & Mrazek, 1994).

Universal intervention programs are designed to reach the general population, such as all students in a given school or school district, through school education or media campaigns, for example. Broadly speaking, universal interventions represent the most widely used approach to drug abuse prevention. A national survey of school administrators revealed that over 90% of middle and high schools report delivering some type of universal program to students (Kumar et al., 2011). From a universal intervention perspective, public health problems and their solutions are inextricably a part of the community social system; solutions are essentially universal, with some types of universal interventions facilitating access to higher-risk groups within the community that may warrant more intensive intervention. Implementation of these types of interventions is typically supported by local community partnerships or coalitions.

Selective and *indicated* interventions specifically target persons identified as at risk of drug abuse, such as those who might already have used a drug and therefore are at higher risk of progression than those not having tried one. Examples of such programs, described below, include programs that screen for youth who have used alcohol and then deliver brief therapeutic interventions to prevent progression in use. Indicated interventions focus more clearly on youth who show signs of serious mental health conditions, such as drug abuse, delinquency, or depression, but have not been diagnosed with a substance use disorder. These programs are more intense than either the universal or selective interventions.

In our review of drug prevention programs, we highlight those classes of interventions that have received the most extensive evaluations, as evidenced by Cochrane or other meta-analyses. Most of these evaluations have appeared since the first edition of this volume. Not surprisingly, the majority of interventions have been universal in scope. In some approaches, universal interventions are used to identify higher-risk youth who are then provided with opportunities to receive more intensive programming.

School-Based Universal Interventions

The most widely adopted universal program in schools is the well-known Drug Abuse Resistance Education (DARE), a school-based primary drug prevention curriculum designed for introduction during the last year of elementary education (Kumar et al., 2013). Despite its popularity, early evaluations of DARE failed to demonstrate its effectiveness (Clayton, Cattarello, & Johnstone, 1996; Lynam et al.,

1999). In response, an enhanced version of DARE was developed and tested, DARE Plus. Additional components added to the original DARE curriculum include a peer-led parental involvement classroom program called "On the VERGE," youth-led extracurricular activities, community adult action teams, and postcard mailings to parents. Evidence suggests that DARE Plus program delivered over two years in seventh and eighth grade produced significant reductions in alcohol, tobacco, and polydrug use among boys but had no effect on girls (Perry et al., 2003). Other versions of the DARE program have evolved, with the adoption of the "Keepin' it REAL" intervention. This program uses interactive exercises that develop skills to Refuse, Explain, Avoid, and Leave situations that encourage drug use. Evaluations of this universal program indicate that it is particularly effective in reducing the uptake of alcohol use (Hecht et al., 2003). It is also effective in reducing the progression of alcohol use among those who have already tried the drug (Kulis, Nieri, Yabiku, Stromwall, & Marsiglia, 2007).

A Cochrane Review of all universal school-based drug prevention programs indicated that programs with an emphasis on decision making, drug resistance, and self-management skills, such as featured in Botvin's life skills training program (Botvin et al., 1995), have shown efficacy, especially in regard to alcohol use (Foxcroft & Tsertsvadze, 2012). A life skills training program implemented in Germany in fifth grade, with boosters in sixth and seventh grades, found reductions in use of alcohol, cigarettes, and illicit drugs over a 2-year follow-up, with effect sizes ranging from 0.34 to 0.44 (Weichold & Blumenthal, 2016). A program delivered in the early elementary school years, the "Good Behavior Game," was also found to be a surprisingly effective program for reducing externalizing behavior in high school, including drug use (Kellam, Reid, & Balster, 2008). Although delivered as a universal program in high-risk schools, this program seems to have its effects by reducing impulsive behavior in children most at risk of later externalizing problems.

A review of school-based prevention programs for illicit drugs conducted by Faggiano et al. (2008) concluded that skill-based programs such the life skills training program were most successful in reducing the use of these drugs, with reductions on the order of 20% in drug use progression. A review of school-based drug education programs focusing on marijuana use found an overall effect size of 0.58 in reduced use, which amounted to a success rate of 28% compared to controls (Porath-Waller, Beasley, & Beirness, 2010). This review also suggested that programs delivered to youth older than 13 were more effective than those for younger youth. A study of potential drug prevention mediators in over 7,000 U.S. students assessed from ninth to 11th grade indicated that apart from attitudes and beliefs about the harms of drugs, youth with better problem-solving skills were more likely to report reduced drug use of alcohol, cigarettes, and marijuana in 11th grade (Stephens et al., 2009). This study supports the strategies employed in the more successful universal school-based drug prevention programs that emphasize skills as well as beliefs and attitudes as targets of intervention.

A more recently developed approach that can potentially reach large audiences without using limited school resources is drug prevention programming delivered over the Internet. A review of these programs found some encouraging evidence of effects on reduction in marijuana use (Tait, Spijkerman, & Riper, 2013). These programs have been tested with adolescents and found to have an effect size of 0.17; however, the follow-up periods have been short. Although the effects are smaller than more intense school-based programs, these interventions are still in the early stages of development and may be a useful approach to consider for further refinement.

Mandatory Random Drug Testing in Schools

Another school-based approach to drug use prevention that has gained popularity in recent years is the use of mandatory random drug testing among students involved in sports and other extracurricular activities. These programs require students who wish to play sports or participate in clubs and organizations to agree to be tested at random with biological assays during the school year. It is estimated that approximately 13% of schools have adopted some version of this policy (CDC, 2015). Although this policy has been challenged in the courts, the U.S. Supreme Court has ruled on two occasions that schools are not barred from implementing such policies. Students who screen positively are referred to treatment and are often excluded from participating in school activities for the school year. Only two trials have been conducted to test this strategy (Goldberg et al., 2007; James-Burdumy, Goesling, Deke, & Einspruch, 2012), and the results have been largely negative. In the one trial that found reductions in reported drug use in the past 30 days (James-Burdumy et al., 2012), there was no evidence that the intervention reduced attitudes or intentions toward drug use. A large analysis of MTF data over a period of 14 years (Terry-McElrath, O'Malley, & Johnston, 2013) found that students in schools that employed drug testing reported less use of marijuana but increased use of other drugs that were not subject to testing. Other surveys have found that schools with better social climates had less drug use but that, apart from this school characteristic, testing was not associated with reduced use of tobacco, alcohol, or marijuana (Sznitman, Dunlop, Nakkur, & Romer, 2012; Sznitman & Romer, 2014).

Environmental Universal Interventions

Another class of universal interventions implements policies that attempt to influence the social and legal environment of entire communities, including schools, parents, drug dispensaries (e.g., bars, shops, and other retail outlets), and police regarding legal purchase age and other restrictions on drug use, such as driving under the influence of alcohol. We first review some environmental strategies that have been implemented through statewide policy and then examine efforts that include greater enforcement of restrictions on drug access and use in local communities.

Mass Media Campaigns

Mass media campaigns represent an environmental approach sometimes combined with school-based programs. The most frequent uses of mass media involve campaigns to reduce the uptake of cigarettes. These programs typically highlight the harms of drug use and the benefits of cessation for those who have already initiated. A Cochrane Review of seven programs that met the best standards of evaluation found evidence to support their efficacy (Brinn, Carson, Esterman, Chang, & Smith, 2010). However, such programs are difficult to evaluate and the evidence was regarded as weak in relation to programs delivered in typical randomized clinical trials. A longstanding campaign implemented in California appears to have had success (Pierce, White, & Gilpin, 2005), and indeed California has among the lowest rates of adolescent smoking in the United States (California Department of Public Health, 2015). Campaigns that raised awareness about the ways that the tobacco industry has misled young people about the hazards of smoking have had success (The Truth campaign). This message, which has been tested both in national samples by the American Legacy Foundation (Thrasher et al., 2004) and in selected states (e.g., Sly, Heald, & Ray, 2001), appears capable of reducing the uptake of smoking in adolescents. Nevertheless, these evaluations relied on quasi-experimental designs that do not meet the highest standards of evidence. With the passage of the Family Smoking Prevention and Tobacco Control Act of 2009, the U.S. Food and Drug Administration, in collaboration with the U.S. Centers for Disease Control and Prevention, has developed smoking cessation media campaigns directed toward both adults and adolescents. Initial results of these efforts in regard to adult outcomes suggest that the campaigns encourage quitting (McAfee et al., 2013). However, effects on youth initiation have not as yet been evaluated.

Other programs have been delivered to reduce the uptake of illegal drugs, such as marijuana. A Cochrane Review of these programs also found some evidence of efficacy; however, the evidence was not consistent (Ferri et al., 2013). The National Youth Anti-Drug Media Campaign, supported by the U.S. Office of National Drug Control Policy (ONDCP), was intensely evaluated. From September 1999 to June 2004, three nationally representative cohorts of U.S. youths ages 9 to 18 years were surveyed at home four times. Main outcomes were self-reported lifetime, past-year, and past-30-day marijuana use and related cognitions. Most analyses showed no effects of the campaign (Hornik, Jacobsohn, Orwin, Piesse, & Kalton, 2008). It was concluded that through June 2004, the campaign was unlikely to have had favorable effects and may have actually had delayed unfavorable effects. In particular, exposure at round three predicted marijuana initiation at round four, potentially because the campaign increased perceptions that peers were using marijuana and that its use was appealing despite the risks.

The failure of the ONDCP media campaign led to the development of a new program that is currently sponsored by the nonprofit Partnership for Drug-Free Kids. This program features a message that encourages youth to live "Above the Influence" of illicit drug use. The campaign does not highlight peer use of drugs but rather features the importance of being in control of one's life. An evaluation of the program using a randomized community design indicated reductions in use of marijuana over a 2-year follow-up period (Slater, Kelly, Lawrence, Stanley, & Comello, 2011). The study was also able to evaluate the concurrent national campaign using the same message strategy. Exposure to both programs was found to produce less use of marijuana. In addition, the message that drug use interferes with personal life aspirations was found to mediate campaign effects.

Raising Drug Prices

Making drugs more costly is another universal approach that can affect adolescent drug use. This approach is most amenable to intervention for legal drugs, such as tobacco and alcohol, for which taxes can be applied that increase the cost to the consumer. Price interventions for cigarettes vary considerably across states, and thus evaluations can be conducted to assess their success. These studies tend to find that price does affect adolescent uptake of cigarettes (Huang & Chaloupka, 2012), although there is some dispute about the breadth of the effect (Fletcher, Deb, & Sindelar, 2009). Price effects on alcohol are similar, but efforts to raise taxes on this product have been much less successful (National Research Council, 2004). Indeed, taxes on alcohol have remained relatively low in comparison to inflation in the United States.

Age of Purchase

Legal age of purchase of alcohol has been aggressively pursued as official policy since 1984, when the U.S. Congress voted to withhold federal funds for highway construction in states that did not adopt 21 as the legal age for purchase of alcohol. This policy has been credited with reducing motor vehicle crashes attributable to alcohol in adolescents (DeJong & Blanchette, 2014). However, it is noteworthy that the policy was adopted following an aggressive media campaign by Mothers Against Drunk Driving, which highlighted the dangers of alcohol use, especially in regard to driving. This campaign was also active in Canada, which also experienced a parallel reduction in adolescent motor vehicle crashes despite having legal purchase ages of 18 and 19, depending on the province (Hedlund, Ulmer, & Preusser, 2001). Thus, at least some of the effects of this policy are likely to be attributed to changes in societal views about the dangers of using alcohol, as reflected in the steady decline in alcohol use among adolescents illustrated in Figure 19.1. At the same time, rates of heavy drinking among college students have been lower in Canada than in the United States (Kuo et al., 2002), suggesting that the lower legal drinking age in Canada has not encouraged excessive drinking in this young transitioning adult group. Adolescent driving habits have also changed, with less reporting of driving while under the influence of alcohol (Terry-McElrath, O'Malley, & Johnston, 2014) and greater use of seatbelts (Carpenter & Stehr, 2008). These changes are also likely to be the result of societal influences apart from the age 21 law (Hedlund et al., 2001).

The legal age for purchase of cigarettes has been 18 in most states. However, efforts are under way at the time of this writing to raise the age to 21, just as for alcohol. Support for this policy also derives from research suggesting that it would deter the progression of cigarette use in adolescents, when most initiate the use of this drug.

Marijuana is now a legally purchased product in several states with the age of purchase set at 21.

Community Environmental Interventions

Community environmental interventions use various strategies to enforce restrictions on the sale of drugs to youth, especially alcohol and cigarettes, or to encourage responsible alcoholic beverage service as a way to reduce the adverse effects of alcohol use in bars and other retail outlets (Saltz, Grube, & Treno, 2015). Based on the evidence that statewide policies regarding purchase and access to alcohol and tobacco can reduce its uptake in young people, the various strategies employed in community environmental interventions attempt to increase the effects of these policies through greater enforcement and awareness of restrictions. In their review of these interventions, Saltz et al. (2015) note that the evidence that has accumulated over time finds that these programs can produce modest reductions in a variety of outcomes, including reductions in alcohol-related injuries and use of alcohol by young people. Here again, however, the studies that have evaluated these interventions tend to require quasi-experimental designs that do not meet the highest standards of evidence. In addition, the interventions tend to combine a variety of strategies, so it is not clear which ones worked or the theoretical processes that mediated the effects (Saltz et al., 2015). Nevertheless, the finding that such programs can reduce the adverse effects of alcohol use and tobacco uptake suggests that communities that wish to address youth access and use of drugs can do so with a variety of strategies.

Family-Focused Interventions

Another important category of universal interventions are family-focused ones. Such programs are designed to strengthen bonds to family, school, and community and facilitate participant development of family-connected skills consistent with etiological research. Educating on the dangers of substance abuse is not the main focus, since, by this model, substance abuse is understood as having important family components, at several levels: parental monitoring, effective parent–child communication and disciplining, and improved conflict resolution. They have been adapted for various age groups and can be used as selective and indicated programs as well. An early version of this approach called the Supporting Families Program is illustrated in the causal model in Figure 19.3. As is evident, the family is only one component of influences on drug use in adolescents. In this social ecology model, family bonding is central to establishing effective supervision of the adolescent, which then influences family and peer norms for drug use. Family bonding also encourages greater attachment to school, which enhances norms against drug use. All of these influences are embedded within the larger community, which also affects peer and family norms. Kumpfer, Alvarado, and Whiteside (2003) argued, based on a literature review at the time, that family-focused interventions are up to nine times more effective than school-based programs in reducing alcohol use. A Cochrane Review found that a majority of family-based programs reduced alcohol use in adolescents (Foxcroft & Tsertsvadze, 2012). A review of the effects of various universal as well as selective family-based interventions in regard to marijuana and other illicit drugs found that these programs have some success in reducing the initiation of marijuana use (Vermeulen-Smit, Verdurmen, & Engels, 2015). However, evidence of success in reducing the uptake of other illicit drugs was less robust.

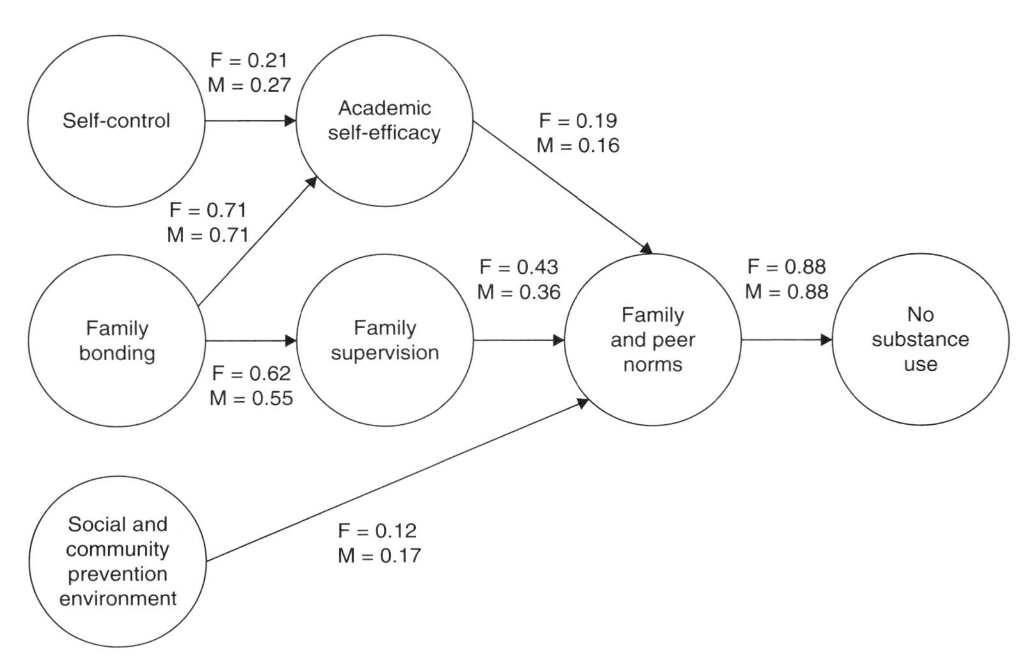

Figure 19.3 Social ecology model of substance abuse by gender (path weights are for males/females). (From Kumpfer, 2014.)

Spoth, Trudeau, Guyll, and Redmond (2009) have produced a shorter version of this intervention that has been rigorously evaluated and found to be effective, the Strengthening Families Program for Parents and Youth Ages 10–14 (SFP 10-14). Implementation of the SFP entails seven weekly sessions. The SFP has separate sessions for parents and children that run concurrently for 1 hour and focus on skills building. During the second hour parents and children participate together in a joint hour-long family session, during which they practice the skills learned in their separate sessions. The family session affords the opportunity for higher-risk families and those with special needs to identify available services. In addition, the family session includes activities designed to encourage family cohesiveness and positive involvement of the child in family activities. For the parental sessions, the essential content and key concepts of the program are also presented on videotape. Further detail regarding the SFP is provided in a recent review (Spoth, Redmond, Mason, Schainker, & Borduin, 2015). A 10-year follow-up of one test of the intervention found reduced levels of illicit drug use at age 21 mediated by reduced progression of drug use produced by the intervention (Spoth, Trudeau, Guyll, & Shin, 2012).

Because family-based interventions have positive effects on family functioning, they can also reduce other outcomes that are associated with drug use, such as internalizing symptoms of depression and anxiety. In a trial that employed SFP approaches, Trudeau et al. (2007) found that the intervention reduced internalizing symptoms, especially in girls, as well as polydrug use over a period of several years. Other crossover effects include reductions in risky sexual behavior and enhanced school performance (reviewed in Spoth et al., 2015). The growing evidence in support of SFP also includes cost-effectiveness analyses showing clear benefits for each dollar spent on the program (Spoth et al., 2015).

Some interventions merge family-focused approaches with other community programs, such as school-based interventions and media programs. An example of this type of expanded program is Project STAR (Pentz et al., 1989).

This intervention model attempts to involve the entire community with a comprehensive school program, a mass media campaign, a parent program, a community organizing component, and a health policy change component. Project STAR has been shown to be effective in terms of reductions in drug use behavior in high school for those youth who began the program in middle school. Another noteworthy example is the program of university–community partnerships developed by Spoth et al. (2011). In this program, communities collaborate with university researchers to implement a menu of effective drug prevention interventions. A demonstration of this approach in 28 school districts in rural Iowa and Pennsylvania found sizeable reductions in drug use compared to controls over a 7.5-year period (Spoth et al., 2011, 2013).

Indicated Intervention Programs

One of the limitations of universal drug prevention programs for schools is their need for multiple sessions over periods of 1 to 2 years (Gottfredson & Wilson, 2003). The review by Porath et al. (2010) found that programs with fewer than 15 sessions were less successful in reducing use of marijuana. Another approach is to implement more concentrated and brief interventions (e.g., 5 hours) that target youth already using drugs. A review of these programs that focus on prevention of alcohol-use progression found that such programs, when delivered individually, can have a positive effect (Hennessy & Tanner-Smith, 2015). Ideally, such programs would be more feasible if they could be delivered in group settings; however, group interventions also can introduce iatrogenic effects resulting from peer modeling among high-risk youth (Dishion & Dodge, 2005). An approach that screens for and then treats higher-risk youth in schools is discussed in Chapter 31.

The Reconnecting Youth Program (Eggert et al., 1994, 1995) is another example of a school-based indicated intervention. This program is for adolescents in grades nine to 12 who show signs of poor school achievement and the potential to drop out. The program teaches skills to build resiliency toward risk factors and to moderate early signs of drug abuse. It consists of several components, such as a Personal Growth Class designed to enhance self-esteem, decision making, personal control, and interpersonal communications; a Social Activities and School Bonding Program to establish drug-free peer relationships; and a School System Crisis Response Plan to address suicide prevention. Evaluations of this intervention have documented only short-term benefits, with long-term studies yet to be done.

Indicated programs for older adolescents and young adults have been developed primarily to address heavy use of alcohol in college students. These programs employ Motivational Interviewing, which is typically delivered individually by a skilled interventionist (e.g., McCambridge & Strang, 2004). Toumbourou et al. (2007) identified these as effective interventions for this age group.

Applying Knowledge of Genetics to Reduce Drug Use

The enormous toll that drug dependence takes may also lead prevention experts to consider ways that genetic risk information might be used to identify high-risk subgroups of youth who might benefit from more intensive or tailored prevention approaches. As reviewed in greater detail elsewhere in regard to the prevention of adolescent smoking (Audrain-McGovern & Tercyak, 2011; Lerman, Patterson, & Shields, 2003; Wilfond et al., 2002), there are many ethical challenges and considerations regarding this strategy. From a scientific perspective, research on genetics and tobacco use is still in its infancy. There is no single "tobacco use gene," as for any other drug, and as such, risk estimates will need to take into account multiple interactions among genetic, social, and psychological factors. Even considering genetic variants with widely validated effects on smoking behavior, these effects are likely to be small, and risk estimates will be highly probabilistic. Additional risks of genetic testing of adolescents include stigmatization, discrimination, and potential adverse psychological effects

(Audrain-McGovern & Tercyak, 2011; Lerman, Patterson, & Shields, 2003).

Multilevel Intervention Programs

Multilevel intervention programs are typically combinations of the above intervention models. They include universal, selected, and indicated strategies gauged to the needs of the adolescent.

The Family Check-Up (Dishion & Kavanagh, 2000) is an example of a multilevel intervention designed to address the needs of families of young adolescents who present with a range of problem behaviors and diverse developmental histories, as illustrated in Figure 19.2. This ambitious program incorporates universal, selective, and indicated prevention components. The universal intervention is offered to all students in middle schools in the form of a school-based family management program. This intervention is a shortened version of Botvin's life skills training program, with only six sessions. Families whose children need further attention are offered the selective intervention, which offers a more intense three-session assessment of family interaction patterns, with suggestions for ways to improve those interactions to support the at-risk youth's healthier development. Motivational Interviewing techniques are used to encourage more adaptive family conflict resolution and parent engagement strategies to prevent the escalation of unhealthy behavior. The program provides a menu of services that includes a brief family intervention, school monitoring system, parent groups, behavioral family therapy, and case management services. In one study, the selective Family Check-Up intervention condition was related to increased levels of students' self-regulation skills from sixth to seventh grades, which in turn reduced the risk for growth in antisocial behavior, involvement with deviant peers, and alcohol, tobacco, and marijuana use through the eighth grade (Fosco, Frank, Stormshak, & Dishion, 2013). A 10-year follow-up study showed that the selective intervention reduced the progression in use of alcohol, tobacco, and marijuana through age 21 (Veronneau, Dishion, & Connell, 2014).

In a review of this program of research, Dishion et al. (2015) emphasized the value of their multilevel approach to drug use prevention for its effectiveness, efficiency, and cost. Families with the lowest-risk children receive only the universal intervention, which saves on resources and time without compromising the benefits of this program. Greater resources are devoted primarily to families with greater needs, and these families show the strongest preventive effects. Thus, the program is able to allocate attention to the children who would otherwise not receive adequate preventive services in a universal-only program. Finally, the selective and indicated interventions are only provided to families who seek those services. However, experience in the program suggests that families recognize the need for those services and willingly accept them. Finally, the program can be tailored to the ethnic background of the families, thus increasing their effectiveness and acceptability.

Another example of a multilevel intervention with a family focus is the Triple-P (Positive Parenting Program) (Sanders, 2012; Sanders et al., 2014). This program employs a mass media intervention to reach and engage parents across the risk spectrum and to identify those at greater need for intervention. Up to five levels of selective and indicated interventions are delivered in various venues to parents (e.g., through face-to-face meetings with a practitioner, phone meetings, self-directed materials, or in small groups). An extensive meta-analysis involving over 16,000 children across the United States, Europe, and Australia found that each level of the program produced improvements in parenting behavior and child outcomes related to the emergence of externalizing behavior in adolescence (Sanders et al., 2014). The program has been replicated in poor urban neighborhoods as well as in larger jurisdictions, thus providing a model of prevention that can be easily brought to scale.

FUTURE CHALLENGES FOR PREVENTIVE INTERVENTIONS

Since the first edition of this book, numerous efforts have been undertaken to identify and disseminate descriptive information about model preventive interventions. Reviews of these interventions typically include descriptions of selection criteria or rules of evidence applied and summaries of the intervention review process. Many also delineate salient characteristics of the types of programs that have proven to be effective. A major issue for the field is the variability in the rules of evidence and intervention selection criteria, with the level of scientific rigor applied varying considerably. A commonly expressed concern in the Cochrane Reviews is the absence of rigor in the evaluation of drug prevention interventions (Foxcroft & Tesertsvadze, 2012). There is concern regarding the presence of bias in many evaluations, with program designers being involved in the tests of their interventions. One review of early school-based drug prevention programs that were evaluated by researchers unconnected with the design of the programs found no evidence of efficacy (Flynn, Falco, & Hocini, 2015). While this is unlikely to explain all of the favorable evidence we have reviewed, it is a source of concern.

Another issue for future development of drug abuse prevention programs is determining the best ages to deliver programs in schools and for families (see Spoth, Greenberg, & Turisi, 2009, for an overview of interventions that target different age groups). Family interventions tend to focus on childhood and early adolescence. School-based programs also tend to be delivered in middle school, with follow-ups that only extend into the middle of high school. These programs were designed in part to prevent the early initiation of drug use. However, given that progression continues well into high school, it is important to deliver programs to youth at these ages as well. One review found that such programs tended to be more effective in reducing the use of marijuana, which is likely to emerge later in high school, than programs delivered in middle school. A family-based program using SFP principles delivered to older adolescents in the rural South was noted to be one of the few designed for older adolescents (Brody et al., 2012).

An issue often noted in the field of prevention research is the absence of theoretical models that distill the essential mechanisms underlying intervention efficacy. Interventions are designed to include multiple components that target important sources of efficacy. However, program effects are often evaluated with a focus on drug use endpoints without assessing the mediating mechanisms. This problem has been noted for the evaluation of tobacco cessation programs by Baker et al. (2011), with a call for greater attention to short-term mediating mechanisms that can help to determine the efficacy of intervention components as they proceed. For example, it is not clear across the various prevention approaches reviewed here what the mediating mechanisms are that underlie program efficacy and the time courses of their influence. Unless we understand those mechanisms, it will be difficult to determine the correct mix and strength of program components. Attempts to isolate such components, such as the Multiphase Optimization Strategy (MOST) of Collins et al. (2011), are important steps that could advance the evaluation of prevention programs. However, to achieve the full benefits of MOST, greater attention to effects on mediating mechanisms will be required.

Prevention professionals have broadened the target of their interventions, going beyond substance abuse to address the global quality of youth development. Advocates of positive youth development approaches emphasize that efforts to address public health concerns by preventing youth problem behaviors must be pursued in concert with youth-related health promotion goals. The need to integrate prevention and youth-related health promotion—or positive youth development—has emerged as a consequence of the observation that problem-free youth are not necessarily fully prepared youth (Pittman, 2000). A review of these programs is presented in Chapter 26.

A final challenge regarding effective interventions is the failure of schools and communities to employ evidence-based programs. An excellent source of evidence-based programs is available in the Blueprints registry (http://www.blueprintsprograms.com/). In addition, both the National Institute on Drug Abuse (NIDA) and the Substance Abuse and Mental Health Services Administration (SAMHSA) maintain lists of effective drug abuse prevention programs. However, schools adopt a wide range of programs that vary in effectiveness (Kumar et al., 2011). They may also resort to strategies that sound effective but have little evidence to support them (e.g., drug testing). The emerging field of implementation science is an attempt to identify the best ways to translate efficacious programs into acceptable and enduring practices in communities (Neta et al., 2015; Pas & Bradshaw, 2015; Spoth et al., 2013). A future challenge in the field of prevention science is to identify methods that encourage adoption of effective programs that can be implemented with fidelity in community settings.

Chapter 30 outlines recent advances in the implementation of evidence-based interventions (EBIs) for child and adolescent healthcare. It is striking how these EBIs have been aided by the need to enhance the cost-effectiveness of medical care across all provider systems. Although significant challenges remain, the successes achieved using Internet education to hasten the dissemination of EBIs to providers suggests that similar strategies will be helpful to prevention specialists. For example, although registries such as Blueprints identify effective programs, they do little to help users select the right program for their specific needs, and they do not always link to resources that can be used to train interventionists to implement the program faithfully. Based on our review of EBIs, it is clear that schools are a major venue for delivery of prevention programs and that health providers in those settings should be a target for the dissemination of EBIs. In addition, community-based prevention activities could be administered by county health officials who are responsible for promoting the health of their localities. A major challenge for the successful dissemination and adoption of EBIs will be the demonstration of return on investment, especially in regard to whatever funds are currently devoted to activities that better prevention practices would curtail (e.g., drug enforcement, school failure, and youth injury). There is some evidence that prevention and health promotion programs are cost-effective (see also Chapter 26). Greater efforts to make these programs attractive to local stakeholders will be a critical element in future efforts to increase adoption of effective prevention programs.

CONCLUSION

It is fitting to close this chapter on prevention by highlighting the need for a national youth development strategy. Planning for a comprehensive strategy to foster positive youth development and to prevent youth substance-related problems necessitates a sustained, well-organized effort, with inputs from a range of community interventionists, scientists, and policymakers at the state and federal levels. One potential contribution to this larger planning effort is a design for universities and communities to partner together to foster a higher prevalence of capable and problem-free youth (Spoth et al., 2011). However, the wide range of tasks for those involved in community–university partnerships, the many barriers to task accomplishment, and the limited resources available highlight the challenges to the design of developmentally appropriate preventive interventions. There are well-known predictors of risk for drug abuse and reliable screening instruments, and some early risk factors can be easily recognized based on clinical presentation, such as fighting or school absence. There are also effective multilevel programs, such as Triple-P, using a public health approach that can serve as a model for the effective delivery of preventive interventions. However, an integrated program of prevention activities, as a national policy, is still lacking.

Concerns about inadequate prevention programming are all the more urgent given trends in drug use that affect adolescents, a prime example being various forms of legalization of marijuana. Although this drug may be less harmful than alcohol, its legalization will create new challenges to prevention programs, which will have to deal with a newly legal but addictive drug (Caulkins, Hawken, Kilmer, & Kleiman, 2012). There are also challenges to the increased use of prescription drugs, with a lifetime prevalence of 18.3%, including narcotics that are often prescribed for the reduction of pain (8.4%) (Johnston et al., 2016a, 2016b). Adolescents are increasingly trying these drugs, sometimes with unfortunate consequences. Finally, there is the new method of delivering nicotine, the electronic cigarette, that is also being tried by adolescents (16.2% past 30-day prevalence) (Johnston et al., 2016a, 2016b). Although use of cigarettes has declined in recent years, overall experimentation with tobacco products still remains high, at around 26% (Arrazola et al., 2015). All of these emerging ways of delivering addictive products will pose new challenges to the field of drug abuse prevention. It is hoped that the potential benefits of efficient and effective intervention strategies that employ the full range of universal, selective, and indicated interventions will become a common feature of an overall positive youth development program delivered through existing community, state, and national structures.

Research Agenda for Substance Use Disorders

Charles O'Brien
Daniel Romer

chapter 20

For a variety of reasons, limited research has been conducted among adolescents with substance dependence. We operate as though the data obtained from studies in adults apply to adolescents, but we know that there are critical differences. Thus, assumptions about adolescents must be empirically tested, and adolescents do not readily volunteer as participants in clinical trials. The following are a series of questions compiled by the Substance Abuse Commission, updated for the second edition.

What We Know

- If not treated, substance use can often progress to addiction and become a lifelong illness.
- There are gender differences in the addiction pathway.
- Heredity increases the vulnerability to addiction.
- Psychiatric comorbidity is common and may add risk for drug addiction.
- Long-term treatment is usually required to arrest addiction.
- Motivation is an important ingredient for successful treatment.
  Changes in lifestyle are required.
  Drug use is a pleasure-reinforced compulsion.
  Drug craving may be stimulated by drug-using environments, which may also provoke relapse.
- Adolescents are different from adults:
  Differences in brain development and plasticity
  Differences in social, personal, academic, and professional challenges.
- Specialized treatment approaches are necessary, including:
  Age-appropriate interventions
  More focus on family treatment
  Longitudinal continuation of treatment
- Availability of drugs and beliefs about the hazards of drug use are key variables in the uptake and progression of drug use.
- Prevention programs do work, although there is no single approach that can succeed for all youth.

What We Do Not Know

- Which psychosocial treatments are most effective? All of the following show some promise:
  Individual therapy (cognitive-behavioral therapy, motivational enhancement therapy)
  Family therapy
  Group therapy
  12-step rehabilitation
- Is group therapy an effective modality for adolescents?
  If so, how should it be structured?
  Should adolescents always be segregated from adults in group treatment?
- What is the neurobiology of adolescent addiction (initiation and progression of addictive pattern, vulnerability to specific agents)?
- What effects do addictive drugs have on brain development in youth, and are they reversible?
- Is harm reduction an acceptable goal for adolescents?
  Does nicotine use impede recovery?
- How can we enhance perceived risk concerning experimenting with drugs?
- How can we best match patients with treatments? Matching problems to treatments has been found effective in small studies but is rarely used in practice.
- Can the judicial system positively influence outcome?

What We Urgently Need To Know: The Priorities

- Which specialized treatments for adolescent addiction provide the best outcomes?
- Which specialized programs can prevent binge drinking in college?
- Which pharmacological treatments work best for adolescents with substance use disorders?
  Pharmaceutical companies have shown little interest in developing medications for adult addictions and none for substance abuse in adolescence. How can we

recruit pharma into the area of prevention and treatment?

- What are the best means of identifying adolescents at risk for addiction?
- How can we recruit scientists into the area of addiction research?
- How can we best respond to the increasing acceptance of cannabis, and what kinds of prevention programs will best avoid the widespread use of this drug in youth?
- How can we best respond to the increasing use of alternative ways of delivering nicotine?
- How can we improve the treatment system?

  How can we obtain adequate reimbursement for treatment providers? Adolescent treatment programs are scarce and underfunded.

  How can we provide an accessible continuum of care with age-appropriate expertise?

    - Medical and psychiatric evaluation capability
    - Inpatient facilities
    - Partial hospitalization/intensive outpatient programs
    - Outpatient treatment with long-term capability

  How can we integrate substance abuse treatment with other mental health treatment?

    - Comorbidity of substance abuse with other mental disorders is very common.
    - Few treatment programs are equipped to treat dual-diagnosis patients.
    - Clinical trials in adolescents do exist, but they are few in number.
    - Clinicians, including psychiatrists, typically have little training in the treatment of patients with substance abuse, especially patients with coexisting psychiatric disorders.

- How can we disseminate scientific evidence supporting the disease concept of addiction? How can we bring effective prevention programs to scale in states and communities?
- How can political initiatives secure appropriate resource allocation?

Youth Suicide and Suicide Attempts

COMMISSION ON ADOLESCENT SUICIDE PREVENTION

Herbert Hendin, *Commission Chair*

Second Edition

Ann P. Haas

Jill Harkavy-Friedman

Maggie G. Mortali

First Edition

David A. Brent

Jack R. Cornelius

Tamera Coyne- Beasley

Madelyn Gould

Ted Greenberg

Ann Pollinger Haas

Jill Harkavy- Friedman

Richard Harrington

Gregg Henriques

First Edition cont.

Douglas G. Jacobs

John Kalafat

Mary Margaret Kerr

Cheryl A. King

Richard Ramsay

David Shaffer

Anthony Spirito

Howard Sudak

Elaine Adams Thompson

part VI

Defining Youth Suicide

Ann P. Haas

chapter 21

SCOPE AND DEMOGRAPHICS

Completed Suicide

In the middle of the last century, suicide among adolescents and young adults was a relatively infrequent event, and suicides in this age group constituted less than 5% of all suicides in the United States. As shown in Figure 21.1, in the 25-year period from 1955 to 1980, the rate of suicide among youth roughly tripled, from around four suicides to over 12 per 100,000 persons ages 15 to 24. By 1980, suicides by 15- to 24-year-olds constituted almost 17% of the almost 27,000 total suicides in the United States (National Center for Health Statistics, n.d.), with males accounting for about 80% of youth suicides.

Rising youth suicide rates continued, albeit at a slower pace, during the 1980s and early 1990s, reaching a peak age-adjusted rate of 13.4 per 100,000 in 1994. In 1995, rates began a general decline, decreasing to a low of 9.6 per 100,000 youth in 2003. Since that year, youth suicide rates have again shown an increasing trend. Between 2004 and 2015 (the last year for which national data are currently available), the youth suicide rate steadily rose from 10.2 to 12.3 per 100,000, with the exception of 2007, when the rate decreased to 9.5. In 2015, the suicide rate among youth ages 15 to 24 approximated what it had been in 1980. The 5,491 suicides that occurred in youth in 2015 represented slightly more than 12% of the 44,193 total suicides in the United States (Centers for Disease Control and Prevention, n.d.a). The decrease from 17% in 1980 was largely attributable to the increased number of suicides occurring in age groups other than youth in recent years. Among youth, suicide is currently the third leading cause of death, with only accidents and homicide claiming more young lives.

Figures available since 1970 (Fig. 21.2) show that the suicide rates among the younger subset of youth (ages 15–19) have been consistently lower than those for the older subset (ages 20–24). In 2015, suicide took the lives of 2,061 youth between the ages of 15 and 19, with a suicide rate of 9.8. This compares to 3,430 suicides occurring among youth ages 20 to 24, for a rate of 15.1 per 100,000. In both age groups, the suicide rate has been trending upward in recent years.

Suicides in youth before the age of 15 are rare, but the rate increases with every year past puberty (CDC, n.d.a). Although suicide

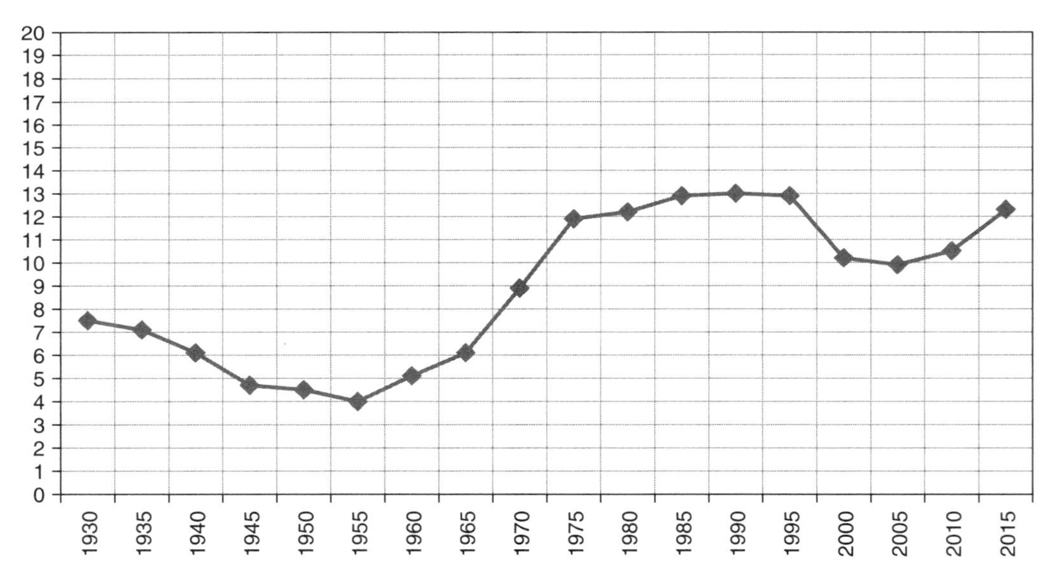

Figure 21.1 Rates of suicide for 15- to 24-year-olds, both sexes, all races. (Source: National Center for Health Statistics)

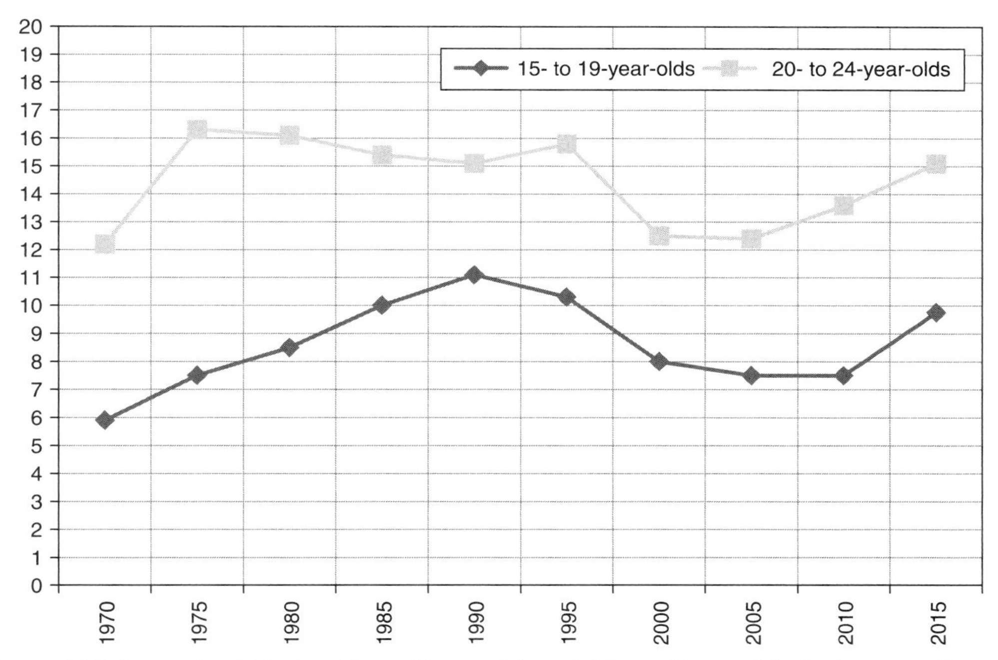

Figure 21.2 Rates of suicide for 15- to 19-year-olds and 20- to 24-year-olds, both sexes, all races. (Source: National Center for Health Statistics)

deaths among preteens have tended to receive considerable media attention, the suicide rate of youth ages 5 to 14 remained well under 1 per 100,000 up until 2014, when it slightly exceeded 1.0. In 2015, the age-adjusted suicide rate for this age group was exactly 1.0 per 100,000.

The previously mentioned gender disparity in youth suicide has continued to be noted. In 2015, the suicide rate for males ages 15 to 24 was 19.1 per 100,000, and the rate for females of the same ages was 5.3. At these rates, young males ages 15 to 24 are almost four times as likely to die by suicide compared to young females. This gender disparity in youth has been decreasing slightly in recent years but continues to be generally maintained across the lifespan.

Youth suicide rates also vary among different racial and ethnic groups. In 2015, American Indians/Alaskan Natives had the highest suicide rate among youth ages 15 to 24, at 20.6 per 100,000. Rates for youth in all other racial and ethnic groups were considerably lower, with white youth having a suicide rate of 13.2, Asian American/Pacific Islander youth 9.9, black youth 8.1, and Hispanic youth 5.2 per 100,000 (CDC, n.d.a). Youth whose race/ethnicity was classified as "other" had a suicide rate of 12.3 per 100,000. In recent years, the suicide rate for youth in all racial and ethnic groups has increased except for Hispanic youth, whose rate has decreased.

Considering young males separately, the highest suicide rate was found among American Indians/Alaskan Natives (48.4 per 100,000), followed by whites (23.0), "other" (19.8), Asian Americans/Pacific Islanders (14.9), blacks (12.8), and Hispanics (12.6). The rank order of suicide rates among young females was American Indians/Alaskan Natives (18.9), "other" (6.8), whites (6.1), Asian Americans/Pacific Islanders (4.7), Hispanics (3.8) and blacks (3.6).

National data are lacking for other demographic characteristics that appear to be related to rates of youth suicide, notably sexual orientation and gender identity. The U.S. Standard Death Certificate, which is the key source of Centers for Disease Control and Prevention (CDC) mortality statistics, does not record information on the deceased person's sexual orientation (e.g., heterosexual, gay, lesbian, bisexual). Additionally, the death certificate includes only two gender categories, male and female, precluding identification of transgender status and decedents whose gender was outside this binary system. Although supplemental data are collected and recorded by the National Violent Death Reporting System, this information is drawn primarily from the records of medical examiners, coroners, and law enforcement personnel, and none of these sources systematically inquire about sexual orientation or gender identity (http://www.cdc.gov/violenceprevention/nvdrs/).

Clearly, identifying young people by sexual orientation and gender identity after death would be challenging. Parents, who typically would be the ones to make this determination, may not know or be willing to share this information with the appropriate officials. And even if all youth who die by suicide could be identified by sexual orientation and gender identity, translating these figures into age-specific suicide rates would require knowing how many sexual and gender minority (SGM) youth there are in the specific locale—information that is not gathered by the U.S. Census.

Lacking official information about suicide rates in SGM populations, psychological autopsy methods have been used to determine whether sexual minority youth are overrepresented among young suicide decedents (Renaud et al., 2010; Shaffer et al., 1995). Although these studies have concluded that youth with a minority sexual orientation were not overrepresented, a reanalysis of the reported data suggested that such youth may be more likely than heterosexual youth to die by suicide (Plöderal et al., 2013). The absence of national confirmatory data, however, limits our efforts to address the underlying problems that may be responsible for this finding.

Also not identified in mortality statistics is whether youth were attending college at the time of death, which may have implications for how suicide prevention interventions might be targeted (Haas, Hendin, & Mann, 2003). An in-depth study of suicides in 12 Midwestern universities (Silverman, Meyer, Sloane, Raffel, & Pratt, 1997) and later analyses (Schwartz, 2011) point to a significantly lower rate of suicide in college students compared to youth of the same ages who are not in school. Despite a rise in previous decades, the overall suicide rate among college students appears to have remained stable or decreased since the early 1990s (Schwartz, 2006, 2011), although a higher risk for suicide has been observed in certain groups, including commuter students, older students, sexual and gender minority students, and international students (Russell, Van Camen, Hoefle, & Boor, 2011). If suicides among students who drop out or were encouraged by schools to take leaves of absence because of mental health problems were consistently counted, college suicide rates might be higher than reported. Even at the reported rate, suicide is thought to be the second leading cause of death among college students, following accidents, since homicide rates on college campuses are extremely low.

Suicide Attempts and Suicidal Ideation

In the United States, trends in the prevalence of nonfatal suicide attempts are tracked primarily through population-based surveys. Caution should be taken when interpreting these data as studies have shown sometimes substantial discrepancies between reported and clinically verified suicide attempts (Bongiovi-Garcia et al., 2009; Kessler et al., 1999; Nock & Kessler, 2006). Because survey questions do not typically define what is meant by a suicide attempt, respondents may include self-harm behaviors that lacked the intent to die, or omit those where intent was present but by chance resulted in minimal harm. Comparing U.S. survey findings on suicide attempts with findings from international studies is further complicated by the common use of the term *self-harm behavior* in some countries, which does not consistently distinguish behaviors with intent to die from what is commonly called non-suicidal self-injury (Nock et al., 2006).

Since 1991, the most systematic data on adolescent suicide attempts and suicidal ideation have come from the national Youth Risk

Behavior Survey (YRBS), conducted by the CDC to monitor behaviors that pose substantial risk to health and mortality, including suicide attempts. The YRBS is administered every other year to a representative sample of public and private school students in grades nine through 12 (http://www.cdc.gov/healthyyouth/yrbs/pdf/ system_overview_yrbs.pdf). The YRBS is a school-based survey and thus may underestimate suicide-related behaviors among youth since those who are not currently attending school have been found to be at a higher risk for suicide attempts than those who are in school (Gould et al., 1996, 2003).

During the first decade of YRBS implementation (1991–2001), the percentage of students who reported making one or more suicide attempts in the past 12 months fluctuated between 7.3% and 8.8%. Beginning in 2002, this percentage began decreasing and reached a low of 6.3% in 2009 before returning to the levels of the 1990s. In 2015, the most recent year for which YRBS data are available, 8.6% of students in grades nine through 12 reported a past-year suicide attempt, with 2.8% saying the attempt required medical attention. Taking into account all data points and adjusting for changes in sex, grade, and race/ethnicity over time, CDC analyses show an overall decrease in the prevalence of reported suicide attempts on the YRBS across the period from 1991 to 2015 (https://www.cdc.gov/healthyyouth/data/yrbs/pdf/2015/ss6506_updated.pdf).

In contrast to completed suicides, which are more prevalent among young males, suicide attempts are reported more frequently by young females. In the 2015 YRBS, 11.6% of female high school students reported a past-year suicide attempt, compared to 5.5% of male students (and 8.6% overall). The percentage of students reporting an attempt in the past year was highest among ninth-grade students (9.9%) and lowest among those in grade 12 (6.2%). Students who identified as Hispanic were more likely to report a past-year suicide attempt (11.3%) than white (6.8%) students (https://www.cdc.gov/healthyyouth/data/yrbs/pdf/2015/ss6506_updated.pdf). Although the YRBS questionnaire provided other racial/ethnic categories, too few students in these categories responded to the suicide attempt question for stable percentages to be reported.

In studies conducted in the United States and abroad, sexual minority adolescents and adults have been found to be significantly more likely to report making a suicide attempt than heterosexual individuals of the same age (King et al., 2008). In some studies, lesbian, gay, and bisexual youth have been found to be three to four times more likely than heterosexual youth to report making a suicide attempt (Marshal et al., 2011; Stone, Luo, Ouyang, Lippy, Hertz, et al., 2014). In 2015, questions added to the national YRBS questionnaire provided the first national estimates of the percentage of sexual minority high school students, as measured by either sexual identity as gay, lesbian, or bisexual (8.0%) or any same-sex sexual contact (6.3%). In addition, the survey found that nationwide 29.4% of sexual minority students had attempted suicide one or more times in the past 12 months, compared to 6.4% of heterosexual students and 13.7% of those who answered "not sure" to the sexual identity question (Kann et al., 2016). Among students who had any same-sex sexual contact, 27.6% reported making a suicide attempt in the past 12 months, compared to 9.7% of students who had sexual contact with only the opposite sex and 4.2% of students who had no sexual contact.

YRBS data likewise provide a clear picture of trends in suicidal ideation among high-school students. During the previous two decades, this survey showed a steady decline in the percentage of high school students saying they had seriously considered attempting suicide in the past year, going from 29.0% in 1991 to 13.8% in 2009. Since then, this percentage has increased, rising to 17.7% in 2015. Prevalence of suicidal ideation is higher in female (23.4%) than male (12.2%) students (https://www.cdc.gov/healthyyouth/data/yrbs/pdf/2015/ss6506_updated.pdf).

Perhaps the best source of data on the prevalence of suicide attempts and suicidal ideation among older youth is the National College Health Assessment (NCHA), conducted every semester since spring 2000 by the American

College Health Association (ACHA). This survey is limited to students enrolled in American colleges and universities and thus almost certainly underestimates the prevalence of these behaviors among the 18- to 24-year-old population as a whole. Findings from the most recent NCHA, conducted in spring 2016, showed that 1.5% of almost 96,000 respondents reported making a suicide attempt in the past 12 months, while 9.8% said they had seriously considered suicide in the past 12 months (American College Health Association, 2016). Although there have been fluctuations over the years, the current figures are almost exactly the same as those found by the spring 2000 ACHA survey.

ETIOLOGY OF YOUTH SUICIDE

There is considerable evidence that attempted and completed suicide in young people are complex, multidimensional behaviors that usually result from many interacting factors rather than a single identifiable cause. In the following pages, we review the factors that have been identified in the research literature as conveying primary risk for suicide and suicide attempts among young people, as well as factors that have been suggested to mediate or protect against suicidal behavior.

Risk Factors

Although true suicide causation is difficult to empirically establish, an accumulated body of research points to a number of individual and environmental factors that have been closely and fairly consistently associated with youth suicidal behaviors. These risk factors are identified and briefly discussed below. Clearly, there is considerable overlap and mutual reinforcement among these factors, although most studies have considered them separately.

Psychiatric Disorders

There is clear evidence that psychiatric or mental disorders are key risk factors for both suicide deaths and suicide attempts among youth. Psychological autopsy studies have determined that up to 90% of adolescents who died by suicide had one or more psychiatric disorders at the time of death (Brent, Perper, Moritz, et al., 1993a; Brent et al., 1999; Groholt, Ekeberg, Wichstrom, & Haldorsen, 1997; Shaffer et al., 1996). The onset of these disorders commonly preceded the suicide by several years.

Studies of samples drawn from both community and clinical settings have likewise consistently found psychiatric disorders to be present in youth who attempt suicide (Brent et al., 1999; Bridge, Goldstein, & Brent, 2006; Goldstein et al., 2005). In both attempted and completed suicide, the most common psychiatric conditions are depressive disorder, bipolar disorder, schizophrenia/psychotic disorders, anxiety disorders, conduct disorder, and substance use disorders. Comorbidity among disorders is common among youth who attempt and complete suicide, and has been found to significantly increase the risk for suicidal behavior (Bridge, Goldstein, & Brent, 2006; Gould et al., 1998; Shaffer et al., 1996).

Among suicidal youth, females are more likely than males to have diagnoses of major depression and anxiety disorders, including panic disorder (Brent et al., 1999; Gould et al., 1996, 1998; Shaffer et al., 1996). Bipolar disorder, which has been found to be strongly associated with both suicide deaths (Brent, Perper, Moritz, et al., 1993b) and suicide attempts (Goldstein et al., 2005) among youth, is generally more common among young males than young females (Moreno et al., 2007). Substance use disorders have been found to be comorbid with bipolar disorder in suicidal youth.

Even without comorbid disorders, there is considerable evidence that substance abuse is associated with suicidal ideation, planning, and attempts among adolescents, in particular those who use illicit substances such as heroin, methamphetamines, and steroids, and those who use multiple substances (Wong, Zhou, Goebert, & Hishinuma, 2013). Especially among older suicidal youth, substance use disorder diagnoses are overall more common among males than females (Gould et al., 1998; Marttunnen, Avo, Henriksson, & Lonnqvist, 1991; Shaffer et al., 1996). Abuse of alcohol and other substances has been strongly linked to suicide attempts among college students (Lamis & Bagge, 2011; Westefeld, 2006). Students who binge drink when they are alone appear to be especially at risk of suicidal behavior (Gonzalez, 2012). Conduct disorder is also more prevalent in young males with suicidal behavior, often comorbid with mood, anxiety, and substance use disorders (Brent, Perper, Moritz, et al., 1993a; Gould et al., 1998; Shaffer et al., 1996). Suicide attempts in sexual minority youth and adults have been related to psychiatric disorders, notably depression, anxiety disorders, and substance abuse (King et al., 2008).

There is increasing evidence that youth with autistic spectrum disorders are at elevated risk for suicide and suicide attempts (Mayes, Gorman, Hillwig-Garcia, & Syed, 2013) as well as other self-destructive behavior (Bodfish, Symons, Parker & Lewis, 2000). Increases in self-destructive behaviors among autistic young people are thought to result in part from limitations in understanding their consequences, although depression is likely a key factor as well.

Behavioral and Personality Factors

Aggressive-impulsive behavior in adolescents has an increased association with suicidal behavior (Apter, Plutchik, & van Praag, 1993; Gould et al., 1998, 2003; McKeown, Garrison, Cuffe, Waller, Jackson, & Addy, 1998; Sourander, Helstela, Haavisto, & Bergroth, 2001), particularly in the context of a mood disorder (Brent, Johnson, et al., 1994; Johnson, Brent, Bridge, & Connolly, 1998). Aggressive-impulsive behavior has been found to discriminate suicide attempters from psychiatric controls, and also appears to be related to familial transmission of suicidal behavior.

Hopelessness has also been implicated as an important factor associated with youth suicidal behavior, although its relationship does not generally appear to be independent of depression and depressed mood (Gould et al., 2003; Rotheram-Borus & Trautman, 1988; Rotheram-Borus, Trautman, Dopkins, & Shrout, 1990). Among depressed youth, hopelessness may be a significant indicator of increased risk for suicide. Depression and hopelessness have been identified as the most significant predictors of suicide attempts in a diverse sample of sexual and gender minority youth (Mustanski & Liu, 2013). Pessimism, a negative cognitive style that may be related to hopelessness, has been found to characterize suicide attempters independent of depression (Lewinsohn, Rhode, & Seeley, 1996).

Previous Suicidal Behavior

A suicide attempt history has been identified in one quarter to one third of adolescents who die by suicide (Brent, Perper, Moritz et al., 1993a; Groholt et al., 1997; Shaffer at al., 1996). As among adults, studies have found that a previous suicide attempt is one of the strongest predictors of subsequent attempts and suicide death among youth (Beautrais, 2004; Shaffer et al., 1996; McKeown et al., 1998; Wichstrom, 2000), especially among those with mood disorders (Brent et al., 1999; Shaffer et al., 1996). A suicide attempt history in a young person has been estimated to increase the risk of future suicidal behavior by three to 17 times (Groholt et al., 1997). Even in a high-risk group of people who have attempted suicide, however, suicide is a relatively rare event, with an absolute risk of about 10% in those who have been followed up for more than 30 years after the attempt (Tidemalm, Långström, Lichtenstein, & Runeson, 2008).

Biological and Genetic Factors

Both attempted suicide and completed suicide have been found to be increased in families in which a parent has attempted suicide or died by suicide, even when controlling for the impact of parents' psychiatric disorders (Brent, Bridge, Johnson, & Connolly, 1996; Brent, Oquendo, Birmaher, Greenhill, Koloko, Stanley, et al., 2002; Glowinski, Bucholz, Nelson, Qiang, Madden, Reich, et al., 2001). This relationship may be mediated by familial transmission of impulsive aggression (Brent, Oquendo, Birmaher, Greenhill, Koloko, Stanley, et al., 2003). Some studies have also linked youth suicidal behavior to mental disorders in parents that did not include suicidal behavior (Brent et al., 1988; Brent, Perper, Moritz, Liotus, Schweers, Balach, et al., 1994; Gould et al., 1996).

The mechanisms through which parental suicidal behavior and psychiatric disorders may influence youth suicidal behavior are not yet fully understood. Although little is currently known about the genetics of youth suicide, adult studies suggest that biological factors play a significant role in suicide. Neurobiological abnormalities, in particular lower levels of central nervous system serotonin (5-HT), have been implicated in aggressive impulsivity and suicidal behavior in adults (Oquendo & Mann, 2000). Postmortem studies of the brains of adult suicide victims have also shown higher levels of serotonin (5-HT) receptors compared to normal controls (Arango, Ernsberger, Marzuk, Chen, Tierney, Stanley, Reis & Mann, 1990; Mann, Stanley, McBride & McEwen, 1986).

Postmortem studies of youth who have died by suicide are rare, and therefore the implications of adult findings for understanding youth suicide are not clear. One postmortem study involving 15 teenage suicide victims and 15 normal matched control subjects found significantly higher levels of 5-HT receptor expression in the prefrontal cortex and hippocampus of those who had died by suicide, suggesting that this abnormality may be a marker of adolescent as well as adult suicide (Pandey, 2002). This study noted that higher levels of serotonin receptor expression have been implicated in alterations in emotion, stress, and cognition, suggesting promising avenues of exploration for understanding the neurobiology of youth suicide. A subsequent study of teenage suicides found that decreased gene expression of glucocorticoid receptors in the prefrontal cortex and amygdala, but not the hippocampus, distinguished the suicide victims from the controls (Pandey, Rizavi, Ren, Dwivedi, & Palkovits, 2013).

Negative Life Events

There is considerable evidence that stressful life events contribute independently to youth suicide (see Wagner, 1997; Wagner et al., 2003) over and above other risk factors (Gould et al., 1996; Johnson, Cohen, et al., 2002). Negative life events have been found to be associated with suicide deaths (Beautrais, 2001; Brent, Perper, Moritz, et al., 1993b; Gould et al., 1996; Marttunnen, Aro, & Lonnqvust, 1993) and suicide attempts (Beautrais, Joyce, & Mulder, 1997; Fergusson, Woodward, & Horwood, 2000; Lewinsohn et al., 1996).

Stressful factors within the family environment have been found to contribute to risk for youth suicidal behavior (Wagner, 1997; Wagner et al., 2003). There is considerable evidence that exposure to suicidal behavior of family members increases the risk for suicidal behavior among youth (Crepeau-Hobson, & Leech, 2014). Particularly among younger youth who die by suicide, parent–child conflict has been identified as a common precipitant to suicidal behavior (Brent et al., 1999; Groholt, Ekeberg, Wichstrom, & Haldorsen, 1998), as has lack of emotional support within the family. Family rejection and lack of support related to sexual orientation and/or nonconforming gender behavior have been found to be strongly related to elevated rates of suicidal ideation and suicide attempts in SGM youth (D'Augelli, Grossman, Salter, et al., 2005; D'Augelli, Hershberger, & Pilkington, 2001; Remafedi et al., 1991; Ryan, Huebner, Diaz, & Sanchez, 2009). SGM youth who experience a high degree of family rejection have been found to be about nine times more likely to make a suicide attempt than those with low or no rejection. Unrealistic parental expectations may be a risk factor for youth in general. One early study of male college students found that those who had attempted suicide were disproportionately characterized by feelings of being a failure for their inability to live up to the expectations their parents had for them, which they themselves had internalized (Hendin, 1975).

Child abuse has been found to increase the risk for posttraumatic stress disorder, major depressive disorder, and suicidal behavior in adolescents. Physical abuse has been demonstrated to increase youth suicide risk in case-control (Brent, Johnson, et al., 1994; Brent et al., 1999) and longitudinal studies (Johnson,

Cohen, Brown, Smailes, & Bernstein, 1999; Johnson et al., 2002; Silverman, Reinherz, & Giaconia, 1996) and has been associated with youth suicidal behavior even after controlling for other contributory factors such as parental psychopathology (Johnson et al., 2002; Wagner, 1997; Wagner et al., 2003).

Childhood sexual abuse has also been found to be associated with an increased risk for suicidal behavior (Brand, King, Olson, Ghaziuddin & Naylor, 1996; Johnson et al., 2002; Silverman et al., 1996), as well as with many other adverse psychological outcomes (Fergusson, Horwood, & Lynskey, 1996.). Girls are significantly more likely to be victims of sexual abuse than boys. Some of the suicide risk conferred by child sexual abuse is likely related more generally to parental psychopathology, although one longitudinal study (Fergusson et al., 1996) identified a unique contribution of this variable to suicidal behavior in youth after taking many other risk factors into account. Studies show that SGM youth are more likely to have experienced sexual abuse than heterosexual youth (Arreola, Neilands, Pollack, et al., 2008; Brady, 2008; Friedman, Marshal, Guadamuz, et al., 2011).

Homelessness among youth resulting from any reason, including poverty, family breakup, family conflict, and rejection, has been associated with an increased risk for suicidal behavior. One study of homeless youth in four Midwestern states found that 54% had suicidal ideation and 26% had attempted suicide in the previous year (Yoder, Hoyt, & Whitbeck, 1998). Associated risk factors among homeless youth include a high prevalence of sexual abuse and use of drugs and alcohol (Rew, Taylor-Seehafer, & Fitzgerald, 2001). It is estimated that SGM youth account for up to 40% of the youth homeless population, with the large majority of these young people leaving their homes because of conflict or rejection related to their sexual orientation or gender identity (Ray, 2006). Studies have also found that youth who were in foster care were twice as likely to die by suicide compared to other youth (Hjern et al., 2004) and four times more likely to have attempted suicide (Pilowsky & Wu, 2006).

Stressful life events related to peers have also been linked to youth suicidal behavior. Especially among older female adolescents, suicidal behavior has been found to be frequently precipitated by interpersonal loss, in particular the loss of a romantic relationship (Brent et al., 1999; Groholt et al., 1998). Interpersonal loss has also been identified as a significant stressor among youth with substance abuse problems (Brent, Perper, Moritz, et al., 1993c; Gould et al., 2003; Marttunen, Aro, Henriksson, & Lönnqvist, 1994). Rather than an independent risk factor, loss appears to precipitate suicidal behavior among youth when it occurs in the context of other risk factors.

Bullying, harassment, and victimization by peers have also been linked to suicidal behavior among a broad range of behavioral, emotional, and social problems (Kim & Leventhal, 2008). Being involved in bullying as either a victim or a perpetrator has been associated with an elevated suicide risk, with youth who are both victims and perpetrators showing the highest risk. One study of a large sample of middle school students, among whom bullying is especially common, found that 60% of bully-victims reported suicidal ideation, compared to 48% of physically aggressive bullies, 32% to 38% of verbal bullies and victims, and 12% of youth who were not involved in bullying (Espelage & Holt, 2013). Similarly, 44% of bully-victims reported deliberately trying to hurt or kill themselves, compared to 35% of physically aggressive bullies, 24% to 28% of verbal bullies and victims, and 8% of uninvolved youth. Higher risk for suicidal ideation and behavior among physically aggressive bullies compared to victims of bullying was thought to be related to higher rates of comorbid symptoms such as impulsivity and anger. After controlling for delinquency and depression, however, only minimal difference among the groups remained, leading the study authors to emphasize the importance of considering other risk factors in assessing suicidality of youth who are involved in bullying.

Youth who are perceived to be gay or lesbian appear to be significantly more likely than other youth to be bullied and harassed (Haas et al., 2011), and being bullied because of perceived sexual orientation has been found to have a greater impact on adolescents' quality of life than being bullied for other reasons (Patrick, Bell, Huang, Lazarakis, & Edwards, 2013). Youth with cross-gender appearance, traits, or behaviors or who identify as gay or transgender at an early age are especially vulnerable to this type of bullying. One longitudinal study (Mustanski & Liu, 2013) has shown, however, that depression and hopelessness are significantly stronger predictors of suicide attempts in SGM youth than is peer victimization. Depression and other mental and developmental disorders have also been found to increase the likelihood of a young person being bullied (Kochel, Ladd, & Rudolph, 2012).

Findings from a longitudinal study (Klomek et al., 2011) of youth who were bullied during high school found that those who were most vulnerable to subsequent negative outcomes, including suicidal ideation and behavior, showed symptoms of depression at the time the bullying occurred. This suggests that increased suicide risk among youth who are involved in bullying may result primarily from the interaction of bullying and depression. This hypothesis is supported by the finding of an analysis of circumstances that precipitated suicide among 1,046 youth ages 10 to 17 years in 16 U.S. states from 2005 to 2008 (Karch, Logan, McDaniel, Floyd, & Vagi, 2013). While mental health factors were identified to be a factor in 37% of youth suicides, bullying was identified as a circumstance in about 3% of the deaths.

Studies have shown that adolescents who have a history of problems with the law are at increased risk for both attempted and completed suicide (Farand, 2004; Thompson, 1995). Legal problems commonly overlap with a range of other problem behaviors such as school truancy, fighting with parents or guardians, and use of alcohol or drugs. There is clear evidence, however, that youth who have contact with the juvenile justice system are significantly more likely than those who do not to engage in suicidal behavior (Hayes, 2004). A systematic review of suicides in U.S. juvenile detention and correctional facilities in the late 1990s found the rate of suicide among youth in these facilities to be more than four times greater than in the general population, with 110 suicides identified over a 4-year period (Hayes, 2004). The largest number of these suicides (42%) took place in secure training schools, and 37% occurred in detention centers; 40% of the suicides occurred in the first 72 hours of detention. Almost three quarters of the youth who died by suicide had a history of mental illness, 71% had a history of prior suicidal behavior, and 45% had made a prior suicide attempt. The elevated suicide risk among youth who are involved with the juvenile justice system is also supported by a study in Utah that found that 63% of male suicide decedents between the ages of 13 and 21 had contact with juvenile courts (Moskos, Halbem, Alder, Kim, & Gray, 2007). Suicide attempts within juvenile justice system facilities are also starkly elevated relative to the general youth population (Battle, 1993; Wasserman, 2002, 2006). Contact with the legal system has been found to precipitate suicidal behavior especially in youth with conduct disorder and other disruptive disorders (Brent, Perper, Moritz, et al., 1993b; Gould et al., 1996).

Being subjected to school disciplinary procedures and being at risk of dropping out of school have also been linked to increased risk for suicidal ideation and behavior (Beautrais, Joyce, & Mulder, 1996; Thompson & Eggert, 1999; Wunderlich et al., 1998). Further, school problems and not being in school or in a work situation have been found to pose considerable risk for suicide death in adolescents (Gould et al., 1996).

Suicide Exposure and Contagion

There is strong evidence that adolescents and young adults are particularly vulnerable to the impact of suicide contagion resulting from media coverage of suicide (Gould, 2001; Gould, Romer, & Jamieson, 2003; Gould, Kleinman, Lake, & Midle, 2014; Stack, 2000, 2005) or exposure to suicidal behavior within the family (Crepeau-Hobson & Leech, 2014). Young people appear to be particularly affected when media accounts include pictures of the decedent or the site of the suicide, present the suicide in a romanticized or glamorized manner, or link the suicide to a common stressful experience, such as bullying or the breakup of a relationship (Gould, 2001; Pirkis & Blood, 2001a, 2001b; Schmidtke & Shaller, 2000; Stack, 2000).

Many different studies support the conclusion that having a friend or acquaintance attempt suicide is likewise significantly related to the risk for suicidal thoughts and behavior among youth (Crepeau-Hobson & Leech, 2014). Research findings have been less consistent with respect to the impact of a peer's death by suicide, with some studies showing an association with subsequent youth suicidal behavior and others not (Crepeau-Hobson & Leech, 2014). Among studies in which contagion following a peer's suicide death has been found, younger adolescents appear to be at the highest risk for adverse outcomes. A large-scale survey of Canadian youth (Swanson & Coleman, 2013) found that youth ages 12 and 13 were especially likely to report suicidal thoughts and suicide attempts following the suicide of a schoolmate or someone they personally knew. Among those who reported a schoolmate's suicide, personally knowing the decedent did not alter the risk of suicidal ideation or behavior, leading the study authors to recommend schoolwide interventions over those that target children closest to the decedent. They also found youth with other risk factors such as mental health problems to have greater risk for suicidal behavior following exposure to the suicide of a peer.

A number of reports have described outbreaks or clusters of suicide deaths among young people following exposure to suicide (Gould, Wallenstein, & Davidson, 1989; Gould, Wallenstein, & Kleinman, 1990; Gould, Wallenstein, Kleinman, O'Carroll, & Mercy, 1990; Gould et al., 2014). Gould et al. found suicide clusters in adolescents to be independently associated with a greater number of newspaper stories about suicidal individuals (as distinct from other stories about suicide) and two specific story characteristics: an accompanying picture displaying sadness and the celebrity status of the suicide decedent (Gould et al., 2014). Other story characteristics found to be associated with cluster suicides, including front-page placement, headlines containing the word "suicide" or the suicide method, detailed descriptions of the decedent and the suicidal act, and mention of a suicide note, did not differentiate cluster and non-cluster suicides independently of the number of stories about suicidal individuals. This study also found no significant differences between cluster and non-cluster suicides regarding their occurrence in a public location or the unusualness of the suicide method, which may have contributed to more media coverage.

Psychological mechanisms such as modeling, suggestion, imitation, identification, and social learning are also thought to affect the formation of youth suicide clusters (Haw, Hawton, Niedzwiedz, & Platt, 2013). The roles of identification and modeling are supported by the finding of Gould et al. (2014) that only stories about individual suicides—especially those occurring in celebrities or other teens—were associated with the occurrence of subsequent suicides. Normalization of suicide through repeated and detailed reporting of suicide cases, along with the resulting reduction of inhibitions against suicide among vulnerable youth, likely contributes to contagion and clusters as well (Lake & Gould, 2014). To date, the impacts of social media on suicide contagion and the development of clusters have not been extensively studied. Thus, the degree to which findings from studies of print media are applicable to the media to which youth are most exposed today is not known.

Clusters of suicide attempts among youth have also been reported (Gould, Petrie, Kleinman, & Wallenstein, 1994). Having a friend who has attempted suicide has been found to discriminate depressed adolescents who make a suicide attempt from those who do not (Lewinsohn, Rohde, & Seeley, 1994). A study using two waves of data from the National Longitudinal Study of Adolescent Health (Add Health) found that knowing someone who attempted suicide commonly preceded an adolescent's own report of engaging in suicidal behavior (Cutler, Glaeser, & Norberg, 2001).

Access to Lethal Means

Access to lethal means for suicide—especially firearms—contributes to suicide among persons of all ages, and youth are no exception. In 2011, 45% of all suicides occurring among youth ages 15 to 24 involved use of a firearm (CDC, 2014). States in which overall gun ownership is high generally show the highest rates of attempted and completed suicide among youth, possibly because community norms affect the likelihood of a young person having immediate access to a gun in the home environment (Birckmayer & Hemenway, 2001; Miller, Lippmann, Azrael, & Hemenway, 2007). Guns have been estimated to be four to five times more prevalent in the homes of youth who have died by suicide compared to controls (Brent, Perper, Moritz, et al., 1993d; Kellermann et al., 1992; Shah et al., 2000). There appears to be a gradient of risk, with loaded guns and handguns posing the greatest risk. In a review of case-control studies, Brent and Bridge (2003) reported that the odds of a youth dying by suicide were 31.3 to 107.9 times higher in homes where a gun was present than in homes without guns. An ecological study by Miller, Barber, White, and Azrael (2013) confirmed that in the population overall, the relationship between household firearm ownership rates and suicide mortality persists after controlling for rates of underlying suicidal behavior as measured by prior suicide attempts.

Youth who use firearms for suicide reportedly have fewer identifiable risk factors, such as expressing suicidal thoughts, suicidal intent, psychopathology, and substance abuse, compared to those using other means (Azrael, 2001; Brent et al., 1999; Groholt et al., 1998), and firearm suicides appear to be more impulsive and spontaneous (Azrael, 2001). Thus, having easy access to guns may contribute to youth suicide, independent of other risk factors (Brent, Perper, Moritz, et al., 1993d; Kellerman et al., 1992).

There is some evidence from an Australian study (De Leo, Dwyer, Firman, & Neulinger, 2003) that efforts to restrict access to guns can reduce the rate of firearm suicide among young males. In that study, however, declines in firearm suicides among males ages 15 to 24 coincided with an increase in the rate of suicide by hanging, which caused a slight increase in the overall suicide rate for young males.

Protective Factors

Considerably less research has been done to identify factors that protect youth against suicidal behavior. Studies to date have identified factors that appear to broadly foster psychological health and well-being in youth, and it is likely that their impact on suicidal behavior is mediated to a considerable extent by reduced levels of depression and other psychiatric disorders. Further, conclusions are limited by the fact that most studies have not simultaneously examined risk and protective factors. Discussed below are the key factors that have been described in the research literature as protecting young people from suicidal behavior.

Family Connectedness and Support

A considerable body of research has found that youth who describe their families as emotionally involved and supportive are much less likely to report suicidal behavior than those who described their families as less supportive and involved (Kaminski et al., 2010; McKeown et al., 1998; Resnick, Berman, Blum, Bauman, Harris, Jones, et al., 1997; Rubenstein, Halton, Kasten, Rubin, & Stechler, 1998; Rubenstein, Heeren, Housman, Rubin, & Stechler, 1989; Ryan at al., 2010; Zhang & Jin, 1996). One large-scale national study of seventh-graders through 12th-graders found that family connectedness was a significantly stronger inverse predictor of suicidal ideation and suicide attempts than connectedness to peers or school (Kaminsky et al., 2010). Family connectedness was also found to be the most potent protective factor for suicidal behavior among youth who were at elevated risk due to a history of sexual abuse (Eisenberg et al., 2007). Among all youth, the presence of supportive siblings appears to have protective impact and may help compensate for a lack of parental support (Simon, 2011).

Family connectedness appears to be an especially important protective factor for SGM youth. One study of a diverse sample of SGM youth suggests that family acceptance of gay/lesbian orientation or transgender identity may reduce the risk of depression and hopelessness and, in turn, suicidal behavior (Mustanski & Liu, 2013). Parental behaviors that demonstrate acceptance and support of SGM adolescents have been linked to their higher self-esteem, better overall health, and lower rates of depression and suicidal ideation and behavior in young adulthood (Ryan et al., 2010). One study in Minnesota found that perceived caring by adult relatives other than parents and other adults in the community was similarly protective of suicide attempts in sexual minority youth (Eisenberg & Resnick, 2007).

School Connectedness and School Safety

School connectedness has also been suggested as a protective factor against youth suicidal behavior (Resnick et al., 1997), although it may be less impactful among high-school youth than connectedness within the family (Kaminsky, 2010). Among college students, several studies have found perceived school support, emotional connections to friends, and involvement in extracurricular activities to be associated with lower rates of suicidal behavior (Marion & Range, 2003; Westefeld et al., 2006).

Perceived safety at school appears to be a protective factor for youth with a history of sexual abuse (Eisenberg at al., 2007) and SGM youth (Eisenberg & Resnick, 2007). One study of youth in Oregon found that a positive school environment that included the presence of Gay-Straight Alliances and nondiscrimination and antibullying policies reduced SGM students' risk of attempting suicide by 20% (Hatzenbuehler, 2011).

Reduced Access to Lethal Means

There is evidence that preventive laws and policies can reduce rates of youth suicide involving the use of firearms (Cummings, Grossman, Rivera, et al., 1997; Webster, Vernick, Zeoli, et al., 2004). One multistate case-control study (Grossman, Mueller, Riedy, et al., 2005) found that in households where firearms are present, certain practices—locking both guns and ammunition, storing guns unloaded, and storing guns and ammunition separately—had a protective effect for intentional and unintentional self-harm with firearms among children and adolescents. The relative absence of firearms on college campuses has been identified as a protective factor for suicide among college students (Schwartz, 2011). These findings are consistent with the conclusion of an international review that restricting access to common means of suicide, including firearms, toxic gas, and pesticides, results in reduced rates of death by suicide for all affected population groups (Sarchiapone, Mandelli, Iosue, et al., 2011).

Social-Behavioral Skills

Based on studies by Jessor (1991), during the 1990s there was considerable interest in the role of decision making, problem solving, healthy coping, and related social-behavioral skills in protecting youth from suicidal behavior. Several studies from that decade found that at-risk students who participated in interventions designed to strengthen these skills and behaviors in vulnerable youth showed decreased depression and suicidal behavior (LaFramboise & Howard-Pitney, 1995; Thompson, Eggert, & Herting, 2000; Thompson, Eggert, Randell, & Pike, 2001). Because these programs included other aspects, however, it was difficult to demonstrate the degree to which decreases in suicidality were specifically due to increases in social-behavioral skills, as opposed to other benefits of the interventions.

Social-behavioral skills have been emphasized as potential protective factors in general populations of young people. There is some evidence that targeted interventions can increase healthy peer-group norms that influence coping practices and problem behaviors, including self-harm, drug use, and unhealthy sexual practices (Wyman et al., 2010).

Youth Suicide Prevention

Since the mid-1980s, significant public attention has been focused on youth suicide prevention. During the 1980s and 1990s, a proliferation of youth suicide prevention programs were developed and implemented, particularly in schools, where they targeted students, parents, teachers, and other school personnel. This coincided with an increase in the recognition of childhood and adolescent depression, and mental health professionals and medical practitioners looking for ways to prevent the tragic loss of young lives to suicide. Many of these early youth suicide prevention efforts were not sustained due to a lack of theoretical foundation, a failure to demonstrate success, and/or a lack of funding.

In 2001, the country's first National Strategy for Suicide Prevention (U.S. Department of Health, 2001) provided renewed attention to the problem of youth suicide. Developed by the Department of Health and Human Services and the Office of the Surgeon General, the National Strategy called for the development of statewide suicide prevention programs to address youth as well as other priority target populations. It also prompted suicide prevention efforts at the national level, including the creation of a Suicide Prevention Resource Center in 2002 (http://www.sprc.org), and the passage of the Garrett Lee Smith Memorial Act, which created a suicide prevention grant program for states, tribes, and college and university campuses.

The revision of the National Strategy in 2012 maintained the previous document's attention to youth while reflecting the accumulated research evidence that suicide risk is concentrated in groups that may include people of different ages. Nine such groups were identified in the revised National Strategy: American Indians/Alaska Natives, individuals bereaved by suicide, individuals in justice and child welfare settings, individuals who engage in non-suicidal self-injury, individuals who have attempted suicide, individuals with mental and/or substance use disorders, individuals with medical conditions, SGM populations, and members of the Armed Forces and veterans. Only two age-specific groups were noted as having increased suicide risk: men in midlife and older men (U.S. Department of Health and Human Services, Office of the Surgeon General, and National Action Alliance for Suicide Prevention, 2012). One of the important questions to emerge from this perspective is whether reducing suicide risk in people at different points in the lifespan requires different approaches to prevention, intervention, and treatment. Although answering this question is beyond our present scope, it is worth considering as we look at recent approaches to youth suicide prevention.

As in the previous edition of the book, our primary goal in this part is to examine current youth suicide prevention strategies and interventions with an eye toward identifying what works, what does not appear to work, and what research needs to be undertaken to move the field forward. Given the multiplicity of risk and protective factors that have been related to youth suicide, it is understandable that many different approaches have been taken in the attempt to prevent this behavior. In the next three chapters, we discuss and critique the major preventive strategies and treatment approaches that have been used. Rather than undertaking an exhaustive review of every program that has been identified, we have selected those we feel best illustrate a general type or approach. Reflecting the strategies that have received the widest application, our review focuses primarily on suicide prevention programs targeting groups of youth, rather than on clinical care or evaluation of individual youth who are potentially suicidal.

Universal Approaches to Youth Suicide Prevention

Maggie G. Mortali

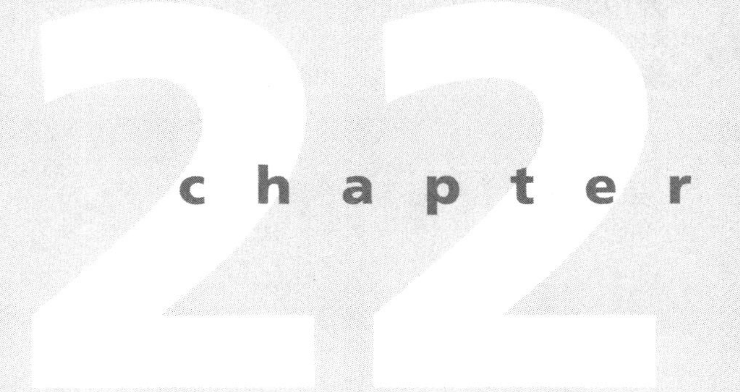

In this chapter, we focus on suicide prevention programs that have taken a universal approach, targeting whole populations of youth regardless of individual risk factors. The aim of universal suicide prevention programs is to reduce risk factors or enhance protective factors across the entire population. One particularly widespread approach targets youth where they are most accessible—in the schools.

There are four types of universal prevention programs that are especially common and continue to be the most widely used approach in schools:

- School-based screening programs
- Adult and peer gatekeeper training programs
- Skills training programs
- Comprehensive or "whole school" programs

Over the past 10 years, the number of school-based suicide programs has expanded considerably. Because of the seriousness and pervasiveness of the problem of youth suicide, and given that youth spend much of their time in schools, school personnel have been asked to take an increasingly prominent role in suicide prevention (Gould & Kramer, 2001; Kalafat, 2003; Miller, Eckert, & Mazza, 2009). Schools have transitioned into an obvious and accepted environment for implementing suicide prevention initiatives for young people. The increase in the number of school-based programs is also due to federal and state policies that call for increased school mental health and the use of evidence-based programs and practices for suicide prevention (George et al., 2013).

In each category, suicide prevention efforts have been separately designed for high school and college students. In the following pages, we summarize these universal programs, identifying for each broad type the underlying assumptions and specific program examples, and providing a summary critique of the approach.

SCREENING PROGRAMS

Assumptions

The primary assumption underlying screening programs is that because anxiety, depression, substance abuse, and suicidal preoccupation among youth often go unnoticed and untreated, a systematic, universally applied effort is needed to improve identification of at-risk individuals. Although not always explicitly stated, screening programs also rest on the assumptions that identification of youth with psychiatric disorders will substantially increase the number receiving treatment, the treatment will be sufficiently effective, and effective treatment will decrease suicides. Universal screening programs as a youth suicide prevention strategy are designed to identify young people who should receive treatment because they are at risk for suicide. Some programs focus specifically on identifying symptoms of psychopathology known to be related to adolescent and young adult suicidal behavior, while others assess specifically for signs of suicidality.

Program Examples

The first widely used screening program was the Columbia TeenScreen Program (CTSP), which was used in high schools between 2003 and 2012. In one variant of the CTSP, students completed a brief, self-report questionnaire, the Columbia Suicide Screen. Those who screened positive on this measure were given a computerized instrument, the Voice DISC 2.3, a version of the Diagnostic Interview Schedule for Children, which has been found to accurately identify a comprehensive range of psychiatric disorders in children and adolescents (Shaffer, Fisher, Lucas, Dulcan, & Schwab-Stone, 2000; Shaffer et al., 2004). This stage of the screen was regarded as particularly important for avoiding overidentification of students at risk. In the final stage, youth who had been identified through Voice DISC 2.3 as meeting specific diagnostic criteria for a psychiatric disorder were evaluated by a clinician, who determined whether the student needed to be referred for treatment or further evaluation. Ideally, the program also included a case manager who contacted the parents of students who were referred and established links with a clinic to facilitate treatment adherence.

Evaluation results indicate that most of the adolescents identified as being at high risk for suicide through the program were not previously recognized as such, and very few had received prior treatment. About half of the students referred for treatment attended at least one treatment visit, however. A study by Husky et al. (2011) found that students that participated in TeenScreen had greater odds of making contact with a student assistance mental health professional and of establishing contact with community-based services. This increase in the rate of referral reflects the superiority of mental health screening over traditional methods for identifying adolescents at risk for clinically significant problems (Brown, Goldstein, & Grumet, 2009; Husky et al., 2011; Scott et al., 2009).

TeenScreen was endorsed by a number of organizations, including the National Alliance for Mental Illness (NAMI), and received federal grant funding and support from the Substance Abuse and Mental Health Services Administration (SAMHSA). TeenScreen became the model for other school-based screening programs that are still used today, including use of the Columbia Suicide Screen in primary care settings (Kreipe, 2013).

Two screening programs used in college and universities are the CollegeResponse program, developed by Screening for Mental Health, and the Interactive Screening Program, developed by the American Foundation for Suicide Prevention. Formerly known as the Comprehensive College Initiative, the CollegeResponse program promotes the prevention, early detection, and treatment of prevalent, often underdiagnosed and treatable mental health disorders and alcohol problems through in-person and online screening. The CollegeResponse program offers kits to host in-person events for National Depression Screening Day, the National Eating Disorders Screening Program, and National Alcohol Screening Day. In addition, CollegeResponse provides access to unlimited, anonymous online screenings and/or confidential screenings at in-person events; tools for help seeking; and immediate results and referrals to on-campus counseling and the health center following the completion of the screening questionnaire.

The second program, the Interactive Screening Program, provides an anonymous, web-based method of outreach that starts with a brief, confidential Stress & Depression Questionnaire. As currently applied, the primary focus of the program is connecting people at risk for suicide to a counselor who provides information and support for help seeking (Garlow, 2008; Haas et al., 2008). This program, which is currently in place at over 100 colleges and universities nationwide, is based on the following principles: anonymity for the user, personalized contact with real counselors, interactive engagement between user and counselor, and identifying and resolving the user's personal barriers to treatment. The program provides a brief online questionnaire to help the user to identify depression or other mental health problems. The instrument is an adaptation of the Patient Health Questionnaire, which has been established to be an effective tool for identifying depression among community samples (Spitzer et al., 1999, 2000). In addition to depression, the questionnaire includes items dealing with current suicidal ideation, past suicide attempts, anxiety and other affective disorders, use of drugs and alcohol, and eating disorders. The questionnaire is housed on a secure website, which is customized for each participating college and university. Students are typically invited to participate via email, and use a self-assigned user ID and password to log in to the website. Those who complete and submit the questionnaire receive a personalized written response from a counselor and are encouraged to exchange follow-up messages online with the counselor without having to identify themselves. The dialogs with the counselor play a critical role in the process of encouraging the student to seek help by facilitating the resolution of barriers to treatment. Students who agree to meet with the counselor in person are further evaluated, and treatment options are discussed.

Two additional publications on the Interactive Screening Program describe its effectiveness in graduate and medical school populations (Moffit et al., 2014; Moutier et al., 2012). The expansion of this program, along with other efforts such as those funded by the SAMHSA Campus Suicide Prevention Grants, should lead to improved knowledge about interventions to increase identification of mental illness and help seeking (Hunt et al., 2010).

Critique

Screening programs as implemented within both high school and college settings closely conform to scientifically validated premises regarding the causes of suicide—that is, that suicide risk is not randomly distributed but rather is conferred by certain factors that are both identifiable and, to a considerable extent, alterable. At the same time, such programs face a number of challenges. Even with acceptable sensitivity and specificity, screening measures will necessarily miss some in the population who will go on to make suicide attempts, while identifying many more as at risk when they are not. The often transient or episodic nature of suicidality among young people makes screening this population even more difficult. Given that costs are involved each time a segment of the target group is screened, most school-based screening programs assess students only once a year, and in some cases, only once during a several-year period. The timing of the screening may increase or decrease the likelihood of identifying students in need of referral.

Both high school and college screening programs report relatively low adherence with treatment recommendations among those identified through the screening instrument to be at risk. Although this is likely due to a range of problems that are beyond the scope of the screening effort (e.g., lack of parental support, perceived quality of available treatment, and attitudes of treatment providers), additional strategies appear to be needed to encourage students at risk to access and make effective use of needed treatment services. In this regard, better integration of skills training programs, gatekeeper training programs, and screening programs may be helpful.

Although it is intuitive that contextual factors such as peer support, residential settings, and the supportiveness of academic personnel would affect student mental health, researchers have yet to examine these relationships rigorously. All school-based suicide screening programs need to be mindful of the availability and quality of mental health services for students who are identified as at risk. On college campuses, this is sometimes a formidable problem. Most colleges and universities limit the number of sessions or offer only group therapy that may not be appropriate for students at risk for suicide. Although many colleges require students to have health insurance, most students (as well as most people in the general population) do not have adequate coverage for acute or long-term mental health services.

Even when implemented under ideal conditions, there is no clear evidence that screening for suicide in general populations improves rate-reduction outcomes. In addition, as yet, no data have been reported on the effectiveness of high school or college screening programs on reducing suicide risk factors, including depression and suicidal ideation, or suicidal behavior at the schools where screening programs are being implemented.

Within high schools, there is evidence that administrators prefer suicide education awareness programs over screening programs (Miller, Eckert, DuPaul, & White, 1999). Many colleges and universities have also expressed reluctance about implementing depression and suicide screening programs. This appears to reflect, in part, concerns about the liability schools may assume in the event that students identified as at risk for suicide do not follow through with treatment recommendations and engage in suicidal behavior.

Parental and community opposition to school-based screening efforts has also been an issue, contributing to the demise of some programs, as in the case of Columbia TeenScreen. Finally, an additional limitation to screening programs is their inability to reach youth who are not in school, and most screening programs directed at young adults are designed specifically for college students. Although screening programs can be expensive to administer and monitor, creative strategies are needed for integrating and supporting screening into existing healthcare settings that reach all youth.

GATEKEEPER TRAINING PROGRAMS

Assumptions

Gatekeeper training is designed to give teens and adults in the school environment the knowledge and skills needed to identify at-risk youth and to take appropriate action (Garland & Zigler, 1993; Gould et al., 2003; Kalafat & Elias, 1995; Lake & Gould, 2011). A common goal of gatekeeper training programs is to increase participants' general knowledge of youth suicide and suicide-related behavior, risk factors, and warning signs, as well as changing attitudes toward suicide intervention to enhance referrals to treatment. Another common theme is to increase gatekeepers' confidence and self-efficacy in relation to working with suicidal students and to apply what they have learned to help someone else (Robinson et al., 2013).

Program Examples

Many states are currently implementing universal youth suicide prevention programs that frequently include gatekeeper training for parents, teachers, and other school personnel, or follow a peer-to-peer model by training youth as gatekeepers. One widely applied program is the Signs of Suicide (SOS) program, developed by Screening for Mental Health, Inc. Although the SOS program contains a screening component, the primary goals are to educate students about mental illness, particularly depression, and teach them to identify symptoms of depression, suicidality, and self-injury in themselves and their peers using the SOS technique. Through video and group discussions, SOS teaches students to ACT: Acknowledge the signs of depression or suicidal thoughts in a friend; let the friend know you Care and want to help; and Tell a responsible adult. Schools in which the program has been implemented have reported substantial increases in students' help-seeking behavior and high satisfaction with the program among school officials (Aseltine, Jacobs, Kopans, & Bloom, 2003). The results of the post-only evaluation involving nine high schools in three states implementing the SOS program confirms and expands the first-year results that demonstrated the program's efficacy in an urban, economically disadvantaged sample of youth. The Aseltine et al. (2007) analysis of 4,133 students, based on a more socially, economically, and geographically diverse group of high school students, found the SOS program to be associated with significantly greater knowledge, more adaptive attitudes about depression and suicide, and significantly fewer suicide attempts reported by intervention youths relative to untreated controls 3 months after the intervention. The impact of the SOS program on knowledge, attitudes, and suicidal behavior was not associated with increased help seeking among emotionally troubled youth.

The broadest and most frequently applied gatekeeper training program is the Applied Suicide Intervention Skills Training (ASIST), developed by LivingWorks Education for application in community settings (Ramsay, Cooke, & Lang, 1990; Rothman, 1980). Although not specifically targeting young people, ASIST provides a model that has been applied to helping teens and young adults, and school personnel have been increasingly targeted by ASIST. Developed in 1983, ASIST is a 2-day gatekeeper training workshop that seeks to develop participants' readiness and ability to use "first-aid" actions to prevent suicidal behavior, and to network with other gatekeepers to improve communication and continuity of care. Evaluations of participants before and after the workshop suggest that it enhances caregivers' sense of readiness for suicide intervention, increases their knowledge about suicidal behavior, increases their willingness to intervene, and improves competence in dealing with suicidal individuals (Eggert et al., 1999; Smith et al., 2013; Tierney, 1994). In one evaluation report of training programs in Australia, more than three quarters of ASIST workshop participants reported using their knowledge and intervention skills directly during the 4 months following their participation in the program (Turley & Tanney, 1998).

Another commonly used gatekeeper training program is Question Persuade Refer (QPR). QPR is a 1- to 2-hour training program delivered by certified instructors in person or online. This brief program is designed to teach parents, teachers, coaches, and other gatekeepers the warning signs of a suicide crisis and how to respond by Questioning the individual's desire or intent regarding suicide, Persuading the person to seek and accept help, and Referring the person to appropriate resources.

Computer-assisted self-study training strategies for school personnel and parents have used audiovisual materials to train school-based gatekeepers. Recent advancements in technology have expanded such strategies and are changing the way that many gatekeepers are being trained. One program getting a lot of attention is At-Risk, developed by Kognito Interactive. The At-Risk program was adapted to meet criteria for use by educators in a variety of settings, including middle schools, high schools, and colleges. The 45-minute to 1-hour online gatekeeper training program seeks to teach school personnel how to identify students exhibiting signs of distress, including depression and thoughts of suicide; approach students to discuss their concern; and make a referral to school support services. Unlike in-person gatekeeper training, participants are guided through virtual conversations with student avatars to learn strategies for broaching the topic of psychological distress to motivate students to seek help.

Recently, At-Risk, QPR, and other gatekeeper programs have gained a lot of attention in colleges.

Critique

Gatekeeper training in schools is one widely used strategy designed to improve early identification of students at risk for suicide and to facilitate timely mental health referrals, responding to the fact that suicidal youth are underidentified and few are using services. Despite their widespread use, gatekeeper training has been largely untested in rigorous evaluations (Wyman et al., 2008). Long-term controlled studies of gatekeeper training programs are needed to determine the frequency and effectiveness of participants' direct interventions during the years following the training. In addition, further evaluation is needed to determine the types of referrals being made, the connection to treatment, and the impact that it may have on the reduction of suicide risk factors and suicidal behavior among youth.

There is some evidence of an increase in referral of youth to treatment through ASIST (Walsh & Perry, 2000); however, evidence of the program's success in preventing suicidal behavior has not been established. School personnel in Washington state, for example, demonstrated increased knowledge about suicide and intervention skills after the ASIST training, showed a mix of intervention behaviors 6 months after training, and showed decreased intervention behaviors 9 and 12 months after training (Guttormsen et al., 2003).

A study by Wyman et al., (2008) used a randomized trial designed to assess the impact of QPR training on school staff members' knowledge, appraisals of willingness to assume a gatekeeper role, and self-reported suicide identification behaviors with students. In addition to assessing overall impact, they tested whether QPR training had a differential effect on gatekeeper surveillance and gatekeeper communication. Researchers found that while the training increased self-reported knowledge, appraisals of efficacy, and service access, the follow-up showed that staff members' increased knowledge and appraisals were not sufficient to increase suicide identification behaviors; when such behaviors did increase, it was mostly for staff members who were already communicating with students about suicide and distress.

SKILLS TRAINING

Skills training programs are designed to enhance protective factors and reduce risk factors for youth suicide through the development of cognitive and social skills (Lake & Gould, 2011). Skills training curricula may be presented universally or may be targeted at a specific population known to be at higher risk for suicide (Lake & Gould, 2011). This section will focus on skills training programs with a universal approach to suicide prevention.

Assumptions

Skills training programs aim to prevent suicide by enhancing problem-solving, coping, and cognitive skills, which have been found to be impaired in suicidal youth (Lake & Gould, 2011). The key assumptions underlying skills training programs are that developing and enhancing these skills may mitigate suicide risk factors such as depression, hopelessness, and drug abuse.

Program Examples

Developed by Barrish et al., (1969) the Good Behavior Game (GBG) is a universal program directed at socializing children for the student role and reducing aggressive, disruptive behavior. In a classroom-based randomized trial examining the GBG intervention for young adult suicide ideation and attempts, Wilcox et al. (2008) found that first-grade students who were assigned to GBG classrooms experienced a lower incidence of suicidality through childhood, adolescence, and young adulthood compared to those who did not. In addition, this group reported half the amount of lifetime rates of suicidal ideation and attempts compared to the matched controls. While this program shows a reduction in suicidal ideation and attempts among the two groups, GBG's effect on suicide attempts was less definitive once researchers controlled for gender and baseline depressive symptoms.

Critique

Most skills training programs continue to involve only one or a limited number of relatively brief sessions focused on suicidal behavior, frequently as part of a larger curricular effort aimed at reducing multiple high-risk behaviors. Although comparing evidence from before and after such programs suggests that they can increase students' knowledge and awareness of suicide risk and improve their help-seeking behaviors, little attention has been paid to determining the scientific accuracy of the program content. Examination of curricular materials used by some of these programs reveals considerable variation in regard to their portrayal of suicide risk factors, in particular the relationship between suicide and mental illness, as well as suicide demographics.

Some concerns have been voiced by high school personnel and parents that overt discussion of suicide in the school curriculum may increase suicidal thoughts and behavior for those at risk. Indeed, one study found statistically significant increases in hopelessness and maladaptive coping resources among some male students after exposure to a suicide awareness curriculum (Overholser, Hemstreet, Spirito, & Vyse, 1989). It is essential that school personnel be made aware of referral sources in the community and for the school to have in place a plan of action for identified students that includes a debriefing component for peers and faculty who are involved in making referrals.

Generalizable conclusions about the efficacy and effectiveness of skills training programs are further limited by the lack of control or comparison groups that would make it possible to differentiate the impact of the program from broader co-occurring trends. For the comprehensive, multilevel skills training programs, insufficient attention has been paid to documenting which program components are responsible for the reported outcomes.

ECOLOGICAL AND COMPREHENSIVE APPROACHES

Comprehensive or "whole school" approaches to school-based youth suicide prevention seek to build a competent school community in which all members are aware of options and resources for preventing youth suicide (Kalafat & Elias, 1995; Lake & Gould, 2011). Comprehensive programs may include the specific goal of transforming the culture, climate, or social ecology of the school to ensure that the school environment is positive and health-promoting (Kalafat, 2003; Kalafat & Elias, 1995).

Assumptions

The key assumptions underlying comprehensive "whole school" programs are that (1) a cohesive and supportive school environment may be protective against suicide risk and

(2) fostering a school climate of open communication may facilitate help seeking on the part of a student in crisis (Lake & Gould, 2011).

Program Examples

Suicide prevention efforts in the Dade County, Florida, public school system provide an example of universal programs applied on a community-wide level. The Youth Suicide Prevention and Intervention Program, which began in 1989, included related curricula across kindergarten through 12th grade, although only 10th-graders received direct discussion of suicide and suicide prevention. In addition to the instructional components, it also included intervention and postvention activities by school-based crisis teams. A 5-year longitudinal study of the Dade County program examined rates of suicide deaths and suicide attempts by youth in the county in the years during which the program was operative (1989–1994), comparing them to comparable rates over the 8-year period preceding the program (Zenere & Lazarus, 1997). One study (Zenere & Lazarus, 2009) was a longitudinal extension of the earlier work, examining the program effects from 1995 to the last data collection period in 2006. The 18-year longitudinal case study showed a significant decrease in the annual suicide rate from an average of 12.9 deaths per 100,000 youth prior to the program to 1.4 per 100,000 in 2006. Known suicide attempt data also showed a decrease from 88 per 100,000 in the program's first year to 9.0 per 100,000 in 2006. This case study is among the first to suggest that comprehensive school-based suicide prevention programs can reduce youth suicidal behavior and sustain this reduction over time. A frequent criticism of many school-based suicide prevention programs is that most of them to date have been largely focused on changing knowledge and attitudes about suicide rather than actual rates of suicide and suicide attempts.

Similar to the first study, the lack of a contemporaneous local control group in this study makes it difficult to determine the linkage between the educational program and the reported decline in suicide rates. Although this report concludes that the comprehensive educational program contributed to the declines, it should be noted that youth suicide rates were declining nationally during the program's implementation, although not as sharply as were reported in this particular county. In addition, the county under study was quite small (330,000 students), so that relatively large fluctuations in suicide rates are not as meaningful as they would be for the national populations.

In its most fully developed form, the Adolescent Suicide Awareness Program (ASAP) includes education for teachers, school staff members, and parents as well as students. Although no controlled evaluations have been reported, the developers cited anecdotal reports of increased referrals of at-risk youth following implementation of ASAP in a number of schools (Kalafat & Ryerson, 1999). This program was one of the first of its kind and has laid the foundation for enhancements in curriculum-based suicide prevention and awareness efforts.

The Lifelines program developed by Hazelden is a comprehensive, schoolwide suicide prevention program for middle and high school students. The goal of the Lifelines program is to promote a caring, competent school community in which help seeking is encouraged and modeled and suicidal behavior is recognized as an issue that cannot be kept secret. A quasi-experimental study by Kalafat et al. (2007) found that the posttest results from the intervention group demonstrated a significantly greater increase in knowledge about suicide and more positive attitudes about seeking help compared to the control group.

Critique

Comprehensive, "whole school" approaches to school-based youth suicide prevention often group together multiple suicide prevention strategies. This presents a challenge for evaluation, and to date, insufficient attention has been paid to documenting which program components are responsible for the reported outcomes. Generalizable conclusions about the efficacy and effectiveness of such comprehensive programs for both high school and college students are further limited by the lack of control or comparison groups that would make it possible to differentiate the program's impact from broader co-occurring trends.

CONCLUSION

The universal suicide prevention programs addressed in this chapter aim to prevent youth suicide by establishing a school community in which all members play a role in supporting youth who may be suicidal or are at risk for suicidal behavior. These programs aim to establish a supportive school environment that promotes students' resilience and well-being and in which all members are aware of options and resources for preventing youth suicide.

Follow-up evaluations on the impact of universal programs have been rare, and thus little is currently known about their impact on reducing suicidal behavior among the targeted group. Longitudinal controlled studies that look at youth several years after participating in educational programs are needed to address the question of long-term behavioral change. This will require addressing the fact that neither high schools nor colleges currently have a reliable system for reporting suicidal behaviors among students, thus hampering the collection of reliable data to determine an educational program's impact. Also, students graduate and leave the school environment, making follow-up difficult.

Targeted Youth Suicide Prevention Programs

Jill Harkavy-Friedman
Herbert Hendin

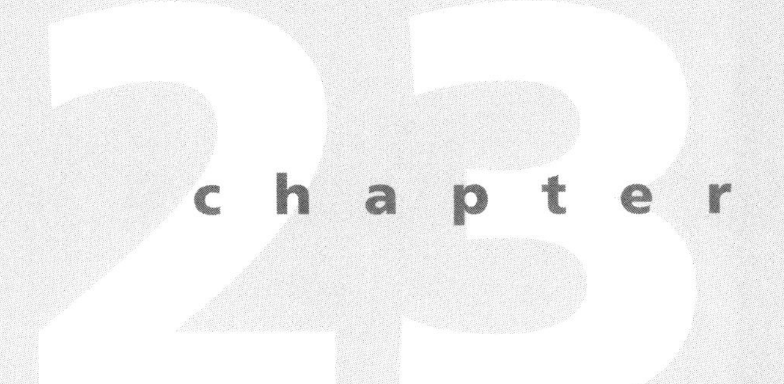

Discussed here are programs for five specific youth populations, each of which has shown elevated rates of suicidal behavior: Native American youth, youth with recent exposure to a suicide in the school or community, youth who have access to firearms in the home, youth who have been detained in the juvenile justice system, and lesbian/gay/bisexual/transgender/questioning (LGBTQ) youth. While there has been considerable research suggesting that adolescents and young adults in these groups are at greater risk for suicide, relatively few intervention programs for these populations have been developed to date.

PROGRAMS FOR NATIVE AMERICAN YOUTH

Assumptions

Based on their research indicating markedly different rates of suicide among different Native American tribes, May and Van Winkle (1994) suggested that high suicide rates among certain tribes were linked to a loosening of social integration within the tribe as members become increasingly acculturated into the broader society. The underlying assumption for a small number of programs is that instilling certain personal traits and social skills in Native American youth will counter the negative effects of the acculturation process and protect these youth against suicidal ideation and behavior.

Program Examples

The Zuni Life Skills Curriculum for preventing suicidal behavior (LaFramboise et al., 1995) is illustrative of programmatic efforts in this category. This program, developed specifically for Zuni youth, featured a 30-week, three-times-a-week course focused on building self-esteem, helping youth identify feelings and stresses, improving communication and problem-solving skills, decreasing self-destructive behavior, and goal setting. The curriculum also provided information about suicide and training regarding intervening with suicidal peers. Results of the program were mixed, with students showing a decrease in hopelessness but not depression after the intervention. Although the program was not specifically addressed to suicidal youth, some of those who participated reported decreased suicidal behaviors. Adult judges rated the impact of the skills training program as positive, but youth overall reported few effects on social functioning. The program was terminated by the school district after 2 years for a variety of reasons outlined by La Framboise and Lewis (2008). They suggest that factors that led to the closing of the program include cultural discomfort with suicide and suicide prevention, privacy concerns, and administrative changes in the community. They report that the program has been adapted for other Native American communities, but these adaptations have not been formally tested.

Critique

Although the Zuni curriculum demonstrated some success, more specific evaluation of program efficacy is needed that incorporates a control-group design and links outcomes to specific program components. In particular, studies that suggest differential acculturation to be pivotal in explaining suicide rates among Native American youth have not controlled for other variables such as psychopathology or family influences. It should also be emphasized that no empirical evidence has been put forth that supports a link between high suicide rates among Native American youth and deficits in personal or social skills.

While adaptations have been reported (La Framboise & Lewis, 2008), the application and the effectiveness of the program have not been studied in other at-risk tribes. Resources available for the development, implementation, and evaluation of suicide prevention programs for Native American youth appear to be limited (Middlebrook, LeMaster, Beals, Novins, & Manson, 2001). An additional observation is that although programs targeting Native American youth are based in part on the premise that external forces in the social and cultural environment contribute to the difficulties these young people face, their strategies focus on changing individuals rather than the external influences. Today's American Indian Reservations, however, vary from modern cities complete with Las Vegas–style casinos, shopping centers, medical and dental offices, police and fire departments, educational centers, museums, and luxury housing, to poverty-stricken Indian Reservations still struggling from generations of governmental and societal neglect. Examining the effects of those differences on suicide rates and behavior would make a valuable contribution to our ability to deal with the problem.

PROGRAMS FOR YOUTH EXPOSED TO SUICIDE

Assumptions

Studies show that adolescents' exposure to the suicide of a family member or peer can trigger new-onset or recurrent major depressive disorder, posttraumatic stress disorder, and suicidal ideation, especially within the month following the suicide (Brent, Perper, Moritz, et al., 1993a,b,c,d,e, 1994). Youth who were already at risk for depression due to family history, a prior episode of depression, or recent interpersonal conflict were found to be at increased risk for suicidal ideation following a suicide, as were those who knew about the victim's plan, felt responsible for the death, or had a conversation with the victim within 24 hours of the suicide. Both the studies by Brent et al. cited above and studies of the contagion effect of suicide (Gould et al., 1990, 1994) reported increased suicidal ideation but not an increase in suicide attempts among exposed youth. A Canadian study, however, of youth ages 13 to 16 found they reported both suicide thoughts and suicide attempts following the death of someone they personally knew (Swanson & Coleman, 2013). Simply knowing the student did not alter the risk for suicidal ideation or behavior, leading the authors to conclude that schoolwide interventions target those closest to the decedent.

Analysis of data on a nationally representative sample of over 10,000 U.S. high school students from the National Longitudinal Study of Adolescent Health (ADD Health) found that "teens who know friends or family members who have attempted suicide are about three times more likely to attempt suicide than are teens who do not know someone who attempted suicide" (Cutler, Glaesen, & Norberg, 2001). In a further analysis of these same data, an effect was also found for exposure to a friend's completed suicide (Feigelman & Gorman, 2008). Having lost a friend to suicide within the previous 12 months increased the odds of a suicide attempt by 2.47 at Wave 1, and by 2.54 at Wave 2, a year later, but this effect was no longer significant at Wave 3, 6 years after that. Of 16 studies reviewed by Insel and Gould (2008) on the impact on adolescents of exposure to a suicidal peer, the majority found a significant association between exposure to the suicidal behavior of an adolescent peer and a subsequent adolescent suicide attempt. Odds ratios ranged from 2.8 to 11.0 for the effects of exposure to attempted suicide, which appeared to confer greater risk than exposure to completed suicide.

The assumption of programs targeting youth exposed to suicide, referred to as "postvention," is that suicide exposure carries increased risk for suicidal ideation, and possibly suicidal behavior, in a school or community where a recent suicide has occurred. Postvention within schools generally seeks to support those grieving the loss, to identify and assist those at risk for developing depression or posttraumatic stress disorder in response to the suicide, and to return the community or school to its normal routines.

Program Examples

The only published evaluation of a postvention program was conducted in Somerville, Massachusetts, after a number of suicides and deaths by drug overdose occurred among 10- to 24-year-olds (Hacker, Collins, Gross-Young, Almeida, & Burke, 2008). The program was initiated by two community groups, Somerville Cares about Prevention (SCAP), a community suicide prevention task force, and a local research group, Institute for Community Health (ICH). To determine the scope of the problem and the needs of the community, the community developed a surveillance system that included death certificates, health records, hospital discharge records, youth surveys, and police and fire department records. Once they established that the community had rates of youth suicides, overdose deaths, and attempts higher than surrounding communities, they investigated whether or not there was a contagion factor. Using family interviews and Internet social websites they discovered connections among most of the deceased. In 2002, with the high rate and possible contagion verified and the support of their newly elected mayor, SCAP and ICH developed a multilevel community-wide prevention/postvention program enlisting many professionals in the community. The intervention involved the development of local support services, working with the media regarding safe reporting, providing targeted education, and beginning several youth leadership programs. The program began in 2003 and continued until 2005. Outcome measures included suicide and overdose death rates, rates of medical treatment for suicidal behavior, and responses to the behavioral surveys administered to youth. From 2002 to 2005 the rates of suicide, overdose, and reported suicidal ideation and attempts on surveys decreased relative to levels before the intervention.

Based on the recommendation of the U.S. Centers for Disease Control and Prevention (CDC, 1988) to develop a community response to suicide that involves all relevant aspects of the community, many postvention programs have been developed and implemented in schools across the country (Askland, Sonnenfeld, & Crosby, 2003; Hazell & Lewin, 1993; Kerr, Brent, & McKain, 1997) as well as abroad (Poijula, Wahlberg, & Dyregrov, 2001). The limited nature of the interventions that were implemented, limited articulation of the intervention models, and the small samples that were studied preclude meaningful conclusions about their impact.

Critique

Although there have been many community postvention programs, only one published study (Hacker et al., 2008) systematically assessed the impact of a postvention program. The program was community-wide and had several components, so it is not possible to identify specific components that were particularly helpful or potentially harmful. Broad guidelines for postvention responses by schools have been in existence for some time (CDC, 1988), but the interventions implemented by individual school districts and communities are varied, each based on some of the interventions recommended by the CDC. The American Foundation for Suicide Prevention, the Suicide Prevention Resource Center, and the Substance Abuse and Mental Health Services Administration (SAMHSA) developed research-based guidelines that are freely available for schools to help them to implement timely and effective postvention programs (*After a Suicide: A Toolkit for Schools* [American Foundation for Suicide Prevention and Suicide Prevention Resource Center, 2011]). These recommendations have not been formally tested.

Staffing for postvention programs and follow-up can be costly for schools both financially and emotionally, and this may be a significant impediment to their implementation. Conducting formal evaluations of the impact of such programs within schools is fraught with difficult ethical issues such as parental consent, confidentiality of data regarding students' emotional and behavioral responses to suicide, and the use of control or comparison groups. As can be seen in the study by Hacker et al. (2008), the development, implementation, and evaluation of postvention programs must be comprehensive and supported by government, municipal, educational, and mental health services as well as the general public.

PROGRAMS REDUCING ACCESS TO LETHAL MEANS

Assumptions

Several different programs have been developed to encourage limiting access to firearms by children and adolescents. The key assumption underlying such programs is that accessibility is a primary risk factor for suicide (Miller, Barber, White, & Azrael, 2013). Grossman, Mueller, Reidy, et al. (2005) demonstrated that youth who died by suicide and accidental death with firearms were significantly more likely to come from homes where guns were less likely to be stored unloaded, less likely to be stored unlocked, less likely to be stored away from ammunition, and less likely to be locked separately from ammunition. In other words, storing guns locked, unloaded, and with ammunition stored and locked elsewhere was associated with a decrease in death by firearms. Programs of this type have been directed primarily to parents.

Program Examples

A core strategy of programs that teach limited access to firearms has involved firearm safety counseling to parents that encourages removal or safe storage of firearms from homes where children reside. One such effort, entitled Love our Kids: Lock Your Guns, was developed by Coyne-Beasley, Schoenbach, and Johnson (2001), following research that documented the presence of unlocked and loaded weapons within many households in which children and adolescents live (Azrael, Miller, & Hemenway, 2000; Brent, Perper, Goldstein, Kolko, Allan, Allman, et al., 1988; Coyne-Beasley et al., 2002; Schuster, Franke, Bastian, Sor, & Halfon, 2000; Senturia, Christoffel, & Donovan, 1994, 1996; Stennies, Ikeda, Leadbetter, Houston, & Sacks, 1999). Prior research by Coyne-Beasley et al. (2002) established that firearm storage practices were frequently lax even among parents who demonstrated high safety consciousness with respect to other potential hazards in the home.

The intervention aimed essentially to reach male gun owners who lived with children, and thus was implemented in an outdoor community setting. Program developers provided firearm safety counseling, distributed free gunlocks, and demonstrated their use on a community-wide basis. Politicians, law enforcement personnel, and the media participated in the program along with youth and their parents; T-shirts and certificates were presented to participants. A 6-month follow-up evaluation found improved safe storage habits among gun owners who had participated in the program. Participants with children, who overall were more likely than other gun owners to store weapons unlocked and loaded at baseline, were found in the post-test to be more likely to have removed guns from the home and to lock the guns that remained. Those who had participated in the counseling were also more likely to report talking with friends about safe storage practices.

A few attempts have been made to deliver firearms and lethal means counseling in mental health settings. One such effort involved education for parents of children who made a visit to an emergency room mental health department of a rural Midwestern hospital (Kruesi, Grossman, Pennington, Woodward, Duda, & Hirsch, 1999). At 6-month follow-up, these investigators found that the education led to decreased youth access to guns, prescription medications, and over-the-counter medication, but not to alcohol. Firm conclusions were limited, however, by the high attrition rate at follow-up.

A similar effort was made with parents of depressed adolescents who participated in a randomized clinical trial of psychotherapy (Brent, Baugher, Birmaher, Kolko, & Bridge, 2000). Parents who reported the presence of firearms in the homes of these adolescents received an intervention designed to encourage removal of firearms. Although compliance with recommendations was more likely in the homes of adolescents with active suicidal ideation and attempts and in single-parent homes, overall less than one third of the targeted parents removed their guns from the home. Urban families and families in which there was marital discord or a father with a drinking problem were less likely to remove guns. The investigators emphasized the need to talk directly with the parent who owned the gun. In addition, 17% of parents who reported no gun in the home at intake and therefore were not targeted by the intervention purchased a gun during the study. This points to the advisability of counseling about lethal means for all parents and not just those who own a firearm at the outset of the intervention.

Looking at soldiers ages 18 to 21, a program instituted by the Israeli army (Lubin, Werbeloff, Halperin, Shmushkevitch, Weiser, & Knobler, 2010) demonstrated that access to firearms affected suicide rates. The Israeli army changed its regulations such that soldiers were no longer allowed to bring their guns home on weekends. In this naturalistic epidemiologic study the suicide rates before and after the policy were compared. The suicide rate dropped 40%, with the reduction primarily for weekend suicides; the rate during the week did not change. This example is a powerful demonstration of the impact of limiting access to lethal means on suicide rates and that individuals did not switch to other means of suicide when access was limited.

The policy statement on firearm safety of the American Academy of Pediatrics (2000) has urged parents to remove firearms from the environment where children live and visit, and if guns remain in the home, to store them unloaded and locked, with ammunition stored separately. One attempt to apply this policy in an intervention program (although not specifically a suicide prevention program) is the Steps to Prevent Firearms Injury Program (STOP) of the American Academy of Pediatrics and the Center to Prevent Handgun Violence. This intervention provides counseling to parents in primary care clinics. Evaluations have not found the program to be effective in reducing firearm safety and removal (Grossman, Cummings, Koepsell, Marshal, D'Ambrosio, Thompson, & Mack, 2000; Oatis, Fenn Buderer, Cummings, & Fleitz, 1999), possibly because it has primarily reached mothers, while fathers and other males in the household are more often responsible for the presence and storage practices of the guns in the home.

Critique

In assessing the effectiveness of lethal means counseling programs on reducing youth suicide, it is important to note that some of the activities described here have been implemented during a period of declining use and ownership of firearms in U.S. homes, notable since 1980. Thus, care must be exercised in drawing conclusions about the impact of specific interventions on reducing the presence of guns in American households. There have been no recent evaluations of the effectiveness of efforts to reduce the access to firearms among youth.

Assessing the impact of firearms removal and firearms safety on youth suicidal behavior is likewise a difficult task. It is not surprising that young people who use guns for self-injury live in a house where there are firearms, and where the firearms are accessible. This does not mean, however, that the presence of firearms has set in motion the lengthy and complex process that leads to suicide. The methodological challenge ultimately facing firearms access programs is to demonstrate that suicide-prone youth survive in firearms-free homes but do not in homes where firearms are accessible. As was noted in Chapter 21, it is not clear the extent to which a decrease in youth suicide deaths from firearms may be offset by increases in the use of other lethal methods (Beautrais, 2001; De Leo et al., 2003), and this possibility needs to be considered in evaluating the impact of firearms access programs. It is noteworthy that this did not happen during the Israel army study (Lubin et al., 2010).

Although comprehensive evaluations of this sort have not yet been undertaken, existing programs suggest the potential of community-based programs that provide lethal means counseling to males within households in which children and youth live. It should be noted that means access have not received widespread funding, in part due to political pressures and in part because they address a more limited audience than universal interventions that can be easily incorporated into public school systems.

PROGRAMS FOR YOUTH IN THE JUVENILE JUSTICE SYSTEM

Based on the findings of a national survey (Juvenile Suicide in Confinement) of the National Center of Institutions and Alternatives (NCIA) commissioned by the U.S. Justice Department's Office of Juvenile Justice and Delinquency Prevention (OJJDP), it was recommended that all correction facilities that house juveniles, regardless of the facility's size, develop and implement suicide prevention programs with the following components (Hayes, 2004). They were published and distributed by the National Commission on Correctional Health Care (2009):

1. Staff training should specifically address juvenile inmate suicide risk factors and potential interventions.
2. Identification of suicide risk should be ongoing among all juvenile inmates, and mental health treatment and day-to-day management plans should be in place for those identified as being at risk.
3. Communication should occur across all staff regarding individuals at risk and appropriate treatment.
4. Housing must be designed to be suicide-resistant, and youth in room confinement must be monitored closely.
5. Levels of monitoring must be based on clinical need rather than resources available, and must include a level of observation appropriate to each inmate's suicide risk.
6. Interventions based on best clinical practices for identification and treatment are to be used.
7. Mortality and morbidity review should be conducted of every suicide and suicide attempt requiring hospitalization by a multidisciplinary team across clinical and management staff. The review should be conducted to determine what factors contributed to the suicide, including personnel behavior and organization policies and procedures, and what changes in protocols are indicated.

Critique

Although the recommendations have been published, the extent to which they are being implemented by juvenile justice institutions across the country is not clear. Follow-up studies are needed to determine compliance with these suicide prevention guidelines, as well as the effectiveness of the recommended procedures in reducing suicide attempts and deaths among juvenile inmates.

PROGRAMS FOR LGBT YOUTH

Assumptions

Programs for LGBT youth have tended to focus on reducing external factors that make these young people especially vulnerable to suicidal ideation and behavior, in particular rejection, antigay discrimination, and victimization. Although there is considerable indication that LGBT youth are at higher risk for suicide attempts (Fergusson, Horwood, & Beautrais, 1999) than heterosexual youth, there is as yet a paucity of suicide prevention programs or interventions designed specifically for this population.

Program Examples

The Trevor Project, founded in 1998, is the leading national organization that provides crisis intervention and suicide prevention services to LGBT youth. Specific services include a 24/7 telephone helpline, an online chat service, an online question-and-answer resource for young people with questions related to sexual orientation and gender identity, and an online social networking community for LGBT youth ages 13 through 24 and their friends and allies. The Trevor Project also educates youth about sexuality and gender identity through its Lifeguard Workshop Program, which also teaches young people to recognize depression and suicide risk among their peers and provides training in suicide prevention skills. No evaluation studies have been undertaken to document the outcomes of any of these services, however.

Gay-Straight Alliances (GSAs) are student-led organizations primarily within high schools, colleges, and universities that are intended to provide a safe, supportive environment for LGBT students (http://en.wikipedia.org/wiki/Gay-straight_alliance). GSAs began in the late 1980s and have been actively promoted by the national organization the Gay, Lesbian and

Straight Education Network (GLSEN) and in California by that state's Gay-Straight Alliance Network. Although systematic evaluation of the impact of GSAs in U.S. schools is lacking, one study showed that students and teachers considered these organizations to be more effective in changing attitudes than any of the educational or training programs offered in the schools (Szalacha, 2003). More recently, a school-based survey of almost 22,000 secondary school students in British Columbia, Canada, showed that the presence of a GSA in a school for at least 3 years was associated with lower odds of reported past-year antigay discrimination, suicidal ideation, and suicide attempts among LGB students (Saewyc, Konishi, Rose, & Homma, 2014). Heterosexual boys, but not girls, also had lower odds of suicidal ideation and attempts in schools with well-established GSAs. Similar outcomes were found in schools that had well-established anti-homophobic bullying policies; however, these policies had a less consistent effect across schools than GSAs.

Critique

The Trevor Project is limited by a lack of outcome data. Despite increasing recognition of the increased suicide risk among LGBT youth, suicide prevention efforts for this population were underdeveloped and underresourced, reflecting a lack of media attention to the problem both by mainstream suicide prevention organizations and agencies and by the LGBT movement. This is beginning to change, and the positive results of the Canadian study should lead other schools to follow suit.

Preventive Interventions and Treatments for Suicidal Youth

Jill Harkavy-Friedman
Herbert Hendin

chapter 24

The last category of youth suicide prevention efforts focuses on indicated interventions and treatments that target those who have already shown signs of suicidal ideation and behavior. Such efforts seek essentially to prevent suicide attempts and suicide completion. The interventions and treatments described in this chapter differ widely in terms of the groups they target, the methods they use, and the settings in which they have been implemented.

SCHOOL-BASED PROGRAMS FOR SUICIDAL STUDENTS

Assumptions

The central underlying assumption of school-based programs for suicidal students is that subsequent suicidal thoughts and behavior can be reduced by enhancing protective factors, in particular students' personal and social support resources.

Program Examples

The most comprehensive school-based programs are those developed and tested by Eggert, Thompson, and their colleagues (1994, 1999, 2000, 2001), as part of the Reconnecting Youth (RY) Prevention Research Program. The interventions are directed to students who are deemed to be at risk of dropping out of high school, based primarily on school attendance data and observations of teachers, counselors, and other gatekeepers. Such students have been reported to have multiple co-occurring problems that, in addition to school performance difficulties, include depression, suicidality, drug involvement, and tendencies toward aggressive and violent behaviors (Eggert, Thompson, Herting, & Nichols, 1994; Lewinsohn, Rohde, & Seeley, 1993).

The interventions are based on a theoretical model that rests essentially on improving the student's personal resources, leading to an enhanced sense of personal control and self-esteem, improved decision making, increased use of social support resources, and reduced suicidal behavior. The early research involved systematic evaluation of a semester-long, school-based small group intervention called the Personal Growth Class (PGC). The intervention included life skills training using strategies of group process, teacher and peer support, goal setting, and weekly monitoring of mood management, school performance, and drug involvement.

Evaluation studies by Thompson, Eggert, and their colleagues (Eggert, Thompson, Herting, & Nicholas, 1994, 1995; Thompson, Eggert, & Herting, 2000) involved approximately 100 high school students at risk for dropping out of high school, as determined by a set of defined criteria, who screened positive for suicidal behavior (as discussed in Chapter 22). The students were randomly assigned to one of three conditions: assessment protocol plus one semester of PGC; assessment protocol plus two semesters of PGC; and assessment protocol only. Participants were assessed at baseline and at 5 and 10 months after the intervention. Participants in all three groups showed significant declines in suicidal behavior. Unlike the students who received the assessment protocol only, PGC participants showed significant improvement in self-perceived ability to manage problem circumstances. Also reported was a significant positive impact of both teacher and peer support in decreasing suicide risk behaviors and depression.

Thompson, Eggert, and their colleagues (2001) subsequently tested two additional school-based prevention programs based on the PGC: a brief one-on-one intervention known as Counselors Care (C-CARE), and a small group skills-building intervention program, Coping and Support Training (CAST), derived directly from the PGC program. Both interventions, compared to a usual care control group, were found to reduce suicide risk behaviors and depression, even at the 9-month follow-up assessment; CAST was most effective in enhancing and sustaining protective factors such as problem-solving ability.

The CARE intervention, expanded to include a parent intervention component, P-CARE (Randell, 1999), is being studied to determine the added benefit of this component to further reduce depression, anger, and suicide risk behaviors. Preliminary results suggest that C-CARE, coupled with the parent intervention, is associated with more rapid rates of decline in suicidal ideation, direct suicide threats, depression, hopelessness, and anxiety when compared to usual care (Thompson, 2003).

CAST, originally designed for high school youth, has been found to be effective with young adults up to age 25 in school settings and other institutions, and as a community-based program. The results compared with treatment as usual showed a significant decrease in positive attitudes toward suicide and suicidal ideation and a significantly greater and swifter decrease in depressive symptoms, feelings of hopelessness, anxiety for female patients, and anger-control problems; there was a significant and greater increase in feelings of personal control and problem-solving and coping skills (Benchmark, 2009).

Critique

These programs for suicidal students at risk of dropping out of high school have demonstrated efficacy in reducing suicidal behavior and depression. There is some indication that prolonged intervention results in the most positive outcomes related to suicide, although it is not clear whether these effects are due to repeated contact with the treatment or to the nature of the treatment itself. As is often the case with programs involving multiple components, it is difficult to identify which component is most responsible for the outcomes reported by these programs. Preliminary reports suggest that including parents in the intervention is particularly effective.

The target groups addressed by the studies of Eggert and Thompson may limit the generalizability of the findings to other populations of suicidal youth. From the outset, the focus of these programs has been on students at risk of dropping out of high school as principally defined through attendance records. There is some evidence that high school dropouts may come from more deviant and neglecting families and thus may not be representative of suicidal adolescents overall. In addition, the inclusion criteria for these programs are somewhat idiosyncratic in their use of gatekeeper identification of problematic students, which may limit the exportability and testing of the model.

In addition, these interventions were designed and implemented by highly skilled, university-based professionals, who devoted considerable attention to ensuring program fidelity, evaluating program results, and making improvements based on empirical findings. Although the results appear promising, replication of the program in schools that do not have such resources may be difficult. The community-based dissemination of the CAST intervention implemented and evaluated in three sites (Randell, Eggert, & Pike, 2001), addressed this problem. Although the study widens the scope of the program, since the data for adolescents among this group are not presented, it limits the conclusions that can be drawn about them from the study.

EMERGENCY DEPARTMENT INTERVENTIONS FOR YOUNG SUICIDE ATTEMPTERS

Assumptions

A considerable number of adolescents who make suicide attempts obtain some form of medical intervention (Grunbaum, Kann, Kinchen, et al., 2002), typically beginning in a hospital emergency department (ED). This suggests that the ED may be a prime location for initiating treatment programs for them. Numerous studies have documented, however, that young suicide attempters' adherence to outpatient treatment recommendations made in the ED is poor, with over 15% never attending any recommended outpatient sessions and fewer than half attending more than a few sessions (Spirito, Plummer, Gispert, et al., 1992; Stewart, Manion, & Cloutier, 2001; Trautman, Stewart, & Morishima, 1993). Poor adherence has been attributed to ED factors such as long waits, repetitive evaluations, and poor communication by ED staff, and also to cultural factors, including the perception that mental health treatment is shameful (Spirito, 2003). The primary assumption underlying ED interventions is that improved treatment adherence will result in decreased suicidal behavior; thus, their goal is to develop mechanisms for engaging suicide attempters in the treatment process.

Program Examples

Rotheram-Borus et al. (1996, 2000) designed an intervention that targeted both the ED staff and families of Latino adolescent females who attempted suicide and followed participants over 18 months. Using videotapes and therapists, this program involved ED staff and families with a focus on encouraging participation in outpatient treatment. In comparison with patients who received family therapy alone, participants who received both family therapy and the ED intervention were found to adhere more frequently to the recommendation to attend a first treatment session. Families receiving the combined intervention also had more favorable outcomes in terms of maternal depression and general psychopathology, patient ideation, and parent-reported family interaction.

Spirito, Boergers, Donaldson, et al. (2002) also developed an adherence enhancement intervention to improve adolescent suicide attempters' engagement in therapy. Treatment expectations, misperceptions, and reasons for treatment dropout were separately presented to adolescents and parents, along with a 1-hour intervention to facilitate problem solving around factors that might impede treatment attendance. After this ED intervention, telephone contacts were made separately to adolescents and their parents at at 1, 2, 4, and 8 weeks. Many service barriers were reported, such as delays in getting an appointment, being placed on a waiting list, and insurance and out-of-pocket expenses. Family barriers to treatment included parental emotional problems, transportation difficulties, language difficulties, and scheduling problems. The adherence enhancement program increased the number of sessions attended, although premature termination of treatment continued to be a problem. The program developers emphasized the importance of reducing service barriers for adolescents who have attempted suicide.

Hospitalization for suicidal behavior, though often securing the safety of the suicidal individual, is quite costly and not always beneficial. In an effort to decrease hospitalization rates and suicidality and improve functioning, Greenfield, Larson, Hechtman, et al. (2002) implemented the Rapid Response (RR) ED intervention for suicidal adolescents who were not considered to require immediate medical or psychiatric hospitalization. The intervention included family therapy, medication, and community intervention, as indicated. Hospitalization rates were decreased and outpatient therapy was initiated more rapidly as a result of the RR intervention when compared with standard care. In addition, adolescents receiving the intervention were less likely to be readmitted to the hospital during the 6 months after their visit to the ED. Neither hospitalization nor RR was found to prevent subsequent suicidal behavior or ED visits.

Asarnow, Baraff, Berk, et al. (2011) conducted a randomized controlled trial in which 181 suicidal youths at two EDs (ages 10–18) were individually assigned to one of two conditions: (1) an enhanced mental health intervention involving a family-based cognitive-behavioral therapy session designed to increase motivation for follow-up treatment and safety, supplemented by telephone contacts after ED discharge, or (2) usual ED care enhanced by provider education. Assessments were conducted at baseline and approximately 2 months after discharge from the ED or hospital. The primary outcome measure was rates of outpatient mental health treatment after discharge. Intervention patients were significantly more likely than usual care patients to attend outpatient treatment (92% vs. 76%; $p = .004$). The intervention group also had significantly higher rates of psychotherapy (76% vs. 49%; $p = .001$), combined psychotherapy and medication (58% vs. 37%; $p = .003$), and psychotherapy visits (mean 5.3 vs. 3.1; $p = .003$). Neither the ED intervention nor community outpatient treatment (in exploratory analyses) was significantly associated with improved clinical or functioning outcomes.

Currier, Fisher, and Caine (2010) sought to determine whether a mobile crisis team (MCT) intervention would be more effective than standard referral to a hospital-based clinic as a means of establishing near-term clinical contact after ED discharge. This objective was based on the premise that increased attendance at the first outpatient mental health appointment would initiate an ongoing treatment course, with subsequent differential improvements in psychiatric symptoms and functioning for patients successfully linked to care. In a rater-blinded, randomized controlled trial, 120 participants who were evaluated for suicidal thoughts, plans, or behaviors, and who were subsequently discharged from an urban ED, were randomized to follow-up either in the community via MCT or an outpatient mental health clinic (OPC). Both MCTs and OPCs offered the same structured array of clinical services and referral options. Successful first clinical contact after ED discharge occurred in 39 of 56 (69.6%) participants randomized to the MCT versus 19 of 64 (29.6%) randomized to the OPC (relative risk =2.35, 95% confidence interval [CI] 1.55–3.56, $p < .001$). No significant differences were detected between the groups in symptom or functional outcome measures at either 2 weeks or 3 months after enrollment, nor were any significant differences found in outcomes between participants who did attend their first prescribed appointment via MCT or OPC versus those who did not. However, divided (MCT vs. OPC, present at first appointment vs. no show), groups showed significant improvements but maintained clinically significant levels of dysfunction and continued to rely on ED services at a similar rate in the 6 months after study enrollment. Community-based mobile outreach was a highly effective method of contacting suicidal patients who were discharged from the ED. However, establishing initial post-discharge contact in the community versus the clinic did not prove more effective at enhancing initial symptomatic or functional outcomes, nor did successful linkage with outpatient psychiatric care. Overall, participants showed some improvement shortly after ED discharge regardless of outpatient clinical contact but nonetheless remained significantly symptomatic and at risk for reported ED presentations.

Critique

The results of the programs implemented to date suggest that some improvement in outpatient treatment adherence by young suicide attempters, as well as reduced hospital admissions, can be achieved by concerted efforts in the ED. Such efforts, however, require educating the ED staff regarding the suicide risks and treatment needs of young suicide attempters. Barriers to outpatient treatment appear to remain significant and difficult to surmount, even for the most cohesive and well-functioning families. It seems essential that ED interventions provide some continuity of contact with the youth beyond the initial ED visit, which will require additional staffing. While this may seem costly, the cost reductions associated with decreasing immediate and future hospital admissions are significant. The fact that there was no significant reduction in suicidal behavior or functional outcomes indicates the need for improvements in community outpatient treatment.

POSTHOSPITALIZATION PROGRAMS FOR SUICIDAL YOUTH

Assumptions

Research has pointed to a lack of posthospital treatment adherence among the many youth who are hospitalized on inpatient psychiatric units following serious suicidal behavior (Cohen-Sandler, Berman, & King, 1982; Spirito, Brown, Overholser, & Fritz, 1989). One result is frequent readmission to the hospital for repeated suicidality (Greenfield et al., 2002; Stewart et al., 2001). The key assumption of posthospitalization programs is that providing consistent support and improving adherence to aftercare recommendations will help to prevent future suicidal behavior.

Program Example

The only fully developed program of this sort is the Youth-Nominated Support Team (YST) intervention, developed by King et al. (King, 2003; King, Preuss, & Krammer, 2001). This program was an outgrowth of the developers' finding that family dysfunction and parental psychopathology significantly impact treatment adherence by suicidal youth after hospitalization (King, Hovey, Brand, Wilson, & Ghaziuddin, 1997). Concentrating on the high-risk period for suicidality immediately following psychiatric hospitalization, the program specifically targets poor treatment adherence and negative perceptions of family support and helpfulness.

Before leaving the hospital, program participants nominate specific adults from their home, school, or community to support them when they are released. YST conducts a psychoeducation session with these adults, then engages them in weekly consultations designed to improve their understanding of the suicidal youngster and how he or she can be effectively supported. A social network is encouraged among the adults, who typically come from diverse settings. The program is designed to supplement usual treatments.

The response to YST by participating youth and the nominated adults has been positive (King, 2003), with 80% of those nominated actually participating in the program. Positive effects have been reported for adolescent females, including reduced suicidal ideation and mood impairment. Similar benefits were not evidenced among male participants, although some described YST as having beneficial effects.

Critique

Since this intervention has only recently been implemented, it is too early to know whether the positive effects found among the suicidal girls will be translated into reductions of suicide attempts and repeat hospital admissions. It will also be important to identify the reasons underlying the lack of clear effects among male participants, and to incorporate the necessary programmatic changes. The fact that the program has been manualized will likely encourage its replication, while permitting independent assessment of specific program components.

PSYCHOTHERAPEUTIC TREATMENTS FOR SUICIDAL YOUTH

As noted in Chapter 21, previous suicidal behavior is the most important factor associated with suicide risk among both adults and youth. Because recognizing that repetition of a suicide attempt vastly increases the risk of a fatal outcome (Arensman et al., 2001), considerable effort has been directed toward developing psychotherapeutic and other psychosocial treatment modalities to prevent subsequent suicidal behavior among identified individuals.

Most of the psychotherapeutic approaches for treating suicidal youth have employed variations of cognitive-behavioral therapy (CBT). The underlying assumption is that the primary focus of treatment should be the suicidal behavior itself, rather than the underlying psychopathology (Brent, Holder, Kolko, Birmaher, Baugher, Roth, et al., 1997; Harrington, Kerfoot, Dyer, McNiven, Gill, Harrington, et al., 1998; Stanley et al., 2009).

Program Examples

Rudd et al. provided the first description of a cognitive-behavioral skills group intervention designed to treat young adults with suicidal ideation or suicidal behavior (Rudd, Rajab, Orman, Stulman, Joiner, & Dixon, 1996). The intervention, an intensive 2-week program that participants attended for 9 hours per day, included an experiential affective group, psychoeducational classes with homework, and a problem-solving and social competence group. A variety of strategies such as behavioral rehearsal, role playing, and modeling were used to improve basic social skills and effective coping. Participants (N = 264) were randomly assigned to either the experimental intervention or a treatment-as-usual condition involving long-term outpatient treatment. In a 2-year follow-up, Rudd et al. found that participants in both groups showed significant reductions in suicidal ideation and behavior and experienced stress, and improvements in self-appraised problem-solving ability. The intensive time-limited intervention was found to be more effective than long-term treatment in retaining the highest-risk participants. Subsequent analyses showed that patients with psychiatric symptomatology experienced the most improvement in response to this intervention (Joiner, Voelz, & Rudd, 2001). The rate of suicide attempts at follow-up was not reported for either the experimental or control group, however, and conclusions were limited by high attrition rates in both the experimental and control group.

Harrington and his colleagues in Great Britain (Byford, Harrington, Torgerson, Kerfoot, Dyer, Harrington, et al., 1999; Harrington et al., 1998; Harrington, Kerfoot, Dyer, M, McNiven, Gill, Harrington, et al., 2000) developed a home-based family intervention for adolescents with a history of deliberate self-poisoning. This intervention used a cognitive-behavioral approach to address family dysfunction assumed to be related to the suicide attempt (Kerfoot, 1988; Kerfoot, Dyer, Harrington, Woodham, & Harrington, 1996), and to improve adherence to treatment by bringing it into the home. The intervention consisted of five highly structured sessions focusing on goal setting, reviewing the self-poisoning episode, communication, problem solving, and issues related to the family. The program included a treatment manual and videotape for training. This brief intervention was found to be effective primarily among those adolescents who were not seriously depressed and had less severe suicidal ideation, who made up about one third of the 85 participants (Harrington et al., 1998, 2000). Adherence and parental satisfaction with treatment were better for participants in this treatment relative to treatment as usual. The intervention was found to be no more costly than routine care alone (Byford et al., 1999).

Wood et al. have developed an additional psychotherapeutic variant, using Developmental Group Therapy (DGT) as an alternative to usual care for adolescents who have repeatedly attempted to harm themselves (Wood, Harrington, & Moore, 1996; Wood, Trainor, Rothwell, Moore, & Harrington, 2001). The group therapy format was hypothesized to be useful in providing an arena for working on social problem-solving and relationship skills that are often considered core to suicidal behavior. Using a developmental approach to address issues unique to adolescents, the intervention combines problem-solving and cognitive-behavioral interventions (Harrington, et al., 1998), Dialectical Behavior Therapy (DBT; Linehan et al., 1991), and psychodynamic approaches. An acute phase focusing on core themes (family and peer relationships, school problems, anger management, depression, self-harm, and hopelessness) is followed by a longer phase that concentrates on group processes. In interviews conducted about 7 months after treatment began, DGT participants reported engaging in less self-harm than did adolescents who received routine care, although depression did not appear to improve. Episodes of self-harm became less frequent as participants attended more sessions of the group therapy, whereas among those in usual care, self-harm behaviors were found to increase compared to baseline. DGT participants, particularly youth who had made multiple suicide attempts, also showed reductions in conduct problems. While DGT shows promise, Hazell et al. (2009) attempted to replicate its effectiveness in a sample of 72 12- to 16-year-olds by comparing this treatment to routine care and assessing youth 6 and 12 months after treatment. Adolescents in the DGT sample reported more self-harm at both follow-up periods. Changes specific to suicide attempts could not be determined since the groups were not equal at baseline. Given the inconsistent findings, further study of this intervention is warranted.

As part of the multisite Treatment of Adolescent Suicide Attempters study, Stanley et al. (2009) developed Cognitive-Behavior Therapy Suicide Prevention (CBT-SP). The goal of this intervention is to prevent future suicidal behavior among adolescents with depression and a previous suicide attempt. The treatment is manual-based and focuses specifically on suicidal behavior and therefore can be applied to adolescents with recent or imminent suicidal behavior. It can accompany other forms of treatment focused on other mental health issues. The stress-diathesis model serves as the theoretical basis for this treatment. The assumption is that an individual is at potential risk for suicidal behavior as the result of a variety of individual and environmental factors, and the individual's risk for suicidal behavior may increase as part of his or her response to a significant stressor. The goal of the treatment is to identify triggers for suicidal behavior and apply cognitive and behavioral tools rather than suicidal behavior when the triggers are present. Parents are involved to the extent that they can learn specific strategies to help reduce suicidal behavior in their adolescent.

The 6-month treatment includes acute and continuation phases. The acute phase includes initial, middle, and end phases and may take up to six family sessions. During the initial acute phase of treatment a chain analysis is conducted to understand the precipitants for the suicidal behavior, a safety plan is developed that includes strategies the patient can use to stay safe, and psychoeducation is provided to the patient and family regarding suicidal behavior, depression, and removal of lethal means. The middle phase of acute treatment takes place after the immediate crisis is over and includes skills development for the individual and the family. Sessions have a specific structure, and the goal is to help the patient and family develop an effective approach to managing stressors and suicidal ideation and behavior if it emerges. The end of the acute treatment phase and the continuation phase are focused on preventing relapse. The suicide attempt and the chain of events, thoughts, feelings, and behaviors that led to it are reviewed, and the patient discusses how he or she can use the new skills under similar circumstances. This reinforces the newly developed skills and problem solving. The 12-week continuation phase focuses on titrating treatment, continued presentation of new skills, and practice of all learned skills.

The investigators reported that 72.4% of participants completed the acute treatment phase but only 28.6% completed the continuation phase. Based on a qualitative interview conducted with 42 participants, the treatment was found to be helpful by 100% of patients, 42% stated that they would not change the treatment if given the opportunity, and 86% said they would recommend the treatment to others. Those who recommended changes focused primarily on procedures such as rewards, assessments, and the research protocol itself. While most found repeated assessments to have no impact (30%) or a positive effect (19%), 30.9% found the repeated assessments to be mildly negative and almost 12% found the repeated assessments aversive. No participant reported increased suicidal ideation of the repeated assessments.

Therapist adherence was also assessed and varied depending on the module being considered. Overall, therapist adherence was good, although modules related to mobilizing supports and social skills for the patients were less likely to be presented.

A 6-month treatment similar to CBT-SP was developed and pilot tested in London (Taylor et al., 2011). Of an original sample of 37 12- to 18-year-olds, 16 adolescents with deliberate self-harm (13 of whom also had an incident of self-harm with suicidal ideation) completed the treatment. The treatment modules were (1) Getting Started; (2) Feelings, Thoughts, and Behaviors; (3) Coping; and (4) On You Go. A parent module was offered, but only two parents agreed to participate. The investigators were only able to obtain follow-up information on the treatment completers, thereby barring comparison with those who did not complete the program. Self-harm and suicidal behavior were greatly reduced, with only one participant having made a suicide attempt at 3-month follow-up. In sum, CBT with a focus on suicidal behavior has demonstrated potential for treating the adolescent with suicide attempts.

In another variation, Miller et al. (1997; Rathus & Miller, 2002) used a modification of DBT in their treatment of adolescent suicide attempters who demonstrated at least three features of borderline personality disorder. The intervention they developed consisted of 12 weeks of twice-weekly individual and family skills training. In one trial (Rathus & Miller, 2002), participants in the DBT group were found to have better adherence to treatment and fewer hospitalizations than those receiving treatment as usual, even though they had greater psychiatric comorbidity than control subjects. DBT treatment was also found to be associated with reduced suicidal ideation, symptom severity, and distress. Although suicide attempts were less likely in the DBT group compared to the controls, this difference was not found to be significant.

The feasibility of DBT with adolescent inpatients admitted because of a suicide attempt or strong preoccupation with suicide was tested with a 2-week inpatient adolescent DBT program and compared with patients with treatment as usual, which used a traditional psychodynamically oriented assessment and treatment model (Katz et al., 2004). Assessments of depressive symptoms, suicidal ideation, hopelessness, parasuicidal behavior, hospitalizations, ED visits, and adherence to follow-up recommendations were conducted before and after treatment and at 1-year follow-up for both groups. In addition, behavioral incidents on the units were evaluated. DBT significantly reduced behavioral incidents during admission when compared with treatment as usual. Both groups demonstrated highly significant reductions in parasuicidal behavior, depressive symptoms, and suicidal ideation at 1 year. The authors concluded that DBT can be effectively implemented in acute-care child and adolescent psychiatric inpatient units (Katz, Cox, Gunasekara, & Miller, 2004).

Fleischhaker et al. (2011) conducted a pilot study of DBT with 12 adolescent females with non-suicidal self-injury, eight of whom also had a suicide attempt. Participants received 16 to 24 weeks of DBT at an outpatient mental health clinic in Germany and were assessed 4 weeks and 1 year after treatment. Non-suicidal self-injury was reduced but persisted. No suicide attempts occurred during the 1-year follow-up period.

Interpersonal Psychotherapy for depressed adolescents (IPT-A; Mufson et al., 2004) has been shown to be equally effective as CBT in treating depression in adolescents (Horowitz et al., 2007). IPT-A works to reduce suicidal behavior by helping adolescents and their families resolve problems between them and deals with the affects that underlie the problems. Its approach is different than that of CBT, which treats maladaptive cognitions as the root of the problem. It is being tested for its ability to reduce suicidal behavior in adolescents.

Mentalization, an important component of DBT, served as the core of an intervention developed by Rossouw and Fonagy (2012) to treat adolescents who engaged in self-harm behavior, including suicide attempts. In a randomized controlled trial, Mentalization-Based Treatment for Adolescents (MBT-A) was compared with treatment as usual among 12- to 17-year-olds presenting at a community health center or hospital ED. To qualify, the youth had to have engaged in self-harm behavior (80% reported at least one suicide attempt). MBT-A was a year-long manualized treatment program that combined attachment theory–based psychoanalytic therapy with monthly family therapy sessions (MBT-F) that focused on impulsivity and affect regulation. The goals of the treatment include more accurate assessment of their own and others' emotions and improved functioning in emotionally challenging situations. The assumption is that reduced self-harming behavior would result. Eighty adolescents were randomized to MBT-A or treatment as usual, and 97% met the criteria for at least one mental disorder. One third of the MBT-A families refused to participate in treatment. While both groups improved, the MBT-A group showed greater reduction in self-harm. By 12 months, depression was reduced for both groups, more so for those receiving MBT-A. It is noteworthy that the rate of self-harm behavior during treatment (MBT-A 43% vs. treatment as usual 68%) and the presence of depression (MBT-A 49% vs. treatment as usual 70%) were still significantly high. Thus, this approach showed reduction in self-harm behavior and depression but not remission.

Family psychotherapeutic approaches for adolescents who have made a suicide attempt have also been developed and are currently being tested. Attachment-Based Family Therapy (ABFT; Diamond et al., 2002), originally developed for the treatment of adolescents with depression, has been found to be effective in reducing suicidal ideation among adolescents who have made a suicide attempt and have at least one parent available for family treatment (Diamond et al., 2010). It has also been adapted and shows promise among lesbian/gay/bisexual/transgender youth who have made a suicide attempt (Diamond et al., 2012). ABFT assumes that problems with attachment, high levels of parental criticism, and lack of emotional attunement in families lead to the development of ineffective coping skills for dealing with stressors that may trigger depression and suicidal ideation and behavior. ABFT also assumes that these disrupted functions are available for reparation, and improved coping and lower risk for depression and suicide are possible. The targets of treatment include parental criticism and hostility, low motivation and engagement in the adolescent, ineffective parenting, family disengagement, and negative self-concept. Specific tasks are provided to assist family members in developing more functional and effective social and attachment skills. The development of these skills allows for improved coping and decreased depression and suicidal ideation and behavior.

A 12-week randomized control trial of ABFT compared with enhanced usual care was conducted with adolescents between the ages of 12 and 17 recruited from emergency and primary care hospital settings who were assessed to have significant suicidal ideation and depression and who had a parent available for participation in treatment (Diamond et al., 2010). A follow-up assessment was conducted at 24 weeks after baseline. While both groups demonstrated improvement with treatment, adolescents who participated in ABFT demonstrated quicker and greater decreases in suicidal ideation and depression, and the reduction of symptoms persisted at follow-up.

An analysis of the data from 18 families for whom treatment videotapes were available (Shpigel et al., 2012) provided evidence that parental factors improved early in treatment and adolescents' attachment, anxiety, depression, and suicidal ideation improved over the entire course of treatment. These findings suggest that parental improvement plays a role in the suicidal teen's improvement. ABFT has been adapted for LGBT adolescents with the addition of a module just with parents that focuses on their feelings about their child's LGBT status, working toward acceptance, and reducing rejecting statements by parents (Diamond et al., 2012). In a pilot study with 10 LGBT adolescents with significant suicidal ideation, the teens reported significantly reduced suicidal ideation after 12 weeks of treatment. There is strong evidence that ABFT is an effective treatment for reducing suicidal ideation in adolescents with parents willing to engage in treatment.

Pineda and Dadds (2013) examined a parent intervention for parents of adolescents between the ages of 12 and 17 who were initially seen in the ED or mental health program in a hospital and had been identified as experiencing suicidal ideation or behavior or non-suicidal self-injurious behavior. The treatment, Resourceful Adolescent Parent Program (RAP-P), is part of a larger program that includes treatment components for the adolescent as well as his or her school. This study examined the impact of the parent program for 24 adolescents treated with RAP-P compared with 24 adolescents who were treated with usual care. The RAP-P program consisted of usual care for the adolescent plus a psychoeducational program for parents, followed by one to three family sessions. The data suggested a strong effect for the RAP-P program for decreasing scores on the Adolescent Suicide Questionnaire (ASQ; Pearce & Martin, 1994), and a mediation analysis suggested that the reduction in suicidal ideation was a function of change in family functioning as measured by the Family Assessment Device (FAD; Epstein, 1983).

The family approach to treating adolescents with suicidal ideation and behavior demonstrates great promise for families with parents willing to engage in treatment. Psychoeducation and effective family functioning appear to be important components for preventing suicide attempts and reducing suicidal ideation.

Critique

Results reported to date suggest the effectiveness of CBT and DBT interventions in improving social functioning and reducing suicidal ideation among suicidal adolescents, particularly those with mild to moderate depression and those with borderline features. In some cases, however, the outcomes of experimental treatments have not been substantially better than those obtained by comparison or standard care treatments. Treatments focusing specifically on suicidal behavior, its precipitants, and strategies for managing suicidal crises seem to fare the best. In addition, when families are available and willing to participate, family treatments have demonstrated efficacy in reducing suicidal ideation and behavior. However, many studies found that most parents are not willing or available to participate in treatment. Long-term effects of psychotherapy interventions on suicidal behavior, particularly suicide, have not yet been reported. Given that maladaptive cognitions and behaviors have likely developed over a long period of time, it is not clear that short-term psychotherapies will ultimately be found to be effective in reducing suicidal behavior.

PROGRAMS FOR COLLEGE STUDENTS

As was noted in a previous chapter, there has been marked reluctance among college and university officials to specifically identify suicidal students or offer treatment services that specifically address this problem. One university-based treatment program has been based on the assumption that students who engage in suicidal threats or behavior will not voluntarily submit to a clinical assessment, and thus that such assessment must be mandated as a condition of the student's continued enrollment at the university.

In the fall of 1984 the University of Illinois instituted a program designed to reduce the rate of suicide among its students. The program has a policy that requires any student who threatens or attempts suicide to attend four sessions of professional assessment—specifically, identified students are required to attend four weekly sessions at the University Counseling Center, during which the student receives a comprehensive clinical assessment and referral for additional treatment if needed (Joffe, 2003). Students who persist in suicidal behavior and refuse to accept counseling can be obliged to withdraw from the college.

Figures for the suicide rates for the 8 years before the project was instituted (1975–1983) were compared with the suicide rates for the 21 years from 1984 to 2004 (Joffe, 2008). The rate dropped 45% during the project period, from 6.9 per 100,000 students to 3.78 per 100,000. That rate is only half what it is at other Big Ten schools. Despite over two thousand reported incidents during this period (96 per year), only one student who participated in the Illinois program was forced to withdraw. Students who resist coming for the four sessions, however, are told that remaining at the university requires that they do so. Almost 10% of the students known to have threatened or attempted suicide withdrew voluntarily. Others have withdrawn for a variety of reasons, often in response to pressure from parents to do so. Few students who withdraw return to the college.

The data on college student suicides are limited at Illinois and all colleges by the lack of knowledge of students who committed suicide off campus. Students who die by suicide at home or elsewhere during the 4 years after the time they entered college are essentially dropouts and would need to be counted to be able accurately to determine the suicide rate. The Illinois program attempted to track these students with no success, although a few were reported by parents. This limitation of college student figures confirmed an earlier study of suicide rates at the same colleges (Silverman, Meyer, Sloane, et al., 1997). Nevertheless, this program seems ahead of other university programs in its methodology and its ability to provide evidence that it has an impact in preventing suicidal behavior.

Although the utilization figures are an achievement, the program is not in a position to tell us how effective the treatment is that students are receiving after their referral. The drop in suicide rates is even more impressive, However, almost 10% of students known to have threatened or attempted suicide withdrew voluntarily because they did not want to participate in the program or because they did not want to wait until they were asked to leave. Their leaving makes it difficult to evaluate the significance of the suicide figures.

More colleges in the country are developing mental health services for students. Many, however, lack the financial resources or are unwilling to spend them on mental health. The problem is aggravated by the numbers of students now seeking those services. The programs discussed have the resources and are able to evaluate utilization of their services, but neither one is in a position to tell us how effective the treatment is that students are receiving after their referral. In addition, when failure to report suicidal behavior is punishable, it may encourage reporting by some and the opposite behavior by others. Anonymous surveys of students would be needed to ascertain that information.

PHARMACOLOGICAL TREATMENTS FOR SUICIDAL YOUTH

The neurobiological underpinnings of suicidal behavior are the subject of considerable research, and new information has broadened our understanding of this complex area. Researchers have identified serotonergic dysfunction, noradrenergic dysfunction, dopaminergic dysfunction, and hypothalamic–pituitary–adrenal axis hyperactivity as the key neurobiological correlates of suicidality (Mann, 2003; Nemeroff, Compton, Berger, et al., 2001).

The most extensively replicated studies have focused on the role of serotonergic dysfunction. Studies have reported that depressed patients who have made suicide attempts have lower levels of 5-hydroxyindoleacetic acid (5-HIAA) in the brain stem and in cerebrospinal fluid compared to depressed non-attempters (Åsberg, Lil Traskman, & Thoren, 1976; Nordstrom & Åsberg, 1992). Decreased CSF 5-HIAA is hypothesized to be a marker of the impulsive, aggressive, and violent nature of suicide and appears to correlate with a high degree of suicidal planning and a high level of lethality of suicide attempts (Stanley, Molcho, & Stanley, 2000). Central nervous system serotonergic dysfunction has also been associated with suicidal behavior. For patients with unipolar depression, selective serotonin reuptake inhibitors (SSRIs) are considered superior to other antidepressants for treating both suicidal behavior and suicidal ideation (Oquendo, Malone, & Mann, 1997).

Although no large randomized controlled trials of SSRIs have included outcomes related to suicide due to the past exclusion of suicidal patients from most pharmaceutical-sponsored trials, there is considerable evidence pointing to the positive effects of such medications on the central nervous system serotonergic dysfunction noted above to be associated with suicidality in adults (Oquendo, Malone, & Mann, 1997).

Subsequently, several European studies reported inverse correlations between use of SSRIs and suicide deaths, suggesting their potential significance for reducing suicide risk in adults (Barbui, Campomori, D'Avanzo, et al., 1999; Carlsten, Waern, Ekedahl, & Ranstam, 2001; Gunnel, Middleton, Whitley, et al., 2003; Isacsson, 2000). Although large randomized controlled trials need to be conducted in order to determine causative linkages, SSRIs appear to be a potent means of treating suicidality. SSRIs have been reported to have less inherent toxicity than the previously widely used tricyclic antidepressants and are thus less likely to be related to death from overdoses. Although side effects such as gastrointestinal upset, insomnia, and sexual dysfunction are fairly common, most SSRIs appear to be well tolerated.

Program Examples

There was accumulating evidence for the effectiveness of fluoxetine, the one SSRI approved by the U.S. Food and Drug Administration in the treatment of young people who are suicidal. An analysis by Olfson, Shaffer, Marcus, and Greenberg (2003) reported an inverse relationship between regional change in the use of antidepressants among youth ages 10 to 19 and suicide mortality. The relationship was found to be significant specifically among male youth ages 15 to 19 and in geographic regions with lower family median incomes. Although this study does not establish that the use of antidepressants is causally linked to decreases in suicide deaths, other studies provide more direct evidence of their effectiveness. An intervention by Cornelius et al. used fluoxetine (Prozac) to treat adolescents with comorbid major depression and an alcohol use disorder, including some who demonstrated suicidal ideation at baseline (Cornelius, Bukstein, Birmaheret, et al., 2001). The intervention was based on findings that reducing depression and problem drinking in adults resulted in a reduction of suicidal behavior (Dinh-Zarr, Diguiseppi, Heitman, & Roberts, 1999). Cornelius et al. also found fluoxetine to be effective in treating suicidal adults with an alcohol use disorder. Such treatment improved, but did not completely eliminate, both depressive symptoms (including suicidal ideations) and level of drinking (Cornelius, Salhoum, Lynch, et al., 2001). In their studies involving youth, all patients receiving fluoxetine improved with respect to depressive symptoms, and over half improved in symptoms of alcohol dependence. Among participants with suicidal ideation at baseline, ideation decreased and these decreases remained 1 year after treatment (Cornelius, 2003). Cornelius reported no serious adverse effects of fluoxetine among youth.

A definitive study supported by the National Institute of Mental Health known as the Treatment of Adolescents with Depression Study (TADS) has provided the strongest evidence of the effectiveness of fluoxetine in treating adolescent depression and suicidality. This study randomly assigned 439 youths ages 12 to 17 diagnosed with moderate to severe depression to one of four treatment conditions for a period of 36 weeks: fluoxetine therapy alone, cognitive-behavioral therapy (CBT) alone, fluoxetine and CBT, and a placebo drug treatment. Based on the results obtained during the first 12 weeks of the study, the highest rate of clinical improvement (71%) was found among those receiving the combination treatment, followed by 61% in those who received fluoxetine alone, 43% in those who received CBT alone, and 35% in those who received the placebo drug treatment (March, Silva, Petrycki, et al., 2004). The most seriously suicidal adolescents were excluded from the TADS sample, and thus only 29% of participants reported having clinically significant suicidal ideation at baseline. This percentage decreased to 10% by week 12. Although no suicides occurred during the trial, the risk of a suicide attempt among study participants during the first weeks on fluoxetine was reported to be twice that for participants not receiving the medication. The study investigators concluded, however, that the benefits of the medication far outweighed any associated risk.

Although fluoxetine is the only antidepressant medication approved by the FDA as effective for the treatment of major depression in children and adolescents, it did not forbid the use of other SSRIs such as sertraline and citalopram. Both have been shown to be effective in the treatment of depression (Papanikolau, Richardson, Pehlivanidis, et al., 2006; Pösel & Hauzinger, 2006; Wagner, 2005) and are used by clinicians ("off-label") where fluoxetine has been ineffective (Taurines, Gerlach, Warnke, et al., 2011).

For depressed adolescents who do not respond to an SSRI, drugs that are noradrenergic as well as serotonergic receptor inhibitors have been found to be effective. These medications reduce anxiety as well as depression; a combination of both symptoms increases the risk of suicide. Venlafaxine (Effexor), which affects both receptors, was the first such drug and is independently approved for the treatment of anxiety disorders (Bailly, 2008; Courtney, 2004; Emslie, Waslick, Weller, et al., 2007; Mandoki, Tapia, Tapia, et al., 1997).

A controlled study of augmentation treatments for treatment-resistant depression enrolled patients who met the DSM-IV criteria for major depression but were not psychotic. Atypical (second-generation) antipsychotics, such as risperidone, olanzapine, and quetiapine, which add the stimulant effects of dopamine to the brain, were shown to cause rapid improvement in the mood of patients with treatment-resistant depression, reflected in dramatic drops in their Hamilton Depression Scale scores (Ostroff & Nelson, 1999). Studies of the effectiveness of atypical antipsychotics in adolescents with treatment-resistant depression have been limited in terms of the number of cases seen because of the danger of side effects, mainly weight gain and drowsiness. In adolescents, these medication are used only when SSRIs have not helped.

A small open-label study of 10 adolescents with treatment-resistant depression treated with adjunctive use of quetiapine showed a significant improvement in mood; three who had engaged in cutting had relief from that symptom. Drowsiness was seen in 40% but usually resolved in the first few weeks of treatment. Eighty percent of patients had insignificant weight gains, but in two of the patients weight gain was significant (Pathak, Johns, & Kowatch, 2005).

Long-term treatment with clozapine, another atypical antipsychotic, has been shown to reduce symptoms among treatment-resistant adolescents with schizophrenia. Its side effects—neutropenia, akathisia, and weight gain—make it a useful line of defense, but only after other atypical antipsychotics have been tried (Gogtay & Rapoport, 2008; Sporn, Vermani, Greenstein, et al., 2007).

Suicidality is decreased among mood-disordered adult patients receiving long-term lithium treatment (Sharma, 2003; Tondo, Jamison, & Baldessarini, 1997). Lithium has been effective in treating severe and persistent aggression among children and adolescents (Malone, Delaney, Luebbert, et al., 2000). Although it is being used to augment SSRIs in treatment-resistant depression, there is no evidence that by itself or in combination it reduces suicidal behavior in adolescents.

Since 2003, concerns have been raised about the safety of the use of SSRIs by children and adolescents, based initially on unpublished data from drug company studies linking use of SSRIs by children and adolescents to suicidal ideation and self-harm behaviors. In late 2003, these reports led the British drug regulatory agency to recommend against the use of all SSRIs except fluoxetine in treating depression among youth under age 18 (Goode, 2003). In 2004, the FDA undertook a review of 23 clinical trials involving the use of nine different antidepressant medications by children and adolescents. There were no completed suicides among the 2,200 children treated with SSRIs. The results of this analysis, however, found that the medications increased the risk of suicidal thinking and behavior (suicidality) in children and adolescents with major depressive disorder or other psychiatric disorders (Hammand, 2004). Specifically, 4% of all youth taking medication reported an "adverse event" (i.e., thoughts of suicide and/or potentially dangerous behavior) compared to 2% of those taking a placebo drug.

On October 15, 2004, the FDA directed pharmaceutical companies to label all antidepressant medications distributed in the United States with a "black box" warning of the danger to young people who are prescribed these medications. The warning states that the increased risk of suicidal thinking and/or behavior occurs in a small proportion of youth and is most likely to occur during the early phases of treatment. In 2007, further review led the FDA to recommend that the warning be extended to include young adults up to age 25. Although the FDA did not prohibit the use of antidepressants by children and adolescents, it called upon physicians and parents to closely monitor youth who are taking the medications for a worsening in symptoms of depression or unusual changes in behavior.

On February 1, 2005, the American Psychiatric Association (APA) and the American Academy of Child and Adolescent Psychiatry (AACAP) released detailed fact sheets for physicians and parents on the use of medications in treating childhood and adolescent depression. The fact sheets were jointly developed by the two organizations and endorsed by more than a dozen leading medical, mental health, and advocacy organizations because of their concern that the FDA black-box warning could have the unintended effect of limiting necessary, appropriate, and effective treatment of depression and other psychiatric disorders in youth. The APA/AACAP statement was particularly critical of the FDA's measurement of suicidality following antidepressant use among young people, which essentially used thoughts of suicide or potentially dangerous behaviors that had been spontaneously shared by the young participants and subsequently recorded in the researchers' "adverse events reports." Although the FDA analysis showed more such spontaneous reports among those taking an antidepressant medication as compared to placebo (4% vs. 2%), this finding was not supported by data from 17 of the 23 studies examined that had systematically asked all participants about their suicidal thoughts and behaviors, using standardized forms and not clinicians' reports. The FDA's analysis of these data concluded that medication neither increased suicidality that had been present before the treatment, nor induced new suicidality in those who were not thinking about suicide at the start of the study. All studies collecting such data reported a reduction in suicidality over the course of treatment. The APA/AACAP statement noted that while the FDA reported both sets of findings, it did not comment on the contradiction between them. The statement further questioned the reliability of the 2% and 4% spontaneous report rates, noting findings from numerous community samples that as many as half of adolescents with major depression were thinking of suicide at the time of diagnosis and 16% to 35% had reported making a suicide attempt. The statement included suggestions for physicians and parents in monitoring youth receiving antidepressant medication and called for the development of a readily accessible registry of clinical trials that could aid in resolving the controversy and conflicting information surrounding the prescribing of antidepressants to children and adolescents.

A comprehensive review of pediatric trials conducted between 1998 and 2006, partly funded by National Institute for Mental Health (NIMH), concluded that the benefits of antidepressant medications likely outweigh their risks to children and adolescents with major depression and anxiety disorders (Bridge, Iyengar, & Salary, 2007). In a meta-analysis published in 2012 (Gibbons, Brown, Hur, et al., 2012), investigators obtained complete longitudinal data for randomized controlled trials conducted by Eli Lilly on their treatment of depressed adolescents with fluoxetine. The patient-level data allowed them to (1) estimate rates of change in suicidal thoughts and behavior during the course of treatment; (2) study the relationship between depression severity and suicidal thoughts and behavior; and (3) determine the extent to which changes in depressive symptoms mediate the relationship between antidepressant treatment and suicidal thoughts and behavior. These analyses substantially expand the original analyses conducted by the FDA in youth by including the complete longitudinal record of each patient, which was not previously reported by the FDA. An unanswered question noted by the investigators was the absence of any statistically significant effect of fluoxetine on the suicide risk of young people despite a large overall reduction in their depressive symptoms. They point out that we do not know why some youths whose depressive symptoms are reduced continue to have suicidal ideation and behavior. Perhaps other psychological factors play a more important role in suicidal behavior and ideation, such as aggressive, impulsive traits in youths (Brent, Oquendo, Birmaher, at al., 2002). Thus, even if antidepressants reduce depressive symptoms overall in youths, it is possible that a subset may retain some level of risk for suicidal ideation or attempt. The overall rate, however, was not significantly greater than that found for youths randomized to placebo. They found no evidence that fluoxetine increased the risk of suicidal thoughts or behavior.

In a comprehensive release of information to parents and caregivers, available online, NIMH supported and referred parents to the 2007 review by Bridges et al. indicating that the benefits of SSRIs outweighed the risks to children and adolescents with major depression and anxiety disorders. That controversy is essentially resolved, at least among mental health professionals.

Until recently, seriously suicidal adolescents (and adults) were excluded from randomized controlled trials conducted by all pharmaceutical companies. In 2010 the FDA mandated that pharmaceutical companies include suicidal patients in all drug trials with depressed patients, a widely welcomed decision that should stimulate needed additional pharmacological research. Many of the medications that are useful in reducing adult suicidal behavior, and have proven successful in treating depression in adolescents, need to be tested for their effect on adolescent suicidal behavior. The avoidance of adolescents at serious risk for suicide has been true of clinical research in medical centers as well. A recent suicide attempt has often been the basis for exclusion from a treatment research project.

Two multisite projects have addressed this problem. The Treatment of Adolescent Suicide Attempters (TASA) study was designed to examine the course of depression during the treatment of adolescents who had made a suicide attempt in the past 90 days (Brent, Greenhill, Compton, et al., 2009; Vitiello, Brent, Greenhill, et al., 2009). At five academic sites, these adolescents entered a 6-month program of treatment with antidepressant medication; a modified CBT focused on suicide prevention; or a combination of both. Treatment assignment was either random or chosen by the study participants. Most patients chose their treatment assignment and, overall, three quarters received the combined treatment.

Among these adolescent attempters, the factors that predicted another suicide attempt or acute suicide ideation requiring emergency referral were higher self-rated depression, suicidal ideation, family income, greater number of previous suicide attempts, lower maximum lethality of previous attempt, history of sexual abuse, and lower family cohesion.

Vitiello et al. reported that, with combined medication and CBT, which was chosen by the majority of patients, rates of improvement and remission of depression were comparable to those in non-suicidal depressed adolescents. Brent et al. reported that allocation to CBT, medication, or the combination lowered the 6-month risks for suicidal events and reattempts. These promising results need to be interpreted in light of the fact that the TASA trial was largely nonrandomized and uncontrolled; that patients with substance abuse (common among suicide attempters) were excluded; that the dropout rate—albeit in the range of other treatment studies and hardly surprising with this adolescent sample—was not small (31%); and that approximately 20% of the subjects displayed suicidal behavior during treatment (Walter, 2009).

The Treatment of SSRI-Resistant Depression in Adolescents study (TORDIA) was designed to inform clinicians as to the best next step in treatment after a depressed adolescent has not responded to an adequate trial with an SSRI. In this six-site study, conducted from 2000 to 2006, 334 treatment-resistant adolescents with major depressive disorder were randomized to one of the four treatment strategies: (a) switch to another SSRI; (b) switch to venlafaxine; (c) switch to another SSRI and CBT; or (d) switch to venlafaxine and add CBT (Emslie et al., 2010). Poorer response across treatments was predicted by greater severity of self-rated depression, hopelessness, suicidal ideation, a history of non-suicidal self-injury, and family conflict. CBT continued to be associated with an increased likelihood of a response, even after controlling for the most salient adverse predictors of response. SSRIs were superior to venlafaxine in those participants with higher self-reported depression. The combination of CBT and medication was superior to medication alone for those with multiple comorbidities, particularly anxiety or attention-deficit/hyperactivity disorder. Participants with a history of substance abuse showed a lower response rate to combination treatment than to medication monotherapy. Those who received pharmacological treatment for sleep difficulties showed a poorer response rate than those who did not receive medication for sleep. Participants whose self-reported drug and alcohol use was high at baseline and remained so, or whose substance use accelerated during the trial, showed a poorer response rate compared to those whose drug and alcohol use either remained or became low.

The TORDIA study found no difference in the rate of suicidal events among treatments, perhaps because the proportion of seriously suicidal participants was much higher than in most studies. Surprisingly, TORDIA found a lower rate of non-suicidal self-harm in the medication-only group. Given that the medication time to a suicidal event in TORDIA was 3 weeks, it is unlikely that CBT as currently delivered could effectively protect against these early events. The TORDIA study demonstrated that highly suicidal individuals can be included and managed in the context of clinical trials. The authors stress the importance of studying high-risk populations if we are going to improve the treatment of these suicidal adolescents.

Critique

In the TASA study, the rates of improvement and remission seen in adolescent suicide attempters treated with CBT, medication, or a combination of both are encouraging. That the study was not randomized or controlled should stimulate efforts to build on it.

The TORDIA study provided guidelines for therapists in choosing options available for treatment-resistant depression in adolescents depending on their symptoms. Still, matching patients to appropriate treatments remains largely a matter of guesswork. The fact that seriously suicidal adolescents could be included in the trials without a problem will encourage further research. The medication options were limited to SSRIs and the noradrenergic receptor inhibitor venlafaxine. There is a need for randomized controlled testing of the atypical antipsychotics that have shown effectiveness in treatment studies of adolescents whose depression is resistant to SSRIs.

Research Agenda for Youth Suicide Prevention

Ann P. Haas
Herbert Hendin
Jill Harkavy-Friedman
Maggie Mortali

25

chapter

WHAT WE KNOW

Youth Suicide

- Between 1955 and 1980, the suicide rate among young people in the United States roughly tripled from about 4 suicides per 100,000 population ages 15 to 24 to over 12 suicides per 100,000. Most of this was due to a startling increase in the suicide rate among young males. Through the 1980s and early 1990s, the youth suicide rate increased much more slowly, reaching a peak rate of over 13 per 100,000 in 1994, and then generally declined to a low of 9.6 in 2003. Since 2004, the youth suicide rate has again been trending upward, rising to 12.3 in 2015, the last year for which national data are available. In 2015, the suicide rate among youth approximated what it was in 1980.
- In 2015, almost 5,500 young people ages 15 to 24 died by suicide.
- Suicide is the currently the third leading cause of death among youth ages 15 to 24.
- Among young people ages 15 to 24, the suicide rate for males is almost four times the rate for females. In recent years, the gender difference in suicide rates has been generally decreasing.
- Youth suicide rates vary widely among different racial and ethnic groups. In 2015, the highest rate was among American Indian and Alaskan Native youth (21 per 100,000), followed by white youth (13 per 100,000), Asian American/Pacific Islander youth (10 per 100,000), and black youth (8 per 100,000). With the exception of Hispanics, youth in all racial and ethnic groups have recently experienced rising suicide rates.
- Like gender differences, racial-ethnic differences have been decreasing somewhat in recent years.
- Although college enrollment is not systematically identified postmortem, studies point to a significantly lower suicide rate in college students compared to youth of the same ages who are not in school.
- In 2015 school-based surveys, 9% of American high school students reported making a suicide attempt within the previous 12 months, with female students more likely than males to report an attempt. Eighteen percent of high school students reported having seriously considered suicide during the previous 12 months.
- Although mortality statistics do not identify sexual orientation or gender identity, studies consistently point to elevated rates of reported suicide attempts among sexual and gender minority (SGM) youth relative to the general youth population. Specific stressors related to SGM status, including rejection, discrimination, and victimization, appear to contribute to higher rates of mental health problems, suicidal ideation, and suicide attempts in SGM youth.
- Among youth (and adults), a prior suicide attempt significantly increases the risk of subsequent attempts and suicide death.
- A large majority of youth (70%–90%) who die by suicide had at least one psychiatric illness at the time of death. The most common diagnoses among youth are depression, substance abuse, and conduct disorders.
- Other factors associated with youth suicide include physical abuse, sexual abuse, serious conflict with parents, interpersonal loss, not being in school or not working, exposure to the juvenile justice system, knowing someone who has attempted suicide or died by suicide, and access to firearms.
- Suicide and suicide attempts are increased in families in which a parent has died by suicide or attempted suicide.
- Factors that appear to protect against suicidal behavior in youth include family connectedness and support, school connectedness, school safety, reduced access to lethal means, and social-behavioral

skills. Among SGM youth, acceptance by family and peers appears to protect against suicidal ideation and behavior.

Youth Suicide Prevention Programs

- Programs that screen high school and college students to identify those at risk for suicide and refer them for treatment can identify some high-risk individuals who were not previously recognized or treated.
- Programs that train teachers and school personnel, counselors, and community gatekeepers about suicide intervention can increase knowledge about suicide and suicide prevention, increase self-confidence and willingness to intervene, and increase referrals to treatment.
- Under adequate conditions of implementation, programs that educate students about suicide can increase students' knowledge of mental health conditions and suicide, encourage more adaptive attitudes about these problems, encourage help-seeking behaviors, and increase referrals of at-risk students to treatment.
- Skills training programs that enhance problem-solving, coping, and cognitive skills, which have been found to be impaired in suicidal youth, may reduce suicide risk factors associated with depression, hopelessness, and substance abuse among at-risk individuals.
- Comprehensive programs that aim to create a supportive school environment by fostering a climate of open communication can serve as a protective factor against suicide risk and increase help-seeking among at-risk students.

Treating Suicidal Ideation and Behavior and Underlying Disorders in Youth

- Under adequate conditions of implementation, intensive school-based programs focusing on improving problem solving and social behavior can reduce rates of depression, suicidal ideation, and suicide attempts in students at risk of dropping out of school.
- Programs that engage young suicide attempters and their families while they are in the emergency department can increase adherence to outpatient treatment and decrease immediate and subsequent hospital admissions.
- Psychotherapies that include a focus on managing suicidal ideation can improve social functioning and reduce suicidal ideation and self-harm behaviors among suicidal youth. When families are available and willing to participate in treatment, family therapy that includes a focus on understanding and managing the adolescent's suicidal behavior has demonstrated effectiveness for reducing suicidal ideation and behavior.
- Cognitive-behavioral therapy (CBT), Dialectical Behavioral Therapy (DBT), and Interpersonal Therapy (IPT) have demonstrated the ability to relieve depression and improve social functioning in adolescents. CBT and DBT have shown some success, at least in the short term, in reducing suicidal ideation and behaviors in suicidal youth.
- There is evidence that treatment with fluoxetine (Prozac) can reduce depression, alcohol dependence, and suicidal ideation in youth.
- Combination treatment involving fluoxetine and psychotherapy appears to result in the most positive outcomes for depressed, suicidal youth.
- There is some evidence that posthospitalization programs for suicidal youth can reduce subsequent suicidal ideation and mood impairment among female participants.

WHAT WE DON'T KNOW

Despite considerable research and program development focusing on youth suicide, there is much we do not yet know about the factors that cause or significantly influence suicidal behavior among youth, and how this behavior can be prevented or treated. Listed below are the key knowledge needs our review has identified, which constitute a future research agenda for youth suicide.

Youth Suicide

- Although psychopathology has been well documented to be the most potent factor underlying suicide among all age groups, relatively little is known about the specific clinical pathways to youth suicide. In particular, more needs to be known about the contribution of bipolar disorder, panic attacks, and posttraumatic stress disorder to suicide deaths among youth. The impact of demographics, including race, ethnicity, sexual orientation, and gender identity, on diagnostic profiles and clinical pathways to suicide likewise needs greater scrutiny. Longitudinal studies of young people with suicidal ideation and behavior are especially needed. In addition, because most people with psychopathology do not engage in suicidal behavior, and suicidal behavior crosses many different psychopathologies, more research is needed on the interactions among specific forms of psychopathology, suicide risk factors other than mental disorders, and factors that protect against suicide.
- Much more needs to be known about the role of neurobiological abnormalities that contribute to youth suicidal behavior, especially the role of genetic processes such as gene expression. Family studies of adults and adolescents who have attempted suicide or died by suicide can provide important information about the interaction between genes and the environment, and it is essential that youth be included in such research.
- The extent to which parental/familial psychopathology influences suicide ideation, attempts, and completions among youth, over and above genetic influences, needs to be examined. Specifically, what is the effect of exposure to parental suicide attempts and completion on the suicide risk among youth? Does childhood physical and sexual abuse confer suicide risk independent of other effects of family psychopathology?
- Because sexual orientation and gender identity are not systematically identified at the time of death, mortality rates cannot be determined for SGM people. Psychological autopsy studies have produced equivocal conclusions about whether SGM youth make up a higher percentage of youth suicides than their prevalence in the population. Although recent analyses of psychological autopsy findings suggest a higher rate of completed suicide in SGM youth, these studies are not an adequate substitute for systematic, routine identification of sexual orientation and gender identity in suicide decedents.
- Although suicide clusters have been identified among youth, the characteristics of those most vulnerable to "contagion" and the mechanisms through which contagion occurs have not been precisely identified.
- More needs to be understood about the role of personal and social skills in protecting youth from suicidal behavior. Do strong problem-solving skills, decision-making abilities, and support from family and schools actually protect young people from developing suicidal impulses, or is the absence of such skills a manifestation of psychopathology that is more directly related to suicidal thoughts or behavior? What is the role of culture, identity, and religious beliefs in reducing suicide risk?
- Both theoretically and in practical programmatic terms, it is essential to have better understanding of which combinations of risk and protective factors have the greatest predictive value for youth suicide. Current research points to the identification and treatment of psychopathology among adolescents as a priority suicide prevention strategy, but better understanding is needed of the

wide range of interpersonal, cultural, and environmental factors that may exacerbate or mitigate the impact of psychopathology among particular groups of high-risk youth. In addition, some treatments have been found to reduce suicidal ideation and behavior without significantly affecting psychopathology. Research to date has focused almost exclusively on looking at relationships between single risk or protective factors and adolescent suicidal behavior. Comprehensive analyses that simultaneously consider a number of individual variables are essential.
- Greater understanding of the suicidal state, including onset, cognitions, access to self-care, and protective factors, is needed to assist youth in managing a suicide crisis.

Youth Suicide Prevention Programs

- Most suicide education programs have not identified the active ingredients responsible for the outcomes they produce.
- Most suicide education programs target outcomes whose relationship to youth suicide has not been precisely identified. Many, for example, have reported increased knowledge of mental health conditions and suicide among students, although the impact of this outcome on suicidal behavior is not known. Greater attention needs to be given to identifying long-term behavioral outcomes among students who have received such education, particularly those with particular risk factors.
- Although increasing the number of referrals to treatment is a key goal of screening programs, there is no clear evidence of a direct linkage between increased referrals and decreased suicidal behavior among youth.
- Screening programs have generally not identified effective mechanisms for encouraging larger numbers of youth identified as being at risk for suicide to enter treatment.
- Few data are currently available about the cost-effectiveness of school-based screening programs.
- Although popular in recent years, the effects of postvention programs, both positive and adverse, on youth exposed to a suicide death have not been clearly documented.
- Despite limited evidence that educational programs directed to parents, particularly fathers, can decrease youth access to firearms, the impact of means restriction programs on decreasing suicide attempts and suicide deaths among youth has not been documented.

Treatment of Suicidality and Underlying Disorders Among Youth

- The active ingredients of comprehensive high school–based programs for treating at-risk students, including those who are depressed and suicidal, have not been clearly identified.
- It has not been demonstrated that students at risk of dropping out of school are representative of suicidal youth generally, and therefore that programs that address this population have wide applicability.
- The replication of such programs, which require considerable personnel and financial resources, has not been established.
- The impact of emergency department programs for young suicide attempters and their families on decreasing suicide deaths has not been established.
- Although studies have demonstrated the success of behavioral and educational treatments in improving the social skills and reducing the aggressive behavior of autistic children and adolescents, their effect on reducing suicidal behavior has not yet been determined.
- Assessment of suicide risk in emergency departments is still challenging, and although new screening approaches are currently being tested, the best method for implementing risk assessment has yet to be determined.

- Engagement in treatment in the emergency department can facilitate treatment and reduce suicidal ideation and behavior in the short term, yet the impact on engagement and effectiveness in longer-term treatment is unclear.
- Although some promising outcomes have been reported, long-term effects of psychotherapy with suicidal youth are not yet known.
- Although fluoxetine (Prozac) and other selective serotonin reuptake inhibitors (SSRIs) have been shown to reduce depression, alcohol dependence, and suicidal ideation in youth, the long-term effects of these drugs on adolescents are not known.
- Much more needs to be known about the combinations of psychotherapeutic and pharmacological treatment that produce the most positive short- and long-term outcomes for depressed, suicidal youth.
- Long-term effects of posthospitalization programs for suicidal youth have not been documented.

METHODOLOGICAL CHALLENGES

Our review has made clear the extent to which scientific evaluation of youth suicide prevention programs has lagged far behind their development and implementation. As a result, efforts may show promise, but very few have been shown with reasonable certainty to be effective in preventing suicidal ideation, suicide attempts, or suicide deaths among youth.

Prospective randomized controlled trials (RCTs) are needed to determine the effectiveness, safety, and active ingredients of universal and targeted suicide prevention programs, including school-based education, screening, and skills development programs, and school and community interventions for at-risk populations, including limiting access to lethal means such as firearms and implementing gatekeeper training programs.

Some suicide prevention programs, in particular universal education programs, have targeted outcome variables whose relationship to youth suicide has not been precisely identified. Clearer hypotheses about variables believed to contribute to suicidal behavior need to be formulated, justified, and addressed in the prevention strategy. Following the intervention, changes in the variable must be specifically measured to determine if in fact it functions as a mediator of suicide-related outcomes. Without such a procedure, findings from many studies are difficult to integrate, leaving the field with an absence of information as to what actually worked, and what directions and models are worthy of further investigation.

Since universal and selective suicide prevention programs focus heavily on encouraging help seeking and on identifying vulnerable youth and referring them to treatment, their impact on reducing youth suicide depends ultimately on the effectiveness of the treatments that are available to such young people. Thus, the single highest priority must be given to determining the relative efficacy and effectiveness of all currently employed treatments and indicated interventions for suicidal youth.

Sampling Strategies

Relatively few suicide prevention programs have systematically studied adequate numbers of representative at-risk youth to allow meaningful conclusions to be reached about program effectiveness, and only rarely have appropriate comparison groups been simultaneously studied. Further, most outcome studies have had access to program participants for a short period of time, which precludes identification of any long-term effects of the program, including adverse effects.

Evaluation

In regard to school-based programs in particular, effective evaluation requires follow-up of students who have participated in curricular or screening activities in order to determine long-term outcomes. To date, sufficient resources for such research programs have not been available. Further, evaluations of youth suicide prevention programs have been largely internal, and objective third-party evaluation of outcomes remains rare. Few youth suicide prevention programs have had the necessary personnel or financial resources to conduct independent program evaluations. If the field is to move forward, however, mechanisms need to be established that mandate and support comprehensive, well-designed outcome studies as a regular part of prevention programming.

Treatment Research

As has been noted, RCTs of treatments used for suicidal youth are seriously lacking, and there are improvements in the approach to suicide prevention that have yet to be systematically tested. Comparative RCTs of clinical treatment are clearly needed to determine the impact of brief interventions with young suicide attempters presenting to emergency departments, psychotherapeutic strategies for suicidal youth, pharmacological treatments for young suicide ideators and attempters, as well as hospitalization, partial hospitalization, and posthospitalization support programs for youth. Psychotherapies that have been found to be effective for suicidal youth have many components, and further study is needed to determine which components are the essential ingredients for effective treatment. Also, while most treatment studies have focused on a particular therapy such as CBT, DBT, or IPT, clinicians who treat suicidal adolescents or adults frequently use aspects of each of these therapies, in addition to psychodynamic techniques and medication when indicated. Although many clinicians believe an "integrative approach" is the best treatment strategy, to date its effectiveness in reducing suicidal ideation and behavior has not been definitively demonstrated, at least in part because of the challenges of clearly specifying and measuring the components of therapies that combine multiple techniques. As part of future research efforts, an integrative treatment for suicidally depressed adolescents should be developed, implemented, and tested for effectiveness, using a treatment like CBT as a control.

In addition to the general evaluation concerns noted above, treatment trials involving high-risk youth need to be especially attentive to building in appropriate safeguards. Although control or comparison groups are essential, the inclusion of such groups necessitates ethical consideration of appropriate "control" treatments. Few studies involving treatments for suicidality among youth have adequately defined or measured the therapeutic effects of treatment as usual.

Many treatment trials involving adolescents deemed to be at risk for suicide eliminate those who have recently made a suicide attempt. Although recent attempters are at increased risk for suicide, they can and need to be included unless they are actively suicidal. Further, youth who engage in suicidal behavior vary considerably with respect to specific forms of psychopathology, substance abuse, and other psychosocial problems, and treatment trials must address this variability (Hawton & Sinclair, 2003). Particular protections must be developed to allow inclusion in such trials of suicidal youth with serious alcohol and drug problems, which confer considerable risk for subsequent attempts and suicide death. Adverse effects of treatment, including medications, also need to be more closely evaluated.

A major problem for suicide research in general, and for research with adolescents in particular, is keeping patients at serious risk for suicide involved in outpatient treatment, and hence in treatment evaluation studies. Innovative approaches need to be developed to engage and sustain troubled youth in treatment, in order both to prevent subsequent suicidal behavior and to allow short- and long-term treatment outcomes to be observed.

The ultimate criteria for effectiveness in suicide prevention remain reduction in suicide attempts and suicide deaths, events for which the population base rate is low. The primary limitation of virtually all studies of the effectiveness of treatments for suicidal patients has been their relatively small size and thus their limited power to detect significant differences between or among alternative strategies (Hawton & Sinclair, 2003). Enrolling adequate numbers of appropriate participants into treatment trials can best be achieved through a number of centrally coordinated treatment research centers that can pursue common studies of treatment effectiveness. The formation of such centers was a primary recommendation of a 2002 Institute of Medicine report on suicide (Goldsmith, Pellmar, Kleinman, & Bunney, 2002), but limited progress has been made toward this goal. The Internet has facilitated virtual collaborations for researchers, and more attention needs to be given to these and other strategies for securing a large enough patient population to reliably determine the impact of specific treatments on suicide-related outcomes, specifically suicidal ideation and behavior.

CONCLUSION

Much has been learned about why suicide occurs in young people and how it can be prevented, but more needs to be done. Based on our review, we offer the following summary conclusions to guide future research and prevention efforts:

1. Suicidal ideation, suicide attempts, and completed suicide are distinct behaviors, and findings about one behavior do not necessarily explicate the others. Thinking about suicide and attempting suicide are indicators of distress and/or limited personal resources, but only infrequently are they markers for completed suicide. Even with recent increases, death by suicide in youth is rare. While relying on expanding understanding of ideation and attempts, research must also seek to learn more about young people who have died by suicide.
2. Suicide is a complex phenomenon with multiple biological, psychological, social, and environmental contributors. How these converge to produce a state of suicide crisis is not well understood. Greater focus on understanding how the suicidal state develops and resolves in youth is critical.
3. To be effective, suicide prevention will need to occur simultaneously on both the individual and community levels, with continued attention to developing, implementing, and evaluating empirically based universal, targeted, and indicated interventions.
4. Limiting access to lethal means is an essential consideration in any effort to prevent suicide.
5. Longitudinal studies of large samples are needed to follow up suicidal and at-risk youth through their young adult, middle adult, and later life years. It is clear that risk factors experienced early in life, including psychopathology, can have long-term impact, and sustained attention to the problems evidenced by vulnerable youth population is needed across the lifespan.

Beyond Disorder

COMMISSION ON POSITIVE YOUTH DEVELOPMENT

Martin E. P. Seligman, *Commission Chair*

Second Edition

Margaret L. Kern

Nansook Park

Daniel Romer

First Edition

Marvin W. Berkowitz

Richard F. Catalano

William Damon

Jacquelynne S. Eccles

Jane E. Gillham

Kristin A. Moore

First Edition cont.

Heather Johnston Nicholson

Nansook Park

David L. Penn

Christopher Peterson

Margaret Shih

Tracy A. Steen

Robert J. Sternberg

Joseph P. Tierney

Roger P. Weissberg

Jonathan F. Zaff

part VII

The Positive Perspective on Youth Development

Margaret L. Kern
Nansook Park
Daniel Romer

chapter 26

OVERVIEW

The things that go right in our lives do predict future successes and the things that go wrong do not damn us forever.

—J. Kirk Felsman
and George E. Vaillant (1987)

How can we promote and sustain the mental health of children and adolescents? Earlier sections in this volume provide one answer to this question: treat and prevent psychological disorders such as anxiety, depression, suicide, substance abuse, eating disorders, and schizophrenia among youth. It is certainly important to prevent and treat these problems, but this alone is insufficient for fostering mental health. Imagine a society in which no young person meets the diagnostic criteria for mental illness. Treatments and prevention have been so pervasively and perfectly implemented that not a single youth reports any symptoms of disorder. This would eliminate considerable amounts of individual suffering and would provide substantial economic benefits. But *such a society is still not a psychological utopia*. There are huge differences between a teenager who is not depressed or anxious versus one who bounds out of bed in the morning with twinkling eyes, or between an adolescent who says no to drugs versus one who says yes to meaningful involvement in family, school, and community activities.

"Mental health" has long been approached from a deficit perspective (Huppert & So, 2013). Effective treatment strategies and risk-based prevention programs like those described earlier in this volume are among our most notable scientific achievements, but they represent only a part of the journey. These traditional approaches—all based on a disease model where well-being is defined only by the absence of distress and disorder—have been challenged. Calls have been made for balanced attention to both the negative *and* the positive aspects of human development. The past decade has produced a profound shift in how mental health is defined, built, and maintained, which highlights the full spectrum of psychosocial function. From a positive psychological perspective, well-being and flourishing are not simply the absence of ill-being, but something more (Huppert & So, 2013; Seligman & Csikszentmihalyi, 2000). The spectrum of mental health ranges from severe psychological disorder to fully thriving in life. From this perspective, even those who are doing well in life can improve and strive to be the best they can be.

The reduction of youth mental disorders has been the priority for good reasons: "positive" outcomes can be a difficult sell when juxtaposed with what appear to be more pressing problems, such as depression, bullying, and suicide. But there has been ample evidence to support the contention that enhancing positive outcomes has the additional effect of reducing negative outcomes. From the positive perspective, the goals of mental health promotion are first to move people beyond deficits in function, and second to maintain good mental health once achieved. To fully prepare youth for the business of life, it is key to develop skills, talents, character, happiness, engagement, and social involvement (Benson & Scales, 2009; Pittman, 1991, 2000). As necessary as it is to reduce or eliminate problems among children and adolescents, it is just as important to help them thrive and form positive connections with the larger world. Parents want their children not only to survive the choppy waters of adolescence but also to truly thrive—being safe, healthy, happy, moral, fully engaged in life, and productive contributors to the communities in which they live (Noddings, 2003; Seligman et al., 2009).

This positive approach to mental health has been increasingly studied, accepted, and implemented across a growing array of fields, including education, counseling, health, business, neuroscience, and public policy (Rusk & Waters, 2013). In this revised chapter, we focus on three predominant approaches that explicitly target youth: (1) *positive youth development*, because of its explicit concern with how to encourage the well-being of children and adolescents; (2) *positive psychology*, because of its interest in the underlying psychological processes leading to well-being and optimal functioning;

and (3) *positive education*, because of its focus on applying positive psychology principles to the classroom and creating positive institutions that support youth well-being.

Our goal is to review the positive perspective and use it to complement the problem-oriented disciplines (cf., Larson, 2000; Maton et al., 2003). A balanced view of youth must acknowledge assets along with problems, including risk factors, protective factors, and promoting factors (Pollard, Hawkins, & Arthur, 1999). As Pittman (1991, 2000) phrased this challenge, "problem-free is not fully prepared." We have three working assumptions, each buttressed by suggestive evidence:

- Psychosocial characteristics are associated with reduced problems *and* increased well-being among youth.
- Youth development programs can encourage positive characteristics.
- Similar features can be incorporated into classrooms and schools to support well-being both inside and outside of the classroom.

Not only are positive characteristics valuable in their own right, but they may also buffer against the development of psychological problems among youth. Attention to positive characteristics may help us promote the full potential of all youth, including those with current or past psychological problems. This contribution therefore addresses positive youth development with respect to mental illness *and* mental health. We discuss positive characteristics of youth and their settings and how these are related to thriving. We summarize what is known about programs and institutions that promote positive development. Finally, we take stock of what is known and what remains unknown within positive-oriented research and practice.

THE POSITIVE PERSPECTIVE ON YOUTH DEVELOPMENT

The positive approach to youth development begins with a vision of a fully able child eager to explore the world, gain competence, and acquire the capacity to contribute to the world. It recognizes the existence of adversities and developmental challenges that may affect children in various ways, but it resists conceiving of the developmental process as mainly an effort to overcome deficits and risk. The goal is to understand, educate, and engage children in productive activities rather than to correct, cure, or treat them for maladaptive tendencies and disabilities. A driving premise is that attention to what is good about a young person provides a foundation on which to base interventions. Further, children and adolescents are not miniature adults; youth have valuable perspectives and need to be understood on their own terms. This perspective thus urges us not to give up on children, no matter what challenges they may have experienced or patterns of behavior they display.

Although positive youth development, positive psychology, and positive education are relatively recent developments, they are not new perspectives (Kristjánsson, 2012). Some of the best-known youth programs in the United States were founded a century or more ago to promote the health and character of young people through structured activities outside of school (Erickson, 1999), including the YWCA (1851) and YMCA (1855), Boys Clubs (1860) and Girls Clubs (1906), Girls Incorporated (1864), American Red Cross (1881), Big Brothers (1903)/Big Sisters (1908), Boy Scouts (1910) and Girl Scouts (1912), Camp Fire (1910), and 4-H (1914). Today's positive perspective is rediscovering and reaffirming the premise of these programs, while increasingly adding empirical evidence for their efficacy and effectiveness (Rhodes, 2014).

Also contributing to the positive perspective on development were humanistic psychology as popularized by Rogers (1951) and Maslow (1970); utopian visions of education like those of Neill (1960); primary prevention programs based on notions of wellness (sometimes called promotion programs) as pioneered by Albee (1982) and Cowen (1994); developmental theories emphasizing person–environment interactions (e.g., Bronfenbrenner, 1979; Lerner &

Kauffman, 1985); work by Bandura (1989) and others on human agency; studies of giftedness, genius, and talent (e.g., Winner, 2000); conceptions of multiple intelligence (e.g., Gardner, 1983; Sternberg, 1985); studies of the quality of life among psychiatric patients that went beyond an exclusive focus on symptoms and diseases (e.g., Levitt, Hogan, & Bucosky, 1990); and health psychology theories and studies on prevention (e.g., Friedman, 2000).

Over the past few decades, the youth development field has had a strong interest in application (Catalano, Berglund, Ryan, Lonczak, & Hawkins, 1999; Durlak, Weissberg, & Pachan, 2010). The focus on application arose from studies in the 1960s through the early 1990s that identified adolescence as an important period of human development, with particular focus on the plasticity of development and dynamic associations that occur between youth and their contexts (Lerner & Steinberg, 2009). From their very beginning, national youth groups embraced promotion goals, but throughout the 20th century, efforts were increasingly directed at youth problems such as school dropout, juvenile crime, alcohol and drug use, and teenage pregnancy (Catalano et al., 2012; Jessor & Jessor, 1977). Positive approaches have thus returned to the promotion-focused goals through individual and universal programs and interventions delivered inside and outside of schools. These programs aim to support youth before problems develop, immunizing and buffering them against life's challenges. The earliest applications were informed more by common sense and intuition than by research. Yet increasingly over the past decade, research and theory have begun to guide practice (Catalano et al., 2012).

Bronfenbrenner's (1977, 1979, 1986) *bioecological approach*, which articulates multiple contexts that impact the individual, has been particularly influential for framing and understanding youth development. Bronfenbrenner's model articulates the importance of the social ecology, including the *microsystem* with which the individual directly interacts (family, peers, school, and neighborhood) and the *exosystem*, which is made up of larger ecologies that indirectly impact development and behavior, like the legal system, the social welfare system, and mass media. At the broadest level, the *macrosystem* consists of ideological and institutional patterns that collectively define a culture. Each youth brings his or her own characteristics to the challenges of life, which influence and are influenced by these different interacting ecologies.

Under the broad umbrella of positive approaches to youth development, several specific areas of research and application have taken root. *Positive youth development* recognizes the good in young people, focusing on each and every child's unique talents, strengths, interests, and potential (Damon, 2004). It is an interdisciplinary field, with roots in developmental psychology, developmental epidemiology, and prevention science (Guerra & Bradshaw, 2008; Larson, 2000), and emphasizes the multiple contexts in which development occurs. For instance, researchers at the Search Institute in Minneapolis have studied what they call *developmental assets*, which include contextual factors like family support and adult role models and personal factors like commitment to learning, positive values, and sense of purpose (Leffert et al., 1998; Scales, Benson, Leffert, & Blyth, 2000). Youth with more of these assets not only show fewer problems but also display other valued outcomes (e.g., school success, leadership, helping others, and physical health).

A major incentive for adopting a positive youth development approach is the recognition that prevention efforts targeting a single problem overlook opportunities to adopt a more integrated approach (Guerra & Bradshaw, 2008; Romer, 2003). Many problems co-occur and have the same risk factors, so multipronged interventions can have broad effects. Part of the broadening of youth development and its applications was a call for studying and eventually cultivating desirable outcomes such as school achievement, vocational aspirations, community involvement, and good interpersonal relations. As Roth and Brooks-Gunn (2003) noted, the positive youth development approach asserts the "belief in youth as resources to be developed rather than problems to be managed" (p. 172).

Here is where positive youth development converges with *positive psychology*, a scientific, strengths-based approach that examines optimal functioning and aims to discover and promote factors that allow individuals, organizations, and communities to thrive (Gable & Haidt, 2005; Seligman & Csikszentmihalyi, 2000). The positive psychology perspective contends that the absence of mental illness is not the same as flourishing; rather, what makes life worth living deserves its own field of inquiry. It does not simply disregard negative emotions and experiences; rather, it aims to provide a more complete and balanced scientific understanding of human experience that incorporates both the positive and negative ends of the mental health spectrum.

Positive psychology has provided an umbrella term for what previously were isolated lines of theory and research. Although officially arising from psychology, it may now more aptly be called "positive science" or "well-being science." Similar concepts and terms are rising across disciplines, including medicine, education, sport science, organizational behavior, neuroscience, social science, and public health (Rusk & Waters, 2013). For example, health becomes not only treating disease and disability that occurs, but also promoting healthy behaviors and wellness (Snyder, Schactman, & Young, 2015). The virtuous workplace is not only a place of business but also a place that enhances the well-being of employees and consumers impacted by that business (Cameron & Caza, 2004; Cameron, Dutton, & Quinn, 2003).

The concerns of positive psychology can generally be parsed into four related domains that reflect different socioecological levels: *positive subjective experiences* (e.g., happiness, pleasure, fulfillment, flow), *positive individual traits* (e.g., character strengths, talents, interests, values), *positive interpersonal relationships* (e.g., relationships between friends, parents and child, and teacher and students), and *positive institutions* (e.g., families, schools, businesses, organizations). Growing interest in applications to public policy has added a fifth domain of *enabling societies*. Studies and scholarship in positive psychology have focused primarily on subjective experiences and individual traits, whereas positive organizational scholarship has focused on enabling institutions. Bridging these multiple domains, *positive education* combines the concepts and ideas of positive psychology with best practice guidelines from education to promote student flourishing within the school environment (Norrish, Williams, O'Connor, & Robinson, 2013).

There are multiple reasons why schools are an important place for implementing positive psychology. Throughout adolescence, youth spend a considerable amount of time at school. Parents and educators generally believe that schools are responsible for developing student character (Cohen, 2006), and student well-being is a core value for many educational institutions (Seligman et al., 2009). Schools are one of the few institutions that consistently provide funds and resources for youth (Clonan, Chafouleas, McDougal, & Riley-Tillman, 2004). In addition, education has a rich history of identifying best practices for learning and teaching.

Early evidence suggests that positive education approaches are building student well-being (see Waters, 2011 for a review), with some links to greater achievement as well (Durlak, Weissberg, Dymnicki, Taylor, & Schellinger, 2011). However, schools are complex organizations, with multiple levels of influence. Although student well-being may be the target, teachers and staff are often the ones who implement curriculum and intervention-type activities. If the staff members are burned out or believe that teaching well-being is just one more thing to add to an already over-packed curriculum, they will be unmotivated to teach positive skills and mindsets. Further, staff members are affected by the leadership and policies of the school, which in turn are affected by educational policies and cultural norms. Beyond incorporating specific activities, change will be most effective when a whole-school approach is taken (Kern, Adler, Waters, & White, 2015; Waters & White, 2015). As Waters (2011) notes, "a school-wide positive education framework is required to ensure that schools move beyond the use of specific programs conducted within selected classrooms to adopting a whole-school approach that becomes the general way of life at the school" (p. 85). Schools need to be enabling institutions, with moral goals that help both students and staff members become responsible, productive citizens of society (Peterson, 2006; Waters & White, 2015).

Positive youth development, positive psychology, and positive education emphasize the importance of creating positive institutions that enable the development of a positive culture, which supports positive relationships, which in turn facilitate positive traits and subjective experiences (Park & Peterson, 2003). The word "enable" avoids strict causal language. It is possible for people to be happy or content even in the absence of character strengths, and good character can operate against the interpersonal and institutional grain, but people are at their best when institutions, relationships, traits, and experiences are in alignment (Lerner & Steinberg, 2009; Lerner et al., 2013). Indeed, doing well in life represents a coming together of all five domains.

The positive perspective can sound at times rather Pollyanna-ish—encapsulating the feel-good parts of life while ignoring life's challenges. Yet beyond simply "doing well," positive youth development and positive education explicitly target building resilience by teaching youth the mindsets, attitudes, skills, and behaviors that will allow them to successfully ride the waves of life. The term *resiliency* is used to describe the quality that enables young people to thrive even in the face of adversity (Masten, 2001; Werner, 1982). Children can and do overcome adversity and thrive (Werner & Smith, 2001). Resiliency is characterized by persistence, hardiness, goal-directedness, an orientation to success, achievement motivation, educational aspirations, a belief in the future, a sense of anticipation, a sense of purpose, and a sense of coherence (Benard, 1991; Luthar, 2006; Luthar, Cicchetti, & Becker, 2000; Masten, 2011, 2014). However, resiliency does not operate in a vacuum: few if any children are impervious to unrelenting adversity, and without appropriate environmental or social support, children will likely succumb to problems. On the flip side, effective parenting and other protective factors can buffer risks (Masten, 2001; Werner & Smith, 2001). Change in the developmental trajectory, for positive or negative, occurs at many different points, and the context can guide youth toward pathology or resilience (Sroufe, 1997). Young people thrive through a combination of individual hardiness *and* protective factors embedded in socializing institutions (cf. Luthar, 2006).

Accordingly, the assets of youth that protect against problems and allow young people to do well include not only individual psychological characteristics like talents, competence, character strengths, and constructive interests, but also characteristics of their social settings such as family support, parental involvement in schooling, adult role models outside the family, high expectations within the community, and the availability of creative activities (e.g., Benson, 1997; Masten, 2001; Wang, 2009). The agenda of the positive approach is to maximize the potential of young people by encouraging both personal and environmental assets. To do so requires recognition of the reciprocal relations among the multiple socioecological levels that surround youth (Agans et al., 2014; Brändstadter, 1998; Bronfenbrenner & Ceci, 1994; Lerner et al., 2010, 2013).

POSITIVE YOUTH DEVELOPMENT: CORE COMPONENTS

Positive approaches to youth developmental take a deliberately broad perspective on the qualities of young people that should be promoted. A wide range of researchers in the positive youth development field (e.g., Catalano et al., 2004; Guerra & Bradshaw, 2008; Lerner et al., 2010; Roth & Brooks-Gunn, 2003) have primarily focused on six domains, which intersect with core concepts of positive psychology and positive education. Perhaps the best-known system, popularized by Lerner et al. (2000) and Roth and Brooks-Gunn (2003), is the *five C's*: Connection, Competence, Confidence, Caring, and Character. Pittman, Irby, and Ferber (2001) added a sixth C,

Contribution, which is believed to result from the other five. We organize our discussion around these concepts inasmuch as Lerner et al. have amply demonstrated that these components are interrelated and subsumed by a higher-order construct of positive youth development across adolescence (Lerner et al., 2005). Furthermore, youth who exhibit high levels of the 5 C's tend to engage in fewer harmful activities such as drug use, experience less depression, and are more closely attached to family and school, among other positive outcomes (Arbeit et al., 2014; Hoyt, Chase-Lansdale, McDade, & Adam, 2012; Lerner, Phelps, Forma, & Bowers, 2009).

Connection

Connection refers to bidirectional emotional and committed bonds between a youth and others in the family, peer group, school, community, or culture (Geldhof et al., 2014). Studies by Ainsworth et al. (1978) and Bowlby (1969, 1973, 1980) have demonstrated the importance of early bonding and attachment processes for the development of social connections with others. The quality of early bonds with caregivers has considerable impact on the manner in which the child later bonds to peers, school, the community, and culture(s) and is an essential aspect of positive development into a healthy adult (Brophy, 1988; Brophy & Good, 1986; Dolan, Kellam, & Brown, 1989; Hawkins, Catalano, & Miller, 1992; Poortinga, 2012). Notably, in Lerner et al.'s (2005) factorial studies of the five C's in adolescents, Connection stands out as the most influential component of positive youth development.

Positive bonding with an adult is crucial to the development of a capacity for adaptive responses to change and has been related to numerous biopsychosocial outcomes throughout childhood and adolescence, including good peer relationships, social-emotional competence, cognition, and physical and mental health (Catalano et al., 2004; Ranson & Urichuk, 2008; Schneider, Atkinson, & Tardif, 2001). Good bonding establishes the child's trust in oneself and others. Poor bonding establishes a fundamental mistrust of others, and insecure attachments can negatively influence peer relationships throughout adolescence, resulting in internalizing or externalizing disorders and behaviors (Allen et al., 2007; Brook, Brook, Gordon, Whiteman, & Cohen, 1990; Mikulincer & Shaver, 2012; Ranson & Urichek, 2008).

Although parents or primary caregivers are often the key point of connection in the early years, relationships with peers, teachers, and other non-parental adults also matter (Bowers et al., 2012; Erickson, McDonald, & Elder, 2009; Greenberger, Chen, & Beam, 1998; Rhodes, Ebert, & Fischer, 1992; Zimmerman, Bingenheimer, & Notaro, 2002). Parents and other adults also interact to have complementary, compensatory, or detrimental effects on youth outcomes (Bowers et al., 2014). Schools in particular can provide a positive environment that can have salutary effects on a range of health outcomes. Adolescents attending schools with better social climates tend to experience less drug use, depression, and bullying (Allen, Kern, Vella-Brodrick, Hattie, & Waters, in press; Cohen, 2006; Larusso, Romer, & Selman, 2007), possibly due to the better relationships that students experience with teachers and peers (Allen et al., in press; Larusso & Selman, 2003) as well as the clear establishment of healthy norms of behavior (Baumrind, 1998). Social-emotional learning curricula that promote positive connections with others along with the development of skills can buffer adolescents at risk for antisocial behavior (Caplan et al., 1992; Dryfoos, 1990; Durlak et al., 2011; Hawkins et al., 1999; Roth & Brooks-Gunn, 2003).

Competence

Competence covers several areas of youth functioning, including social, emotional, cognitive, and vocational skills that are basic to healthy behavior (Lerner et al., 2009; Roth & Brooks-Gunn, 2003). While the enhancement of competence can help to prevent negative outcomes (Botvin, Baker, Dusenbury, Botvin, & Diaz, 1995), competence can also be specified and measured as an important outcome in its own right, indicative of positive development (Weissberg & Greenberg, 1997).

In an early study of the importance of competencies for mental health, Kornberg and Caplan (1980) reviewed research on biopsychosocial risk factors for mental disorder and concluded that competence training to promote adaptive behavior and mental health was one of the most significant developments in primary prevention. In the education space, growing focus has been given to social and emotional learning, which focuses on teaching students a range of interpersonal skills that help youth integrate feelings, thinking, and actions in order to achieve specific social and interpersonal goals (Caplan et al., 1992; Durlak et al., 2011; Weissberg, Caplan, & Sivo, 1989). For instance, the Collaborative for Academic, Social, and Emotional Learning (CASEL) provides strategies to teach students how to recognize, interpret, and respond to social and emotional cues, including accurately interpreting those cues; generating effective solutions to interpersonal problems; realistically anticipating consequences and potential obstacles to one's actions; and translating social decisions into effective behavior.

Some research has focused on particular cognitive competencies involved in the development of self-control (Guerra & Bradshaw, 2008). For example, Rothbart and Posner (2006) have identified effortful self-control as a critical competence in children, and Moffitt et al. (2013) have observed its beneficial effects across the lifespan in their study of the Dunedin birth cohort. Children and adolescents with greater self-control tend to experience fewer problems with impulse control, such as drug use and early sexual activity (Duckworth, Gendler, & Gross, 2014). Greater self-control is also associated with less persistence of negative affect and better academic performance (Duckworth et al., 2014; Duckworth & Seligman, 2005).

Character

Character refers to a moral and ethical disposition that respects cultural and societal values (Geldhof et al., 2014). Following in the Piagetian tradition (1965), Kohlberg (1963, 1969) defined moral development as a multistage process through which children acquire increasingly advanced powers of reasoning regarding society's standards of right and wrong. Gilligan (1982) countered that morality is as much about relationships and caring about the welfare of others as about obeying abstract rules, and Hoffman (1981) proposed that the roots of morality lie in empathy, which has a neurological basis and can be either fostered or suppressed by environmental influences (Feshbach & Feshbach, 2009). Several scholars have argued that character is core to moral competence—good character drives an individual to do what is right (Baumrind, 1998; Park & Peterson, 2006). To acknowledge, measure, and build moral competencies, much of the research and application in positive psychology and positive education centers around strengths of character, as described in greater detail below.

Caring

Caring refers to the ability to sympathize and empathize with others (Geldhof et al., 2014). Empathic concern for others is regarded as a necessary condition for understanding others and resolving conflicts with them (Eisenberg, Huerta, & Michalska, 2012). Related to the personality trait of agreeableness, caring individuals are more likely to have high-quality and harmonious relationships with others, good school performance, less bullying and victimization, and lower levels of depression (Jensen-Campbell, Knack, & Gomez, 2010; Kern et al., 2013). Caring thus is an important foundation for establishing positive relationships with peers, teachers, and others.

Confidence

Confidence refers to an internal sense of self-efficacy and self-worth (Geldhof et al., 2014). Although Bandura (1993) regarded self-efficacy as domain-specific, youth who understand their capabilities and feel confident in their ability to act on them are more likely to engage in appropriate levels of goal striving and achievement (Deci & Ryan, 2000, 2011).

Contribution

Arising from the 5 C's, *Contribution* to one's community is seen as an outgrowth of successful development (Lerner et al., 2009; Pitman et al., 2001). Indeed, Lerner et al. (2013) find that programs such as the 4-H club encourage activities that contribute to community and civic engagement. In the National Longitudinal Study of Adolescent Health, connections with parents, schools, and the community related to greater likelihood of being a good citizen in young adulthood—voting, volunteering in the community, and being involved socially (Duke, Skay, Pettingell, & Borowsky, 2009). Other research indicates that schools also play a role in encouraging civic engagement (Torney-Purta, Richardson, & Barber, 2004).

ADDITIONAL COMPONENTS FROM POSITIVE PSYCHOLOGY

Positive psychology has added components that characterize or contribute to youth well-being. Whereas positive youth development has maintained a strong theoretical base centered on the 6 C's, positive psychology scholarship includes a broader range of constructs, which are less structured, speaking to the diversity of scholars and perspectives that fall under the positive psychology umbrella. Over the past two decades, scholarship in the field has focused primarily on adults, but it is increasingly focusing on youth and adolescents, through the lens of positive education.

Subjective Well-Being and Flourishing

A core focus in positive psychology is the theoretical understanding of *subjective well-being* (also commonly referred to as flourishing, thriving, optimal functioning, and so forth). At its most basic level, flourishing can be defined as "feeling good and functioning well" (Huppert & So, 2013, p. 839). It is a combination of high levels of mental health and low levels of mental illness (Keyes, 2002). Scholarship surrounding well-being has generally encompassed two traditions: hedonic happiness, which centers on positive emotions, and eudaimonic happiness, or the good life, encompassing aspects such as purpose in life, self-acceptance, mastery, and relationships with others (Deci & Ryan, 2008; Forgeard et al., 2011; Ryff & Keyes, 1995; Seligman, 2011). Early in the field, scholars primarily discussed happiness and well-being from the hedonic perspective, in part because emotions are easier to measure, manipulate, and change than the more abstract eudaimonic components (Biswas-Diener, 2015). As the field has matured, definitions and measures of well-being have become increasingly multidimensional, with flourishing defined in terms of a profile across mental, physical, social, and functional domains (Forgeard et al., 2011; Seligman, 2011). Notably, this returns to the World Health Organization's (1946) definition of health as "a state of complete physical, mental, and social well-being and not merely the absence of disease or infirmity."

Within and across the broader hedonic and eudaimonic domains, there are multiple (often overlapping) models of well-being and flourishing. Across models, *positive emotions*, such as joy, excitement, and contentment, are central. Positive emotions feel good, but seemingly have other benefits as well. Fredrickson (2001) proposed that whereas negative emotions narrow our focus, positive emotions broaden and build cognitive, psychological, and social skills and abilities (see also Fredrickson, 2013a). They help connect us to others (Fredrickson, 2013b) and have been linked with greater creativity, financial gain, better physical health, and even longevity (Diener & Chan, 2011; Howell, Kern, & Lyubormirsky, 2007; Lyubomirsky, King, & Diener, 2005; Pressman & Cohen 2005; Tugade, Fredrickson, & Feldman Barrett, 2004). Emotions vary throughout the day and across contexts, but evidence suggests that up to a point, it may be most adaptive to have a greater proportion of positive versus negative emotions during the day (Fredrickson, 2013c).

Diener et al. (1985) defined subjective well-being in terms of high positive affect, low negative affect, and high *life satisfaction*, thus adding a cognitive component to the affective evaluation. Life satisfaction refers to the overall judgment that one's life is going well (Diener, 1984). Measures of general satisfaction have been used for decades and are increasingly being considered as a complement to economic measures in public policy for evaluating how a nation is doing (Diener, Inglehart, & Tay, 2012). Life satisfaction among youth is pervasively associated with the presence of desirable psychological characteristics (e.g., self-esteem, resiliency, health-promoting habits, and pro-social behavior) and the absence of negative characteristics (anxiety, depression, loneliness, school discipline problems, drug and alcohol use, teenage pregnancy, and violence) (Gilman & Huebner, 2003; Huebner, 2004; Huebner, Funk, & Gilman, 2000; Park, 2004).

On the eudaimonic side, *meaning in life* is a core part of most models of flourishing. Meaning in life includes two dimensions: *comprehension*, or having a sense of direction in life and feeling connected to something larger than oneself, and *purpose*, or long-term aspirations that align with one's values and motivate activity (Steger, 2012). With youth, definitions have focused on the purpose sub-domain, and some evidence suggests that adolescents define purpose in life similar to adults (Hill, Burrow, O'Dell, & Thornton, 2011). In adults, a sense of purpose in life is associated with reduced mortality risk (Boyle et al., 2009; Hill & Turiano, 2014), and in adolescents, purpose relates to well-being and hope (Bronk et al., 2009; Burrow, O'Dell, & Hill, 2010).

A sense of meaning is something that must be developed over time; young adults are more likely to be searching for a sense of meaning than older adults (Steger, Oishi, & Kasdan, 2009). The presence of meaning in life has been related to greater reported life satisfaction, more positive affect, higher levels of optimism, better self-esteem, and fewer psychological problems (Damon, 2008; Mariano & Going, 2011; Steger et al., 2009). However, although positive emotion and meaning often are positively correlated, the meaningful life is not always a happy one (Baumeister, Vohs, Aaker, & Garbinsky, 2013). It is possible that positive youth development programs might help youth discover a sense of meaning and purpose at an earlier age, reducing the struggle to find meaning that often occurs in young adulthood.

Adding in the social component, most models of flourishing include *positive relationships with others*. There is considerable evidence for the importance of social relationships (cf., Taylor, 2011). Put simply, "other people matter" (Peterson, 2006, p. 249). On the flip side, loneliness is a major risk factor for physical morbidity, mental illness, poor cognitive function, and mortality (Cacioppo, Hawley, & Berntson, 2003; Hawkley & Cacioppo, 2010). This again is where positive youth development sets the stage for positive adult outcomes; both connection and caring feed into better perceptions of social relationships and better interactions with others, reducing loneliness and improving physical, mental, and cognitive outcomes.

Other components of flourishing depend on the theoretical model. For instance, Seligman (2011) adds accomplishment and engagement in life to positive emotion, relationships, and meaning. Other scholars include constructs such as self-acceptance, mastery/competence, optimism, vitality, self-esteem, resilience, and engagement in life (e.g., Diener et al., 2010; Huppert & So, 2013; Ryff & Keyes, 1995).

Although well-being is treated at times as a predictor of other outcomes (e.g., happiness leading to health and longevity outcomes; Diener & Chan, 2011; Howell et al., 2007), it is a multidimensional outcome that results from attitudes, behaviors, skills, circumstances, and experiences that occur through life (Friedman & Kern, 2014). It can be measured at a point in time but is also fluid and shifts, depending on mood, circumstance, and a host of other factors. As an analogy, consider a flower garden. When in full bloom, it is flourishing and provides us with a sense of pleasure. But it requires care to continue to thrive. Weeds that threaten the blossoms must be removed, and water and nutrients need to be provided. Likewise, thriving in life does not simply occur but needs support and care, removing ill-being and supporting wellness. Flourishing in life (however it is defined), then, is an outcome that ideally will result from the personal strengths developed in adolescence through positive youth development and positive education programs.

Individual Characteristics

Positive psychology and positive education also highlight various individual characteristics that contribute to well-being. Positive youth development explicitly suggests that to promote positive outcomes in youth, alignment between individual strengths and contextual assets is critical (Agans et al., 2014).

One of the most dominant areas of research and application has focused on *character strengths*. Peterson and Seligman (2004) suggested 24 strengths that are valued across cultures: appreciation of beauty and excellence, bravery, capacity to love and be loved, creativity, curiosity, fairness, forgiveness/mercy, gratitude, honesty, hope/optimism, humor, kindness, judgment/open-mindedness, leadership, love of learning, modesty/humility, perseverance, perspective/wisdom, prudence, self-regulation/self-control, social intelligence, spirituality, teamwork, and zest. The Values in Action (VIA) survey was developed to assess the strengths, and millions of people have completed the measure. Across over one million participants from 75 nations, there is considerable consistency across nations (McGrath, 2015a), and the characteristics cluster into three higher-order factors: caring, inquisitiveness, and self-control (McGrath, 2015b).

Character strengths have been linked to numerous positive outcomes (see Niemiec, 2014, for a summary of research findings). Among young people, such strengths have been linked to higher well-being, life satisfaction, achievement, school performance, and social functioning, and reduced behavior problems (Park & Peterson, 2009; Shoshani & Slone, 2013; Toner, Haslam, Robinson, & Williams, 2012; Weber & Ruch 2012). Strengths form a main component of most positive education programs (e.g., Norrish et al., 2013; Seligman et al., 2009; White & Waters, 2015). In many of these programs, students learn to identify and use their top strengths and practice spotting strengths in others. Strengths-based language might be incorporated into the curriculum and extracurricular activities. Strengths-focused positive education programs have been linked with improved skills, school engagement, life satisfaction, and school success (Proctor et al., 2011; Seligman et al., 2009). Although such programs show early signs of success, research is needed on the contextual nature of strengths; depending on the goal and circumstances, a different combination of strengths may be best (Hogan, 2008).

A growing amount of research has centered on specific strengths, and we focus here on those that have been most directly applied to youth through positive education. *Gratitude* is both a positive emotion and a life orientation that involves noticing and appreciating positives in the world (Morgan, Gulliford, & Kristjánsson, 2016; Wood, Froh, & Geraghty, 2010). In adults, gratitude relates to lower levels of depression and negative affect, greater life satisfaction and positive affect, good social relationships, and pro-social behavior (see Wood et al., 2010, for a review), with a similar pattern of positive associations in youth (Froh, Yurkewicz, & Kashdan, 2009; Waters, 2011). Some evidence suggests that gratitude is an important part of recovering from traumatic experiences (Davis, Nolen-Hoeksema, & Larson, 1998; Joseph & Linley, 2005; Linley & Joseph, 2004). Various interventions have been developed to increase gratitude, such as listing what one is grateful for (e.g., "what went well" exercises, gratitude boards), counting one's blessings, and writing and giving a gratitude letter to someone else, and generally boost positive affect, at least temporarily.

Kindness includes the motivation to be kind to others, recognition of kindness of others, and regularly behaving in kind ways. Engaging in acts of kindness has been related to greater well-being and happiness (Aknin et al., 2012; Lyubomirsky, Sheldon, & Schkade, 2005; Parks

& Biswas-Diener, 2013). Across 19 classrooms in Vancouver, acts of kindness were found to be related to positive social outcomes, such as better emotional adjustment, increased cooperation, reduced likelihood of being bullied, and more satisfying friendships (Layous & Lyubomirsky, 2014).

Hope involves having goals for the future, motivation or agency to move toward those goals (willpower), and pathways to achieve those goals (waypower) (Snyder, 1994). In youth, hope relates to greater life satisfaction, self-esteem, and perceived competence (Valle, Huebner, & Suldo, 2006). Underlying this future-minded drive is *optimism*, a generalized favorable expectation about the future. Optimism is the road that says the future will be positive, and hope is the vehicle that drives the individual there. Optimism is a relatively stable individual difference and relates to better physical health, longer life, proactive coping strategies, persistence in educational and occupational domains, and better social relationships (cf., Carver, Scheier, & Segerstrom, 2010). Cognitive-behavioral techniques appear to be the most effective approach for shifting levels of optimism, although it is questionable how much change can be expected as patterns of thought and behavior become more ingrained and habitual over time (Friedman, 2000). Adolescence is a core period in which relatively stable levels of hope and optimism are developed. Programs such as BounceBack! (McGrath & Noble, 2003) and the Penn Resiliency Program (Gillham, Jaycox, Reivich, Seligman, & Silver, 1990) embed optimistic thinking into curriculum units, teaching mindsets and behaviors within the classroom.

The character strengths of perseverance and self-regulation are particularly relevant for achievement and success. Both are part of the Big Five personality construct of conscientiousness, which predicts better physical and mental health, longer life, healthy behaviors, academic and professional success, and good social relationships (Kern & Friedman, 2008; Roberts, Kuncel, Shiner, Caspi, & Goldberg, 2007; Roberts et al., 2014). *Perseverance* refers to the ability to focus on longer-term or superordinate goals, and to stick with the pursuit of these goals over time, despite setbacks and obstacles that occur along the way. Applied to education, academically tenacious students tend to be more engaged in their learning, work hard, seek challenges, and are not derailed by difficulties (Dweck, Walton, & Cohen, 2014). *Self-control* refers to the ability to regulate attention, emotion, and/or behavior, despite temptation (Duckworth & Gross, 2014). It involves voluntarily regulating oneself in the moment to align with personal or societal values, standards, or goals (Duckworth & Kern, 2011). Combining elements of perseverance and self-control, Duckworth et al. have popularized the concept of *grit*, in which an individual tenaciously pursues an overarching goal, despite setbacks that might occur along the way (Duckworth, Peterson, Matthews, & Kelly, 2007). Self-control involves "resisting the hourly temptations," whereas grit involves "passion and effort sustained over years," pursuing a particular goal (Duckworth & Gross, 2014, pp. 319–320). Grit is particularly relevant for academic and professional outcomes, characterizing those who achieve at the highest levels and remain in school and teaching (Duckworth et al., 2007; Duckworth & Seligman, 2005).

Beyond character strengths, two other individual characteristics appear to be particularly important for academic achievement. First, the capacity to engage in learning contributes to success both in and out of the classroom. Like well-being, *engagement* is multidimensional, with cognitive, affective, and behavioral domains, and is inconsistently defined and measured (Appleton, Christenson, & Furlong, 2008). Definitions include a capacity to become absorbed in and focused on what one is doing (cognitive engagement), involvement in interesting life activities and tasks (behavioral engagement), and commitment, passion, enthusiasm, focused effort, and energy (psychological/affective engagement). Both the quality and amount of support received at home and school, along with the student's levels of intrinsic and extrinsic motivation, influence levels of engagement in the classroom, which in turn impact academic, social, and emotional outcomes (Appleton et al., 2008; Connell & Wellborn, 1991). The positive psychology literature has focused primarily on the psychological domain. In particular, Csikszentmihalyi (1990) introduced the idea of *flow*, a state of extremely high psychological engagement where one is completely focused on and immersed in the task at hand, such that time seemingly stands still. Flow occurs when both challenge and skill levels are high. Frequent experience of flow during adolescence foreshadows long-term desirable consequences, such as achievement in creative domains (Rathunde & Csikszentmihalyi, 1993), reduction of delinquency, and academic achievement (Nakamura & Csikszentmihalyi, 2009).

A second core characteristic is mindset. Those with a *fixed mindset* tend to see intellectual ability as something that one either does or does not have, and worry about proving their intellectual ability. This can lead to destructive thoughts, feelings, and behaviors when that ability is threatened or challenged (Dweck et al., 2014). In contrast, those with a *growth mindset* view intelligence as malleable and developed through effort and learning, and tend to respond to challenges with more constructive thoughts, feelings, and behaviors. One's mindset impacts goal selection, the extent to which one seeks help and support, and achievement and motivation both in the classroom and beyond, and it ultimately can impact self-esteem, perceived competence, hope, and perseverance toward future goals (Dweck, 2006). Notably, mindset is malleable. Feedback by others matters; constructive praise focuses on the process of learning, including effort given and strategies involved (e.g., "you worked hard, making great revision notes"), whereas destructive praise focuses on the person and the outcome (e.g., "you are smart and kind").

In sum, positive psychology emphasizes numerous concepts relevant for youth. Strengths, mindsets, and other individual characteristics contribute to the 5 C's of positive youth development, and positive education is applying these concepts to the classroom and school environment. By developing such characteristics, behaviors, and attitudes in youth, both within schools through positive education approaches and outside of school through positive youth development programs, a foundation is laid for youth to develop into flourishing, contributing adults.

PROGRAMS THAT CULTIVATE POSITIVE DEVELOPMENT

Researchers have identified many of the precursors of the aforementioned positive youth characteristics and are now turning their attention to their deliberate cultivation (Seligman, 2011; Seligman, Steen, Park, & Peterson, 2005). One of the early demonstrations of the positive youth development approach was the work of Hawkins and Catalano in their Seattle Youth Development Project (Hawkins et al., 1992). This project applied positive youth development principles to build competencies in children and bonding to both teachers and parents across the elementary school years. The project produced favorable outcomes that lasted over at least 15 years, with enhancements in educational outcomes and community engagement and reductions in mental health disorders and sexual risk outcomes (Hawkins et al., 2008). Notably, the program has been estimated to produce a benefit-to-cost ratio of greater than 2 to 1 (Catalano et al., 2012).

Another notable program led by Botvin (1998) developed a competency-based intervention for middle school youth that built life skills for healthier decision making by teaching drug resistance, self-management, and social skills. This program has been shown to reduce drug and substance use and violence by 40% to 80%, with effects that last for several years beyond the program; however, careful and complete implementation of the program is important, and booster sessions may be needed to maintain gains (Botvin, 2000). This program has been estimated to produce a sizeable benefit-to-cost ratio of greater than 40 to 1 (Catalano et al., 2012).

The most direct test of the positive youth development model comes from the 4-H Study of Positive Youth Development, led by Lerner et al. at Tufts University. Beginning in 2002–2003, the study has prospectively followed a sample of diverse youth and their parents to understand individual and environmental factors that influence positive, healthy development (Lerner et al., 2005). The study aims to empirically understand the individual and contextual processes through which positive youth development emerges. Many findings have arisen from the study (see Lerner et al., 2009, and the 2014 special issue of *The Journal of Youth & Adolescence* for detailed findings and discussions of the study). For instance, participation in sports and youth development programs helps promote positive youth development and prevent youth problems. Further, promoting positive youth development is not the same as preventing problem behaviors.

Perhaps one of the most significant developments in the field of positive development over the last decade has been the proliferation of school-based programs designed to promote *social and emotional learning* (SEL) of children and youth, led primarily by CASEL (www.casel.org). Extensive research shows that social and emotional competencies are associated with success in school and life. That is, students who appreciate themselves and their abilities realistically (confidence), who recognize and regulate their emotions and behaviors appropriately (self-control), who are able to take the perspective of and care about others (caring), who handle conflicts effectively and build and maintain good relationships (relationship and problem-solving skills), and who make ethical and sensible decisions (character) are more likely perform better academically and less likely to engage in problem behaviors. Durlak et al.'s (2011) meta-analysis confirmed the effectiveness of school-based interventions to promote these competencies with effect sizes in the range of $r = .30$. They have also identified effects of after-school programs, especially those with a clear focus on SEL objectives, but with smaller effect sizes, in the range of $r = .15$. These programs tend to have positive effects on a range of outcomes, including improved academic performance and reduced problem behaviors and emotional distress.

A growing number of positive education programs have been developed, many of which draw together different positive psychology concepts into the curriculum. The Penn Resiliency Program, spearheaded by Gillham et al., developed a positive education curriculum based on cognitive-behavioral therapy for increasing mental resilience. The intervention strategies have been shown to reduce depression and associated conditions in adolescents by as much as 50% (Gilham et al., 2013; Seligman et al., 2005; Sin & Lyubomirsky, 2009). A modification of the program has been developed for the U.S. Army, following a train-the-trainer approach (i.e., train the masters in command, who in turn train army personnel under their command; Reivich, Seligman, & McBride, 2011). Evidence suggests that the program has reduced diagnoses of mental health problems and substance abuse after deployment (Harms, Herian, Krasikova, Vanhove, & Lester, 2013).

Schools are incorporating positive psychology concepts into their curricular and extracurricular areas. For instance, a secondary education program at Strath Haven High School in suburban Philadelphia integrated various positive activities into the language and literature curriculum, with a focus on developing positive emotions, meaning, and purpose and identifying and using signature strengths (Seligman et al., 2009). Wellington College in the United Kingdom includes biweekly lessons on thriving and practical living skills (Green, Oades, & Robinson, 2011). The BounceBack! program in Australia has developed various curricula for primary schools focused on coping and resilience, courage, optimism, emotion regulation, social relationships, and skills for achieving success (McGrath & Noble, 2011). Numerous programs focus on identifying, reinforcing, and using character strengths, including Happy Classrooms in Spain (Rey, Valero, Paniello, & Monge, 2012), Celebrating Strengths in the United Kingdom (Fox Eades, 2008), and Strengths Gym (Proctor et al., 2011), Strong Planet (Fox, 2008), and SMART Strengths in the United States (Yeager, Fisher, & Shearon, 2011).

Although mostly focused on curriculum, some schools are starting to approach positive education from a whole-school approach, more directly addressing the context and system of the school. For example, beginning in 2008, Geelong Grammar School in Victoria, Australia, began applying the concepts of positive psychology, focusing on six domains: positive emotions, engagement, accomplishment, purpose, relationships, and health, underpinned by character strengths (Norrish et al., 2013). Following a "live it, teach it, and embed it" framework, the program focuses first on training staff and supporting their well-being, next teaching well-being to students implicitly and explicitly, and then embedding well-being across the multiple stakeholders and policies of the school to create a culture centered on well-being. St. Peter's College, Adelaide, South Australia, similarly has incorporated a whole-school strategy by incorporating well-being into the strategy of the school, working with leadership to build top-down support, training and supporting teachers and staff, and incorporating well-being and strengths education implicitly and explicitly into curricular and extracurricular activities (Kern et al., 2015; Waters & White, 2015).

To date, few data are available that evaluate the long-term effects of these programs, but the results are promising in terms of reducing youth problems and promoting positive outcomes such as academic achievement and mental health (Gillham et al., 2013). Many of these positive strategies and positive interventions (e.g., counting our blessings exercise) are simple and ordinary and thus could be easily incorporated into various interventions, preventions, or promotion efforts in the classrooms; after-school programs; and mental health service settings. Such strategies can successfully influence emotions, peer relationships, and classroom behaviors, although what works best, for whom, when, and where is unknown. It is unlikely that a simple exercise will have much lasting impact, but as such exercises become part of the culture of the school or program, it may have an influence on mindsets, attitudes, and behaviors, with lasting impact.

Of the many thousands of youth development programs worldwide, at most several hundred have been evaluated, and only a few dozen of these evaluations satisfy rigorous methodological standards (Durlak et al., 2011). Often, the reviews conclude by identifying a small number of model programs (as judged by rigorous evaluations) that are then described in detail. Box 26.1 lists some of the frequently cited model programs and their design features. (More detailed descriptions of most of these programs as well as many others are available at http://www.casel.org/guide/programs.) These programs are not the only ones that work, but the evidence for their effectiveness is especially solid because it usually involved evaluation with random assignment, multiple outcome measures, and long-term follow-up.

Box 26.2 summarizes some of the major reviews of empirical studies of the effectiveness of youth development programs in reducing problems and/or promoting well-being. As can be seen, each of the reviews was able to point to empirical evidence that at least some programs achieved one or more of their stated goals, as shown by demonstrable effects on the outcomes of interest. These are largely consistent with the summary reports provided by Eccles and Gootman (2002), Nation et al. (2003), Park and Peterson (2004), and Durlak et al. (2011). The core messages stemming from these reviews is that well-designed and well-executed youth development programs can promote the positive and reduce the negative. However, caution is needed as there are inconsistent measures across studies, especially for positive outcomes, and in most cases long-term follow-up data (i.e., years after the program is done) are lacking. Program evaluations rarely assess fidelity of implementation; when the program turns out as not effective, it is difficult to know whether it is because the program was not implemented as intended or if there were problems with the design of the program. Further, returning to the contextual nature of positive youth development, consideration of personal and social factors that moderate program effects are needed.

In general, various youth development programs have produced positive results, but not all programs are effective. Indeed, in one large evaluation of seven youth development programs delivered to students in third through fifth grade, there was little evidence of positive

Box 26.1 Model Youth Development Programs

Big Brothers/Big Sisters (Tierney & Grossman, 2000)

- Ongoing community-based mentoring program (3–5 contact hours per week) that matches low-income children and adolescents, many from single-parent homes, with adult volunteers with the expectation that a caring and supportive relationship will develop
- Evaluated with random-assignment design, long-term follow-up
- Outcome measures included academic achievement, parental trust, violence, alcohol and drug use, truancy.

Caring School Community (Solomon, Battistich, Watson, Schaps, & Lewis, 2000)

- 25-session school-based program that targets drug use and violence through community-building exercises
- Evaluated with quasi-experimental design using multiple comparison groups, long-term follow-up
- Outcome measures included social acceptance, alcohol and drug use, loneliness, social anxiety, antisocial behavior (weapon carrying, vehicle theft).

Communities That Care (CTC) (Hawkins et al., 2007)

- A coalition-based community system operating through a five-phase process to help decision makers in the community select and implement tested, effective prevention policies and programs to be implemented
- Evaluated with random-assignment design, long-term follow-up
- Outcome measures included academic success, substance abuse, delinquency.

Penn Resiliency Program (Gillham & Reivich, 2004)

- 12-session school-based program for preventing depression among children and adolescents by teaching cognitive-behavioral skills, especially those involved in optimistic thinking
- Evaluated with random-assignment design, long-term follow-up
- Outcome measures included depression and anxiety (symptoms and diagnoses), physical health, violence, optimism.

Positive Action Program (Flay & Allred, 2010)

- A comprehensive school-based social-emotional and character development (SACD) program that consists of 140 lessons of K–12 classroom lessons (15–20 minutes daily) as well as school climate development and family and community involvement
- Evaluated with quasi-experimental and experimental design, long-term follow-up
- Outcome measures included academic achievement, problem behaviors, problem-solving skills, pro-social behavior, healthy school climate.

Promoting Alternative Thinking Strategies (PATHS) (Greenberg & Kusche, 1998)

- Multiple-year school-based program to promote social and emotional competencies and reduce problem behaviors for young children to sixth-graders from various backgrounds, such as regular education students, deaf children, and at-risk students. It has both classroom/school and parent components.
- Evaluated with a randomized controlled trial design, long-term follow-up
- Outcome measures included emotional knowledge, self-control, positive behaviors, conduct problems, skills for social planning, and social problem solving.

Quantum Opportunities Program (Hahn, Leavitt, & Aaron, 1994)

- Year-round multiple-year community-based program (750 contact hours per year) for very poor adolescents that provides educational, community service, and development activities and financial incentives for participation
- Evaluated with random-assignment design, long-term follow-up
- Outcome measures included high school graduation, college attendance, positive attitudes, volunteer work, criminal activity.

Seattle Social Development Project (Hawkins, Kosterman, Catalano, Hill, & Abbott, 2008)

- School-based program for grades one through six to promote healthy behaviors and positive social development; provides teacher training in classroom instruction and management, child social and emotional skill development, and parent training
- Evaluated with nonrandom-assignment design, 15-year long-term follow-up
- Outcome measures included functioning in school and work, mental health, sexual behavior, crime, substance use, court records.

Skills, Opportunities, and Recognition (Hawkins, Catalano, Kosterman, Abbott, & Hill, 1999)

- Multiple-year school-based program infused into the entire curriculum that targets positive development and academic competence by reducing risk factors and increasing connections to school and family; provides teacher training in classroom instruction and management, child social and emotional skill development, and parent training
- Evaluated with random-assignment design, long-term follow-up
- Outcome measures included pro-social bonds, academic achievement, commitment to school, violence, substance use, sexual behavior.

impacts, especially for high-risk students (Social and Character Development Research Consortium, 2010). Thus, there is room for improvement within current programs. Too little is known about what the critical components of successful programs are, and what the process and mechanisms are that lead to effective outcomes. Most of the programs do not separate the effects of each component of the program and do not evaluate different combinations of components. Also, although reviews found that programs benefited children from diverse geographic, socioeconomic, and racial, ethnic, and cultural backgrounds, more research is needed to understand how programs uniquely work for children with special challenges such as parent divorce, poverty, and disabilities and how to improve their effectiveness for the children's social and emotional well-being.

And what about communities? Epidemiologic research tells us that problems are more likely to occur in some communities than others, but the studies are not fine-grained, and in any event we know that problems co-occur. Not enough is known about the features of community settings that help youth thrive in all the ways that we have described, with a few exceptions (e.g., Theokas & Lerner, 2006). It is disappointing that in the extensive study of positive youth development in youth participating in various after-school activities, greater participation in school and after-school activities in resource-poor communities was associated with increased risky behavior in boys and greater depression in girls (Phelps et al., 2007). These findings suggest that despite the best efforts of positive youth development programs, the obstacles posed by poor communities can outweigh the potential benefits of those programs.

TAKING STOCK OF WHAT WE KNOW

Over the past three decades, advances in research and practices have bolstered our understanding of various individual and contextual factors linked to youth's health and well-being, as well as effective ways to cultivate them. Labels vary, but there is general agreement about the positive characteristics of youth. These characteristics exist in degrees, not types. Children and adolescents are not simply doing well or doing poorly; they range and move along a spectrum. Accordingly, we need to take a broad and nuanced view of the goals of positive youth development. Indicators and indices of positive youth development must do more than ascertain the absence of disorder and distress; they must also promote the existence and cultivation of wellness and hope. Much more work needs to be done to craft generally useful measures of positive constructs, and to see that these are routinely used in evaluations of youth programs (Lippman, Moore, & Mcintosh, 2011; Moore, Lippman, & Brown, 2004).

Box 26.2 Reviews of Empirical Studies of Youth Development Programs

Berkowitz & Bier (2007)

- Reviewed 78 studies of different character education programs; included only studies with character-relevant outcomes, comparison groups, and pre-to-post (change) data
- Results: Total 51% of targeted outcomes were significantly impacted by programs, with 62% of "head" (knowledge and reasoning), 49% of "hand" (action), and 45% of "heart" (caring) outcomes.

CASEL (2003)

- Reviewed 242 school-based programs whose descriptions were rated by experts as satisfying the principles of how to impart social and emotional intelligence, and in particular the 80 programs that covered multiple years
- Results: The review identified the 22 most effective and comprehensive SEL programs. Effective programs improved sense of connection to school, self-regulation, character development, responsibility, skills for goal setting and problem solving, and academic achievement.

Catalano, Berglund, Ryan, Lonczak, & Hawkins (2004)

- Reviewed 77 promotion programs for youth, and 25 in detail; included only programs with comparison groups and at least one significant result
- Results: 76% of programs improved positive behaviors, including interpersonal skills, quality of relationships, self-control, problem solving, competencies, self-efficacy, commitment to schooling, and academic achievement. 96% of programs reduced problem behaviors, including smoking, drug and alcohol use, school misbehavior, aggressive behavior, truancy, and high-risk sexual behavior. Two thirds of the effective programs operated in multiple settings including the school, the family, and the community. Programs with multiple methods, multiple components, and longer, structured, and consistent delivery were more effective.

Durlak, Weissberg, & Pachan (2010)

- Reviewed 68 after-school programs that offer activities between the ages of 5 and 18; included only programs with comparison groups and with the promotion of personal and social development as goals, about 35% with randomized design
- Results: Only SAFE (sequenced, active, focused, and explicit) programs were associated with significant reductions in conduct problems and drug use, and improvements in self-perceptions, school bonding, positive social behaviors, school attendance, and academic achievement. Of the 68 programs, 60% were identified as SAFE programs.

Durlak, Weissberg, Dymnicki, Taylor, & Schellinger (2011)

- Reviewed 213 school-based, universal SEL programs for youth between the ages of 5 and 18 without adjustment or learning problems; included only programs with comparison groups, about 47% with random assignment
- Results: Programs improved students' social and emotional skills, attitudes toward self and others, positive social behaviors, and academic performance, and decreased problem behaviors and emotional distress. The SAFE (sequenced, active, focused, and explicit) practices moderated program outcomes.

Gavin, Catalano, David-Ferdon, Gloppen, & Markham (2010)

- Reviewed 30 positive youth development programs that offer activities to foster general positive youth development outcomes in multiple socialization domains; included studies with experimental or quasi-experimental evaluation design
- Results: 50% of programs had evidence of moderate and sustained effects on improving adolescent sexual and reproductive health outcomes. Effective programs significantly strengthened the school context and delivered activities in a supportive way. Effective programs

also tended to empower youth, engage youth in real activities, improve relationships and bonding, strengthen the family, build new skills, and communicate expectations clearly, and were relatively longer in duration.

Greenberg, Domitrovich, & Bumbarger (1999)

- Started with 130 prevention programs that were either universal (targeting all youth), selective (targeting at-risk youth), or indicated (targeting youth showing early signs of disorders but not meeting diagnostic criteria) and reviewed 34 in detail that included a comparison group, pre- and post-test measures, and a written manual specifying theory and procedures
- Results: Short-term prevention programs produce short-term benefits, while multiple-year programs fostered lasting effects on reducing internal and external problems. For at-risk or serious problems groups, ongoing programs starting in the preschool and early elementary years were more effective at reducing resistance and morbidity. Programs focusing on risk and protective factors were more effective than categorical problem behaviors. Effective programs were directed at changing multiple domains including family, school, and community as well as individuals.

Hattie, Neill, & Richards (1997)

- Reviewed 96 evaluations of adventure programs (e.g., Outward Bound) and excluded nine as being of poor scientific quality. Also excluded school-based programs as insufficiently challenging. Included only programs that had comparison groups, adequate measures, and detailed methodological descriptions.
- Results: The greatest effects on outcomes related to a sense of control, self-regulation, self-confidence, self-understanding, decision making, and responsibility; the effects were long-lasting and the gains were sustained. Selective programs with older participants, longer program length, and quality of instructors were effective.

Nelson, Westhues, & Macleod (2004)

- Reviewed 34 programs for at-risk preschoolers in terms of positive and negative outcomes classified as cognitive or socioemotional. Included studies with comparison groups and long-term follow-ups.
- Results: Cognitive impacts were at kindergarten to eighth grade, with the greatest in the preschool period. Socioemotional impacts were at kindergarten to eighth grade and high school, and parent/family wellness impacts were at preschool and kindergarten to eighth grade.

Roth & Brooks-Gunn (2003)

- Drawing on earlier reviews to identify programs, these researchers evaluated 48 studies of programs that targeted one or more of these positive youth outcomes; notable was the attempt to categorize programs according to program goals, program atmosphere, and program activities, and relate these features to effectiveness.
- Results: All programs with enhancing competency, character building, and caring goals, 68% of programs with confidence goals, and 54% of programs with connections goals were met with success. For the success of programs, atmosphere and activities of programs were not important, but modest goals of programs were.

Roth, Brooks-Gunn, Murray, & Foster (1998)

- Reviewed 60 community-based prevention and intervention programs for youth and selected 15 for their final review; included only studies with comparison groups
- Results: Long-term programs with more elements that engaged youth and viewed young people as resources were the most effective. Resistance skills-based prevention programs were the least effective. A caring adult–adolescent relationship was proven to be important in the positive youth development outcomes.

Importantly for the purpose of this volume, positive characteristics *can* buffer against the development of the most common psychological disorders among youth (Gillham et al., 2013; Pollard et al., 1999). There is the potential to immunize youth against ever experiencing mental disorder, or at least minimizing the severity of disorders that might occur. SEL programs and early successes in positive education further suggest the value of incorporating positive development within and outside of schools. Empirical reviews and meta-analyses suggest that comprehensive and well-integrated positive youth development programs contribute to youth well-being and health by reducing unhealthy behaviors and emotional problems, while cultivating and improving social skills, pro-social behaviors, competencies, positive relationships, and learning (Durlak et al., 2010, 2011). Furthermore, there is agreement that we can encourage optimal development through youth programs, either those that already exist (e.g., Big Brothers/Big Sisters) or those explicitly designed by psychologists, prevention scientists, and youth development practitioners for this purpose.

Despite some limitations, there are several common threads across reviews about what makes programs more effective. There is generally agreement that programs are apt to be most successful—increasing positive outcomes and reducing negative outcomes—if they have the following features:

1. **More is better.** Longer-term programs are more effective. Hour-long or weekend workshops are not effective interventions; however, programs in which youth spend more extended periods of time are likely to be more effective in reducing negative outcomes and encouraging positive outcomes. However, the frequency and the intensity of intervention needed to achieve success is unknown. This is important to resolve, given the limited resources typically available in schools and other settings (Roth, Malone, & Brooks-Gunn, 2010).
2. **Begin early, but with appropriate timing**. In general, the most effective programs do not wait for their participants to enter adolescence, but begin with younger children (cf. Zigler & Berman, 1983). As a preventive approach, the more that youth can learn before entering rocky periods of life, the greater skills and resources they will have to buffer and face stresses that occur. However, the optimal range of ages remains unclear (Nelson, Westhues, & MacLeod, 2004). Interventions and programs need to be developmentally appropriate. Any program that requires metacognitive skills on the part of participants needs to be sure that these skills exist (e.g., Gillham & Reivich, 2004). In the preschool years, for instance, it might be most beneficial to target parents and caregivers rather than the youth themselves. Care needs to be taken that youth do not become bored, lest the programs backfire and lead to rebellion. And some preventive programs might be best at the ages when youth are encountering triggers. For example, one meta-analysis found that eating disorder prevention programs had larger effects for participants over age 15 (Stice & Shaw, 2004).
3. **Structured and accurate.** Effective programs have a clear plan that is monitored on an ongoing basis, and are implemented with fidelity. Practices that use the sequenced, active, focused, and explicit (SAFE) approach (i.e., they provide youth with an opportunity for active involvement, have explicit goals, and focus on reaching them) tend to be more effective (Bond & Hauf, 2004; Durlak, 1997; Durlak et al., 2011; Dusenbury & Falco, 1995). Manuals that spell out the program components in detail are helpful for maintaining program fidelity.
4. **Supportive.** The best programs are those in which youth have at least one supportive relationship with an adult. Successful programs focus on building supportive

relationships between youth participants and group leaders, teachers, and parents.

5. **Active.** The most effective programs actively teach skills related to the target outcome through hands-on and minds-on engagement. Youth need to be empowered to take control of their own learning, well-being, and development.
6. **Broad.** The most effective programs target several systems simultaneously, such as home and school. General life skills provide a broader base of influence than specific resistance skills. Programs that work best provide ways for youth to think differently and also to act differently.
7. **Contextually relevant.** Programs work best when they are tailored to the cultural background of their participants and take a sophisticated "person-in-environment" approach. They do not address just internal factors like character strengths, and they do not address just external factors like school safety. Instead, they address both.
8. **Theory-based.** Programs work best when guided by explicit theories about the causes of outcomes and the mechanisms of change. A working theory or model informs the structure of the program, the activities used, outcomes of interest, and measures of success.
9. **Multipronged.** Effective programs use multiple components that intervene at various levels: individual, teacher, family, friends, school, and community. They also use various strategies (e.g., classroom learning, after-school programs, activities) that enhance social, emotional, behavioral, cognitive, and moral competencies.

WHAT WE NEED TO KNOW

These broad principles of "what works" give some guidance, but there is much we do not know, in large part due to lack of rigorous evaluations, inadequate measurement, and the complexity of factors involved in development. Although evaluations suggest statistically significant improvements, the size of such effects is unclear. We do not know which features are more versus less important in producing outcomes, which combination might be needed, the timing involved, or individual and social moderators. We do not know if promotion programs help troubled youth as much as they help youth in general, although violence prevention programs and eating disorder prevention programs seem more successful when they target at-risk individuals (e.g., Stice & Shaw, 2004). Further, almost nothing is known about the cost-effectiveness of different programs (or program features) with respect to various outcomes (see Newman, Smith, & Murphy, 2000).

To provide guidance for future research, we propose two areas of studies that would advance our knowledge and practice of positive youth development vis-à-vis mental health and mental illness.

The Natural History of Positive Youth Development

What is a healthy and thriving youth? We have concluded that the positive perspective provides a consensual answer to this question, but it is only a snapshot. We know relatively little about who these young people are except that they can be found in all walks of life. We need detailed descriptions of youth who are naturally doing well—where they come from, where they go, what choices they make, and what routes they take in between. A good first step has been taken by studies already under way that use existing samples followed over many years (e.g., Hawkins et al., 1992). For example, the Terman Life Cycle Study (a prospective longitudinal study that followed gifted individuals from childhood through death; Friedman & Martin, 2011) and the Harvard Grant Study (a prospective study of Harvard graduates followed across their lives; Vaillant, 2012) have provided in-depth descriptions of people's lives, with in-depth characterizations of factors that influence health, well-being, career success, societal contribution, and social relationships.

Numerous archival datasets, with both quantitative and qualitative information, large samples, longitudinal designs, and multiwave assessments, are increasingly available. Secondary analysis of archival data will be useful for understanding trajectories, key turning points, and mechanisms and moderators of positive development. However, it will be important for studies to incorporate youth from a broad range of socioeconomic backgrounds.

Beyond existing data, additional measures can be added to ongoing longitudinal studies. Such studies should include measures of positive characteristics (positive emotions, flow, character strengths, positive relationships, skills, talents, and life purposes), measures of risk, and measures of problems (negative emotions, risky behaviors, symptoms, and psychological disorders). That is, the full spectrum of psychosocial function and behaviors should be included. It would be a shame if the positive psychology perspective leads researchers to repeat the error of business-as-usual psychology by ruling out a balanced view of youth and the adults they become. Including both positive and negative measures over time allows the critical questions we have posed to be answered with hard data (cf. deVries, 1992). Do positive characteristics preclude recurrence of problems? Do they limit them? Do they allow youth to learn lessons from crises, episodes of disorder, and misfortunes? Which positive characteristics provide the best buffers against depression, substance abuse, or anxiety disorders?

The data from such studies can be productively examined with the techniques of causal modeling that use statistical techniques to evaluate the adequacy of causal relationships between variables (e.g., Connell, Gambone, & Smith, 2000; Gambone, 1997; Halpern, Barker, & Mollard, 2000; Walker, 2001). Sample sizes must be large enough, especially to discern interactions between and among variables. But with adequately powered designs, these models allow inferences about what might prevent what and why. As already emphasized, explicit theory is imperative to specify hypothesized links prior to causal modeling.

Although studies often rely on quantitative data, qualitative information can highlight narratives of life. Realistic portrayals of young people, including their flaws and problems and how they cope with them, might inspire other teenagers to focus on what they do well and to eschew a victim mentality (Shih, 2004). There are plenty of examples, in the past and the present, of people who live successful personal and professional lives while they live with mental disorders. Deserving of study are the more mundane among us who go to school or show up at work or raise our families even when we are depressed or anxious. What is their everyday life like? How do they deal with challenges and difficulties? How and why are some people with mental disorders better adapted than the others?

Dissemination of information about youth who are thriving might help combat negative stereotypes about teenagers. For example, a retrospective study conducted with several thousand adults asked respondents if they had ever experienced a severe psychological disorder, and if so, how well they had recovered from it (Peterson, Park, & Seligman, 2006). The study also measured their life satisfaction and various strengths of character. Individuals who had fully recovered from a disorder were just as satisfied with their lives as those who had never experienced a disorder. At least for some, there is light at the end of the psychopathology tunnel: "'Tis an ill wind that blows no good." And individuals who had fully recovered from a disorder also reported higher levels of appreciation of beauty, bravery, creativity, curiosity, forgiveness, gratitude, love of learning, and spirituality, compared to those who had never experienced a psychological disorder. Whether these character strengths were in place before the disorder and helped in recovery or whether they represent lessons learned during difficult days is unclear from the research design, but the need for a richer prospective study is implied.

Positive Interventions for At-Risk and Troubled Youth

With respect to needed intervention studies, we believe that there are two promising research avenues to pursue. First, *positive prevention* would use already-established best-practice youth development interventions to help at-risk youth. Although we know that these interventions in general make disorder less likely, we need to know more about why and how prevention works when it does, especially among those at risk. We have proposed that positive prevention programs are effective because they cultivate the ingredients of the good life, such as positive emotions, strengths of character, competencies, and social engagement. An opposing hypothesis is that prevention only works when it undoes biological risks to disorder. By this view, the cultivation of the positive should be irrelevant in predicting who benefits from prevention programs, especially in the long run.

The questions of immediate interest are who does or does not develop a disorder and whether some disorders are more easily prevented than others. But we are also interested in what happens to those youth who do develop a disorder in spite of the interventions. Some will show recurrent problems, and some will not. What predicts differing courses following initial episodes? The positive psychology prediction is that even if cultivated positive characteristics do not prevent a disorder, they might well limit recurrence and allow the eventual achievement of a good life.

Second, *positive rehabilitation* again uses existing best-practice youth development programs with troubled teens during or after an episode. With adults, numerous reviews find that psychotherapy is as effective, if not more so, than pharmacological approaches, depending on the type of disorder, therapy, and drug (e.g., Anderson et al., 2008; Casacalenda, Perry, & Looper, 2002; Steinbrueck, Maxwell, & Howard, 1983). However, most adults with serious mental disorders can also expect to be in and out of treatment for the rest of their lives. At its worst, this phenomenon is dubbed "revolving-door psychiatry." Even at its best, this phenomenon leads to perpetual aftercare in the form of support groups, booster psychotherapy sessions, and/or prophylactic medication (Weissman, 1994). Further, among adults, it seems clear that prognosis worsens with age for almost all psychological disorders (e.g., Seivewright, Tyrer, & Johnson, 1998). Although the apparent magnitude of this effect may be an artifact of studying patient samples rather than community samples, past psychological problems remain the best predictor of future psychological problems.

Matters may be different for young people. A depressed middle-aged adult will likely become depressed again, no matter how effective treatment may be in the short term, but young people who become depressed may not become depressed again if early intervention takes place (e.g., Birmaher, Arbelaez, & Brent, 2002; Clarke et al., 2001; Lewinsohn, Pettit, Joiner, & Seeley, 2003; but cf. Weissman et al., 1999). The same is true for many other problems, such as anxiety disorders (Dadds et al., 1999). Indeed, among adolescents showing early (prodromal) symptoms of schizophrenia, early intervention may help stave off the full-blown disorder (Cannon et al., 2002; Harrigan, McGorry, & Krstev, 2003; McGorry et al., 2002; Phillips, Yung, Yuen, Pantelis, & McGorry, 2002). And it is clear that many teenagers experiment with drugs or alcohol without dooming themselves to a life in recovery (Spooner, Mattick, & Noffs, 2001). At least for some young people and for some disorders, it becomes meaningful to speak of curing mental illness, which provides a powerful rationale for the focus on youth taken by this volume.

We know that some youth who enter the mental health system are successfully treated and are never seen again, just as we know that the majority of young people who enter the juvenile justice system never return again (Snyder & Sickmund, 1999). The skeptic might argue that these cases are not really cures—maybe the initial diagnoses were simply wrong, maybe the problems recurred but further treatment was not sought, and so on. The positive perspective suggests that we take this phenomenon at face value and fill in its details with the facts. The natural history studies we have proposed would begin to yield critical information about single-episode individuals.

Why are young people different? We speculate that it is not age per se that is the crucial factor but rather the number of untreated episodes someone experiences and the psychosocial consequences of these episodes that determine long-term prognosis—the doors closed by lost time, missed opportunities, and pervasive stigma. Indeed, the more episodes of a disorder, the greater the likelihood of still more episodes and the worse the prognosis for an individual. If this downward spiral can be interrupted early enough, perhaps the business of life can take over as a curative agent.

Consistent with this analysis, Joiner (2000) grappled with the self-propagating nature of depression and argued that interpersonal processes like excessive reassurance seeking and conflict avoidance are largely responsible for its persistence and/or recurrence. Other interpersonal processes by implication set the person on a different course that entails true recovery. Perhaps youth development programs and positive interventions can preclude recurrence of depression—and other psychological problems—by imparting appropriate strengths and competencies on which the person can rely when troubled. To the degree that young people have more life satisfaction, greater character strengths, and better social support and are more engaged with learning and new experiences, they may be set for an upward spiral of positive life experiences and experience fewer problems in the wake of difficulties.

The studies of positive rehabilitation that we propose would go further in trying to influence prognosis by deliberately cultivating the ingredients of a healthy life. In the field of positive psychology, there has been some success with positive psychotherapy, which incorporates positive psychology concepts into clinical work. Positive psychotherapy accentuates the positive resources that clients have for treating psychopathology (Rashid, 2015; Seligman, Rashid, & Parks, 2006). It assumes that people inherently desire growth and happiness, that strengths are authentic and real, and that therapeutic relationships can focus on strengths and use of resources, not just weakness and distress. Validation studies to date provide early evidence for the effectiveness of this approach.

Further, studies of *psychosocial rehabilitation* for troubled youths add additional support for such an approach. Psychosocial rehabilitation embraces an educational model, as opposed to a disease model, attempting to teach psychological and social skills that facilitate productive community reintegration of youth following treatment (Byalin, Smith, Chatkin, & Wilmot, 1987; Fruedenberger & Carbone, 1984). Such programs are effective in reducing recurrence of a variety of problems and appear to be cost-effective (e.g., Barasch, 1994; Mishna, Michalski, & Cummings, 2001; Rund et al., 1994). The positive psychology perspective goes beyond typical psychosocial rehabilitation to specify the active ingredients that allow imparted skills to be deployed to best effect.

Studies of positive rehabilitation would use the same general research design already sketched for studies of positive prevention: randomly assign research participants—in this case adolescents with disorders—to intervention and comparison groups, and do a thorough assessment of both positive and negative characteristics before, during, and after the intervention. Measures of perceived stigma would be an informative addition to the assessment battery. Those in comparison groups would of course receive conventional (business-as-usual) aftercare. Both specific and general programs should be included. It might also be of interest to see if the timing of positive rehabilitation matters: should it begin during treatment of a disorder (in the middle of the episode) or following symptom relief (after the episode)?

Studies of positive prevention and especially positive rehabilitation for youth would represent a strong test of the perspective put forward here. If the positive perspective on youth development has legs, it should be able to move young people not only from +2 to +5, but also from −3 to +5—and to keep them there.

CONCLUSION

Research findings over the past three decades have brought empirical support for key premises of positive youth development and provided important insights into what constitutes positive youth development and what individual and contextual factors might relate to youth thriving. The goal of positive youth development goes beyond merely surviving in the face of adversity to thriving. Evidence is accumulating that positive characteristics play important roles in positive youth development, not only as protective factors, preventing or mitigating psychological and behavior problems, but also as enabling conditions that promote resilience and a flourishing life. These sets of positive characteristics can be cultivated by appropriate parenting, schooling, various youth development programs, and caring communities.

Future studies will continue to refine measures and to use empirical findings to understand its development, effective interventions, and the processes that give rise to positive development. All young people with or without problems have unique strengths and the capacity to grow. It is our responsibility to help them to realize their potentials and build a life worth living for themselves and for society.

GLOSSARY

5 C's – system of five positive qualities (connection, competence, character, caring, and confidence) that should be promoted in young people, according to positive youth development theory and scholarship, resulting in a sixth C, contribution

Bioecological approach – Bronfenbrenner's approach to development emphasizing the multiple contexts in which behavior occurs

Caring – the ability to sympathize and empathize with others

Character – a moral and ethical disposition that respects cultural and societal values

Character strengths – positive traits (individual differences) like curiosity, kindness, hope, and teamwork that contribute to fulfillment

Competence – having a positive view of oneself across social, emotional, cognitive, and vocational domains

Competencies – social, emotional, cognitive, behavioral, and moral abilities

Confidence – an internal sense of self-efficacy and self-worth

Connection – bidirectional emotional and committed bonds between a youth and others in the family, peer group, school, community, or culture

Contribution – productive involvement in the community, which is seen as an outgrowth of successful development

Engagement – a multidimensional characteristic, with definitions including a capacity to become absorbed and focused on what one is doing (cognitive), involvement and interesting life activities and tasks (behavioral), and commitment, passion, enthusiasm, focused effort, and energy (psychological/ affective)

Flourishing – feeling good and functioning well, which combines high levels of mental health and low levels of (or absent) mental illness

Flow – psychological state that accompanies highly engaging activities

Gratitude – a positive emotion or a life orientation that involves noticing and appreciating positives in the world

Grit – the tenacious pursuit of an overarching goal, despite setbacks that might occur along the way

Growth mindset – a tendency to view intelligence as malleable and developed through effort and learning

Hope – a characteristic that involves having goals for the future, motivation or agency to move toward them, and pathways to achieve them

Life satisfaction – overall judgment that one's life is going well

Meaning in life – having a sense of direction in life, feeling connected to something larger than oneself, or long-term aspirations that align with one's values and motivate activity

Optimism – a generalized favorable expectation about the future

Perseverance – the ability to focus on longer-term or superordinate goals and stick with the pursuit of these goals over time, despite setbacks and obstacles that occur along the way

Positive education – application of positive psychology in educational settings; combines positive psychology concepts with best-practice guidelines from education and learning

Positive emotions – emotions like joy, contentment, and love that are thought to "broaden and build" cognitive and behavioral repertoires

Positive prevention – positive youth development programs that prevent problems by encouraging assets

Positive psychology – a scientific, strengths-based approach that examines optimal functioning and aims to discover and promote factors that allow individuals, organizations, and communities to thrive

Positive rehabilitation – positive youth development programs that promote recovery by encouraging assets

Positive youth development – umbrella term for approaches that recognize and encourage what is good in young people

Prevention programs – interventions that prevent problems

Promotion programs – interventions that promote well-being

Resiliency – quality that enables young people to thrive in the face of adversity

Self-control – the ability to regulate attention, emotion, and/or behavior, despite temptation

Social-emotional learning (SEL) – the process of acquiring social and emotional skills in five domains: self-awareness, social awareness, responsible decision making, self-management, and relationships management

Subjective well-being – often used interchangeably with flourishing; high life satisfaction and positive affect and low negative affect

ACKNOWLEDGMENTS

Remembering Christopher Peterson: "Other People Matter" On October 9, 2012, the world lost a distinguished scholar, inspirational teacher, and wonderful human being. Chris Peterson provided much of the initial vision, contents, and structure of this chapter. The Commission on Positive Youth Development is indebted to him for his leadership, intellectual contribution, generosity, and, most of all, friendship. He not only studied and taught but also lived out positive psychology—the scientific study of "what makes life worth living"—in all that he did. He had a rare combination of intellectual rigor, warmth, generosity, integrity, humility, and a gentle sense of humor. Although his sudden passing was a great loss for the field of positive psychology and all those who were touched through his life, his scholarly and personal contributions will continue to inspire and guide all those who care about studying and living the life worth living. He coined the phrase "Other people matter" as a vital ingredient for good life. Other people matter to him, and he to others.

Other Behavioral Disorders

Amy Bleakley
Jeffrey L. Derevensky
Lynette Gilbeau
Sunhee Park
Daniel Romer

VIII

part

Adolescent Gambling

Jeffrey L. Derevensky
Lynette Gilbeau

chapter 27

OVERVIEW

The landscape of gambling throughout the world continues to evolve, with more states and countries expanding gambling opportunities. This has resulted in a significant increase in availability, more diversity, and alternative types of gambling opportunities, with easier accessibility for both adults and youth. What began with state-sponsored lotteries in the United States (44 states currently operate a lottery) and a limited number of casinos in Nevada and New Jersey has mushroomed, with the number of gambling opportunities (lotteries, casinos, poker parlors, gambling machines, horse and dog tracks, sports wagering, online gambling) throughout the United States and worldwide increasing exponentially during the past decade. No longer do individuals have to travel considerable distances or even venture outside of their homes to place a wager. Gamblers can bet on a wide diversity of activities and games via the Internet on their computer or smartphone using gambling apps, online wagering, and state-supported games. During the past decade, gambling has been one of the fastest changing and growing industries in the world. While some jurisdictions (e.g., Atlantic City) have showed declines in gambling revenues, these revenues have been accounted for by increases in neighboring states. Gambling opportunities have become so widespread that it is difficult to find jurisdictions in which some form of gambling is not controlled, regulated, organized, or owned by the government. Internationally, gambling has become a socially acceptable pastime and form of entertainment despite the recognized social and personal costs associated with excessive problematic gambling.

ADOLESCENT GAMBLING

While gambling has been traditionally viewed as an adult activity, there is a growing body of research suggesting its popularity among adolescents (Derevensky, 2012; Volberg, Gupta, Griffiths, Olason, & Delfabbro, 2010). This is likely a result of gambling's general social acceptability, governmental support and regulation, advertisements, the glitz and glamour associated with casinos, and the way in which gambling has been positively portrayed in the media. With television shows and movies depicting its glamour and excitement (e.g., *21*, *Runner Runner*, *Casino Royale*, *Rounders*, *Vegas*, *The Gambler*) and televised world championship poker tournaments where young people win millions of dollars (the recent World Series of Poker multimillion-dollar tournament winners have most often been in their twenties), gambling has grown in popularity among youth. The perceived ease of becoming wealthy without working has resulted in gambling taking on a new level of status among adolescents. Even though almost all jurisdictions prohibit children and adolescents from engaging in government-sponsored and/or -regulated forms of gambling (e.g., lottery, casinos, horse racing, machine gambling, online wagering), many young people continue to be actively engaged in both regulated and nonregulated (e.g., card games and sports wagering among peers, fantasy sports leagues) forms of gambling.

Research studies throughout North America, Europe, Asia, and Australasia all suggest gambling's popularity among adolescents. Survey and prevalence findings examining youth gambling behavior have consistently revealed that adolescents (12–17 years of age) have managed to participate, to some degree, in practically all forms of social, government-sanctioned, and nonregulated gambling available in their homes and communities (Volberg et al., 2010). Typical forms of gambling among teens include card playing for money (poker, while waning, is still popular), sports wagering, dice, and board games with family and friends; betting with peers on games of personal skill (e.g., pool, bowling, basketball and other sports); playing arcade or video games for money; and purchasing lottery tickets (especially scratch-off tickets). While some youth engage in other forms of gambling, such as wagering at horse and dog tracks, gambling in bingo halls and card rooms, gambling on electronic gambling machines (slot machines, video poker machines), sports wagering through a bookmaker, and wagering via Internet gambling sites, these are more often limited due to age and accessibility (Derevensky, 2012; Derevensky & Gupta, 2007; Griffiths & Parke, 2010; Griffiths & Wood, 2007; Jacobs, 2004; Jackson, Dowling, Thomas, Bond & Patton, 2008; Productivity Commission, 2010; Volberg et al., 2010; Wardle et al., 2011; Welte, Barnes, Tidwell & Hoffman, 2008). A recent study from the United Kingdom suggests that one in six children ages 11 to 15 had spent their own money on gambling in the last week; however, the overall self-reported rate of gambling among 11- to 15-year-olds has remained relatively static over time despite the increased availability of different forms of gambling (Ipsos MORI, 2014). In the United Kingdom, "fruit machines" (low-cost slot machines that are legal without any age restrictions) remain the most popular form of gambling among youngsters, followed by placing a bet and playing cards for money with friends. A relatively small percentage of youth participate in lottery activities (6%).

Adolescents' wagering behaviors have often been found to depend on a number of factors, including the following:

- Local availability and accessibility of games
- Geographic proximity of gaming locations
- Gender (male teens tend to gamble more frequently and for larger amounts of money and are more actively engaged in sports wagering, whereas female adolescents prefer purchasing lottery tickets and playing bingo)
- Age restrictions (lottery purchases typically have a lower age limit than casino entry; older adolescents and young adults prefer machine gambling, poker, and casino games)
- Cultural ethnicity (see Abbott, Volberg, Bellringer, & Reith, 2004; National Research Council, 1999; Productivity Commission, 2010; Volberg et al., 2010; Wardle et al., 2011)

While there is ample research suggesting that adolescents typically have gambled for money sometime before reaching 18 years of age, most teens do so occasionally with few gambling and/or gambling-related problems. Adolescent gambling behavior, similar to adult gambling behavior, can be viewed on a continuum ranging from not gambling at all, to social/occasional/recreational gambling, to problem/pathological/disordered gambling (DSM-5 now refers to the most serious form of gambling problems as *disordered gambling*). In the adolescent gambling literature, the terms *social, occasional, nonproblematic,* and *recreational gambling* have typically been used to denote occasional, infrequent use where the individual is experiencing relatively few gambling-related problems. Those adolescents deemed to be at risk for a gambling disorder begin exhibiting some gambling-related problems yet fail to reach the clinical level identified in the DSM-5. The terms *disordered, problem, pathological,* and *compulsive gambling* are used to denote behaviors reaching the clinical criteria and most often result in severe psychosocial, behavioral, economic, interpersonal, mental health, and legal difficulties.

ADOLESCENT PROBLEM/DISORDERED GAMBLING

While most adolescents gamble occasionally for money and don't experience significant problems, there is a large body of research suggesting that adolescents as a developmental group constitute a high-risk population for gambling problems (Abbott et al., 2004; Derevensky, 2012; National Research Council, 1999; Volberg et al., 2010; Wardle et al., 2011; Welte et al., 2008). Volberg et al. (2010), while noting significant methodological differences in prevalence studies, concluded that between 60% and 80% of adolescents report having engaged in some form of gambling for money during the past year (depending on age and accessibility), with most of these adolescents being social, recreational, and occasional gamblers. However, they also noted that prevalence studies have revealed that between 2% and 8% of adolescents report experiencing serious gambling problems, with another 10% to 15% being at risk for the development of a gambling problem. The prevalence rates for adolescent problem gambling are two to four times that of adults. Further, there is considerable research pointing to young adults (ages 18–25) experiencing the highest prevalence of gambling problems among adults (National Research Council, 1999; Productivity Commission, 2010).

Interestingly, despite the increased diversity of gambling activities and their increased availability and accessibility, these prevalence rates have remained relatively constant for the past two decades and in some cases may have actually declined. There is certainly evidence that cultural, regional, and ethnic differences may impact the prevalence rates (Volberg et al., 2010). However, as the population of young people increases, the absolute number of individuals with gambling problems increases despite stable prevalence rates.

Adolescents with gambling problems have been reported to experience a wide range of social, economic, personal, academic, mental health, familial, criminal, delinquent, and legal problems. They also have increased rates of suicide ideation and attempts, and difficult peer relationships resulting from their gambling. All of these behaviors place the adolescent with gambling problems at high risk for a diversity of mental health issues (Derevensky, 2012; Derevensky & Gupta, 2004; Derevensky, Pratt, Hardoon, & Gupta, 2007; Dickson, Derevensky, & Gupta, 2008; Felsher, Derevensky, & Gupta, 2010; Griffiths, King, & Delfabbro, 2009; Hardoon et al., 2002, 2004; Petry, 2005; Shead et al., 2010; Winters & Anderson, 2000).

Problem gambling among adolescents is typically marked by the following:

- Being preoccupied with gambling
- Attempting to recoup losses
- Increasing wagers
- Lying to family members, peers, and friends about their gambling
- Exhibiting anxiety and/or depression when trying to reduce their gambling

Adolescents with a severe gambling disorder frequently report using gambling as a coping mechanism to escape daily problems (familial, peer, and school-related). Given that gambling by its nature requires increasing amounts of money, many youth acquire their funds illegally, often stealing money from family members (who are reluctant to report such thefts to the police) and sometimes resorting to criminal behavior outside of their home. These adolescents may also borrow large sums of money from friends, peers, and loan sharks. The adolescent's preoccupation with gambling and the necessity to recoup losses becomes paramount. Other behaviors can include a preoccupation with watching TV shows or movies with gambling themes, playing online social casino games for virtual currency (to improve their skills), and reading books related to gambling strategies (Derevensky, 2012).

Pathological/disordered gamblers are not a homogeneous group; for instance, sports gamblers are often different from poker players, who are different from casino gamblers. Also, some types or forms of gambling, due to their structural or situational factors, may be more problematic and symptomatic of problem gamblers. Slot machines and electronic gambling machines, for example, have been called the "crack cocaine" of gambling because they are designed to result in repetitive play (Schüll, 2012).

There is little doubt that the vast majority of adolescent gamblers will ultimately wind up losing their money. Why, then, do some individuals continue to gamble in spite of repeated losses? In a number of studies, we found that the predominant reason youth report gambling is for the enjoyment, excitement, and entertainment associated with gambling. While making money is not necessarily the primary reason initially given for gambling, it often propels problem gamblers to keep wagering in order to recoup their losses and "get even." Similarly, as the thrill and exhilaration associated with gambling plateau, to keep it exciting and maintain or enhance the adrenaline rush derived from gambling, gamblers must increase both the frequency and amounts of money wagered. This typically accounts for the increasing escalation of wagers, which ultimately results in increased losses (Derevensky, 2012; Derevensky & Gupta, 2004).

Other factors have also been shown to account for gamblers' continued play. Stinchfield (2000) has suggested that adolescents may be engaging in this behavior as a form of experimenting with adult behaviors. Derevensky (2012) has speculated that gambling in general may be conceived as a rite of passage. Most adolescents report gambling for multiple reasons (see Derevensky, 2012; Shead, Derevensky, & Gupta, 2010 for reviews), such as the following:

For the competition
As a potential profession
To fulfill mental health needs (e.g., coping with adversity, escaping from daily stressors, reducing anxiety and depression)
To facilitate peer relationships and socialization
To escape from boredom
To relieve loneliness
To pass time
To help with financial pressures or difficulties

Adolescent problem gamblers typically report an early age of onset (approximately 10 or 11 years of age) compared with peers who report gambling but have few gambling-related problems (Derevensky & Gupta, 2001; Gupta & Derevensky, 1997, 1998b; Productivity Commission, 2010; Vitaro, Wanner, Ladouceur, et al., 2004; Volberg et al., 2010; Wynne et al., 1996). Among adolescents, there often is a rapid movement from social/occasional/recreational gambling to problem/disordered gambling (Derevensky & Gupta, 1999; Gupta & Derevensky, 1998a; Volberg et al., 2010). These youth frequently report having had an early "big win" during their early gambling experiences (the size of the win can vary considerably, and the perception of a "big win" often depends on age and socioeconomic status) (Gupta & Derevensky, 1997; Productivity Commission, 1999; Wynne et al., 1996).

Pathological/disordered gamblers' initial gambling experiences often occur with family members at home (Gupta & Derevensky, 1997), with both parents and older siblings having an early influence. It is not atypical for parents to report giving their children a scratch-off lottery ticket for holidays or special occasions (Campbell et al., 2011). As children get older, the peer group becomes more important. Problem gamblers also begin seeking out peers with similar gambling behaviors (Derevensky, 2012).

CORRELATES AND RISK FACTORS ASSOCIATED WITH PROBLEM GAMBLING

Problem gambling, similar to other mental health disorders, has been shown to have multiple associated risk factors. Given the general acceptance that adolescent problem or disordered gamblers are not a homogeneous group, there is no single constellation of risk factors that alone can predict with certainty that an individual will develop a gambling disorder. Nevertheless, considerable research during the past 25 years has focused on identifying those risk factors associated with excessive gambling problems and has identified possible protective factors as a way to minimize problems through early prevention strategies as well as informing evidence-based treatment strategies (Derevensky, 2012; Dickson, Derevensky, & Gupta, 2002, 2004; Shead et al., 2010).

While there are multiple constellations of risk factors that, in conjunction with a lack of specific protective factors, likely place certain adolescents at high risk for a specific problem, the etiology underlying gambling problems is not universal. Risk factors may be different for individuals, and a number of distinct pathways may exist that lead to pathological gambling (Gupta, Nower, Derevensky, Blaszczynski, Faregh, & Temcheff, 2013; Nower & Blaszczynski, 2004). These pathways also have implications for the treatment of gambling disorders.

Gupta et al. (2013) have suggested that adopting a biopsychosocial–environmental framework may facilitate our understanding of the onset and developmental course of gambling problems. In spite of the adoption of the framework, understanding the risk factors may better influence our prevention and treatment programs. The reviews by Derevensky (2012) and Shead et al. (2010) point to the empirical studies supporting behavioral patterns, correlates, and risk factors associated with adolescent gambling and problem gambling.

The following risk factors have been identified and will be discussed: gender; parents and peers; attitudes toward gambling; cultural and regional factors; personality traits; mental health disorders; and behavioral, situational, and environment influences.

Gender Differences

In adolescence, gambling remains more popular among males than females, with more adolescent males than females exhibiting severe gambling-related behaviors (Abbott et al., 2004; Derevensky & Gupta, 2004; National Research Council, 1999; Ipsos MORI, 2014; Productivity Commission, 2010; Volberg et al, 2010; Wardle et al., 2011; Welte et al., 2008). Disordered gambling can be two to four times more common among males than females (Derevensky & Gupta, 2004; Gupta & Derevensky, 1998a; Stinchfield, 2000; Volberg et al., 2010). In general, males have been found to make larger gross wagers (Derevensky et al., 1996), gamble on more diverse activities, gamble more frequently, spend more time and money, have an earlier age of onset, and experience more gambling-related problems than females (Jacobs, 2000, 2004). Whereas males prefer sports betting and wagering on games of skill, females tend to prefer gambling on the lottery and bingo (Derevensky, 2012; Wilson & Ross, 2011). While there is speculation that there is a greater genetic component among males, parents have been found to be more likely to encourage their son's gambling, and males report gambling more often with their parents (Campbell, Derevensky, Meerkamper, & Cutajar, 2011; Ladouceur et al., 1994).

Parental and Peer Influences

Adolescents with gambling problems often report having parents whom they perceive gamble excessively, are involved in other addictive behaviors, and/or have been involved in illegal activities (Abbott & Volberg, 2000; Campbell et al, 2011; Hardoon et al., 2004; Raylu & Oei, 2002; Ipsos MORI, 2014). As previously noted, for older adolescents the peer group plays an important role in endorsing or promoting gambling (King, Abrams, & Wilkinson, 2010). Dickson, Derevensky, and Gupta (2008) reported that 40% of disordered gamblers indicated that they had friends with similar gambling interests. Adolescents who were taught to maintain a budget, save money, and be financially responsible were less likely to show an interest in gambling (Delfabbro & Thrupp, 2003).

Attitudes Toward Gambling

Adolescents in general and especially those with gambling problems report positive attitudes toward gambling. Gambling is viewed as a highly socially acceptable behavior and recreational pastime (Derevensky, 2012). While these youth typically fail to comprehend both the immediate and long-term negative consequences of *their* gambling behaviors, many are cognizant of the problems associated with excessive gambling. Hardoon et al. (2003) reported that even though adolescent problem gamblers scored exceedingly high on gambling severity indices, they nevertheless did not perceive *themselves* as having a gambling problem. As such, the risks associated with disordered gambling are viewed as a long-term consequence and not of immediate concern (Gillespie, Gupta, Derevensky, et al., 2005). In an interesting study, Hanss et al. (2014) reported that in addition to gender, degree of sensation seeking, agreeableness, a family history of gambling, and family and peer approval of gambling were the most powerful influences on adolescents' attitudes toward gambling.

Cultural and Regional Factors

Overall prevalence rates of gambling and problem gambling vary between countries (Volberg et al., 2010). These differences may be due to differing data collection methodologies (telephone surveys, school-based survey), situational factors (e.g., availability, ease of accessibility, age restrictions), advertisements, or cultural/attitudinal factors. Arndt and Palmer (2013) reported significant racial/ethnic differences among students who have gambled, with white (26.0%) and Asian (25.8%) adolescents having had the least lifetime exposure and Latino (30.1%), African-American (32.6%), and American Indian (34.1%) adolescents having the highest exposure. In Canada, Ellenbogen, Gupta, and Derevensky (2007) reported significant cultural differences in adolescents' gambling behaviors among Francophones (French-speaking families), Anglophones (English-speaking families), and allophones (neither English nor French was their mother tongue), with allophones exhibiting the highest rates of problem gambling.

Personality Traits

A number of studies have identified personality traits and clusters associated with adolescent problem gambling. Problem gamblers have been found to score more highly on measures of excitability and extroversion, they tend to have difficulty conforming to societal norms, and they experience difficulties with self-discipline (Gupta, Derevensky, & Ellenbogen, 2006; Hardoon et al., 2002, 2003, Ste-Marie, Gupta, & Derevensky, 2006). They have been similarly shown to exhibit higher state and trait anxiety scores (Gupta & Derevensky, 1998b; Ste-Marie, Gupta, & Derevensky 2002), are more impulsive (Derevensky et al., 2007; Gupta, Nower, Derevensky, et al., 2013; Nower, Derevensky, & Gupta, 2004; Vitaro, Ferland, Jacques, & Ladouceur, 1998; Vitaro et al., 2001), are greater risk takers (Abbott et al., 2004; Nower, Derevensky, & Gupta, 2004; Zuckerman, 1994), and are more self-blaming and guilt-prone (Gupta & Derevensky, 2000).

Adolescent problem gamblers exhibit higher scores on measures of disinhibition, boredom susceptibility, and other self-regulatory behaviors (e.g., conformity to norms, self-indulgence) (Gupta, Nower, Derevensky, et al., 2013; Nower, Derevensky & Gupta, 2004; Shead et al., 2010).

Mental Health Disorders

Consistent with the Pathways Model (the theoretical integration of biological, personality, developmental, cognitive, learning theory, and environmental factors) that describes the etiology of different subtypes of problem gamblers (see Gupta et al., 2013; Nower & Blaszczynski, 2004), adolescents with gambling disorders report multiple mental health problems, including high levels of anxiety and depressive symptomatology (Bergevin, Gupta, Derevensky, & Kaufman, 2006; Felsher, Derevensky, & Gupta, 2010; Gupta & Derevensky, 1998b; Gupta, Derevensky, & Ellenbogen, 2006). Other research, using latent class analyses (Kong et al., 2014), as well as two recent longitudinal research projects with adults, has strongly supported these findings (el-Guebaly et al., 2015; Williams et al., 2015). Youth with gambling problems are at heightened risk for suicide ideation and attempts (Nower, Gupta, Blaszczynski, & Derevensky, 2004), they exhibit an increased frequency of substance abuse and psychosomatic problems, and they tend to be involved in a wide variety of risky behaviors (Gupta & Derevensky, 1998a; Hammond et al., 2014; Jacobs et al., 1989; Leeman et al., 2014; Lesieur & Rothschild, 1989; Rahman et al., 2012).

Behavioral, Situational, and Environmental Factors

Today's social acceptability of gambling, prolific advertisements, and ease of accessibility has enabled young people to gamble on a greater variety of activities in spite of prohibitions on regulated forms of gambling. Whether buying a lottery ticket at a convenience store, entering gambling establishments when they are underage, or gambling online, most adolescents have figured out a way to circumvent restrictions. Major reviews have in general concluded that the greater the availability and accessibility of gambling, the greater gambling participation and gambling-related problems (Ariyabuddhiphongs, 2013; Blinn-Pilke et al., 2010; Derevensky, 2012; Raylu & Oie, 2002; St-Pierre, Walker, Derevensky, & Gupta, 2014). While an alternative gambling exposure and adaptation model has been presented (Laplante & Shaffer, 2007), there is ample evidence to suggest that gambling among adolescents will not dissipate, especially in light of social casino gambling, online gambling, and mobile gambling (Derevensky & Gainsbury, 2016). However, despite the proliferation of gambling internationally, new technological forms of gambling, and widespread advertising and the glamorization of gambling, prevalence rates of problem/disordered gambling among adolescents and adults have not risen dramatically. Indeed, there is some evidence that in certain jurisdictions the prevalence rates of both gambling and problem gambling among adolescents have decreased somewhat, supporting Shaffer et al.'s (2007) contention of adaptation. Others have argued that stricter enforcement of age restrictions, more punitive fines and sanctions for gambling establishments that permit underage gambling, and increased prevention interventions may have accounted for these decreases.

PROTECTIVE FACTORS

While most studies have focused on the risk factors associated with adolescent problem gambling, a number of studies have sought to identify those attributes thought to protect youth from developing a gambling problem. Such studies have focused on identifying the protective and buffering factors thought to reduce and minimize the incidence of adolescent disordered gambling. While there are some unique risk factors associated with problem gambling compared with other adolescent high-risk and addictive behaviors (e.g., substance and alcohol abuse), Dickson, Derevensky, and Gupta (2008), using multiple self-report measures, concluded that poor family and school connectedness was symptomatic of adolescent problem gambling, with family cohesion playing a significant role as a protective factor. If one also looks at the attitudinal research, there is evidence that familial and peer disapproval of gambling may be a reliable protective factor (Hanss et al., 2014). Research by Kundu et al. (2013; see also Rahman et al., 2012) suggests that giving lottery tickets to underage minors has been associated with more permissive attitudes toward gambling. This has resulted in the annual Holiday Campaign, a collaborative initiative of McGill University's International Centre for Youth Gambling Problems and High Risk Behaviors and the U.S. National Council on Problem Gambling designed to educate parents on the relationship between an early onset of gambling and later gambling problems.

In several studies, Lussier, Derevensky, and Gupta (2004) and Lussier, Derevensky, Gupta, and Vitaro (2014) sought to examine the role of resilience in the presence of identified risk factors as a possible protective factor for youth gambling problems and other adolescent high-risk behaviors (this was also addressed in a study of the impact of physical, sexual, and mental abuse upon disordered gambling by Felsher et al., 2010). Early findings revealed that adolescents perceived to be *Vulnerable* (high risk/low protective factors) had a mean gambling severity score nine times larger than the *Resilient* group (high risk/high protective factors), eight times larger than the *Fortunate* group (low risk/low protective factor), and 13 times larger than the *Ideal* group (low risk/high protective factors). The *Vulnerable* group were at the greatest risk for experiencing gambling problems. All of the adolescents identified as pathological/disordered gamblers and 87% of those identified as being at risk for problem gambling (exhibiting a number of clinical difficulties but not reaching the clinical criteria for a formal diagnosis of pathological gambling) scored on the resilience measure as being *Vulnerable*, while only 4.3% of the youth categorized as *Resilient* were identified as at-risk gamblers, and none of them were pathological gamblers despite their reporting high levels of risk exposure. Thus, the construct of resilience appears to be a key protective factor and should be addressed in mental health initiatives and problem gambling prevention initiatives (Felsher et al., 2010; Lussier, Derevensky, Gupta, & Vitaro, 2014; Nower et al., 2004).

ASSESSING AND MEASURING GAMBLING SEVERITY

Despite advances in our understanding of the etiology, correlates, and risk and protective factors associated with adolescent problem gambling, our ability to accurately assess and measure gambling severity has been limited. While a number of instruments have been developed to identify adolescent problem gamblers, most have been adapted from adult instruments (using adult criteria while modifying or replacing questions to make them more age-appropriate) and none of the instruments have undergone rigorous psychometric evaluation (Stinchfield, 2010). The most commonly used instruments include the South Oaks Gambling Screen-Revised for Adolescents (SOGS-RA; Winters, Stinchfield, & Fulkerson, 1993), DSM-IV-J (Fisher, 1992) and its revision the DSM-IV-MR-J (Fisher, 2000), the Massachusetts Adolescent Gambling Screen (MAGS; Shaffer, LaBrie, Scanlan, & Cummings, 1994; Stinchfield, 2010), and the Canadian Adolescent Gambling Inventory (CAGI; Wiebe, Wynne, Stinchfield, & Tremblay, 2005, 2007). A number of studies of older adolescents have employed the GA-20 (Gamblers Anonymous) questions (Blinn-Pike et al., 2010).

Among these instruments, only the CAGI was originally developed for adolescents. The CAGI, which has been used in only a limited number of studies to date, moves beyond a single scale of measurement (one score) to include multiple domains of problem gambling severity; it measures gambling behavior itself as well as problem gambling severity (Stinchfield, 2010). Using a more limited timeframe for assessing gambling behavior (3 months; most instruments assess past-year gambling-related problems), it assesses and identifies behavior in five distinct areas:

1. Types of gambling behaviors/activities in which the individual engages
2. Frequency of participation in each of these behaviors/activities
3. Time spent on each of the gambling activities
4. Money wagered
5. Severity of gambling problems

Similar to adult instruments (the DSM-5 being the new gold standard), a number of common constructs underlie most of the instruments, including both psychological factors and the negative financial and behavioral costs associated with excessive gambling. Stealing money to support gambling (this item no longer exists in DSM-5), occupational/school-related problems, disrupted relationships, chasing losses, lying or deception about one's gambling problems, disrupted familial relationships, the need to increase the frequency and amount wagered, preoccupation with gambling, and concern/criticism from others are common constructs examined by these instruments. Derevensky (2012) concluded after considerable research that the DSM-IV-MR-J seems to be a more conservative measure of gambling severity. (For a more comprehensive description of the instruments, see Blinn-Pike et al., 2010; Derevensky, 2012; and Stinchfield, 2010. An online search can also produce these instruments.)

TREATMENT OF YOUTH WITH GAMBLING DISORDERS

As there remains no single identifiable cause or universally accepted theoretical model for understanding problem gambling, treatment approaches have differed. Individuals' motivations to gamble and gamble excessively vary greatly, thus necessitating different treatment approaches. The current treatment approaches for adolescents have been based upon a wide variety of theoretical approaches paralleling those used for adults, including the following:

Psychoanalytic or psychodynamic (Rosenthal, 1987; Rugle & Rosenthal, 1994)

Behavioral (Blaszczynski & McConaghy, 1993; Petry & Roll, 2001; Walker, 1993)

Cognitive and cognitive-behavioral (Blaszczynski & Nower, 2013; Bujold, Ladouceur, Sylvain, & Boisvert, 1994; Dowling, 2013; Ladouceur & Walker, 1998; Toneatto & Sobell, 1990; Walker, 1993)

Pharmacological (Grant, Chambers, & Potenza, 2004; Grant, Kim, & Potenza, 2003; Haller & Hinterhuber, 1994; Hollander, Sood, Pallanti, et al., 2005) (although few adolescent treatment approaches include psychopharmacological interventions)

Physiological (Blaszczynski, Winter, & McConaghy, 1986)
Biological/genetic (DeCaria, Hollander, & Wong, 1997; Hollander et al., 1992; Saiz, 1992)
Addiction-based models (Lesieur & Blume, 1991)
Self-help models (Brown, 1986, 1987; Ferentzy, Skinner, & Antze, 2013; Lesieur, 1990)

For a more comprehensive overview of these various therapeutic models and their efficacy in treating gambling problems, see reviews by Grant and Potenza (2011), Hodgins, Stea, and Grant (2011), Ladouceur and Shaffer (2005), Petry (2005), and Richard et al. (2013).

There is unequivocal evidence that most adults and adolescents learn from their past mistakes. While most individuals occasionally exceed their preset gambling limits (time and/or money) and may suffer some short-term negative consequences, most individuals eventually refrain from excessive gambling. Some individuals may stop gambling altogether; others regain control of their behavior, curtailing their gambling in terms of both frequency and money wagered. Yet for some individuals, their physiological and psychological needs, perceived skill and knowledge, erroneous cognitions, and/or need for escape from daily and long-term stressors and mental health issues lead them to increase the frequency and intensity of their gambling even though they know that their odds of winning are limited.

Paradigms for the treatment of gambling problems in youth have traditionally incorporated a relatively narrow focus depending on the therapist's theoretical orientation and conceptualization of the etiology of a gambling disorder, the therapist's background work in the field of addictions, and whether the therapist believes in "controlled gambling" versus abstinence (Derevensky, 2012). The development of empirically based prevention programs has been hampered by a lack of theoretical understanding of the etiology underlying problem gambling (the biomedical model, arguing that there is a strong underlying biological basis for disordered gambling, dominates the treatment community in the United States), the lack of public awareness of the needs for such programs, and the resistance of adolescents to recognize the severity of their problem and to seek treatment. Problem/disordered gambling has often been referred to as a "hidden addiction" (Derevensky, Shek, & Merrick, 2011). Unlike a drug, alcohol, or tobacco addiction, it is often difficult to detect a gambling disorder; there are also no blood or urine tests to confirm it. Denial of the problem is common by teens, even though they score high on gambling severity measures and acknowledge that their parents, siblings, and/or peers view their behavior as problematic. While adolescents in general typically do not want to seek help for any addiction or mental health disorder, this is likely even more common among adolescent problem gamblers.

The fact that only a very small percentage of individuals (both adolescents and adults) with a severe gambling disorder perceive themselves as having a problem helps account for the low turnout of adolescents seeking help for a gambling disorder (Derevensky, Temcheff, & Gupta, 2011; Hardoon, Derevensky, & Gupta, 2003). Even among adults with gambling disorders, the fact that only approximately 10% of these individuals present for treatment is a serious concern (Hodgins, 2014; Hodgins, Stea, & Grant, 2011; Slutske, Blaszczynski, & Martin, 2009). Perceived barriers to seeking treatment include a desire to manage the problem themselves, denial, and shame (Suurvali, Hodgins, & Cunningham, 2010). For the adolescent, logistical travel considerations and their unwillingness to acknowledge a problem to their parents place them at an even greater disadvantage.

There is considerable empirical support suggesting that gambling involves a complex and dynamic interaction between ecological, psychophysiological, developmental, cognitive, and behavioral components, with environmental issues (e.g., accessibility, availability, and game type) being important considerations (Hodgins et al., 2011). Derevensky (2012), Derevensky, Temcheff, and Gupta (2011), Gupta and Derevensky (2000, 2004), and Gupta, Nower, Derevensky, Blaszczynski, Faregh, and Temcheff (2013) have long asserted that in the absence of empirically validated treatment programs and the varying underlying reasons for gambling, a dynamic interactive approach needs to take into account the multiplicity of interacting factors in a treatment paradigm for youth with significant gambling problems. Empirical support for Jacobs' General Theory of Addiction and a Pathways Model approach (see Gupta et al., 2013) for adolescent problem gamblers (Gupta & Derevensky, 1998b) suggests that adolescent pathological gamblers exhibit evidence of abnormal physiological resting states, report significantly greater emotional distress and anxiety, have increased levels of dissociation when gambling, demonstrate erroneous cognitions when gambling (e.g., they believe that they can predict the outcome of the game even when the outcome is based purely on randomness, they report exaggerated levels of skill, they have little pragmatic understanding of randomness and independence of events), and display depressive symptomatology and other mental health issues. As such, Gupta and Derevensky (2004) contend that treating gambling problems in isolation from other social, psychological, developmental, cognitive, and emotional difficulties may lead only to limited, short-term success. Their clinical experience has suggested that ultimately many of these adolescents will relapse, sometimes with concomitant substance abuse disorders (Ledgerwood, Loree, & Lundahl, 2013).

Derevensky, Temcheff, and Gupta (2011) and Gupta and Derevensky (2000, 2004) have presented a treatment model predicated on their research and clinical findings with youth problem gamblers. Their results suggest that adolescent pathological gamblers generally exhibit depressive symptomatology, somatic disorders, anxiety, impulsivity, attention deficits, mood disorders, high risk taking, and poor coping skills along with a host of academic, social, personal, and familial problems. The vast majority of adolescent problem gamblers use gambling as a distraction to escape from daily problems. It becomes a way to fill a void, to deal with boredom and multiple problems, and to reduce stress and anxiety.

While Gupta and Derevensky acknowledge that adolescent pathological gamblers experience numerous erroneous cognitive beliefs and distortions, they strongly recommend that clinicians simultaneously address underlying psychological problems as well as the presenting gambling problem. This is especially true in light of many comorbid factors, such as attention-deficit/hyperactivity disorder, substance abuse, and legal and antisocial problems. Understanding the causes and triggers of the gambling behavior remains crucial.

While many clinicians view pathological/disordered gambling as a continuous and progressive disorder, there is some clinical and empirical support suggesting that it in fact may be episodic: individuals may gamble excessively for a limited time, experience difficulties, and then stop for undetermined amounts of time. This may be viewed as binge gambling; see Gupta and Derevensky (2011) for a discussion of adolescent binge gambling.

Combinations of behavioral and psychopharmacological therapies have been shown to be successful for youth with other addictive disorders, but there are currently no drugs approved by the U.S. Food and Drug Administration for the treatment of adolescent gambling disorders. Gupta et al. (2013) contend that best practices for helping teens with gambling problems cannot be achieved until we refine our ability to match treatment strategies with gambler typologies.

PREVENTION

Unlike prevention programs for substance abuse and other mental health issues, gambling prevention programs have been hindered by a number of beliefs and common misconceptions, such as (1) age restrictions on gambling activities deter adolescent participation and (2) adolescents have little available discretionary funds for gambling. Nevertheless, the need for the early development and implementation of prevention programs is predicated upon the fact that youth often begin gambling at a young age.

Abstinence Versus Harm-Minimization Approaches

Prevention approaches can be categorized into two general paradigms: abstinence and harm minimization (sometimes referred to as harm reduction). While these two approaches are not mutually exclusive, they are predicated on different goals and processes. A harm-reduction framework encompasses policies, programs, or strategies that help individuals to reduce the harmful, negative consequences incurred through involvement in a risky behavior without requiring abstinence (Ariyabuddhiphongs, 2013; Dickson, Derevensky, & Gupta, 2004). In most jurisdictions, youth are prohibited to enter government-regulated gambling venues, supporting an abstinence approach. However, is abstinence a realistic goal for youth when the majority of adolescents report having gambled and report that their peers take part in unregulated gambling activities? This highlights both the paradox and the confusion as to which primary prevention approach to promote, abstinence or harm reduction (Dickson et al., 2004)

Harm-Minimization Programs

In general, universal adolescent harm-reduction programs are intended to modify inappropriate attitudes toward risky behaviors, enhance positive decision making, and educate youth about the short- and long-term risks associated with a particular behavior (Derevensky & Gupta, 2011). Most youth gambling prevention programs foster a harm-minimization framework and emphasize responsible gambling (Derevensky & Gupta, 2011). Ample research highlights that the age of onset of gambling is a significant factor associated with problem gambling (Dickson et al., 2002, 2004; Jacobs, 2004; National Research Council. 1999; Productivity Commission, 1999; Volberg et al., 2010). As such, delaying the age of onset may well be beneficial in minimizing gambling-related harm.

The available gambling prevention programs designed for youth have typically incorporated the following harm-minimization and educational objectives:

1. Highlight the difference between games of chance and games of skill
2. Educate participants about probability and the independence of events
3. Dispel erroneous cognitions concerning the "illusion of control" regarding random events
4. Address issues of independence of events
5. Articulate the characteristics and warning signs of problem gambling
6. Provide resources to aid individuals either experiencing a gambling problem or who are at risk for a gambling problem (Derevensky, 2012; Ladouceur, Goulet, & Vitaro, 2013; Turner, Macdonald, & Somerset, 2008)

Some more comprehensive prevention curricula seek to encourage the development of interpersonal skills, foster effective coping strategies, provide techniques to improve self-esteem, and offer ideas for resisting peer pressure (Derevensky & Gupta, 2011).

Comprehensive and substantive elementary and high school prevention programs for problem gambling are relatively uncommon but do exist in some jurisdictions (Williams, West, & Simpson, 2012). Several adolescent gambling prevention and awareness initiatives currently in use internationally are presented in Table 27.1.

As the role of and the interaction of risk and protective factors become better understood, a complementary understanding of resiliency is achieved (Shead, Derevensky, & Gupta, 2010). Research suggests that resilient youth possess a constellation of skills including competent problem-solving abilities, social competence (effective communication skills, flexibility, concern for others), autonomy, and a sense of purpose (Masten, Best, & Garmezy, 1990). One of the central goals of science-based prevention initiatives is to promote resilience (Dickson et al., 2002). Lussier et al. (2007), using Jessor's (1998) Adolescent Risk Behavior model, explored the concept of resilience and its relationship to youth problem gambling. Their findings suggest that a variety of risk and protective factors interact uniquely to contribute to the predictive model of gambling problems. The promotion and development of resilience should, therefore, be among the factors included in mental health initiatives and prevention programs.

Evaluating Prevention Programs

Evaluating the success or effectiveness of prevention programs is fundamental to improving public

Table 27.1 Youth Gambling Prevention Programs

Prevention Program	*School Level*	*Developer*	*Website*
Amazing Chateau	Grades 4–6	International Centre for Youth Gambling Problems and High-Risk Behaviors, McGill University	www.youthgambling.com
Clean Break	Grades 8–12	International Centre for Youth Gambling Problems and High-Risk Behaviors, McGill University	www.youthgambling.com
Don't Bet on It	Grades 10–12	Responsible Gambling Council	http://curriculum.org/resources/dont-bet-on-it-8211-a-youth-problem-gambling-prevention-program
Facing the Odds	Grades 5–8	Harvard Medical School, Division of Addictions	http://www.divisiononaddictions.org/curr/facing_the_odds.htm
Hooked City	Grades 6–8	International Centre for Youth Gambling Problems and High-Risk Behaviors, McGill University	www.youthgambling.com
Stacked Deck	Grades 9–12	Robert Williams and Robert Wood	http://www.uleth.ca/research/alberta-gambling-research-institute-agri
Wanna Bet?	Grades 3–8	Minnesota Council on Compulsive Gambling	http://www.nati.org/prevention_tools/youth.aspx
Youth Gambling: An Awareness and Prevention Workshop—Level I	Grades 4–6	International Centre for Youth Gambling Problems and High-Risk Behaviors, McGill University	www.youthgambling.com
Youth Gambling: An Awareness and Prevention Workshop—Level II	Grades 7–10	International Centre for Youth Gambling Problems and High-Risk Behaviors, McGill University	www.youthgambling.com
Youth Making Choices: A Curriculum-Based Gambling Prevention Program	Grades 10–12	Centre for Addiction and Mental Health (CAMH)	http://www.problemgambling.ca/EN/ResourcesForProfessionals/Pages/CurriculumYouthMakingChoices.aspx

health (Dickson-Gillespie, Rugle, Rosenthal, & Fong, 2008). There have been relatively few published evaluations of youth gambling prevention or intervention programs (Blinn-Pike, Worthy, & Jonkman, 2010). Ladouceur, Goulet, and Vitaro (2013), in their review of youth gambling prevention program evaluations, concluded that the majority of the evaluative studies did not include measures of gambling behaviors or long-term outcomes. Short-term benefits of these prevention programs point to improved knowledge and a reduction in misconceptions about gambling among youth (Ladouceur et al., 2013; Lupu & Lupu, 2013). However, without follow-up evaluations and measurement of gambling behaviors, it is unclear whether gambling behavior is actually affected in the long term (Ladouceur et al., 2013).

Future Directions

There is a real need to raise awareness among the general public, parents, teachers, and mental health professionals about the extent of adolescent problem gambling (Campbell et al., 2011; Derevensky, St-Pierre, Temcheff, & Gupta, 2014; Hayer, Griffiths, & Meyer, 2005; Temcheff, Derevensky, St-Pierre, Gupta, & Martin, 2014). It makes intuitive sense to incorporate gambling-related information and prevention efforts into existing and effective mental health and education programs to form a more comprehensive mental health curriculum (Derevensky, 2012; Hayer, Griffiths, & Meyer, 2005).

CONCLUSION

The landscape of gambling is continually changing with technological advances, new forms of gambling, and ever-increasing ease of access. The thrill, excitement, and entertainment associated with gambling contribute to the positive perception of gambling. This changing landscape, with a heavy emphasis on online and mobile gambling, the inclusion of social casino games, and the normalization and social acceptability of gambling, represents a renewed challenge to help minimize problems.

Clinicians and researchers studying adolescence have long suggested that it is a developmental stage marked by significant physical, social, cognitive, and emotional changes. The continued expansion of gambling, the enticing advertisements, the glitz and glamour associated with gambling, and the social acceptance of the industry's expansion may spell trouble for our youth. Research is only beginning to highlight the determinants of both the risk and protective factors associated with different forms of gambling. Researchers and clinicians have not yet realized best practices for treatment or prevention. Nevertheless, youth gambling, like so many other risky behaviors among teens, is an important public health issue that needs to be addressed. Incorporating youth gambling into a public health framework (Messerlian & Derevensky, 2005; Messerlian, Derevensky, & Gupta, 2005), using a multidimensional perspective recognizing the individual and social determinants while simultaneously drawing upon health promotion principles, represents a plausible approach for better addressing the issues of youth gambling and problem gambling.

Internet Addiction

Amy Bleakley
Sunhee Park
Daniel Romer

chapter 28

OVERVIEW

The Internet has transformed the way youth communicate, learn, and network, with implications for their broader social, psychological, and physical health and well-being. For example, according to the Pew Research Center, 95% of adolescents (ages 12–17) and young adults (ages 18–29) in the United States are online, which is a figure that has for the most part remained stable for nearly a decade (Madden, Lenhart, Duggan, Cortesi, & Gasser, 2013). Differences in Internet access based on income and race are not as steep as previously noted, especially among younger adults (Smith, 2014). Among youth in the United States, estimates of time spent on a computer, but not necessarily online, range from an average of 1.4 hours per day among 15- to 18-year-olds (Rideout, Foehr, & Roberts, 2010) to 2.6 hours per day among 12- to 17-year-olds (Bleakley, Vaala, Jordan, & Romer, 2014). Mobile technologies like smartphones have made the Internet more accessible, and ownership of such devices among youth has increased (Madden et al., 2013). Of course, Internet use among youth is a global phenomenon, and not limited to Western countries, but together these trends provide mere snapshots of the time some youth spend online and the technologies that make it possible to do so.

WHAT IS INTERNET ADDICTION?

With the ability to access the Internet from anywhere, at any time, paired with the enormous variety of Internet activities in which youth engage (e.g., social networking, chatting, streaming videos, playing games, watching television content), instances of problematic Internet behavior have emerged. The term "Internet addiction" is often used to describe compulsive Internet use similar to clinically diagnosable behavioral and substance use addictions. However, there is widespread disagreement about basic terminology and definitions pertaining to the idea of Internet addiction, and whether it is actually a diagnosable condition or disorder (Mitchell, 2000). The DSM-5 (American Psychiatric Association, 2013) included Internet gaming disorder as a condition for further study. Although the focus of this disorder is the "persistent and recurrent use of the Internet to engage in games, often with other players," the authors point out that Internet gaming disorder is also referred to as "Internet use disorder, Internet addiction, or gaming addiction." Obviously, two of these terms are not specific to Internet gaming and appear to conflate different concepts under the rubric of Internet overuse. While inclusion in the DSM was recommended by several scholars (Block, 2008; Petry & O'Brien, 2013; Pies, 2009), in their current form the proposed criteria seem to do little to clarify any differences.

In addition to "Internet addiction," synonymous terms include "cyberspace addiction, online addiction, net addiction, Internet addicted disorder, and high Internet dependency" (Douglas et al., 2008). Terms used in the literature to describe closely related phenomena include "Internet addiction disorder," "pathological Internet use," "problematic Internet use," "excessive Internet use," and "compulsive Internet use" (Douglas et al., 2008). In general these terms share conceptual notions of underlying pathology but may vary with regard to diagnostic criteria (Petry et al., 2014), the extent to which Internet addiction should be characterized as a psychiatric disorder or a problematic behavior pattern (Yellowlees & Marks, 2007), and whether the problems associated with Internet use arise from the medium itself or specific uses of it (e.g., social networking, gaming; van Rooij, Schoenmakers, Van de Eijnden, & van de Mheen, 2010).

HOW IS INTERNET ADDICTION ASSESSED?

Internet addiction as a measurable concept emerged through the work of Young (1996, 1998), who pioneered much of the early Internet addiction research. Young contended that Internet addiction is an impulse control disorder, similar to pathological gambling. The terms "impulse control disorder" and "addiction" are often used interchangeably but are defined using different, although overlapping, criteria (Potenza, 2006). The main difference between "addiction" disorders and "impulse control" disorders is that impulse control disorders do not involve a substance or intoxicant. Because of similarities between pathological gambling and Internet addiction, Young adapted the DSM-IV criteria used to diagnose pathological gambling for the identification of Internet addiction. Some modifications (to be discussed below) have been proposed and to some extent implemented since.

Young (1996) specified eight screening criteria to classify (if at least five were answered affirmatively) respondents as Internet addicts:

1. Preoccupation or salience: Do you feel preoccupied with the Internet (think about previous online activity or anticipate next online session)?
2. Tolerance: Do you feel the need to use the Internet for increasing amounts of time to achieve satisfaction?
3. Loss of control: Have you repeatedly made unsuccessful efforts to control, cut back, or stop your Internet use?
4. Withdrawal: Do you feel restless, moody, depressed, or irritable when attempting to cut down or stop your Internet use?
5. Loss of control: Do you stay online longer than originally intended?
6. Interference with work or career: Have you jeopardized or risked the loss of a significant relationship, job, or educational or career opportunity because of the Internet?
7. Need to conceal behavior: Have you lied to family members, a therapist, or others to conceal the extent of your involvement with the Internet?
8. Escape: Do you use the Internet as a way of escaping from problems or of relieving a dysphoric mood (e.g., feelings of helplessness, guilt, anxiety, depression)?

In 2003, Shapira et al. proposed more diagnostic criteria that were consistent with Young's thinking of Internet addiction as an impulse control disorder but were not as broad "as to ignore other known psychiatric disorders that may account for patient's symptomology" (Shapira et al., 2003). In particular, they suggested that a diagnosis of Internet addiction should not be made if excessive use occurred exclusively during periods of hypomania or mania and therefore would be better accounted for by other disorders. The DSM-5 focuses on one form of Internet use: playing games either alone or with others, such as in massive multiplayer online games (MMOGs). It includes one additional criterion that is also common in addictive disorders: loss of interest in other activities, which in the case of gaming includes other forms of entertainment.

Young's eight diagnostic criteria, referred to as the Diagnostic Questionnaire for Internet Addiction, have been treated as a scale with eight yes-or-no items, with some reports of reliability exceeding .70 (standardized alpha = .76 [Johansson & Goetstam, 2004]; 0.72 [Cao et al., 2007]). Eventually, however, Young (1998) developed an expanded 20-item instrument scored on a 0-to-100 scale, called the Internet Addiction Test, which elaborated on the original criteria based on the diagnostic criteria for compulsive gambling and alcoholism (Beard & Wolf, 2001). The Internet Addiction Test was intended to identify two groups: those exhibiting Internet addictive behavior (scores ≥ 70) and those not clearly addicted but for whom Internet use may be problematic (scores 40–69). This test is considered a reliable and valid scale based on initial psychometric testing (Widyanto & McMurran, 2004). More information on the factors underlying the items (salience, anticipation, excessive use, lack of control, and neglect of work or social life) and the items themselves can be found in Widyanto and McMurran (2004). A recent review of research specifically related to Internet gaming disorder (Petry, Rehbein, Ko, & O'Brien, 2015) noted that the most diagnostic symptoms were those related to giving up other activities and exhibiting tolerance to gaming.

There are many other standardized instruments used to assess problematic or addicted Internet use, and subdimensions are not identical across the tools. Lortie and Guitoon (2013) reviewed 14 questionnaires used to assess excessive Internet use and provided an overview of their psychometric properties. They concluded that there is great variation in assessment methods as well as study methodology, and that social aspects of the behavior, such as social motivation for overuse, are often missing from these scales (Lortie & Guitton, 2013). The three dominant dimensions among the assessment tools they reviewed were compulsive use, negative outcomes, and salience. It is also important to recognize that instruments such as the Internet Addiction Test rely on self-reports of symptoms on questionnaires and thus may be less sensitive than clinical interviews (Beard, 2005).

DOES INTERNET ADDICTION RESEMBLE OTHER ADDICTIONS?

Griffiths (2005) argues that the characteristics of substance use addiction apply equally well to behaviors such as Internet addiction (Kuss, Shorter, van Rooij, Griffiths, & Schoenmakers, 2014). In particular, Griffiths (2000, 2005) proposes that core components of addiction, including preoccupation, mood modification, tolerance, withdrawal, conflict, and relapse, are all evident to various degrees in excessive Internet users. Kuss et al. (2014) assessed these criteria in two samples of adolescents and young adults using self-reports and found support for the components model in classifying Internet addiction as a disorder similar to substance use addiction. That Internet addiction shares features with other impulse control disorders has also been supported by other research (Shapira, Goldsmith, Keck, Khosla, & McElroy, 2000; Shapira et al., 2003).

Researchers who study gambling disorders (e.g., Kuss & Griffiths, 2012; Shaffer et al., 2004) argue that all addictions, including behavioral addictions such as pathological gambling, are manifestations of an underlying addiction syndrome with similar behavioral and neurobiological characteristics. Although research examining brain correlates of persons with Internet addiction is still emerging and has focused more heavily on Internet gaming, a review by Brand, Young, and Laier (2014) found that "the brain of Internet addicted individuals reacts with craving to the confrontation with Internet-related cues in the same way as the brain of substance-dependent individuals reacts on substance-related stimuli." There is also growing evidence that persons with Internet addiction exhibit impulse control problems similar to those with substance use disorders (Brand et al., 2014). A study of young men with Internet gaming disorder found differential ventral versus dorsal striatal brain responses to gaming cues that were similar to those of persons unable to control their substance use (Liu et al., 2016). This evidence suggests that the same executive function weaknesses that characterize drug use in adolescents also apply to youth engaging in problematic Internet use, including online gaming (Billieux et al., 2015).

Despite the ability to classify persons regarding their problematic Internet use, controversy surrounds the meaning of the classification. In particular, some argue that rather than being a unique disorder, it is more useful to consider it a coping mechanism for other problems (e.g., Davis, 2001). Others question whether the behavior is truly an addiction to the Internet per se or merely a convenient outlet for behavior that would otherwise occur offline, such as gambling, gaming, or use of pornography (e.g., Griffiths & Pontes, 2014).

COGNITIVE-BEHAVIORAL MODEL OF INTERNET ADDICTION

One model of problematic Internet use introduced by Davis (2001) uses a cognitive-behavioral approach that labels the behavior as "pathologic Internet use" (PIU) rather than Internet addiction. This model posits the pre-existence of other mental disorders as a diathesis for PIU. In particular, the model suggests that persons with depression, anxiety, or substance use disorders may retreat to the Internet as a way of coping with their disorder, especially as a substitute for offline social activity. Furthermore, certain maladaptive cognitions that accompany these disorders can enhance attraction to the Internet, such as beliefs of low self-worth that incline the user to retreat to more satisfying online forms of interaction with persons unknown to the individual, such as gaming or certain types of social networking. Social isolation and lack of social support in the offline world, often associated with other disorders, are likely to increase attraction to such online forms of social interaction.

The major difference between the Davis model and addiction models is that the Davis model does not require an addictive process to motivate excessive and compulsive use of the Internet. The person with PIU is using the Internet as an ineffective coping mechanism for other disorders characterized by maladaptive beliefs about the self and the world (Caplan, 2010; King & Delfabbro, 2014). Nevertheless, the symptoms of PIU are largely the same as those of systems that consider compulsive Internet use as an addiction (Davis, 2001). Thus, as with many other disorders in the DSM, symptom clusters for one diagnosis may overlap with those of other disorders, and heterogeneity in underlying pathogenesis may be masked by apparently similar symptoms (Insel & Cuthbert, 2015).

Caplan (2010) attempted to integrate the Davis model with impulse control disorders. In his model, social anxiety associated with face-to-face interaction is proposed as a diathesis for PIU, with persons exhibiting this condition preferring to socialize on the Internet rather than in offline activity. In addition, persons with this characteristic find online interaction effective for regulating their moods and reducing loneliness. These preferences for online social interaction are said to lead to the inability to regulate online behavior. Tests of the model have shown that it can explain considerable variation in PIU in both Internet gamers (Haagsma, Caplan, Peters, & Pieterse, 2013) and users of the Internet in general (Caplan, 2010). A meta-analysis of the relation between social anxiety and PIU found support for the cognitive-behavioral models, with an effect size of r = .20 (Prizant-Passal, Shechner, & Aderka, 2016). Another meta-analysis of the relation between PIU and reports of loneliness found the two significantly related, r = .32 (Tokunaga & Rains, 2016). Nevertheless, it is likely that the individuals who experience difficulty in regulating their online behavior experience deficits in self-control that increase their risk for PIU.

Research examining comorbidities between Internet addiction and other psychiatric disorders suggests that the condition exhibits a profile similar to substance use disorders (Ho et al., 2014). A meta-analysis of 1,641 patients with Internet addiction and 11,210 controls, primarily in Asian countries, found rates of comorbidity ranging from 13% to 26%. The highest comorbidity in adolescents was with alcohol abuse (25%), followed by attention-deficit/hyperactivity disorder (ADHD; 20%), anxiety (20%), and depression (14%). The meta-analysis by Tokunaga and Rains (2016) found a correlation of r = .42 between PIU and depressive symptoms. It is difficult to determine the source of these comorbidities, because attempts to withdraw from Internet use may produce problems of their own. On the other hand, onset of ADHD is likely to predate the appearance of Internet addiction, consistent with evidence that persons with Internet addiction exhibit executive control deficits (Brand et al., 2014).

A large prospective study of Chinese adolescents ages 13 to 18 found that about 6% of the youth exhibited moderate to severe levels of PIU using Internet Addiction Test criteria (Lam & Peng, 2010). This group was 2.5 times more likely to develop symptoms of depression 9 months later. However, there was no increase in symptoms of anxiety. This study suggests that depression is a potential consequence of Internet addiction in adolescents, while anxiety and alcohol use may more likely be correlates or precursors. A longitudinal study of third- to eighth-grade students in Singapore (Gentile et al., 2011) found that continued pathological use of videogames predicted increased symptoms of depression and anxiety. Consistent with the cognitive-behavioral model, youth with poor social skills were more likely to be classified as pathological gamers. However, consistent with addiction models, youth with impulse control problems were overrepresented as pathological gamers. A longitudinal study of adolescents and young adults in the United States found that heavy Internet use, including gaming, was both a consequence and a precursor of depressive symptoms (Romer et al., 2013). Similarly, a longitudinal study of adolescents in Spain found that prior depressive symptoms predicted later Internet use and symptoms of Internet addiction and that prior symptoms of Internet addiction predicted later depression symptoms (Garmez-Guadix, 2014). Thus, bidirectional relations between depression and Internet addiction are likely to characterize the condition in adolescents.

A recent study of 1,057 primarily young, European MMOG players (mean age 26) attempted to disentangle the sources of Internet gaming disorder (Billieux et al., 2015). The authors found that about half reported relatively high levels of Internet addiction symptoms. However, it was possible to identify three subtypes with this condition. In support of the cognitive-behavioral model, one type was characterized by low self-esteem, high impulsivity, and high needs for escape from life problems. These players appeared to play MMOGs as a coping mechanism for life problems. However, two other groups did not display deficits in self-esteem as predicted by the Davis model. One group appeared to be motivated by the achievement opportunities afforded by the game, but the members of this group were also highly impulsive, suggesting that they also had problems controlling their behavior. The members of the third group were also highly impulsive but very controlled in other ways (high levels of perseverance), suggesting that their play was more characteristic of a compulsive disorder. These divergent patterns suggest that although Internet gaming disorder is characterized by impulse control problems (see also Gentile et al., 2011), it is a complex behavior that may reflect very different underlying motivations. Among those who did not display symptoms of Internet addiction but who played at high rates, there was evidence that the games were attractive for their social value. Other studies of online MMOG players have found that many can be characterized as highly social and interested in gaming for both its social rewards and its opportunity for achievement (Herodotou et al., 2014). Thus, simply spending time on MMOGs does not imply disorder.

DOES THE TYPE OF INTERNET USE MATTER?

In his development of the cognitive-behavioral model, Davis argued for a distinction between two types of pathological Internet use (PIU): specific use and generalized use. In specific use the user has an addictive disorder, such as pathological gambling, and then migrates to the Internet to satisfy the addiction. In that case, PIU is restricted to a behavior that would otherwise occur offline. Alternatively, generalized use is a broader condition that refers exclusively to online activities, for example social media. In such instances, the Internet may be used to overcome problems in maintaining satisfying social relationships offline. Griffiths, too (1999, 2010, 2012; Widyanto & Griffiths, 2006), has maintained that the concept of Internet addiction is too broad to be useful. He notes that we should distinguish between "addictions *on* the Internet" and "addictions *to* the Internet." The former merely represent the use of the Internet to satisfy addictions (perhaps more conveniently) that are also pursued offline, such as gambling, video gaming, or use of pornography. However, if the behavior is particularly attached to the Internet (e.g., social networking or playing MMOGs), this might suggest that it truly is a form of addiction to the Internet, at least for the uses to which it is put. This distinction is less about the breadth of Internet use than the need to use the Internet to satisfy a particular addiction.

Research supports the notion that specific uses often dominate PIU (see Lam, 2014). For example, in a longitudinal sample of Dutch adolescents, van Rooij et al. (2010) found that time spent on the specific Internet application of online gaming (both MMOGs and casual, or simple and free, games) was most strongly associated with PIU in their sample. Nevertheless, PIU was also associated with downloading, social networking, chatting, instant messaging, and blogging (van Rooij et al., 2010). Several studies have demonstrated an association between online gaming and PIU (e.g., Billieux et al., 2015; Kiraly et al., 2014), but the relation between social anxiety and gaming appears to be stronger than between some forms of online social interaction, such as instant messaging and using email (Prizant-Passal et al., 2016).

Despite the prevalence of online gaming in Internet addiction, it is not always the most dominant activity associated with the condition. Kuss et al. (2013) found that social networking rather than online gaming was the activity most closely associated with PIU in British college students. A study of 4,875 16-year-old Hungarian high school students reported rates of PIU as well as problematic online gaming (Kiraly et al., 2014). The study found that 15.5% could be classified as engaging in PIU; however, less than half of this group (6.7%) engaged in problematic online gaming. In contrast, more than half of the problematic gamers were also classified as engaging in PIU. Thus, it appears that problematic gaming is an important subset of PIU in adolescents but that PIU can encompass a broader set of problematic Internet activities, a finding observed in other studies (e.g., van Rooj et al., 2010).

In sum, it is difficult to determine the exact nature of the behavior variously labeled as Internet addiction, PIU, or Internet gaming disorder. There is very little research designed to determine whether youth who use the Internet excessively do so primarily to satisfy a preexisting addiction, such as gambling. These ambiguities extend to the interpretation of prevalence rates of problematic Internet behavior.

HOW WIDESPREAD IS INTERNET ADDICTION?

Competing definitions and theoretical approaches to Internet addiction, in addition to inconsistent measurement, have led to a range of estimates on the prevalence of PIU (Moreno et al., 2011). Two studies on Internet behavior among adolescents from Europe are worth mentioning because of their cross-national samples. A study by Durkee et al. (2012) included 11,956 participants (mean age 14.9 [SD 0.89]) from 11 European countries and found that the overall prevalence of what they called PIU was 4.4%. Estimates varied by gender and country, with males exhibiting greater PIU than females. A later study by Tsitsika et al. (2014) found that 1% of 13,284 adolescents from seven European countries exhibited Internet addiction based on the Internet Addiction Test, with 12.7% exhibiting problematic Internet behavior. The authors concluded that 13.9% showed "dysfunctional" Internet behavior, defined as the sum of the two Internet Addiction Test classifications. Similar to the Durkee et al. (2012) study, differences were found in rates by gender and country, once again with boys displaying greater Internet addiction than girls.

The DSM-5 states that the prevalence of Internet addiction seems to be highest in Asian countries (American Psychiatric Association, 2013), although rates vary from study to study and between countries. A meta-analysis of studies across 31 countries (Cheng & Li, 2014), which included samples of respondents ages 12 to 41 (average age 18.4), did not find lower rates of Internet addiction in the United States (8.0%) compared to Asia (7.1%) or northern and western Europe (2.6%). A large study across six Asian countries (China, Hong Kong, Japan, the Republic of Korea, Malaysia, and the Philippines) involving a randomly selected sample of over 5,000 adolescents ages 12 to 17 found rates ranging from 1.2% in the Republic of Korea to 4.9% in the Philippines using Internet Addiction Test cutoffs (Mak et al., 2014). The authors noted that their rates were higher than those observed in Europe, which as noted above tended to have rates closer to 1% using the Internet Addiction Test. However, it is in the category of problematic Internet use (the less serious form of Internet addiction according to Young's classification) that Asian youth appear to be at greater risk. In the Mak et al. study, these rates ranged from 12.5% in the Republic of Korea to over 40% in Japan and the Philippines. Rates in college students may be even higher. In a survey of 3,616 college students in Taiwan, Internet addiction prevalence measured using the Chen Internet

Addiction Scale—Revision (CIAS-R) was 15.3% (Lin, Ko, & Wu, 2011).

There is evidence that youth who exhibit symptoms of Internet addiction will no longer show signs of the disorder within a year's time. A remission rate of 50% was observed in samples of Taiwanese adolescents (Ko et al., 2007). On the other hand, Gentile et al. (2011) observed a much lower rate of remission for Internet gaming disorder in Singapore (16%). Whether these differences are due to the type of behavior (gaming vs. other forms of online behavior) or to other factors is difficult to determine. Nevertheless, the evidence suggests that at least some forms of the condition may be relatively temporary and that it can remit on its own without intervention. This also has implications for evaluating treatment interventions that do not assess long-term outcomes.

CHARACTERISTICS AND CORRELATES OF PROBLEMATIC INTERNET USE IN U.S. ADOLESCENTS

Using data from a national survey of adolescents and their parents in spring 2012 (the Annenberg Media Environment Survey), we investigated problematic Internet behavior and its various correlates in an effort to gain a more comprehensive understanding of U.S. youth who report symptoms of Internet addiction. Data were obtained from an online survey of 629 adolescents ages 12 to 17 and one of their parents who were members of an Internet research panel maintained by the survey firm Gfk (see Bleakley et al., 2014, for details of the procedure). The panel comprised parents recruited through random-digit dialing or address-based sampling procedures in an effort to reach as representative a sample of U.S. adolescents as possible. We present findings here weighted to be representative of the U.S. population of 12- to 17-year-olds based on age, gender, race/ethnicity, region, metro status, and household income.

Adolescents were asked to answer four questions about their Internet use, irrespective of whether it was accessed through a computer or a cellphone. These items were adapted from Young's original criteria (described above) and, using a 4-point scale ranging from 0 (never) to 3 (often), measured the frequency with which adolescents had the following experiences when using the Internet:

1. You stay on the Internet (online) longer that you thought you would
2. You find yourself thinking about when you will go online again
3. You have trouble trying to cut down on the amount of time you spend online
4. Your grades or schoolwork have suffered because of the amount of time you spend online

A composite problematic Internet scale was created for analytic purposes (Cronbach's alpha = 0.82; mean: 1.20, SE: 0.04). Distributions

Table 28.1 Frequencies for Symptoms of Problematic Internet Use

Item	*Never* %	*Rarely* %	*Sometimes* %	*Often* %
Stay online longer than you thought you would	6.1	17.6	54.7	21.6
Think about when you will go online again	25.7	37.4	28.0	9.0
Have trouble cutting down the amount of time you spend online	32.1	37.4	21.1	9.3
Grades or school have suffered because of amount of time online	60.0	24.2	12.4	3.3

Weighted estimates.

From Bleakley et al., 2016.

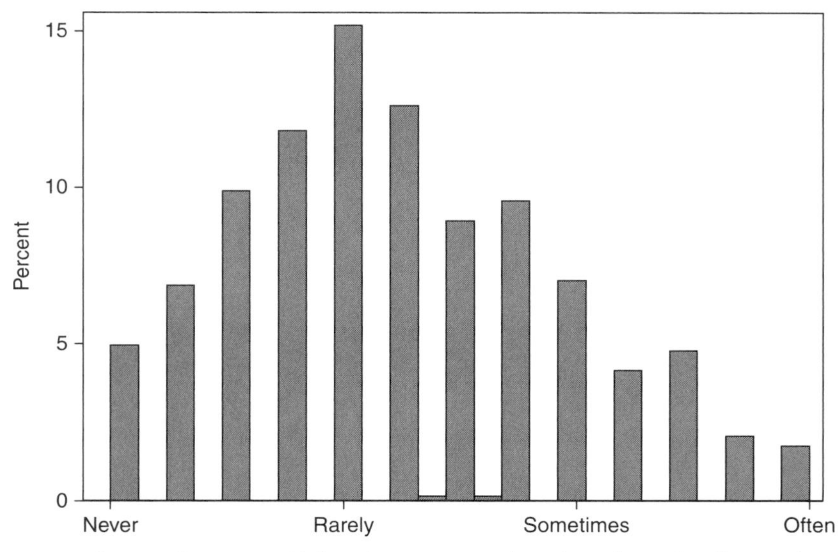

Figure 28.1 Unweighted distribution of problematic Internet use scale. (Four items, alpha = .82) (From Bleakley et al., 2016)

of these items are shown in Table 28.1, with the distribution of the index presented in Figure 28.1.

The most commonly reported behavior was staying online longer than anticipated. As seen in Figure 28.1, only 15.7% of the sample reported experiencing the symptoms on average more often than sometimes. Nevertheless, the problematic Internet index was correlated with reports of weaker grades at school (r = .18). Surprisingly, neither age nor gender was related to the index.

We asked about various uses of the Internet that might be related to our index. The strongest relation with the index was for socializing with friends, including using instant messaging or chatting (r = .40), which about 23% of the adolescents reported doing most days of the week. Also related were other social activities, such as using social networks (r = .25), playing MMOGs (r = . 30), and blogging (r = .28). Accessing YouTube was also common and related to problematic use (r = .29). Using the Internet for schoolwork (r = .05) or as a source of news (r = .17) were less related to problematic use. Use of other entertainment media, namely watching television and playing videogames, was unrelated (r's = −.02 and .07, respectively). These patterns are consistent with other research showing that heavy use of the Internet can be separated from other forms of entertainment and that using the Internet for school and acquiring information is not associated with unhealthy outcomes (Romer et al., 2013). Youth who scored higher on the index were also somewhat less likely to participate in school activities, such as sports (r = −.10), clubs (r = −.14), and voluntary community service (r = −.12). All of these relations are consistent with the finding that PIU is associated with a wide range of Internet activity and that youth with PIU are more socially isolated offline.

Youth scoring higher on the index appeared to experience greater stress in their lives, including less favorable relations with parents and greater exposure to both online and offline harassment from peers. An index of recent experience of stress was correlated (r = .31) with the problematic Internet index. Youth with higher scores also reported receiving less support from their parents, such as praise for doing well in school and getting help with schoolwork. Indeed, they reported receiving more criticism and blame from their parents than youth with lower scores on the index. This pattern is consistent with findings from studies of both Asian (Chng, Li, Liau, & Khoo, 2015; Liu, Fang, Deng, & Zhang, 2012) and European (Siomos et al., 2012) adolescents exhibiting PIU, who also report less favorable relations with parents. In addition, adolescents with higher scores on the index reported less parental monitoring of their behavior outside the home (r = –.33), a pattern consistent with their also experiencing more harassment both online and offline. Other research with the same sample found that adolescents with less parental monitoring experienced greater harassment online, such as receiving upsetting emails or instant messages and having rumors posted about them on social media (Khurana et al., 2015).

The associations we observed with problematic Internet use among U.S. adolescents suggest that youth who engage in this behavior have a less favorable social environment both at home and school. This pattern is consistent with the Davis model, which emphasizes poor social support and other adverse conditions as precursors to PIU. It is not surprising, therefore, that those who reported feeling "sad or hopeless for a period of at least two weeks during the past year" were more likely to report problematic Internet use than those who did not. Nevertheless, this could also be an outcome of Internet use. Finally, in a further analysis of the data from this survey, Bleakley et al. (2016) found that motor impulsivity was a significant correlate of the index controlling for parenting behavior, time spent online, and demographic characteristics. Thus, our findings suggest that PIU in youth is bound up with a constellation of risks for poor mental health, including the family, the peer group, individual characteristics, and excessive use of the Internet.

OTHER HEALTH CORRELATES

Another health-related outcome associated with problematic Internet use is lack of sleep. A review by Lam (2014) of four studies (all conducted in East Asia) found that problematic Internet use was associated with sleep problems, such as insomnia, short sleep duration, and poor sleep quality. The Annenberg Media Environment Survey also supports an association between problematic Internet use and sleep outcomes. For example, the problematic index was positively correlated with using media in the hour before bed, which is related to poor sleep (Cain & Gradisar, 2010), and time spent at night using media (from 6 p.m. to bedtime). Similarly, the index was negatively correlated (r = –.15) with reported average number of hours spent sleeping per night. Furthermore, self-reports of general health status on a scale of very poor to excellent were also negatively correlated (r = –.23) with the index, such that youth with more problematic use of the Internet had poorer self-reported health.

More general societal indicators have also been linked to Internet addiction. The meta-analysis across 31 countries conducted by Cheng and Li (2014) found that various quality-of-life indices were related to Internet addiction, in particular time spent commuting to work and levels of air pollution. In addition, countries with lower life satisfaction ratings were likely to report higher levels of Internet addiction. The authors suggested that people living in high-stress, poor-quality environments may be more inclined to spend time on the Internet, leading to higher levels of Internet addiction.

THERAPEUTIC INTERVENTIONS

The cognitive-behavioral approach described by Davis (2001) suggests that cognitive symptoms often associated with PIU actually precede the use, which is in contrast to other models that contend that PIU results in adverse cognitive symptoms, such as "feelings of self-consciousness, low self-worth, a depressogenic cognitive style, low self-esteem, and social anxiety" (Davis, 2001). This model suggests that the treatment of PIU, namely cognitive-behavioral therapy (CBT), should focus on the underlying adverse cognitive symptoms that promote the condition. Huang et al. (2010) describe some of the CBT strategies that have been applied. These include recognizing maladaptive cognitions, identifying triggers that lead to excessive use, learning how to control impulses and to manage time, and learning relaxation techniques. This approach could also reduce the symptoms that co-occur with the condition, such as depression and anxiety. A demonstration study by Young (2007) using CBT to treat adults with Internet addiction provided initial support for this approach.

Several studies have tested the efficacy of various therapeutic interventions for persons with Internet addiction. For example, a study that provided 8 weeks of stimulant medication to children with ADHD who also displayed excessive use of Internet videogames found reductions in Internet use (Han et al., 2009). A meta-analytic review by Winkler et al. (2013) reached a somewhat optimistic conclusion that CBT as well as pharmacological treatments could reduce symptoms of Internet addiction, such as time spent online, as well as associated depression and anxiety; however, they also concluded that CBT was more effective than pharmacotherapy in reducing Internet addiction. The review did not find that age moderated the effectiveness of the therapies studied.

A somewhat less optimistic review by King and Delfabbro (2014) with a focus on Internet gaming disorder primarily in adolescents noted that studies to date have not examined the effects of therapeutic interventions with sufficient follow-up periods to conclude that therapy produces lasting benefit. As noted above, Internet addiction may resolve within a year's time (Ko et al., 2007). Nevertheless, based on current evidence, there is reason to be optimistic that CBT may be an effective treatment approach for adolescents with Internet addiction. Przepiorka et al. (2014), in their recent review of treatment for Internet addiction, suggested that use of both pharmacological and psychological approaches may be most effective in treating this very heterogeneous disorder. Future research with youth displaying different forms of Internet overuse and receiving different forms of placebo-controlled therapy will be needed to identify the most effective treatment modalities. To be useful, these studies will require the use of consistent measures of outcomes and long-term evaluations of treatment success.

CONCLUSION

Evidence is gradually accumulating regarding the various forms of Internet addiction. Although several related yet different measurement tools have been used across various populations, making it difficult to generalize findings, evidence suggests that Internet addiction (and its various manifestations) is a real phenomenon that is associated with many adverse outcomes among youth. Whether Internet addiction is truly a form of addiction or the attempt to cope with other problems is, at this point, still a matter of dispute. Nevertheless, irrespective of the theoretical approach to the condition, the symptoms appear to be the same, suggesting that some form of poor impulse control is involved. In addition, the condition may exhibit high rates of remission, perhaps reflecting the heterogeneous nature of its genesis, with some sources reflecting more serious and chronic influence (e.g., impulse control problems) and others reflecting more transient factors (e.g., weak social support). The methodological rigor of the studies on this topic is not sufficient to draw causal conclusions or to elucidate the etiological pathways that lead to the condition. Nevertheless, research to answer these questions is quite active, with greater understanding imminent.

Conclusions, Recommendations, Priorities

Second Edition
John Cacciola
Ka Ho Brian Chor
Kimberly E. Hoagwood
Patrick E. Jamieson
Kathleen Meyers
Su-Chin Serene Olin
Daniel Romer
Suzanne Ward
Abigail Woodworth

First Edition
Joyce Garczynski
Michael Hennessy
Kimberly Hoagwood
Kathleen Hall Jamieson
Patrick E. Jamieson
Abigail Judge
Mary McIntosh
A. Thomas McLellan
Kathleen Meyers
David Penn
Daniel Romer

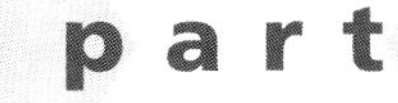

IX

Stigma

Patrick E. Jamieson
Daniel Romer

chapter 29

The *Oxford English Dictionary* (2016) defines stigma as a "mark of disgrace or infamy; a sign of severe censure or condemnation ... impressed on a person or thing." Stigma occurs when a person or group, such as those with mental illness, is stereotyped in a pejorative way that sets those individuals apart from the majority and treats them as socially unacceptable. Dissatisfied with the notion that stigma is merely an attribute that an individual possesses, and aware that social processes are at work in labeling, Link and Phelan (2001) apply the term "stigma" when "elements of labeling, stereotyping, separation, status loss, and discrimination co-occur in a power situation that allows them to unfold." For some, stigma becomes internalized (also known as self-stigma), with further harmful consequences to health and well-being (Corrigan, 2004). The Surgeon General's Report on Mental Illness from 1999 highlighted the importance of reducing the stigma of mental illness in order to increase the rate of diagnoses and improve the treatment and well-being of those with mental disorders in the United States (USDHS, 1999).

Stigma has serious consequences. For example, those with severe mental illness are less likely to have apartments leased to them (Page, 1995), be given job opportunities (Farina & Felner, 1973; Link & Phelan, 2001), or be provided with adequate healthcare (Lawrie, 1999) relative to individuals without such illness. Furthermore, for the mentally ill, stigmatization is associated with a lowered quality of life (Mechanic, McAlpine, Rosenfield, & Davis, 1994), reduced self-esteem (Link, Struening, Neese-Todd, Asmussen, & Phelan, 2001; Wright, Gronfein, & Owens, 2000), and increased symptoms and stress (Markowitz, 1998). To manage stigma, those with mental illness may use strategies that lead to social isolation (Perlick et al., 2001), such as avoiding others or engaging in secrecy (Link, Mirotznik, & Cullen, 1991), which in turn could lower their social support and increase their likelihood of relapsing. Therefore, stigma poses a significant threat to the recovery of persons with severe mental illness.

The stigma attached to mental illness can affect the likelihood that those with symptoms of mental health disorders will seek treatment. Fear of disclosing one's mental or substance use disorder is the most commonly reported reason for not seeking help, especially in youth (Gulliver et al., 2010). In adults, both treatment-related and internalized stigma were frequently associated with failure to seek help (Clement et al., 2015). Label avoidance can also be harmful when it results in nondisclosure to an employer and hence a lack of access to the protections afforded by the Americans with Disabilities Act (Cummings et al., 2013). A national survey found that about 10% of adult respondents reported not having sought or having avoided mental health treatment because of fear of negative social or work consequences (SAMHSA, 2013).

Reluctance to seek treatment is especially critical for adolescents, because numerous disorders, such as major depression, bipolar disorder, anxiety disorders, anorexia and bulimia, and schizophrenia, emerge in adolescence or early adulthood. Because those with a greater number of affective episodes prior to receiving pharmacotherapy have a less favorable prognosis than those with fewer episodes (Post, Leverich, Xing, & Weiss, 2001), such delays in seeking treatment have important implications for youth. In schizophrenia, the duration of untreated psychotic episodes may also be linked with poorer long-term prognosis (Lieberman et al., 2001; Norman & Malla, 2001).

A study from the Annenberg Public Policy Center at the University of Pennsylvania that was described in the first edition of this volume concluded that young people attach less stigma to help seeking when the source of help is seen as more effective, as it is in the case of seeing a doctor/nurse or taking medication (Penn et al., 2005, p. 535). On the other hand, for sources of help perceived to be less effective, stigma tended to be negatively related to help seeking, particularly for the least effective sources, the Internet and telephone help lines. For the subsample of youth who reported symptoms of depression, poorer perceptions of treatment effectiveness were present for all but one of the sources of help. The findings are consistent with results from a large (N = 1,387) U.K. national adult survey, which concluded that the most common reason individuals with "neurotic disorders" (22%) did not seek treatment was that they didn't think any action or individual could help them (Meltzer et al., 2003).

Once in treatment, perceived stigma may be a barrier to medication compliance and treatment continuation (Buck, Baker, Chadwick, & Jacoby, 1997; Pugatch, Bennett, & Patterson, 2002; Sirey et al., 2001a, 2001b). A 2010 meta-analysis identified strong relationships between internalized stigma and psychiatric symptom severity and treatment nonadherence (Livingston & Boyd, 2010). These findings indicate that stigma may affect the course of the illness by interfering with treatment compliance.

COMMUNITY ATTITUDES TOWARD PERSONS WITH MENTAL ILLNESS

Stigmatizing attitudes toward persons with severe mental illness have a number of recurring themes: they are viewed as dangerous, unpredictable, irresponsible, and childlike (Brockington, Hall, Levings, & Murphy, 1993; Levey & Howells, 1995) and unable to manage their own treatment needs (Pescosolido, Monahan, Link, Stueve, & Kikuzawa, 1999). For example, a significant percentage of adult Australian respondents reported that those with mental disorders such as depression or schizophrenia were unpredictable and dangerous and were less likely to be hired for employment (Reavley and Jorm, 2011). A survey of U.S. adults found that 81% considered children with depression to be dangerous to others (Pescosolido et al., 2007).

Unfavorable attitudes toward persons with mental illness are not only held by those in the community but also may be present among mental health professionals and trainees. Specifically, there is evidence that some mental health professionals, including psychiatrists (Chaplin, 2000; Miller, Shepard, & Magen, 2001), social workers (Dudley, 2000; Minkoff, 1987), general mental health providers (Ryan, Robinson, & Hausmann, 2001; Sartorius, 2002), and medical and mental health graduate students (Hasui, Sakamoto, Sugiura, & Kitamua, 2000; Mukherjee, Fialho, Wijetunge, Checinski, & Surgenor, 2002; Werrbach & DePoy, 1993), may hold stigmatizing beliefs about those with mental disorders. These findings suggest that efforts to destigmatize mental illness should not be limited to community members but also should include mental health/medical training professionals.

The tendency to stigmatize individuals with mental illness often has its roots in childhood. In a review of the literature, Wahl (2002) concluded that negative attitudes toward persons with mental illness are evident as early as third grade. In general, those with mental illness are viewed more negatively and with more fear than are individuals with physical disabilities (Wahl, 2002). Wahl reported evidence that these negative attitudes increase over time, suggesting a longitudinal process in which negative stereotypes become increasingly ingrained, culminating in potentially discriminatory behaviors in adulthood.

The presence of stigmatizing beliefs in young people was documented in a 2002 Annenberg Public Policy Center survey of U.S. adolescents ages 14 to 22 that was reported in this volume's first edition (Penn et al., 2005, p. 533). It found that large proportions of young people believed that peers with major depression, bipolar disorder, schizophrenia, and eating disorders are different from other people. For example, over half of respondents reported that persons with major depression are more likely to be violent; over 90% reported that they are more prone to suicide, and about three quarters said they are less likely to be good in school than other people. In that survey, violence was most associated with schizophrenia and depression was most associated with doing poorly in school, while eating disorders were less associated with violence than the other disorders (Penn et al., 2005, p. 533).

FACTORS THAT CONTRIBUTE TO STIGMA

The role of stigma in reducing help-seeking behavior in youth increases the importance of understanding the factors that contribute to stigma. In this section, we summarize the research on this topic for both the general population and among youth. In general, factors contributing to stigma include (a) pejorative labels for the symptoms and/or anomalous behaviors associated with mental illness; (b) causal attributions about mental illness; (c) misinformation about mental illness and negative images promulgated by the mass media; and (d) lack of contact with persons who have been successfully treated for mental illness.

Labels

Labels are so powerful that those with mental illness "are faced with recovering not just from mental illness, but also from the effects of being labeled mentally ill" (Deegan, 1993). Many labels commonly capsulizing mental illness contribute to stigma, including such pejorative terms as "schizo," "psycho," and "wacko," all of which connote violent or erratic behavior. The meanings attached to such labels are shaped and reinforced in media accounts as well as personal encounters (Link & Phelan, 1999; Phelan & Link, 1999).

Labels do not exist in a vacuum but derive meaning from their relationship with characteristics of the disorder, both real (e.g., hearing voices) and portrayed in the media culture (e.g., being homicidal). Thus, the behaviors associated with mental illness may be stigmatizing in their own right. Evidence in support of this hypothesis comes from studies showing that the social behaviors of individuals with depression can elicit negative reactions from others (Segrin, 2000) and that the social skill deficits present in patients with schizophrenia (Mueser & Bellack, 1998) may increase stigma even beyond the contribution of symptoms (Penn, Kohlmaier, & Corrigan, 2000).

Modified labeling theory explains how stigma can shape people's lives through their acceptance of being labeled as mentally ill or disordered and the resulting experiences of social rejection and loss of social support (Link et al., 1989). Such effects lead to the acceptance of the label and the resulting sense of self-stigma. Thoits (2006) proposed a version of modified labeling theory suggesting that some individuals with mental illness "do exercise their personal agency by resisting the devaluation tied to stigmatization."

Causal Attributions

Attributions are thought to play a role in the creation of stigma because our explanations for mental and physical illness (i.e., in terms of controllability and responsibility) affect our attitudes toward these disorders (Weiner, 1993; Weiner, Perry, & Magnusson, 1988). Tests of this model applied to severe mental illnesses, such as schizophrenia, indicate that when such conditions are seen as under the person's control and something for which she or he is responsible, the tendency to blame and stigmatize that individual increases (Corrigan, 2000).

One approach to counteracting these attributional biases has been to educate the public about the role of brain processes in the etiology of mental disorders (Pescosolido et al., 2010). The President's New Freedom Commission on Mental Health (2003) advocated this educational strategy in predicting that attributing mental illness to brain dysfunction would reduce stigma. While the strategy appears to have increased public support for services to treat mental disorders, it has not resulted in reductions in stigma toward persons with these disorders (Pescosolido et al., 2010). Also, while attributing causality to biological factors, such as genetics, can decrease attributions of responsibility, it may also increase beliefs that the problem cannot be changed or that relatives of the person may have similar problems (i.e., a courtesy stigma; Phelan, Cruz-Rojas, & Reiff, 2002).

Misinformation

The fact that the mass media are the most frequent source of information about mental illness for people in the United States (Wahl, 1995) may account in part for widespread misinformation about mental illness, especially in regard to the supposed violent characteristics of persons with severe mental disorders. Although there has been little research that directly links stigma with media images of mental illness, there is evidence that greater exposure to television viewing is associated with heightened intolerance toward persons with mental illness (Granello & Pauley, 2000). In addition, persons with mental illness are disproportionately portrayed in films, television, and newspapers as violent, erratic, and dangerous (Angermeyer & Schulze, 2001; Diefenbach, 1997; Granello, Pauley, & Carmichael, 1999; Hyler, Gabbard, & Schneider, 1991, Monahan, 1992; Nairn, Coverdale, & Claasen, 2001; Wahl 1995; Wahl & Roth, 1982; Williams & Taylor, 1995). As noted by Wahl (2002), entertainment media depictions of violence committed by persons with a mental disorder are more graphic and disturbing than depictions of violence in persons without a mental disorder. Nevertheless, despite the stereotypes promulgated by the media, mental health status contributes only slightly to violent behavior (Appelbaum, 2013; Monahan, 1992).

Examination of newspaper reports suggests that mental illness is more frequently associated with criminality in U.S. media than in other Western countries. An analysis of two decades of research concluded that "descriptions of mental illness and the mentally ill are distorted due to inaccuracies, exaggerations, or misinformation" and that those with mental illness are often presented as peculiar, different, and dangerous (Klin & Lemish, 2008; Ma, 2017). U.S. newspaper stories exaggerate the incidence of violence in persons with mental illness. Violence was associated with bipolar disorder 29.1% of the time and with depression, 15.2% (Silver, 2001). Conrad and Schneider (1992) found that in the United States, newspaper coverage associated mental illness with criminality 34% of the time, while in Germany and Iceland the rate was only 20%. These negative depictions are not limited to adult media but also are present in children's programming (Wahl, 2002, 2003; Wahl, Wood, Zaveri, Drapalski, & Mann, 2003; Wilson, Nairn, Coverdale, & Panapa, 2000).

REDUCING THE STIGMA OF MENTAL ILLNESS

Approaches to reducing the stigmatization of mental disorders have included education and promotion of personal contact. Consistent with earlier research, a 2012 meta-analysis of data from 72 outcome studies in 14 countries (Corrigan et al., 2012) concluded that education about mental illness and contact with people who have mental illness are both effective, with contact more effective at reducing stigma among adults (Couture & Penn, 2003) and education more so among adolescents (Corrigan et al., 2014). Thornicroft et al.'s (2016) more recent review of antistigma and antidiscrimination interventions found that the most effective programs for adults without mental illness involved contact with those diagnosed with mental illness. In addition, indirect evidence demonstrates the effectiveness of information about psychiatric/psychological treatments, either through direct instruction (Esters et al., 1998) or via role modeling (Schulze et al., 2003).

Interventions to reduce self-stigma have also been undertaken with varying degrees of success (Mittal et al., 2012). These have involved small-group sessions involving educational and cognitive-behavioral approaches. However, the sustainability of effects has not been evaluated, which suggests the need for further research. While the long-term effects of these programs remain unstudied, assessments of the Opening Minds program in Canada (described below) indicate that school-based programs can be successful. However, there is less evidence of intervention efficacy for programs delivered in primary and secondary schools, with evidence on important outcomes often lacking (Mellor, 2014).

Healthcare providers are another important audience for stigma-reduction efforts. A recent review of programs implemented in Canada revealed that such interventions have greater success when they involve multiple forms of direct contact with presenters who have recovered from mental disorders and when those contacts focus on disproving stereotypes and myths about these conditions (Knaak et al.,

2014). Providing training in best practices for interacting with patients was also found to be helpful, but more long-term outcome evaluations are needed.

Promoting personal contact between a stigmatized group and community members is based on the "contact hypothesis," which has an extensive history in the study of racism (Jackson, 1993; Kolodziej & Johnson, 1996). Pettigrew and Tropp (2006) suggested that contact could disconfirm negative stereotypes about mental illness and reduce discrimination. According to this hypothesis, contact effects will be strongest when the individuals meet as equals and have a chance to work cooperatively rather than competitively on a task, and when the target person mildly disconfirms the stereotype. The last criterion refers to the finding that encountering someone who greatly disconfirms a stereotype may result in categorizing that target as an "exception" to the rule; therefore, positive experiences with the target individual may not generalize to the broader group (Johnstone & Hewstone, 1992). Nevertheless, Sadow and Ryder (2008) found that a personal presentation from a person who is recovering that includes elements of personal relevance and inspiration can reduce stigmatizing attitudes held by future health professionals. In addition, other research suggests that if multiple examples of disconfirming evidence about a stereotype are received, the stereotyped group may no longer be seen as homogeneous, thereby opening the potential for greater acceptance of the group (Brewer, 1981).

Most interpersonal contact studies have been conducted either with college-age students or with adults in the community. In addition, there have been numerous grassroots and community efforts to reduce stigma, some focused on children and adolescents (Estroff, Penn, & Toporek, 2004; WPA, 2005). For interventions to reduce the stigma of mental illness, contact has occurred through volunteer activities, classroom experiences, job training, and simulated laboratory encounters (Couture & Penn, 2003; Kolodziej & Johnson, 1996). Consistent with results from studies of interethnic contact (Pettigrew, 2016), the findings suggest that interpersonal contact effects are robust (Corrigan, 2002; Couture & Penn, 2003); an early meta-analysis of the literature reported that the average effect size of contact on attitudes was .34 (Kolodziej & Johnson, 1996). These effects were greater when the contact was provided for students, rather than professionals, especially if the contact was not a required part of the classroom or training experience (Kolodziej & Johnson, 1996).

The message that mental disorders can be successfully treated is another strategy that appears to hold success in reducing stigma. An experiment conducted with youth ages 14 to 22 found that evidence about treatment efficacy (namely that a depressed peer had fully recovered thanks to treatment) reduced harmful stereotypes about the peer (Romer & Bock, 2008). This effect extended to those who reported recent symptoms of depression, suggesting that "treatment efficacy" is a powerful message even for those most affected by stigma. A second more recent study with adults replicated more favorable responses to vignettes of mentally ill persons if they were described as having received successful treatment for their condition (McGinty et al., 2015). In this study, effects were evident for persons described as diagnosed with schizophrenia, depression, and drug addiction. These studies suggest that interventions to reduce stigma should focus on the potential for successful treatment, such that mental disorders are seen as more similar to other health conditions from which recovery is possible.

Media exposure may influence negative and/or positive beliefs about mental illness in adolescents. A qualitative study with 12- to 14-year-olds found that television was their primary source of information about mental illness (Secker, Armstrong, & Hill, 1999). Adolescents are heavy consumers of mass media (total media use for 8- to 18-year-olds per day was reported as 7 hours and 38 minutes by Rideout, Foehr, & Roberts, 2010), and their attitudes and behaviors are influenced by such exposure. Reviews of the literature indicate a relationship between media exposure and the formation of gender stereotypes (Signorielli, 2001); aggression and desensitization to violence (Bushman & Anderson, 2001), particularly among children and young adolescents (Roberts & Foehr, 2004); and body image in adolescent women (Groesz, Levine, & Murnen, 2002). Furthermore, the media serve as a source of information for youth; over half of teenage women report learning about sex and birth control from TV, movies, and magazines (Brown & Witherspoon, 2001).

The Entertainment Industries Council supports efforts by film and television producers to portray mental illness and substance use in educationally helpful ways and to reduce harmful stereotypes associated with these conditions. However, little is known about the effectiveness of these efforts on the general public. The belief of adolescents that they cannot get effective treatment for mental illness was greater in depressed as well as suicidal adolescents the more they reported having watched films that portrayed mentally ill characters (Jamieson, Romer, & Jamieson, 2006). As noted earlier, such beliefs may be linked with mental illness stigma. This raises the question of whether stigma reduction could be achieved with films that emphasize the recovery of persons with mental illness. For example, the film *A Beautiful Mind* (2002) did well at the box office (IMDB, 2016), won four Oscars, and was given the year's "Most Outstanding Contribution to Public Understanding of Mental Illness" award from the National Alliance for the Mentally Ill (NAMI, 2002). The film was based on the life of Princeton mathematician John Nash (1928–2015) (played by Russell Crowe), whose academic work in an era before helpful treatments for mental illness were available later earned him a Nobel Prize.

EXAMPLES OF SUCCESSFUL STIGMA-REDUCTION PROGRAMS

Beginning in 2007, Great Britain's anti-stigma "Time to Change" (TTC) program included a national marketing effort, community outreach, and endorsements by celebrities. In addition to its antistigma marketing campaign, TTC sponsored exercise events, such as "Time to Get Moving," in order to increase contact with people who had experienced long-term mental health problems. A phone survey conducted in 2009 reported significantly less discrimination among friends and family and the inability to find and keep employment (Henderson et al., 2012). A 2009–2012 evaluation also found positive effects, concluding that in England "important gains were made in reducing public stigma and discrimination" (Evans-Lacko, 2014).

Under the auspices of California's Mental Health Services Act of 2004, the state undertook an ambitious program of stigma and discrimination reduction in 2011. The program involved 10 projects focused on various groups, including segments of the general public and healthcare providers (Clark et al., 2013). A major component was a social marketing campaign involving the dissemination of an hour-long film entitled *A New State of Mind: Ending the Stigma of Mental Illness*, as well as media programming directed to adolescents and young adults. A website, EachMindMatters.org, provided a central location for dissemination of program materials and discussion forums.

The RAND Corporation evaluated the program in 2014 using a statewide survey of over 1,000 adults who had indicated in an earlier survey that they experienced moderate to severe symptoms of psychological distress. Approximately 35% of this sample reported exposure to either the film or other aspects of the campaign. Compared to a matched subsample who did not see the campaign, those with some campaign exposure were more likely to have sought professional help for a mental or behavioral health condition in the past 12 months (49.7% vs. 34.3%). RAND attributed half of this difference to the campaign and estimated that as a result over 120,000 adults received treatment for their condition. A cost–benefit analysis that took into account the cost of the campaign, state expenses for treatment, and time away from work, the program delivered $35 in benefit to the state budget for every dollar spent on the campaign. Thus, on a cost–benefit basis, the campaign was considered a success (Ashwood et al., 2016).

A program of stigma-reduction projects has been ongoing in Canada since 2007. The Opening Minds program targets adolescents, healthcare providers, the workforce, and the news media in various educational programs (Mental Health Commission of Canada, 2015). The communication strategy has focused on in-person interventions featuring contact between audiences and persons with mental illness. Preliminary results indicate that the school-based programs for adolescents increase knowledge about mental illness; however, the effectiveness of the programs in increasing social acceptance of persons with mental illness has varied. The programs that increased knowledge the most were also more successful in reducing stigma. However, long-term follow-up has not yet been assessed. Nevertheless, going forward, the project aims to focus on those programs for youth that have exhibited the strongest outcomes.

CONCLUSION

This chapter reviewed evidence that addressing the stigma of mental illness in adolescence is an important endeavor. It is likely that adolescents who are informed about mental illness, both in terms of facts and the dispelling of myths, will be less likely to stigmatize others and more likely to seek and stay in treatment for their own mental health symptoms. In particular, there is evidence that increasing awareness of the efficacy of treatment can reduce harmful stereotypes and discrimination against those who experience mental illness.

This chapter has also highlighted the potential role of the mass media in destigmatizing mental illness, a role that will be more effective in partnerships with mental health professionals. Destigmatization also depends on mental health educators. Promoting positive contact by inviting persons with mental illness to classrooms as guest speakers and/or providing opportunities for adolescents to volunteer with persons with mental illness has been shown to be beneficial (Couture & Penn, 2003).

A recent report from the National Academy of Science (2016) on strategies to reduce stigma laid out an ambitious national agenda for the reduction of mental illness stigma. Indeed, that report and the review of successful programs in this chapter suggest that, if they are consistently pursued over the long term, such efforts can succeed. Part of the challenge involved in facilitating early intervention for mental illness is promoting and developing liaisons between mental health professionals and gatekeepers, such as general practitioners and school teachers and counselors, who are often the first to identify adolescent mental health problems. Such contact facilitates mental health referrals and reduces the time from symptom onset to treatment. In addition, to address the stigma or shame of seeking treatment for physical disorders (e.g., AIDS; Gewirtz & Gossart-Walker, 2000) or psychiatric disorders (prodromal symptoms; McGorry, Yung, & Phillips, 2001), there have been efforts to provide treatment at home or in settings that are not identified as psychiatric facilities. These approaches, coupled with increased education and contact opportunities with those diagnosed with mental disorders and efforts to provide accurate and helpful views of mental illness in media, are important steps in minimizing harm from stigma and ensuring that adolescents get early treatment for their developing or active mental disorders.

An Update on Evidence-Based Practices for Children and Adolescents in the Context of Policy, Research, and Practice: A Systems Perspective

Ka Ho Brian Chor
Kimberly E. Hoagwood
Su-Chin Serene Olin

chapter 30

OVERVIEW

In the past decade, the policy, research, and practice contexts of evidence-based practices (EBPs) for children and adolescents have undergone significant transformation. While hundreds of potentially effective treatments have been developed (Chorpita, Daleiden, et al., 2011), their translation into real-world settings has been stymied by challenges at multiple levels (Fixsen, Blase, Metz, & van Dyke, 2013; Fixsen, Naoom, Blase, Friedman, & Wallace, 2005). The purpose of this chapter is to provide a 10-year update on our last synthesis by describing the major changes in the policy, research, and practice contexts that have highlighted systems issues in the dissemination and implementation of EBPs. We first provide an overview of the system issues surrounding the three contexts.

Since the early 1990s the treatment development literature has yielded both breadth and depth in knowledge about EBPs for major child and adolescent disorders (Silverman & Hinshaw, 2008). The focus of EBP has extended beyond DSM-bound disorders and specialty mental health contexts, as reviews have identified effective home-based (Chaffin, Hecht, Bard, Silovsky, & Beasley, 2012), school-based (Langley, Nadeem, Kataoka, Stein, & Jaycox, 2010), and family engagement interventions (Kim, Munson, & McKay, 2012). Further, there has been an accompanying shift away from treatment efficacy trials toward the dissemination and implementation of EBPs in child mental health systems (Bruns & Hoagwood, 2008; Fixsen et al., 2013; Kazak et al., 2010). This shift has been fueled by two troublesome findings. First, there is a 17-year gap between publishing research findings and having those findings translated into practice. Second, of research findings that are published, only 14% are ultimately used to change practice (Green, 2001, 2007).

States have undertaken the monumental task of installing EBPs in their delivery systems (Fixsen et al., 2013; Gleacher et al., 2011). At least 20 states have invested over $100 million in EBP rollouts in the past decade (Bruns & Hoagwood, 2008), with some states further supported by contracts with purveyors (Fixsen et al., 2005) and by federal assistance in implementation (Substance Abuse and Mental Health Services Administration, 2013). Despite such investments, many state systems find themselves rolling out EBPs through trial and error (McHugh & Barlow, 2010) with limited impact on service delivery (Fixsen et al., 2013); only 10% of public systems in California, for example, deliver any kind of EBP (Wang, Saldana, Brown, & Chamberlain, 2010).

Major policy changes in healthcare are reframing the research and practice contexts for implementation of EBPs for children. Unlike the political climate a decade ago, when reports from the Institute of Medicine (IOM, 2001, 2006), the Surgeon General's Report on Mental Health (U.S. Public Health Service, 1999), and the National Action Plan on Children's Mental Health (U.S. Public Health Service, 2000) converged on the research–practice gaps in mental health, the current healthcare reform is presenting a new set of opportunities. The Children's Health Insurance Program Reauthorization Act of 2009 (CHIPRA; P.L. 111-3), the Paul Wellstone and Pete Domenici Mental Health Parity and Addiction Equity Act of 2008 (MHPAEA; P.L. 110-343), and the Patient Protection and Affordable Care Act of 2010 (ACA; P.L. 111-148) are changing the infrastructure, financing policies, and provider accountability standards for the mental health system. These policies have also repositioned mental health within a broader public health and prevention framework (Hoagwood, Olin, & Cleek, 2013; IOM, 2006; 2009).

PARADIGM SHIFTS IN POLICY

The system changes consequent to the ACA and broader healthcare policies include continued attention to the installation of EBPs, but they extend beyond this. Integration of the behavioral health and the healthcare systems is happening across the country in part to address problems of costly service duplication and fragmentation. Increasingly, payers are demanding monitoring and tracking of mental health outcomes. This requires the development of specific quality indicators and measures. New financing systems and business practices are also needed to sustain these changes and to maintain fiscal solvency. These changes are described below.

Integrated Care and Care Coordination

The traditional specialty mental health system is being replaced by mental health services delivered within regionalized networks of healthcare providers (Hoagwood, 2013; Kelleher, 2010). In the ACA, this paradigm shift translates to accountable care organizations (ACOs) on the system level and patient-centered medical homes (PCMHs)/health homes on the individual practitioner level. Both models aim to improve the quality and outcomes of care (Katon & Unützer, 2013). A key example is the Nationwide Children's Hospital Partners for Kids ACO, which serves 300,000 Medicaid children in Ohio. Partners for Kids uses a capitated arrangement with three Medicaid managed care plans. For each child, Partner for Kids is paid a set fee and is held responsible for managing and providing quality care, including mental health care (Allen, 2010; Vecchione, 2012). In the PCMH model, primary care physicians function as treatment leaders and are responsible for providing comprehensive and coordinated care with other professionals, including mental health professionals (Gabel, 2010). Many ACO and PCMH models are still being tested. Measuring their success will likely depend on the integration of clinical and administrative data and the performance of provider networks (Landon et al., 2013; Lewis & Fisher, 2012).

Standalone mental health clinics are being replaced by integrated health and behavioral health service agencies. This poses benefits and challenges. Since the ACA is incentivizing the integration of services through the co-location of primary and specialty care in community-based health settings, the overall quality and linkage of services for children, especially in rural areas, is likely to improve (Gabel, 2010). However, an integrated health and behavioral health system does not address the coordination of other child-serving sectors, most notably child welfare, juvenile justice, and education. These sectors operate under independent definitional and fiscal arrangements. Unless a broader reorganization is created to manage the behavioral health needs of children in these sectors, the fragmentation that has characterized mental health services for children for decades is likely to persist.

Quality Indicators

Quality indicators addressing children's health needs are being developed to hold the healthcare system accountable for improving the quality of care and for targeting the needs of all children (Institute of Medicine & National Research Council, 2011). Quality indicators addressing behavioral or mental health needs are new and relatively undeveloped, lagging behind those developed for adults (Pincus, Spaeth-Rublee, & Watkins, 2011; Zima & Mangione-Smith, 2011). To initiate this work, CHIPRA (P.L. 111-3) awarded $55 million to the Agency for Healthcare Research and Quality in 2010 to fund seven national Centers of Excellence over 4 years. These Centers of Excellence are tasked with developing core quality indicators across all areas of children's health (Zima et al., 2013). One priority area is the development of behavioral and mental health quality measures (Institute of Medicine & National Research Council, 2011). Specifically, one of the centers, the National Collaborative for Innovation in Quality (Scholle, principal investigator), is developing and testing quality indicators in child and adolescent depression (Lewandowski et al., 2013) and antipsychotic prescribing practices (Kealey et al., 2014). These quality indicators will help to align children's behavioral health services with broader healthcare services. However, this is only a small start. Much larger efforts are needed to develop measures of quality addressing mental health services for children (Zima et al., 2013).

The establishment of quality indicators facilitates tracking, reporting, and communicating outcomes (Berenson, Pronovost, & Krumholz, 2013). Although electronic health records

(EHRs) can support these functions, they are generally used to collect data on day-to-day operations and may not be transferrable from one record system to another. Further, their "meaningful use" for recording quality has not been a priority until the introduction of the Health Information Technology for Economic and Clinical Health (HITECH) Act under the American Recovery and Reinvestment Act of 2009 (P. L. 111-5). Moving forward, EHR-based quality measures will have vast potential to identify outcome patterns and trends to inform decision making (Zima et al., 2013) and to initiate quality improvement (Torda & Tinoco, 2013).

Financing Policies

Financing policies for mental health services are shaped by payment reforms that accompany care coordination. The ACO model employs a flexible payment infrastructure (e.g., capitation, shared losses and savings) to control the total cost of care and to incentivize networked providers with reimbursements that are tied to quality measures (Center for Medicare & Medicaid Services, 2013). In mental health, incentivized outcomes may provide additional flexibility for networked providers to innovate their practices by incorporating EBPs. Adoption of specific EBPs, however, will be a function of economic resources, network mission, and whether an EBP will cover a large portion of clients within the network, especially high-need and high-cost clients.

Payment reforms are also occurring on the state level. Mirroring the impetus of the ACA, New York State, for example, has initiated a Medicaid Redesign Team to rein in Medicaid spending, the largest payment source for child mental health services (New York State Department of Health, 2011). A key initiative stemming from Medicaid Redesign is contracting with behavioral health organizations to provide mental health services. The services include direct delivery and administrative, monitoring, and management functions using standard quality indicators such as inpatient admission rates, engagement with follow-up outpatient services, and use of EHR (NYSOMH, 2012). The behavioral health organization initiative will affect both inpatient and outpatient providers serving Medicaid populations, with one goal being cost reduction. Under this payment system shift, the viability of EBPs will depend on their goodness-of-fit with standard quality indicators and financing parameters (e.g., length of treatment allowed). It will also depend on providers' ability to improve their business practices (e.g., setting and reaching productivity benchmarks, redesigning financial structure, and improving operational flow) in order to fiscally and operationally support EBP integration into their routine services. EBPs that yield measurable outcomes and long-term cost reductions will be particularly valuable (Saldana, Chamberlain, Bradford, Campbell, & Landsverk, 2015).

PARADIGM SHIFTS IN RESEARCH

To improve care quality, practitioners, states, and healthcare systems are increasingly motivated to translate the knowledge base for EBP (Silverman & Hinshaw, 2008) into service systems (Kazdin, 2013). Their efforts to adopt and routinize EBPs depend on many factors that are relevant to the fit of EBPs to the context of their system (Fixsen et al., 2013; McHugh & Barlow, 2010). In short, there is a strong need for a complementary knowledge base in dissemination and implementation research.

The research funding climate in the past 10 years has reflected this shift. In 2001, the National Institute of Mental Health (NIMH) released a funding announcement specifically for Dissemination Research in Mental Health and funded three grants; this number surged to over 40 grants from 2005 to 2009. On average 50 to 60 grant applications are now reviewed per funding cycle (Chambers, 2010, 2012). These funded studies increasingly target sustainability, adaptability, scaling up systems, and organizational decision making (Chambers, 2010, 2012). The recently established Patient-Centered Outcomes Research Institute (PCORI, 2013) funded 50 pilot projects to address five priorities in research to help patients and healthcare providers make informed decisions. These funding opportunities look beyond treatment development in a laboratory setting, focusing instead on aligning effective services and treatments with the demands of healthcare reform. A key funding priority is the communication and dissemination of research results to patients, caregivers, and clinicians to improve decision making (PCORI, 2013).

Below we highlight some of the progress and challenges in the models, designs, and measures surrounding dissemination and implementation (D&I) research.

D&I Models

Creating a scientific knowledge base on the effectiveness of services that can be readily adopted within different contexts requires a different paradigm from the typical efficacy to effectiveness model that has guided much research in the past. Two models designed to short-circuit the unnecessary delays in translating research findings into practice were developed and have been used to guide intervention development: the Deployment-Focused Model (Weisz, 2004) and the Clinic-Community Intervention Model (Hoagwood, Burns, & Weisz, 2002). Both models suggest that researchers attend to multilevel contextual variables through the development and testing of new interventions, even in the initial efficacy phase. These variables might include characteristics of practitioners, organizations, communities, and families.

There has been significant growth in the refinement of D&I-specific frameworks, as well as efforts to synthesize these models (Damschroder et al., 2009). Comprehensive D&I models such as the Consolidated Framework for Implementation Research (Damschroder et al., 2009), the Practical, Robust Implementation and Sustainability Model (Feldstein & Glasgow, 2008), and the Advanced Conceptual Model of EBP Implementation (Aarons, Hurlburt, & Horwitz, 2011) converge on the multiphase (i.e., from intervention development, to adoption, to implementation) and multilevel (e.g., from individual, organization, to system) nature of EBP delivery. Each model is useful in delineating information about facilitators and barriers to D&I (Damschroder et al., 2009; Durlak & DuPre, 2008). These models have been applied to health and mental health intervention implementation across diverse settings and sectors (Aarons et al., 2011; Damschroder et al., 2009; Feldstein & Glasgow, 2008).

In contrast to the traditional EBP focus on client-treatment factors, a key feature of D&I models is an emphasis on the organizational context in which changes, outcomes, and services take place. Organization-level variables such as leadership, operational capacity, and vertical and horizontal networks are influential in the different phases of D&I (Aarons et al., 2011; Wisdom, Chor, Hoagwood, & Horwitz, 2014). Organizational social context (e.g., culture and climate) has been found to influence a range of outcomes and quality practices (Glisson, 2007; Glisson & Schoenwald, 2005; Olin, Kutash, et al., 2014; Olin, Williams, et al., 2014).

D&I Designs and Measures

To expand the science base of D&I research, D&I designs are needed to study large system changes. For this purpose, Curran, Bauer, Mittman, Pyne, and Stetler (2012) propose three hybrid designs:

1. Testing a clinical intervention and gathering implementation data at the same time
2. Testing a clinical intervention and testing implementation strategies at the same time
3. Testing an implementation and gathering data on a clinical intervention's impact on relevant outcomes.

Hybrid type 1 is best for reducing the time gap between efficacy and effectiveness research (e.g., during a randomized controlled trial, data on barriers and facilitators to implementation are gathered). Hybrid type 2 is most appropriate when there are clear clinical outcomes (e.g., patient-level improvement) and implementation outcomes (e.g., clinic-level adoption of EBP). For example, feasibility pilots or preliminary, small-scale randomized controlled trials prior to large-scale implementation are best suited for Hybrid type 2. Hybrid type 3 is best used when the focus is on implementation without necessarily completing the full portfolio of effectiveness studies so that the clinical effectiveness of an EBP can be tested under different conditions. Each hybrid design has different units of analysis (e.g., patient, clinic, system) and evaluation methods (e.g., quantitative, qualitative, mixed, formative, or summative methods).

Beyond individual interventions, D&I designs have been applied to several large-scale experiments that address healthcare system changes, with promising evidence. The Depression Improvement Across Minnesota—Offering a New Direction (DIAMOND) initiative partnered health plans with clinics to evaluate the implementation impact of a collaborative care model for depression on patient outcomes and stakeholder engagement (Solberg et al., 2010). The Community Partners in Care model, which promotes community engagement and planning and interagency collaboration, was found to be superior to a technical assistance and outreach approach in implementing depression quality improvement programs across community service sectors (Wells et al., 2013). A third study has focused on implementation strategies that are effective in communities, such as the Communities That Care coalition-based strategy targeted toward the adoption of prevention EBPs (Shapiro et al., 2013).

Optimal D&I designs also need to be compatible with evolving technologies in interventions. The Continuous Evaluation of Evolving Behavioral Intervention Technology (CEEBIT) is an evaluation framework tailored specifically to web-based and mobile interventions (Mohr, Cheung, Schueller, Brown, & Duan, 2013). Based on electronic data, the CEEBIT framework involves simultaneous evaluations of multiple interventions, eliminates those with inferior outcomes, and incorporates new interventions for further evaluation. Thus, this framework can empirically accelerate the validation of interventions that have the capacity to spread, a luxury that conventional, time-consuming D&I evaluations often cannot afford (Mohr et al., 2013).

Although effective and efficient D&I designs are important, few systematic measures assess the implementation processes and mechanisms to identify when and how implementation fails or succeeds. The Stages of Implementation Completion (Chamberlain, Brown, & Saldana, 2011) and the Reach Effectiveness Adoption Implementation (Glasgow, Lichtenstein, & Marcus, 2003) represent focused measurement efforts to derive useful and communicable metrics for implementation studies. Other complementary efforts include construction of measures associated with predictors of implementation outcomes. The Seattle Implementation Research Collaborative (2013) Instrument Review Project and the Grid-Enabled Measures database (National Cancer Institute, 2013) centralize measures for implementation-related factors (e.g., community, organization, provider, individual, and innovation characteristics). The measurement of implementation factors means that essential data at each stage of the implementation process are collected. This effort will improve the understanding of implementation thresholds, advance program evaluations, and refine D&I study designs (Durlak & DuPre, 2008).

PARADIGM SHIFTS IN PRACTICE

Trends in practice are driven by the prevalence of psychiatric disorders, service delivery characteristics, and the needs of the populations being served. The occurrence of a DSM disorder associated with severe impairment is unfortunately common, affecting one in 10 children and adolescents (ages 8–15) every year (Merikangas, He, Brody, et al., 2010), and one in five adolescents (ages 13–18) in their lifetime (Merikangas, He, Burstein, et al., 2010). Among two nationally representative samples, 50% to 63% did not access mental health services (Mechanic, McAlpine, & Rochefort, 2014; Merikangas, He, Brody, et al., 2010; Merikangas et al., 2011). Racial/ethnic minorities also received significantly fewer services than their white counterparts. Adolescents diagnosed with mood, anxiety, and attention-deficit/hyperactivity disorders (ADHD) also received limited services (Merikangas et al., 2011). The underuse of mental health services, however, masks the needs of specific child-serving sectors with high rates of mental health problems (Farmer et al., 2010), including children in out-of-home placements (Substance Abuse and Mental Health Services Administration, 2007), foster care (Administration for Children and Families, 2013), and juvenile justice systems (Office of Juvenile Justice and Delinquency Prevention, 2009). These sectors continue to demonstrate high needs for mental health services (Desai et al., 2006; Farmer et al., 2010).

For clinicians, EBPs are the means to meet the population needs for mental health services. Pragmatic tools and resources help clinicians and consumers assess treatment options and select appropriate treatment. Public EBP registries facilitate this goal. The National Registry of Evidence-based Programs and Practices contains 195 mental health and substance abuse EBPs for children ages 0 to 17 (SAMHSA, 2013); the National Child Traumatic Stress Network (NCTSN, 2013) summarizes 48 EBPs and promising practices for trauma. EBP registries are also tailored to child-serving sectors. The California Evidence-based Clearinghouse (2013) contains 173 child welfare EBPs for children ages 0 to 17. The Office of Juvenile Justice and Delinquency Prevention (OJJDP, 2013) Model Programs Guide is a database of 142 EBPs that cover the continuum of services for youth in juvenile justice. Although review methods for evidence may vary across registries, treatments that are considered EBPs are relatively consistent. The underlying constant among diverse EBPs is the integration of best research evidence, clinical expertise, and patient values to produce specific, desired outcomes (IOM, 2001; Sexton et al., 2010).

Below we outline some of the significant changes in clinical practice that have occurred in the past decade.

Pediatric Psychopharmacology and the Role of Primary Care Physicians in Mental Health

Increasingly, mental health services for children and adolescents include use of psychotropic medications, especially for mood disorders and ADHD (Merikangas, He, Rapoport, Vitiello, & Olfson, 2013). Although antipsychotic use is infrequent in the general population (Merikangas, He, Rapoport, Vitiello, & Olfson, 2013), it has increased threefold between 1999 and 2008 among pediatric Medicaid recipients and has created a significant financial burden on Medicaid spending (Lagnado, 2013). These concerns prompted the Department of Health and Human Services to launch a five-state probe to review antipsychotic prescriptions for Medicaid children (Lagnado, 2013).

Since primary care physicians (e.g., pediatricians and family physicians) are often the first-line treatment providers for children with mental health needs, there is a high need to train these providers in identifying and managing mental health conditions in children, beyond prescribing psychotropic medications (Gabel, 2010; Pidano & Honigfeld, 2012). Twenty-six states have formed the National Network of Child Psychiatry Access Programs to exchange technical assistance in supporting child psychiatry training in primary care, developing documentation and outcome tools (Straus & Sarvet, 2012). Key state training efforts include the Massachusetts Child Psychiatry Access Project (Sarvet et al., 2010), the Washington Partnership Access Line (Hilt, McDonell, Rockhill, Golombek, & Thompson, 2009), and the New York State Training and Education for the Advancement of Children's Health (Gabel, 2010). These concurrent efforts will likely result in improved identification and diagnosis of children with mental health disorders, leading to greater access and linkage to mental health services for these children who presented in primary care settings.

Large-Scale EBP Training and Use of Technology for Training

Major national and state initiatives have invested in large-scale EBP training to increase public access to EBPs and strengthen the professional workforce (Bruns & Hoagwood, 2008; McHugh & Barlow, 2010). They use a combination of didactics, workshops, supervision, and expert consultation to facilitate sustainability of adoption (Comer & Barlow, 2013; McHugh & Barlow, 2010). The SAMHSA-funded NCTSN has invested $377 million in 180 centers to train 901,411 professionals in 41 trauma-informed EBPs and promising practices between 2001 and 2009 (B. J. Burns, personal communication, October 17, 2013). States have also scaled up training in multiple EBPs (Bruns & Hoagwood, 2008; McHugh & Barlow, 2010). New York is a leading state in this training effort (McHugh & Barlow, 2010). In 2004, New York State Office of Mental Health funded the Evidence-Based Treatment Dissemination Center to train frontline clinicians and supervisors in outpatient and inpatient settings to provide EBPs. To date, more than 1,300 clinicians and 200 supervisors have been trained in functional family therapy and cognitive-behavioral therapy for trauma, depression, and disruptive behaviors (Gleacher et al., 2011).

The increased availability of webinars and online training has facilitated large-scale training initiatives. Webinars and online training can reach clinicians who want to keep abreast of current treatments. For clinicians with varying experiences, web- or computer-based training offers self-paced learning, standardization, and consistency of quality (Kendall, Khanna, Edson, Cummings, & Harris, 2011; Sigel et al., 2013). For others who are limited by cost and the inability to attend live training, free, web-based learning sanctioned by EBP developers becomes a feasible alternative (Sigel et al., 2013). The Medical University of South Carolina (2013) has partnered with trauma-focused cognitive-behavioral therapy (TF-CBT) developers to create TF-CBTWeb (http://tfcbt.musc.edu), which offers free resources for key treatment components, printable scripts, handouts, and instructions on handling challenging situations. To supplement TF-CBTWeb, Washington University in St. Louis and the University of Missouri have formed the Missouri Therapy Network (2013) to offer free TF-CBT training webinars, demonstration videos, and manuals (https://motherapynetwork.wustl.edu). National and state technical assistance centers also offer clinical webinars on a variety of topics. SAMHSA (2013) has funded the Disaster Technical Assistance Center (www.samhsa.gov/dtac) to offer webcasts on behavioral health training; the New York State Clinic Technical Assistance Center (2013) offers free webinars (www.ctacny.com) on important clinical topics, including cognitive-behavioral therapy, trauma assessment, and Motivational Interviewing.

Technology Advances in Practice

Technology advances are also revolutionizing the delivery of treatment to address patient needs and improve engagement. The structure and sequence of cognitive-behavioral therapy makes for a natural transition to interactive, computer, or web-based platforms (Baum, Epstein, & Kelleher, 2013). Cognitive-behavioral therapy for depression (e.g., Stressbuster) and anxiety (e.g., Camp-Copa-A-Lot) are available in CD-ROM packages and are associated with symptom reductions (Abeles et al., 2009; Khanna & Kendall, 2010). Online EBPs are appealing to children and families who are unable or unwilling to seek in-person treatment (Baum et al., 2013). For example, Triple P Online derives from the Triple P Positive Parenting Program, an EBP for parents of children with disruptive behavior. This online version allows parents to proceed through electronic modules at their own pace, and empirical evidence now exists for child behavioral outcomes and parent satisfaction (Sanders, Baker, & Turner, 2012). Effective online cognitive-behavioral treatments for depression include Master Your Mood Online (Gerrits, van der Zanden, Visscher, & Conijn, 2007) and MoodGYM (O'Kearney, Gibson, Christensen, & Griffiths, 2006). For anxiety, the BRAVE-ONLINE program exists (March, Spence, & Donovan, 2009). Diverse online peer support groups have also emerged in recent years to expand ancillary support for substance abuse in adolescents (Mermelstein

& Turner, 2006) and children coping with parents' medical conditions (Giesbers, Verdonck-de Leeuw, van Zuuren, Kleverlaan, & van der Linden, 2010). This trend in using digital technologies to deliver treatments, educational trainings, and supportive services will likely continue (Donovan, Spence, & March, 2013).

To support EBPs delivered in different technological modalities, web and mobile software applications are available for psychoeducation, symptom assessment, tracking of treatment progress, and communication between patients and clinicians (Baum et al., 2013; Luxton, McCann, Bush, Mishkind, & Reger, 2011). The myADHDportal.com, developed by Cincinnati Children's Hospital Medical Center, offers training in office ADHD workflow and registers a child's ADHD and side effect ratings by parents and teachers to aid diagnosis and monitoring of treatment (Baum et al., 2013). The portal also maintains secure communications among parents, teachers, and pediatricians during the treatment process (Baum et al., 2013). To improve self-awareness in adolescent depression, the Murdoch Children Research institute created the mobiletype program (Mobile Tracking Young People's Experiences), a phone application that reminds users to monitor their daily mood, stress, and activities. These data are uploaded to a secure website and shared with the users' physicians (Kauer et al., 2012). Although web and mobile data collection platforms may create ethical and confidentiality concerns (Luxton et al., 2011), their potential to streamline individual patient–clinician experiences and assist quality improvement should not be minimized (Baum et al., 2013).

Evidence-Based Clinical Decision Making

Given the EBP knowledge base in children's mental health (Chorpita, Bernstein, & Daleiden, 2011; Silverman & Hinshaw, 2008), the field is turning to evidence-based clinical decision making to reach a larger portion of children with diverse clinical case mixes (Gomory, 2013) and to use electronic measurement systems to improve the quality of clinical decision making. Several scalable innovations have shown promising evidence.

The Modular Approach to Therapy for Children with anxiety, depression, trauma, or conduct problems (MATCH-ADTC; Chorpita & Weisz, 2009; Weisz et al., 2012) enables clinicians to conceptualize EBPs collectively rather than singly by offering a treatment package that consists of a guiding protocol for each problem area and 33 practice modules (e.g., a decision flowchart guiding module selection and sequencing for self-calming). In a two-state randomized controlled trial involving 84 clinicians and 174 treated children, MATCH-ADTC was compared with standard cognitive-behavioral psychotherapy and usual care. Results indicated that MATCH-ADTC produced significantly faster improvement, fewer diagnoses after treatment, and a balanced flexibility that resulted in more evidence-based treatment (Weisz et al., 2012).

An outgrowth of MATCH-ADTC is the Managing Adaptive Practice (MAP) tool, which provides clinicians access to the most updated scientific treatment information and detailed evidence-based treatment recommendations for specific problems (Southam-Gerow et al., 2014). The MAP web-based dashboard feedback system allows data collection on client outcomes. It also records the clinician's use of practice elements throughout a client's treatment trajectory. In Los Angeles County, youth treated by practitioners trained in the MAP tool demonstrated large effect sizes in the improvement of trauma and depression symptoms (Southam-Gerow et al., 2014).

Another clinical decision-making tool is the Contextualized Feedback System (CFS), which promotes clinicians' practice through session-to-session documentation of psychometrically and clinically sound measures (e.g., client functioning) (Bickman, Kelley, Breda, de Andrade, & Riemer, 2011). Multisite trials of the CFS over a 2-year period showed that youths treated by clinicians who received weekly feedback from CFS improved faster than youths treated by clinicians who did not use CFS (Bickman et al., 2011). Another study examined the implementation challenges of embedding CFS into community-based mental health clinics in New York State (Hoagwood et al., 2014). Strategies for integrating CFS in routine use included mandating clinical documentation, developing site-specific project plans to manage implementation, and using weekly consultation calls to strengthen the appropriate use of the system (Hoagwood et al., 2014).

Treatment innovations such as MATCH-ADTC, MAP, and CFS can enhance client outcomes and can be adapted to fit the real-world context of divergent practices and settings. Their scalability in state systems can be extended to other kinds of systems, including healthcare systems, and even countries.

Task Shifting and Use of Peers in Family Support Services

A systemic approach to improving EBP delivery and care coordination not only is driven by policy mandates, but is also influenced by evolution of the clinical workforce. Changes in healthcare are leading to workforce shifts that redistribute specialist tasks to nonspecialists. Task shifting has a long history in global health and mental health initiatives in developing countries. It has transferred the roles previously assumed by more experienced and expensive providers to others with less formal training to provide therapeutic and support services. Task shifting has direct implications for the delivery of mental health services in both developed and underdeveloped countries (Kazdin & Rabbitt, 2013). The U.S. public mental health system is largely supported by bachelor's-level counselors and social workers who are supervised by advanced mental health professionals. It entails the use of standardized trainings and simplified treatment protocols geared toward lay counselors, with a built-in model of monitoring and evaluation to ensure fidelity (Kazdin & Rabbitt, 2013).

An example of task shifting in children's mental health is the employment of parents or caregivers who have raised a child with a mental health problem in working directly—family to family—with other parents/caregivers seeking services. These peer parents may deliver a range of services, including family support, intake, screening, referral, and group interventions (Hoagwood et al., 2010). One group treatment employs peer parents along with social workers in the Multiple Family Group intervention (McKay et al., 2011).

Family support services have become billable under Medicaid or federal block grants in 16 states (Center for Health Care Strategies Inc., 2012). In addition, family advocacy organizations report a national trend to certify family support specialists (Hoagwood et al., 2008). The evidence base for peer/parent-delivered services in children's mental health is emerging (Hoagwood et al., 2010), but evidence for its impact on youth outcomes is needed (Blau et al., 2010; Hoagwood et al., 2010; Kutash, Duchnowski, Green, & Ferron, 2011).

One major challenge is the integration of family support services into agencies that provide an array of child-centered services. A study is under way in New York State to assist in understanding methods for integrating and assessing the quality of these services. To characterize 21 organizations that provide family support services in New York State, this study identified 14 organization-level and 27 family support services–level quality indicators (Olin, Kutash, et al., 2014). These indicators were significantly associated with organizational climate and culture (Olin, Williams, et al., 2014). The relationship between these quality indicators and the organizational social context suggests that some contextual aspects of agencies (role clarity, stress, decision making, job attitudes) may be malleable and could be improved to facilitate integration of high-quality family support services. These quality indicators may also be a useful tool for aligning family support services with other health services in the new healthcare context, as they provide metrics for monitoring quality.

SUMMARY

Significant—even tectonic—shifts in healthcare policy, research, and practice have occurred in the past decade and have laid a new foundation for the work that lies ahead. ACA marks a significant policy shift; ACA and MHPAEA restructure mental health services under the umbrella of general health services. MHPAEA ensures that all individuals with mental health and substance abuse problems are given equitable care, care that is equivalent in value (i.e., in its financial requirements and treatment limitations) to medical benefits. The ACA's emphasis on integrating and coordinating care, use of EHR, ACOs, health homes, and quality benchmarks holds providers accountable for outcomes. This is a major change for health and behavioral health systems. Under these new mandates, requirements, and structures, networks of service providers integrated within larger structures will be responsible for the health of the population under their purview.

The foci of research on children's mental health during the decade 1990 to 2000 emphasized efficacy and effectiveness studies designed to strengthen the knowledge base on interventions and services that improved children's outcomes. The emphasis in the past decade has advanced a broader set of aims, focusing on the translation of effective interventions and services into different contexts, settings, and systems. This shift has called for a different set of frameworks and theories that are oriented toward broader public health impact. This is the crux of the new scientific agenda in dissemination and implementation. It is leading to a set of research projects and a portfolio that tests strategies, methods, and designs to support large-scale system changes. The D&I research agenda, by definition, has to be practical and innovative with respect to partnerships with system designers, practitioners, and consumers/families. Studies of interventions targeted at organizational, policy, and even system changes will also be important. These include how to embed and implement effective practices into primary care, schools, child welfare systems, juvenile justice facilities, communities, and the healthcare system. With the latest funding interest in global mental health research, D&I studies will be needed to address, for example, the World Health Organization's global development agenda after 2015 to improve mental health services research in low- and middle-income countries (NIMH, 2013). Further, as the National Institutes of Health (2012) awarded $100 million to fund 11 Autism Centers of Excellence, research on diagnosis and treatment will reflect a stronger focus on genetics and neuroscience in the coming years (Insel, 2013).

As major changes in emphasis and direction have been shaped by advances in policy and research, the practice of mental health services is also shifting. Training models to install EBPs in the hands of front-line practitioners (i.e., primary care physicians, nurses, social workers, teachers, case managers, peer/parent partners) have been developed and are being tested. Yet, unmet service needs persist. Child-serving sectors (e.g., primary care, schools, mental health clinics, child welfare agencies, juvenile justice facilities) face significant challenges: heavy caseloads, long waiting lists, more distressed families, and changes in reimbursement structures away from volume only (as in fee-for-service environments) and toward accountability for outcomes. To adapt to this new environment, clinicians need tools and resources to provide effective and efficient services. These include tele-health consultation, supervision models that attend to specific changes in outcomes, and clinical decision-making tools. The behavioral health workforce will continue to expand as states and healthcare systems expand Medicaid services and health insurance coverage under the ACA. Workforce expansion will include training individuals who enter the workforce with less formal training and require more targeted skills. These workforce changes will also require different trainings not only on specific EBP skills but also on organizational issues related to the culture and climate of the work environment. These may include team building (Kutash et al., 2014), organizational problem solving (Glisson, Hemmelgarn, et al., 2012; Glisson & Schoenwald, 2005), and use of quality indicators (Olin, Kutash, et al., 2014; Olin, Williams, et al., 2014).

CONCLUSION

The policy, research, and practice changes that have occurred in the past decade are altering the fundamental infrastructure of mental health services for children and adolescents. These changes necessitate that policymakers, researchers, practitioners, and consumers/families form new alliances and partnerships among themselves and with healthcare systems. These new alliances and networks, if structured correctly, have the potential to provide, for the first time, quality health and mental health care to the millions of children and their families who suffer unnecessarily. Aligning policy, research, and practice in the service of improved quality of life for children with mental health needs should be our horizon line.

The American Treatment System for Adolescent Substance Use Disorders in the 21st Century: Challenges Remain But Change Is on the Horizon

Kathleen Meyers
John Cacciola
Suzanne Ward
Abigail Woodworth

31

chapter

OVERVIEW

The number of youth in need of various levels of substance abuse intervention is staggering. There are 1.7 million U.S. youth (ages 12–17 years) struggling with a substance use disorder, with an additional 1.65 million new adolescent substance use initiators (Substance Abuse and Mental Health Services Administration [SAMHSA], 2012). These data are cause for concern as at no other point in an individual's development are the stakes for addiction so high: adolescence is the at-risk period for developing a substance use disorder (Dennis, 2009; Hingson, Heeren, Winter, & Wechsler, 2003; Hingson & Zha, 2009; Hingson, Zha, & Weitzman, 2009; Kandel, Yamaguchi, & Chen, 1992; Wagner & Anthony, 2002), with youth five times more likely to develop a substance use disorder compared to adults (Hingson, Heeren, & Winter, 2006; Miller, Naimi, Brewer, & Jones, 2007). To make matters worse, only 8.4% of the 1.7 million youth (ages 12–17 years) in need of addiction treatment are receiving specialty care (SAMHSA, 2012).

There are many reasons why adolescents do not access treatment. At the individual level, adolescents (perhaps even more than adults) minimize or fail to recognize an alcohol or other drug problem (Melnick, De Leon, Hawke, Jainchill, & Kressel, 1997). Moreover, adolescent concerns about disclosing sensitive information to parents and competing priorities for families with multiple problems render access problematic (Cheng, Savageau, Sattler, & DeWitt, 1993; Cornelius, Pringle, Jernigan, Kirisci, & Clark, 2001; Ford, Millstein, Halpern-Felsher, & Irwin, 1997). While these individual problems are significant, there are efforts to bring about problem recognition and motivation for change through parent-focused interventions (Rahdert & Czechowicz, 1995; Wagner & Waldron, 2001).

The purpose of this chapter is to discuss an additional complicating factor that impacts adolescent treatment and goes beyond the individual youth and his or her family: the service delivery system. While adolescent substance use represents a continual national concern, the American substance abuse treatment system continues to underperform in terms of its ability to prevent, identify, treat, and support substance-abusing youth despite numerous scientific advances (e.g., Adolescent Community Reinforcement Approach [A-CRA], cognitive-behavioral therapy [CBT], Motivational Enhancement Therapy [MET], Multisystemic Therapy, Multidimensional Family Therapy [MDFT], Seeking Safety, and Seven Challenges; Jainchill, 2012; Muck, et al., 2001; Rahdert & Czechowicz, 1995; Segal, Morral, & Stevens, 2014; Wagner & Waldron, 2001). The focus on the acute phases of the disease, coupled with the limited number of adolescent specialty programs, the quality concerns of programs that do exist, and the fact that only small proportions of youth access any type of treatment including continuing care, means that youth who use and/or abuse alcohol or other drugs as well as those with a substance use disorder cannot take advantage of scientific developments within a full continuum of care (Meyers, Cacciola, Ward, Kaynak, & Woodworth, 2014).

Fortunately, we are at a watershed moment in the way in which substance use disorders are perceived and are about to be managed in this country. We have the real opportunity to open service doors to increasing numbers of youth with varying degrees of substance use (e.g., mild, moderate, severe), but we must improve the treatment system (e.g., screening, early intervention, treatment, and recovery) so that these scientific advances can be capitalized upon.

HEALTH INSURANCE REFORM AND PARITY LEGISLATION

Two pieces of legislation make it possible to finally integrate substance use and mental health disorders into the rest of healthcare and to ensure that these illnesses are cared for at par with other medical disorders. Specifically, the Affordable Care Act (ACA) requires providers and insurers to implement and cover the full range of prevention, early intervention, and care management services for substance use disorders in virtually all healthcare organizations, and it extends dependent coverage under a parent's healthcare plan until the age of 26 years. Given that substance use disorders typically develop during adolescence and manifest as serious problems among emerging adults, preventing and treating this disease in its early form should prove most cost-effective, benefiting not only adolescents, their families, and society, but insurers as well. In addition to the ACA, the Paul Wellstone and Pete Domenici Mental Health Parity and Addiction Equity Act of 2008 requires that care for substance use disorders must have generally the same type, duration, range of service options, and patient financial burden as the care currently available to patients with comparable physical illnesses. This combined legislation requires a change in the national discourse and approach to the treatment and financing of substance use disorders (including in adolescents): they are to be treated like other chronic illnesses, and health plans are to offer care for the full spectrum of substance use disorders at par with other medical disorders. The time has come to address system inadequacies so that important and sustained changes occur in the way care is delivered to adolescents and young adults who are at risk for substance use disorders, who have used alcohol or other drugs, and who are recovering from substance use disorders.

ACUTE VERSUS CHRONIC CARE

The number of youth in need of varying levels of treatment is staggering. Yet, in many ways, the American system of substance abuse treatment for adolescents is antiquated as it has not kept pace with numerous scientific advances. For example, scientific evidence clearly indicates that addiction is similar to other chronic conditions (e.g., asthma, hypertension, type 2 diabetes) necessitating a chronic disease model for management (McLellan et al., 2000; Saitz et al., 2008). This means identifying and treating this disease (or its pre-disease state) as early as possible, and treating and managing the full expression of the disease over time (McLellan et al., 2000; Saitz et al., 2008). Despite this knowledge, acute care dominates the system for treating substance use disorders in adolescents: failing to recognize or ignoring warning signs, treating only the acute expression of this chronic disease, and failing to provide any follow-up monitoring or care. Reimbursement for care is generally restricted to adolescents who are already "in deep" with a disorder, usually with associated juvenile justice and/or mental health problems. This is in direct contrast to informed public health approaches to other chronic conditions.

Like other chronic illnesses with social, biological, and environmental determinants, substance use disorders are best addressed with a full continuum of care, including screening, early intervention, treatment, and continuing care and supportive services. Unfortunately, the currently used approaches to screening and early intervention are largely inadequate. The availability and the quality of adolescent treatment are insufficient, and continuing care and supportive services are basically nonexistent. However, there are systematic opportunities to transform the adolescent substance abuse treatment system at every point on the service continuum.

SCREENING

Adolescents with varying degrees of substance use can be found throughout U.S. communities, coming into contact with a variety of settings and service systems. Identification of these teens by their levels of use is important because different stages of substance use require qualitatively different types of targeted interventions (e.g., brief interventions, outpatient treatment, long-term residential treatment, continuing care services; Wagner & Waldron, 2001; Winters, 1999). This has the potential to halt the trajectory to addiction and reduce the morbidity and mortality related to this condition. Thus, screening for risk factors, early use, or early disease presence is one of the first lines of defense against a disease that begins in adolescence and is routinely associated with a costly combination of social, physical, mental, and public health problems (Meyers et al., 2014). Unfortunately, there is a pervasive failure to identify substance use as well as the emerging signs of a developing disorder. As a result, youth are *not* treated early, their substance use and other problems escalate, and more intensive and expensive care is needed.

Adolescents should be screened within all treatment and social services systems that they come in contact with (e.g., mental health system, foster care system, juvenile justice system). However, there are two settings that are ideal for early case finding: healthcare settings (e.g., primary care facilities) and schools. Large numbers of "general population" youth can be found at each these sites.

Screening in Healthcare Settings

The majority of adolescents see a healthcare provider at least annually, making healthcare settings particularly good sites for case finding (Freeborn, Polen, & Mullooly, 1995; National Association of State Alcohol and Drug Abuse Directors [NASADAD], 1998, 2002; Newacheck, Brindis, Cart, Marchi, & Irwin, 1999; Sterling & Weisner, 2007). There are now federally supported Screening, Brief Intervention, and Referral to Treatment (SBIRT) projects (Madras et al., 2009) designed to encourage school nurses and primary care physicians to screen, conduct a brief intervention for a positive screen, and when necessary refer adolescents with substance use problems to treatment. A growing body of evidence demonstrates the utility and/or efficacy of SBIRT in reducing adolescent substance use in emergency rooms, primary care settings, and federal qualified healthcare centers (Bernstein et al., 2010; Knight et al., 2005; Madras et al., 2009; Mitchell, Gryczynski, O'Grady, & Schwartz, 2013; Mitchell et al., 2016; Monti et al., 1999; Spirito et al., 2004; Tait, Hulse, Robertson, & Sprivulis, 2005; Tanner-Smith, Wilson, & Lipsey, 2013; Walton et al., 2010). It is not surprising, then, that SBIRT is endorsed by the National Institute of Alcohol Abuse and Alcoholism, the National Institute on Drug Abuse, the Substance Abuse and Mental Health Services Administration, and most importantly the American Academy of Pediatrics (Levy & Kokotailo, 2011) and the American Medical Association.

While promising, all three components of adolescent SBIRT are challenging for healthcare providers. This will be discussed below.

Screening in Schools

Schools are a logical location to identify and appropriately intervene with youth at various points on the addiction continuum. Unfortunately, random drug testing and zero-tolerance policies are the predominant school-based approach to identifying and addressing adolescent substance use. Introduced in 1994 to address weapons in schools, with Elementary and Secondary Education Act funding contingent upon their enactment (Martin, 2000; McAndrews, 2001), zero-tolerance policies quickly expanded to include a wide range of disciplinary issues such as drug use (through school drug-testing practices). While the original intent of school drug-testing policies was substance use identification and early intervention, they have not increased access to care and thus have made limited contributions to the subsequent well-being of adolescents (Lear, 2002; Wagner, Kortlander, & Morris, 2001).

While advocates of school drug testing do not encourage reports to law enforcement or breaks in student confidentiality, the on-the-ground reality tends to be harsh punishment, including reports to law enforcement, suspension from athletic teams, and school suspension and expulsion (National Center on Addiction and Substance Abuse [CASA], 2011; Ringwalt et al., 2009). All of these are contraindicated by federal advisory guides.

The negative psychosocial outcomes of such policies are compounded by the real potential for physical harm, given (1) the toxicity, overdose potential, and dangerous electrolyte imbalances associated with detection-avoidance techniques used to "clean" urine; (2) the adolescent's move to using drugs with metabolites that remain in the body far less than marijuana to avoid detection; and (3) the move toward use of illicit drugs not included in the testing panel (Centers for Disease Control and Prevention, 2007; Chaloupka & Laixuthal, 2002; Terry-McElrath, O'Malley, & Johnston,

2013; Yamaguchi, Johnston, & O'Malley, 2003a, 2003b; Zeese, 2002).

It is not surprising that the American Academy of Pediatrics (Levy et al., 2015) and the American Bar Association (Henault, 2001) do not support drug testing and zero-tolerance policies in schools. This does not mean, however, that schools are not relevant to the early detection and intervention of adolescent substance use: quite the contrary. There are three reasons why schools are uniquely positioned to implement screening and targeted intervention:

1. At least 60% of high school students report that drugs are used, kept, or sold on school grounds, over half (52%) say that there is a place on school grounds or near their school where students go to get high, and over one third (36%) report that it is easy for students to smoke, drink, or use drugs during the day at their school without getting caught (Center for Substance Abuse Research, 2012).
2. The National Association of School Nurses (2015) has been vocal about school nurses' role as agents for substance use prevention in school communities, specifically addressing marijuana and prescription opiate use and the need for onsite naloxone at schools throughout the country. (Naloxone is an opioid overdose antidote that reverses life-threatening respiratory depression [Hardesty, 2014]).
3. School health services—delivered in school-based health centers or the school nurse's office—are a "normalized" part of the school community, thus destigmatizing visits and ensuring anonymity for the specific service received.

SBIRT services could naturally be imbedded within school-based health centers. More than half of the roughly 1,930 school-based health centers in 50 states already provide substance abuse counseling (53.2%), with nearly one in 10 having a trained alcohol and drug counselor on staff (Lofink et al., 2013), making them exceptionally suited to SBIRT services. Their ability to increase access to behavioral health services; decrease emergency room visits; reduce funding, stigma, and confidentiality concerns (Clayton, Chin, Blackburn, & Echeverria, 2010; Santelli, Kouzis, & Newcomer, 1996; Sterling, Valkanoff, Hinman, & Weisner, 2012); and even increase school attendance and student achievement (Walker, Kerns, Lyon, Bruns, & Cosgrove, 2010) adds to the appeal of embedding screening protocols into their day-to-day operations.

While the inclusion of SBIRT services would clearly have the best fit within schools that have school-based health centers, there is evidence (although limited) that these programs can also be incorporated into schools without health centers provided that a substance use counselor from a local treatment provider works within the school (Curtis, McLellan, & Gabellini, 2014). The extent of alcohol and other drug accessibility in schools, coupled with the large numbers of teens who attend school, makes schools practical locations to implement SBIRT and related protocols that include follow-up, case management, and the delivery of preventive care and brief interventions (Clayton et al., 2010; Sterling, Valkanoff, et al., 2012). While more work is clearly needed in both settings, routinely incorporating SBIRT or other substance use screening and referral services into various school-based protocols is a much needed and clearly achievable step in expanding screening, early intervention, and treatment.

Barriers to Adolescent SBIRT

It is clear that the research on SBIRT and the future increase of dependent coverage for a variety of medical and behavioral screenings holds great promise: early risk and use can be identified and reduced, decreasing the likelihood of a future substance use disorder. There are, however, challenges that could hinder bringing SBIRT services to scale.

While there is a growing body of evidence supporting SBIRT for adolescents (Tanner-Smith et al., 2013), gaps in evidence remain such that it has yet to be endorsed by the U.S. Preventive Services Task Force, a critical entity in garnering service coverage among private and public insurers. Second, workforce issues impede widespread implementation of SBIRT. The limited number of certificates in adolescent medicine (466 certificates awarded over a 10-year period), the dearth of pediatric residency programs with an approved adolescent medicine fellowship (only 12% of residency programs), and the belief among pediatricians that they are not well trained to care for adolescents (83%) limit the ability of the healthcare system to meet even the basic medical needs of the estimated 40 million adolescents in this country (Cullen & Salganicoff, 2011). In terms of screening for and addressing adolescent substance use disorders, workforce issues are even more pronounced. For example, nurse practitioner graduate programs include less than 3 hours of addictions education (Campbell-Heider et al., 2009). Among physicians and other healthcare providers, over half (56%) do not feel equipped to discuss (or comfortable when discussing) adolescent substance use issues, and less than half stay current on related literature (Sterling, Kline-Simon, Wibbelsman, Wong, & Weisner, 2012). In fact, they are less concerned about alcohol and marijuana versus other drugs (e.g., opiates) even though (1) alcohol and marijuana are typically the substances of use and abuse among teenagers (Sterling, Weisner, Hinman, & Parthasarathy, 2010) and (2) alcohol and marijuana are *not* benign substances of abuse, particularly on the developing adolescent brain. At a most basic level, the adolescent brain is more susceptible to the addictive effects of substances, making use in and of itself a risky proposition. Also, marijuana, alcohol, and all other drugs of abuse show diverse neurotoxic effects, adversely affecting brain development and maturation in the areas related to motivation, memory and learning, and inhibition (Brown & Tapert, 2004; CASA, 2011; Squeglia, Jacobus, & Tapert, 2009; Squeglia, Spadoni, Infante, Myers, & Tapert, 2009; White & Swartzwelder, 2005).

These perspectives are compounded by the fact that many healthcare providers feel unprepared to address a positive drug screen (Van Hook et al., 2007). It is not surprising, then, that adolescents who screen positive or show early signs of substance use problems rarely receive recommended levels of preventive care through primary care visits (American Academy of Pediatrics, Division of Child Health Research, 1998; Bethell, Klein, & Peck, 2001). For those who require and receive a treatment referral, healthcare staff typically provide the contact information of potential treatment providers, requiring families to navigate networks of services and insurers on their own (Sterling et al., 2010).

SBIRT is further hampered by a lack of information about available adolescent treatment programs designed to treat substance use disorders that are appropriate, effective, and of high quality once the need for treatment is established (Cacciola et al., 2015). When referral sources are unaware of which programs actually treat adolescents with substance use disorders, timely, efficient, and appropriate referrals are compromised. This lack of information is compounded by the fact that the quality of care provided within the adolescent treatment system is variable and often inadequate, as few scientific advances have made it into adolescent community treatment programs (see Kaminer, Burleson, & Burke, 2008; Knudsen, 2009; Mark et al., 2006; McLellan & Meyers, 2004; Meyers & McLellan, 2005a, 2005b; Roman & Johnson, 2002; Young, Dembo, & Henderson, 2007). This reduces confidence in the treatment system. Healthcare providers who do not have the resources or confidence in the system to make a quality referral have been shown to skip the screening process completely (Horwitz et al., 2007).

Finally, while school-based health centers are uniquely positioned to embed SBIRT services into their array of health services, not all schools have health centers. The one study that examined SBIRT services in general school settings is not enough to demonstrate its feasibility or effectiveness in schools without health centers.

The Future of Screening

The future of adolescent screening is promising, as federal and private initiatives are in place to address screening-related limitations and gaps in knowledge. First, increases in healthcare provider training about substance use disorders are being driven by SAMHSA. Since 2003, SAMHSA has funded 17 medical residency cooperative agreements (SAMHSA, 2015a) and will invest an additional $3.75 million in SBIRT health professions student training grants (SAMHSA, 2008). These are designed to develop and implement training programs to teach students in the health professions (physician assistants, dentists, psychologists, pharmacists, nurses, social workers, counselors, and medical students and residents) the skills necessary to provide SBIRT services, with the ultimate goal of helping clients avoid substance use disorders (SAMHSA, 2015b). In the private sector, a web-based medical school curriculum on substance use disorders incorporates lectures, case presentations, and fieldwork designed to integrate substance use education into the general medicine curriculum (McLellan, Curtis, Nordstrom, & Skrajewski, 2014). A module on SBIRT in general and adolescent SBIRT specifically could be easily integrated into the course. Within the nursing field, specialized certification programs are available and could be expanded (e.g., Certified Addictions Registered Nurse [CARN] and Certified Addictions Registered Nurse—Advanced Practice [CARN-AP]). Further, family nurse practitioner programs include specialty courses in addiction nursing (Finnell, Garbin, & Scarborough, 2004), which could be enhanced with specialty courses in adolescent addiction nursing; this could benefit school-based health centers and other school nursing programs.

A comprehensive strategy to address training, financing, and SBIRT implementation is being funded by the Hilton Foundation. Projects are working to identify effective healthcare training models (with the American Board of Addiction Medicine Foundation and the American Academy of Pediatrics), to enact policy changes needed to sustain SBIRT financing, and to advance learning to improve SBIRT implementation. Finally, the ACA contains numerous provisions to encourage public health, including the Prevention and Public Health Fund ($15 billion) to support screenings, prevention, wellness, and public health activities.

While all of this is good news in terms of case-finding efforts, other system-of-care components (i.e., early intervention, treatment, continuing care, and supports) require improvement to provide an adequate and effective response.

EARLY INTERVENTION

Hundreds of billions of dollars are spent annually to treat diseases that are preventable (Robert Wood Johnson Foundation, 2013). Far too often healthcare providers in general, and behavioral health providers in particular, focus on treating the full expression (vs. the early signs) of disease. Treating early disease states is the most commonsense and cost-effective approach for most disorders, and adolescent substance use disorders are no exception. In fact, early intervention targeted at substance use and emerging signs of substance use disorders has the real potential to minimize the future utilization of high-cost residential/inpatient treatment programs, to increase the probability of a positive outcome, and to arrest the trajectory of addiction—thereby reducing downstream social, personal, and financial costs (Doherty et al., 2011; Meyers et al., 2014). This level of service is essential not only because early intervention can forestall addiction, but also because not all adolescents who have experienced serious consequences as a result of substance use will meet the diagnostic criteria for a substance use disorder due to the short-term nature of their history with substances (Martin & Winters, 1998; Pollock & Martin, 1999). Although they do not have a diagnostic label, the immediate and long-term consequences of substance use can be detrimental to the developing brain, to educational attainment, and to social relationships.

Unfortunately, the early stages of adolescent substance use disorders are often not addressed, in part because early intervention services are not accessible and higher-level interventions are not yet appropriate. Hence, targeted intervention that addresses early signs before the youth meets the criteria for a DSM diagnosis (i.e., preclinical levels of service) is basically nonexistent and nonreimbursable within financing systems and funding streams. Model development in terms of intervention specifics and financing strategies is needed.

The American Society for Addiction Medicine (ASAM) has established an early intervention level of care referred to as the ASAM .5 Level of Care (Mee-Lee, Shulman, Fishman, Gastfriend, & Miller, 2013). Operationalized with professionally vetted criteria to determine eligibility for this level of care, this ASAM level-of-care code is ready for justifying and receiving reimbursement for service provision. However, ASAM's .5 Level of Care is rarely reimbursed or funded.

Inroads in the funding and provision of early intervention services could be made in two ways. First, the ACA can address critical service gaps if reimbursement streams for this level of care can be identified. One possibility is the repurposing of a portion of block grant dollars, the funding mechanism currently used to treat the uninsured. Since more Americans should have insurance coverage under the ACA either through Medicaid expansion or employer-based healthcare insurance expansion, block grant dollars could be redirected to fund early intervention services. This underutilized service (which exists largely in theory rather than in practice) could then become available and accessible.

Second, the American Academy of Pediatrics has shown tremendous leadership in developing, promoting, and disseminating health supervision guidelines through its Bright Futures initiative for health promotion and disease prevention. If early intervention services for substance use could be included within the Bright Futures framework, they would no longer be overlooked, and the potential for service reimbursement would be increased.

Screening coupled with early intervention services has the potential to reduce the number of adolescents requiring the next component on the service delivery continuum: treatment.

ADOLESCENT SUBSTANCE ABUSE TREATMENT

Lack of Specialty Adolescent Substance Abuse Treatment

We have discussed the multiple and complex system-level problems associated with identifying and intervening early with adolescents who use and/or abuse substances. One might think that it would be comparatively easy for adolescents with substance use disorders to access treatments suited to their needs, as "treatment" fits within the acute-care approach that dominates the treatment of addiction, but this is not the case.

First, there have always been few adolescent treatment programs (White, 1998). In the early 1980s, when it became apparent that adolescents with substance use disorders were a unique client group requiring specific assessment and particular therapeutic approaches (see Deas, Riggs, Langenbucher, Goldman, & Brown, 2000, for a discussion; Poulin, Dishion, & Burraston, 2001), traditional substance abuse treatment facilities had to adapt their adult-oriented programs if they were to accept and appropriately treat an adolescent clientele (Winters, Stinchfield, Opland, Weller, & Latimer, 2000). Few responded to this challenge then, and the numbers are equally discouraging now. Less than 30% of the roughly 13,600 substance abuse treatment programs in this country now offer special programming for adolescents (Mericle et al., 2015), and only 8.4% of the 1.7 million youth in need of addiction treatment are receiving specialty care (SAMHSA, 2012). This limited number of adolescent treatment programs, coupled with problems of access, can only worsen if the screening phase (demand side) of the system improves without parallel improvements in the treatment phase (supply side) of the system. However, even if the treatment component of the system could absorb additional adolescents, the quality of treatment for adolescents is of concern.

Varying Quality of Treatment

A substantial body of evidence demonstrates that providing adequate and appropriate evidence-based practices and evidence-based treatments can improve substance use outcomes (e.g., reduce alcohol or other drug use) and have a positive impact on other life domains (e.g., interpersonal functioning) (Jainchill, 2012). Substance abuse treatment can lessen the rate, duration, and intensity of many health and behavioral health problems and cut or at least control the growth of overall healthcare costs (Hutchings & King, 2009). Societal costs can also be lessened by increases in productivity (e.g., academic success) and reductions in public health threats (Hutchings & King, 2009).

Unfortunately, the relatively limited number of adolescent treatment programs within the substance abuse treatment system is further encumbered by a lack of treatment quality in the programs that exist. In other words, there is great variability in the availability, provision, and quality of those treatment practices and features that have been shown to be effective in combating this disease (Brannigan, Schackman, Falco, & Millman, 2004; Ducharme, Mello, Roman, Knudsen, & Johnson, 2007; Kaminer et al., 2008; Knudsen, 2009; Mark et al., 2006; Roman & Johnson, 2002; Young et al., 2007), making a bad situation worse.

Specifically, there are 10 broad principles with 64 corresponding discrete practices (evidence-based practices) that have strong empirical, clinical, and expert support as being associated with reductions in substance use and co-occurring problems among adolescents with substance use disorders (Brannigan et al., 2004; Cacciola et al., 2015). For example, attention to mental health practices (e.g., onsite mental health services or linkages to mental health assessment, treatment, and/or medication management), family involvement in treatment (e.g., providing family intervention and multiple-family education and support groups), and continuing care and recovery supports (e.g., continuing care plan complements treatment plan) are a few of the practice indicators of the quality of adolescent substance abuse treatment.

There are also evidence-based treatments that, when implemented with fidelity, improve the outcome of adolescents with substance use disorders. For example, extensive research has shown that family-based treatment (e.g., MDFT, functional family therapy), psychosocial treatment (e.g., CBT, MET), pharmacotherapies, and integrative models (CBT/MET) reduce substance use among teenagers (CASA, 2011; Jainchill, 2012; Kaminer, 1994; Lipsey, Tanner-Smith, & Wilson, 2010). In fact, research is clear that adolescents exhibit significant reductions in substance use shortly after the end of treatment provided they complete treatment in quality treatment programs that implement evidence-based practices well (Lipsey et al., 2010). Family therapy and multiple-service packages yield greater reductions in overall substance use than most other types of treatment.

Despite the importance of evidence-based care for adolescent substance use disorders, studies conducted over the past 10 years identified underutilization of evidence-based practices and treatments within and between general community programs, high- and low-cost programs, "highly regarded programs," and programs for juvenile offenders (Brannigan et al., 2004; Ducharme et al., 2007; Kaminer et al., 2008; Knudsen, 2009; Mark et al., 2006; Roman & Johnson, 2002; Young et al., 2007). In other words, the majority of adolescent treatment programs in this country offer very few of the clinical and social support services that have been demonstrated to be effective. Without quality and targeted intervention (and adequate post-acute care, as discussed in the following section), relapse and retreatment are essentially ensured. The same youth is more likely to cycle in and out of multiple systems of care (Soler, 1992), with each intervention "failure" accompanied by a "repeat" cost to some sector of the system, a truly inefficient use of public health resources (Meyers & McLellan,

2005a, 2005b). The use of evidence-based practices and treatments, with subsequent improvement in quality within the already limited adolescent treatment system, is vital.

Credentialing Staff

Since knowledge of adolescent development and skill and interest in treating youth are of paramount importance (Deas et al., 2000; Winters et al., 2000), staff credentialing processes should require adolescent-specific knowledge. The National Association of Alcoholism and Drug Abuse Counselors' certification program recently added a National Certified Adolescent Addictions Counselor certification to their credentialing portfolio. Recognizing the different set of competencies and clinical practices needed to treat adolescents with substance use disorder, this group's competency-based tiered system now includes adolescent-specific specialization credentials and endorsements. To be eligible for this certification, applicants must have (1) a bachelor's degree or higher degree from an accredited college or university in addiction or a counseling-related field (e.g., psychology, social work); (2) a current credential or license as a substance use disorder/addiction counselor issued by a state or credentialing authority; (3) at least 5 years of supervised experience working as a licensed addiction counselor, with 2.5 of these years with adolescents; and (4) at least 70 contact hours of training related to adolescent treatment, with 50% or more face to face. They must also pass a certification exam. There are no data available on the number of such certified counselors in the country, making it difficult to assess whether staff in adolescent treatment programs have this certification.

When one looks at state credentialing practices, there is an average of 6.5 certification programs per state. In addition to the traditional alcohol and drug counselor certifications, states also offer specialization certifications. Of these, certifications related to serving patients involved in the criminal justice system (35%) and those with co-occurring disorders (33%) are most common. Only one state in the country even came close to adolescent credentialing: Illinois offers an adolescent treatment endorsement certificate that documents an individual's specialization in services to adolescents.

The Future of Adolescent Substance Abuse Treatment

The limited number of adolescent substance abuse treatment providers would be less worrisome if youth were treated in quality programs offering the constellation of services they need. Efficiencies would be created as unnecessarily intensive treatment and repeat treatments (and associated costs) could be avoided. It stands to reason, then, that improving the quality of adolescent substance abuse treatment has been—and remains—a national priority (Institute of Medicine, 1989, 2006; National Institute of Mental Health, 2001; New Freedom Commission on Mental Health, 2003). To this end, the Network for the Improvement of Addiction Treatment (NIATx) has designed a model of process improvement in addiction treatment. The NIATx quality improvement model focuses on improving access to and retention in treatment by reducing waiting times and missed appointments, and increasing treatment admissions and retention. The underlying premise is that when individuals have (and take advantage of) opportunities to receive beneficial dosages of treatment, the cost and the effectiveness of the care delivery system are improved. NIATx strategies have enhanced the quality of care for adult substance use disorders (i.e., reduction in days to treatment, increases in retention in care), and participating programs were able to institutionalize the changes that led to enhanced performance (Ford et al., 2008; McCarty et al., 2007).

Specifically designed to drive quality improvement in adolescent substance use treatment; to support optimal specialty care referrals by pediatric, primary care, and family practice physicians and the justice system; and to improve the performance of programs (e.g., retention rates) and patients (e.g., reduced substance use), a web-based prototype of the Consumer Guide to Adolescent Treatment (Cacciola et al., 2015;

Meyers et al., 2014) has been designed. It uses a systematic methodology to measure treatment quality across 10 dimensions of care and translates the data into a practical and science-based "report card." It includes comparative treatment program information, consumer education, and a navigator function to guide users to treatment options. Program-specific management reports highlight quality scores across the 10 programmatic areas, with recommendations of ways to improve quality in problematic areas. The use of the Consumer Guide's web-based system of data dissemination should enhance quality improvement efforts because publicly reported performance stimulates quality improvements (Robert Wood Johnson Foundation, 2011) and informed consumers are essential to improving the quality of services, particularly in healthcare (Hibbard, Stockard, & Tusler, 2005; Hirth, 1999; Ippolito, 1992). This kind of consumer information can immediately inform and direct an individual consumer's choice and increase the chances that a young person arrives at an appropriate treatment door at an earlier stage in his or her disease. Over time, receipt of treatment that is related to the adolescent's problems/needs and is of higher quality should result in more success and ultimately less treatment and associated costs.

CONTINUING CARE

Evidence-based adolescent substance abuse treatment works, at least in the short term, if the youth attends and completes treatment. As mentioned above, research from 29 unique treatment samples (yielding 489 effect size estimates) is clear: adolescents with substance use disorders exhibit significant reductions in substance use shortly after the end of treatment (Tanner-Smith et al., 2013). Observed reductions are strongest for those youth completing treatment and for youth who attend quality programs that implement evidence-based practices well. Unfortunately, approximately 40% of youth do not complete treatment (Mutter, Ali, Smith, & Strashny, 2015). Further, treatment gains significantly and rapidly diminish following treatment. Generally within 3 to 6 months after care, between 66% and 79% of youth return to substance use (Brown, Vik, & Creamer, 1989; Cornelius et al., 2003; Myers, Brown, & Mott, 1995). For youth with comorbid conditions, median survival time to relapse (i.e., first use after 7 days of nonuse) is just 19 days, less than 3 weeks (Cornelius et al., 2004).

Driven by research supporting the view that addiction is similar to other chronic conditions (e.g., asthma, hypertension, type 2 diabetes), it is not surprising that relapse occurs: continuing care and monitoring are needed to sustain treatment gains (McLellan et al., 2000; Saitz et al., 2008). Importantly, there is a growing literature illustrating the protective effect of continuing care on longer-term rates of abstinence among adolescents who receive it (Garner et al., 2009; Godley & Godley, 2012). However, for adolescents who have a substance use disorder, find themselves at the end of an acute treatment, and are not in research protocols, little to no monitoring or continuing care is provided (Meyers et al., 2014). These posttreatment services are rarely available in adequate quantity or quality to forestall a relapse.

For adolescents, there are three approaches to the traditional continuing care paradigm (e.g., stepdown treatment) that have yet to truly penetrate the field: (1) recovery high schools (followed by collegiate recovery services, including sober college housing), (2) youth development programs such as A-CRA and alternative peer groups, and (3) technology check-ins. Each can help youth with different challenges and needs and can help in different ways; all can substantially add to the sparse continuing care that is currently in place.

Emerging research indicates that attending a recovery school for at least 3 months enabled students to (1) maintain sobriety for an average of eight times longer than before they attended a sober school, (2) decrease negative feelings and delinquent and offending behavior, and (3) increase interest in school, work, family, and friends (Moberg & Finch, 2008). Continuing care through youth development is realized through A-CRA (Godley et al., 2001) and alternative peer groups (Morrison & Bailey, 2011). Both approaches have found positive outcomes

(Godley & Godley, 2011; Godley, Godley, Dennis, Funk, & Passetti, 2002) and recognize that for recovery to have a chance it has to be fun and developmentally appropriate, that peer relationships are as important to recovery as they are to the initiation and continued support of substance use, and that skill-building activities that are engaging and challenging and focus on how to have fun without the use of alcohol and other drugs are necessary.

The use of technology as a continuing care approach with adolescents is gaining momentum, undoubtedly due to the prominence of it in the life of adolescents and the seminal work of McKay et al.'s telephone follow-ups (McKay, Lynch, Shepard, & Pettinati, 2005; McKay et al., 2004), Scott and Dennis's recovery checkups (Scott, Dennis, & Foss, 2005), Cacciola et al.'s clinical monitoring (Cacciola, Camilleri, Kolwicz, Brooks, & Alterman, 2012), and Gustafson et al.'s automated Addiction-Comprehensive Health Enhancement Support System (Gustafson et al., 2014). In a pilot study conducted by Trudeau et al. (2012), 86% of counselors (n = 16) and 84% of adolescents (n = 24) found an online relapse-prevention program easy to use, rated the content as relevant to recovery (e.g., setting boundaries with peers, following through with decisions), and reported interest in using this type of technology to meet and manage recovery challenges. Gonzales et al. (2014) took this early work further, developing and testing Educating & Supporting Inquisitive Youth in Recovery (ESQYIR), an automated mobile monitoring and feedback aftercare intervention for youth. Pilot data demonstrated significantly better substance use and recovery behavior outcomes among ESQYIR youth compared to an aftercare-as-usual condition.

Taken together, recovery high schools, continuing care through youth development, and technology should have a place in the future of continuing care.

PRIVACY

Adolescents in all states and the District of Columbia are protected by minor-consent laws wherein adolescents as young as 14 can consent to treatment for drug use, pregnancy and pregnancy prevention, sexually transmitted infections, mental health issues, and emergencies without parental consent or knowledge (English, Gold, Nash, & Levine, 2012). However, the complex maze of insurance-related billing procedures and electronic health records may inadvertently compromise confidentiality, thereby preventing already reluctant youth from agreeing to care (or seeking it in the first place) even within a well-functioning system of care.

Insurance companies normally communicate with, and send explanation of benefits (EOB) statements to, the policyholder (generally a parent). While EOBs were designed to increase transparency of the health insurance process, mitigate insurance fraud, and reduce medical identify theft, EOBs unintentionally violate confidentiality, especially for services rendered to individuals insured as dependents (English et al., 2012). EOBs typically identify the individual who received the service, the type of service received, the healthcare provider who delivered the service, the cost of the service, insurance coverage of the service, and the remaining cost balance (e.g., policyholder's financial liability).

Electronic health records were designed to improve information sharing and care within a clinical system. Impressively, they have been shown to improve treatment for adolescents with attention-deficit/hyperactivity disorder and depression, to increase human papillomavirus vaccination rates, and to reduce unnecessary antibiotic prescribing (Co et al., 2010; Fiks et al., 2013; Gonzales et al., 2013; Valuck et al., 2012). Despite these benefits, many electronic health records do not have default privacy settings for adolescents, allowing parents access to online personal health information of their minor child (Gray et al., 2014). Currently, 60% of American children's hospitals (Nakamura, Harper, & Jha, 2013) and 69% of primary care practices have an electronic health record (Schoen et al., 2012).

Tebb et al. (2014) summarize eight current attempts (including the pros and cons of each) to address the tension between healthcare transparency and confidentiality (e.g., applies a generic Current Procedural Terminology [CPT] code to sensitive services). While no strategy has emerged as "the strategy" to adopt, it provides valuable options as the best way forward is determined.

SUMMARY

If we are to reduce the burden of substance use disorders, the most humane and cost-effective time to do so is during adolescence, the developmental stage in which they so frequently present. Treatment and policies are poised to be positively transformed in the coming years by both the current state of scientific knowledge and the legislative changes to the healthcare system. Legislative advances have brought us ever closer to parity and integrated care, the research base is expanding so that we can better address the social and biological determinants of these disorders, and mechanisms for system improvements exist, if only in small-scale, pilot, or prototype form. The necessary elements for change are now in place, and with proper alignment and leveraging of these forces, there is an enormous opportunity to have a significant impact on the adolescent substance abuse treatment system.

This chapter has described the challenges that our field must address in order to quell the tide of adolescent substance abuse in this country. The changes that are needed will not be simple or quick, and they will require coordinated efforts. But necessary changes are achievable, with an actual possibility that they will result in important and sustained modifications in the way care is delivered to adolescents who are at risk for substance use disorder, who have used or abused alcohol or other drugs, and who are recovering from substance use.

ACKNOWLEDGMENTS

This work was supported in part by the National Institute on Drug Abuse (NIDA) grant P50-DA02784 and the Bridge Foundation.

Conclusion: Successes Since the First Edition and Pressing Issues for the Future of Adolescent Mental and Behavioral Health

Daniel Romer

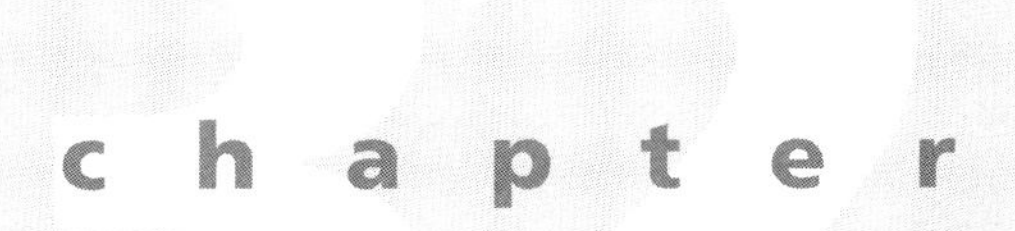

OVERVIEW

Our concluding chapter of the first edition of *Treating and Preventing Adolescent Mental Health Disorders* presented a number of pressing concerns about the status of adolescent mental and behavioral health in the United States. In looking back, it is clear that for some of the concerns, progress has been made. As noted by Timothy Walsh in the introduction to this edition, we have greater evidence of the effectiveness of various treatments for adolescents than at the time of the first edition. In addition, the Affordable Care Act and the Mental Health Parity and Addiction Equity Act (MHPAEA) have increased access to healthcare for millions of Americans, including about a third of the population that is under age 26. In particular, healthcare coverage for children through age 25 has been required as part of any health insurance policy. And the MHPAEA has required coverage for mental health and substance use disorder treatment that is comparable to physical health conditions. Greater coordination of pediatric care under the "medical home" model should also enhance access to appropriate health providers (see Chapter 30 in this volume). Initial examination of the effectiveness of greater integration of behavioral health into primary care suggests that this strategy will yield benefits (Asarnow et al., 2015; Kolko, 2015). Whether these changes in access to healthcare services will lead to improvements in population mental and behavioral health in children and adolescents remains to be seen. Nevertheless, these policy changes are no small achievement, and it is difficult to see how they could not improve the health and welfare of children and families in the United States. It is distressing therefore to consider the possibility that many of these advances in healthcare may be abandoned. As this book goes to press, the new administration in Washington is proposing to dismantle the Affordable Care Act. This change in healthcare policy would do considerable damage to the progress that has been made and would threaten the ability to address continued shortfalls in mental health care in the United States.

Despite improvements in the delivery and financial coverage of healthcare, there remain notable deficiencies in the U.S. healthcare system. The first edition noted weaknesses in the major service delivery systems for adolescents, namely the schools and primary care. In particular, neither system has personnel trained to identify, much less treat, major forms of mental and behavioral disorders (Meyers & McLellan, 2005; Romer & McIntosh, 2005a, 2005b). The schools are woefully unequipped to serve this purpose not only due to lack of personnel tasked with this objective but also because training for school staff, even professionals such as counselors, is not directed toward this goal. Similarly, pediatricians and family medicine providers are not trained to recognize or treat common adolescent mental disorders (with the possible exception of attention-deficit/hyperactivity disorder). Finally, there are hardly sufficient numbers of psychiatrists and psychologists trained to treat adolescent mental and behavioral disorders even if they could be correctly identified. Progress has been made in developing resources for improving the identification and treatment of substance use disorders (see Chapter 31 in this volume), and evidence-based practices continue to be disseminated in primary care (see Chapter 30). However, more resources need to be directed toward the training of personnel and medical providers in all of the various services for children (schools, primary care, foster care, juvenile justice) so that adolescents receive the support needed to advance their mental and behavioral health. It is a hopeful sign that the recently signed legislation to improve mental health care in the United States (the 21st Century Cures Act of 2016) will devote resources to the training of more mental health practitioners.

Despite various signs of progress, one of the main conclusions from this edition is the insufficient evidence base on effective treatments for adolescent presentations of the disorders covered in this volume. We find it disconcerting that these gaps remain despite the fact that all of these disorders inflict a heavy toll on adolescents. Although we have considerable evidence regarding treatments for adults, there remain many unanswered questions about how best to treat adolescents. It is hoped that the National Institutes of Health that support research on adolescent mental health will work to overcome these deficits.

PERVASIVE EFFECTS OF POVERTY ON PARENTS AND CHILDREN

Even if we could do a better job of identifying and treating mental disorders in adolescents, the effects of poverty, a major source of poor health outcomes, would continue to affect adolescents. Since the first edition of this volume, poverty levels have increased in children and adults ages 18 to 64 largely due to the financial crisis of 2008 (DeNavas-Walt & Proctor, 2015). The financial status of families has become all the more precarious since that event, with over 20% of children living in poverty. Although suicide rates had been declining at the time of the first edition, following the financial crisis, those rates have increased in adolescents and young adults (Romer & Rich, 2016). In addition, there is some evidence of a recent increase in symptoms of major depression among adolescents (Center for Behavioral Health Statistics and Quality, 2015). Although the reasons for these increases are probably complex, they are coincident with increases in suicide among adults in the parent age range that were evident even before the financial crisis (Curtin et al., 2016). While suicide is only the tip of the iceberg, so to speak, youth with poor mental health are disproportionately located at the bottom of the economic ladder (Reiss, 2013). The effects of financial distress undoubtedly compromise the ability of parents to provide appropriate care, with a multitude of effects on children's mental health, including greater risk for maltreatment, mood disorders, and externalizing behavior (Choe et al., 2013; Reiss, 2013; Roberts et al., 2009).

One approach introduced since the first edition to reduce the effects of impaired parenting, nurse visitation for first-time mothers living in poverty, has been expanded with additional support from the Affordable Care Act. It is a tribute to the government for expanding this program, which has a substantial evidence base in its support. However, other approaches to ameliorating the effects of poverty are also supported by evidence (AAP Council on Community Pediatrics, 2016; Yoshikawa et al., 2012). For example, the study by Copeland and Costello (2010) of Indian reservations in which poor families received a cash supplement that substantially increased their resources found dramatic improvements in child externalizing behavior that were attributable to better parenting. There are many ways to improve the financial security of families (AAP Council on Community Pediatrics, 2016; Yoshikawa et al., 2012), but evidence suggests that reducing the financial hardship of poverty for families with children is a cost-effective intervention for enhancing child and adolescent health and well-being.

GUN VIOLENCE

It is disconcerting that the effects of violence in youth continue to dominate national attention. Although rates of death involving gun violence in youth have declined since the peak of the 1990s, rates of youth injury from guns treated in emergency departments have increased (Planty & Truman, 2013), and death by suicide in youth is heavily attributable to the use of guns (Wintemute, 2015). Efforts to reduce exposure to unsecured guns in homes is an important policy objective, and laws that restrict access to guns appear to reduce their use in suicide (Mann & Michel, 2016). Continued pressure to pass such laws will be needed if the United States is ever going to achieve success in reducing the harm from this highly potent means.

At the time of this writing, new legislation to reform mental health care confronts the harmful use of guns by focusing on persons with mental disorders as an important source of the problem. While this strategy may be well intentioned if it helps to reduce the mental health conditions that predispose to suicide, it is unlikely to have much impact on the role of gun violence in assaults and homicides. Those forms of gun violence are much more heavily related to the ill effects of poverty and the ready access to guns in high-poverty locations (Harrell et al., 2014). Nevertheless, reforms that increase the number of providers and other resources for greater access to care represent a welcome development. Continued efforts to reform the juvenile justice system should also be pursued in view of the high rates of mental disorder in the juvenile population that is ensnared in this system (Bushman et al., 2016).

RESEARCH ON THE GENESIS AND TREATMENT OF MENTAL DISORDERS

In the first edition, we noted the need for a national study of youth development that could follow a large cohort of children into and beyond adolescence to identify trajectories of healthy and unhealthy development and potential influences on those outcomes. Although a large children's health study was eventually abandoned by National Institute of Health, another effort to study brain development in a cohort of 10,000 early adolescents into adulthood (the Adolescent Brain Cognitive Development [ABCD] study) may provide a mechanism to identify such trajectories (Reardon, 2014). Although this study focuses on drug use, it should also provide evidence regarding the development of a wide range of mental and behavioral disorders that are comorbid with drug use and that potentially encourage its use. We look forward to the findings from this ambitious effort and hope that it will shed light on the factors that influence adolescent mental health.

The National Institute of Health has also embarked on a new effort to study mental health conditions that partially abandons reliance on DSM classifications of disorder as the route to discovery. This effort, known as the Research Domain Criteria (RDoC) approach, emphasizes research on more general processes that appear to underlie a wide range of disorders, including negative and positive valence systems, cognitive systems, social processes, and arousal systems. To the extent this approach recognizes the considerable comorbidity that characterizes mental health conditions, it should shed light on the pathogenesis of these disorders. Recent research suggests that just as tests of cognitive ability share considerable variation, the same may be true to some extent of mental disorders (Kim & Eaton, 2015; Lahey et al., 2015). The RDoC approach may help to identify the processes that underlie such general predispositions and advance our understanding of their development.

A NATIONAL YOUTH DEVELOPMENT STRATEGY

As outlined in Chapter 19 on substance abuse prevention, the United States does not have a national strategy to enhance the development of youth. Many evidence-based practices sit in repositories but go unused in a concerted fashion. The challenges posed by persistent poverty leave many youth in jeopardy of school failure (Sznitman et al., 2011), which has deleterious effects on the future productivity and health of the population (Muennig, 2015). There is evidence that early intervention, such as nurse visitation and preschool attendance, produces large dividends (Campbell et al., 2014), and many states and localities are moving ahead with these strategies. However, a coordinated strategy of resources to assist families with children from birth to young adulthood should be a national priority.

Most of the developed world has such policies in place (see http://www.youthpolicy.org/nationalyouthpolicies/). A good example is the plan put forth by the government of Australia, which includes objectives for a variety of youth health and education needs and specific programs to advance the objectives (http://www.youthpolicy.org/national/Australia_2010_National_Youth_Strategy.pdf). Some steps toward a coordinated youth development plan for the United States were initiated in 2013 with Pathways for Youth (http://www.youthpolicy.org/national/United_States_2013_Pathways_for_Youth.pdf). The federal government also hosts a website with resources for program planners (youth.gov). We look forward to further progress in that initiative.

Despite the challenges noted, we would like to end on a positive note. In recent years, many indicators of adolescent mental and behavioral health have shown marked improvement. For example, use of many drugs and cigarettes is down, rates of death due to homicide have declined, as have birth rates among adolescents (Romer & Rich, 2016). However, there is little evidence that major forms of adolescent mental health disorders have declined, and thus greater efforts to reduce these conditions are clearly needed. Suicide remains well above the levels of the 1960s, when those rates began to rise, and, as noted above, in recent years those rates have increased. A national agenda that focuses on adolescent mental and behavioral health across the spectrum of disorder would be a welcome addition to our public health priorities.

References

Introduction

Merikangas, K. R., Nakamura, E. F., & Kessler, R. C. (2009). Epidemiology of mental disorders in children and adolescents. *Dialogues in Clinical Neuroscience, 11*, 7–20.

Part I: Depression and Bipolar Disorder

Abbass, A., & Driessen, E. (2010). The efficacy of short-term psychodynamic psychotherapy for depression: A summary of recent findings. *Acta Psychiatrica Scandinavica, 121*(5), 398–398.

Aber, J. L., Bennett, N. G., Conley, D. C., & Li, J. (1997). The effects of poverty on child health and development. *Annual Review of Public Health, 18*, 463–483.

Abramson, L. Y., Metalsky, G. I., & Alloy, L. B. (1989). Hopelessness depression: A theory-based subtype of depression. *Psychological Review, 96*, 358–372.

Abramson, L. Y., Seligman, M. E. P., & Teasdale, I. (1978). Learned helplessness in humans: Critique and reformulation. *Journal of Abnormal Psychology, 87*, 49–59.

Agency for Health Care Policy and Research. (1993). Treatment of major depression: Clinical Guidelines, vol 5, number 2: AHCPR Publication No. 93-0551. Rockville, MD, US Department of Health and Human Services.

Agerup, T., Lydersen, S, Wallander, J., & Sund, A. M. (2015). Maternal and paternal psychosocial risk factors for clinical depression in a Norwegian community sample of adolescents. *Nordic Journal of Psychiatry, 69*(1), 35–41.

Akiskal, H. S., Downs, J., et al. (1985). Affective disorders in referred children and younger siblings of manic-depressives: Mode of onset and prospective course. *Archives of General Psychiatry, 42*, 996–1003.

Akiskal, H. S., & McKinney, W. T. (1975). Overview of recent research in depression: Integration of ten conceptual models into a comprehensive clinical frame. *Archives of General Psychiatry, 32*, 285–305.

Allgood-Merten, B., Lewinson, P. M., & Hops, H. (1990). Sex differences and adolescent depression. *Journal of Abnormal Psychology, 99*, 55–63.

Altmann, E. O., & Gotlib, I. H. (1988). The social behavior of depressed children: An observational study. *Journal of Abnormal Child Psychology, 16*, 29–44.

American Psychiatric Association. (2013). *Diagnostic and statistical manual of mental disorders* (5th ed.). Arlington, VA: American Psychiatric Association.

Amick, H. R., Gartlehner, G., Gaynes, B. N., Forneris, C., Asher, G. N., Morgan, L. C., ... Lohr, K. N. (2015). Comparative benefits and harms of second generation antidepressants and cognitive behavioral therapies in initial treatment of major depressive disorder: Systematic review and meta-analysis. *BMJ, 351*, h6019.

Andrews, B. (1995). Bodily shame as a mediator between abusive experiences and depression. *Journal of Abnormal Psychology, 104*, 277–285.

Angold, A., & Costello, E. J. (1993). Depressive comorbidity in children and adolescents: Empirical, theoretical and methodological issues. *American Journal of Psychiatry, 150*(12), 1779–1791.

Angold, A., Costello, E. J., & Erkanli, A. (1999). Comorbidity. *Journal of Child Psychology and Psychiatry, 40*, 57–87.

Angold, A., Costello, E. J., et al. (1998). Puberty and depression: The roles of age, pubertal status and pubertal timing. *Psychological Medicine, 28*(1), 51–61.

Angold, A., Erkanli, A., Farmer, E. M., Fairbank, J. A., Burns, B. J., Keeler, G., & Costello, E. J. (2002). Psychiatric disorder, impairment, and service use in rural African American and white youth. *Archives of General Psychiatry, 59*(10), 893.

Arean, P. A., Perri, M. G., Nezu, A. M., Schein, R. L., Christopher, F., & Joseph, T. X. (1993). Comparative effectiveness of social problem-solving therapy and reminiscence therapy as treatments for depression in older adults. *Journal of Consulting and Clinical Psychology, 61*(6), 1003–1010.

Arnarson, E. Ö., & Craighead, W. E. (2009). Prevention of depression among Icelandic adolescents. *Behaviour Research and Therapy, 47*(7), 577–585.

Arnarson, E. Ö., & Craighead, W. E. (2011). Prevention of depression among Icelandic adolescents: A 12-month follow-up. *Behaviour Research and Therapy, 49*(3), 170–174.

Arnold, L. E., et al. (2011). Pediatric bipolar spectrum disorder and ADHD: Comparison and comorbidity in the LAMS clinical sample. *Bipolar Disorders, 13*, 509–521.

Aronson, R., Offman, H. J., Joffe, R. T., & Naylor, C. D. (1996). Triiodothyronine augmentation in the treatment of refractory depression: A meta-analysis. *Archives of General Psychiatry, 53*(9), 842–848.

Asarnow, J. R., Baraff, L. J., Berk, M., et al. (2011b). An emergency department intervention for linking pediatric suicidal patients to follow-up mental health treatment. *Psychiatric Services, 62*, 1303–1309.

Asarnow, J. R., Carlson, G. A., & Guthrie, D. (1987). Coping strategies, self-perceptions, hopelessness, and perceived family environments in depressed and suicidal children. *Journal of Consulting and Clinical Psychology, 55*, 361–366.

Asarnow, J. R., Emslie, G., Clarke, G., et al. (2009). Treatment of selective serotonin reuptake inhibitor-resistant depression in adolescents: Predictors and moderators of treatment response. *Journal of the American Academy of Child and Adolescent Psychiatry, 48*, 330–339.

Asarnow, J. R., Goldstein, M. J., Tompson, M., & Guthrie, D. (1993). One-year outcomes of depressive disorders in child psychiatric inpatients: Evaluation of the prognostic power of a brief measure of expressed emotion. *Journal of Child Psychology and Psychiatry, 34*, 129–137.

Asarnow, J. R., Porta, G., Spirito, A., et al. (2011a). Suicide attempts and nonsuicidal self-injury in the treatment of resistant depression in adolescents: Findings from the TORDIA study. *Journal of the American Academy of Child and Adolescent Psychiatry, 50*, 772–781.

Aseltine, R. H., Jr., Gore, S., & Colten, M. E. (1994). Depression and the social developmental context of adolescence. *Journal of Personality and Social Psychology, 67*, 252–263.

A study of DVS SR in treatment of children and adolescent outpatients with MDD. ClinicalTrials.gov Identifier: NCT01372150.

Atkinson, S. D., Prakash, A., Zhang, Q., Pangallo, B. A., Bangs, M. E., Emslie, G. J., & March, J. S. (2014). A double-blind efficacy and safety study of duloxetine flexible dosing in children and adolescents with major depressive disorder. *Journal of Child and Adolescent Psychopharmacology, 24(4),* 180–189.

Axelson, D. A., Birmaher, B., Strober, M. A., Goldstein, B. I., Ha, W., Gill, M. K., et al. (2011). Course of subthreshold bipolar disorder in youth: Diagnostic progression from bipolar disorder not otherwise specified. *Journal of the American Academy of Child and Adolescent Psychiatry, 50*(10), 1001–1016.

Axelson, D., et al. (2006). Phenomenology of children and adolescents with bipolar spectrum disorders. *Archives of General Psychiatry, 63*(10), 1139–1148.

Axelson, D., Findling, R. L., Fristad, M. A., Kowatch, R. A., Youngstrom, E. A., Horwitz, S. M., et al. (2012). Examining the proposed disruptive mood dysregulation disorder diagnosis in children in the Longitudinal Assessment of Manic Symptoms study. *Journal of Clinical Psychiatry, 73*(10), 1342–1350.

Bakr, A., Amr, M., Sarhan, A., Hammad, A., Ragab, M., El-Refaey, A., & El-Mougy, A. (2007). Psychiatric disorders in children with chronic renal failure. *Pediatric Nephrology (Berlin), 22*(1), 128–131.

Baldessarini, R. J., Lau, W. K., Sim, J., Sum, M. Y., & Sim, K. (2015) Duration of initial antidepressant treatment and subsequent relapse of major depression. *Journal of Clinical Psychopharmacology, 35*, 75–76.

Bandura, A. (1977). *Social learning theory.* Englewood Cliff, NJ: Prentice Hall.

Barbe, R. P., Bridge, J. A., Birmaher, B., Kolko, D. J,. & Brent, D. A. (2004). Lifetime history of sexual abuse, clinical presentation, and outcome in a clinical trial for adolescent depression. *Journal of Clinical Psychiatry, 65*, 77–83.

Barber, B. K. (1996). Parental psychological control: Revisiting a neglected construct. *Child Development, 67*, 3296–3319.

Barber, J. P., Barrett, M. S., Gallop, R., Rynn, M. A., & Rickels, K. (2012). Short-term dynamic psychotherapy versus pharmacotherapy for major depressive disorder: A randomized, placebo-controlled trial. *Journal of Clinical Psychiatry, 73*(1), 66–73.

Barkham, M., Rees, A., Shapiro, D. A., Stiles, W. B., Agnew, R. M., Halstead, J., Culverwell, A., & Harrington, V. M. (1996). Outcomes of time-limited psychotherapy in applied settings: Replicating the Second Sheffield Psychotherapy Project. *Journal of Consulting & Clinical Psychology, 64*(5), 1079–1085.

Barzman, D. H., DelBello, M. P., Kowatch, R. A., Warner, J., Rofey, D., Stanford, K., . . . Strakowski, S. M. (2005). Adjunctive topiramate in hospitalized children and adolescents with bipolar disorders. *Journal of Child and Adolescent Psychopharmacology, 15*, 931–937.

Bassuk, E. L., Buckner, J. C., Perloff, J. N., & Bassuk, S. S. (1998). Prevalence of mental health and substance use disorders among homeless and low-income housed mothers. *American Journal of Psychiatry, 155*, 1561–1564.

Bauer, M. S., McBride, L., Chase, C., Sachs, G., & Shea, N. (1998). Manual-based group psychotherapy for bipolar disorder: A feasibility study. *Journal of Clinical Psychiatry, 59*(9), 449–455.

Baumann, P. (1996). Pharmacology and pharmacokinetics of citalopram and other SSRIs. *International Clinical Psychopharmacology, 11*(Suppl 1), 5–11.

Beardslee, W. R., Brent, D. A., Weersing, V. R., Clarke, G. N., Porta, G., Hollon, S. D., ... Garber, J. (2013). Prevention of depression in at-risk adolescents: Longer-term effects. *JAMA Psychiatry, 70*(11), 1161–1170.

Beardslee, W. R., Gladstone, T. R. G., & O'Connor, E. E. (2011). Transmission and prevention of mood disorders among children of affectively ill parents: A review. *Journal of the American Academy of Child & Adolescent Psychiatry, 50*(11), 1098–1109.

Beardslee, W. R., Gladstone, T. R., Wright, E. J., & Cooper, A. B. (2003). A family-based approach to the prevention of depressive symptoms in children at risk: Evidence of parental and child change. *Pediatrics, 112*, e119–131.

Beardslee, W. R., Keller, M. B., Seifer, R., Lavori, P. W., Staley, J., Podorefsky, D., & Shera, D. (1996). Prediction of adolescent affective disorder: Effects of prior parental affective disorders and child psychopathology. *Journal of the American Academy of Child & Adolescent Psychiatry, 35*, 279–288.

Beardslee, W. R., & Podorefsky, D. (1988). Resilient adolescents whose parents have serious affective and other psychiatric disorders: Importance of self-understanding and relationships. *American Journal of Psychiatry, 145*(1), 63–69.

Beardslee, W. R., Versage, E. M., & Gladstone, T. R. G. (1998). Children of affectively ill parents: A review of the past ten years. *Journal of the American Academy of Child and Adolescent Psychiatry, 37*, 1134–1141.

Beck, A. T. (1967). *Depression: Clinical experimental and theoretical aspects*. New York: Harper and Row.

Beck, A. T., Rush, A. J., Shaw, B. F., & Emery, G. (1979). *Cognitive therapy of depression*. New York: Guilford Press.

Bell, A. C., & D'Zurilla, T. J. (2009). Problem-solving therapy for depression: A meta-analysis. *Clinical Psychology Review, 29*, 348–353.

Benazzi, F. (2006). Symptoms of depression as possible markers of bipolar II disorder. *Progress in Neuro-Psychopharmacology and Biological Psychiatry, 30*(3), 471–477.

Bennett, D. S., Pendley, J. S., & Bates, J. E. (1995). Daughter and mother report of individual symptoms on the Children's Depression Inventory. *Journal of Adolescent Health, 20*, 51–57.

Berard, R., Fong, R., Carpenter, D. J., Thomason, C., & Wilkinson, C. (2006) An international, multicenter, placebo-controlled trial of paroxetine in adolescents with major depressive disorder. *Journal of Child and Adolescent Psychopharmacology, 16*, 59–75.

Biederman, J. (1998). Resolved: Mania is mistaken for ADHD in prepubertal children. *Journal of the American Academy of Child and Adolescent Psychiatry, 37*(10), 1091–1093.

Biederman, J., Faraone, S. V., Chu, M. P., & Wozniak, J. (1999). Further evidence of a bidirectional overlap between juvenile mania and conduct disorder in children. *Journal of the American Academy of Child and Adolescent Psychiatry, 38*(4), 468–476.

Biederman, J., Faraone, S., Hatch, M., Mennin, D., Taylor, A., & George, P. (1997). Conduct disorder with and without mania in a referred sample of ADHD children. *Journal of Affective Disorders, 44*(2-3), 177–188.

Biederman, J., Faraone, S. V., Marrs, A., Moore, P., Garcia, J., Ablon, S., ... Kearns, M. E. (1997). Panic disorder and agoraphobia in consecutively referred children and adolescents. *Journal of the American Academy of Child and Adolescent Psychiatry, 36*(2), 214–223.

Biederman, J., Faraone, S., Mick, E., & Lelon, E. (1995). Psychiatric comorbidity among referred juveniles with major depression: Fact or artifact? *Journal of the American Academy of Child and Adolescent Psychiatry, 34*(5), 579–590.

Biederman, J., Faraone, S. V., Mick, E., Wozniak, J., Chen, L., Ouellette, C., ... Lelon, E. (1996). Attention deficit hyperactivity disorder and juvenile mania: An overlooked comorbidity? *Journal of the American Academy of Child and Adolescent Psychiatry, 35*(8), 997–1008.

Biederman, J., Faraone, S., Wozniak, J., Mick, E., Kwon, A., & Aleardi, M. (2004). Further evidence of unique developmental phenotypic correlates of pediatric bipolar disorder: Findings from a large sample of clinically referred preadolescent children assessed over the last 7 years. *Journal of Affective Disorders, 82*, S45–S58.

Biederman, J., Faraone, S. V., Wozniak, J., & Monuteaux, M. C. (2000). Parsing the association between bipolar, conduct, and substance use disorders: A familial risk analysis. *Biological Psychiatry, 48*(11), 1037–1044.

Biederman, J., Mick, E., Wozniak, J., Monuteaux, M. C., Galdo, M., & Faraone, S. V. (2003). Can a subtype of conduct disorder linked to bipolar disorder be identified? Integration of findings from the Massachusetts General Hospital Pediatric Psychopharmacology Research Program. *Biological Psychiatry, 53*(11), 952–960.

Biederman, J., Rosenbaum, J. F., Hirshfeld, D. R., Faraone, S. V., Bolduc, E. A., Gersten, M., et al. (1990). Psychiatric correlates of behavioral inhibition in young children of parents with and without psychiatric disorders. *Archives of General Psychiatry, 47*, 21–26.

Biederman, J., Wilens, T. E., et al. (1997). Is ADHD a risk factor for psychoactive substance use disorders? Findings from a four-year prospective follow-up study. *Journal of the American Academy of Child and Adolescent Psychiatry, 36*(1), 21–29.

Biederman, J., Wozniak, J., Kiely, K., Ablon, S., Faraone, S., Mick, E., Mundy, E., & Kraus, I. (1995). CBCL clinical scales discriminate prepubertal children with structured-interview derived diagnosis of mania from those with ADHD. *Journal of the American Academy of Child and Adolescent Psychiatry, 34*, 464–471.

Bifulco, A., Brown, G. W., & Adler, Z. (1991). Early sexual abuse and clinical depression in adult life. *British Journal of Psychiatry, 159*, 115–122.

Billings, A. G., & Moos, R. H. (1983). Comparisons of children of depressed and nondepressed parents: A social–environmental perspective. *Journal of Abnormal Child Psychology, 11*, 463–485.

Bird, H. R., Canino, G., Rubio-Stipec, M., Gould, M. S., Ribera, J., Sesman, M., . . . Moscoso, M. (1988). Estimates of the prevalence of childhood maladjustment in a community survey in Puerto Rico: The use of combined measures. *Archives of General Psychiatry, 45*(12), 1120.

Birmaher, B. (2007). Longitudinal course of pediatric bipolar disorder. *American Journal of Psychiatry, 164*, 537–539.

Birmaher, B. (2012). Pediatric bipolar disorder: Clinical picture and longitudinal course. *International Clinical Psychopharmacology, 28*, e27.

Birmaher, B. (2013). Bipolar disorder in children and adolescents. *Child and Adolescent Mental Health, 18*(3), 140–148.

Birmaher, B., Arbelaez, C., & Brent, D. (2002). Course and outcome of child and adolescent major depressive disorder. *Child and Adolescent Psychiatric Clinics of North America, 11*(3), 619–637.

Birmaher, B., Axelson, D., Goldstein, B., et al. (2009). Four-year longitudinal course of children and adolescents with bipolar spectrum disorders: The Course and Outcome of Bipolar Youth (COBY) study. *American Journal of Psychiatry, 166*, 795–804.

Birmaher, B., Axelson, D., Monk, K., Kalas, C., Goldstein, B., Hickey, M. B., . . . Brent, D. (2009). Lifetime psychiatric disorders in school-aged offspring of parents with bipolar disorder: The Pittsburgh Bipolar Offspring study. *Archives of General Psychiatry, 66*(3), 287–296.

Birmaher, B., Axelson, D., Strober, M., et al. (2006). Clinical course of children and adolescents with bipolar spectrum disorders. *Archives of General Psychiatry, 63*, 175–183.

Birmaher, B., Brent, D., AACAP Work Group on Quality Issues, Benet, W., Bukstein, O., Benson, R. S. . . . Medicus, J. (2007). Practice parameter for the assessment and treatment of children and adolescents with depressive disorders. *Journal of American Academy of Child and Adolescent Psychiatry, 46*, 1503–1526.

Birmaher, B., Brent, D. A., Kolko, D., Baugher, M., Bridge, J., Holder, D., Iyengar, S., & Ulloa, R. E. (2000). Clinical outcome after short-term psychotherapy for adolescents with major depressive disorder. *Archives of General Psychiatry, 57*, 29–36.

Birmaher, B., Neal, R. D., Williamson, D. E., Brent, D. A., Kaufman, J., Dahl, R. E., Perel, J., & Nelson, B. (1996). Childhood and adolescent depression: A review of the past 10 years. Part I. *Journal of the American Academy of Child and Adolescent Psychiatry, 35*(11), 1427–1439.

Birmaher, B., Williamson, D. E., Dahl, R. E., Axelson, D. A., Kaufman, J., Dorn, L. D., et al. (2004). Clinical presentation and course of depression in youth: Does onset in childhood differ from onset in adolescence? *Journal of the American Academy of Child and Adolescent Psychiatry, 43*(1), 63–70.

Blackburn, I. M., Eunson, K. M., & Bishop, S. (1986). A two-year naturalistic follow-up of depressed patients treated with cognitive therapy, pharmacotherapy and a combination of both. *Journal of Affective Disorders, 10*(1), 67–75.

Blackburn, I. M., & Moore, R. G. (1997). Controlled acute and follow-up trial of cognitive therapy and pharmacotherapy in out-patients with recurrent depression. *British Journal of Psychiatry, 171*(4), 328–334.

Blatt, S. J., Quinlan, D. M., Chevron, E. S., McDonald, C., & Zuroff, D. (1982). Dependency and self-criticism: Psychological dimensions of depression. *Journal of Consulting and Clinical Psychology, 50*, 113–124.

Blumberg, H. P., Martin, A., Kaufman, J., Leung, H.-C., Skudlarski, P., Lacadie, C., ... Peterson, B. S. (2003). Frontostriatal abnormalities in adolescents with bipolar disorder: Preliminary observations from functional MRI. *American Journal of Psychiatry, 160*(7), 1345–1347.

Bolton, P., Bass, J., Neugebauer, R., Verdeli, H., Clougherty, K. F., Wickramaratne, P., ... Weissman, M. (2003). Group interpersonal psychotherapy for depression in rural Uganda. *Journal of the American Medical Association, 289*(23), 3117–3124.

Borchardt, C. M., & Bernstein, G. A. (1995). Comorbid disorders in hospitalized bipolar adolescents compared with unipolar depressed adolescents. *Child Psychiatry and Human Development, 26*(1), 11–18.

Bowen, R., South, M., & Hawkes, J. (1994). Mood swings in patients with panic disorder. *Canadian Journal of Psychiatry, 39*(2), 91–94.

Bowlby, J. (1980). By ethology out of psychoanalysis: An experiment in interbreeding. *Animal Behavior, 28*(Pt 3), 649–656.

Brauner, C. B., & Stephens, C. B. (2006). Estimating the prevalence of early childhood serious emotional/behavioral disorders: Challenges and recommendations. *Public Health Reports, 121*(3), 303.

Brent, D. A., Baugher, M., Bridge, J., Chen, T., & Chiappetta, L. (1999). Age- and sex-related risk factors for adolescent suicide. *Journal of the American Academy of Child and Adolescent Psychiatry, 38*, 1497–1505.

Brent, D. A., Brunwasser, S. M., Hollon, S. D., Weersing, V. R., Clarke, G. N., Dickerson, J. F., ... Garber, J. (2015). Effect of a cognitive-behavioral prevention program on depression 6 years after implementation among at-risk adolescents: A randomized clinical trial. *JAMA Psychiatry, 72*(11), 1110–1118.

Brent, D., Emslie, G., Clarke, G., et al. (2008). Switching to another SSRI or to venlafaxine with or without cognitive behavioral therapy for adolescents with SSRI-resistant depression: The TORDIA randomized controlled trial. *Journal of the American Medical Association, 299*, 901–913.

Brent, D. A., Holder, D., Kolko, D., et al. (1997). A clinical psychotherapy trial for adolescent depression comparing cognitive, family, and supportive therapy. *Archives of General Psychiatry, 54*, 877–885.

Brent, D. A., Kolko, D. J., Birmaher, B., et al. (1998). Predictors of treatment efficacy in a clinical trial of three psychosocial treatments for adolescent depression. *Journal of the American Academy of Child and Adolescent Psychiatry, 37*, 906–914.

Brent, D., Melhem, N., Ferrell, R., Emslie, G., Wagner, K. D., Ryan, N., ... Keller, M. (2010). Association of FKBP5 polymorphisms with suicidal events in the Treatment of Resistant Depression in Adolescents (TORDIA) study. *American Journal of Psychiatry, 167*(2), 190–197.

Brent, D. A., Perper, J. A., Goldstein, C. E., Kolko, D. J., Allan, M. J., Allman, C. J., & Zelenak, J. P. (1988). Risk factors for adolescent suicide: A comparison of adolescent suicide victims with suicidal inpatients. *Archives of General Psychiatry, 45*(6), 581–588.

Brent, D. A., Perper, J. A., Moritz, G., et al. (1993). Psychiatric risk factors for adolescent suicide: A case-control study. *Journal of the American Academy of Child and Adolescent Psychiatry, 32*, 521–529.

Breslau, N., & Davis, G. C. (1992). Posttraumatic stress disorder in an urban population of young adults: Risk factors for chronicity. *American Journal of Psychiatry, 149*, 671–675.

Breslau, N., Davis, G. C., & Andreski, P. (1995). Risk factors for PTSD-related traumatic events: A prospective analysis. *American Journal of Psychiatry, 152*, 529–535.

Bridge, J. A., Iyengar, S., Salary, C. B., Barbe, R. P., Birmaher, B., Pincus, H. A., Ren, L., Brent, D. A. (2007). Clinical response and risk for reported suicidal ideation and suicide attempts in pediatric antidepressant treatment: A meta-analysis of randomized controlled trials. *Journal of the American Medical Association, 297*, 1683–1696.

Brody, D., Roper, M., & Narrow, W. E. (2003). Prevalence of mood disorders in a national sample of young American adults. *Social Psychiatry and Psychiatric Epidemiology, 38*(11), 618–624.

Brown, G. W., & Moran, P. M. (1997). Single mothers, poverty and depression. *Psychological Medicine, 27*(1), 21–33.

Brown, L. K., Lourie, K. J., & Pao, M. (2000). Children and adolescents living with HIV and AIDS: A review. *Journal of Child Psychology & Psychiatry, 41*(1), 81–96.

Browne, A., & Finkelhor, D. (1986). Impact of child sexual abuse: A review of the research. *Psychological Bulletin, 99*(1), 66–77.

Bruce, M. L., Takeuchi, D. T., & Leaf, P. J. (1991). Poverty and psychiatric status: Longitudinal evidence from the New Haven Epidemiologic Catchment Area Study. *Archives of General Psychiatry, 48*, 470–474.

Brunson, K. L., Eghbal-Ahmadi, M., Bender, R., Chen, Y., & Baram, T. Z. (2001). Long-term, progressive hippocampal cell loss and dysfunction induced by early-life administration of corticotropin-releasing hormone reproduce the effects of early-life stress. *Proceedings of the National Academy of Sciences of the United States of America, 98*, 8856–8861.

Brunwasser, S. M., Gillham, J. E., & Kim, E. S. (2009). A meta-analytic review of the Penn Resiliency Program's effect on depressive symptoms. *Journal of Consulting and Clinical Psychology, 77*(6), 1042.

Buka, S. L., Monuteaux, M., & Earlsi, F. (2002). The epidemiology of child and adolescent mental disorders. In M. T. Tsuang & M. Tohen, eds. *Textbook in Psychiatric Epidemiology* (2nd ed., pp. 629–655). West Sussex: John Wiley & Sons.

Buka, S. L., Stichick, T. L., Birdthistle, I., & Earls, F. J. (2001). Youth exposure to violence: Prevalence, risks, and consequences. *American Journal of Orthopsychiatry, 71*, 298–310.

Burge, D., & Hammen, C. (1991). Maternal communication: Predictors of outcome at follow-up in a sample of children at high and low risk for depression. *Journal of Abnormal Psychology, 100*(2), 174–180.

Burge, D., Hammen, C., Davila, J., Daley, S. E., Paley, B., Lindberg, N., et al. (1997). The relationship between attachment cognitions and psychological adjustment in late adolescent women. *Development and Psychopathology, 9*, 151–167.

Burnam, M. A., Wells, K. B., Leake, B., & Landsverk, J. (1988). Development of a brief screening instrument for detecting depressive disorders. *Medical Care, 26*, 775–789.

Burnand, Y., Andreoli, A., Kolatte, E., Venturini, A., & Rosset, N. (2002). Psychodynamic psychotherapy and clomipramine in the treatment of major depression. *Psychiatric Services, 53*(5), 585–590.

Cairns, K. E., Yap, M. B. H., Pilkington, P. D., & Jorm, A. F. (2014). Risk and protective factors for depression that adolescents can modify: A systematic review and meta-analysis of longitudinal studies. *Journal of Affective Disorders, 169*, 61–75.

Canino, G., Shrout, P. E., Rubio-Stipec, M., Bird, H. R., Bravo, M., Ramirez, R., ... Martinez-Taboas, A. (2004). The DSM-IV rates of child and adolescent disorders in Puerto Rico: Prevalence, correlates, service use, and the effects of impairment. *Archives of General Psychiatry, 61*(1), 85.

Caplan, R. (2012). Depressive disorders in children and adolescents with neurologic disorders. In *Depression in neurologic disorders: Diagnosis and management* (p. 77).

Caplan, R., Arbelle, S., Magharious, W., Guthrie, D., Komo, S., Shields, W. D., et al. (1998). Psychopathology in pediatric complex partial and primary generalized epilepsy. *Developmental Medicine & Child Neurology, 40*(12), 805–811.

Cardemil, E. V., Reivich, K. J., Beevers, C. G., Seligman, M. E., & James, J. (2007). The prevention of depressive symptoms in low-income, minority children: Two-year follow-up. *Behaviour Research and Therapy, 45*(2), 313–327.

Cardemil, E. V., Reivich, K. J., & Seligman, M. E. (2002). The prevention of depressive symptoms in low-income minority middle school students. *Prevention & Treatment, 5*(1), 8a.

Carlson, G. A. (1983). Bipolar affective disorders in childhood and adolescence. In D. P. Cantwell and G. A. Carlson (Eds.), *Affective disorders in childhood and adolescence* (pp. 61–83). New York: Spectrum Publications.

Carlson, G. A. (1984). Classification issues of bipolar disorders in childhood. *Psychiatric Developments, 2*(4), 273–285.

Carlson, G. A. (1999). Juvenile mania versus ADHD. *Journal of the American Academy of Child and Adolescent Psychiatry, 38*(4), 353–354.

Carlson, G. A., & Blader, J. C. (2011). Diagnostic implications of informant disagreement for manic symptoms. *Journal of Child and Adolescent Psychopharmacology, 21*(5), 399–405.

Carlson, G. A., Bromet, E. J., et al. (2000). Phenomenology and outcome of subjects with early- and adult-onset psychotic mania. *American Journal of Psychiatry, 157*(2), 213–219.

Carlson, G. A., & Kelly, K. L. (1998). Manic symptoms in psychiatrically hospitalized children: What do they mean? *Journal of Affective Disorders, 51*, 123–135.

Carlson, G. A., Loney, J., Salisbury, H., & Volpe, R. J. (1998). Young referred boys with DICA-P manic symptoms vs. two comparison groups. *Journal of Affective Disorders, 51*(2), 113–121.

Carlson, G. A., & Strober, M. (1979), Affective disorders in adolescence. *Psychiatric Clinics of North America, 2*, 511–526.

Caspi, A., Moffitt, T. E., Newman, D. L., & Silva, P. A. (1996). Behavioral observations at age 3 years predict adult psychiatric disorders. Longitudinal evidence from a birth cohort. *Archives of General Psychiatry, 53,* 1033–1039.

Caspi, A., Sugden, K., Moffitt, T. E., Taylor, A., Craig, I. W., Harrington, H., et al. (2003). Influence of life stress on depression: Moderation by a polymorphism in the 5-HTT gene. *Science, 301*(5631), 386–389.

Catalan, J., Gath, D. H., Anastasiades, P., Bond, S. A., Day, A., & Hall, L. (1991). Evaluation of a brief psychological treatment for emotional disorders in primary care. *Psychological Medicine, 21*(4), 1013–1018.

Center for Behavioral Health Statistics and Quality. (2015). *Behavioral health trends in the United States: Results from the 2014 National Survey on Drug Use and Health* (HHS Publication No. SMA 15-4927, NSDUH Series H-50). Retrieved from http://www.samhsa.gov/data/

Chang, K., Adleman, N. E., Dienes, K., Simeonova, D. I., Menon, V., & Reiss, A. (2004). Anomalous prefrontal-subcortical activation in familial pediatric bipolar disorder: A functional magnetic resonance imaging investigation. *Archives of General Psychiatry, 61*(8), 781–792.

Chang, K. D., Steiner, H., & Ketter, T. A. (2000). Psychiatric phenomenology of child and adolescent bipolar offspring. *Journal of the American Academy of Child and Adolescent Psychiatry, 39,* 453–460.

Chen, Y., & Dilsaver, S. (1995). Comorbidity of panic disorder in bipolar illness: Evidence from the epidemiologic catchment area survey. *American Journal of Psychiatry, 152*(2), 280–283.

Chentsova-Dutton, Y., & Tsai, J. (2009). Culture and depression. In R. E. Ingram (Ed.), *International encyclopedia of depression* (pp. 194–199). New York: Springer Publishing.

Cheung, A., Kusumakar, V., Kutcher, S., Dubo, E., Garland, J., Weiss, M., Kiss, A., Levitt, A. (2008). Maintenance study for adolescent depression. *Journal of Child and Adolescent Psychopharmacology, 18,* 389–394.

Children's Defense Fund—Minnesota (2011). *Zero to three research to policy project: Maternal depression and early childhood.* Retrieved from http://http://www.cdf-mn.org/research-library/maternal-depression-report.pdf

Cicchetti, D., Rogosch, F. A., & Toth, S. L. (1998). Maternal depressive disorder and contextual risk: Contributions to the development of attachment insecurity and behavior problems in toddlerhood. *Development & Psychopathology, 10*(2), 283–300.

Cicchetti, D., & Toth, S. L. (1998). The development of depression in children and adolescents. *American Psychologist, 53*(2), 221–241.

Clark, L. A., Vittengl, J., Kraft, D., & Jarrett, R. B. (2003). Separate personality traits from states to predict depression. *Journal of Personality Disorders, 17*(2), 152–172.

Clark, L. A., Watson, D., & Mineka, S. (1994). Temperament, personality, and the mood and anxiety disorders. *Journal of Abnormal Psychology, 103,* 103–116.

Clarke, A. S., & Schneider, M. L. (1993). Prenatal stress has long-term effects on behavioral responses to stress in juvenile rhesus monkeys. *Developmental Psychobiology, 26,* 293–304.

Clarke, A. S., Wittwer, D. J., Abbott, D. H., & Schneider, M. L. (1994). Long-term effects of prenatal stress on HPA axis activity in juvenile rhesus monkeys. *Developmental Psychobiology, 27,* 257–269.

Clarke, G., Debar, L., Lynch, F., et al. (2005). A randomized effectiveness trial of brief cognitive-behavioral therapy for depressed adolescents receiving antidepressant medication. *Journal of the American Academy of Child & Adolescent Psychiatry, 44,* 888–898.

Clarke, G. N., Hawkins, W., Murphy, M., Sheeber, L. B., Lewinsohn, P. M., & Seeley, J. R. (1995). Targeted prevention of unipolar depressive disorder in an at-risk sample of high school adolescents: A randomized trial of a group cognitive intervention. *Journal of the American Academy of Child & Adolescent Psychiatry, 34,* 312–321.

Clarke, G. N., Hornbrook, M., Lynch, F., Polen, M., Gale, J., Beardslee, W., et al. (2001). A randomized trial of a group cognitive intervention for preventing depression in adolescent offspring of depressed parents. *Archives of General Psychiatry, 58,* 1127–1134.

Clarke, G. N., Lewinsohn, P. N., & Hops, H. (1990). *Instructor's manual for the adolescent: Coping with depression course.* Portland, OR: Kaiser Permanente Center for Health Research. Available at: http// www.kpchr.org/acwd/acwd.html.

Clarke, K., Mayo-Wilson, E., Kenny, J., & Pilling, S. (2015). Can non-pharmacological interventions prevent relapse in adults who have recovered from depression? A systematic review and meta-analysis of randomised controlled trials. *Clinical Psychology Review, 39,* 58–70.

Clarkin, J. F., Glick, I. D., Haas, G. L., Spencer, J. H., Lewis, A. B., Peyser, J., et al. (1990). A randomized clinical trial of inpatient family intervention. Results for affective disorders. *Journal of Affective Disorders, 18*, 17–28.

ClinicalTrials.gov. A Study in the Treatment of Children and Adolescents with Major Depressive Disorder, Clinicaltrials.gov Study NCT00849901 and Study NCT00849693. Accessed March 13, 2014.

Cloninger, C. R. (1987). A systematic method for clinical description and classification of personality variants: A proposal. *Archives of General Psychiatry, 44*, 573–588.

Cohen, P., Cohen, J., Kasen, S., Velez, C. N., Hartmark, C., Johnson, J., ... Streuning, E. L. (1993). An epidemiological study of disorders in late childhood and adolescence. I. Age- and gender-specific prevalence. *Journal of Child Psychology & Psychiatry, 34*, 851–867.

Cohn, J. F., & Tronick, E. (1989). Specificity of infants' response to mothers' affective behavior. *Journal of the American Academy of Child and Adolescent Psychiatry, 28*, 242–248.

Cole, D. A., & Rehm, L. P. (1986). Family interaction patterns and childhood depression. *Journal of Abnormal Child Psychology, 14*, 297–314.

Cole, D. A., & Turner, J. E., Jr. (1993). Models of cognitive mediation and moderation in child depression. *Journal of Abnormal Psychology, 102*(2), 271–281.

Commission on Chronic Illness. (1957). *Chronic illness in the United States, Vol. 1.* Cambridge, MA: Harvard University Press.

Committee and Pediatric Advisory Committee. September 13–14, 2004. Available at: http:www.fda.gov/ohrms/dockets/as/04/briefing/2004-4065b1.htm. Accessed January 2011.

Compas, B. E., Forehand, R., Thigpen, J. C., et al. 2011. Family group cognitive-behavioral preventive intervention for families of depressed parents: 18- and 24-month outcomes. *Journal of Consulting and Clinical Psychology, 79*, 488–499.

Compas, B. E., Grant, K. E., & Ey, S. (1994). Psychosocial stress and child and adolescent depression: Can we be more specific? In W. M. Reynolds & H. F. Johnston (Eds.), *Handbook of depression in children and adolescents* (pp. 509–523). New York: Plenum Press.

Compas, B. E., Howell, D. C., Phares, V., Williams, R. A., & Giunta, C. T. (1989). Risk factors for emotional/behavioral problems in young adolescents: A prospective analysis of adolescent and parental stress and symptoms. *Consulting & Clinical Psychology, 57*(6), 732–740.

Connolly Gibbons, M. B., Gallop, R., Thompson, D., Luther, D., Crits-Christoph, K., Jacobs, J., ... Crits-Christoph, P. (2016). Comparative effectiveness of cognitive and dynamic therapies for major depressive disorder in a community mental health setting: A randomized non-inferiority trial. *JAMA Psychiatry*, 73, 904–911.

Copeland, W. E., Shanahan, L., Costello, E. J., & Angold, A. (2009). Childhood and adolescent psychiatric disorders as predictors of young adult disorders. *Archives of General Psychiatry, 66*(7), 764–772.

Coplan, J. D., Andrews, M. W., Rosenblum, L. A., Owens, M. J., Friedman, S., Gorman, J. M., et al. (1996). Persistent elevations of cerebrospinal fluid concentrations of corticotropin-releasing factor in adult nonhuman primates exposed to early-life stressors: Implications for the pathophysiology of mood and anxiety disorders. *Proceedings of the National Academy of Sciences of the United States of America, 93*, 1619–1623.

Costa, P. T., & McCrae, R. R. (1980). Influence of extraversion and neuroticism on subjective well-being: Happy and unhappy people. *Journal of Personality and Social Psychology, 38*, 668–678.

Costello, E. J., Angold, A., Burns, B. J., Erkanli, A., Stangl, D. K., & Tweed, D. L. (1996). The Great Smoky Mountains Study of Youth. Functional impairment and serious emotional disturbance. *Archives of General Psychiatry, 53*, 1137–1143.

Costello, E. J., Costello, A. J., Edelbrock, C., Burns, B. J., Dulcan, M. K., Brent, D., & Janiszewski, S. (1988). Psychiatric disorders in pediatric primary care: Prevalence and risk factors. *Archives of General Psychiatry, 45*(12), 1107.

Costello, E. J., Farmer, E. M., Angold, A., Burns, B. J., & Erkanli, A. (1997). Psychiatric disorders among American Indian and white youth in Appalachia: The Great Smoky Mountains Study. *American Journal of Public Health, 87*(5), 827–832.

Costello, E. J., Mustillo, S., Erkanli, A., Keeler, G., & Angold, A. (2003). Prevalence and development of psychiatric disorders in childhood and adolescence. *Archives of General Psychiatry, 60*(8), 837.

Costello, E. J., Pine, D. S., Hammen, C., March, J. S., Plotsky, P. M., Weissman, M. M., ... Leckman, J. F. (2002). Development and natural history of mood disorders. *Biological Psychiatry, 52*(6), 529–542.

Cox, G. R., Callahan, P., Churchill, R., et al. (2012). Psychological therapies versus antidepressant medication, alone and in combination for depression in children and adolescents. *Cochrane Database of Systematic Reviews, 11*, CD008324.

Cox, G. R., Fischer, C. A., DeSilva, S., Phelan, M., Akinwale, O. P., Simmons, M. B., & Hetrick, S. E. (2012). Interventions for preventing relapse and recurrence of depressive disorder in children and adolescents. *Cochrane Database of Systematic Reviews, 11*, CD007504.

Cox, L. J., Stanley, B. H., Melhem, N. M., et al. (2012). A longitudinal study of nonsuicidal self-injury in offspring at high risk for mood disorder. *Journal of Clinical Psychiatry, 73*, 821–828.

Coyne, J. C., Kessler, R. C., Tal, M., Turnbull, J., Wortman, C. B., & Greden, J. F. (1987). Living with a depressed person. *Journal of Consulting & Clinical Psychology, 55*(3), 347–352.

Craddock, N., Davé, S., & Greening, J. (2001). Association studies of bipolar disorder. *Bipolar Disorders, 3*(6), 284–298.

Craighead, W. E., Miklowitz, D. J., Vajk, F. C., & Frank, E. (2002). Psychosocial treatments for bipolar disorder. In P. E. Nathan & J. M. Gorman (Eds.), *A guide to treatments that work* (2nd ed., pp. 263–275). New York: Oxford University Press.

Cross-National Collaborative Group. (1992), The changing rate of major depression: Cross-national comparisons. *Journal of the American Medical Association, 268*, 3098–3106.

Cuijpers, P., Beekman, A. T., & Reynolds, C. F. (2012). Preventing depression: A global priority. *Journal of the American Medical Association, 307*(10), 1033–1034.

Cuijpers, P., Berking, M., Andersson, G., Quigley, L., Kleiboer, A., & Dobson, K. S. (2013). A meta-analysis of cognitive-behavioural therapy for adult depression, alone and in comparison with other treatments. *Canadian Journal of Psychiatry, 58*(7), 376–385.

Cuijpers, P., Geraedts, A. S., van Oppen, P., Markowitz, J. C., & van Straten, A. (2011). Interpersonal psychotherapy for depression: A meta-analysis. *American Journal of Psychiatry, 168*(6), 581–592.

Cullen, K. R., Gee, D. G., et al. (2009). A preliminary study of functional connectivity in comorbid adolescent depression. *Neuroscience Letters, 460*(3), 227–231.

Cullen, K. R., Klimes-Dougan, B., et al. (2010). Altered white matter microstructure in adolescents with major depression: A preliminary study. *Journal of the American Academy of Child and Adolescent Psychiatry, 49*(2), 173–183.

Curry, J., Rohde, P., Simons, A., et al. (2006). Predictors and moderators of acute outcome in the Treatment for Adolescents with Depression Study (TADS). *Journal of the American Academy of Child and Adolescent Psychiatry, 45*, 1427–1439.

Curry, J., Silva, S., Rohde, P., Ginsburg, G., Kratochvil C., Simons, A., ... March, J. (2011). Recovery and recurrence following treatment for adolescent major depression. *Archives of General Psychiatry, 68*, 263–270.

Dahl, R. E. (2001). Affect regulation, brain development, and behavioral/emotional health in adolescence. *CNS Spectrums, 6*, 60–72.

Davies, S., Heyman, I., & Goodman, R. (2003). A population survey of mental health problems in children with epilepsy. *Developmental Medicine & Child Neurology, 45*(5), 292–295.

Decina, P., Kestenbaum, C. J., Farber, S., Kron, L., Gargan, M., Sackeim, H. A., & Fieve, R. R. (1983), Clinical and psychological assessment of children of bipolar probands. *American Journal of Psychiatry, 140*, 548–553.

de Jonghe, F., Kool, S., van Aalst, G., Dekker, J., & Peen, J. (2001). Combining psychotherapy and antidepressants in the treatment of depression. *Journal of Affective Disorders, 64*(2), 217–229.

DelBello, M. P., Chang, K., Welge, J. A., Adler, C. M., Rana, M. , Howe M, ... Strakowski, S. M. (2009). A double-blind, placebo-controlled pilot study of quetiapine for depressed adolescents with bipolar disorder. *Bipolar Disorders, 11*, 483–493.

DelBello, M. P., et al. (2011). A double-blind, placebo-controlled study of selegeline transdermal system (EMSAS) in depressed adolescents. Presented at Annual Meeting of American Academy of Child and Adolescent Psychiatrists Annual Meeting. Toronto, Canada.

DelBello, M. P., Findling, R. L., Kushner, S., Wang, D., Olson, W. H., Capece, J. A., Fazzio, L., & Rosenthal, N. R. (2005). A pilot controlled trial of topiramate for mania in children and adolescents with bipolar disorder. *Journal of the American Academy of Child and Adolescent Psychiatry, 44*, 539–547.

DelBello, M., Hanseman, D., Adler, C. M., Fleck, D. E., & Strakowski, S. M. (2007). Twelve-month outcome of adolescents with bipolar disorder following first hospitalization for a manic or mixed episode. *American Journal of Psychiatry, 164*(4), 582–590.

DelBello, M. P., Schwiers, M. L., Rosenberg, H. L., & Strakowski, S. M. (2002). A double-blind, randomized, placebo-controlled study of quetiapine as adjunctive treatment for adolescent mania. *Journal of the American Academy of Child and Adolescent Psychiatry, 41*, 1216–1223.

DelBello, M. P., Zimmerman, M. E., Mills, N. P., Getz, G. E., & Strakowski, S. M. (2004). Magnetic resonance imaging analysis of amygdala and other subcortical brain regions in adolescents with bipolar disorder. *Bipolar Disorders, 6*(1), 43–52.

DeMulder, E. K., & Radke-Yarrow, M. (1991). Attachment with affectively ill and well mothers: Concurrent behavioral correlates. *Development and Psychopathology, 3*, 227–242.

DeRubeis, R. J., Gelfand, L. A., Tang, T. Z., & Simons, A. D. (1999). Medications versus cognitive behavior therapy for severely depressed outpatients: Mega-analysis of four randomized comparisons. *American Journal of Psychiatry, 156*(7), 1007–1013.

DeRubeis, R. J., Hollon, S. D., Amsterdam, J. D., Shelton, R. C., Young, P. R., Salomon, R. M., ... Gallop, R. (2005). Cognitive therapy vs medications in the treatment of moderate to severe depression. *Archives of General Psychiatry, 62*(4), 409–416.

Detke, H. C., DelBello, M., Landry, J., Usher, R., & Dingankar, M. (2012). Safety and efficacy of olanzapine/fluoxetine combination vs. placebo in patients ages 10 to 17 in the acute treatment of major depressive episodes associated with bipolar I disorder. Presented at the American College of Neuropsychopharmacology 51st Annual Meeting; Hollywood Florida, December 2–6.

Devine, D., Kempton, T., & Forehand, R. (1994). Adolescent depressed mood and young adult functioning: A longitudinal study. *Journal of Abnormal Child Psychology, 22*, 629–640.

Devries, K. M., Mak, J. Y., Bacchus, L. J., Child, J. C., Falder, G., Petzold, M., ... Watts, C. H. (2013). Intimate partner violence and incident depressive symptoms and suicide attempts: A systematic review of longitudinal studies. *PLoS Medicine, 10*(5): 31001439.

Diamond, G. S., Reis, B. F., Diamond, G. M., Siqueland, L., & Isaacs, L. (2002). Attachment-based family therapy for depressed adolescents: A treatment development study. *Journal of the American Academy of Child and Adolescent Psychiatry, 41*, 1190–1196.

Diamond, G. S., Wintersteen, M. B., Brown, G. K., et al. (2010). Attachment-based family therapy for adolescents with suicidal ideation: A randomized controlled trial. *Journal of the American Academy of Child and Adolescent Psychiatry, 49*, 122–131.

Dickstein, D. P., Milham, M. P., Nugent, A. C., Drevets, W. C., Charney, D. S., Pine, D. S., & Leibenluft, E. (2005b). Frontotemporal alterations in pediatric bipolar disorder: Results of a voxel-based morphometry study. *Archives of General Psychiatry, 62*, 734–741.

Dickstein, D. P., Rich, B. A., Binstock, A. B., Pradella, A. G., Towbin, K. E., Pine, D. S., & Leibenluft, E. (2005a). Comorbid anxiety in phenotypes of pediatric bipolar disorder. *Journal of Child and Adolescent Psychopharmacology, 15*, 534–548.

Diekstra, R. F. W. (1995). Depression and suicidal behaviors in adolescence: Sociocultural and time trends. In M. Rutter (ed.), *Psychosocial disturbances in young people: Challenges for prevention* (pp. 212–243). Cambridge: Cambridge University Press.

Diflorio, A., & Jones, I. (2010). Is sex important? Gender differences in bipolar disorder. *International Review of Psychiatry (Abingdon, England), 22*(5), 437–452.

Digman, J. M. (1989). Five robust trait dimensions: Development, stability, and utility. *Journal of Personality, 57*, 195–214.

Digman, J. M., & Inouye, J. (1986). Further specification of the five robust factors of personality. *Journal of Personality and Social Psychology, 50*, 116–123.

Digman, J. M., & Shmelyov, A. G. (1996). The structure of temperament and personality in Russian children. *Journal of Personality and Social Psychology, 71*(2), 341–351.

Diler, R. S. (ed.). (2007). *Pediatric bipolar disorder: A global perspective*. Hauppage, NY: Nova Publishers, 2007.

Diler, R. S., & Birmaher, B. (2012). Bipolar disorder in children and adolescents. In *IACAPAP e-Textbook of Child and Adolescent Mental Health*. Geneva: International Association for Child and Adolescent Psychiatry and Allied Professions.

Dimidjian, S., Hollon, S. D., Dobson, K. S., Schmaling, K. B., Kohlenberg, R. J., Addis, M. E., ... Jacobson, N. S. (2006). Randomized trial of behavioral activation, cognitive therapy, and antidepressant medication in the acute treatment of adults with major depression. *Journal of Consulting and Clinical Psychology, 74*(4), 658–670.

Dixon, J. F., & Ahrens, A. H. (1992). Stress and attributional style as predictors of self-reported depression in children. *Cognitive Therapy and Research, 16*, 623–634.

Dobson, K. S. (1989). A meta-analysis of the efficacy of cognitive therapy for depression. *Journal of Consulting and Clinical Psychology, 57*(3), 414–419.

Dobson, K. S., Hollon, S.D., Dimidjian, S., Schmaling, K. B., Kohlenberg, R. J., Gallop, R., ... Jacobson, N. S. (2008). Randomized trial of behavioral activation, cognitive therapy, and antidepressant medication in the prevention of relapse and recurrence in major depression. *Journal of Consulting and Clinical Psychology, 76*(3), 468–477.

Dohrenwend, B. P., Levav, I., Shrout, P. E., Schwartz, S., Naveh, G., Link, B. G., et al. (1992). Socioeconomic status and psychiatric disorders: The causation-selection issue. *Science, 255*, 946–952.

Dong, J., & Blier, P. (2001). Modification of norepinephrine and serotonin, but not dopamine, neuron firing by sustained bupropion treatment. *Psychopharmacology (Berlin), 155*(1), 52–57.

Dougherty, L. R., Smith, V. C., Olino, T. M., Dyson, M. W., Bufferd, S. J., Rose, S. A., & Klein, D. N. (2013). Maternal psychopathology and early child temperament predict young children's salivary cortisol 3 years later. *Journal of Abnormal Child Psychology, 41*(4), 531–542.

Downey, G., & Coyne, J. C. (1990). Children of depressed parents: An integrative review. *Psychological Bulletin, 108*(1), 50–76.

Dowrick, C., Dunn, G., Ayuso-Mateos, J. L., Dalgard, O. S., Page, H., Lehtinen, V., ... Wilkinson, G. (2000). Problem solving treatment and group psychoeducation for depression: Multicentre randomised controlled trial. *BMJ, 321*(7274), 1450.

Driessen, E., Cuijpers, P., de Maat, S. C. M., Abbass, A. A., de Jonghe, F., & Dekker, J. J. M. (2010). The efficacy of short-term psychodynamic psychotherapy for depression: A meta-analysis. *Clinical Psychology Review, 30*(1), 25–36.

Driessen, E., Hegelmaier, L. M., Abbass, A. A., Barber, J. P., Dekker, J .J. M., Henricus, L. V., Jansma, E. P., & Cuijpers, P. (2015). The efficacy of short-term psychodynamic psychotherapy for depression: A meta-analysis update. *Clinical Psychology Review, 42*, 1–15.

Driessen, E., Van, H. L., Don, F. J., Peen, J., Kool, S., Westra, D., ... Dekker, J. J. M. (2013). The efficacy of cognitive–behavioral therapy and psychodynamic therapy in the outpatient treatment of major depression: A randomized clinical trial. *American Journal of Psychiatry, 170*(9), 1041–1050.

Duax, J. M., Youngstrom, E. A., Calabrese, J. R., & Findling, R. L. (2007). Sex differences in pediatric bipolar disorder. *Journal of Clinical Psychiatry, 68*(10), 1565–1573.

Dube, S. R., Anda, R. F., Felitti, V. J., Chapman, D. P., Williamson, D. F., & Giles, W. H. (2001). Childhood abuse, household dysfunction, and the risk of attempted suicide throughout the life span: findings from the Adverse Childhood Experiences Study. *Journal of the American Medical Association, 286*, 3089–3096.

Dubicka, B., Carlson, G. A., Vail, A., & Harrington, R. (2008). Prepubertal mania: Diagnostic differences between US and UK clinicians. *European Child & Adolescent Psychiatry, 17*(3), 153–161.

Dubicka, B., Elvins, R., Roberts, C., et al. (2010). Combined treatment with cognitive-behavioural therapy in adolescent depression: Meta-analysis. *British Journal of Psychiatry, 197*, 433–440.

DuBois, D. L., Felner, R. D., Brand, S., & George, G. R. (1999). Profiles of self-esteem in early adolescence: Identification and investigation of adaptive correlates. *American Journal of Community Psychology, 27*, 899–932.

Earls, F. (1982). Epidemiology and child psychiatry: Future prospects. *Comprehensive Psychiatry, 23*(1), 75–84.

Egeland, J. A., Shaw, J. A., Endicott, J., Pauls, D. L., Allen, C. R., Hostetter, A. M., & Sussex, J. N. (2003). Prospective study of prodromal features for bipolarity in well Amish children. *Journal of the American Academy of Child and Adolescent Psychiatry, 42*(7), 786–796.

Egger, H. L., & Angold, A. (2006). Common emotional and behavioral disorders in preschool children: Presentation, nosology, and epidemiology. *Journal of Child Psychology & Psychiatry, 47*(3-4), 313–337.

Ehlers, C. L., Frank, E., & Kupfer, D. J. (1988). Social zeitgebers and biological rhythms: A unified approach to understanding the etiology of depression. *Archives of General Psychiatry, 45*, 948–952.

Ekers, D., Richards, D., & Gilbody, S. (2008). A meta-analysis of randomized trials of behavioural treatment of depression. *Psychological Medicine, 38*(5), 611–623.

Elliott, R., Greenberg, L. S., Watson, J. C., Timulak, L., & Freire, E. (2013). Research on humanistic-experiential psychotherapies. In M. Lambert (Ed.), *Bergin & Garfield's handbook of psychotherapy and behavior change* (pp. 495–538). New York: John Wiley & Sons.

Emiroglu, F. N. I., Gencer, O., & Ozbek, A. (2006). Adjunctive olanzapine treatment in bipolar adolescents responding insufficiently to mood stabilizers: four case reports. *European Child and Adolescent Psychiatry, 15*, 500–503.

Emslie, G. J., Findling, R. L., Yeung, P. P., Kunz, N. R., & Li, Y. (2007). Venlafaxine ER for the treatment of pediatric subjects with depression: Results of two placebo-controlled trials. *Journal of the American Academy of Child and Adolescent Psychiatry, 46*, 479–488.

Emslie, G. J., Heiligenstein, J. H., Wagner, K. D., et al. (2002). Fluoxetine for acute treatment of depression in children and adolescents: A placebo-controlled, randomized clinical trial. *Journal of the American Academy of Child and Adolescent Psychiatry, 41*, 1205–1215.

Emslie, G. J., Kennard, B. D., & Kowatch, R. A. (1995). Affective disorders in children: Diagnosis and management. *Journal of Child Neurology, 10*(Suppl 1), S42–49.

Emslie, G. J., Mayes, T., Porta, G., Vitiello, B., Clarke, G., Wagner, K. D., . . . Brent, D. (2010). Treatment of resistant depression in adolescents (TORDIA): Week 24 outcomes. *American Journal of Psychiatry, 167*, 782–791.

Emslie, G. J., Prakash, A., Zhang, Q., Pangallo, B. A., Bangs, M. E., & March, J. S. (2014). A double-blind efficacy and safety study of duloxetine fixed doses in children and adolescents with major depressive disorder. *Journal of Child and Adolescent Psychopharmacology, 24*(4), 170–179.

Emslie, G. J., Rush, A. J., Weinberg, W. A., et al. (1997). A double-blind, randomized, placebo-controlled trial of fluoxetine in children and adolescents with depression. *Archives of General Psychiatry, 54*, 1031–1037.

Emslie, G. J., Ventura, D., Korotzer, A., et al. (2009). Escitalopram in the treatment of adolescent depression: A randomized placebo-controlled multisite trial. *Journal of the American Academy of Child and Adolescent Psychiatry, 48*, 721–729.

Emslie, G. J., Wagner, K. D., Kutcher, S., et al. (2006). Paroxetine treatment in children and adolescents with major depressive disorder: A randomized, multicenter, double-blind, placebo-controlled trial. *Journal of the American Academy of Child and Adolescent Psychiatry, 45*, 709–719.

England, M. J., & Sim, L. J. (Eds.). (2009). *Depression in parents, parenting, and children: Opportunities to improve identification, treatment, and prevention*. Washington, DC: National Academies Press.

Esposito-Smythers, C., Spirito, A., Kahler, C. W., Hunt, J., & Monti, P. (2011). Treatment of co-occurring substance abuse and suicidality among adolescents: A randomized trial. *Journal of Consulting & Clinical Psychologoy, 79*, 728–739.

Evans, M. D., Hollon, S. D., DeRubeis, R. J., Piasecki, J. M., Grove, W. M., Garvey, M. J., & Tuason, V. B. (1992). Differential relapse following cognitive therapy and pharmacotherapy for depression. *Archives of General Psychiatry, 49*(10), 802–808.

Expert Panel (2001). Expert Panel on Detection, Evaluation, and Treatment of High Blood Cholesterol in Adults. Executive summary of the third report of the national cholesterol education program (NCEP) expert panel on detection, evaluation, and treatment of high blood cholesterol in adults (Adult Treatment Panel III). *Journal of the American Medical Association, 285*, 2486–2497.

Eysenck, H. J. (1947). *Dimensions of personality*. London: Kegan Paul.

Faedda, G., Baldessarini, R., et al. (1995). Pediatric-onset bipolar disorder: A neglected clinical and public health problem. *Harvard Review of Psychiatry, 3*(4), 171–195.

Fagiolini, A., Frank, E, Scott, J. A., Turkin, S., & Kupfer, D. J. (2005). Metabolic syndrome in bipolar disorder: Findings from the Bipolar Disorder Center for Pennsylvanians. *Bipolar Disorders, 7*, 424–430.

Faraone, S. V., Biederman, J., Mennin, D., & Russel, R. I. (1998). Bipolar and antisocial disorders among relatives of ADHD children: Parsing familial subtypes of illness. *Neuropsychiatric Genetics, 81*, 108–116.

Faraone, S. V., Biederman, J., Mennin, D., Wozniak, J., & Spencer, T. (1997). Attention-deficit hyperactivity disorder with bipolar disorder: A familial subtype? *Journal of American Academy of Child and Adolescent Psychiatry, 36*, 1378–1387.

Faraone, S. V., Biederman, J., & Monuteaux, M. C. (2000). Attention-deficit disorder and conduct disorder in girls: Evidence for a familial subtype. *Biological Psychiatry, 48*(1), 21–29.

Faraone, S. V., Biederman, J., Wozniak, J., Mundy, E., Mennin, D., & O'Donnell, D. (1997). Is comorbidity with ADHD a marker for juvenile-onset mania? *Journal of American Academy of Child and Adolescent Psychiatry, 36*, 1046–1055.

Faraone, S. V., Glatt, S. J., & Tsuang, M. T. (2003). The genetics of pediatric-onset bipolar disorder. *Biological Psychiatry, 53*, 970–977.

Faraone, S. V., & Tsuang, M. T. (1995). Methods in psychiatric genetics. In M. Tohen, M. T. Tsuang, & G. E. P. Zahner (eds.), *Textbook in psychiatric epidemiology* (pp. 81–134). New York: John Wiley.

Faraone, S. V., Tsuang, D., et al. (1999). *Genetics and mental disorders: A guide for students, clinicians, and researchers*. New York: Guilford.

Farvolden, P., Kennedy, S. H., & Lam, R. W. (2003). Recent developments in the psychobiology and pharmacotherapy of depression: Optimising existing treatments and novel approaches for the future. *Expert Opinion on Investigational Drugs, 12*, 65–86.

Fava, G. A. (1999). Subclinical symptoms in mood disorders: Pathological and therapeutic implications. *Psychological Medicine, 29*, 47–61.

Fava, G. A., Grandi, S., Zielezny, M., & Rafanelli, C. (1996). Four-year outcome for cognitive behavioral treatment of residual symptoms in major depression. *American Journal of Psychiatry, 153*(7), 945–947.

Fava, G. A., Rafanelli, C., Grandi, S., Conti, S., & Belluardo, P. (1998). Prevention of recurrent depression with cognitive behavioral therapy: Preliminary findings. *Archives of General Psychiatry, 55*(9), 816–820.

Feinstein, S. C., & Wolpert, E. A. (1973). Juvenile manic-depressive illness: Clinical and therapeutic considerations. *Journal of the American Academy of Child and Adolescent Psychiatry, 12*(1), 123–136.

Felitti, V. J., Anda, R. F., Nordenberg, D., Williamson, D. F., Spitz, A. M., Edwards, V., et al. (1998). Relationship of childhood abuse and household dysfunction to many of the leading causes of death in adults: The Adverse Childhood Experiences (ACE) Study. *American Journal of Preventive Medicine, 14*, 245–258.

Fendrich, M., Warner, V., & Weissman, M. M. (1990). Family risk factors, parental depression and psychopathology in offspring. *Developmental Psychology, 25*, 40–50.

Fergusson, D. M., & Horwood, L. J. (2001). The Christchurch Health and Development Study: Review of findings on child and adolescent mental health. *Australian and New Zealand Journal of Psychiatry, 35*(3), 287–296.

Fergusson, D. M., & Woodward, L. J. (2002). Mental health, educational, and social role outcomes of adolescents with depression. *Archives of General Psychiatry, 59*(3), 225–231.

Ferrari, A. J., Charlson, F. J., Norman, R. E., Patten, S. B., Freedman, G., Murray, C. J., Vos, T., & Whiteford, H. A. (2013). Burden of depressive disorders by country, sex, age, and year: Findings from the global burden of disease study 2010. *PLoS Medicine, 10*, e1001547.

Field, T. (1995). Massage therapy for infants and children. *Journal of Developmental and Behavioral Pediatrics, 16*, 105–111.

Findling, R. L., Correll, C. U., Nyilas, M., Forbes, R. A., McQuade, R. D., Jin, N., . . . Carlson, G. A. (2013). Aripiprazole for the treatment of pediatric bipolar I disorder: A 30-week, randomized, placebo-controlled study. *Bipolar Disorders, 15*, 138–149.

Findling, R. L., & Ginsberg, L. D. (2012). A phase IV, multi-center, open-label study of extended-release carbamazepine in the treatment of manic or mixed states in youths aged 10-17 years. Poster presented at the American Psychiatry Association Annual Meeting, Philadelphia, May 5–9.

Findling, R. L., Gracious, B. L., McNamara, N. K., Youngstrom, E. A., Demeter, C. A., Branicky, L. A., & Calabrese, J. R. (2001). Rapid, continuous cycling and psychiatric co-morbidity in pediatric bipolar I disorder. *Bipolar Disorders, 3*, 202–210.

Findling, R. L., Kafantaris, V., Pavuluri, M., McNamara, N. K., McClellan, J., Frazier, J. A., . . . Taylor-Zapata, P. (2011). Dosing strategies for lithium monotherapy in children and adolescents with bipolar I disorder. *Journal of Child and Adolescent Psychopharmacology, 21*, 195–205.

Findling, R. L., Landersdorfer, C. B., Kafantaris, V., Pavuluri, M., McNamara, N. K., McClellan, J., . . . Jusko, W. J. (2009). First dose pharmacokinetics of lithium carbonate in children and adolescents. *Journal of Clinical Psychopharmacology, 30*, 404–410.

Findling, R. L., McNamara, N. K., Gracious, B. L., Youngstrom, E. A., Stansbrey, R. J., Reed, M. D., . . . Calabrese, J. R. (2003). Combination lithium and divalproex sodium in pediatric bipolarity. *Journal of the American Academy of Child and Adolescent Psychiatry, 42*, 895–901.

Findling, R. L., McNamara, N. K., Youngstrom, E. A., Stansbrey, R., Gracious, B. L., Reed, M. D., & Calabrese, J. R. (2005). Double-blind 18-month trial of lithium versus divalproex maintenance treatment in pediatric bipolar disorder. *Journal of the American Academy of Child and Adolescent Psychiatry, 44*, 409–417.

Findling, R. L., & Pavuluri, M. N. (2008). Lithium. In B. Geller & M. P. DelBello (Eds.), *Treatment of bipolar disorder in children and adolescents*. New York: Guilford Press.

Findling, R. L., Robb, A., & Bose, A. (2013). Escitalopram in the treatment of adolescent depression: A randomized, double-blind, placebo-controlled extension trial. *Journal of Child and Adolescent Psychopharmacology, 23*(7), 468–480.

Findling, R. L., Robb, A., McNamara, N. K., Pavuluri, M. N., Kafantaris, V., Scheffer, R., ... Taylor-Zapata, P. (2015). Lithium in the acute treatment of bipolar I disorder: a double-blind, placebo-controlled study. *Pediatrics, 136*(5), 885–894.

Findling, R. L., Youngstrom, E. A., Fristad, M. A., Birmaher, B., Kowatch, R. A., Arnold, L. E., ... Horwitz, S. M. (2010). Characteristics of children with elevated symptoms of mania: The Longitudinal Assessment of Manic Symptoms (LAMS) study. *Journal of Clinical Psychiatry, 71*(12), 1664–1672.

Fine, S., Forth, A., Gilbert, M., & Haley, G. (1991). Group therapy for adolescent depressive disorder: A comparison of social skills and therapeutic support. *Journal of the American Academy of Child and Adolescent Psychiatry, 30*, 79–85.

Fleming, T., Dixon, R., Frampton, C., & Merry, S. (2012). A pragmatic randomized controlled trial of computerized CBT (SPARX) for symptoms of depression among adolescents excluded from mainstream education. *Behavioral and Cognitive Psychotherapy, 40*, 529–541.

Flemming, J. E., Offord, D. R., & Boyle, M. H. (1989). Prevalence of childhood and adolescent depression in the community: Ontario Child Health Study. *British Journal of Psychiatry, 155*, 647–654.

Flores, D. L., Alvarado, I., Wong, M. L., Licinio, J., & Flockhart, D. (2004). Clinical implications of genetic polymorphism of CYP2D6 in Mexican Americans. *Annals of Internal Medicine, 140*(11), W71.

Forbes, E. E., & Dahl, R. E. (2012). Research review: Altered reward function in adolescent depression: What, when and how? *Journal of Child Psychology & Psychiatry, 53*(1), 3–15.

Frank, E., Kupfer, D. J., Perel, J. M., Cornes, C., Jarrett, D. B., Mallinger, A. G., ... Grochocinski, V. J. (1990). Three-year outcomes for maintenance therapies in recurrent depression. *Archives of General Psychiatry, 47*(12), 1093–1099.

Frazier, J. A., Chiu, S., Breeze, J. L., Makris, N., Lange, N., Kennedy, D. N., ... Biederman, J. (2005). Structural brain magnetic resonance imaging of limbic and thalamic volumes in pediatric bipolar disorder. *American Journal of Psychiatry, 162*(7), 1256–1265.

Frazier, J. A., Meyer, M. C., Biederman, J., Wozniak, J., Wilens, T. E., Spencer, T. J., Kim, G. S., & Shapiro, S. (1999). Risperidone treatment for juvenile bipolar disorder: A retrospective chart review. *Journal of the American Academy of Child & Adolescent Psychiatry, 38*, 960–965.

Frazier, T. W., Youngstrom, E. A., Horwitz, S. M., Demeter, C. A., Fristad, M. A., Arnold, L. E., ... Findling, R. L. (2011). Relationship of persistent manic symptoms to the diagnosis of pediatric bipolar spectrum disorders. *Journal of Clinical Psychiatry, 72*(6), 846–853.

Freemantle, N., Anderson, I. M., & Young, P. (2000). Predictive value of pharmacological activity for the relative efficacy of antidepressant drugs: Meta-regression analysis. *British Journal of Psychiatry, 177*, 292–302.

Fride, E., Dan, Y., Feldon, J., Halevy, G., & Weinstock, M. (1986). Effects of prenatal stress on vulnerability to stress in prepubertal and adult rats. *Physiology & Behavior, 37*(5), 681–687.

Fride, E., & Weinstock, M. (1988). Prenatal stress increases anxiety related behavior and alters cerebral lateralization of dopamine activity. *Life Sciences, 42*(10), 1059–1065.

Friedman, R. A. (2014). Antidepressants' black-box warning—10 years later. *New England Journal of Medicine, 371*, 1666–1668.

Fristad, M. A., Verducci, J. S., Walters, K., & Young, M. E. (2009). Impact of multifamily psychoeducational psychotherapy in treating children aged 8 to 12 years with mood disorders. *Archives of General Psychiatry, 66*, 1013–1021.

Frombonne, E., Wostear, G., Cooper, V., Harrington, R., & Rutter, M. (2001). The Maudsley long-term follow-up of child and adolescent depression. I. Psychiatric outcomes in adulthood. *British Journal of Psychiatry, 179*, 210–217.

Frost, A. K., Reinherz, H. Z., Pakiz-Camra, B., Fiaconia, R. M., & Lekowitz, E. S. (1999). Risk factors for depressive symptoms in late adolescence: A longitudinal community study. *American Journal of Orthopsychiatry, 69*(3), 370–381.

Gaensbauer, T. J., Harmon, R. J., Cytryn, L., & McKnew, D. H. (1984). Social and affective development in infants with a manic-depressive parent. *American Journal of Psychiatry, 141*, 223–229.

Gaensbauer, T. J., & Sands, K. (1979). Distorted affective communications in abused/neglected infants and their potential impact on caretakers. *Journal of the American Academy of Child Psychiatry, 18*(2), 236–250.

Gaffan, E. A., Tsaousis, J., & Kemp-Wheeler, S. M. (1995). Researcher allegiance and meta-analysis: The case of cognitive therapy for depression.

Journal of Consulting and Clinical Psychology, 63(6), 966–980.

Gallagher, D.E., & Thompson, L.W. (1982). Treatment of major depressive disorder in older adult outpatients with brief psychotherapies. *Psychotherapy: Theory, Research & Practice, 19*(4), 482–490.

Gallagher-Thompson, D., & Steffen, A. M. (1994). Comparative effects of cognitive-behavioral and brief psychodynamic psychotherapies for depressed family caregivers. *Journal of Consulting and Clinical Psychology, 62*(3), 543–549.

Garber, J., Clarke, G. N., Weersing, V. R., Beardslee, W. R., Brent, D. A., Gladstone, T. R., . . . Iyengar, S. (2009). Prevention of depression in at-risk adolescents: A randomized controlled trial. *Journal of the American Medical Association, 301*(21), 2215–2224.

Garber, J., & Hilsman, R. (1992). Cognition, stress, and depression in children and adolescents. *Child and Adolescent Psychiatric Clinics of North America, 1*, 129–167.

Garber, J., Keiley, M. K., & Martin, N.C. (2002). Developmental trajectories of adolescents' depressive symptoms: Predictors of change. *Journal of Consulting and Clinical Psychology, 70*, 79–95.

Garber, J., Kriss, M. R., Koch, M., & Lindholm, L. (1988). Recurrent depression in adolescents: A follow-up study. *Journal of the American Academy of Child and Adolescent Psychiatry, 27*(1), 49–54.

Garber, J., & Little, S. (1999). Predictors of competence among offspring of depressed mothers. *Journal of Adolescent Research, 14*, 44–71.

Garber, J., Martin, N. C., & Keiley, M. K. (2002, September). *Predictors of the first onset of major depressive disorder.* Presented at the Society for Research on Psychopathology, San Francisco, CA.

Garber, J., & Robinson, N. S. (1997). Cognitive vulnerability in children at risk for depression. *Cognitions and Emotions, 11*, 619–635.

Garber, J., Weiss, B., & Shanley, N. (1993). Cognitions, depressive symptoms, and development in adolescents. *Journal of Abnormal Psychology, 102*, 47–57.

Garrison, C. Z., Jackson, K. L., Marsteller, F., McKeown, R., & Addy, C. (1990). A longitudinal study of depressive symptomatology in young adolescents. *Journal of the American Academy of Child and Adolescent Psychiatry, 29*, 581–585.

Gaynes, B. N., Dusetzina, S. B., Ellis, A. R., Hansen, R. A., Farley, J. F., Miller, W. C., & Stürmer, T. (2012). Treating depression after initial treatment failure: Directly comparing switch and augmenting strategies in STAR*D. *Journal of Clinical Psychopharmacology, 32*(1), 114–119.

Ge, X., Conger, R. D., Lorenz, F. O., & Simons, R. L. (1994). Parents' stressful life events and adolescent depressed mood. *Journal of Health and Social Behavior, 35*(1), 28–44.

Geller, B., Badner, J. A., Tillman, R., Christian, S. L., Bolhofner, K., & Cook, E. H. (2004). Linkage disequilibrium of the brain-derived neurotrophic factor Val66Met polymorphism in children with a prepubertal and early adolescent bipolar disorder phenotype. *American Journal of Psychiatry, 161*(9), 1698–1700.

Geller, B., Bolhofner, K., Craney, J. L., Williams, M., DelBello, M. P., & Gundersen, K. (2000). Psychosocial functioning in a prepubertal and early adolescent bipolar disorder phenotype. *Journal of the American Academy of Child & Adolescent Psychiatry, 39*(12), 1543–1548.

Geller, B., & Cook, E. H. (1999). Serotonin transporter gene (HTTLPR) is not in linkage disequilibrium with prepubertal and early adolescent bipolarity. *Biological Psychiatry, 45*(9), 1230–1233.

Geller, B., & Cook, E. H. (2000). Ultradian rapid cycling in prepubertal and early adolescent bipolarity is not in transmission disequilibrium with val/met COMT alleles. *Biological Psychiatry, 47*(7), 605–609.

Geller, B., Fox, L., et al. (1994). Rate and predictors of prepubertal bipolarity during follow-up of 6-to 12-year-old depressed children. *Journal of the American Academy of Child and Adolescent Psychiatry, 33*(4), 461–468.

Geller, B., & Luby, J. (1997). Child and adolescent bipolar disorder: A review of the past 10 years. *Journal of the American Academy of Child and Adolescent Psychiatry, 36*, 1168–1176.

Geller, B., Luby, J. L., Joshi, P., Wagner, K. D., Emslie, G., Walkup, J. T., . . . Lavori, P. (2012). A randomized controlled trial of risperidone, lithium, or divalproex sodium for initial treatment of bipolar I disorder, manic or mixed phase, in children and adolescents. *Archives of General Psychiatry, 69*(5), 515–528.

Geller, B., Sun, K., et al. (1995). Complex and rapid-cycling in bipolar children and adolescents: A preliminary study. *Journal of Affective Disorders, 34*, 259–268.

Geller, B., Tillman, R., Bolhofner, K., Zimerman, B., Strauss, N. A., & Kaufmann, P. (2006). Controlled, blindly rated, direct-interview family study of a prepubertal and early-adolescent bipolar I disorder phenotype: Morbid risk, age at onset, and comorbidity. *Archives of General Psychiatry, 63*(10), 1130–1138

Gershon, E. S., Hamovit, N. J., Guroff, J. J., & Nurnberger, J. I. (1987). Birth cohort changes in manic and depressive disorders in relatives of bipolar and schizoaffective patients. *Archives of General Psychiatry, 44*, 314–319.

Gershon, E. S., McKnew, D., Cytryn, L., Hamovit, J., Schreiber, J., Hibbs, E., & Pelligrini, D. (1985). Diagnoses in school-age children of bipolar affective disorder patients and normal controls. *Journal of Affective Disorders, 16*, 167–179.

Gershuny, B. S., & Sher, K. J. (1998). The relation between personality and anxiety: Findings from a 3-year prospective study. *Journal of Abnormal Psychology, 107*, 252–262.

Gibbons, R. D., Hur, K., Bhaumik, D. K., & Mann, J. J. (2006). The relationship between antidepressant prescription rates and rate of early adolescent suicide. *American Journal of Psychiatry, 163*(11), 1898–1904.

Gillham, J. E., & Reivich, K. J. (1999). Prevention of depressive symptoms in school children: A research update. *Psychological Science, 10*, 461–462.

Gillham, J. E., Reivich, K. J., Brunwasser, S. M., Freres, D. R., Chajon, N. D., Kash-MacDonald, V., ... Seligman, M. P. (2012). Evaluation of a group cognitive-behavioral depression prevention program for young adolescents: A randomized effectiveness trial. *Journal of Clinical Child and Adolescent Psychology, 41*(5), 621–639.

Gillham, J. E., Reivich, K. J., & Jaycox, L. H. (2008). The Penn Resiliency Program (also known as the Penn Depression Prevention Program and the Penn Optimism Program). Unpublished manuscript, University of Pennsylvania.

Gillham, J. E., Reivich, K. J., Jaycox, L. H., & Seligman, M. E. P. (1995). Prevention of depressive symptoms in school children: Two-year follow-up. *Psychological Science, 6*, 343–351.

Gilman, S. E., Kawachi, I., Fitzmaurice, G. M., & Buka, S. L. (2002). Socioeconomic status in childhood and the lifetime risk of major depression. *International Journal of Epidemiology, 31*, 359–367.

Gilman, S. E., Kawachi, I., Fitzmaurice, G. M., & Buka, S. L. (2003). Socio-economic status, family disruption and residential stability in childhood: Relation to onset, recurrence and remission of major depression. *Psychological Medicine, 33*(8), 1341–1355.

Gilman, S. E., Ni, M. Y., Dunn, E. C., Breslau, J., McLaughlin, K. A., Smoller, J. W., & Perlis, R. H. (2014). Contributions of the social environment to first-onset and recurrent mania. *Molecular Psychiatry* [Epub April 22].

Gladstone, T. R., & Kaslow, N. J. (1995). Depression and attributions in children and adolescents: A meta-analytic review. *Journal of Abnormal and Child Psychology, 23*, 597–606.

Goldberg, L. R. (1992). The development of markers for the Big-Five factor structure. *Psychological Assessment, 4*, 26–42.

Goldhagen, S., Harbin, V., & Forry, N. (2013). *Maryland child care choices study: Maternal depression among applicants for temporary cash assistance*. Retrieved from http://www.childtrends.org/wp-content/uploads/2013/07/2013-30ChildCareChioicesDepression.pdf.

Goldman-Mellor, S., Hamer, M., & Steptoe, A. (2012). Early-life stress and recurrent psychological distress over the lifecourse predict divergent cortisol reactivity patterns in adulthood. *Psychoneuroendocrinology, 37*(11), 1755–1768.

Goldstein, B. I. (2012). Recent progress in understanding pediatric bipolar disorder. *Archives of Pediatric and Adolescent Medicine, 166*, 362–371.

Goldstein, T. R., Birmaher, B., Axelson, D., Goldstein, B. I., Gill, M. K., Esposito-Smythers, C., et al. (2009). Psychosocial functioning among bipolar youth. *Journal of Affective Disorders, 114*(1-3), 174–183.

Goldstein, B. I., & Levitt, A. J. (2007). Prevalence and correlates of bipolar I disorder among adults with primary youth-onset anxiety disorders. *Journal of Affective Disorders, 103*(1), 187–195.

Goldstein, B. I., Shamseddeen, W., Axelson, D. A., Kalas, C., Monk, K., Brent, D. A., Kupfer, D. J., & Birmaher, B. (2010). Clinical, demographic, and familial correlates of bipolar spectrum disorders among offspring of parents with bipolar disorder. *Journal of the American Academy of Child and Adolescent Psychiatry, 49*(4), 388–396.

Goldstein, B. I., Strober, M. A., Birmaher, B., Axelson, D. A., Esposito-Smythers, C., Goldstein, T. R., ...Keller, M. B. (2008). Substance use disorders among adolescents with bipolar spectrum disorders. *Bipolar Disorders, 10*(4), 469–478.

Goleman, D. (1995). *Emotional intelligence*. New York: Bantam Books.

Goodman, S. H., Adamson, L. B., Riniti, J., & Cole, S. (1994). Mothers' expressed attitudes: Associations with maternal depression and children's self-esteem and psychopathology. *Journal* of the American Academy of Child & Adolescent Psychiatry, 33(9), 1265–1274.

Goodman, S. H., & Gotlib, I. H. (1999). Risk for psychopathology in the children of depressed mothers: A developmental model for understanding mechanisms of transmission. *Psychological Review, 106*, 458–490.

Goodman, S. H., Hoven, C. W., Narrow, W. E., Cohen, P., Fielding, B., Alegria, M., ... Dulcan, M. K. (1998). Measurement of risk for mental disorders and competence in a psychiatric epidemiologic community survey: The National Institute of Mental Health Methods for the Epidemiology of Child and Adolescent Mental Disorders (MECA) Study. *Social Psychiatry and Psychiatric Epidemiology, 33*(4), 162–173.

Goodyer, I. M., Bacon, A., Ban, M., Croudace, T., & Herbert, J. (2009). Serotonin transporter genotype, morning cortisol and subsequent depression in adolescents. *British Journal of Psychiatry, 195*(1), 39–45.

Goodyer, I., Dubicka, B., Wilkinson, P., Kelvin, R., Roberts, C., Byford, S., ... Harrington, R. (2007). Selective serotonin reuptake inhibitors (SSRIs) and routine specialist care with and without cognitive behaviour therapy in adolescents with major depression: Randomised controlled trial. *BMJ, 335*, 142.

Goodyer, I. M., Dubicka, B., Wilkinson, P., Kelvin, R., Roberts, C., Byford, S., ... Harrington, R. (2008). A randomized controlled trial of cognitive behaviour therapy in adolescents with major depression treated by selective serotonin reuptake inhibitors: The ADAPT trial. *Health Technology Assessment, 12*(14).

Goodyer, I. M., Germany, E., Gowrusankur, J., & Altham, P. (1991). Social influences on the course of anxious and depressive disorders in school-age children. *British Journal of Psychiatry, 158*, 676–684.

Goodyer, I. M., Herbert, J., & Altham, P. M. (1998). Adrenal steroid secretion and major depression in 8to 16-year-olds, III. Influence of cortisol/DHEA ratio at presentation on subsequent rates of disappointing life events and persistent major depression. *Psychological Medicine, 28*, 265–273.

Goodyer, I. M., Wright, C., & Altham, P. M. (1988). Maternal adversity and recent stressful life events in anxious and depressed children. *Journal of Child Psychology and Psychiatry, 29*, 651–667.

Gordon, D., Burge, D., Hammen, C., Adrian, C., Jaenicke, C., & Hiroto, D. (1989). Observations of interactions of depressed women with their children. *American Journal of Psychiatry, 146*, 50–55.

Gordon, R. (1983). An operational classification of disease prevention. *Public Health Reports, 98*, 107–109.

Gordon, R. (1987). An operational classification of disease prevention. In J. Steinberg & M. Silverman (Eds.), *Preventing mental disorders: A research perspective* (pp. 20–26). Rockville, MD: Dept. of Health and Human Services.

Gore, S., & Aseltine, R. H., Jr. (2003). Race and ethnic differences in depressed mood following the transition from high school. *Journal of Health and Social Behavior, 44*(3), 370–389.

Gotlib, I. H., & Hammen, C. (1992). Psychological aspects of depression: Toward a cognitiveinterpersonal integration. In: *The Wiley series in clinical psychology*. Chichester, UK: John Wiley & Sons.

Gotlib, I. H., LeMoult, J., Colich, N. L., Foland-Ross, L. C., Hallmayer, J., Joormann, J., ... Wolkowitz, O. M. (2015). Telomere length and cortisol reactivity in children of depressed mothers. *Molecular Psychiatry, 20*(5), 615–620.

Gould, M., King, R., et al. (1998). Psychopathology associated with suicidal ideation and attempts among children and adolescents. *Journal of the American Academy of Child and Adolescent Psychiatry 37*(9), 915–923.

Grant, B. F., Stinson, F. S., Hasin, D. S., Dawson, D. A., Chou, S. P., Ruan, W., & Huang, B. (2005). Prevalence, correlates, and comorbidity of bipolar I disorder and axis I and II disorders: Results from the National Epidemiologic Survey on Alcohol and Related Conditions. *Journal of Clinical Psychiatry, 66*(10), 1205–1215.

Grant, K. E., Compas, B. E., Stuhlmacher, A. F., Thurm, A. E., McMahon, S. D., & Halpert, J. A. (2003). Stressors and child and adolescent psychopathology: Moving from markers to mechanisms of risk. *Psychological Bulletin, 129*, 447–466.

Gray, J. A. (1982). *The neuropsychology of anxiety: An enquiry into the functions of the septo-hippocampal system*. New York: Oxford University Press.

Graziano, W. G., & Ward, D. (1992). Probing the big five in adolescence: Personality and adjustment during a developmental transition. *Journal of Personality, 60*(2), 425–439.

Green, J. M., Wood, A. J., Kerfoot, M. J., et al. (2011). Group therapy for adolescents with repeated self harm: Randomised controlled trial with economic evaluation. *BMJ, 342*, d682.

Grillon, C., Warner, V., Hille, J., Merikangas, K. R., Bruder, G. E., Tenke, C. E., ... Weissman, M. M.

(2005). Families at high and low risk for depression: A three-generation startle study. *Biological Psychiatry, 57*(9), 953–960.

Guiao, I., & Adams Thompson, E. (2004). Ethnicity and problem behaviors among adolescent females in the United States. *Health Care for Women International, 25*(4), 296–310.

Gunlicks-Stoessel, M., Mufson, L., Jekal, A., & Turner, J. B. (2010). The impact of perceived interpersonal functioning on treatment for adolescent depression: IPT-A versus treatment as usual in school-based health clinics. *Journal of Consulting and Clinical Psychology, 78*, 260–267.

Gutiérrez, B., Bellón, J. Á., Rivera, M., Molina, E., King, M., Marston, L., & Cervilla, J. (2015). The risk for major depression conferred by childhood maltreatment is multiplied by BDNF and SERT genetic vulnerability: A replication study. *Journal of Psychiatry & Neuroscience, 40*(3), 187–196.

Hakim-Larson, J., & Essau, C. A. (1999). Protective factors and depressive disorders. In C. A. Essau & F. Petermann F (Eds.), *Depressive disorders in children and adolescents: Epidemiology, risk factors, and treatment*. New York: Jason Aronson Inc.

Halpert, M., & Rosenfeld, E. (2014, May 21). Depressed, but not ashamed. *New York Times*. Retrieved from http://www.nytimes.com.

Hammad, T. A., Laughren, T., & Racoosin, J. (2006). Suicidality in pediatric patients treated with antidepressant drugs. *Archives of General Psychiatry, 63*(3), 332–339.

Hammen, C. (1991). Generation of stress in the course of unipolar depression. *Journal of Abnormal Psychology, 100*, 555–561.

Hammen, C., Burge, D., Burney, E., & Adrian, C. (1990). Longitudinal study of diagnosis in children of women with unipolar and bipolar affective disorder. *Archives of General Psychiatry, 47*, 1112–1117.

Hammen, C., Ellicott, A., Gitlin, M., & Jamison, K. R. (1989). Sociotropy/autonomy and vulnerability to specific life events in patients with unipolar depression and bipolar disorders. *Journal of Abnormal Psychology, 98*(2), 154–160.

Hankin, B. L., Abramson, L. Y., Moffitt, T. E., Silva, P. A., McGee, R., & Angell, K. E. (1998). Development of depression from preadolescence to young adulthood: Emerging gender differences in a 10-year longitudinal study. *Journal of Abnormal Psychology, 107*(1), 128–140.

Hankin, B. L., Young, J. F., Abela, J. R. Z., Smolen, A., Jenness, J. L., Gulley, L. D., . . . Oppenheimer, C. W. (2015). Depression from childhood into late adolescence: Influence of gender, development, genetic susceptibility, and peer stress. *Journal of Abnormal Psychology, 124*(4), 803–816.

Harkness, K. L., Stewart, J. G., & Wynne-Edwards, K. E. (2011). Cortisol reactivity to social stress in adolescents: Role of depression severity and child maltreatment. *Psychoneuroendocrinology, 36*(2), 173–181.

Harrington, R., Fudge, H., Rutter, M., Pickles, A., & Hill, J. (1990). Adult outcomes of childhood and adolescent depression. *Archives of General Psychiatry, 47*, 465–473.

Harrington, R., Kerfoot, M., Dyer, E., McNiven, F., Gill, J., Harrington, V., et al. (1998). Randomized trial of a home-based family intervention for children who have deliberately poisoned themselves. *Journal of the American Academy of Child and Adolescent Psychiatry, 37*, 512–518.

Harrington, R., & Myatt, T. (2003). Is preadolescent mania the same condition as adult mania? A British perspective. *Biological Psychiatry, 53*(11), 961–969.

Hart, A. B., Craighead, W. E., & Craighead, L. W. (2001). Predicting recurrence of major depressive disorder in young adults: A prospective study. *Journal of Abnormal Psychology, 110*, 633–643.

Hawton, K., Bergen, H., Kapur, N., et al. (2012). Repetition of self-harm and suicide following self-harm in children and adolescents: Findings from the Multicentre Study of Self-harm in England. *Journal of Child Psychology & Psychiatry, 53*, 1212–1219.

Hayden, E. P., Olino, T. M., Mackrell, S. V., Jordan, P. L., Desjardins, J., & Katsiroumbas, P. (2013). Cognitive vulnerability to depression during middle childhood: Stability and associations with maternal affective styles and parental depression. *Personality and Individual Differences, 55*(8), 892–897.

Hayward, C., Gotlib, I. H., Schraedley, P. K., & Litt, I. F. (1999). Ethnic differences in the association between pubertal status and symptoms of depression in adolescent girls. *Journal of Adolescent Health, 25*, 143–149.

Hayward, C., Killen, J. D., Kraemer, H. C., & Taylor, C. B. (2000). Predictors of panic attacks in adolescence. *Journal of the American Academy of Child & Adolescent Psychiatry, 39*, 207–214.

Hazel, N. A., Oppenheimer, C. W., Technow, J. R., Young, J. F., & Hankin, B. L. (2014). Parent relationship quality buffers against the effect of peer stressors on depressive symptoms from middle childhood to adolescence. *Developmental Psychology, 50*, 2115–2123.

Hazell, P. L., Martin, G., McGill, K., et al. (2009). Group therapy for repeated deliberate self-harm in adolescents: Failure of replication of a randomized trial. *Journal of the American Academy of Child & Adolescent Psychiatry, 48*, 662–670.

Hebrani, P., Behdani, F., & Manteghi, A. A. (2009). Double-blind, randomized, clinical trial of topiramate versus sodium valproate for the treatment of bipolar disorder in adolescents. *Pakistan Journal of Medical Sciences, 25*(2), 247–252.

Heim, C., & Nemeroff, C. B. (2001). The role of childhood trauma in the neurobiology of mood and anxiety disorders: Preclinical and clinical studies. *Biological Psychiatry, 49*(12), 1023–1039.

Heim, C., Newport, D. J., Heit, S., Graham, Y. P., Wilcox, M., Bonsall, R., ... Nemeroff, C. B. (2000). Pituitary-adrenal and autonomic responses to stress in women after sexual and physical abuse in childhood. *Journal of the American Medical Association, 284*(5), 592–597.

Heim, C., Newport, D. J., Mletzko, T., Miller, A. H., & Nemeroff, C. B. (2008). The link between childhood trauma and depression: Insights from HPA axis studies in humans. *Psychoneuroendocrinology, 33*(6), 693–710.

Heim, C., Shugart, M., Craighead, W. E., & Nemeroff, C. B. (2010). Neurobiological and psychiatric consequences of child abuse and neglect. *Developmental Psychobiology, 52*(7), 671–690.

Helzer, J. E., Robins, L. N., & McEvoy, L. (1987). Post-traumatic stress disorder in the general population: Findings of the epidemiologic catchment area survey. *New England Journal of Medicine, 317*, 1630–1634.

Henin, A., Biederman, J., Mick, E., Hirshfeld-Becker, D. R., Sachs, G. S., Wu, Y., ... Nierenberg, A. A. (2007). Childhood antecedent disorders to bipolar disorder in adults: A controlled study. *Journal of Affective Disorders, 99*, 51–57.

Henin, A., Biederman, J., Mick, E., Sachs, G. S., Hirshfeld-Becker, D. R., Siegel, R. S., ... Nierenberg, A. A. (2005). Psychopathology in the offspring of parents with bipolar disorder: A controlled study. *Biological Psychiatry, 58*, 554–561.

Hilsman, R., & Garber, J. (1995). A test of the cognitive diathesis–stress model of depression in children: Academic stressors, attributional style, perceived competence, and control. *Journal of Personality and Social Psychology, 69*, 370–380.

Hirshfeld, D. R., Rosenbaum, J. F., Biederman, J., Bolduc, E. A., Faraone, S. V., Snidman, N., et al. (1992). Stable behavioral inhibition and its association with anxiety disorder. *Journal of the American Academy of Child and Adolescent Psychiatry, 31*, 103–111.

Hoek, W., Schuurmans, J., Koot, H. M., & Cuijpers, P. (2012). Effects of Internet-based guided self-help problem-solving therapy for adolescents with depression and anxiety: A randomized controlled trial. *PLoS One, 7*, e43485.

Hoffman, K. B., Cole, D. A., Martin, J. M., Tram, J., & Serocynski, A. D. (2001). Are the discrepancies between self and others' appraisals of competence predictive or reflective of depressive symptoms in children and adolescents: A longitudinal study, Part II. *Journal of Abnormal Psychology, 109*, 651–662.

Hollenstein, T., Allen, N. B., & Sheeber, L. (2016). Affective patterns in triadic family interactions: Associations with adolescent depression. *Development and Psychopathology, 28*, 85–96.

Hollon, S. D., DeRubeis, R. J., Shelton, R. C., Amsterdam, J. D., Salomon, R. M., O'Reardon, J. P., ... Gallop, R. (2005). Prevention of relapse following cognitive therapy versus medications in moderate to severe depression. *Archives of General Psychiatry, 62*(4), 417–422.

Hollon, S. D., & Ponniah, K. (2010). A review of empirically supported psychological therapies for mood disorders in adults. *Depression and Anxiety, 27*(10), 891–932.

Horesh, N., Apter, A., & Zalsman, G. (2011). Timing, quantity and quality of stressful life events in childhood and preceding the first episode of bipolar disorder. *Journal of Affective Disorders, 134*(1-3), 434–437.

Horowitz, J. L., & Garber, J. (2006). The prevention of depressive symptoms in children and adolescents: A meta-analytic review. *Journal of Consulting and Clinical Psychology, 74*(3), 401–415.

Horowitz, J. L., Garber, J., Ciesla, J. A., Young, J. F. & Mufson, L. (2007). Prevention of depressive symptoms in adolescents: A randomized trial of cognitive-behavioral and interpersonal prevention programs. *Journal of Consulting & Clinical Psychology, 75*, 693–706.

Huey, S. J., Jr., Henggeler, S. W., Rowland, M. D., et al. (2004). Multisystemic therapy effects on attempted suicide by youths presenting psychiatric emergencies. *Journal of the American Academy of Child & Adolescent Psychiatry, 43*, 183–190.

Hughes, C. W., Emslie, G. J., Crismon, M. L., Posner, K., Birmaher, B., Ryan, N., ... Trivedi, M. H., and the Texas Consensus Conference

Panel on Medication. (2007). Texas Children's Medication Algorithm Project: Update from Texas Consensus Conference Panel on Medication Treatment of Childhood Major Depressive Disorder. *Journal of the American Academy of Child & Adolescent Psychiatry, 46*(6), 667–686.

Hulvershorn, L., Cullen, K., & Anand, A. (2011). Toward dysfunctional connectivity: A review of neuroimaging findings in pediatric major depressive disorder. *Brain Imaging and Behavior, 5*(4), 307–328.

Ingram, R. E., Miranda, J., & Segal, Z. V. (1998). *Cognitive vulnerability to depression.* New York: Guilford Press.

Institute of Medicine (IOM). (1994). *Reducing risks for mental disorders: Frontiers for preventive intervention research.* Washington, DC: National Academy Press.

Isacsson, G., Holmgren, P., & Ahlner, J. (2005). Selective serotonin reuptake inhibitor antidepressants and the risk of suicide: A controlled forensic database study of 14,857 suicides. *Acta Psychiatrica Scandinavica, 111*(4), 286–290.

Jacobson, N. S., Dobson, K. S., Truax, P. A., Addis, M. E., Koerner, K., Gollan, J. K., Gortner, E., & Prince, S. E. (1996). A component analysis of cognitive-behavioral treatment for depression. *Journal of Consulting and Clinical Psychology, 64*(2), 295–304.

Jaenicke, C., Hammen, C., Zupan, B., Hiroto, D., Gordon, D., Adrian, C., & Burge, D. (1987). Cognitive vulnerability in children at risk for depression. *Journal of Abnormal Child Psychology, 15*(4), 559–572.

Jakobsen, J. C., Hansen, J. L., Storebø, O. J., Simonsen, E., & Gluud, C. (2011a). The effects of cognitive therapy versus "no intervention" for major depressive disorder. *PloS One, 6*(12), e28299.

Jakobsen, J. C., Hansen, J. L., Storebø, O. J., Simonsen, E., & Gluud, C. (2011b). The effects of cognitive therapy versus "treatment as usual" in patients with major depressive disorder. *PloS One, 6*(8), e22890.

Jarrett, R. B., Kraft, D., Doyle, J., Foster, B. M., Eaves, G. G., & Silver, P. C. (2001). Preventing recurrent depression using cognitive therapy with and without a continuation phase: A randomized clinical trial. *Archives of General Psychiatry, 58*(4), 381–388.

Jaycox, L. H., Reivich, K. J., Gillham, J., & Seligman, M. E. P. (1994). Prevention of depressive symptoms in school children. *Behaviour Research and Therapy, 32*, 801–816.

Jayson, D., Wood, A., Kroll, L., Fraser, J., & Harrington, R. (1998). Which depressed patients respond to cognitive-behavioral treatment? *Journal of the American Academy of Child and Adolescent Psychiatry, 37*, 35–39.

Jenness, J. L., Hankin, B. L., Young, J. F., & Gibb, B. E. (2015). Misclassification and identification of emotional facial expressions in depressed youth: A preliminary study. *Journal of Clinical Child & Adolescent Psychology, 44*(4), 559–565.

Jerrell, J. M., & McIntyre, R. S. (2010). Metabolic, digestive, and reproductive adverse events associated with antimanic treatment in children and adolescents: A retrospective cohort study. *Primary Care Companion to The Journal of Clinical Psychiatry, 12*(4), PCC.09m00891.

Johnson, J. G., Cohen, P., Dohrenwend, B. P., Link, B. G., & Brook, J. S. (1999). A longitudinal investigation of social causation and social selection processes involved in the association between socioeconomic status and psychiatric disorders. *Journal of Abnormal Psychology, 108*, 490–499.

Johnson, J., Weissman, M. M., & Klerman, G. L. (1992). Service utilization and social morbidity associated with depressive symptoms in the community. *Journal of the American Medical Association, 267*, 1478–1483.

Johnston, J. A., Lineberry, C. G., Ascher, J. A., Davidson, J., Khayrallah, M. A., Feighner, J. P., et al. (1991). A 102-center prospective study of seizure in association with bupropion. *Journal of Clinical Psychiatry, 52*, 450–456.

Joiner, T. E., Jr., & Wagner, K. D. (1995). Attributional style and depression in children and adolescents: A meta-analytic review. *Clinical Psychology Review, 8*, 777–798.

Jolin, E. M., Weller, R. A., & Weller, E. B. (2012). Occurrence of affective disorders compared to other psychiatric disorders in children and adolescents with 22q11.2 deletion syndrome. *Journal of Affective Disorders, 136*(3), 222–228.

Jonas, B. S., Brody, D., Roper, M., & Narrow, W. E. (2003). Prevalence of mood disorders in a national sample of young American adults. *Social Psychiatry and Psychiatric Epidemiology, 38*(11), 618–624.

Jorm, A. F., Christensen, H., Henderson, A. S. & Jacomb, P. A. (2000). Predicting anxiety and depression from personality: Is there a synergistic effect of neuroticism and extraversion? *Journal of Abnormal Psychology, 109*, 145–149.

Joshi, G., Petty, C., Wozniak, J., Faraone, S. V., Spencer, A. E., Woodworth, K. Y., . . . Biederman, J. (2013). A prospective open-label trial of paliperidone monotherapy for the treatment of bipolar spectrum disorders in children and adolescents. *Psychopharmacology, 227*, 449–458.

Judd, L. L., & Akiskal, H. S. (2003) Depressive episodes and symptoms dominate the longitudinal course of bipolar disorder. *Current Psychiatry Reports 5*(6), 417–418.

Judd, L. L., Akiskal, H. S., & Paulus, M. P. (1997). The role and clinical significance of subsyndromal depressive symptoms (SSD) in unipolar major depressive disorder. *Journal of Affective Disorders, 45*, 5–18.

Kafantaris, V., Coletti, D. J., Dicker, R., Padula, G., & Kane, J. M. (2001). Adjunctive antipsychotic treatment of adolescents with bipolar psychosis. *Journal of the American Academy of Child and Adolescent Psychiatry, 40*, 1448–1456.

Kagan, J., & Snidman, N. (1991). Temperamental factors in human development. *American Psychologist, 46*, 856–862.

Kagan, J., Reznick, J.S., & Snidman, N. (1987). The physiology and psychology of behavioral inhibition in children. *Child Development, 55*, 1459–1473.

Kalin, N. H., & Carnes, M. (1984). Biological correlates of attachment bond disruption in humans and nonhuman primates. *Progress in Neuropsychopharmacology and Biological Psychiatry, 8*, 459–469.

Kaslow, N. J., Rehm, L. P., & Siegel, A. W. (1984). Social-cognitive and cognitive correlates of depression in children. *Journal of Abnormal Child Psychology, 12*, 605–620.

Kaslow, N. J,. & Thompson, M. P. (1998). Applying the criteria for empirically supported treatments to studies of psychosocial interventions for child and adolescent depression. *Journal of Clinical Child Psychology, 27*, 146–155.

Katainen, S., Raikkonen, K., Keskivaara, P., & Keltikangas-Jarvinen, L. (1999). Maternal childrearing attitudes and role satisfaction and children's temperament as antecedents of adolescent depressive tendencies: Follow-up study of 6- to 15-year-olds. *Journal of Youth and Adolescence, 2*, 139–163.

Katon, W., Lozano, P., Russo, J., McCauley, E., Richardson, L., & Bush, T. (2007). The prevalence of DSM-IV anxiety and depressive disorders in youth with asthma compared with controls. *Journal of Adolescent Health, 41*(5), 455–463.

Katona, C. L., Robertson, M. M., Abou-Saleh, M. T., Nairac, B. L., Edwards, D. R., Lock, T., et al. (1993). Placebo-controlled trial of lithium augmentation of fluoxetine and lofepramine. *International Clinical Psychopharmacology, 8*, 323.

Kaufman, J., Martin, A., King, R. A., & Charney, D. (2001), Are child-, adolescent-, and adult-onset depression one and the same disorder? *Biological Psychiatry, 49*, 980–1001.

Kaufman, J., Yang, B.-Z., Douglas-Palumberi, H., Grasso, D., Lipschitz, D., Houshyar, S., ... Gelernter, J. (2006). Brain-derived neurotrophic factor-5-HTTLPR gene interactions and environmental modifiers of depression in children. *Biological Psychiatry, 59*(8), 673–680.

Kazdin, A. E., & Weisz, J. R. (1998). Identifying and developing empirically supported child and adolescent treatments. *Journal of Consulting & Clinical Psychology, 66*, 19–36.

Keller, M. B., Ryan, N. D., Strober, M., Klein, R. G., Kutcher, S. P., ... McCafferty, J. P. (2001). Efficacy of paroxetine in the treatment of adolescent major depression: A randomized, controlled trial. *Journal of the American Academy of Child and Adolescent Psychiatry, 40*, 762–772.

Kendler, K. S., Gardner, C. O., & Prescott, C. A. (2002). Toward a comprehensive developmental model for major depression in women. *American Journal of Psychiatry, 159*, 1133–1145.

Kendler, K. S., Kessler, R. C., Neale, M. C., Heath, A. C., & Eaves, L. J. (1993). The prediction of major depression in women: Toward an integrated etiologic model. *American Journal of Psychiatry, 150*, 1139–1148.

Kendler, K. S., Neale, M. C., et al. (1992). Childhood parental loss and adult psychopathology in women: A twin study perspective. *Archives of General Psychiatry, 49*, 109–116.

Kennard, B. D., Emslie, G. J., Mayes, T. L., Nakonezny, P. A., Jones, J. M., Foxwell, A. A., & King, J. (2014). Sequential treatment with fluoxetine and relapse-prevention CBT to improve outcomes in pediatric depression. *American Journal of Psychiatry, 171*, 1083–1090.

Kennard, B. D., Emslie, G. J., Mayes, T. L., Nightingale-Teresi, J., Nakonezny, P. A., Hughes, J. L., ... Jarrett, R. B. (2008). Cognitive-behavioral therapy to prevent relapse in pediatric responders to pharmacotherapy for major depressive disorder. *Journal of the American Academy of Child and Adolescent Psychiatry, 47*, 1395–1404.

Kennard, B. D., Silva, S. G., Tonev, S., Rohde, P., Hughes, J. L., Vitiello, B., ... March, J. (2009). Remission and recovery in the Treatment for Adolescents with Depression Study (TADS), acute and long-term outcomes. *Journal of the American Academy of Child and Adolescent Psychiatry, 48*(2), 186–195.

Kennard, B., Silva, S., Vitiello, B., et al. (2006). Remission and residual symptoms after short-term treatment in the Treatment of Adolescents with Depression Study (TADS). *Journal of the American Academy of Child and Adolescent Psychiatry, 45*, 1404–1411.

Kenny, M. E., Moilanen, D. M., Lomax, R., & Brabeck, M. D. (1993). Contributions of parental attachment to view of self and depressive symptoms among early adolescents. *Journal of Youth and Adolescence, 13*, 408–430.

Kerestes, R., Davey, C. G., Stephanou, K., Whittle, S., & Harrison, B. J. (2013). Functional brain imaging studies of youth depression: A systematic review. *NeuroImage Clinical, 4*, 209–231.

Kersun, L. S., & Elia, J. (2007). Depressive symptoms and SSRI use in pediatric oncology patients. *Pediatric Blood & Cancer, 49*(7), 881–887.

Kessler, R. C., Avenevoli, S., & Merikangas, K. R. (2001). Mood disorders in children and adolescents: An epidemiologic perspective. *Biological Psychiatry, 49*, 1002–1014.

Kessler, R. C., Berglund, P., Demler, O., Jin, R., Koretz, D., Merikangas, K. R., ... Wang, P. S. (2003). The epidemiology of major depressive disorder. *Journal of the American Medical Association, 289*(23), 3095–3105.

Kessler, R. C., Foster, C., Webster, P. S., & House, J. S. (1992). The relationship between age and depressive symptoms in two national surveys. *Psychology & Aging, 7*(1), 119–126.

Kessler, R. C., McGonagle, K. A., Zhao, S., Nelson, C. B., Hughes, M., Eshleman, S., Wittchen, H. U., & Kendler, K. S. (1994). Lifetime and 12-month prevalence of DSM-III-R psychiatric disorders in the United States: Results from the National Comorbidity Survey. *Archives of General Psychiatry, 51*(1), 8–19.

Kessler, R. C., & Merikangas, K. R. (2004). The National Comorbidity Survey Replication (NCS-R): background and aims. *International Journal of Methods in Psychiatric Reseach, 13*(2), 60–68.

Kessler, R. C., Petukhova, M., Sampson, N. A., Zaslavsky, A. M., & Wittchen, H. U. (2012). Twelve-month and lifetime prevalence and lifetime morbid risk of anxiety and mood disorders in the United States. *International Journal of Methods in Psychiatric Research, 21*(3), 169–184.

Kessler, R. C., Rubinow, D. R., Holmes, C., Abelson, J. M., & Zhao, S. (1997), The epidemiology of DSM-III-R bipolar I disorder in a general population survey. *Psychological Medicine, 27*, 1079–1089.

Kessler, R., & Walters, E. E. (1998). Epidemiology of DSM-III-R major depression and minor depression among adolescents and young adults in the National Comorbidity Survey. *Depression and Anxiety, 7*(1), 3–14.

Khantzian, E. (1997). The self-medication hypothesis of substance use disorders: A reconsideration and recent applications. *Harvard Review of Psychiatry, 4*, 231–244.

Kiely, K. M., & Butterworth, P. (2013). Social disadvantage and individual vulnerability: A longitudinal investigation of welfare receipt and mental health in Australia. *Australian and New Zealand Journal of Psychiatry, 47*(7), 654–666.

Kilpatrick, D. G., Ruggiero, K. J., Acierno, R., Saunders, B. E., Resnick, H. S., & Best, C. L. (2003). Violence and risk of PTSD, major depression, substance abuse/dependence, and comorbidity: Results from the National Survey of Adolescents. *Journal of Consulting and Clinical Psychology, 71*, 692–700.

King, C. A., Klaus, N., Kramer, A., et al. (2009). The Youth-Nominated Support Team-Version II for suicidal adolescents: A randomized controlled intervention trial. *Journal of Consulting & Clinical Psychology, 77*, 880–893.

King, C. A., Kramer, A., Preus, L., et al. (2006). Youth-Nominated Support Team for suicidal adolescents (Version 1): A randomized controlled trial. *Journal of Consulting & Clinical Psychology, 77*, 199–206.

Kistner, J., Balthazor, M., Risi, S., & Burton, C. (1999). Predicting dysphoria in adolescence from actual and perceived peer acceptance in childhood. *Journal of Clinical Child Psychology, 28*, 94–104.

Kistner, J. A., David-Ferdon, C. F., Lopez, C. M., & Dunkel, S. B. (2007). Ethnic and sex differences in children's depressive symptoms. *Journal of Clinical Child and Adolescent Psychology, 36*(2), 171–181.

Klein, D. N., Depue, R. A., & Slater, J. F. (1985). Cyclothymia in the adolescent offspring of parents with bipolar affective disorder. *Journal of Abnormal Psychology, 94*, 115–127.

Klein, D. N., Durbin, C. E., Shankman, S. A., & Santiago, N. J. (2002). Depression and personality. In I. H. Gotlib & C. L. Hammen (Eds.), *Handbook of depression and its treatment* (pp. 115–140). New York: Guilford Press.

Klein, R. G., Pine, D. S., et al. (1998). Resolved: Mania is mistaken for ADHD in prepubertal children. Negative. *Journal of the American Academy of Child and Adolescent Psychiatry 37*(10), 1093–1095.

Klengel, T., & Binder, E. B. (2013). Gene-environment interactions in major depressive disorder. *Canadian Journal of Psychiatry, 58*(2), 76–83.

Klengel, T., Mehta, D., Anacker, C., Rex-Haffner, M., Pariante, C. M., Pace, T. W., ... Binder, E. B. (2013). Epigenetic modification as mediator of gene-childhood trauma interactions [Abstract]. *Biological Psychiatry, 73*(9), 15S.

Klerman, G. L., & Weissman, M. M. (1989). Increasing rates of depression. *Journal of the American Medical Association, 261*, 2229–2235.

Klerman, G. L., Weissman, M. M., Rounsaville, B. J., & Chevron, E. (1984). *Interpersonal psychotherapy of depression*. New York: Basic Books.

Kochanska, G., & Kuczynski, L. (1991). Maternal autonomy granting: Predictors of normal and depressed mothers' compliance and noncompliance with the requests of five-year-olds. *Child Development, 62*, 1449–1459.

Kochanska, G., Kuczynski, L., Radke-Yarrow, M., & Welsh, J. D. (1987). Resolutions of control episodes between well and affectively ill mothers and their young children. *Journal of Abnormal Child Psychology, 15*, 441–456.

Kocsis, J. H., Rush, A. J., Markowitz, J. C., Borian, F. E., Dunner, D. L., Koran, L. M., ... Keller, M. B. (2003). Continuation treatment of chronic depression: A comparison of nefazodone, cognitive behavioral analysis system of psychotherapy, and their combination. *Psychopharmacology Bulletin, 37*(4), 73–87.

Koh, H. K., Blakey, C. R., & Roper, A. Y. (2014). Healthy people 2020: A report card on the health of the nation. *Journal of the American Medical Association, 311*(24), 2475–2476.

Kolko, D. J., Brent, D. A., Baugher, M., Bridge, J., & Birmaher, B. (2000). Cognitive and family therapies for adolescent depression: Treatment specificity, mediation, and moderation. *Journal of Consulting & Clinical Psychology, 68*, 603–614.

Kondo, D. G., Hellem, T. L., Shi, X.-F., Sung, Y. H., Prescot, A. P., Kim, T. S., ... Renshaw, P. F. (2014). A review of MR spectroscopy studies of pediatric bipolar disorder. *American Journal of Neuroradiology, 35*(6 Suppl), S64–80.

Kovacs, M. (1990). Comorbid anxiety disorders in childhood-onset depression. In J. D. Maser & C. R. Cloninger (Eds.), *Comorbidity of mood and anxiety disorders* (pp. 271–282). Washington, DC: American Psychiatric Press.

Kovacs, M. (1996). Presentation and course of major depressive disorder during childhood and later years of the life span. *Journal of the American Academy of Child and Adolescent Psychiatry, 35*(6), 705–715.

Kovacs, M., Akiskal, H., et al. (1994). Childhood-onset dysthymic disorder: Clinical features and prospective naturalistic outcome. *Archives of General Psychiatry, 51*(5), 365–374.

Kovacs, M., Feinberg, T. L., Crouse-Novak, M., Paulauskas, S. L., Pollack, M., & Finkelstein, R. (1984). Depressive disorders in childhood. II. A longitudinal study of the risk source for a subsequent major depression. *Archives of General Psychiatry, 41*(7), 643–649.

Kovacs, M., & Gatsonis, C. (1994). Secular trends in age at onset of major depressive disorders in a clinical sample of children. *Journal of Psychiatric Research, 28*, 319–329.

Kovacs, M., Goldston, D., Obrosky, D. S., & Bonar, L. K. (1997). Psychiatric disorders in youths with IDDM: Rates and risk factors. *Diabetes Care 20*(1), 36–44.

Kovacs, M., Paulaskas, S., Gatsonis, C., & Richards, C. (1988). Depressive disorders in childhood. III. A longitudinal study of comorbidity with risk for conduct disorders. *Journal of Affective Disorders, 15*(3), 205–217.

Kovacs, M., & Pollock M. (1995). Bipolar disorder and comorbid conduct disorder in childhood and adolescence. *Journal of the American Academy of Child and Adolescent Psychiatry, 34*(6), 715–723.

Kovacs, M., Rottenberg, J., & George, C. (2009). Maladaptive mood repair responses distinguish young adults with early-onset depressive disorders and predict future depression outcomes. *Psychological Medicine, 39*(11), 1841–1854.

Kovacs, M., Rush, A. J., Beck, A. T., & Hollon, S. D. (1981). Depressed outpatients treated with cognitive therapy or pharmacotherapy. *Archives of General Psychiatry, 38*(1), 33–39.

Kowatch, R. A., Findling, R. L., Scheffer, R. E., & Stanford, K. (2007). Placebo controlled trial of divalproex versus lithium for bipolar disorder. Presented at the Annual Meeting of the American Academy of Child and Adolescent Psychiatry. Boston, October 23–28.

Kowatch, R. A., Fristad, M., Birmaher, B., Wagner, K. D., Findling, R. L., Hellander, M., Child Psychiatric Workgroup on Bipolar Disorder. (2005). Treatment guidelines for children and adolescents with bipolar disorder. *Journal of the American Academy of Child & Adolescent Psychiatry, 44*(3), 213–235.

Kowatch, R. A., Youngstrom, E. A., Danielyan, A., & Findling, R. L. (2005). Review and meta-analysis of the phenomenology and clinical characteristics of mania in children and adolescents. *Bipolar Disorders, 7*(6), 483–496

Kramer, R. A, Warner, V., Olfson, M., Ebanks, C. M., Chaput, F., & Weissman, M. M. (1998). General medical problems among the offspring of depressed parents: A ten-year follow-up. *Journal of the American Academy of Child & Adolescent Psychiatry, 37*(6), 602–611.

Kratochvil, C., Emslie, G., Silva, S., McNulty, S., Walkup, J., Curry, J., . . . March, J., & the TADS Team. (2006). Acute time to response in the Treatment for Adolescents with Depression study (TADS). *Journal of the American Academy of Child and Adolescent Psychiatry, 45*, 1412–1418.

Kroll, L., Harrington, R., Jayson, D., Fraser, J., & Gowers, S. (1996). Pilot study of continuation cognitive-behavioral therapy for major depression in adolescent psychiatric patients. *Journal of the American Academy of Child and Adolescent Psychiatry, 35*, 1156–1161.

Krueger, R. F., Caspi, A., Moffitt, T. E., Silva, P., et al. (1996). Personality traits are differentially linked to mental disorders: A multitrait-multidiagnosis study of an adolescent birth cohort. *Journal of Abnormal Psychology, 105*, 299–312.

Kutcher, S., & Gardner, D. M. (2008). Use of selective serotonin reuptake inhibitors and youth suicide: Making sense from a confusing story. *Current Opinion in Psychiatry, 21*(1), 65–69.

Kutcher, S. P., Marton, P., & Korenblum, M. (1989). Relationship between psychiatric illness and conduct disorder in adolescents. *Canadian Journal of Psychiatry, 34*(6), 526–529.

Labelle, R., Pouliot, L., & Janelle, A. (2015). A systematic review and meta-analysis of cognitive behavioral treatments for suicidal and self-harm behaviors in adolescence. *Canadian Psychology, 56*(4), 368–378.

Ladd, C. O., Huot, R. L., Thrivikraman, K. V., Nemeroff, C. B., Meaney, M. J., & Plotsky, P. M. (2000). Long-term behavioral and neuroendocrine adaptations to adverse early experience. *Progress in Brain Research, 122*, 81–103.

Lahey, B. B., Flagg, E. W., Bird, H. R., Schwab-Stone, M. E., Canino, G., Dulcan, M. K.. . . Regier, D. A. (1996). The NIMH Methods for the Epidemiology of Child and Adolescent Mental Disorders (MECA) Study: Background and methodology. *Journal of the American Academy of Child & Adolescent Psychiatry, 35*, 855–864.

Larson, R. J. (1992). Neuroticism and selective encoding and recall of symptoms: Evidence from a combined concurrent retrospective study. *Journal of Personality and Social Psychology, 62*, 480–488.

Lazarus, R. S., DeLongis, A., Folkman, S., & Gruen, R. (1985). Stress and adaptational outcomes. The problem of confounded measures. *American Psychologist, 40*, 770–785.

Leadbeater, B. J., Kuperminc, G. P., Blatt, S. J., & Hertzog, C. (1999). A multivariate model of gender differences in adolescents' internalizing and externalizing problems. *Developmental Psychology, 35*(5), 1268–1282.

Lefkowitz, M. M., & Tesiny, E. P. (1985). Depression in children: Prevalence and correlates. *Journal of Consulting & Clinical Psychology, 53*(5), 647–656.

Leibenluft, E. (2011). Severe mood dysregulation, irritability, and the diagnostic boundaries of bipolar disorder in youths. *American Journal of Psychiatry, 168*, 129–142.

Leibenluft, E., Charney, D. S., Towbin, K. E., Bhangoo, R. K., & Pine, D. S. (2003). Defining clinical phenotypes of juvenile mania. *American Journal of Psychiatry, 160*, 430–437.

Lejuez, C. W., Hopko, D. R., Acierno, R., Daughters, S. B., & Pagoto, S. L. (2011). Ten year revision of the brief behavioral activation treatment for depression: Revised treatment manual. *Behavior Modification, 35*(2), 111–161.

Leon, A. C., Marzuk, P. M., Tardiff, K., Bucciarelli, A., Markham Piper, T., & Galea, S. (2006). Antidepressants and youth suicide in New York City, 1999–2002. *Journal of the American Academy of Child and Adolescent Psychiatry, 45*(9), 1054–1058.

Levenson, M. R., Aldwin, C. M., Bosse, R., & Spiro, A. (1988). Emotionality and mental health: Longitudinal findings from the normative aging study. *Journal of Abnormal Psychology, 97*, 94–96.

Leventhal, T., & Brooks-Gunn, J. (2000). The neighborhoods they live in: The effects of neighborhood residence on child and adolescent outcomes. *Psychological Bulletin, 126*, 309–337.

Levitan, R. D., Parikh, S. V., Lesage, A. D., Hegadoren, K. M., Adams, M., Kennedy, S. H., & Goering, P. N. (1998). Major depression in individuals with a history of childhood physical or sexual abuse: Relationship to neurovegetative features, mania, and gender. *American Journal of Psychiatry, 155*(12), 1746–1752.

Lewinsohn, P. M. (1974). A behavioral approach to depression. In R. J. Friedman & M. M. Katz (Eds.), *The psychology of depression: Contemporary theory and research* (pp. 176–178). Washington: Winston-Wiley.

Lewinsohn, P. M., Hops, H., Roberts, R. E., Seeley, J. R., & Andrews, J. A. (1993). Adolescent psychopathology. I. Prevalence and incidence of depression and other DSM-III-R disorders in high school students. *Journal of Abnormal Psychology, 102*, 133–144.

Lewinsohn, P. M., Klein, D. N., & Seeley, J. R. (1995). Bipolar disorders in a community sample of older adolescents: Prevalence, phenomenology, comorbidity and course. *Journal of the American Academy of Child & Adolescent Psychiatry, 34*, 454–463.

Lewinsohn, P. M., Klein, D. N., & Seeley, J. R. (2000). Bipolar disorder during adolescence and young adulthood in a community sample. *Bipolar Disorders, 2*(3p2), 281–293.

Lewinsohn, P. M., Rohde, P., Klein, D. N., & Seeley, J. R. (1999). Natural course of adolescent major depressive disorder: I. Continuity into young adulthood. *Journal of the American Academy of Child and Adolescent Psychiatry, 38*(1), 56–63.

Lewinsohn, P. M., Rohde, P., & Seeley, J. R. (1998). Major depressive disorder in older adolescents: Prevalence, risk factors, and clinical implications. *Clinical Psychology Review, 18*(7), 765–794.

Lewinsohn, P. M., Rohde, P., Seeley, J. R., & Fischer, S. A. (1993). Age-cohort changes in the lifetime occurrence of depression and other mental disorders. *Journal of Abnormal Psychology, 102*, 110–120.

Lewinsohn, P. M., Rohde, P., Seeley, J. R., Klein, D. N., & Gotlib, I. H. (2000). Natural course of adolescent major depressive disorder in a community sample: Predictors of recurrence in young adults. *American Journal of Psychiatry, 157*, 1585–1591.

Lewinsohn, P. M., Seeley, J. R., Buckley, M. E., & Klein, D. N. (2002). Bipolar disorder in adolescence and young adulthood. *Child and Adolescent Psychiatric Clinics of North America, 11*(3), 461–475.

Lewinsohn, P. M., Solomon, A., Seeley, J. R., & Zeiss, A. (2000). Clinical implications of "subthreshold" depressive symptoms. *Journal of Abnormal Psychology, 109*, 345–351.

Lopez-Duran, N. L., Kuhlman, K. R., George, C., & Kovacs, M. (2013). Facial emotion expression recognition by children at familial risk for depression: High-risk boys are oversensitive to sadness. *Journal of Child Psychology & Psychiatry, 54*(5), 565–574.

Lorant, V., Deliège, D., Eaton, W., Robert, A., Philippot, P., & Ansseau, M. (2003). Socioeconomic inequalities in depression: A meta-analysis. *American Journal of Epidemiology, 157*(2), 98–112.

Lou, H. C., Hansen, D., Nordentoft, M., Pryds, O., Jensen, F., Nim, J., et al. (1994). Prenatal stressors of human life affect fetal brain development. *Developmental Medicine and Child Neurology, 36*, 826–832.

Lovejoy, M. C. (1991). Maternal depression: Effects on social cognition and behavior in parent–child interactions. *Journal of Abnormal Child Psychology, 19*, 693–706.

Luby, J. L. (2010). Preschool depression: The importance of identification of depression early in development. *Currents Directions in Psychological Science, 19*(2), 91–95.

Luby, J. L., Belden, A. B., & Tandon, M. (2010). Bipolar disorder in the preschool period: Focus of development and differential diagnosis. In D. J. Miklowitz & D. Cicchetti (Eds.), *Understanding bipolar disorder: A developmental psychopathology prespective* (pp. 391–403). New York: Guilford Press.

Luby, J. L., Belden, A. C., Jackson, J. J., et al. (2016). Early childhood depression and alterations in the trajectory of gray matter maturation in middle childhood and early adolescence. *JAMA Psychiatry, 73*(1), 31–38.

Luby, J. L., Gaffrey, M. S., Tillman, R., April, L. M., & Belden, A. C. (2014). Trajectories of preschool disorders to full DSM depression at school age and early adolescence: Continuity of preschool depression. *American Journal of Psychiatry, 171*(7), 768–776.

Lustman, P. J., et al. (2000). Fluoxetine for depression in diabetes: A randomized double-blind placebo-controlled trial. *Diabetes Care, 23*(5), 618–623.

Ma, D., Zhang, Z., Zhang, X., & Li, L. (2014). Comparative efficacy, acceptability, and safety of medicinal, cognitive-behavioral therapy, and placebo treatments for acute major depressive disorder in children and adolescents: A multiple-treatments meta-analysis. *Current Medical Research and Opinion, 30*(6), 971–995.

MacMillan, H. L., Fleming, J. E., Streiner, D. L., Lin, E., Boyle, M. H., Jamieson, E., et al. (2001). Childhood abuse and lifetime psychopathology in a community sample. *American Journal of Psychiatry, 158*, 1878–1883.

Mann, J. J., Aarons, S. F., Wilner, P. J., Keilp, J. G., Sweeney, J. A., Pearlstein, T., et al. (1989). A controlled study of the antidepressant efficacy and side effects of (-)-deprenyl. A selective monoamine oxidase inhibitor. *Archives of General Psychiatry, 46*, 45–50.

Mannuzza, S., Klein, R. G., Bessler, A., Malloy, P., & LaPadula, M. (1993). Adult outcome of hyperactive boys: Educational achievement, occupational rank, and psychiatric status. *Archives of General Psychiatry, 50*(7), 565–576.

March, J., Silva, S., Petrycki, S., et al. (2004). Fluoxetine, cognitive-behavioral therapy, and their combination for adolescents with depression: Treatment for Adolescents With Depression Study (TADS) randomized controlled trial. *Journal of the American Medical Association, 292*, 807–820.

March, J. S., Silva, S., Petrycki, S., et al. (2007). The Treatment for Adolescents With Depression Study (TADS): Long-term effectiveness and safety outcomes. *Archives of General Psychiatry, 64*, 1132–1143.

Martell, C. R., Dimidjian, S., & Herman-Dunn, R. (2013). *Behavioral activation for depression: A clinician's guide*. New York: Guilford Press.

Masi, G., et al. (2006). Attention-deficit hyperactivity disorder–bipolar comorbidity in children and adolescents. *Bipolar Disorders, 8*(4), 373–381.

Matas, L., Arend, R., & Sroufe, L. (1978). Continuity of adaptation in the second year: The relationship between quality of attachment and later competence. *Child Development, 49*, 547–556.

Mathers, C. D., & Loncar, D. (2006). Projections of global mortality and burden of disease from 2002 to 2030. *PLoS Medicine, 3*(11), e442.

Matos, A. P., Cherpe, S., & Pinheiro, M. R. (2013). Description of the pilot implementation of a study of depression prevention in adolescence. VIII National Symposium of Scientific Research, 20–22 July, Aveiro, PT.

McCauley, E., Myers, K., Mitchell, J., Calderon, R., Schloredt, K., & Treder, R. (1993). Depression in young people: Initial presentation and clinical course. *Journal of the American Academy of Child and Adolescent Psychiatry, 32*(4), 714–722.

McCauley, J., Kern, D. E., Kolodner, K., Dill, L., Schroeder, A. F., DeChant, H. K., ... Bass, E. B. (1997). Clinical characteristics of women with a history of childhood abuse: Unhealed wounds. *Journal of the American Medical Association, 277*(17), 1362–1368.

McCrae, R. R., & Costa, P. T. (1987). Validation of the five-factor model of personality across instruments and observers. *Journal of Personality & Social Psychology, 52*, 81–90.

McElroy, S. L., Keck, P. E., et al. (1992). Clinical and research implications of the diagnosis of dysphoric or mixed mania or hypomania. *American Journal of Psychiatry, 149*(12), 1633–1644.

McElroy, S. L., Strakowski, S. M., West, S. A., Keck, P. E., & McConville, B. J. (1997). Phenomenology of adolescent and adult mania in hospitalized patients with bipolar disorder. *American Journal of Psychiatry, 154*, 44–49.

McFarlane, A. H., Bellissimo, A., & Norman, G. R. (1995). The role of family and peers in social self-efficacy: Links to depression in adolescence. *American Journal of Orthopsychiatry, 65*, 402–410.

McGlashan, T. (1988). Adolescent versus adult onset of mania. *American Journal of Psychiatry, 145*(2), 221–223.

McGrath, C. L., Kelley, M. E., Dunlop, B. W., Holtzheimer, P. E., Craighead, W. E., & Mayberg, H. S. (2014). Pretreatment brain states identify likely nonresponse to standard treatments for depression. *Biological Psychiatry, 76(7)*, 527–535.

McGrath, C. L., Kelley, M. E., Holtzheimer, P. E., Dunlop, B. W., Craighead, W. E., Franco, A. R., Craddock, R. C., & Mayberg, H. S. (2013). Toward a neuroimaging treatment selection biomarker for major depressive disorder. *JAMA Psychiatry, 70*(8), 821–829.

McLaughlin, K. A., Hilt, L. M., & Nolen-Hoeksema, S. (2007). Racial/ethnic differences in internalizing and externalizing symptoms in adolescents. *Journal of Abnormal Child Psychology, 35*(5), 801–816.

McLean, P. D., & Hakstian, A. R. (1979). Clinical depression: Comparative efficacy of outpatient treatments. *Journal of Consulting and Clinical Psychology, 47*(5), 818–836.

McLoyd, V. C. (1998). Socioeconomic disadvantage and child development. *American Psychologist, 53*, 185–204.

Meeker, A. S., Herink, M. C., Haxby, D. G., & Hartung, D. M. (2015). The safety and efficacy of vortixetine for acute treatment of major depressive disorder: A systematic review and meta-analysis. *Systematic Reviews, 4*, 21.

Mellins, C. A., Brackis-Cott, E., Leu, C. S., Elkington, K. S., Donezal, C., Wiznia, A., ... Abrams, E. J. (2009). Rates and types of psychiatric disorders in perinatally human immunodeficiency virus-infected youth and seroreverters. *Journal of Child Psychology and Psychiatry, 50*(9), 1131–1138.

Mellins, C. A., Elkington, K. S., Bauermeister, J. A., Brackis-Cott, E., Dolezal, C., McKay, M., et al. (2009). Sexual and drug use behavior in perinatally HIV-infected youth: Mental health and family influences. *Journal of the American Academy of Child and Adolescent Psychiatry, 48*(8), 810–819.

Melvin, G. A., Tonge, B. J., King, N. J., Heyne, D., Gordon, M. S., & Klimkeit, E. (2006). A comparison of cognitive-behavioral therapy, sertraline, and their combination for adolescent depression. *Journal of American Academy of Child and Adolescent Psychiatry, 45*, 1151–1161.

Merali, Z., Du, L., Hrdini, P., Palkovits, M., Faludi, G., Poulter, M. O., et al. (2004). Dysregulation in the suicide brain: mRNA expression of corticotrophin-releasing hormone receptors and GABAA receptor subunits in frontal cortical brain region. *Journal of Neuroscience, 24*, 1478–1485.

Merikangas, K. R., Akiskal, H. S., Angst, J., Greenberg, P. E., Hirschfeld, R., Petukhova, M., & Kessler, R. C. (2007). Lifetime and 12-month prevalence of bipolar spectrum disorder in the National Comorbidity Survey replication. *Archives of General Psychiatry, 64*(5), 543.

Merikangas, K. R., Avenevoli, S., Costello, E. J., Koretz, D., & Kessler, R. C. (2009). National Comorbidity Survey Replication Adolescent Supplement (NCS-A), I. Background and measures. *Journal of the American Academy of Child & Adolescent Psychiatry, 48*(4), 367–379.

Merikangas, K. R., Avenevoli, S., Dierker, L., & Grillon, C. (1999). Vulnerability factors among children at risk for anxiety disorders. *Biological Psychiatry, 46*, 1523–1535.

Merikangas, K. R., Cui, L., Heaton, L., Nakamura, E., Roca, C., Ding, J., ... Angst J. (2014). Independence of familial transmission of mania and depression: Results of the NIMH family study of affective spectrum disorders. *Molecular Psychiatry, 19*(2), 214–219.

Merikangas, K. R., He, J. P., Brody, D., Fisher, P. W., Bourdon, K., & Koretz, D. S. (2010a). Prevalence and treatment of mental disorders among US children in the 2001–2004 NHANES. *Pediatrics, 125*(1), 75–81.

Merikangas, K. R., He, J. P., Burstein, M., Swanson, S. A., Avenevoli, S., Cui, L., ... Swendsen, J. (2010b). Lifetime prevalence of mental disorders in US adolescents: Results from the National Comorbidity Survey Replication–Adolescent Supplement (NCS-A). *Journal of the American Academy of Child & Adolescent Psychiatry, 49*(10), 980–989.

Merikangas, K. R., & Nakamura, E. F. (2011). The epidemiology of depression and anxiety in children and adolescents. In M. T. Tsuang, M. Tohen, & P. B. Jones (Eds.), *Textbook of psychiatric epidemiology* (3rd ed., pp. 435–448). Hoboken, NJ: John Wiley & Sons.

Merikangas, K. R., Nakamura, E. F., & Kessler, R. C. (2009). Epidemiology of mental disorders in children and adolescents. *Dialogues in Clinical Neuroscience, 11*, 7–20.

Merikangas, K. R., & Pato, M. (2009). Recent developments in the epidemiology of bipolar disorder in adults and children: Magnitude, correlates, and future directions. *Clinical Psychology: Science and Practice, 16*(2), 121–133.

Merikangas, K. R., & Tohen, M. (2011). Epidemiology of bipolar disorder in adults and children. In M. T. Tsuang, M. Tohen, & P. B. Jones (Eds.), *Textbook of psychiatric epidemiology* (3rd ed., pp. 329–342). Hoboken, NJ: John Wiley & Sons.

Merikangas, K., & Yu, K. (2002). Genetic epidemiology of bipolar disorder. *Clinical Neuroscience Research, 2*(3), 127–141.

Merry, S. N., Hetrick, S. E., Cox, G. R., Brudevold-Iverson, T., Bir, J. J., & McDowell, H. (2011). Psychological and educational interventions for preventing depression in children an adolescents. *Cochrane Database of Systematic Reviews, 12*, CD003380.

Mervaala, E., Föhr, J., Könönen, M., Valkonen-Korhonen, M., Vainio, P., Partanen, K., et al. (2000). Quantitative MRI of the hippocampus and amygdala in severe depression. *Psychological Medicine, 30*, 117–125.

Michl, L. C., McLaughlin, K. A., Shepherd, K., & Nolen-Hoeksema, S. (2013). Rumination as a mechanism linking stressful life events to symptoms of depression and anxiety: Longitudinal evidence in early adolescents and adults. *Journal of Abnormal Psychology, 122*(2), 339–352.

Mick, E., et al. (2003). A preliminary meta-analysis of the Child Behavior Checklist in pediatric bipolar disorder. *Biological Psychiatry, 53*(11), 1021–1027.

Miklowitz, D. J. (2008). *Bipolar disorders: A family-focused treatment approach* (2nd ed.). New York: Guilford Publications.

Miklowitz, D. J., Axelson, D. A., Birmaher, B., George, E. L., Taylor, D. O., Schneck, C. D., ... Brent, D. A. (2008). Family-focused treatment for adolescents with bipolar disorder: Results of a 2-year randomized trial. *Archives of General Psychiatry, 65*(9), 1053–1061.

Miklowitz, D. J., George, E. L., Axelson, D. A., Kim, E. Y., Birmaher, B., Schneck, C., ... Brent, D. A. (2004). Family-focused treatment for adolescents with bipolar disorder. *Journal of Affective Disorders, 82*(Suppl 1), S113–128.

Miklowitz, D. J., Goldstein, M. J., Nuechterlein, H., Snyder, K. S., & Mintz J. (1988). Family factors and the course of bipolar affective disorder. *Archives of General Psychiatry, 45*, 225–231.

Miklowitz, D. J., Schneck, C. D., Singh, M. K., Taylor, D. O., George, E. L., Cosgrove, V. E., ... Chang, K. D. (2013). Early intervention for symptomatic youth at risk for bipolar disorder: A randomized trial of family-focused therapy. *Journal of the American Academy of Child & Adolescent Psychiatry*, 52(2), 121–131.

Miklowitz, D. J., Simoneau, T. L., George, E. L., Richards, J. A., Kalbag, A., Sachs-Ericsson, N., et al. (2000). Family-focused treatment of bipolar disorder: 1 year effects of a psychoeducational program in conjunction with pharmacotherapy. *Biological Psychiatry, 48*, 582–592.

Miklowitz, D. J., & Taylor, D. O. (2006). Family-focused treatment of the suicidal bipolar patient. *Bipolar Disorders, 8*(5 Pt 2), 640–651.

Milberger, S., Biederman, J., Faraone, S. V., Murphy, J., & Tsuang, M. T. (1995). Attention deficit hyperactivity disorder and comorbid disorders: Issues of overlapping symptoms. *American Journal of Psychiatry, 152*(12), 1793–1799.

Miller, B., & Taylor, J. (2012). Racial and socioeconomic status differences in depressive symptoms among black and white youth: An examination of the mediating effects of family structure, stress and support. *Journal of Youth and Adolescence, 41*(4), 426–437.

Miller, M., Swanson, S. A., Azrael, D., Pate, V., & Stürmer, T. (2014). Antidepressant dose, age, and the risk of deliberate self-harm. *JAMA Internal Medicine, 174*(6), 899–909.

Monroe, S. M., & Harkness, K. L. (2011). Recurrence in major depression: A conceptual analysis. *Psychological Review, 118*(4), 655–674.

Monroe, S. M., Rohde, P., Seeley, J. R., & Lewinsohn, P. M. (1999). Life events and depression in adolescence: Relationship loss as a prospective risk factor for first onset of major depressive disorder. *Journal of Abnormal Psychology, 108*, 606–614.

Monroe, S. M., & Simons, A. D. (1991). Diathesis-stress theories in the context of life stress research: Implications for the depressive disorders. *Psychological Bulletin, 110*(3), 406–425.

Moreno, C., Laje, G., Blanco, C., Jiang, H., Schmidt, A. B., & Olfson, M. (2007). National trends in the outpatient diagnosis and treatment of bipolar disorder in youth. *Archives of General Psychiatry, 64*(9), 1032.

Morgan, J. K., Olino, T. M., McMakin, D. L., Ryan, N. D., & Forbes, E. E. (2013). Neural response to reward as a predictor of increases in depressive symptoms in adolescence. *Neurobiological Disease, 52*, 66–74.

Morgan, J. K., Shaw, D. S., & Forbes, E. E. (2014). Maternal depression and warmth during childhood predict age 20 neural response to reward. *Journal of the American Academy of Child and Adolescent Psychiatry, 53*(1), 108–117.

Mrazek, D. A., Schuman, W. B., & Klinnert, M. (1998). Early asthma onset: Risk of emotional and behavioral difficulties. *Journal of Child Psychology and Psychiatry, 39*, 247–254.

Mueller, C., & Orvaschel, H. (1997). The failure of "adult" interventions with adolescent depression: What does it mean for theory, research, and practice? *Journal of Affective Disorders, 44*(2-3), 203–215.

Mufson, L., Dorta, K. P., Wickramaratne, P., et al. (2004). A randomized effectiveness trial of interpersonal psychotherapy for depressed adolescents. *Archives of General Psychiatry, 61*, 577–584.

Mufson, L., Moreau, D., Weissman, M. M., et al. (1994). Modification of interpersonal psychotherapy with depressed adolescents (IPT-A): Phase I and II studies. *Journal of the American Academy of Child and Adolescent Psychiatry, 33*, 695–705.

Mufson, L., Weissman, M. M., Moreau, D., & Garfinkel, R. (1999). Efficacy of interpersonal psychotherapy for depressed adolescents. *Archives of General Psychiatry, 56*, 573–579.

Muñoz, R. F., Beardslee, W. R., & Leykin, Y. (2012). Major depression can be prevented. *American Psychologist, 67*(4), 285–295.

Mynors-Wallis, L. M., Gath, D. H., Lloyd-Thomas, A. R., & Tomlinson, D. B. M. J. (1995). Randomised controlled trial comparing problem solving treatment with amitriptyline and placebo for major depression in primary care. *BMJ, 310*(6977), 441–445.

Nanni, V., Uher, R., & Danese, A. (2012). Childhood maltreatment predicts unfavorable course of illness and treatment outcome in depression: A meta-analysis. *American Journal of Psychiatry, 169*(2), 141–151.

National Institute of Mental Health (NIMH). (1998). Priorities for prevention research at NIMH: A report by the National Advisory Mental Health Council Workgroup on Mental Disorders Prevention Research, National Institutes of Health. Bethesda, MD: Author.

Nezu, A. M. (1986). Efficacy of a social problem-solving therapy approach for unipolar depression. *Journal of Consulting and Clinical Psychology, 54*, 196–202.

Nezu, A. M., & Perri, M. G. (1989). Social problem-solving therapy for unipolar depression: An initial dismantling investigation. *Journal of Consulting and Clinical Psychology, 57*(3), 408-413.

Niranjan, A., Corujo, A., Ziegelstein, R. C., & Nwulia, E. (2012). Depression and heart disease in US adults. *General Hospital Psychiatry, 34*, 254–261.

Nivoli, A. M. A., Pacchiarotti, I., Rosa, A. R., Popovic, D., Murru, A., Valenti, M., ... Colom, F. (2011). Gender differences in a cohort study of 604 bipolar patients: The role of predominant polarity. *Journal of Affective Disorders, 133*(3), 443–449.

Nolan, S. A., Flynn, C., & Garber, J. (2003). Prospective relations between rejection and depression in young adolescents. *Journal of Personality and Social Psychology, 85*(4), 745–755.

Nolen-Hoeksema, S. (2000). The role of rumination in depressive disorders and mixed anxiety/depressive symptoms. *Journal of Abnormal Psychology, 109*, 504–511.

Nolen-Hoeksema, S., Girgus, J. S., & Seligman, M. E. (1986). Learned helplessness in children: A longitudinal study of depression, achievement, and explanatory style. *Journal of Personality and Social Psychology, 51*, 435–444.

Nolen-Hoeksema, S., Girgus, J. S., & Seligman, M. E. P. (1992). Predictors and consequences of childhood depressive symptoms: A 5-year longitudinal study. *Journal of Abnormal Psychology, 101*, 405–422.

Nomura, Y., Wickramaratne, P. J., Warner, V., Mufson, L., & Weissman, M. M. (2002). Family discord, parental depression and psychopathology in offspring: 10-year follow-up. *Journal of the American Academy of Child and Adolescent Psychiatry, 41*(4),402–409.

Nottelmann, E., & Jensen, P. S. (1998), Current issues in childhood bipolarity. *Journal of Affective Disorders, 51*, 77–80.

Nurnberger, J. I., Hamovit, J., Hibbs, E. D., Pelligrini, D., Guroff, J. J., Maxwell, M. E., Smith, A., & Gershon, E. S. (1988). A high-risk study of primary affective disorder: Selection of subjects, initial assessment, and 1- to 2-year follow-up. In D. L. Dunner, E. S. Gershon, & J. E. Barrett (Eds.), *Relatives at risk for mental disorder* (pp. 161–177). New York: Raven Press, Ltd.

O'Connell, M. E., Boat, T., & Warner, K. E. (Eds.). (2009). *Preventing mental, emotional, and behavioral disorders among young people: Progress and possibilities*. Washington, DC: National Academies Press.

Offord, D. R., Boyle, M. H., Szatmari, P., Rae-Grant, J. I., Links, P. S., Cadman, D. T., et al. (1987). Ontario Child Health Study. II. Six-month prevalence of disorder and rates of service utilization. *Archives of General Psychiatry, 44*, 832–836.

O'Hara, M. W., Stuart, S., Gorman, L. L., & Wenzel, A. (2000). Efficacy of interpersonal psychotherapy for postpartum depression. *Archives of General Psychiatry, 57*(11), 1039–1045.

Olfson, M., Shaffer, D., Marcus, S. C., & Greenberg, T. (2003). Relationship between antidepressant medication treatment and suicide in adolescents. *Archives of General Psychiatry, 60*(10), 978–982.

Ormel, J., Jeronimus, B. F., Kotov, R., Riese, H., Bos, E. H., Hankin, B., & Oldehinkel, A. J. (2013). Neuroticism and common mental disorders: Meaning and utility of a complex relationship. *Clinical Psychology Review, 33*(5), 686–697.

Orth, U., Robins, R. W., Widaman, K. F., & Conger, R. D. (2014). Is low self-esteem a risk factor for depression? Findings from a longitudinal study of Mexican-origin youth. *Developmental Psychology, 50*(2), 622–633.

Ospina-Duque, J., Duque, C., Carvajal-Carmona, L., Ortiz-Barrientos, D., Soto, I., Pineda, N., & Ruiz-Linares, A. (2000). An association study of bipolar mood disorder (type I) with the 5-HTTLPR serotonin transporter polymorphism in a human population isolate from Colombia. *Neuroscience Letters, 292*(3), 199–202.

Ott, D., et al. (2001). Measures of psychopathology in children with complex partial seizures and primary generalized epilepsy with absence. *Journal of the American Academy of Child and Adolescent Psychiatry, 40*(8), 907–914.

Ougrin, D., Boege, I., Stahl, D., Banarsee, R., & Taylor, E. (2013). Randomised controlled trial of therapeutic assessment versus usual assessment in adolescents with self-harm: 2-year follow-up. *Archives of Disease in Childhood, 98*(10), 772–776.

Ougrin, D., Zundel, T., Kyriakopoulos, M., et al. (2012). Adolescents with suicidal and nonsuicidal self-harm: Clinical characteristics and response to therapeutic assessment. *Psychological Assessment, 24*, 11–20.

Ougrin, D., Zundel, T., Ng, A., et al. (2011). Trial of Therapeutic Assessment in London: Randomised controlled trial of Therapeutic

Assessment versus standard psychosocial assessment in adolescents presenting with self-harm. *Archives of Disease in Childhood, 96,* 148–153.

Panak, W. F., & Garber, J. (1992). Role of aggression, rejection, and attributions in the prediction of depression in children. *Development and Psychopathology, 4,* 145–165.

Pao, D., Fisher, M., Hue, S., Dean, G., Murphy, G., Cane, P. A., et al. (2005). Transmission of HIV-1 during primary infection: Relationship to sexual risk and sexually transmitted infections. *AIDS, 19*(1), 85–90.

Parker, G. (1993). Parental rearing style: Examining for links with personality vulnerability factors for depression. *Social Psychiatry and Psychiatric Epidemiology, 28,* 97–100.

Parry-Langdon, N., Clements, A., Fletcher, D., & Goodman, R. (2008). *Three years on: Survey of the development and emotional well-being of children and young people.* Office for National Statistics.

Pathak, S., Findling, R. L., Earley, W. R., Acevedo, L. D., Stankowski, J., & Delbello, M. P. (2013). Efficacy and safety of quetiapine in children and adolescents with mania associated with bipolar I disorder: A 3-week, double-blind, placebo-controlled trial. *Journal of Clinical Psychiatry, 74*(1), e100–109.

Pathak, S., Johns, E. S., & Kowatch, R. A. (2005) Adjunctive quetiapine for treatment-resistant adolescent major depressive disorder: A case series. *Journal of Child and Adolescent Psychopharmacology, 15,* 696–702.

Patten, S. B., Wilkes, T. C. R., Williams, J. V. A., Lavorato, D. H., el-Guebaly, N., Schopflocher, D., ... Bulloch, A. G. M. (2015). Retrospective and prospectively assessed childhood adversity in association with major depression, alcohol consumption and painful conditions. *Epidemiology and Psychiatric Sciences, 24*(2), 158–165.

Pavuluri, M. N., Henry, D. B., Carbray, J. A., Sampson, G., Naylor, M. W., & Janicak, P. G. (2004). Open-label prospective trial of risperidone in combination with lithium or divalproex sodium in pediatric mania. *Journal of Affective Disorders, 82S,* S103–S111.

Pavuluri, M. N., Henry, D. B., Carbray, J. A., Sampson, G. A., Naylor, M., & Janicak, P. (2006). A one-year open-label trial of risperidone augmentation in lithium nonresponder youth with preschool-onset bipolar disorder. *Journal of Child and Adolescent Psychopharmacology, 16,* 336–350.

Paykel, E. S., Scott, J., Teasdale, J. D., Johnson, A. L., Garland, A., Moore, R., ... Pope, M. (1999). Prevention of relapse in residual depression by cognitive therapy: A controlled trial. *Archives of General Psychiatry, 56*(9), 829–835.

Perlis, R. H., Miyahara, S., Marangell, L. B., Wisniewski, S. R., Ostacher, M., DelBello, M. P., ... STEP-BD Investigators. (2004). Long-term implications of early onset in bipolar disorder: Data from the first 1000 participants in the Systematic Treatment Enhancement Program for Bipolar Disorder (STEP-BD). *Biological Psychiatry, 55*(9), 875–881.

Perlis, R. H., Nierenberg, A. A., Alpert, J. E., Pava, J., Matthews, J. D., Buchin, J., Sickinger, A. H., & Fava, M. (2002). Effects of adding cognitive therapy to fluoxetine dose increase on risk of relapse and residual depressive symptoms in continuation treatment of major depressive disorder. *Journal of Clinical Psychopharmacology, 22*(5), 474–480.

Petersen, T., Gordon, J. A., Kant, A., Fava, M., Rosenbaum, J. F., & Nierenberg, A. A. (2001). Treatment resistant depression and axis I comorbidity. *Psychological Medicine, 31,* 1223–1229.

Peterson, L., Mullins, L. L., & Ridley-Johnson, R. (1985). Childhood depression: Peer reactions to depression and life stress. *Journal of Abnormal Child Psychology, 13,* 597–609.

Pettit, J. W., Hartley, C., Lewinsohn, P. M., Seeley, J. R., & Klein, D. N. (2013). Is liability to recurrent major depressive disorder present before first episode onset in adolescence or acquired after the initial episode? *Journal of Abnormal Psychology, 122*(2), 353–358.

Pettit, J. W., Lewinsohn, P. M., & Joiner T. E., Jr. (2006). Propagation of major depressive disorder: Relationship between first episode symptoms and recurrence. *Psychiatry Research, 141*(3), 271–278.

Piet, J., & Hougaard, E. (2011). The effect of mindfulness-based cognitive therapy for prevention of relapse in recurrent major depressive disorder: A systematic review and meta-analysis. *Clinical Psychology Review, 31*(6), 1032–1040.

Piko, B. F., Luszczynska, A., & Fitzpatrick, K. M. (2013). Social inequalities in adolescent depression: The role of parental social support and optimism. *International Journal of Social Psychiatry, 59*(5), 474–481.

Pine, D. S., Cohen, P., & Brook, J. (1996). The association between major depression and headache: Results of a longitudinal epidemiologic study in youth. *Journal of Child & Adolescent Psychopharmacology, 6,* 153–164.

Pine, D. S., Cohen, E., Cohen, P., & Brook, J. (1999). Adolescent depressive symptoms as predictors of adult depression: Moodiness or mood disorder? *American Journal of Psychiatry, 156*, 133–135.

Pine, D. S., Cohen, E., Gurley, D., Brook, J., & Ma, Y. (1998). The risk for early-adulthood anxiety and depressive disorders in adolescents with anxiety and depressive disorders. *Archives of General Psychiatry, 55*, 56–64.

Pine, D. S., Goldstein, R. B., Wolk, S., & Weissman, M. M. (2001). The association between childhood depression and adulthood body mass index. *Pediatrics, 107*, 1049–1056.

Pineda, J., & Dadds, M. R. (2013). Family intervention for adolescents with suicidal behavior: A randomized controlled trial and mediation Analysis. *Journal of the American Academy of Child and Adolescent Psychiatry, 52*, 851–862.

Plotsky, P. M., & Meaney, M. J. (1993). Early, postnatal experience alters hypothalamic corticotropin-releasing factor (CRF) mRNA, median eminence CRF content and stress-induced release in adult rats. *Brain Research. Molecular Brain Research, 18*, 195–200.

Poltyrev, T., Keshet, G. I., Kay, G., & Weinstock, M. (1996). Role of experimental conditions in determining differences in exploratory behavior of prenatally stressed rats. *Developmental Psychobiology, 29*, 453–462.

Pribor, E. F., & Dinwiddie, S. H. (1992). Psychiatric correlates of incest in childhood. *American Journal of Psychiatry, 149*(1), 52–56.

Quiggle, N. L., Garber, J., Panak, W. F., & Dodge, K. A. (1992). Social information processing in aggressive and depressed children. *Child Development, 63*, 1305–1320.

Rao, O., Ryan, N. D., Birmaher, B., Dahl, R. E., Williamson, D. E., Kaufman, J., et al. (1995). Unipolar depression in adolescents: Clinical outcome in adulthood. *Journal of the American Academy of Child and Adolescent Psychiatry, 34*, 566–578.

Rao, U., Hammen, C., & Daley, S. E. (1999). Continuity of depression during the transition to adulthood: A 5-year longitudinal study of young women. *Journal of the American Academy of Child and Adolescent Psychiatry, 38*(7), 908–915.

Rapee, R. M. (1997). Potential role of childrearing practices in the development of anxiety and depression. *Clinical Psychology Review, 17*, 47–67.

Rehm, L. P. (1977). A self-control model of depression. *Behavior Therapy, 8*, 787–804.

Reinherz, H. A., Giaconia, R. M., Hauf, A. M., Wasserman, M. S., & Silverman, A. B. (1999). Major depression in the transition to adulthood: Risk and impairments. *Journal of Abnormal Psychology, 108*, 500–510.

Reinherz, H., Giaconia, R. M., Pakiz, B., Silverman, A. B., Frost, A. K., & Lefkowitz, E. S. (1993). Psychosocial risks for major depression in late adolescence: A longitudinal community study. *Journal of the American Academy of Child and Adolescent Psychiatry, 32*(6), 1155–1163.

Reiss, D., Neiderhiser, J. M., Hetherington, E. M., & Plomin, R. (2000). *The relationship code: Deciphering genetic and social patterns in adolescent development*. Cambridge, MA: Harvard University Press.

Reynolds C. F., III, Frank, E., Perel, J. M., Imber, S. D., Cornes, C., Miller, M. D., ... Kupfer, D. J. (1999). Nortriptyline and interpersonal psychotherapy as maintenance therapies for recurrent major depression. *Journal of the American Medical Association, 281*(1), 39–45.

Rice, F., Harold, G., & Thapar, A. (2002). The genetic aetiology of childhood depression: A review. *Journal of Child Psychology and Psychiatry, and Allied Disciplines, 43*(1), 65–79.

Rice, S. M., Hickie, I. B., Yung, A. R., Mackinnon, A., Berk, M., Davey, C., ... Amminger, G. P. (2014). Youth depression alleviation: The Fish Oil Youth Depression Study (YoDA-F), A randomized, double-blind, placebo-controlled treatment trial. *Early Intervention in Psychiatry*. [Epub Aug. 13]

Rimay, T., Benak, I., Kiss, E., Baji, I., Feher, A., Juhasz, A., ... Kapornai K; International Consortium of Childhood-Onset Mood disorders. (2015). BDNF Val66Met polymorphism and stressful life events in melancholic childhood-onset depression. *Psychiatric Genetics, 25*(6), 249–255.

Roberts, R. E., & Chen, Y. W. (1995). Depressive symptoms and suicidal ideation among Mexican-origin and Anglo adolescents. *Journal of the American Academy of Child and Adolescent Psychiatry, 34*(1), 81–90.

Roberts, R. E., Roberts, C. R., & Chen, Y. R. (1997). Ethnocultural differences in prevalence of adolescent depression. *American Journal of Community Psychology, 25*(1), 95–110.

Roberts, R. E., Roberts, C. R., & Xing, Y. (2007). Rates of DSM-IV psychiatric disorders among adolescents in a large metropolitan area. *Journal of Psychiatric Research, 41*(11), 959–967.

Roberts, S. B., & Kendler, K. S. (1999). Neuroticism and self-esteem as indices of the vulnerability to major depression in women. *Psychological Medicine, 29*, 1101–1109.

Robins, L. N., Locke, B. Z., & Regier, D. A. (1991). An overview of psychiatric disorders in America. In L. N. Robins & D. A. Regier (Eds.), *Psychiatric disorders in America: The Epidemiologic Catchment Area Project* (pp. 328–366). New York: The Free Press.

Robins, L., & Price, R. (1991). Adult disorders predicted by childhood conduct problems: Results from the NIMH epidemiologic catchment area project. *Psychiatry, 54*(2), 116–132.

Robinson, N. S., Garber, J., & Hilsman, R. (1995). Cognitions and stress: Direct and moderating effects on depressive versus externalizing symptoms during the junior high school transition. *Journal of Abnormal Psychology, 104*, 453–463.

Romero, S., Birmaher, B., Axelson, D. A., Iosif, A. M., Williamson, D. E., Gill, M. K., et al. (2009). Negative life events in children and adolescents with bipolar disorder. *Journal of Clinical Psychiatry, 70*(10), 1452–1460.

Rossello, J., & Bernal, G. (1999). The efficacy of cognitive-behavioral and interpersonal treatments for depression in Puerto Rican adolescents. *Journal of Consulting & Clinical Psychology, 67*, 734–745.

Rossello, J., Bernal, G., & Rivera-Medina, C. (2008). Individual and group CBT and IPT for Puerto Rican adolescents with depressive symptoms. *Cultural Diversity & Ethnic Minority Psychology, 14*, 234–245.

Rossouw, T. I., & Fonagy, P. (2012). Mentalization-based treatment for self-harm in adolescents: a randomized controlled trial. *Journal of the American Academy of Child and Adolescent Psychiatry, 51*, 1304–1313.

Rubin, K., Booth, L., Zahn-Waxler, C., Cummings, M., & Wilkinson, M. (1991). Dyadic play behaviors of children of well and depressed mothers. *Development and Psychopathology, 3*, 243–251.

Rudolph, K. D., Hammen, C., & Burge, D. (1994). Interpersonal functioning and depressive symptoms in childhood: Addressing the issues of specificity and comorbidity. *Journal of Abnormal Child Psychology, 22*, 355–371.

Rueter, M. A., Scaramella, L., Wallace, L. E., & Conger, R. D. (1999). First onset of depressive or anxiety disorders predicted by the longitudinal course of internalizing symptoms and parent–adolescent disagreements. *Archives of General Psychiatry, 56*, 726–732.

Rush, A. J., Fava, M., Wisniewski, S. R., Lavori, P. W., Trivedi, M. H., Sackeim, H. A., . . . Niederehe, G. (2004). Sequenced Treatment Alternatives to Relieve Depression (STAR*D), rationale and design. *Controlled Clinical Trials, 25*, 119–142.

Rush, A. J., Trivedi, M. H., Wisniewski, S. R., Nierenberg, A. A., Stewart, J. W., Warden, D., . . . Fava, M. (2006). Acute and longer-term outcomes in depressed outpatients requiring one or several treatment steps: A STAR*D report. *American Journal of Psychiatry, 163*, 1905–1917.

Rutter, M. (1996), Connections between child and adult psychopathology. *European Child & Adolescent Psychiatry, 5*(Suppl 1), 4–7.

Rynn, M. A., Findling, R. L., Emslie, G. J., & Marcus, R. N. (2002). Efficacy and safety of nefazodone in adolescent with MDD (Abstract NR57). Proceedings of the 155th Annual Meeting of the American Psychiatric Association (Philadelphia, PA, May 18–23): New Research. American Psychiatric Press.

Sachs, G. S., Baldassano, C. F., et al. (2000). Comorbidity of attention deficit hyperactivity disorder with early and late-onset bipolar disorder. *American Journal of Psychiatry, 157*(3), 466–468.

Safer, D. J., & Zito, J. M. (2006). Treatment-emergent adverse events from selective serotonin reuptake inhibitors by age group: Children versus adolescents. *Journal of Child and Adolescent Psychopharmacology, 16*(1-2), 159–169.

Sala, R., et al. (2010). Comorbid anxiety in children and adolescents with bipolar spectrum disorders: Prevalence and clinical correlates. *Journal of Clinical Psychiatry, 71*(10), 1344.

Salminen, J. K., Karlsson, H., Hietala, J., Kajander, J., Aalto, S., Markkula, J., Rasi-Hakala, H., & Toikka, T. (2008). Short-term psychodynamic psychotherapy and fluoxetine in major depressive disorder: A randomized comparative study. *Psychotherapy & Psychosomatics, 77*(6), 351–357.

Saulsberry, A., Marko-Holguin, M., Blomeke, K., et al. (2013). Randomized clinical trial of a primary care Internet-based intervention to prevent adolescent depression: One-year outcomes. *Journal of the Canadian Academy of Child & Adolescent Psychiatry, 22*, 106–117.

Sawyer, M. G., Harchak, T. F., Spence, S. H., Bond, L., Graetz, B., Kay, D., Patton, G., & Sheffield, J. (2009). School-based prevention of depression: A 2-year follow-up of a randomized controlled trial of the beyondblue schools research initiative. *Journal of Adolescent Health, 47*, 297–304.

Sawyer, M. G., Pfeiffer, S., Spence, S. H., Bond, L., Graetz, B., Kay, D., Patton, G., & Sheffield, J. (2010). School-based prevention of depression: A randomised controlled study of the beyondblue schools research initiative. *Journal of Child Psychology and Psychiatry, 51*, 199–209.

Scambler, P. J., Kelly, D., Lindsay, E., Williamson, R., Goldberg, R., Shprintzen, R., ... Burn, J. (1992). Velo-cardio-facial syndrome associated with chromosome 22 deletions encompassing the DiGeorge locus. *Lancet, 339*(8802), 1138–1139.

Schneider, L. S., Cooper, T. B., Staples, F. R., & Sloane, R. B. (1987). Prediction of individual dosage of nortriptyline in depressed elderly outpatients. *Journal of Clinical Psychopharmacology, 7*(5), 311–314.

Schoenbach, V. J., Kaplan, B. H., Grimson, R. C., & Wagner, E. H. (1982). Use of a symptom scale to study the prevalence of a depressive syndrome in young adolescents. *American Journal of Epidemiology, 116*(5), 791–800.

Schürhoff, F., Bellivier, F., Jouvent, R., Mouren-Siméoni, M. C., Bouvard, M., Allilaire, J. F., & Leboyer, M. (2000). Early and late onset bipolar disorders: Two different forms of manic-depressive illness? *Journal of Affective Disorders, 58*(3), 215–221.

Schwarz, J. C., Barton-Henry, M. L., & Pruzinsky, T. (1985). Assessing child-rearing behaviors: a comparison of ratings made by mother, father, child, and sibling on the CRPBI. *Child Development, 56*(2), 462–479.

Sedlack, A. J., & Broadhurst, D. D. (1996). *Executive summary of the Third National Incidence Study of Child Abuse and Neglect.* Washington, DC: U.S. Department of Health and Human Services, Administration for Children and Families, Administration on Children, Youth and Families, National Center on Child Abuse and Neglect.

Severus, E., Taylor, M. J., Sauer, C., Pfennig, A., Ritter, P., Bauer, M., & Geddes, J. R. (2014). Lithium for prevention of mood episodes in bipolar disorders: Systematic review and meta-analysis. *International Journal of Bipolar Disorder, 2*, 15.

Shaffer, D., Gould, M., et al. (1996). Psychiatric diagnosis in child and adolescent suicide. *Archives of General Psychiatry, 53*(4), 339–348.

Shapiro, D. A., Barkham, M., Rees, A., Hardy, G. E., Reynolds, S., & Startup, M. (1994). Effects of treatment duration and severity of depression on the effectiveness of cognitive-behavioral and psychodynamic-interpersonal psychotherapy. *Journal of Consulting and Clinical Psychology, 62*(3), 522–534.

Shaw, B. F. (1977). Comparison of cognitive therapy and behavior therapy in the treatment of depression. *Journal of Consulting and Clinical Psychology, 45*(4), 543–551.

Sheeber, L., Hops, H., Albert, A., Davis, B., & Andrews, J. (1997). Family support and conflict: Prospective relations to adolescent depression. *Journal of Abnormal Child Psychology, 25*, 333–344.

Sheeber, L., Hops, H., & Davis, B. (2001), Family processes in adolescent depression. *Clinical Child and Family Psychology Review, 4*(1), 19–35.

Sheets, E. S., Craighead, L. W., Brosse, A. L., Hauser, M., Madsen, J. W., & Craighead, W. E. (2013). Prevention of recurrence of major depression among emerging adults by a group cognitive-behavioral/interpersonal intervention. *Journal of Affective Disorders, 147*(1), 425–430.

Shirk, S. R., Boergers, J., Eason, A., & Van Horn, M. (1998). Dysphoric interpersonal schemata and preadolescents' sensitization to negative events. *Journal of Clinical Child Psychology, 27*(1), 54–68.

Shochet, I. M., Dadds, M. R., Holland, D., Whitefield, K., Harnett, P. H., & Osgarby, S. (2001). The efficacy of a universal school-based program to prevent adolescent depression. *Journal of Clinical Child Psychology, 30*, 303–315.

Shpigel, M. S., Diamond, G. M., & Diamond, G. S. (2012). Changes in parenting behaviors, attachment, depressive symptoms, and suicidal ideation in attachment-based family therapy for depressive and suicidal adolescents. *Journal of Marital & Family Therapy, 38*(Suppl 1), 271–283.

Silberg, J., Pickles, A., Rutter, M., Hewitt, J., Simonoff, E., Maes, H., ... Eaves, L. (1999). The influence of genetic factors and life stress on depression among adolescent girls. *Archives of General Psychiatry, 56*(3), 225–232.

Sim, K., Lau, W. K., Sim, J., Sum, M. Y., & Baldessarini, R. J. (2015). Prevention of relapse and recurrence in adults with major depressive disorder: Systematic review and meta-analyses of controlled trials. *International Journal of Neuropsychopharmacology*, July, 1–13.

Simeonova, D. I., et al. (2009). Subcortical volumetric correlates of anxiety in familial pediatric bipolar disorder: A preliminary investigation. *Psychiatry Research: Neuroimaging, 173*(2), 113–120.

Simons, A. D., Murphy, G. E., Levine, J. L., & Wetzel, R. D. (1986). Cognitive therapy and pharmacotherapy for depression: Sustained improvement over one year. *Archives of General Psychiatry, 43*(1), 43–48.

Smoller, J. W., & Finn, C. T. (2003). Family, twin, and adoption studies of bipolar disorder. *American Journal of Medical Genetics Part C: Seminars in Medical Genetics*, *123*(1), 48–58.

Smoller, J. W., & Gardner-Schuster, E. (2007). Genetics of bipolar disorder. *Current Psychiatry Reports*, *9*(6), 504–511.

Solantaus, T., & Toikka, S. (2006). The Effective Family Programme: Preventive services for children of mentally ill parents in Finland. *International Journal of Mental Health Promotion*, *8*, 37–44.

Soutullo, C. A., Chang, K. D., Díez-Suárez, A., Figueroa-Quintana, A., Escamilla-Canales, I., Rapado-Castro, M., & Ortuño, F. (2005). Bipolar disorder in children and adolescents: International perspective on epidemiology and phenomenology. *Bipolar Disorders*, *7*(6), 497–506.

Spence, S., Najman, J. M., Bor, W., O'Callaghan, M. J., & Williams, G. M. (2002). Maternal anxiety and depression, poverty and marital relationship factors during early childhood as predictors of anxiety and depressive symptoms in adolescence. *Journal of Child Psychology and Psychiatry and Allied Disciplines*, *43*, 457–469.

Spence, S. H., Sawyer, M. G., Sheffield, J., Patton, G., Bond, L., Graetz, B., & Kay, D.(2014). Does the absence of a supportive family environment influence the outcome of a universal intervention for the prevention of depression? *International Journal of Environmental Research and Public Health*, *11*, 5113–5132.

Spence, S. H., Sheffield, J. K., & Donovan, C. L. (2003). Preventing adolescent depression: An evaluation of the problem solving for life program. *Journal of Consulting and Clinical Psychology*, *71*, 3–13.

Spence, S. H., & Shortt, A. L. (2007). Research review: Can we justify the widespread dissemination of universal, school-based interventions for the prevention of depression among children and adolescents? *Journal of Child Psychology and Psychiatry*, *48*(6), 526–542.

Spencer, T. J. (2006). ADHD and comorbidity in childhood. *Journal of Clinical Psychiatry*, *67*(Suppl 8), 27–31.

Spencer, T., Biederman, J., & Wilens, T. (1999). Attention-deficit/hyperactivity disorder and comorbidity. *Pediatrics Clinics of North America*, *46*(5), 915–927.

Spinelli, M. G., & Endicott, J. (2003). Controlled clinical trial or interpersonal psychotherapy versus parenting education program for depressed pregnant women. *American Journal of Psychiatry*, *160*(3), 555–562.

Stanger, C., McConaughy, S. H., & Achenbach, M. (1992). Three-year course of behavioral/emotional problems in a national sample of 4- to 16-year-olds: II. Predictors of syndromes. *Journal of the American Academy of Child and Adolescent Psychiatry*, *31*, 941–950.

Stark, K. D., Humphrey, L. L., Crook, K., & Lewis, K. (1990). Perceived family environments of depressed and anxious children: Child's and maternal figure's perspectives. *Journal of Abnormal Child Psychology*, *18*(5), 527–547.

St. Clair, M. C., Croudace, T., Dunn, V. J., Jones, P. B., Herbert, J., & Goodyer, I. M. (2015). Childhood adversity subtypes and depressive symptoms in early and late adolescence. *Development and Psychopathology*, *27*, 885–899.

Stein, D., Williamson, D. E., Birmaher, B., Brent, D. A., Kaufman, J., Dahl, R. E., et al. (2000). Parent–child bonding and family functioning in depressed children and children at high risk and low risk for future depression. *Journal of the American Academy of Child and Adolescent Psychiatry*, *39*, 1387–1395.

Steingard, R. J., Renshaw, P. F., Hennen, J., Lenox, M., Cintron, C. B., Young, A. D., ... Yurgelun-Todd, D. A. (2002). Smaller frontal lobe white matter volumes in depressed adolescents. *Biological Psychiatry*, *52*(5), 413–417.

Stice, E., Shaw, H., Bohon, C., Marti, C. N., & Rohde, P. (2009). A meta-analytic review of depression prevention programs for children and adolescents: Factors that predict magnitude of intervention effects. *Journal of Consulting and Clinical Psychology*, *77*, 486–503.

Strober, M. (1992). Relevance of early age-of-onset in genetic studies of bipolar affective disorder. *Journal of the American Academy of Child and Adolescent Psychiatry*, *31*(4), 606–610.

Strober, M., & Carlson, G. (1982). Bipolar illness in adolescents with major depression: Clinical, genetic, and psychopharmacologic predictors in a threeto four-year prospective follow-up investigation. *Archives of General Psychiatry*, *39*, 549–555.

Strober, M., Morrell, W., Burroughs, J., Lampert, C., Danforth, H., & Freeman, R. (1988). A family study of bipolar I disorder in adolescence: Early onset of symptoms linked to increased familial loading and lithium resistance. *Journal of Affective Disorders*, *15*, 255–268.

Strober, M., Morrell, W., Lampert, C., & Burroughs, J. (1990). Relapse following discontinuation of lithium maintenance therapy in adolescents with bipolar I illness: A naturalistic study. *American Journal of Psychiatry*, *147*, 457–461.

Takahashi, L. K., Baker, E. W., & Kalin, N. H. (1990). Ontogeny of behavioral and hormonal responses to stress in prenatally stressed male rat pups. *Physiology and Behavior, 47*, 357–364.

Tang, T. C., Jou, S. H., Ko, C. H., Huang, S. Y., & Yen, C. F. (2009). Randomized study of school-based intensive interpersonal psychotherapy for depressed adolescents with suicidal risk and parasuicide behaviors. *Psychiatry & Clinical Neurosciences, 63*, 463–470.

Tanner, J. M. (1962). *Growth at adolescence: With a general consideration of effects of hereditary and environmental factors upon growth and maturation from birth to maturity.* Oxford: Blackwell Scientific Publications.

Tatro, E. T., Everall, I. P., Kaul, M., & Achim, C. L. (2009). Modulation of glucocorticoid receptor nuclear translocation in neurons by immunophilins FKBP51 and FKBP52: Implications for major depressive disorder. *Brain Research, 1286*, 1–12.

Teasdale, J. D., Segal, Z. V., Williams, J. M. G., Ridgeway, V. A., Soulsby, J. M., & Lau, M. A. (2000). Prevention of relapse/recurrence in major depression by mindfulness-based cognitive therapy. *Journal of Consulting and Clinical Psychology, 68*(4), 615–623.

Teicher, M. H. (2002). Scars that won't heal: The neurobiology of child abuse. *Scientific American, 286*(3), 68–75.

Teti, D. M., Gelfand, D. M., Messinger, D., & Isabella, R. (1995). Maternal depression and the quality of early attachment: An examination of infants, preschoolers and their mothers. *Developmental Psychology, 31*, 364–376.

Thase, M. E., Entsuah, A. R., & Rudolph, R. L. (2001). Remission rates during treatment with venlafaxine or selective serotonin reuptake inhibitors. *British Journal of Psychiatry, 178*, 234–241.

Thompson, L. W., Gallagher, D., & Breckenridge, J. S. (1987). Comparative effectiveness of psychotherapies for depressed elders. *Journal of Consulting and Clinical Psychology, 55*(3), 385–390.

Thompson, R. D., Craig, A., Crawford, E. A., et al. (2012). Longitudinal results of cognitive behavioral treatment for youths with inflammatory bowel disease and depressive symptoms. *Journal of Clinical Psychology in Medical Settings, 19*, 329–337.

Tillman, R., & Geller, B. (2006). Controlled study of switching from attention-deficit/hyperactivity disorder to a prepubertal and early adolescent bipolar I disorder phenotype during 6-year prospective follow-up: Rate, risk, and predictors. *Development and Psychopathology, 18*(4), 1037–1053.

Tillman, R., Geller, B., Bolhofner, K., Craney, J. L., Williams, J. L., & Zimerman, B. (2003). Ages of onset and rates of syndromal and subsyndromal comorbid DSM-IV diagnoses in a prepubertal and early adolescent bipolar disorder phenotype. *Journal of the American Academy of Child and Adolescent Psychiatry, 42*(12), 1486–1493.

Todd, R., Neuman, R., et al. (1993). Genetic studies of affective disorders: Should we be starting with childhood onset probands? *Journal of the American Academy of Child and Adolescent Psychiatry, 32*(6), 1164–1171.

Todd, R. D., Reich, W., Petti, T. A., Joshi, P., DePaulo, J. R., Nurneberger, J., & Reich, T. (1996). Psychiatric diagnoses in the child and adolescent members extended families identified through adult bipolar affective disorder probands. *Journal of the American Academy of Child and Adolescent Psychiatry, 35*, 664–671.

Trad, P. V. (1987). *Infant and childhood depression: Developmental factors.* New York: John Wiley & Sons.

Trad, P. V. (1994). Save our children. *American Journal of Psychotherapy, 48*, 175–178.

Treatment for Adolescents With Depression Study Team. (2003). Rationale, design, and methods. *Journal of the American Academy of Child and Adolescent Psychiatry, 42*, 531–542.

Treatment for Adolescents With Depression Study Team. (2004). Fluoxetine, cognitive-behavioral therapy, and their combination for adolescents with depression. *Journal of the American Medical Association, 292*, 807–820.

Treatment for Adolescents With Depression Study Team. (2009). Outcomes over 1 year of naturalistic follow-up. *American Journal of Psychiatry, 166*(10), 1141–1149.

Turner, R. J., & Lloyd, D. A. (1999). The stress process and the social distribution of depression. *Journal of Health and Social Behavior, 40*, 374–404.

Twenge, J. M., & Nolen-Hoeksema, S. (2002). Age, gender, race, socioeconomic status, and birth cohort difference on the Children's Depression Inventory: A meta-analysis. *Journal of Abnormal Psychology, 111*(4), 578.

Velez, C. N., Johnson, J., & Cohen, P. (1989). A longitudinal analysis of selected risk factors for childhood psychopathology. *Journal of the American Academy of Child & Adolescent Psychiatry, 28*(6), 861–864.

Vincent, J. B., Paterson, A. D., Strong, E., Petronis, A., & Kennedy, J. L. (2000). The unstable trinucleotide repeat story of major psychosis. *American Journal of Medical Genetics, 97*(1), 77–97.

Vitaro, F., Pelletier, D., Gagnon, C., & Baron, P. (1995). Correlates of depressive symptoms in early adolescence. *Journal of Emotional and Behavioral Disorders, 3*, 241–251.

Vittengl, J. R., Clark, L. A., Dunn, T. W., & Jarrett, R. B. (2007). Reducing relapse and recurrence in unipolar depression: A comparative meta-analysis of cognitive–behavioral therapy's effects. *Journal of Consulting and Clinical Psychology, 75*(3), 475–488.

Vythilingam, M., Heim, C., Newport, J., Miller, A. H., Anderson, E., Bronen, R., et al. (2002). Childhood trauma associated with smaller hippocampal volume in women with major depression. *American Journal of Psychiatry, 159*, 2072–2080.

Wagner, K. D., & Ambrosini, P. J. (2001). Childhood depression: Pharmacological therapy/treatment (pharmacotherapy of childhood depression). *Journal of Clinical Child Psychology, 30*(1), 88–97.

Wagner, K. D., Jonas, J., Findling, R. L., Ventura, D., & Saikali, K. (2006). A double-blind, randomized, placebo-controlled trial of escitalopram in the treatment of pediatric depression. *Journal of the American Academy of Child and Adolescent Psychiatry, 45*, 280–288.

Wagner, K. D., Kowatch, R. A., Emslie, G. J., Findling, R. L., Wilens, T. E., McCague K, ... Linden, D. (2006). A double-blind, randomized, placebo-controlled trial of oxcarbazepine in the treatment of bipolar disorder in children and adolescents. *American Journal of Psychiatry, 163*, 1179–1186.

Wagner, K. D., Robb, A. S., Findling, R. L., et al. (2004). A randomized, placebo-controlled trial of citalopram for the treatment of major depression in children and adolescents. *American Journal of Psychiatry, 161*, 1079–1083.

Walker, L. S., Garber, J., & Greene, J. W. (1993). Psychosocial correlates of recurrent childhood pain: A comparison of pediatric patients with recurrent abdominal pain, organic illness, and psychiatric disorders. *Journal of Abnormal Psychology, 102*, 248–258.

Warner, V., Weissman, M. M., Mufson, L., & Wickramaratne, P. J. (1999). Grandparents, parents, and grandchildren at high risk for depression: A three-generation study. *Journal of the American Academy of Child & Adolescent Psychiatry, 38*(3), 289–296.

Watson, D., & Tellegen, A. (1985). Toward a consensual structure of mood. *Psychological Bulletin, 98*, 219–235.

Webster-Stratton, C., & Hammond, M. (1988). Maternal depression and its relationship to life stress, perceptions of child behavior problems, parenting behaviors, and child conduct problems. *Journal of Abnormal Child Psychology, 16*, 299–315.

Weersing, V. R., & Brent, D. A. (2006). Cognitive behavioral therapy for depression in youth. *Child and Adolescent Psychiatric Clinics of North America, 15*, 939–957.

Wegbreit, E., Cushman, G. K., Puzia, M. E., et al. (2014), Developmental meta-analyses of the functional neural correlates of bipolar disorder. *JAMA Psychiatry, 71*(8), 926–935.

Weissman, M. M., Berry, O. O., Warner, V., Gameroff, M. J., Skipper, J., Talati, A., . . . Wickramaratne, P. (2016). A 30-year study of 3 generations at high risk and low risk for depression. *JAMA Psychiatry*, 73, 970–977.

Weissman, M. M., Wolk, S., Goldstein, R. B., Moreau, D., Adams, P., Greenwald, S., ... Wickramaratne, P. J. (1999a). Depressed adolescents grown up. *Journal of the American Medical Association, 281*, 1707–1713.

Weissman, M. M., Wolk, S., Wickramaratne, P., Goldstein, R. B., Adams, P., Greenwald, S., ... Steinberg, D. (1999). Children with prepubertal-onset major depressive disorder and anxiety grown up. *Archives of General Psychiatry, 56*(9), 794–801.

Weisz, J. R., Kuppens, S., Eckshtain, D., Ugeto, A. M., Hawley, K. M., & Jensen-Doss, A. (2013). Performance of evidence-based youth psychotherapies compared with usual clinical care: A multilevel meta-analysis. *JAMA Psychiatry, 70*, 750–761.

Weisz, J. R., McCarty, C. A., & Valeri, S. M. (2006). Effects of psychotherapy for depression in children and adolescents: A meta-analysis. *Psychological Bulletin, 132*, 132–149.

Weisz, J. R., Southam-Gerow, M. A., Gordis, E. B., et al. (2009). Cognitive-behavioral therapy versus usual clinical care for youth depression: An initial test of transportability to community clinics and clinicians. *Journal of Consulting and Clinical Psychology, 77*, 383–396.

Weisz, J. R., Southam-Gerow, M. A., & McCarty, C. A. (2001). Control-related beliefs and self-reported depressive symptoms in clinic-referred children and adolescents. *Journal of Abnormal Psychology, 110*, 97–109.

Weller, R. A., & Weller, E. B. (1986). Tricyclic antidepressants in prepubertal depressed children: Review of the literature. *Hillside Journal of Clinical Psychiatry*, *8*(1), 46–55.

Weller, R. A., Weller, E. B., et al. (1986). Mania in prepubertal children: Has it been underdiagnosed? *Journal of Affective Disorders*, *11*, 151–154.

Wen, X. J., Wang, L. M., Liu, Z. L., Huang, A., Liu, Y. Y., & Hu, J. Y. (2014). Meta-analysis on the efficacy and tolerability of the augmentation of antidepressants with atypical antipsychotics in patients with major depressive disorder. *Brazilian Journal of Medical and Biological Research*, *47*(7), 605–616.

West, A. E., & Pavuluri, M. N. (2009). Psychosocial treatment for childhood and adolescent bipolar disorder. *Child and Adolescent Psychiatric Clinics of North America*, *18*, 471–482.

West, S., McElroy, S., Strakowski, S., Keck, P., & McConville, B. (1995). Attention deficit hyperactivity disorder in adolescent mania. *American Journal of Psychiatry*, *152*(2), 271–274.

West, S. A., Strakowski, S. M., et al. (1996). Phenomenology and comorbidity of adolescents hospitalized for the treatment of acute mania. *Biological Psychiatry*, *39*, 458–460.

Whiffen, V. E., & Clark, S. E. (1997). Does victimization account for sex differences in depressive symptoms? *British Journal of Clinical Psychology*, *36*(Pt 2), 185–193.

Wicki, W., & Angst, J. (1991). The Zurich study. X. Hypomania in a 28- to 30-year-old cohort. *European Archives of Psychiatry and Clinical Neuroscience*, *240*, 339–348.

Wickrama, K. A. S., Noh, S., & Elder, G. H. (2009). An investigation of family SES-based inequalities in depressive symptoms from early adolescence to emerging adulthood. *Advances in Life Course Research*, *14*(4), 147–161.

Wilens, T., Biederman, J., Abrantes, A. M., & Spencer, T. J. (1997). Clinical characteristics of psychiatrically referred adolescent outpatients with substance use disorder. *Journal of the American Academy of Child and Adolescent Psychiatry*, *36*(7), 941–947.

Wilens, T. E., Biederman, J., Kwon, A., Ditterline, J., Forkner, P., Moore, H., . . . Faraone, S. V. (2004). Risk of substance use disorders in adolescents with bipolar disorder. *Journal of the American Academy of Child & Adolescent Psychiatry 43*(11), 1380–1386.

Wilens, T. E., Biederman, J., Mick, E., Faraone, S. V., & Spencer, T. (1997). Attention deficit hyperactivity disorder (ADHD) is associated with early-onset substance use disorders. *Journal of Nervous and Mental Diseases*, *185*(8), 475–482.

Wilens, T., Biederman, J., Millstein, R. B., Wozniak, J., Hahesy, A. L., & Spencer, T. J. (1999). Risk for substance use disorders in youths with childand adolescent-onset bipolar disorder. *Journal of the American Academy of Child and Adolescent Psychiatry*, *36*(6), 680–685.

Wilkinson, P., Kelvin, R., Roberts, C., Dubicka, B., & Goodyer, I. (2011). Clinical and psychosocial predictors of suicide attempts and nonsuicidal self-injury in the Adolescent Depression Antidepressants and Psychotherapy Trial (ADAPT). *American Journal of Psychiatry*, *168*, 495–501.

Wood, A., Harrington, R., & Moore, A. (1996). Controlled trial of a brief cognitive-behavioural intervention in adolescent patients with depressive disorders. *Journal of Child Psychology and Psychiatry*, *37*, 737–746.

World Health Organization. (2008). *The global burden of disease: 2004 update*. Geneva, Switzerland: WHO Press.

Wozniak, J., Biederman, J., Faraone, S. V., Blier, H., & Monuteaux, M. C. (2001). Heterogeneity of childhood conduct disorder: Further evidence of a subtype of conduct disorder linked to bipolar disorder. *Journal of Affective Disorders*, *64*, 121–131.

Wozniak, J., Crawford, M. H., Biederman, J., et al. (1999). Antecedents and complications of trauma in boys with ADHD: Findings from a longitudinal study. *Journal of the American Academy of Child and Adolescent Psychiatry*, *38*, 48–55.

Young, J. F., Gallop, R., & Mufson, L. (2009). Mother-child conflict and its moderating effects on depression outcomes in a preventive intervention for adolescent depression. *Journal of Clinical Child and Adolescent Psychology*, *38*, 696–704.

Young, L., Cooke, R., et al. (1993). Anxious and non-anxious bipolar disorder. *Journal of Affective Disorders*, *29*(1), 49–52.

Youngstrom, E. A., Birmaher, B., & Findling, R. L. (2008). Pediatric bipolar disorder: Validity, phenomenology, and recommendations for diagnosis. *Bipolar Disorders*, *10*(p2), 194–214.

Youngstrom, E., Meyers, O., Demeter, C., Youngstrom, J., Morello, L., Piiparinen, R., . . . Findling, R. L. (2005). Comparing diagnostic checklists for pediatric bipolar disorder in academic and community mental health settings. *Bipolar Disorders*, *7*(6), 507–517.

Zeni, C. P., Mwangi, B., Cao, B., Hasan, K. M., Walss-Bass, C., Zunta-Soares, G., & Soares, J. C. (2016). Interaction between BDNF rs6265 Met allele and low family cohesion is associated with smaller left hippocampal volume in pediatric bipolar disorder. *Journal of Affective Disorders, 189*, 94–97.

Zhou, X., Hetrick S. E., Cuipers, P., Qin, B., Barth, J., Whittington, C. G., ... Xie, P. (2015). Comparative efficacy and acceptability of psychotherapies for depression in children and adolescents: A systematic review and network meta-analysis. *World Psychiatry, 14*, 207–222.

Part II: Schizophrenia

Addington, A., & Rapoport, J. (2009) The genetics of childhood-onset schizophrenia: When madness strikes the prepubescent. *Current Psychiatry Reports, 11*, 156–161.

Addington, D., Addington, J., & Patten, S. (1998). Depression in people with first-episode schizophrenia. *British Journal of Psychiatry Suppl, 172*, 90–92.

Addington, J. (2002). Draft consensus statement: Principles and practice in early psychosis. In J. Edwards & P. McGorry (Eds.), *Implementing early intervention in psychosis: A guide to establishing early psychosis services* (1st ed., pp. 145–155). London: Martin Dunitz.

Addington, J., & Addington, D. (1998). Effect of substance misuse in early psychosis. *British Journal of Psychiatry Suppl, 172*, 134–136.

Addington, J., & Heinssen, R. (2012). Prodromal risk syndrome: Prediction and prevention. *Annual Review of Clinical Psychology, 8*, 269–289.

Addington, J., Penn, D., Woods, S. W., Addington, D., & Perkins, D. (2008). Facial affect recognition in individuals at clinical high risk for psychosis. *British Journal of Psychiatry, 192*, 67–68.

Adler, L. E., & Waldo, M. C. (1991). Counterpoint: Sensory gating-hippocampal model of schizophrenia. *Schizophrenia Bulletin, 17*, 19–24.

Adler, L. E., Waldo, M. C., & Freeman, R. (1985). Neurophysiological studies of sensory gating in schizophrenia: Comparison of auditory and visual responses. *Biological Psychiatry, 20*, 1284–1296.

Agid, O., Arenovich, T., Sajeev, G., Zipursky, R. B., Kapur, S., Foussias, G., & Remington, G. (2011). An algorithm-based approach to first-episode schizophrenia: Response rates over 3 antipsychotic trials with a retrospective data analysis. *Journal of Clinical Psychiatry, 72*, 1439–1944.

Ahn, K., Gogtay, N., Andersen, T., Anvari, A., Gochman, P., Lee,Y., ... Rapoport, J. (2014). High rate of disease-related copy number variations in childhood-onset schizophrenia. *Molecular Psychiatry, 19*(5), 568–572.

Akil, M., Kolachana, B. S., Rothmond, D. A., Hyde, T. M., Weinberger, D. R., & Kleinman, J. E. (2003). Catechol-O-methyltransferase genotype and dopamine regulation in the human brain. *Journal of Neuroscience, 23*, 2008–2013.

Alaghband-Rad, J., McKenna, K., Gordon, C. T., Albus, K. E., Hamburger, S. D., Rumsey, J. M., ... Rapoport, J. L. (1995). Childhood-onset schizophrenia: The severity of premorbid course. *Journal of the American Academy of Child and Adolescent Psychiatry, 34*, 1273–1283.

Alexander, G. E., & Crutcher, M. D. (1990). Functional architecture of basal ganglia circuits: Neural substrates of parallel processing [Review]. *Trends in Neuroscience, 13*, 266–271.

Ambelas, A. (1992). Preschizophrenics: Adding to the evidence, sharpening the focus. *British Journal of Psychiatry, 160*, 401–404.

Amin, S., Singh, S. P., Brewin, J., Jones, P. B., Medley, I., & Harrison, G. (1999). Diagnostic stability of first-episode psychosis. Comparison of ICD-10 and DSM-III-R systems. *British Journal of Psychiatry, 175*, 537–543.

An, S. K., Kang, J. I., Park, J. Y., Kim, K. R., Lee, S. Y., & Lee, E. (2010). Attribution bias in ultra-high risk for psychosis and first-episode schizophrenia. *Schizophrenia Research, 118*, 54–61.

Andreasen, N. C. (1986). *Can schizophrenia be localized in the brain?* Washington, DC: American Psychiatric Press, Inc.

Andreasen, N. C. (1999). A unitary model of schizophrenia: Bleuler's "fragmented phrene" as schizencephaly. *Archives of General Psychiatry, 56*, 781–787.

Andreasen, N. C., Arndt, S., Alliger, R., Miller, D., & Flaum, M. (1995a). Symptoms of schizophrenia: Methods, meanings, and mechanisms. *Archives of General Psychiatry, 52*, 341–351.

Andreasen, N. C., Nopoulos, P., Magnotta, V., Pierson, R., Ziebell, S., & Ho, B. C. (2011). Progressive brain change in schizophrenia: A prospective longitudinal study of first-episode schizophrenia. *Biological Psychiatry, 70*, 672–679.

Andreasen, N. C., O'Leary, D. S., Arndt, S., Cizadlo, T., Rezai, K., Watkins, G. L., Ponto, L. L., & Hichwa, R. D. (1995b). I. PET studies of memory: Novel and practiced free recall of complex narratives. *Neuroimage, 2*, 284–295.

Andreasen, N. C., O'Leary, D. S., Flaum, M., Nopoulos, P., Watkins, G. L., Boles Ponto, L. L., & Hichwa, R. D. (1997). Hypofrontality in schizophrenia: Distributed dysfunctional circuits in neuroleptic-naive patients. *Lancet, 349*, 1730–1734.

Andreasen, N. C., Olsen, S. A., & Dennert, J. W. (1982). Ventricular enlargement in schizophrenia: Relationship to positive and negative symptoms. *American Journal of Psychiatry, 139*, 297–302.

Andreasen, N. C., Rajarethinam, R., Cizadlo, T., Arndt, S., Swayze, V. W., Flashman, L. A., ... Yuh, W. T. (1996). Automatic atlas-based volume estimation of human brain regions from MR images. *Journal of Computer Assisted Tomography, 20*, 98–106.

Antshel, K. M., Fremont, W., Roizen, N. J., Shprintzen, R., Higgins, A. M., Dhamoon, A., & Kates, W. R. (2006). ADHD, major depressive disorder, and simple phobias are prevalent psychiatric conditions in youth with velo-cardio-facial syndrome. *Journal of the American Academy of Child & Adolescent Psychiatry*, 45, 596–603.

Arad, M., & Weiner, I. (2009). Disruption of latent inhibition induced by ovariectomy can be reversed by estradiol and clozapine as well as by co-administration of haloperidol with estradiol but not by haloperidol alone. *Psychopharmacology, 206*, 731–740.

Arndt, S., Alliger, R. J., & Andreasen, N. C. (1991). The distinction of positive and negative symptoms: The failure of a two-dimensional model. *British Journal of Psychiatry, 158*, 317–322.

Arndt, S., Andreasen, N. C., Flaum, M., Miller, D., & Nopoulos, P. (1995). A longitudinal study of symptom dimensions in schizophrenia: Prediction and patterns of change. *Archives of General Psychiatry, 52*, 352–360.

Arseneault, L., Cannon, M., Poulton, R., Murray, R., Caspi, A., & Moffitt, T. E. (2002). Cannabis use in adolescence and risk for adult psychosis: Longitudinal prospective study. *British Medical Journal, 325*, 1212–1213.

Arseneault, L., Cannon, M., Witton, J., & Murray, R. (2004). Causal association between cannabis and psychosis: Examination of the evidence. *British Journal of Psychiatry, 184*, 110–117.

Asarnow, J. (1988). Children at risk for schizophrenia: Converging lines of evidence. *Schizophrenia Bulletin, 14*, 613–631.

Asarnow, J. R. (1994). Annotation: Childhood-onset schizophrenia. *Journal of Child Psychology and Psychiatry, and Allied Disciplines, 35*, 1345–1371.

Asarnow, J. R., & Goldstein, M. J. (1986). Schizophrenia during adolescence and early adulthood: A developmental perspective on risk research. *Clinical Psychology Review, 6*, 211–235.

Asarnow, J. R., Tompson, M. C., & Goldstein, M. J. (2001). Psychosocial factors: The social context of child and adolescent-onset schizophrenia. In H. Remschmidt (Ed.), *Schizophrenia in children and adolescents (pp. 168–181)*. Cambridge, UK: Cambridge University Press.

Asarnow, J. R., Tompson, M., Hamilton, E. B., Goldstein, M. J., & Guthrie, D. (1994). Family-expressed emotion, childhood-onset depression, and childhood-onset schizophrenia spectrum disorders: Is expressed emotion a nonspecific correlate of child psychopathology or a specific risk factor for depression? *Journal of Abnormal Child Psychology, 22*, 129–146.

Asarnow, R. (1983). Schizophrenia. In R. Tartar (Ed.), *The child at psychiatric risk* (pp. 150–194). New York: Oxford University Press.

Asarnow, R., Brown W., & Strandburg, R. (1995). Children with a schizophrenic disorder: Neurobehavioral studies. *European Archives of Psychiatry and Clinical Neuroscience, 245*, 70–79.

Asarnow, R. F., Nuechterlein, K. H., Fogelson, D., Subotnik, K. L., Payne, D. A., Russell, ... Kendler, K. S. (2001). Schizophrenia and schizophrenia-spectrum personality disorders in the first-degree relatives of children with schizophrenia: The UCLA family study. *Archives of General Psychiatry, 58*, 581–588.

Asarnow, R., Steffy, R., MacCrimmon, D., & Cleghorn, J. (1978). An attentional assessment of foster children at risk for schizophrenia. In L. Wynne, R. Cromwell, & S. Matthysse (Eds.), *The nature of schizophrenia: New approaches to research and treatment* (p. 356). New York: John Wiley & Sons, Inc.

Asarnow, R., Tanguay, P., Bott, L., & Freeman, B. (1987). Patterns of intellectual functioning in non-retarded autistic and schizophrenic children. *Journal of Child Psychology and Psychiatry, and Allied Disciplines, 28*, 273–280.

Axelsson, R., & Lagerkvist-Briggs, M. (1992). Factors predicting suicide in psychotic patients. *European Archives of Psychiatry and Clinical Neuroscience, 241*, 259–266.

Aylward, E., Walker, E., & Bettes, B. (1984). Intelligence in schizophrenia: Meta-analysis of the research. *Schizophrenia Bulletin, 10*, 430–459.

Badenhop, R. F., Moses, M. J., Scimone, A., Mitchell, P. B., Ewen-White, K. R., Rosso, A., ... Schofield, P. R. (2002). A genome screen of 13 bipolar affective disorder pedigrees provides evidence for susceptibility loci on chromosome 3 as well as chromosomes 9, 13 and 19. *Molecular Psychiatry, 7*, 594–603.

Badner, J., & Gershon, E. (2002). Meta-analysis of whole-genome linkage scans of bipolar disorder and schizophrenia. *Molecular Psychiatry, 7*, 405–411.

Barbee, J. G., Mancuso, D. M., Freed, C. R., & Todorov, A. A. (1992). Alprazolam as a neuroleptic adjunct in the emergency treatment of schizophrenia. *American Journal of Psychiatry, 149*, 506–510.

Barch, D. M., & Ceaser, A. (2012). Cognition in schizophrenia: Core psychological and neural mechanisms. *Trends in Cognitive Science, 16*, 27–33.

Baribeau-Braun J., Picton T., & Gosselin J. (1983). Schizophrenia: A neurophysiological evaluation of abnormal information processing. *Science, 219*, 874–876.

Bassett, A. S., Chow, E. W., AbdelMalik, P., Gheorghiu, M., Husted, J., & Weksberg, R. (2003). The schizophrenia phenotype in 22q11 deletion syndrome. *American Journal of Psychiatry, 160*, 1580–1586.

Battaglia, J., Moss, S., Rush, J., Kang, J., Mendoza, R., Leedom, L., ... Goodman, L. (1997). Haloperidol, lorazepam, or both for psychotic agitation? A multicenter, prospective, double-blind, emergency department study. *American Journal of Emergency Medicine, 15*, 335–340.

Bauer, M., Praschak-Rieder, N., Kasper, S., & Willeit, M. (2012). Is dopamine neurotransmission altered in prodromal schizophrenia? A review of the evidence. *Current Pharmaceutical Design, 18*(12), 1568–1579.

Beck, A. T., Sokol, L., Clark, D. A., Berchick, R., & Wright, F. (1992). A crossover study of focused cognitive therapy for panic disorder. *American Journal of Psychiatry, 149*, 778–783.

Becker, H. E., Nieman, D. H., Wiltink, S., Dingemans, P. M., van de Fliert, J. R., Velthorst, E., ... Linszen, D. H. (2010). Neurocognitive functioning before and after the first psychotic episode: Does psychosis result in cognitive deterioration? *Psychological Medicine, 40*, 1599–1606.

Bellack, A. S., & Brown, S. A. (2001). Psychosocial treatments for schizophrenia. *Current Psychiatry Reports, 3*, 407–412.

Bellack, A. S., & Mueser, K. T. (1993). Psychosocial treatment for schizophrenia. *Schizophrenia Bulletin, 19*, 317–336.

Bentsen, H. (2003). Correspondence. *Psychological Medicine, 33*, 755.

Berenbaum, S. A., & Beltz, A. M. (2011). Sexual differentiation of human behavior: Effects of prenatal and pubertal organizational hormones. *Frontiers in Neuroendocrinology, 32*(2), 183–200.

Berk, M., Ichim, C., & Brook, S. (2001). Efficacy of mirtazapine add on therapy to haloperidol in the treatment of the negative symptoms of schizophrenia: A double-blind randomized placebo-controlled study. *International Clinical Psychopharmacology, 16*, 87–92.

Berman, K. F., Torrey, E. F., Daniel, D. G., & Weinberger, D. R. (1992). Regional cerebral blood flow in monozygotic twins discordant and concordant for schizophrenia. *Archives of General Psychiatry, 49*, 927–934.

Bertolino, A., Breier, A., Callicott, J. H., Adler, C., Mattay, V. S., Shapiro, M., ... Weinberger, D. R. (2000). The relationship between dorsolateral prefrontal neuronal N-acetylaspartate and evoked release of striatal dopamine in schizophrenia. *Neuropsychopharmacology, 22*, 125–132.

Bhana, N., Foster, R. H., Olney, R., & Plosker, G. L. (2001). Olanzapine: An updated review of its use in the management of schizophrenia. *Drugs, 61*, 111–161.

Bilder, R. M., Goldman, R. S., Robinson, D., Reiter, G., Bell, L., Bates, J. A., ... Lieberman, J. A. (2000). Neuropsychology of first-episode schizophrenia: Initial characterization and clinical correlates. *American Journal of Psychiatry, 157*, 549–559.

Bilder, R. M., Mukherjee, S., Rieder, R. O., & Pandurangi, A. K. (1985). Symptomatic and neuropsychological components of defect states. *Schizophrenia Bulletin, 11*, 409–491.

Birchwood, M., Todd, P., & Jackson, C. (1998). Early intervention in psychosis. The critical period hypothesis. *British Journal of Psychiatry Suppl, 172*, 53–59.

Blatter, D. D., Bigler, E. D., Gale, S. D., Johnson, S. C., Anderson, C. V., Burnett, B. M., ... Horn, S. D. (1995). Quantitative volumetric analysis of brain MR: Normative database spanning 5 decades of life. *American Journal of Neuroradiology, 16*, 241–251.

Bleuler, E. (1908). Die Prognose der Dementia Praecox. *Schizophreniegruppe. Allgemeine Zeitschrift fur Psychiatrie, 65*, 436–464. Translated in: J. Cutting & M. Shepherd, *The Clinical Roots of the Schizophrenia Concept* (1987), pp. 59–74. Cambridge: Cambridge University Press.

Bleuler, E. (1911). *Dementia praecox oder Gruppe der Schizophrenien*. Leipzig, Vienna: Deuticke. Translated as: Bleuler E. (1950). *Dementia Praecox or the group of schizophrenias*. New York: International University Press.

Bleuler, M. (1980). Schizophrenia-neurosis. *Deutsche Medizinische Wochenschrift, 105*, 209–212.

Bleuler, M. (1978). *The schizophrenic disorders: Long-term patient and family studies*. New Haven, CT: Yale University Press.

Bloemen, O. J., de Koning, M. B., Gleich, T., Meijer, J., de Haan, L., Linszen, D. H., ... van Amelsvoort, T. A. (2013). Striatal dopamine D2/3 receptor binding following dopamine depletion in subjects at ultra high risk for psychosis. *European Neuropsychopharmacology*, 23, 126–132.

Bloemen, O. J., de Koning, M. B., Schmitz, N., Nieman, D. H., Becker, H. E., de Haan, L., Dingemans, P., Linszen, D. H., & van Amelsvoort, T. A. (2010). White-matter markers for psychosis in a prospective ultra-high-risk cohort. *Psycholological Medicine, 40*, 1297–1304.

Booth, A., Johnson, D. R., Granger, D. A., Crouter, A., & McHale, S. (2003). Testosterone and child and adolescent adjustment: The moderating role of parent-child relationships. *Developmental Psychology, 39*, 85–98.

Borgwardt, S. J., Riecher-Rossler, A., Dazzan, P., Chitnis, X., Aston, J., Drewe, M., ... McGuire, P. K. (2007). Regional gray matter volume abnormalities in the at-risk mental state. *Biological Psychiatry, 61*, 1148–1156.

Botto, L. D., May, K., Fernhoff, P. M., Correa, A., Coleman, K., Rasmussen, S. A., ... Campbell, R. M. (2003). A population-based study of the 22q11. 2 deletion: Phenotype, incidence, and contribution to major birth defects in the population. *Pediatrics, 112*, 101–107.

Bourdon, K. H., Rae, D. S., Locke, B. Z., Narrow, W. E., & Regier, D. A. (1992). Estimating the prevalence of mental disorders in U.S. adults from the Epidemiologic Catchment Area Survey. *Public Health Report, 107*, 663–668.

Bracha, H. S., Torrey, E. F., Gottesman, I. I., Bigelow, L. B., & Cunniff, C. (1992). Second-trimester markers of fetal size in schizophrenia: A study of monozygotic twins. *American Journal of Psychiatry, 149*, 1355–1361.

Braff, D., Stone, C., Callaway, E., Geyer, M., Glick, I., & Bali, L. (1978). Prestimulus effects on human startle reflex in normals and schizophrenics. *Psychophysiology, 15*, 339–343.

Brent, B. K., Thermenos, H. W., Keshavan, M. S., & Seidman, L. J. (2013). Gray matter alterations in schizophrenia high-risk youth and early-onset schizophrenia: A review of structural MRI findings. *Child and Adolescence Psychiatric Clinics of North America, 22*, 689–714.

Brewer, W. J., Francey, S. M., Wood, S. J., Jackson, H. J., Pantelis, C., Phillips, L. J., ... McGorry, P. D. (2005). Memory impairments identified in people at ultra-high risk for psychosis who later develop first-episode psychosis. *American Journal of Psychiatry, 162*, 71–78.

Brown, G. W., Monck, E. M., Carstairs, G. M., & Wing, J. K. (1962). Influence of family life on the course of schizophrenic illness. *British Journal of Preventative and Social Medicine, 16*, 55–68.

Browne, S., Clarke, M., Gervin, M., Waddington, J. L., Larkin, C., & O'Callaghan E. (2000). Determinants of quality of life at first presentation with schizophrenia. *British Journal of Psychiatry, 176*, 173–176.

Bustillo, J. R., Lauriello, J., Horan, W. P., & Keith, S. J. (2001). The psychosocial treatment of schizophrenia: An update. *American Journal of Psychiatry, 158*, 163–175.

Bustillo, J. R., Lauriello, J., & Keith, S. J. (1999). Schizophrenia: Improving outcome. *Harvard Review of Psychiatry, 6*, 229–240.

Butzlaff, R. L., & Hooley, J. M. (1998). Expressed emotion and psychiatric relapse: A meta-analysis. *Archives of General Psychiatry, 55*, 547–552.

Callicott, J. H., Bertolino, A., Mattay, V. S., Langheim, F. J., Duyn, J., Coppola, R., ... Weinberger, D. R. (2000). Physiological dysfunction of the dorsolateral prefrontal cortex in schizophrenia revisited. *Cerebral Cortex, 10*, 1078–1092.

Cannon, M., Caspi, A., Moffitt, T. E., Harrington, H., Taylor A., & Murray, R. M. (2002). Evidence for early-childhood, pan-developmental impairment specific to schizophreniform disorder: Results from a longitudinal birth cohort. *Archives of General Psychiatry, 59*, 449–456.

Cannon, M., Jones, P., Gilvarry, C., Rifkin, L., McKenzie, K., Foerster, A., & Murray, R. (1997). Premorbid social functioning in schizophrenia and bipolar disorder. Similarities and differences. *American Journal of Psychiatry, 154*, 1544–1550.

Cannon, M., Jones, P., Huttunen, M., Tanskanen A., Huttunen, T., Rabe-Hesketh, S., & Murray, R. M. (1999). School performance in Finnish children and the later development of schizophrenia: A population-based longitudinal study. *Archives of General Psychiatry, 56*, 457–463.

Cannon, M., Jones, P., Huttunen, M., Tanskanen, A., & Murray, R. M. (1999). Motor coordination deficits as predictors of schizophrenia among Finnish school children. *Human Psychopharmacology, 14*, 491–497.

Cannon, T. D., Cadenhead, K., Cornblatt, B., Woods, S. W., Addington, J., Walker, E., ... Heinssen, R. (2008). Prediction of psychosis in youth at high clinical risk: A multisite longitudinal study in North America. *Archives of General Psychiatry, 65*, 28–37.

Cannon, T. D., Mednick, S. A., Parnas, J., Schulsinger, F., Praestholm, J., & Vestergaard, A. (1993). Developmental brain abnormalities in the offspring of schizophrenic mothers. I. Contributions of genetic and perinatal factors. *Archives of General Psychiatry, 50*, 551–564.

Cannon-Spoor, H. E., Potkin, S. G., & Wyatt, R. J. (1982). Measurement of premorbid adjustment in chronic schizophrenia. *Schizophrenia Bulletin, 8*, 470–484.

Cardno, A. G., Marshall, E. J., Coid, B., Macdonald, A. M., Ribchester, T. R., Davies, N. J., ... Murray, R. M. (1999). Heritability estimates for psychotic disorders. *Archives of General Psychiatry, 56*, 162–168.

Carletti, F., Woolley, J. B., Bhattacharyya, S., Perez-Iglesias, R., Fusar-Poli, P., Valmaggia, L., ... McGuire, P. K. (2012). Alterations in white matter evident before the onset of psychosis. *Schizophrenia Bulletin, 38*, 1170–1179.

Carpenter, W. T., Jr., Buchanan, R. W., Kirkpatrick, B., & Breier, A. F. (1999). Diazepam treatment of early signs of exacerbation in schizophrenia. *American Journal of Psychiatry, 156*, 299–303.

Caviness, V. S., Jr., Kennedy, D. N., Richelme, C., Rademacher, J., & Filipek, P. A. (1996). The human brain age 7–11 years: A volumetric analysis based on magnetic resonance images. *Cerebral Cortex, 6*, 726–736.

Censits, D. M., Ragland, J. D., Gur, R. C., & Gur, R. E. (1997). Neuropsychological evidence supporting a neurodevelopmental model of schizophrenia: A longitudinal study. *Schizophrenia Research, 24*, 289–298.

Chakos, M. H., Mayerhoff, D. I., Loebel, A. D., Alvir, J. M., & Lieberman, J. A. (1992). Incidence and correlates of acute extrapyramidal symptoms in first episode of schizophrenia. *Psychopharmacological Bulletin, 28*, 81–86.

Chouljian, T. L., Shumway, M., Balancio, E., Dwyer, E. V., Surber, R., & Jacobs, M. (1995). Substance use among schizophrenic outpatients: Prevalence, course, and relation to functional status. *Annals of Clinical Psychiatry, 7*, 19–24.

Chowdari, K. V., Mirnics, K., Semwal, P., Wood, J., Lawrence, E., Bhatia, T., ... Nimgaonkar, V. L. (2002). Association and linkage analyses of RGS4 polymorphisms in schizophrenia. *Human Molecular Genetics, 11*, 1373–1380.

Christison, G. W., Kirch, D. G., & Wyatt, R. J. (1991). When symptoms persist: Choosing among alternative somatic treatments for schizophrenia. *Schizophrenia Bulletin, 17*, 217–245.

Chumakov, I., Blumenfeld, M., Guerassimenko, O., Cavarec, L., et al. (2002). Genetic and physiological data implicating the new human gene G72 and the gene for D-amino acid oxidase in schizophrenia. *Proceedinsg of the National Academy of Science, U S A, 99*, 13675–13680.

Chung, Y. S., Kang, D. H., Shin, N. Y., Yoo, S. Y., & Kwon, J. S. (2008). Deficit of theory of mind in individuals at ultra-high-risk for schizophrenia. *Schizophrenia Research, 99*, 111–118.

Citrome, L., Levine, J., & Allingham, B. (2000). Changes in use of valproate and other mood stabilizers for patients with schizophrenia from 1994 to 1998. *Psychiatric Service, 51*, 634–638.

Clemmensen, L., Vernal, D. L., & Steinhausen, H. C. (2012). A systematic review of the long-term outcome of early onset schizophrenia. *BMC Psychiatry, 12*, 150–165.

Clouston, T. S. (1892). *Clinical lectures on mental diseases* (3rd ed.). London: Churchill.

Cohen, R. (1990). Event-related potentials and cognitive dysfunction in schizophrenia. In H. Hafner & W. Gattaz (Eds.), *Search for the causes of schizophrenia,* Vol. II. (pp. 342–360). New York/Berlin/Heidelberg: Springer.

Cohen, S., Lavelle, J., Rich, C. L., & Bromet, E. (1994). Rates and correlates of suicide attempts in first-admission psychotic patients. *Acta Psychiatrica Scandinavica, 90*, 167–171.

Connor, C., Birchwood, M., Freemantle, N., Palmer, C., Channa, S., Barker, C., ... Singh, S. (2016). Don't turn your back on the symptoms of psychosis: The results of a proof-of-principle, quasi-experimental intervention to reduce duration of untreated psychosis. *BMC Psychiatry, 16*, 127.

Cormac, I., Jones, C., & Campbell, C. (2002). Cognitive behaviour therapy for schizophrenia.

Cochrane Database of Systematic Reviews, (1):CD000524.

Cormac, I., Jones, C., Campbell, C., & Silveira da Mota Neto, J. (2004). Cognitive behaviour therapy for schizophrenia (Cochrane Review). In: *The Cochrane Library*, Issue 2. Oxford: Update Software.

Cornblatt, B. A. (2002). The New York high-risk project to the Hillside recognition and prevention (RAP) program. *American Journal of Medical Genetics, 114*, 956–966.

Cornblatt, B. A., Lencz, T., & Kane, J. M. (2001). Treatment of the schizophrenia prodrome: Is it presently ethical? *Schizophrenia Research, 51*, 31–38.

Cornblatt, B., Lenzenweger, M., Dworkin, R., & Erlenmeyer-Kimling, L. (1992). Childhood attentional dysfunctions predict social deficits in unaffected adults at risk for schizophrenia. *British Journal of Psychiatry, 161*, 59–64.

Cornblatt, B., & Obuchowski, M. (1997). Update of high-risk research: 1987–1997. *International Review of Psychiatry, 9*, 437–447.

Correll, C. U., Hauser, M., Auther, A. M., & Cornblatt, B. A. (2010). Research in people with psychosis risk syndrome: A review of the current evidence and future directions. *Journal of Child Psycholology and Psychiatry, 51*, 390–431.

Cosway, R., Byrne, M., Clafferty, R., Hodges, A., Grant, E., Abukmeil, S. S., . . . Johnstone, E. C. (2000). Neuropsychological change in young people at high risk for schizophrenia: Results from the first two neuropsychological assessments of the Edinburgh High Risk Study. *Psychological Medicine, 30*, 1111–1121.

Craddock, N., & Owen, M. J. (2010). The Kraepelinian dichotomy—going, going . . . but still not gone. *British Journal of Psychiatry, 196*, 92–95.

Crossley, N. A., Mechelli, A., Fusar-Poli, P., Broome, M. R., Matthiasson, P., Johns, L. C., . . . McGuire, P. K. (2009). Superior temporal lobe dysfunction and frontotemporal dysconnectivity in subjects at risk of psychosis and in first-episode psychosis. *Human Brain Mapping, 30*, 4129–4137.

Crow, T. J., Done, D. J., & Sacker, A. (1995). Childhood precursors of psychosis as clues to its evolutionary origins. *European Archives of Psychiatry & Clinical Neuroscience, 245*, 61–69.

Crow, T. J., MacMillan, J. F., Johnson, A. L., & Johnstone, E. C. (1986). A randomized controlled trial of prophylactic neuroleptic treatment. *British Journal of Psychiatry, 148*, 120–127.

Cullberg, J. (1999). Integrating intensive psychosocial therapy and low-dose medical treatment in a total material of first-episode psychotic patients compared to "treatment as usual," a 3-year follow-up. *Medicinski Arhiv, 53*, 167–170.

Cuthbert, B. N., & Insel, T. R. (2010). Toward new approaches to psychotic disorders: The NIMH Research Domain Criteria project. *Schizophrenia Bulletin, 36*, 1061–1062.

David, A. S., & Cutting, J. (1994). *The neuropsychology of schizophrenia*. Hove: Lawrence Erlbaum.

David, A. S., Malmberg, A., Brandt, L., Allebeck, P., & Lewis, G. (1997). IQ and risk for schizophrenia: A population-based cohort study. *Psychological Medicine, 27*, 1311–1323.

David, C., Greenstein, D., Clasen, L., Gochman, P., Miller, R., Tossell, J., . . . Rapoport, J. (2011). Childhood-onset schizophrenia: High rate of visual hallucination. *Journal of the American Academy of Child and Adolescent Psychiatry, 50*, 681–686.

Davidson, M., Reichenberg, A., Rabinowitz, J., Weiser, M., Kaplan, Z., & Mark, M. (1999). Behavioral and intellectual markers for schizophrenia in apparently healthy male adolescents. *American Journal of Psychiatry, 156*, 1328–1335.

DeGrazia, D. (2001). Ethical issues in early-intervention clinical trials involving minors at risk for schizophrenia. *Schizophrenia Research, 51*, 77–86.

de Haan, L., Linszen, D. H., Lenior, M. E., de Win, E. D., & Gorsira, R. (2003). Duration of untreated psychosis and outcome of schizophrenia: Delay in intensive psychosocial treatment versus delay in treatment with antipsychotic medication. *Schizophrenia Bulletin, 29*, 341–348.

DeLisi, L. E. (1997). Is schizophrenia a lifetime disorder of brain plasticity, growth and aging? *Schizophrenia Research, 23*, 119–129.

DeQuardo, J. R., Carpenter, C. F., & Tandon, R. (1994). Patterns of substance abuse in schizophrenia: Nature and significance. *Journal of Psychiatric Research, 28*, 267–275.

Dickerson, F. B. (2000). Cognitive behavioural psychotherapy for schizophrenia: A review of recent empirical studies. *Schizophrenia Research, 43*, 71–90.

Dickson, H., Laurens, K. R., Cullen, A. E., & Hodgins, S. (2012). Meta-analyses of cognitive and motor function in youth aged 16 years and younger who subsequently develop schizophrenia. *Psychological Medicine, 42*, 743–1498.

Done, D., Crow, T., Johnson, E., & Sacker, A. (1994). Childhood antecedents of schizophrenia and affective illness: Social adjustment at ages 7 and 11. *British Medical Journal, 309*, 699–703.

Dorn, L. D., & Chrousos, G. P. (1997). The neurobiology of stress: Understanding regulation of affect during female biological transitions. *Seminars in Reproductive Endocrinology, 15*, 19–35.

Dorn, L. D., Hitt, S. F., & Rotenstein, D. (1999). Biopsychological and cognitive differences in children with premature vs. on-time adrenarche. *Archives of Pediatrics and Adolescent Medicine, 153*, 137–146.

Dubertret, C., Gorwood, P., Ades, J., Feingold, J., Schwartz, J. C., & Sokoloff, P. (1998). Meta-analysis of DRD3 gene and schizophrenia: Ethnic heterogeneity and significant association in Caucasians. *American Journal of Medical Genetics, 81*, 318–322.

Dworkin, R. H., Cornblatt, B. A., Friedmann, R., Kaplansky, L. M., Lewis, J. A., Rinaldi, A., ... Erlenmeyer-Kimling, L. (1993). Childhood precursors of affective vs. social deficits in adolescents at risk for schizophrenia. *Schizophrenia Bulletin, 19*, 563–577.

Eaton, W. W. (1985). Epidemiology of schizophrenia. *Epidemiologic Reviews, 7*, 105–126.

Eaton, W. W., Badawi, M., & Melton, B. (1995). Prodromes and precursors: Epidemiologic data for primary prevention of disorders with slow onset. *American Journal of Psychiatry, 152*, 967–972.

Eckman, T. A., Wirshing, W. C., Marder, S. R., Liberman, R. P., Johnston-Cronk, K., Zimmermann, K., & Mintz, J. (1992). Technique for training schizophrenic patients in illness self-management: A controlled trial. *American Journal of Psychiatry, 149*, 1549–1555.

Edwards, J., & McGorry, P. (2002). *Implementing early intervention in psychosis: A guide to establishing early psychosis services*. London: Martin Dunitz.

Egan, M. F., Goldberg, T. E., Kolachana, B. S., Callicott, J. H., Mazzanti, C. M., Straub, R. E., ... Weinberger, D. R. (2001). Effect of COMT Val108/158 Met genotype on frontal lobe function and risk for schizophrenia. *Proceedings of the National Academy of Sciences, U S A, 98*, 6917–6922.

Egerton, A., Chaddock, C. A., Winton-Brown, T. T., Bloomfield, M. A., Bhattacharyya, S., Allen, P., ... Howes, O. D. (2013). Presynaptic striatal dopamine dysfunction in people at ultra-high risk for psychosis: Findings in a second cohort. *Biological Psychiatry*, 74, 2, 106–112.

Elvevag, B., & Goldberg, T. E. (2000). Cognitive impairment in schizophrenia is the core of the disorder. *Critical Reviews in Neurobiology, 14*, 1–21.

Emsley, R. A. (1999). Risperidone in the treatment of first-episode psychotic patients: A double-blind multicenter study. Risperidone Working Group. *Schizophrenia Bulletin, 25*, 721–729.

Erickson, D. H., Beiser, M., Iacono, W. G., Fleming, J. A., & Lin, T. Y. (1989). The role of social relationships in the course of first-episode schizophrenia and affective psychosis. *American Journal of Psychiatry, 146*, 1456–1461.

Erlenmeyer-Kimling, L. (2001). Early neurobehavioral deficits as phenotypic indicators of the schizophrenia genotype and predictors of later psychosis. *American Journal of Medical Genetics, 105*, 23–24.

Erlenmeyer-Kimling, L., & Cornblatt, B. A. (1992). Summary of attentional findings in the New York high-risk project. *Journal of Psychiatric Research, 26*, 405–426.

Erlenmeyer-Kimling, L., Cornblatt, B., Friedman, D., Marcuse, Y., Rutschmann, J., Simmens, S., & Devi, F. (1982). Neurological, electrophysiological and attentional deviations in children at risk of schizophrenia. In: F. A. Henn & H. Nasrallah (Eds.), *Schizophrenia as a brain disease* (pp. 61–98). New York: Oxford University Press.

Erlenmeyer-Kimling, L., Rock, D., Roberts, S., Jamal, M., Kestenbaum, C., Cornblatt, B., ... Gottesman, I. I. (2000). Attention, memory, and motor skills as childhood predictors of schizophrenia-related psychoses: The New York high-risk project. *American Journal of Psychiatry, 157*, 1416–1422.

Falloon, I. R. H., Boyd, J. L., & McGill, C. W. (1984). *Family care of schizophrenia.* New York: Guilford Press.

Falloon, I. R. H., Kydd, R. R., Coverdale, J. H., & Laidlaw, T. M. (1996). Early detection and intervention for initial episodes of schizophrenia. *Schizophrenia Bulletin, 22*, 271–282.

Faraone, S. V., Kremen, W. S., Lyons, M. J., Pepple, J. R., Seidman, L. J., & Tsuang, M. T. (1995). Diagnostic accuracy and linkage analysis: How useful are schizophrenia spectrum phenotypes? *American Journal of Psychiatry, 152*, 1286–1290.

Feinberg, I. (1982a). Schizophrenia and late maturational brain changes in man. *Psychopharmacology Bulletin, 18*, 29–31.

Feinberg, I. (1982b). Schizophrenia: Caused by a fault in programmed synaptic elimination during adolescence? *Journal of Psychiatric Research, 17*, 319–334.

Filipek, P. A., Richelme, C., Kennedy, D. N., & Caviness, V. S., Jr. (1994). The young adult human brain: An MRI-based morphometric analysis. *Cerebral Cortex, 4*, 334–360.

Fish, B. (1977). Neurobiological antecedents of schizophrenia in children. *Archives of General Psychiatry, 34*, 1297–1313.

Fish, B. (1984). Characteristics and sequelae of the neurointegrative disorder in infants at risk for schizophrenia: 1952–1982. In N. Watt, E. Anthony, L. Wynne, & J. Rolf (Eds.), *Children at risk for schizophrenia: A longitudinal perspective* (pp. 423–439). New York: Cambridge University Press.

Fish, B. (1987). Infant predictors of the longitudinal course of schizophrenic development. *Schizophrenia Bulletin, 13*, 395–409.

Fish, B., Marcus, J., Hans, S. L., & Auerbach, J. G. (1993). Infants at risk for schizophrenia: Sequelae of a genetic neurointegrative defect: A review and replication analysis of pandysmaturation in the Jerusalem Infant Development Study. *Annual Progress in Child Psychiatry & Child Development*, 153–190.

Fish, B., Marcus, J., Hans, S. L., Auerbach, J. G., & Perdue, S. (1992). Infants at risk for schizophrenia: Sequelae of a genetic neurointergrative defect. *Archives of General Psychiatry, 49*, 221–235.

Fitzsimmons, J., Kubicki, M., & Shenton, M. E. (2013). Review of functional and anatomical brain connectivity findings in schizophrenia. *Current Opinion in Psychiatry, 26*, 172–187.

Flaum, M., O'Leary, D. S., Johnson, D., Arndt, S., Cizadlo, T., Hichwa, R., & Andreasen, N. C. (1997). Relationship between symptom dimensions and cerebral blood flow in schizophrenia as assessed by 15H2O PET. *Schizophrenia Research, 24*, 165.

Flaum, M., O'Leary, D. S., Swayze, V. W. 2nd, Miller, D. D., Arndt, S., & Andreasen, N. C. (1995). Symptom dimensions and brain morphology in schizophrenia and related psychotic disorders. *Journal of Psychiatric Research, 29*, 261–276.

Foerster, A., Lewis, S. W., Owen, M. J., & Murray, R. M. (1991). Pre-morbid adjustment and personality in psychosis: Effects of sex and diagnosis. *British Journal of Psychiatry, 158*, 171–176.

Ford, J. M., White, P. M., Csernansky, J. G., Faustman, W. O., Roth, W. T., & Pfefferbaum, A. (1994). ERPs in schizophrenia: Effects of antipsychotic medication. *Biological Psychiatry, 36*, 153–170.

Freedman, L., Rock, D., Roberts, S., Cornblatt, B., & Erlenmeyer-Kimling, L. (1998). The New York high- risk project: Attention, anhedonia, and social outcome. *Schizophrenia Research, 30*, 1–9.

Freedman, R. F., Adler, L. E., Bickford, P., Byerley, W., Coon, H., Cullum, C. M., ... Waldo, M. (1994). Schizophrenia and nicotinic receptors. *Harvard Review of Psychiatry, 2*, 179–192.

Freedman, R., Adler, L., Waldo, M., Oachtman, E., & Franks, R. (1983). Neurophysiological evidence for a defect in inhibitory pathways in schizophrenia: Comparison of medicated and drug-free patients. *Biological Psychiatry, 18*, 537–551.

Friis, S., Vaglum, P., Haahr, U., et al. (2005). Effect of an early detection programme on duration of untreated psychosis: Part of the Scandinavian TIPS study. *British Journal of Psychiatry Supplement, 48*, s29–s32.

Fromer, M., Pocklington, A. J., Kavanagh, D. H., et al. (2014). De novo mutations in schizophrenia implicate synaptic networks. *Nature, 506*, 179–184.

Fusar-Poli, P., Borgwardt, S., Bechdolf, A., Addington, J., Riecher-Rössler, A., Schultze-Lutter, F., ... Yung, A. (2013a). The psychosis high-risk state: A comprehensive state-of-the-art review. *JAMA Psychiatry, 70*, 107–120.

Fusar-Poli, P., Deste, G., Smieskova, R., Barlati, S., Yung, A. R., Howes, O., ... Borgwardt, S. (2012b). Cognitive functioning in prodromal psychosis: A meta-analysis. *Archives of General Psychiatry, 69*(6), 562–571.

Fusar-Poli, P., McGuire, P., et al. (2012). Mapping prodromal psychosis: A critical review of neuroimaging studies. *European Journal of Psychiatry, 27*, 181–191.

Fusar-Poli, P., & Meyer-Lindenberg, A. (2013). Striatal presynaptic dopamine in schizophrenia, Part I: Meta-analysis of dopamine active transporter (DAT) density. *Schizophrenia Bulletin, 39*, 22–32.

Gershon, E. S., Badner, J. A., Goldin, L. R., Sanders, A. R., Cravchik, A., & Detera-Wadleigh, S. D. (1998). Closing in on genes for manic-depressive illness and schizophrenia. *Neuropsychopharmacology, 18*, 233–242.

Gervin, M., Browne, S., Lane, A., Clarke, M., Waddington, J. L., Larkin, C., & O'Callaghan, E. (1998). Spontaneous abnormal involuntary movements in first episode schizophrenia and schizophreniform disorder: Baseline rate in a group of patients from an Irish catchment area. *American Journal of Psychiatry, 155*, 1202–1206.

Giedd, J. N., Blumenthal, J., Jeffries, N. O., Castellanos, F. X., Liu, H., Zijdenbos, A., ... Rapoport, J. L. (1999). Brain development during childhood and adolescence: A longitudinal MRI study. *Nature Neuroscience, 2,* 861–863.

Giedd, J. N., & Rapoport, J. L. (2010). Structural MRI of pediatric brain development: What have we learned and where are we going? *Neuron, 67,* 728–734.

Giedd, J. N., Snell, J. W., Lange, N., Rajapakse, J. C., Casey, B. J., Kozuch, P. L., ... Rapoport, J. L. (1996). Quantitative magnetic resonance imaging of human brain development: Ages 4–18. *Cerebral Cortex, 6,* 551–560.

Gitlin, M., Nuechterlein, K., Subotnik, K. L., Ventura, J., Mintz, J., Fogelson, D. L., ... Aravagiri, M. (2001). Clinical outcome following neuroleptic discontinuation in patients with remitted recent-onset schizophrenia. *American Journal of Psychiatry, 158,* 1835–1842.

Gittleman-Klein, R., & Klein, D. F. (1969). Premorbid social adjustment and prognosis in schizophrenia. *Journal of Psychiatric Research, 7,* 35–53.

Giuliano, A. J., Li, H., Mesholam-Gately, R. I., Sorenson, S. M., Woodberry, K. A., & Seidman, L. J. (2012). Neurocognition in the psychosis risk syndrome: A quantitative and qualitative review. *Current Pharmaceutical Design, 18,* 399–415.

Glatt, S. J., Faraone, S. V., & Tsuang, M. T. (2003). Meta-analysis identifies an association between the dopamine D2 receptor gene and schizophrenia. *Molecular Psychiatry, 8,* 911–915.

Glausier, J. R., & Lewis, D. A. Dendritic spine pathology in schizophrenia. (2013). *Neuroscience, 251,* 90–107.

Gothelf, D., Schneider, M., Green, T., Debbané, M., Frisch, A., Glaser, B., ... Eliez, S. (2013). Risk factors and the evolution of psychosis in 22q11.2 deletion syndrome: A longitudinal 2-site study. *Journal of the American Academy of Child and Adolescent Psychiatry, 52,* 1192–1203.

Gottesman, I. I. (1991). *Schizophrenia genesis: The origin of madness.* New York: W. H. Freeman.

Gottesman, I. I., & Erlenmeyer-Kimling, L. (2001). Family and twin strategies as a head start in defining prodromes and endophenotypes for hypothetical early interventions in schizophrenia. *Schizophrenia Research, 51,* 93–102.

Gottesman, I. I., & Gould, T. D. (2003). The endophenotype concept in psychiatry: Etymology and strategic intentions. *American Journal of Psychiatry, 160,* 636–645.

Gottesman, I. I., & Shields, J. (1973). Genetic theorizing and schizophrenia. *British Journal of Psychiatry, 122,* 15–30.

Gottesman, I. I., & Shields, J. (1982). *Schizophrenia: The epigenetic puzzle.* Cambridge, UK: Cambridge University Press.

Green, A. I., & Schildkraut, J. J. (1995). Should clozapine be a first-line treatment for schizophrenia? The rationale for a double-blind clinical trial in first-episode patients. *Harvard Review of Psychiatry, 3,* 1–9.

Green, M. F. (1996). What are the functional consequences of neurocognitive deficits in schizophrenia? *American Journal of Psychiatry, 153,* 321–330.

Green, M. F. (1998). *Schizophrenia from a neurocognitive perspective. Probing the impenetrable darkness.* Needham Heights, MA: Allyn & Bacon.

Green, M. F., Bearden, C. E., Cannon, T. D., Fiske, A. P., Hellemann, G. S., Horan, W. P., ... Nuechterlein, K.H. (2012). Social cognition in schizophrenia, part 1: Performance across phase of illness. *Schizophrenia Bulletin, 38,* 854–864.

Green, M. F., Satz, P., Gaier, D. J., Ganzell, S., & Kharabi, F. (1989). Minor physical anomalies in schizophrenia. *Schizophrenia Bulletin, 15,* 91–99.

Green, T., Gothelf, D., Glaser, B., Debbane, M., Frisch, A., Kotler, M., ... Eliez, S. (2009). Psychiatric disorders and intellectual functioning throughout development in velocardiofacial (22q11.2 deletion) syndrome. *Journal of the American Academy of Child and Adolescent Psychiatry, 48,* 1060–1068.

Greenwood, T. A., Lazzeroni, L. C., Murray, S. S., Cadenhead, K. S., Calkins, M. E., Dobie, D. J., ... Braff, D. L. (2011). Analysis of 94 candidate genes and 12 endophenotypes for schizophrenia from the Consortium on the Genetics of Schizophrenia. *American Journal of Psychiatry, 168,* 930–946.

Gualtieri, C. T., Adams, A., Shen, C. D., & Loiselle, D. (1982). Minor physical anomalies in alcoholic and schizophrenic adults and hyperactive and autistic children. *American Journal of Psychiatry, 139,* 640–643.

Gulsuner, S., Wash, T., Watts, A. C., Lee, M. K., Thornton, A. M., Casadei, S., ... McClellan, J. M. (2013). Spatial and temporal mapping of de novo mutations in schizophrenia to a fetal prefrontal cortical network. *Cell, 154,* 518–529.

Gupta, S., Hendricks, S., Kenkel, A. M., Bhatia, S. C., & Haffke, E. A. (1996). Relapse in schizophrenia: Is there a relationship to substance abuse? *Schizophrenia Research, 20,* 153–156.

Gur, R. C., & Gur, R. E. (2013). Memory in health and in schizophrenia. *Dialogues in Clinical Neuroscience, 15*, 399–410.

Gur, R. C., Ragland, J. D., Moberg, P. J., Bilker, W. B., Kohler, C., Siegel, S. J., & Gur, R. E. (2001). Computerized neurocognitive scanning II: The profile of schizophrenia. *Neuropsychopharmacology, 25*, 777–788.

Gur, R. C., Ragland, J. D., Mozley, L. H., Mozley, P. D., Smith, R., Alavi, A., ... Gur, R. E. (1997). Lateralized changes in regional cerebral blood flow during performance of verbal and facial recognition tasks: Correlations with performance and "effort." *Brain and Cognition, 33*, 388–414.

Gur, R. C., Turetsky, B. I., Matsui, M., Yan, M., Bilker, W., Hughett, P., & Gur, R. E. (1999). Sex differences in brain gray and white matter in healthy young adults. *Journal of Neuroscience, 19*, 4065–4072.

Gur, R. E., Cowell, P. E., Latshaw, A., Turetsky, B. I., Grossman, R. I., Arnold, S. E., ... Gur, R. C. (2000a). Reduced dorsal and orbital prefrontal gray matter volumes in schizophrenia. *Archives of General Psychiatry, 57*, 761–768.

Gur, R. E., Cowell, P., Turetsky, B. I., Gallacher, F., Cannon, T., Bilker, W., & Gur, R. C. (1998a). A followup MRI study of schizophrenia: Relationship of neuroanatomic changes with clinical and neurobehavioral measures. *Archives of General Psychiatry, 55*, 145–152.

Gur, R. E., & Gur, R. C. (2010). Functional magnetic resonance imaging in schizophrenia. *Dialogues in Clinical Neuroscience, 12*, 333–343.

Gur, R. E., Maany, V., Mozley, P. D., Swanson, C., Bilker, W., & Gur, R. C. (1998b). Subcortical MRI volumes in neuroleptic-naive and treated patients with schizophrenia. *American Journal of Psychiatry, 155*, 1711–1717.

Gur, R. E., Mozley, P. D., Resnick, S. M., Levick, S., Erwin, R., Saykin, A. J., & Gur R. C. (1991). Relations among clinical scales in schizophrenia. *American Journal of Psychiatry, 148*, 472–478.

Gur, R. E., Turetsky, B. I., Bilker, W. B., & Gur, R. C. (1999). Reduced gray matter volume in schizophrenia. *Archives of General Psychiatry, 56*, 905–911.

Gur, R. E., Turetsky, B. I., Cowell, P. E., Finkelman, C., Maany, V., Grossman, R. I., ... Gur, R. C. (2000b). Temporolimbic volume reductions in schizophrenia. *Archives of General Psychiatry, 57*, 769–775.

Guy, J. D., Majorski, L. V., Wallace, C. J., & Guy, M. P. (1983). The incidence of minor physical anomalies in adult male schizophrenics. *Schizophrenia Bulletin, 9*, 571–582.

Hafner, H., Loffler, W., Maurer, K., Hambrecht, M., & an der Heiden, W. (1999). Depression, negative symptoms, social stagnation and social decline in the early course of schizophrenia. *Acta Psychiatrica Scandinavica, 100*, 105–118.

Hafner, H., Maurer, K., Loffler, W., & Riecher-Rossler, A. (1993). The influence of age and sex on the onset and early course of schizophrenia. *British Journal of Psychiatry, 162*, 80–86.

Hambrecht, M., & Hafner, H. (2000). Cannabis, vulnerability, and the onset of schizophrenia: An epidemiological perspective. *Australian and New Zealand Journal of Psychiatry, 34*, 468–475.

Hans, S., Marcus, J., Nuechterlein K., Asarnow, R., Styr, B., & Auerbach, J. (1999). Neurobehavioral deficits at adolescence in children at risk for schizophrenia: The Jerusalem infant development study. *Archives of General Psychiatry, 56*, 741–748.

Hare, E. H. (1987). Epidemiology of schizophrenia and affective psychoses. *British Medical Bulletin, 43*, 514–530.

Harrison, G., Hopper, K., Craig, T., Laska, E., Siegel, C., Wanderling, J., ... Wiersma, D. (2001). Recovery from psychotic illness: A 15- and 25-year international follow-up study. *British Journal of Psychiatry, 178*, 506–517.

Harrison, P. J., & Owen, M. J. (2003). Genes for schizophrenia? Recent findings and their pathophysiological implications. *Lancet, 361*, 417–419.

Heckers, S., Rausch, S. L., Goff, D., Savage, C. R., Schacter, D. L., Fischman, A. J., & Alpert, N. M. (1998). Impaired recruitment of the hippocampus during conscious recollection in schizophrenia. *Nature Neuroscience, 1*, 318–323.

Helgason, T. (1964). Epidemiology of mental disorders in Iceland: A psychiatric and demographic investigation of 5395 Icelanders. *Acta Psychiatrica Scandinavica, Supplement, 40*, 173.

Hessl, D., Glaser, B., Dyer-Friedman, J., Blasey, C., Hastie, T., Gunnar, M., & Reiss, A. L. (2002). Cortisol and behavior in fragile X syndrome. *Psychoneuroendocrinology, 27*, 855–872.

Hill, S. K., Reilly, J. L., Keefe, R. S., Gold, J. M., Bishop, J. R., Gershon, E. S., ... Sweeney, J. A. (2013). Neuropsychological impairments in schizophrenia and psychotic bipolar disorder: Findings from the Bipolar and Schizophrenia Network on Intermediate Phenotypes (B-SNIP) study. *American Journal of Psychiatry, 170*, 1275–1284.

Hillyard, S., & Hansen, J. (1986). Attention: Electrophysiological approaches. In: M. Coles, E. Donchin, & S. Porges (Eds.), *Psychophysiology: Systems, processes, and applications* (pp. 227–243). New York: Guilford.

Hillyard, S., & Kutas, M. (1983). Electrophysiology of cognitive processing. *Annual Review of Psychology,* 34, 33–61.

Ho, B. C., Alicata, D., Ward, J., Moser, D. J., O'Leary, D. S., Arndt, S., & Andreasen N. C. (2003). Untreated initial psychosis: Relation to cognitive deficits and brain morphology in first-episode schizophrenia. *American Journal of Psychiatry, 160,* 142–148.

Hogarty, G., Anderson, C., Reiss, D., Kornblith, S., Greenwald, D., Ulrich, R., & Carter, M. (1997). Family psychoeducation, social skills training and maintenance chemotherapy in the aftercare treatment of schizophrenia, II: Two-year effects of a controlled study on relapse and adjustment. *Archives of General Psychiatry, 48,* 340–347.

Hogarty, G. E., McEvoy, J. P., Ulrich, R. F., DiBarry, A. L., Bartone, P., Cooley, S., ... Perel, J. (1995). Pharmacotherapy of impaired affect in recovering schizophrenic patients. *Archives of General Psychiatry, 52,* 29.

Holcomb, H. H., Cascella, N. G., Thaker, G. K., Medoff, D. R., Dannals, R. F., & Tamminga, C. A. (1996). Functional sites of neuroleptic drug action in the human brain: PET/FDG studies with and without haloperidol. *American Journal of Psychiatry, 153,* 41–49.

Holcomb, H. H., Lahti, A. C., Medoff, D. R., Weiler, M., Dannals, R. F., & Tamminga, C. A. (2000). Brain activation patterns in schizophrenic and comparison volunteers during a matched-performance auditory recognition task. *American Journal of Psychiatry, 157,* 1634–1645.

Hollis, C., & Rapoport, J. (2011). Child and adolescent schizophrenia. In: D. R. Weinberger & P. Harrison (Eds.), *Schizophrenia* (3rd ed., pp. 24–46). Hoboken, NJ: Wiley-Blackwell.

Holmén, A., Juuhl-Langseth, M., Thormodsen, R., Ueland, T., Agartz, I., Sundet, K., ... Melle, I. (2012). Executive function in early-and adult onset schizophrenia. *Schizophrenia Research, 142,* 177–182.

Holtzman, C. W., Trotman, H. D., Goulding, S. M., Ryan, A. T., Macdonald, A. N., Shapiro, D. I., Brasfield, J. L., & Walker, E. F. (2013). Stress and neurodevelopmental processes in the emergence of psychosis. *Neuroscience, 249,* 172–191.

Howes, O. D., Bose, S. K., Turkheimer, F., Valli, I., Egerton, A., Valmaggia, L. R., ... McGuire, P. (2011). Dopamine synthesis capacity prior to the subsequent onset of psychosis: An [18F]-DOPA PET imaging study. *American Journal of Psychiatry, 168,* 1311–1317.

Huber, T. J., Rollnik, J., Wilhelms, J., von zur Muhlen, A., Emrich, H. M., & Schneider, U. (2001). Estradiol levels in psychotic disorders. *Psychoneuroendocrinology, 26,* 27–35.

Huston, P. E., & Shakow, D. (1946). Studies of motor function in schizophrenia: III. Steadiness. *Journal of General Psychology, 34,* 119–126.

Huttenlocher, P. R. (1984). Synaptic elimination and plasticity in developing human cerebral cortex. *American Journal of Mental Deficiency, 88,* 488–496.

Huttenlocher, P. R., de Courten, C., Garey, L. J., & Van der Loos, H. (1982). Synaptogenesis in human visual cortex: Evidence for synapse elimination during normal development. *Neuroscience Letters, 33,* 247–252.

Ingraham, L., Kugelmass, S., Frankel, E., Nathan, M., & Mirsky, A. (1995). Twenty-five-year follow-up of the Israeli high-risk study: Current and lifetime psychopathology. *Schizophrenia Bulletin, 21,* 183–192.

Insel, T.R. Cuthbert, B.N. (2015). Brain disorders? Precisely. *Science, 348,* 499–500.

Ioannidis, J. P., Ntzani, E. E., Trikalinos, T. A., & Contopoulos-Ioannidis, D. G. (2001). Replication validity of genetic association studies. *Nature Genetics, 29,* 306–309.

Isohanni, M., Jones, P. B., Moilanen, K., Rantakallio, P., Veijola, J., Oja, H., ... Järvelin, M-R. (2001). Early developmental milestones in adult schizophrenia and other psychoses: A 31-year follow-up of the north Finland 1966 birth cohort. *Schizophrenia Research, 52,* 1–19.

Iyegbe, C., Desmond Campbell, D., Butler, A., Ajnakina, O., & Sham, P. (2014). The emerging molecular architecture of schizophrenia, polygenic risk scores and the clinical implications for G×E research. *Social Psychiatry and Psychiatric Epidemiology,* 49, 169–182.

Jablensky, A. (1986). Epidemiology of schizophrenia: A European perspective. *Schizophrenia Bulletin, 12,* 52–73.

Jackson, H., McGorry, P., Henry, L., Edwards, J., Hulbert, C., Harrigan, S., ... Power, P. (2001). Cognitively oriented psychotherapy for early psychosis (COPE): A 1-year follow-up. *British Journal of Clinical Psychology, 40,* 57–70.

Jacobsen, L. K., Giedd, J. N., Castellanos, F. X., Vaituzis, A. C., Hamburger, S. D., Kumra, S., ... Rapoport, J. L. (1998). Progressive reduction of temporal lobe structures in childhood-onset schizophrenia. *American Journal of Psychiatry, 155*, 678–685.

Jacobson, K. C., Prescott, C. A., & Kendler, K. S. (2002). Sex differences in the genetic and environmental influences on the development of antisocial behavior. *Development & Psychopathology, 14*, 395–416.

Jarbin, H., Yngve, O., & Von Knorring, A. (2003). Adult outcome of social function in adolescent-onset schizophrenia and affective psychosis. *Journal of the American Academy of Child and Adolescent Psychiatry, 42*, 176–183.

Jernigan, T. L., & Tallal, P. (1990). Late childhood changes in brain morphology observable with MRI. *Developmental Medicine and Child Neurolology, 32*, 379–385.

Johannesen, J. K., O'Donnell, B. F., Shekhar, A., McGrew, J. H., & Hetrick, W. P. (2013). Diagnostic specificity of neurophysiological endophenotypes in schizophrenia and bipolar disorder. *Schizophrenia Bulletin, 39*, 1219–1229.

Johannessen, J. L., McGlashan, T. H., Larsen, T. K., Horneland, M., Joa, I., Mardal, S., ... Vaglum, P. (2001). Early detection strategies for untreated first-episode psychosis. *Schizophrenia Research, 51*, 39–46.

Johns, A. (2001). Psychiatric effects of cannabis. *British Journal of Psychiatry, 178*, 116–122.

Jones, P. B. (1999). Longitudinal approaches to the search for the causes of schizophrenia: Past, present and future. In W. F. Gattaz & H. Hafner (Eds.), *Search for the causes of schizophrenia* (Vol. 4). Berlin, Germany: Springer.

Jones, P., & Done, D. (1997). From birth to onset: A developmental perspective of schizophrenia in two national birth cohorts. In M. Keshavan & R. Murray (Eds.), *Neurodevelopment and adult psychopathology* (pp. 119–136). Cambridge, UK: Cambridge University Press.

Jones, P. B., & Murray, R. M. (1991). The genetics of schizophrenia is the genetics of neurodevelopment. *British Journal of Psychiatry, 158*, 615–623.

Jones, P. B., Rodgers, B., Murray, R. M., & Marmot, M. G. (1994). Child developmental risk factors for adult schizophrenia in the British 1946 birth cohort. *Lancet, 344*, 1398–1402.

Jones, P., & Tarrant, J. (1999). Specificity of developmental precursors to schizophrenia and affective disorders. *Schizophrenia Research, 39*, 121–125.

Jones, P. B., & van Os, J. J. (2000). Commentary on Davidson, M., Reichenberg, A., Rabinowitz, J., Weiser, M., Kaplan, Z., & Mark, M. (1999). Behavioural and intellectual markers for schizophrenia in apparently healthy male adolescents. *American Journal of Psychiatry*, 156, 1328–1335; *Evidence-Based Mental Health, 3*, 89.

Kahn, R. S., Fleischhacker, W. W., Boter, H., Davidson, M., Vergouwe, Y., Keet, I. P., et al. (2008). Effectiveness of antipsychotic drugs in first-episode schizophrenia and schizophreniform disorder: An open randomised clinical trial. *Lancet, 371*, 1085–1097.

Kahn, R. S., & Keefe, R. S. (2013). Schizophrenia is a cognitive illness: Time for a change in focus. *JAMA Psychiatry, 70*, 1107–1112.

Kane, J. M. (1996). Treatment-resistant schizophrenic patients. *Journal of Clinical Psychiatry, 57*, 35–40.

Kane, J. M., Rifkin, A., Quitkin, F., Nayak, D., & Ramos-Lorenzi, J. (1982). Fluphenazine vs. placebo in patients with remitted, acute first-episode schizophrenia. *Archives of General Psychiatry, 39*, 70–73.

Kasai, K., Shenton, M. E., Salisbury, D. F., Hirayasu, Y., Lee, C. U., Ciszewski, A. A., ... McCarley, R.W. (2003). Progressive decrease of left superior temporal gyrus gray matter volume in patients with first-episode schizophrenia. *American Journal of Psychiatry, 160*, 156–164.

Kasai, K., Shenton, M. E., Salisbury, D. F., Hirayasu, Y., Onitsuka, T., Spencer, M., ... McCarley, R.W. (2003). Progressive decrease of left Heschl's gyrus and planum temporale gray matter volume in schizophrenia: A longitudinal MRI study of first-episode patients. *Archives of General Psychiatry, 60*, 766–775.

Kelleher, I., & Cannon, M. (2011). Psychotic-like experiences in the general population: Characterizing a high-risk group for psychosis. *Psychological Medicine, 41*, 1–6.

Kellner, R., Wilson, R. M., Muldawer, M. D., & Pathak, D. (1975). Anxiety in schizophrenia. The responses to chlordiazepoxide in an intensive design study. *Archives of General Psychiatry, 32*, 1246–1254.

Kemp, R., Hayward, P., Applewhaite, G., Everitt, B., & David, A. (1996). Compliance therapy in psychotic patients: Randomised controlled trial. *British Medical Journal, 312*, 345–349.

Kemp, R., Kirov, G., Everitt, B., Hayward, P., & David, A. (1998). Randomised controlled trial of compliance therapy: 18-month follow-up. *British Journal of Psychiatry, 172*, 413–419.

Kendler, K. S. (2000). Schizophrenia: Genetics. In B. J. Sadock & V. A. Sadock (Eds.), *Comprehensive textbook of psychiatry* (7th ed., pp. 1147–1159). New York: Lippincott, Williams, & Wilkins.

Kendler, K. S., & O'Donovan, M. C. (2014). A breakthrough in schizophrenia genetics. *JAMA Psychiatry, 71*, 1319–1320.

Keshavan, M. S., Anderson, S., & Pettegrew, J. W. (1994). Is schizophrenia due to excessive synaptic pruning in the prefrontal cortex? The Feinberg hypothesis revisited. *Journal of Psychiatric Research, 29*, 239–265.

Keshavan, M. S., Clementz, B. A., Pearlson, G. D., Sweeney, J. A., & Tamminga, C. A. (2013). Reimagining psychoses: An agnostic approach to diagnosis. *Schizophrenia Research, 146*,10–16.

Keshavan, M. S., & Hogarty, G. E. (1999). Brain maturational processes and delayed onset in schizophrenia. *Development and Psychopathology, 11*, 525–543.

Keshavan, M. S., & Schooler, N. (1992). First episode studies of schizophrenia: Criteria and characterization. *Schizophrenia Bulletin, 18*, 491–513.

Kety, S. S., Wender, P., Jacobsen, B., Ingraham, L. J., Jansson, L., Faber, B., & Kinney, D. K. (1994). Mental illness in the biological and adoptive relatives of schizophrenic adoptees: Replication of the Copenhagen study in the rest of Denmark. *Archives of General Psychiatry, 51*, 442–455.

Kim-Cohen, J., Caspi, A., Moffitt, T., Harrington, H., Milene, B., & Poulton, R. (2003). Prior juvenile diagnoses in adults with mental disorder: Developmental follow-back of a prospective-longitudinal cohort. *Archives of General Psychiatry, 60*, 709–717.

Klorman, R. (1991). Cognitive event-related potentials in attention deficit disorder. *Journal of Learning Disabilities, 24*, 130–140.

Knight, R. T., Hillyard, S. A., Woods, D. L., & Neville, H. J. (1981). The effects of frontal cortex lesions on event-related potentials during auditory selective attention. *Electroencephalography and Clinical Neurophysiology, 52*, 571–582.

Ko, G. N., Korpi, E. R., Freed, W. J., Zalcman, S. J., & Bigelow, L. B. (1985). Effect of valproic acid on behavior and plasma amino acid concentrations in chronic schizophrenic patients. *Biological Psychiatry, 20*, 209–215.

Kohler, C. G., Richard, J. A., Brensinger, C. M., Borgmann-Winter, K. E., Conroy, C. G., Moberg, P. J., ... Calkins, M. E. (2014). Facial emotion perception differs in young persons at genetic and clinical high-risk for psychosis. *Psychiatry Research, 216*, 206–212.

Kohler, C. G., Turner, T. H., Bilker, W. B., Brensinger, C. M., Siegel, S. J., Kanes, S. J., ... Gur, R. C. (2003). Facial emotion recognition in schizophrenia: Intensity effects and error pattern. *American Journal of Psychiatry, 160*, 1768–1774.

Kohn, M. I., Tanna, N. K., Herman, G. T., Resnick, S. M., Mozley, P. D., Gur, R. E., ... Gur, R. C. (1991). Analysis of brain and CSF volumes from magnetic resonance imaging: Methodology, reliability and validation. *Radiology, 178*, 115–122.

Kopala, L. C., Fredrikson, D., Good, K. P., & Honer, W. G. (1996). Symptoms in neuroleptic-naive, first-episode schizophrenia: Response to risperidone. *Biological Psychiatry, 39*, 296–298.

Koreen, A. R., Siris, S. G., Chakos, M., Alvir, J., Mayerhoff, D., & Lieberman, J. (1993). Depression in first-episode schizophrenia. *American Journal of Psychiatry, 150*, 1643–1648.

Koutsouleris, N., Davatzikos, C., Bottlender, R., Patschurek-Kliche, K., Scheuerecker, J., Decker, P., ... Meisenzahl, E.M. (2012). Early recognition and disease prediction in the at-risk mental states for psychosis using neurocognitive pattern classification. *Schizophrenia Bulletin, 38*, 1200–1215.

Kovacs, M., Rush, A. J., Beck, A. T., & Hollon, S. D. (1981). Depressed outpatients treated with cognitive therapy or pharmacotherapy. A one-year follow-up. *Archives of General Psychiatry, 38*, 33–39.

Kraepelin, E. (1896). Dementia Praecox. Psychiatrie (5th ed., pp. 426–441). Leipzig: Barth. Translated in J. Cutting & M. Shepherd (Eds.) (1987), *The clinical roots of the schizophrenia concept* (pp. 13–24). Cambridge, UK: Cambridge University Press.

Kraepelin, E. (1919). *Dementia praecox and paraphrenia*. Edinburgh, Scotland: Livingstone.

Kramer, M. (1969). Cross-national study of diagnosis of the mental disorders: Origin of the problem. *American Journal of Psychiatry, 10*, 1–11.

Kravariti, E., Dazzan, P., Fearon, P., & Murray, R. (2004). Can one identify preschizophrenic children? In M. Keshavan, J. L. Kennedy, & R. Murray (Eds.), *Neurodevelopment and schizophrenia* (pp. 415–431). Cambridge, UK: Cambridge University Press.

Kring, A. M., Barrett, L. F., & Gard, D. E. (2003). On the broad applicability of the affective circumplex: Representations of affective knowledge among schizophrenia patients. *Psychological Science, 14*, 207–214.

Kubicki, M., McCarley, R. W., Nestor, P. G., Huh, T., Kikinis, R., Shenton, M. E., & Wible, C. G. (2003). An fMRI study of semantic processing in schizophrenia. *NeuroImage, 20*, 1923–1933.

Kubicki, M., & Shenton, M. E. (2014). Diffusion tensor imaging findings and their implications in schizophrenia. *Current Opinion in Psychiatry, 27*, 179–184.

Kuepper, R., Skinbjerg, M., & Abi-Dargham, A. (2012). The dopamine dysfunction in schizophrenia revisited: New insights into topography and course. In *Current antipsychotics* (pp. 1–26). Berlin/Heidelberg: Springer.

Kulhara, P., Kota, S. K., & Joseph, S. (1986). Positive and negative subtypes of schizophrenia: A study from India. *Acta Psychiatrica Scandinavica, 74*, 353–359.

Kumra, S., Frazier, J. A., Jacobsen, L. K., McKenna, K., Gordon, C. T., Lenane, M. C., ... Rapoport, J. L. (1996). Childhood-onset schizophrenia: A double-blind clozapine-haloperidol comparison. *Archives of General Psychiatry, 53*, 1090–1097.

Kumra, S., Giedd, J. N., Vaituzis, A. C., Jacobsen, L. K., McKenna, K., Bedwell, J., ... Rapoport, J. L. (2000). Childhood-onset psychotic disorders: Magnetic resonance imaging of volumetric differences in brain structure. *American Journal of Psychiatry, 157*, 1467–1474.

Kumra, S., Jacobsen, L. K., Lenane, M., Smith, A., Lee, P., Malanga, C. J., ... Rapoport, J. L. (1998). Case series: Spectrum of neuroleptic-induced movement disorders and extrapyramidal side effects in childhood-onset schizophrenia. *Journal of the American Academy of Child and Adolescent Psychiatry, 37*, 221–227.

Kwon, J. S., O'Donnell, B. F., Wallenstein, G. V., Greene, R. W., Hirayasu, Y., Nestor, P. G., ... McCarley, R.W. (1999). Gamma frequency-range abnormalities to auditory stimulation in schizophrenia. *Archives of General Psychiatry, 56*, 1001–1005.

Kyriakopoulos, M., & Frangou, S. (2009). Recent diffusion tensor imaging findings in early stages of schizophrenia. *Current Opinion in Psychiatry, 22*, 168–176.

Lambe, E. K., Krimer, L. S., & Goldman-Rakic, P. S. (2000). Differential postnatal development of catecholamine and serotonin inputs to identified neurons in prefrontal cortex of rhesus monkey. *Journal of Neuroscience, 20*, 8780–8787.

Lammers, C. H., Garcia-Borreguero, D., Schmider, J., Gotthardt, U., Dettling, M., Holsboer, F., & Heuser, I. J. (1995). Combined dexamethasone/corticotropin-releasing hormone test in patients with schizophrenia and in normal controls. *Biological Psychiatry, 38*, 803–807.

Lane, A., Kinsella, A., Murphy, P., Byrne, M., Keenan, J., Colgan, K., ... O'Callaghan, E. (1997). The anthropometric assessment of dysmorphic features in schizophrenia as an index of its developmental origins. *Psychological Medicine, 27*, 1155–1164.

Langeveld, J., Joa, I., Friis, S., ten Velden Hegelstad, W., Melle, I., Johannessen, J. O., ... Larsen, T. K. (2012). A comparison of adolescent-and adult-onset first-episode, non-affective psychosis: 2-year follow-up. *European Archives of Psychiatry and Clinical Neuroscience, 262*(7), 599–605.

Laruelle, M. (2000). The role of endogenous sensitization in the pathophysiology of schizophrenia: Implications from recent brain imaging studies. *Brain Research. Brain Research Reviews, 31*, 371–384.

Lay, B., Blanz, B., Hartmann, M., & Schmidt, M. H. (2000). The psychosocial outcome of adolescent-onset schizophrenia: A 12-year follow-up. *Schizophrenia Bulletin, 26*, 801–816.

Lee, J. H., Woo, J. I., & Meltzer, H. Y. (2001). Effects of clozapine on sleep measures and sleep-associated changes in growth hormone and cortisol in patients with schizophrenia. *Psychiatry Research, 103*, 157–166.

Lee, Y., & Styne, D. (2013). Influences on the onset and tempo of puberty in human beings and implications for adolescent psychological development. *Hormones and Behavior, 64*(2), 250–261.

Leff, J., Kuipers, L., Berkowitz, R., Eberlein-Vries, R., & Sturgeon, D. (1982). A controlled trial of social intervention in the families of schizophrenic patients. *British Journal of Psychiatry, 141*, 121–134.

Lehman, A. F., & Steinwachs, D. M. (1998). Translating research into practice: The Schizophrenia Patient Outcomes Research Team (PORT) treatment recommendations. *Schizophrenia Bulletin, 24*, 1–10.

Lenior, M. E., Dingemans, P. M., Schene, A. H., Hart, A. A., & Linszen, D. H. (2002). The course of parental expressed emotion and psychotic episodes after family intervention in recent-onset schizophrenia: A longitudinal study. *Schizophrenia Research, 57*, 183–190.

Lenzenweger, M., Dworkin, R., & Wethington, E. (1989). Models of positive and negative symptoms in schizophrenia: An empirical evaluation of latent structures. *Journal of Abnormal Psychology, 98*, 62–70.

Leonard, S., Adams, C., Breese, C. R., Adler, L. E., Bickford, P., Byerley, W., . . . Freedman, R. (1996). Nicotinic receptor function in schizophrenia. *Schizophrenia Bulletin*, *22*, 431–445.

Leonard, S. C., Gault, J., Hopkins, J., et al (2002). Association of promoter variants in the alpha 7 nicotinic acetylcholine receptor subunit gene with an inhibitory deficit found in schizophrenia. *Archives of General Psychiatry*, *59*, 1085–1096.

Leucht, S., McGrath, J., White, P., & Kissling, W. (2002). Carbamazepine augmentation for schizophrenia: How good is the evidence? *Journal of Clinical Psychiatry*, *63*, 218–224.

Levine, S. Z., & Rabinowitz, J. (2010). Trajectories and antecedents of treatment response over time in early-episode psychosis. *Schizophrenia Bulletin*, *36*, 624–632.

Levinson, D. F., Lewis, C. M., et al. (2002). Meta-analysis of genome scans for schizophrenia. *American Journal of Medical Genetics (Neuropsychiatric Genetics)*, *114*, 700.

Lewis, C. M., Levinson, D. F., Wise, L. H., Delisi, L., Straub, R. E., Hovatta, I., . . . Helgason, T. (2003). Genome scan meta-analysis of schizophrenia and bipolar disorder, Part II: Schizophrenia. *American Journal of Human Genetics*, *73*, 34–48.

Lewis, R. (1998). Typical and atypical antipsychotics in adolescent schizophrenia: Efficacy, tolerability, and differential sensitivity to extrapyramidal symptoms. *Canadian Journal of Psychiatry*, *43*, 596–604,

Lewis, S. W., Reveley, A. M., Reveley, M. A., Chitkara, B., & Murray, R. M. (1987). The familial/sporadic distinction as a strategy in schizophrenia research. *British Journal of Psychiatry*, *151*, 306–313.

Lewis, S., Tarrier, N., Haddock, G., Bentall, R., Kinderman, P., Kingdon, D., et al. (2002). Randomised controlled trial of cognitive-behavioural therapy in early schizophrenia: Acute-phase outcomes. *British Journal of Psychiatry*, *43*, s91–s97.

Liddle, P. (1987). The symptoms of chronic schizophrenia. A re-examination of the positive-negative dichotomy. *British Journal of Psychiatry*, *151*, 145–151.

Liddle, P. F., Spence, S. A., & Sharma, T. (1995). A PET study of obligate carriers of the predisposition to schizophrenia. *Schizophrenia Research*, *15*, 90.

Lieberman, J. A. (1996). Atypical antipsychotic drugs as a first-line treatment of schizophrenia: A rationale and hypothesis. *Journal of Clinical Psychiatry*, *57*, 68–71.

Lieberman, J. A. (1999). Is schizophrenia a neurodegenerative disorder? A clinical and neurobiological perspective. *Biological Psychiatry*, *46*, 729–739.

Lieberman, J. A., Alvir, J. M., Koreen, A., Geisler, S., Chakos, M., Sheitman, B., & Woerner M. (1996). Psychobiologic correlates of treatment response in schizophrenia. *Neuropsychopharmacology*, *14*, 13S–21S.

Lieberman, J., Chakos, M., Wu, H., Alvir, J., Hoffman, E., Robinson, D., & Bilder, R. (2001). Longitudinal study of brain morphology in first episode schizophrenia. *Biological Psychiatry*, *49*, 487–499.

Lieberman, J. A., Gu, H., Stroup, S., Zhang, P., Kong, L., Ji, Z., . . . Hamer, R. M. (2003). Atypical and conventional antipsychotic drugs in first-episode schizophrenia: Comparison of clozapine versus chlorpromazine in a 52-week randomized double-blind trial. *Neuropsychopharmacology*, *28*, 995–1003.

Lieberman, J., Jody, D., Geisler, S., Alvir, J., Loebel, A., Szymanski, S., Woerner, M., & Borenstein, M. (1993). Time course and biologic correlates of treatment response in first-episode schizophrenia. *Archives of General Psychiatry*, *50*, 369–376.

Lieberman, J. A., Perkins, D., Belger, A., Chakos, M., Jarskog, F., Boteva, K., & Gilmore, J. (2001). The early stages of schizophrenia: Speculations on pathogenesis, pathophysiology, and therapeutic approaches. *Biological Psychiatry*, *50*, 884–897.

Lieberman, J. A., Tollefson, G., Tohen, M., Green, A. I., Gur, R. E., Kahn, R., . . . Hamer, R. M. (HGDH Study Group). (2003). Comparative efficacy and safety of atypical and conventional antipsychotic drugs in first-episode psychosis: A randomized double-blind trial of olanzapine vs. haloperidol. *American Journal of Psychiatry*, *160*, 1396–1404.

Linnoila, M., & Viukari, M. (1979). Sodium valproate and tardive dyskinesia. *British Journal of Psychiatry*, *134*, 223–224.

Linszen, D. H., Dingemans, P. M., & Lenior, M. E. (1994). Cannabis abuse and the course of recent-onset schizophrenic disorders. *Archives of General Psychiatry*, *51*, 273–279.

Linszen, D., Dingemans, P., & Lenior, M. (2001). Early intervention and a five-year follow-up in young adults with a short duration of untreated psychosis: Ethical implications. *Schizophrenia Research*, *51*, 55–61.

Linszen, D., Dingemans, P., Van der Does, J. W., Nugter, A., Scholte, P., Lenoir, R., & Goldstein,

M. J. (1996). Treatment, expressed emotion and relapse in recent-onset schizophrenic disorders. *Psychological Medicine, 26*, 333–342.

Lohr, J. B., & Flynn, K. (1993). Minor physical anomalies in schizophrenia and mood disorders. *Schizophrenia Bulletin, 19*, 551–556.

Loiselle, D., Stamm, J., Maitinsky, S., & Whipple, S. (1980). Evoked potential and behavioral signs of attention dysfunction in hyperactive boys. *Psychophysiology, 17*,193–201.

Malmberg, A., Lewis, G., David, A., & Allebeck, P. (1998). Premorbid adjustment and personality in people with schizophrenia. *British Journal of Psychiatry, 172*, 308–313.

Manschreck, T. C., Maher, B. A., Rucklos, M. E., & Vereen, D. R. (1982). Disturbed voluntary motor activity in schizophrenic disorder. *Psychological Medicine, 12*, 73–84.

Marcus, J., Hans, S., Auerbach, J., & Auerbach, A. (1993). Children at risk for schizophrenia: The Jerusalem infant development study: II. Neurobehavioral deficits at school age. *Archives of General Psychiatry, 50*, 797–809.

Marcus, J., Hans, S., Nagler, S., Auerbach, J., Mirsky, A., & Aubrey, A. (1987). Review of the NIMH Israeli Kibbutz-city study and the Jerusalem infant development study. *Schizophrenia Bulletin, 13*, 425–438.

Marenco, S., & Weinberger, D. R. (2000). The neurodevelopmental hypothesis of schizophrenia: following a trail of evidence from cradle to grave. *Development and Psychopathology, 12*, 501–527.

Markham, J. A. (2012). Sex steroids and schizophrenia. *Reviews in Endocrine and Metabolic Disorders, 13*, 187–207.

Matsuzawa, J., Matsui, M., Konishi, T., Noguchi, K., Gur, R. C., Bilker, W., & Miyawaki, T. (2001). Age-related volumetric changes of brain gray and white matter in healthy infants and children. *Cerebral Cortex, 11*, 335–342.

May, P. R., Tuma, A. H., Yale, C., Potepan, P., & Dixon, W. J. (1976). Schizophrenia—a follow-up study of results of treatment. *Archives of General Psychiatry, 33*, 481–486.

McCarley, R. W., Hsiao, J. K., Freedman, R., Pfefferbaum, A., & Donchin, E. (1996). Neuroimaging and the cognitive neuroscience of schizophrenia. *Schizophrenia Bulletin, 22*, 703–725.

McCarley, R. W., Salisbury, D. F., Hirayasu, Y., Yurgelun-Todd, D. A., Tohen, M., Zarate, C., ... Shenton, M. E. (2002). Association between smaller left posterior superior temporal gyrus MRI volume and smaller left temporal P300 amplitude in first episode schizophrenia. *Archives of General Psychiatry, 59*, 321–331.

McCarley, R. W., Shenton, M. E., O'Donnell, B. F., Faux, S. F., Kikinis, R., Nestor, P. G., & Jolesz, F.A. (1993) Auditory P300 abnormalities and left posterior superior temporal gyrus volume reduction in schizophrenia. *Archives of General Psychiatry, 50*, 190–197.

McCreadie, R. G., Wiles, D., Grant, S., Crockett, G. T, Mahmood, Z., Livingston, M. G., et al. (1989). The Scottish first episode schizophrenia study. VII. Two-year follow-up. Scottish Schizophrenia Research Group. *Acta Psychiatrica Scandinavica, 80*, 597–602.

McEvoy, J. P., Hogarty, G. E., & Steingard, S. (1991). Optimal dose of neuroleptic in acute schizophrenia. A controlled study of the neuroleptic threshold and higher haloperidol dose. *Archives of General Psychiatry, 48*, 739–745.

McFarlane, W. R., Lukens, E., Link, B., Dushay, R., Deakins, S. A., Newmark, M., ... Toran, J. (1995). Multiple family groups and psychoeducation in the treatment of schizophrenia. *Archives of General Psychiatry, 52*, 679–687.

McGlashan, T. H. (1996). Early detection and intervention in schizophrenia: Research. *Schizophrenia Bulletin, 22*, 327–345.

McGlashan, T. H. (1988). A selective review of recent North American long-term follow-up studies of schizophrenia. *Schizophrenia Bulletin, 14*, 515–542.

McGorry, P. D., & Killackey, E. J. (2002). Early intervention in psychosis: A new evidence-based paradigm. *Epidemiologia e Psichiatria Sociale, 11*, 237–247.

McGorry, P. D., Yung, A. F., Phillips, L. J., Yuen, H. P., Francey, S., Cosgrave, E. M., ... Jackson, H. (2002a). Randomized controlled trial of interventions designed to reduce the risk of progression to first-episode psychosis in a clinical sample with subthreshold symptoms. *Archives of General Psychiatry, 59*, 921–928.

McGrath, J. J., van Os, J., Hoyos, C., Jones, P. B., Harvey, I., & Murray, R. M. (1996). Minor physical abnormalities in psychoses: Associations with clinical and putative aetiological variables. *Schizophrenia Research, 18*, 9–20.

McNeil, T., Harty, B., Blennow, G., & Cantor-Graae, E. (1993). Neuromotor deviation in offspring of psychotic mothers: A selective developmental deficiency in two groups of children at heightened psychiatric risk? *Journal of Psychiatric Research, 27*, 39–54.

Mednick, S. A., Parnas, J., & Schulsinger, R. (1987). The Copenhagen high-risk project. *Schizophrenia Bulletin, 13,* 485–495.

Mednick, S., & Schulsinger, F. (1968). Some premorbid characteristics related to breakdown in children with schizophrenic mothers. In D. Rosenthal & S. Kety (Eds.), *The transmission of schizophrenia* (pp. 267–291). Oxford: Pergamon Press.

Medoff, D. R., Holcomb, H. H., Lahti, A. C., & Tamminga, C. A. (2001). Probing the human hippocampus using rCBF: Contrasts in schizophrenia. *Hippocampus, 11,* 543–550.

Meltzer, H. Y., Alphs, L., Green, A. I., Altamura, A. C., Anand, R., Bertoldi, A., ... Potkin, S. (2003). Clozapine treatment for suicidality in schizophrenia: International Suicide Prevention Trial (InterSePT). *Archives of General Psychiatry, 60,* 82–91.

Meltzer, H. Y., & Okayli, G. (1995). Reduction of suicidality during clozapine treatment of neuroleptic-resistant schizophrenia: Impact on risk-benefit assessment. *American Journal of Psychiatry, 152,* 183–190.

Merlo, M. C., Hofer, H., Gekle, W., Berger, G., Ventura, J., Panhuber, I., ... Marder, S. R. (2002). Risperidone, 2 mg/day vs. 4 mg/day, in first-episode, acutely psychotic patients: Treatment efficacy and effects on fine motor functioning. *Journal of Clinical Psychiatry, 63,* 885–891.

Meyer-Lindenberg, A., Miletich, R. S., Kohn, P. D., Esposito, G., Carson, R. E., Quarantelli, M., ... Berman, K. F. (2002). Reduced prefrontal activity predicts exaggerated striatal dopaminergic function in schizophrenia. *Nature Neuroscience, 5,* 267–271.

Michie, P., Fox, A., Ward, P., Catts, S., & McConaghy, N. (1990). Event-related potential indices of selective attention and cortical lateralization in schizophrenia. *Psychophysiology, 27,* 207–227.

Miklowitz, D. J., Goldstein, M. J., Doane, J. A., Nuechterlein, K. H., Strachan, A. M., Snyder, K. S., & Magana, A. M. (1989). Is expressed emotion an index of a transactional process? Relative's affective style. *Family Process, 28,* 153–167.

Millar, J. K., Wilson-Annan, J. C., Anderson, S., Christie, S., Taylor, M.S., Semple, C. A., ... Porteous, D. J. (2000). Disruption of two novel genes by a translocation co-segregating with schizophrenia. *Human Molecular Genetics, 9,* 1415–1423.

Miller, D. D., Arndt, S., & Andreasen, N. C. (1993). Alogia, attentional impairment, and inappropriate affect: Their status in the dimensions of schizophrenia. *Comprehensive Psychiatry, 34,* 221–226.

Miller, P., Byrne, M., Hodges, A., Lawrie, S. M., Owens, D. G., & Johnstone, E. C. (2002). Schizotypal components in people at high risk of developing schizophrenia: Early findings from the Edinburgh High-Risk Study. *British Journal of Psychiatry, 180,* 179–184.

Miller, T. J., McGlashan, T. H., Rosen, J. L., et al. (2003). Prodromal assessment with the structured interview for prodromal syndromes and the scale of prodromal symptoms: Predictive validity, interrater reliability, and training to reliability. *Schizophrenia Bulletin, 29,* 703–715.

Mittal, V. A., Neumann, C., Saczawa, M., & Walker, E. F. (2008). Longitudinal progression of movement abnormalities in relation to psychotic symptoms in adolescents at high risk of schizophrenia. *Archives of General Psychiatry, 65*(2), 165.

Mittal, V. A., & Walker, E. F. (2007). Movement abnormalities predict conversion to Axis I psychosis among prodromal adolescents. *Journal of Abnormal Psychology, 116*(4), 796.

Mizrahi, R., Addington, J., Rusjan, P. M., Suridjan, I., Ng, A., Boileau, I., ... Wilson, A. A. (2012). Increased stress-induced dopamine release in psychosis. *Biological Psychiatry, 71*(6), 561–567.

Moises, H. W., Yang, L., Kristbjarnarson, H., Wiese, C., Byerley, W., Macciardi, F., et al. (1995). An international two-stage genome-wide search for schizophrenia susceptibility genes. *Nature Genetics, 11,* 321–324.

Muck-Seler, D., Pivac, N., Jakovljevic, M., & Brzovic, Z. (1999). Platelet serotonin, plasma cortisol, and dexamethasone suppression test in schizophrenic patients. *Biological Psychiatry, 45,* 1433–1439.

Murray, G., Isohanni, M., Isohanni, I., & Jones, P. (2003). School and schizophrenia. In A. Grispini (Ed.), *Prevention strategies for schizophrenic disorders.* Rome: Giovanni Fioriti Editore.

Murray, R. M. (1994). Neurodevelopmental schizophrenia: The rediscovery of dementia praecox. *British Journal of Psychiatry, 165,* 6–12.

Murray, R. M., & Jones, P. B. (1995). Schizophrenia: Disease or Syndrome? In H. Hafner & W. F. Gattaz (Eds.), *Search for the causes of schizophrenia, Vol. III* (pp. 186–192). Heidelberg/Berlin: Springer-Verlag.

Murray, R., & Lewis, S. (1987). Is schizophrenia a neurodevelopmental disorder? [editorial]. *British Medical Journal Clinical Research Edition, 295,* 681–682.

Myin-Germeys, I., Krabbendam, L., Delespaul, P., & van Os, J. (2003a). Can cognitive deficits explain differential sensitivity to life events in psychosis? *Social Psychiatry and Psychiatric Epidemiology, 38*, 262–268.

Myin-Germeys, I., Krabbendam, L., Delespaul, P. A., & van Os, J. (2003b). Do life events have their effect on psychosis by influencing the emotional reactivity to daily life stress? *Psychological Medicine, 33*, 327–333.

Myin-Germeys, I., Peeters, F., Havermans, R., Nicolson, N. A., DeVries, M. W., Delespaul, P., & van Os, J. (2003). Emotional reactivity to daily lie stress in psychosis and affective disorder: An experience sampling study. *Acta Psychiatrica Scandinavica, 107*, 124–131.

Naatanen, R. (1982). Processing negativity: An evoked potential reflection of selective attention. *Psychological Bulletin, 92*, 605–640.

Nagy, J., & Szatmari, P. (1986). A chart review of schizotypal personality disorders in children. *Journal of Autism & Developmental Disorders, 16*, 351–367.

National Institute for Clinical Excellence. (2002). *Clinical Guideline I: Schizophrenia. Core interventions in the treatment and management of schizophrenia in primary and secondary care*. London: NICE.

Neumann, C. S., Grimes, K., Walker, E. F., & Baum, K. (1995). Developmental pathways to schizophrenia: Behavioral subtypes. *Journal of Abnormal Psychology, 104*, 558–566.

Nicolson, R., Lenane, M., Singaracharlu, S., Malaspina, D., Giedd, J. N., Hamburger, S. D., ... Rapoport, J. L. (2000). Premorbid speech and language impairments in childhood-onset schizophrenia: Association with risk factors. *American Journal of Psychiatry, 157*, 794–800.

Nicolson, R., & Rapoport, J. L. (1999). Childhood-onset schizophrenia: Rare but worth studying. *Biological Psychiatry, 46*, 1418–1428.

Niemi, L. T., Suvisaari, J. M., Tuulio-Henriksson, A., & Loennqvist, J. K. (2003). Childhood developmental abnormalities in schizophrenia: Evidence from high-risk studies. *Schizophrenia Research, 60*, 239–258.

Niwa, M., Jaaro-Peled, H., Tankou, S., Seshadri, S., Hikida, T., Matsumoto, Y., ... Sawa, A. (2013). Adolescent stress-induced epigenetic control of dopaminergic neurons via glucocorticoids. *Science, 339*, 335–339.

Norman, R. M., & Malla, A. K. (2001). Duration of untreated psychosis: A critical examination of the concept and its importance. *Psychogical Medicine, 31*, 381–400.

Nottelmann, E. D., Susman, E. J., Inoff-Germain, G., Cutler, G. B., Jr., Loriaux, D. L., & Chrousos, G. P. (1987). Developmental processes in early adolescence: Relationships between adolescent adjustment problems and chronologic age, pubertal stage, and puberty-related serum hormone levels. *Journal of Pediatrics, 110*, 473–480.

Nuechterlein, K. H., Dawson, M. E., Ventura, J., Gitlin, M., Subotnik, K. L., Snyder, K. S., ... Bartzokis, G. (1994). The vulnerability/stress model of schizophrenic relapse: A longitudinal study. *Acta Psychiatrica Scandinavica Supplement, 382*, 58–64.

Nugter, A., Dingemans, P., Van der Does, J. W., Linszen, D., & Gersons, B. (1997). Family treatment, expressed emotion and relapse in recent-onset schizophrenia. *Psychiatry Research, 72*, 23–31.

O'Donnell, C., Donohoe, G., Sharkey, L., Owens, N., Migone, M., Harries, R., ... O'Callaghan, E. (2003). Compliance therapy: A randomised controlled trial in schizophrenia. *British Medical Journal, 327*, 834.

O'Leary, D. S., Flaum, M., Kesler, M. L., Flashman, L. A., Arndt, S., & Andreasen, N. C. (2000). Cognitive correlates of the negative, disorganized, and psychotic symptom dimensions of schizophrenia. *Journal of Neuropsychiatry and Clinical Neurosciences, 12*, 4–15.

Owen, M. J., Craddock, N., & O'Donovan, M. C. (2010). Suggestion of roles for both common and rare risk variants in genome-wide studies of schizophrenia. *Archives of General Psychiatry, 67*, 667–673.

Pantelis, C., Velakoulis, D., McGorry, P. D., Wood, S. J., Suckling, J., Phillips, L. J., ... McGuire, P. K. (2003). Neuroanatomical abnormalities before and after onset of psychosis: A cross-sectional and longitudinal MRI comparison. *Lancet, 361*, 281–288.

Parnas, J. (1982). Behavioral precursors of schizophrenia spectrum: A prospective study. *Archives of General Psychiatry, 39*, 658–664.

Paus, T., Keshavan, M., & Giedd, J. N. (2008). Why do many psychiatric disorders emerge during adolescence? *Nature Reviews Neuroscience, 9*, 947–957.

Paus, T., Zijdenbos, A., Worsley, K., Collins, D. L., Blumenthal, J., Giedd, J. N., ... Evans, A. C. (1999). Structural maturation of neural pathway in children and adolescents: In vivo study. *Science, 283*,1908–1911.

Peper, J. S., Hulshoff Pol, H. E., Crone, E. A., & van Honk, J. (2011). Sex steroids and brain structure in pubertal boys and girls: A mini-review of neuroimaging studies. *Neuroscience, 191*, 28–37.

Peters, B. D., & Karlsgodt, K. H. (2015). White matter development in the early stages of psychosis. *Schizophrenia Research, 161*, 61–69.

Pfefferbaum, A., Mathalon, D. H., Sullivan, E. V., Rawles, J. M., Zipursky, R. B., & Lim, K. O. (1994). A quantitative magnetic resonance imaging study of changes in brain morphology from infancy to late adulthood. *Archives of Neurolology, 51*, 874–887.

Philippe, A., Martinez, M., Guilloud-Bataille, M., Gillberg, C., Rastam, M., Sponheim, E., ... van Malldergerme, L. (1999). Genome-wide scan for autism susceptibility genes. Paris Autism Research International Sibpair Study. *Human Molecular Genetics, 8*, 805–812.

Phillips, L. J., Yung, A. R., Yuen, H. P., Pantelis, C., & McGorry, P. D. (2002). Prediction and prevention of transition to psychosis in young people at incipient risk for schizophrenia. *American Journal of Medical Genetics (Neuropsychiatric Genetics), 114*, 929–937.

Pidgeon, D. A. (1964). Tests used in the 1954 and 1957 surveys. In J. W. B. Douglas. (Ed.), *The home and the school* (pp. 129–132). London: MacGibbon & Kee.

Pidgeon, D. A. (1968). Appendix: Details of the fifteen-year tests. In J. W. B. Douglas, J. M. Ross, & H. R. Simpson. (Eds.), *All our futures* (pp. 194–197). London: Peter Davies.

Pilling, S., Bebbington, P., Kuipers, E., Garety, P., Geddes, J., Orbach, G., & Morgan, C. (2002). Psychological treatments in schizophrenia: I. Meta-analysis of family intervention and cognitive behaviour therapy. *Psychological Medicine, 32*, 763–782.

Pinkham, A. E., Penn, D. L., Perkins, D. O., Graham, K. A., & Siegel, M. (2007). Emotion perception and social skill over the course of psychosis: A comparison of individuals "at-risk" for psychosis and individuals with early and chronic schizophrenia spectrum illness. *Cognitive Neuropsychiatry, 12*(3), 198–212.

Plocka-Lewandowska, M., Araszkiewicz, A., & Rybakowski, J. K. (2001). Dexamethasone suppression test and suicide attempts in schizophrenic patients. *European Psychiatry, 16*, 428–431.

Plomin, R., Reiss, D., Hetherington, E. M., & Howe, G. W. (1994). Nature and nurture: Genetic contributions to measures of the family environment. *Developmental Psychology, 30*, 32–43.

Pogue-Geile, M. F. (1997). Developmental aspects of schizophrenia. In M. S. Keshavan & R. M. Murray. (Eds.), *Neurodevelopment and adult psychopathology* (pp. 137–154). Cambridge, UK: Cambridge University Press.

Poulton, R., Caspi, A., Moffitt, T. E., Cannon, M., Murray, R., & Harrington, H. (2000). Children's self-reported psychotic symptoms and adult schizophreniform disorder: A 15-year longitudinal study. *Archives of General Psychiatry, 57*, 1053–1058.

Pritchard, W. (1986). Cognitive event-related potential correlates of schizophrenia. *Psychological Bulletin, 100*, 43–66.

Pukrop, R., Ruhrmann, S., Schultze-Lutter, F., Bechdolf, A., Brockhaus-Dumke, A., & Klosterkötter, J. (2007). Neurocognitive indicators for a conversion to psychosis: Comparison of patients in a potentially initial prodromal state who did or did not convert to a psychosis. *Schizophrenia Research, 92*, 116–125.

Purcell, S. M., Moran, J. L., Fromer, M., ... Sklar, P. (2014). A polygenic burden of rare disruptive mutations in schizophrenia. *Nature, 506*, 185–190.

Rabinowitz, J., Bromet, E. J., Lavelle, J., Carlson, G., Kovasznay, B., & Schwartz, J. E. (1998). Prevalence and severity of substance use disorders and onset of psychosis in first-admission psychotic patients. *Psychological Medicine, 28*, 1411–1419.

Rantakallio, P. (1969). Groups at risk in low birth weight infants and perinatal mortality. *Acta Paediatrica Scandinavica, 193*, 1–71.

Rapoport, J. L., Giedd, J., Kumra, S., Jacobsen, L., Smith, A., Lee, P., Nelson, J., & Hamburger, S. (1997). Childhood-onset schizophrenia. Progressive ventricular change during adolescence. *Archives of General Psychiatry, 54*, 897–903.

Raux, G., Bonnet-Brilhault, F., Louchart, S., Houy, E., Gantier, R., Levillain, D., ... Campion, D. (2002). The -2 bp deletion in exon 6 of the 'alpha 7-like' nicotinic receptor subunit gene is a risk factor for the P50 sensory gating deficit. *Molecular Psychiatry, 7*, 1006–1011.

Rector, N. A., & Beck, A. T. (2002). Cognitive therapy for schizophrenia: From conceptualization to intervention. *Canadian Journal of Psychiatry, 47*, 41–50.

Reid, W. H., Mason, M., & Hogan, T. (1998). Suicide prevention effects associated with clozapine therapy in schizophrenia and schizoaffective disorder. *Psychiatric Service, 49*, 1029–1033.

Reiss, A. L., Abrams, M. T., Singer, H. S., Ross, J. L., & Denckla, M. B. (1996). Brain development, gender and IQ in children: A volumetric imaging study. *Brain, 119*, 1763–1774.

Reite, M., Teale, P., & Rojas, D. C. (1999). Magnet oencephalography: Applications in psychiatry. *Biological Psychiatry, 45*, 1553–1563.

Reveley, A. M., Reveley, M. A., & Clifford, R. M. (1982). Cerebral ventricular size in twins discordant for schizophrenia. *Lancet, 1*, 540–541.

Riecher-Rossler, A., Pflueger, M. O., Aston, J., Borgwardt, S. J., Brewer, W. J., Gschwandtner, U., & Stieglitz, R. D. (2009). Efficacy of using cognitive status in predicting psychosis: A 7-year follow-up. *Biological Psychiatry, 66*, 1023–1030.

Ripke, S., O'Dushlaine, C., Chambert, K., ... Sullivan, P. F. (2013). Genome-wide association identifies 13 new risk loci for schizophrenia. *Nature Genetics, 45*, 1150–1159.

Roalf, D. R., Ruparel, K., Verma, R., Elliott, M. A., Gur, R. E., & Gur, R. C. (2013). White matter organization and neurocognitive performance variability in schizophrenia. *Schizophrenia Research, 143*, 172–178.

Robins, L. N. (1966). *Deviant children grown up. A sociological and psychiatric study of sociopathic personality.* Baltimore: Williams and Wilkins.

Robins, L. N., Helzer, J. E., Weissman, M. M., Orvaschel, H., Gruenberg, E., Burke, J. D. Jr., & Regier, D. A. (1984). Lifetime prevalence of specific psychiatric disorders in three sites. *Archives of General Psychiatry, 41*, 949–958.

Robinson, D., Woerner, M. G., Alvir, J. M., Bilder, R., Goldman, R., Geisler, S., ... Lieberman, J. A. (1999a). Predictors of relapse following response from a first episode of schizophrenia or schizoaffective disorder. *Archives of General Psychiatry, 56*, 241–247.

Robinson, D. G., Woerner, M. G., Alvir, J. M., Geisler, S., Koreen, A., Sheitman, B., ... Lieberman, J. A. (1999b). Predictors of treatment response from a first episode of schizophrenia or schizoaffective disorder. *American Journal of Psychiatry, 156*, 544–549.

Rodriguez, E., George, N., Lachaux, J-P., Martinerie, J., Renault, B., & Varela, F. J. (1999). Perception's shadow: Long-distance synchronization of human brain activity. *Nature, 397*, 430–433.

Rohrbaugh, J., McCallum, W., Galliard, A., Simons, R., Birbaumer, N., & Papakostopoulos, D. (1986). ERPs associated with preparatory and movement-related processes: A review. In M. McCallum, R. Zappoli, & F. Denoth (Eds.), *Cerebral psychophysiology: Studies in event-related potentials* (pp. 189–229). EEG Suppl 38, Amsterdam: Elsevier.

Rose, V. L. (1997). APA practice guideline for the treatment of patients with schizophrenia. *American Family Physician, 56*, 1217–1220.

Rupprecht, R., & Holsboer, F. (1999). Neuroactive steroids: Mechanisms of action and neuropsychopharmacological perspectives. *Trends in Neurosciences, 22*, 410–416.

Saint-Cyr, J. (2003). Frontal-striatal circuit functions: Context, sequence, and consequence. *Journal of the International Neuropsychological Society, 9*, 103–128.

Salisbury, D. F., Bonner-Jackson, A., Griggs, C. B., Shenton, M. E., & McCarley, R. W. (2001). Mismatch negativity in schizophrenia: Does MMN amplitude decline with disease duration? *Biological Psychiatry, 49* (Suppl.), 85S.

Salisbury, D. F., Shenton, M. E., Griggs, C. B., Bonner-Jackson, A., & McCarley, R. W. (2002). Mismatch negativity in chronic schizophrenia and first-episode schizophrenia. *Archives of General Psychiatry, 59*, 686–694.

Salzman, C., Solomon, D., Miyawaki, E., Glassman, R., Rood, L., Flowers, E., & Thayer, S. (1991). Parenteral lorazepam versus parenteral haloperidol for the control of psychotic disruptive behavior. *Journal of Clinical Psychiatry, 52*, 177–180.

Sanger, T. M., Lieberman, J. A., Tohen, M., Grundy, S., Beasley, C., Jr., & Tollefson, G. D. (1999). Olanzapine versus haloperidol treatment in first-episode psychosis. *American Journal of Psychiatry, 156*, 79–87.

Sartorius, N., Fleischhacker, W., Gjerris, A., Kern, U., Knapp, M., Leonard, B. E., ... Twomey, E. (2002). The usefulness and use of second-generation antipsychotic medications. *Current Opinion in Psychiatry, 15*, S1–S51.

Satterfield, J., Schell, A., Nicholar, T., Satterfield, B., & Freese, T. (1990). Ontogeny of selective attention effects on event-related potentials in attention-deficit hyperactivity disorder and normal boys. *Biological Psychiatry, 28*, 879–903.

Satterthwaite, T. D., Vandekar, S. N., Wolf, D. H., Bassett, D. S., Ruparel, K., Shehzad, Z., ... Gur, R. E. (2015). Connectome-wide network analysis of youth with psychosis-spectrum symptoms. *Molecular Psychiatry, 20*, 1508–1515.

Satterthwaite, T. D., Wolf, D. H., Erus, G., Ruparel, K., Elliott, M. A., Gennatas, E. D., ... Gur, R. E. (2013). Functional maturation of the executive system during adolescence. *Journal of Neuroscience, 33*, 16249–16261.

Saykin, A. J., Shtasel, D. L., Gur, R. E., Kester, D. B., Mozley, L. H., Stafiniak, P., & Gur, R. C. (1994). Neuropsychological deficits in neuroleptic-naive, first-episode schizophrenic patients. *Archives of General Psychiatry*, *51*,124–131.

Schaffner, K. F., & McGorry, P. D. (2001). Preventing severe mental illnesses—new prospects and ethical challenges. *Schizophrenia Research*, *51*, 3–15.

Schizophrenia Working Group of the Psychiatric Genomics Consortium. (2014). Biological insights from 108 schizophrenia-associated genetic loci. *Nature*, *511*, 421–427.

Schmidt, A., Lenz, C., Smieskova. R., Harrisberger, F., Walter, A., Riecher-Rössler, A., . . . Borgwardt, S.J. (2015). Brain diffusion changes in emerging psychosis and the impact of state-dependent psychopathology. *Neurosignals*, *23*, 71–83.

Schooler, N., Keith, S., Severe, J., Matthews, S., Bellack, A., Glick, I., . . . Woerner, M. (1997). Relapse and rehospitalization during maintenance treatment of schizophrenia. *Archives of General Psychiatry*, *54*, 453–463.

Schreiber, H., Stolz-Born, G., Heinrich, H., & Kornhuber, H. H. (1992). Attention, cognition, and motor perseveration in adolescents at genetic risk for schizophrenia and control subjects. *Psychiatry Research*, *44*, 125–140.

Schwab, S. G., Knapp, M., Mondabon, S., Hallmayer, J., Borrmann-Hassenbach, M., Albus, M., . . . Wildenauer, D. B. (2003). Support for association of schizophrenia with genetic variation in the 6p22.3 gene, dysbindin, in sib-pair families with linkage and in an additional sample of triad families. *American Journal of Human Genetics*, *72*, 185–190.

Scottish Schizophrenia Research Group. (1987). The Scottish First Episode Schizophrenia Study. II. Treatment: Pimozide versus flupenthixol. *British Journal of Psychiatry*, *150*, 334–338.

Seeman, M. V. (1997). Psychopathology in women and men: Focus on female hormones. *American Journal of Psychiatry*, *154*, 1641–1647.

Seidman, L. J., Faraone, S. V., Goldstein, J. M., Goodman, J. M., Kremen, W. S., Matsuda, G., . . . Tsuang, M. T. (1997). Reduced subcortical brain volumes in nonpsychotic siblings of schizophrenic patients: A pilot MRI Study. *American Journal of Medical Genetics*, *74*, 507–514.

Seidman, L. J., Giuliano, A. J., Meyer, E. C., Addington, J., Cadenhead, K. S., Cannon, T. D., . . . Cornblatt, B. A. (2010). Neuropsychology of the prodrome to psychosis in the NAPLS Consortium: Relationship to family history and conversion to psychosis. *Archives of General Psychiatry*, *67*, 578–588.

Selemon, L. D. (2013) A role for synaptic plasticity in the adolescent development of executive function. *Translational Psychiatry*, *3*, e238.

Selemon, L., & Goldman-Rakic, P. (1999). The reduced neuropil hypothesis: A circuit based model of schizophrenia. *Biological Psychiatry*, *45*, 17–25.

Sernyak, M. J., Desai, R., Stolar, M., & Rosenheck, R. (2001). Impact of clozapine on completed suicide. *American Journal of Psychiatry*, *158*, 931–937.

Shansky, R. M., & Lipps, J. (2013). Stress-induced cognitive dysfunction: Hormone–neurotransmitter interactions in the prefrontal cortex. *Frontiers in Human Neuroscience*, *7*, 123.

Sharma, S., & Lal, R. (1986). Minor physical anomalies in schizophrenia. *International Journal of Neuroscience*, *31*, 138.

Shenton, M., Kikinis, R., Jolesz, F., Pollak, S., LeMay, M., Wible, C., . . . McCarley, R. (1992). Abnormalities of the left temporal lobe and thought disorder in schizophrenia: A quantitative magnetic resonance imaging study. *New England Journal of Medicine*, *327*, 604–612.

Shifman, S., Bronstein, M., Sternfeld, M., Pisante-Shalom, A., Lev-Lehman, E., Weizman, A., . . . Darvasi, A. (2002). A highly significant association between a COMT haplotype and schizophrenia. *American Journal of Human Genetics*, *71*, 1296–1302.

Shinkai, T., Ohmori, O., Hori, H., & Nakamura, J. (2002). Allelic association of the neuronal nitric oxide synthase (NOS1) gene with schizophrenia. *Molecular Psychiatry*, *7*, 560–563.

Silberg, J., Pickles, A., Rutter, M., Hewitt, J., Simonoff, E., Maes, H., . . . Eaves, L. (1999). The influence of genetic factors and life stres on depression among adolescent girls. *Archives of General Psychiatry*, *56*, 225–232.

Silbersweig, D. A., Stern, E., Frith, C., Cahill, C., Holmes, A., Grootoonk, S., . . . Frackowiak, R. S. J. (1995). A functional neuroanatomy of hallucinations in schizophrenia. *Nature*, *378*, 176–179.

Silver, H., Barash, I., Aharon, N., Kaplan, A., & Poyurovsky, M. (2000). Fluvoxamine augmentation of antipsychotics improves negative symptoms in psychotic chronic schizophrenic patients: A placebo-controlled study. *International Clinical Psychopharmacololgy*, *15*, 257–261.

Silver, H., & Nassar, A. (1992). Fluvoxamine improves negative symptoms in treated chronic schizophrenia: An add-on double-blind, placebo-controlled study. *Biological Psychiatry, 31*, 698–704.

Smieskova, R., Fusar-Poli, P., Allen, P., Bendfeldt, K., Stieglitz,R. D., Drewe, J., ... Borgwardt, S. J. (2010). Neuroimaging predictors of transition to psychosis: A systematic review and meta-analysis. *Neuroscience and Biobehavior Review, 38*, 1207–1222.

Smoller, J. W., Craddock, N., Kendler, K., Lee, P. H., Neale, B. M., Nurnberger, J. I., ... Sullivan, P. F. (2013). Cross-Disorder Group of the Psychiatric Genomics Consortium. Identification of risk loci with shared effects on five major psychiatric disorders: A genome-wide analysis. *Lancet, 38*, 1371–1379.

Sørensen, H. J., Mortensen, E. L., Reinisch, J. M., & Mednick, S. A. (2009). Parental psychiatric hospitalization and offspring schizophrenia. *World Journal of Biological Psychiatry, 10*, 571–575.

Sowell, E. R., Thompson, P. M., Holmes, C. J., Jernigen, T. L, & Toga, A. W. (1999). In vivo evidence for post-adolescent brain maturation in frontal and striatal regions. *Nature Neuroscience, 2*, 859–861.

Sporn, A., Clasen, L. S., Greenstein, D., Giedd, J. N., Lenane, M., Gochman, P. A., ... Rapoport, J.L. (2003). Progressive brain volume loss during adolescence in childhood-onset schizophrenia. *American Journal of Psychiatry, 160*, 2181–2189.

Srihari, V. H., & Shah, J. (2012). Is early intervention for psychosis feasible and effective? *Psychiatric Clinics of North America, 35*, 613–631.

Srihari, V. H., Tek, C., Pollard, J., et al. (2014). Reducing the duration of untreated psychosis and its impact in the U.S.: The STEP-ED study. *BMC Psychiatry, 14*, 335.

Stefansson, H., Sarginson, J., Kong, A., Yates, P., Steinthorsdottir, V., Gudfinnsson, E., ... St. Clair, D. (2003). Association of neuregulin 1 with schizophrenia confirmed in a Scottish population. *American Journal of Human Genetics, 72*, 83–87.

Stefansson, H., Sigurdsson, E., Steinthorsdottir, V., Bjornsdottir, S., Sigmundsson, T., Ghosh, S., ... Stefansson, K. (2002). Neuregulin 1 and susceptibility to schizophrenia. *American Journal of Human Genetics, 71*, 877–892.

Steinert, T., Wiebe, C., & Gebhardt, R. P. (1999). Aggressive behavior against self and others among first-admission patients with schizophrenia. *Psychiatric Services, 50*, 85–90.

Stevens, J. R. (2002). Schizophrenia: Reproductive hormones and the brain. *American Journal of Psychiatry,159*, 713–719.

Strandburg, R., Marsh, J., Brown, W., Asarnow, R., & Guthrie, D. (1984). Event-related potentials concomitants of information processing dysfunction in schizophrenic children. *Electroencephalography and Clinical Neurophysiology, 57*, 236–253.

Strandburg, R., Marsh, J., Brown, W., Asarnow, R., Guthrie, D., & Higa, J. (1990). Event-related potential correlates of impaired attention in schizophrenic children. *Biological Psychiatry, 27*, 1103–1115.

Strandburg, R., Marsh, J., Brown, W., Asarnow, R., Guthrie, D., & Higa, J. (1994a). Continuity of information processing deficits across childhood- and adult-onset schizophrenia: ERP correlates. *Schizophrenia Bulletin, 20*, 685–696.

Strandburg, R., Marsh, J., Brown, W., Asarnow, R., Guthrie, D., & Higa, J. (1994b). Reduced attention-related negative potentials in schizophrenic adults. *Psychophysiology, 31*, 272–281.

Strandburg, R., Marsh, J., Brown, W., Asarnow, R., Higa, J., & Guthrie, D. (1994c). Continuous processing-related ERPs in schizophrenic and normal children. *Biological Psychiatry,* 35, 525–538.

Straub, R. E., Jiang, Y., MacLean, C. J., Ma, Y., Webb, B. T., Myakishev, M. V., ... Kendler, K. S. (2002a). Genetic variation in the 6p22.3 gene DTNBP1, the human ortholog of the mouse dysbindin gene, is associated with schizophrenia. *American Journal of Human Genetics, 71*, 337–348.

Straub, R. E., MacLean, C. J., Ma, Y., Webb, B. T., Myakishev, M. V., Harris-Kerr, C., ... Kendler, K. S. (2002b). Genome-wide scans of three independent sets of 90 Irish multiplex schizophrenia families and follow-up of selected regions in all families provides evidence for multiple susceptibility genes. *Molecular Psychiatry, 7*, 542–559.

Strelzyk, F., Hermes, M., Naumann, E., Oitzl, M., Walter, C., Busch, H. P., ... Schachinger, H. (2012). Tune it down to live it up? Rapid, non-genomic effects of cortisol on the human brain. *Journal of Neuroscience, 32*, 616–625.

Suarez, B. K., Hampe, C. L., & Van Eerdewegh, P. (1994). Problems of replicating linkage claims in psychiatry. In E. S. Gershon, C. R. Cloninger, & J. E. Barrett (Eds.), *Genetic approaches in nental disorders* (pp. 23–46). Washington, DC: American Psychiatric Press.

Susman, E. J., Inoff-Germain, G., Nottelmann, E. D., Loriaux, D. L., Cutler, G. B., Jr., & Chrousos, G. P. (1987). Hormones, emotional dispositions, and aggressive attributes in young adolescents. *Child Development, 58*, 1114–1134.

Szily, E., & Keri, S. (2009). Anomalous subjective experience and psychosis risk in young depressed patients. *Psychopathology, 42*, 229–235.

Szymanski, S., Masiar, S., Mayerhoff, D., Loebel, A., Geisler, S., Pollack, S., ... Lieberman, J. (1994). Clozapine response in treatment-refractory first-episode schizophrenia. *Biological Psychiatry, 35*, 278–280.

Tada, M., Nagai, T., Kirihara, K., Koike, S., Suga, M., Araki, T., ... Kasai, K. (2016). Differential alterations of auditory gamma oscillatory responses between pre-onset high-risk individuals and first-episode schizophrenia. *Cerebral Cortex, 26*(3), 1027–1035.

Tallon-Baudry, C., & Bertrand, O. (1999). Oscillatory gamma activity in humans and its role in object representation. *Trends in Cognitive Science, 3*,151–162.

Tamminga, C. A., Ivleva, E. I., Keshavan, M. S., Pearlson, G. D., Clementz, B. A., Witte, B., ... Sweeney, J. A. (2013). Clinical phenotypes of psychosis in the bipolar and schizophrenia network on intermediate phenotypes (B-SNIP). *American Journal of Psychiatry, 170*, 1263–1274.

Tamminga, C. A., Thaker, G. K., & Medoff, D. R. (2002). Neuropsychiatric aspects of schizophrenia. In S. C. Yudofsky & R. E. Hales (Eds.), *The American Psychiatric Publishing textbook of neuropsychiatry and clinical neurosciences* (4th ed., pp. 989–1020). Washington, DC: American Psychiatric Publishing, Inc.

Tang, S. X., Yi, J. J., Calkins, M. E., Whinna, D. A., Kohler, C. G., Souders, M. C., ... Gur, R. E. (2014). Psychiatric disorders in 22q11.2 deletion syndrome are prevalent but under-treated. *Psychological Medicine, 44*, 1267–1277.

Tarrant, C., & Jones, P. (1999). Precursors to schizophrenia: Do biological markers have specificity? *Canadian Journal of Psychiatry, 44*, 335–349.

Thakore, J. H., Mann, J. N., Vlahos, I., Martin, A., & Reznek R. (2002). Increased visceral fat distribution in drug-naive and drug-free patients with schizophrenia. *International Journal of Obesity & Related Metabolic Disorders, 26*, 137–141.

Thompson, K. N., McGorry, P. D., & Harrigan, S. M. (2001). Reduced awareness of illness in first-episode psychosis. *Comprehensive Psychiatry, 42*, 498–503.

Thompson, P. M., Vidal, C., Giedd, J. N., Gochman, P., Blumenthal, J., Nicolson, R., ... Rapoport, J. L. (2001). Mapping adolescent brain change reveals dynamic wave of accelerated gray matter loss in very early-onset schizophrenia. *Proceedings of the National Academy of Sciences, U S A, 98*, 11650–11655.

Tkachev, D., Mimmack, M. L., Ryan, M. M., Wayland, M., Freeman, T., Jones, P. B., ... Bahn, S. (2003). Oligodendrocyte dysfunction in schizophrenia and bipolar disorder. *Lancet, 362*, 798–805.

Tompson, M. C., Asarnow, J. R., Hamilton, E. B., Newell, L. E., & Goldstein, M. J. (1997). Children with schizophrenia-spectrum disorders: Thought disorder and communication problems in a family interactional context. *Journal of Child Psychology and Psychiatry, 38*, 421–429.

Trotman, H. D., Holtzman, C. W., Ryan, A. T., Shapiro, D. I., MacDonald, A. N., Goulding, S. M., ... Walker, E. F. (2013). The development of psychotic disorders in adolescence: A potential role for hormones. *Hormones and Behavior, 64*, 411–419.

Tsuang, M. T., Stone, W. S., Tarbox, S. I., & Faraone, S. V. (2002). An integration of schizophrenia with schizotypy: Identification of schizotaxia and implications for research on treatment and prevention. *Schizophrenia Research, 54*, 169–175.

Tucker, D., & Williamson, P. (1984). Asymmetric neural control systems in human self-regulation. *Psychological Review, 91*, 185–215.

Ueland, T., & Rund, B. R. (2004a). A controlled randomised treatment study: The effects of a cognitive training program on adolescents with early onset psychosis. *Acta Psychiatrica Scandinavica, 109*(1), 70–74.

Ueland, T., Rund, B., Borg, N., Newton, E., Purvis, R., & Wykes, T. (2004b). Modification of performance on the Span of Apprehension Task in a group of young people with early onset psychosis. *Scandinavian Journal of Psychology, 45*(1), 55–60.

Umbricht, D., Javitt, D. C., Bates, J., Kane, J., & Lieberman, J. A. (2002). Auditory event-related potentials (ERP): Indices of both premorbid and illness-related progressive neuropathology in schizophrenia? *Schizophrenia Research, 53*, 18.

Umbricht, D., Javitt, D. C., Novak, G., Pollack, S., Liberman, J., & Kane, J. (1998). Effects of clozapine on auditory event-related potentials in schizophrenia. *Biological Psychiatry, 44*, 716–725.

van Oel, C. J., Sitskoorn, M. M., Cremer, M. P. M., & Kahn, R. S. (2002). School performance as a premorbid marker for schizophrenia: A twin study. *Schizophrenia Bulletin, 28*, 401–414.

Van Os, J., Jones, P., Lewis, G., Wadsworth, M., & Murray, R. (1997). Developmental precursors of affective illness in a general population birth cohort. *Archives of General Psychiatry, 54*, 625–631.

van Os, J., Linscott, R. J., Myin-Germeys, I., Delespaul, P., & Krabbendam, L. (2009). A systematic review and meta-analysis of the psychosis continuum: Evidence for a psychosis proneness-persistence impairment model of psychotic disorder. *Psychological Medicine, 39*(2), 179–195.

van Rijn, S., Aleman, A., de Sonneville, L., Sprong, M., Ziermans, T., Schothorst, P., ... Swaab, H. (2011). Misattribution of facial expressions of emotion in adolescents at increased risk of psychosis: The role of inhibitory control. *Psychological Medicine, 41*, 499–508.

Walder, D. J., Walker, E. F., & Lewine, R. J. (2000). Cognitive functioning, cortisol release, and symptom severity in patients with schizophrenia. *Biological Psychiatry, 48*, 1121–1132.

Waldo, M. C., Carey, G., Myles-Worsley, M., Cawthra, E., Adler, L. E., Nagamoto, H. T., ... Freedman, R. (1991). Codistribution of a sensory gating deficit and schizophrenia in multi-affected families. *Psychiatry Research, 39*, 257–268.

Walker, E. (1991). Research on life-span development in schizophrenia. In E. Walker (Ed.), *Schizophrenia: A life-course developmental perspective* (pp. 1–6). San Diego: Academic Press, Inc.

Walker, E. F. (1994). Developmentally moderated expressions of the neuropathology underlying schizophrenia. *Schizophrenia Bulletin, 20*, 453–480.

Walker, E. F. (2002). Adolescent neurodevelopment and psychopathology. *Current Directions in Psychological Science, 11*, 24–28.

Walker, E., & Bollini, A-M. (2002). Pubertal neurodevelopment and the emergence of psychotic symptoms. *Schizophrenia Research, 54*, 17–23.

Walker, E. F., Brennan, P. A., Esterberg, M., Brasfield, J., Pearce, B., & Compton, M. T. (2010). Longitudinal changes in cortisol secretion and conversion to psychosis in at-risk youth. *Journal of Abnormal Psychology, 119*(2), 401.

Walker, E. F., & Diforio, D. (1997). Schizophrenia: A neural diathesis-stress model. *Psychological Review, 104*, 667–685.

Walker, E., & Emory, E. (1985). Infants at risk for psychopathology: Offspring of schizophrenic parents. *Child Development, 54*, 1269–1285.

Walker, E. F., Grimes, K. E., Davis, D. M., & Smith, A. J. (1993). Childhood precursors of schizophrenia: Facial expressions of emotion. *American Journal of Psychiatry, 150*, 1654–1660.

Walker, E., & Lewine, R. J. (1990). Prediction of adult-onset schizophrenia from childhood home movies of the patients. *American Journal of Psychiatry, 147*, 1052–1056.

Walker, E. F., Lewine, R. R. J., & Neumann, C. (1996). Childhood behavioral characteristics and adult brain morphology in schizophrenia. *Schizophrenia Research, 22*, 93–101.

Walker, E., Lewis, N., Loewy, R., & Palyo, S. (1999). Motor dysfunction and risk for schizophrenia. *Development & Psychopathology, 11*, 509–523.

Walker, E., Mittal, V. & Tessner, K. (2008). Stress and the hypothalamic pituitary adrenal axis in the developmental course of schizophrenia. *Annual Review of Clinical Psychology, 4*, 189–216.

Walker, E. F., Savoie, T., & Davis, D. (1994). Neuromotor precursors of schizophrenia. *Schizophrenia Bulletin, 20*, 441–451.

Walker, E. F., Trotman, H. D., Goulding, S. M., Holtzman, C. W., Ryan, A. T., McDonald, A., ... Brasfield, J. L. (2013). Developmental mechanisms in the prodrome to psychosis. *Developmental Psychopatholology, 25*(4 Pt 2), 1585–1600.

Walker, E. F., Trotman, H. D., Pearce, B. D., Addington, J., Cadenhead, K. S., Cornblatt, B. A., ... Woods, S. W. (2013). Cortisol levels and risk for psychosis: Initial findings from the North American Prodrome Longitudinal Study. *Biological Psychiatry, 74*(6), 410–417.

Walker, E. F., Walder, D. J., & Reynolds, F. (2001). Developmental changes in cortisol secretion in normal and at-risk youth. *Development & Psychopathology, 13*, 721–732.

Wassef, A. A., Dott, S. G., Harris, A., Brown, A., O'Boyle, M., Meyer, W. J., 3rd, & Rose, R. M. (2000). Randomized, placebo-controlled pilot study of divalproex sodium in the treatment of acute exacerbations of chronic schizophrenia. *Journal of Clinical Psychopharmacology, 20*, 357–361.

Watkins, J., Asarnow, R., & Tanguay, P. (1988). Symptom development in childhood-onset schizophrenia. *Journal of Child Psychology and Psychiatry, 29*, 865–878.

Watt, N. F. (1978). Patterns of childhood social development in adult schizophrenics. *Archives of General Psychiatry, 35*, 160–165.

Watt, N., Grubb, T., & Erlenmeyer-Kimling, L. (1982). Social, emotional, and intellectual behavior at school among children at high risk for schizophrenia. *Journal of Consulting and Clinical Psychology*, *50*, 171–181.

Watt, N., & Lubensky, A. (1976). Childhood roots of schizophrenia. *Journal of Consulting and Clinical Psychology*, *44*, 363–375.

Watt, N., & Saiz, C. (1991). Longitudinal studies of premorbid development of adult schizophrenics. In E. Walker (Ed.), *Schizophrenia: A life-course developmental perspective* (pp. 158–185). San Diego: Academic Press, Inc.

Weinberger, D. (1986). The pathogenesis of schizophrenia: A neurodevelopmental theory. In H. Nasrallah & D. Weinberger (Eds.), *The neurobiology of schizophrenia* (pp. 397–406). Amsterdam: Elsevier Science Publishers.

Weinberger, D. R. (1987). Implications of normal brain development for the pathogenesis of schizophrenia. *Archives of General Psychiatry*, *44*, 660–669.

Weinberger, D. R. (1995). From neuropathology to neurodevelopment. *Lancet*, *346*, 552–557.

Weinberger, D. R., Berman, K. F., Suddath, R., & Torrey, E. F. (1992). Evidence of dysfunction of a prefrontal-limbic network in schizophrenia: A magnetic resonance imaging and regional cerebral blood flow study of discordant monozygotic twins. *American Journal of Psychiatry*, *149*, 890–897.

Weinberger, D. R., DeLisi, L. E., Neophytides, A. N., & Wyatt, R. J. (1981). Familial aspects of CT scan abnormalities in chronic schizophrenic patients. *Psychiatry Research*, *4*, 65–71.

Weinberger, D. R., Egan, M. F., Bertolino, A., Calicott, J. H., Mattay, V. S., Lipska, B. K., ... Goldberg, T. E. (2001). Prefrontal neurons and the genetics of schizophrenia. *Biological Psychiatry*, *50*, 825–844.

Weinstein, D. D., Diforio, D., Schiffman, J., Walker, E., & Bonsall, R. (1999). Minor physical anomalies, dermatoglyphic asymmetries, and cortisol levels in adolescents with schizotypal personality disorder. *American Journal of Psychiatry*, *156*, 617–623.

Werry, J. S. (1981). Drugs and learning. *Journal of Child Psychology and Psychiatry*, *22*, 283–290.

Werry, J. S., McClellan, J. M., & Chard, L. (1991). Childhood and adolescent schizophrenic, bipolar, and schizoaffective disorders: A clinical and outcome study. *Journal of the American Academy of Child and Adolescent Psychiatry*, *30*, 457–465.

Whitford, T. J., Kubicki, M., Pelavin, P. E., Lucia, D., Schneiderman, J. S., Pantelis, C., ... Shenton, M. E. (2015). Cingulum bundle integrity associated with delusions of control in schizophrenia: Preliminary evidence from diffusion-tensor tractography. *Schizophrenia Research*, *161*, 36–41.

Wible, C. F., Kubicki, M., Yoo, S-S, Kacher, D. F., Salisbury, D. F., Anderson, M. C., ... McCarley, R. W. (2001). A functional magnetic resonance imaging study of auditory mismatch in schizophrenia. *American Journal of Psychiatry*, *158*, 938–943.

Wiersma, D., Wanderling, J., Dragomirecka, E., Ganev, K., Harrison, G., an der Heiden, W., ... Walsh, D. (2000). Social disability in schizophrenia: its development and prediction over 15 years in incidence cohorts in six European centres. *Psychological Medicine*, *30*, 1155–1167.

Wiersma, D., Nienhuis, F. J., Slooff, C. J., & Giel, R. (1998). Natural course of schizophrenic disorders: A 15-year follow-up of a Dutch incidence cohort. *Schizophrenia Bulletin*, *24*, 75–85.

Williams, J., McGuffin, P., Nothen, M., & Owen, M. J. (1997). Meta-analysis of association between the 5-HT2a receptor T102C polymorphism and schizophrenia. EMASS Collaborative Group. European Multicentre Association Study of Schizophrenia. *Lancet*, *349*, 1221.

Wolff, A. L., & O'Driscoll, G. A. (1999). Motor deficits and schizophrenia: The evidence from neuroleptic-naive patients and populations at risk. *Journal of Psychiatry & Neuroscience*, *24*, 304–314.

Wood, S. J., Pantelis, C., Proffitt, T., Phillips, L. J., Stuart, G. W., Buchanan, J.-A., ... McGorry, P. D. (2003). Spatial working memory ability is a marker of risk-for-psychosis. *Psychological Medicine*, *33*, 1239–1247.

Woodberry, K. A, Seidman, L. J, Giuliano, A. J., Verdi, M. B., Cook, W. L., & McFarlane, W. R. (2010). Neuropsychological profiles in individuals at clinical high risk for psychosis: Relationship to psychosis and intelligence. *Schizophrenia Research*, *123*, 188–198.

Woods, S. W., Miller, T. J., Davidson, L., Hawkins, K. A., Sernyak, M. J., & McGlashan, T. H. (2001). Estimated yield of early detection of prodromal or first episode patients by screening first-degree relatives of schizophrenic patients. *Schizophrenia Research*, *52*, 21–27.

Woods, S., Zipursky, R., Perkins, D., Addington, J., Marquez, E., Breier, A., & McGlashan, T. H. (2002). Olanzapine vs. placebo for prodromal symptoms. *Acta Psychiatrica Scandinavica*, *106*, 43.

Wykes, T., Reeder, C., Williams, C., Corner, J., Rice, C., & Everitt, B. (2001). Are the effects of cognitive remediation therapy (CRT) durable? Results from an exploratory trial in schizophrenia. *Schizophrenia Research, 61*, 163–174.

Wykes, T., & van der Gaag, M. (2001). Is it time to develop a new cognitive therapy for psychosis—cognitive remediation therapy (CRT)? *Clinical Psychology Review, 21*, 1227–1256.

Yakovlev, P. L., & Lecours, A. R. (1967). The myelogenetic cycles of regional maturation of the brain. In A. Minkowski (Ed.), *Regional development of the brain in early life* (pp. 3–70). Oxford: Blackwell.

Yap, H. L., Mahendran, R., Lim, D., Liow, P. H., Lee, A., Phang, S., & Tiong, A. (2001). Risperidone in the treatment of first episode psychosis. *Singapore Medical Journal, 42*, 170–173.

Yarden, P. E., & Discipio, W. J. (1971). Abnormal movements and prognosis in schizophrenia. *American Journal of Psychiatry, 128*, 317–323.

Yi, J. J., Calkins, M. E., Tang, S. X., Kohler, C. K., McDonald-McGinn, D. M., Zackai, E. H., ... Gur, R. E. (2015). Impact of psychiatric comorbidity and cognitive deficit on function in 22q11.2 deletion syndrome. *Journal of Clinical Psychiatry, 76*, 1262–1270.

Yung, A. R., & McGorry, P. D. (1996). The prodromal phase of first-episode psychosis: Past and current conceptualizations. *Schizophrenia Bulletin, 22*, 353–370.

Yung, A. R., Phillips, L. J., Yuen, H. P., Francey, S. M., McFarlane, C. A., Hallgren, M., & McGorry, P. D. (2003). Psychosis prediction: 12-month follow up of a high-risk ("prodromal") group. *Schizophrenia Research, 60*, 21–32.

Zammit, S., Allebeck, P., Andreasson, S., Lunberg, I., & Lewis, G. (2002). Self-reported cannabis use as a risk factor for schizophrenia in Swedish conscripts of 1969: Historical cohort study. *British Medical Journal, 325*, 1199–1201.

Zhang-Wong, J., Zipursky, R. B., Beiser, M., & Bean, G. (1999). Optimal haloperidol dosage in first-episode psychosis. *Canadian Journal of Psychiatry, 44*, 164–167.

Zornberg, G. L., Buka, S. L., & Tsuang, M. T. (2000). Hypoxic-ischemia-related fetal/neonatal complications and risk of schizophrenia and other nonaffective psychoses: A 19-year longitudinal study. *American Journal of Psychiatry, 157*, 196–202.

Part III: Anxiety Disorders

Abramowitz, J. S., Whiteside, S. P., & Deacon, B. J. (2005). The effectiveness of treatment for pediatric obsessive-compulsive disorder: A meta-analysis. *Behavior Therapy, 36*, 55–63.

Achenbach, T. M. (1991). *Manual for the Child Behavior Checklist/4-18 and 1991 Profile.* Burlington, VT: University of Vermont Department of Psychiatry.

Achenbach, T. M., & Edelbrock, C. S. (1984). Psychopathology of childhood. *Annual Review of Psychology, 35*, 227–256.

Achiam-Montal, M., Tibi, L., & Lipsitz, J. D. (2013). Panic disorder in children and adolescents with noncardiac chest pain. *Child Psychiatry and Human Development, 44*(6), 742–750.

Ainsworth, M. D. S., Blehar, M. C., Waters, E., & Wall, E. (1978). *Patterns of attachment: A psychological study of the strange situation.* Hillsdale, NJ: Lawrence Erlbaum Associates.

Albano, A. M., Chorpita, B. F., & Barlow, D. H. (2003). *Childhood anxiety disorders.* New York: Guilford Press.

Alderman, J., Wolkow, R., Chung, M., & Johnston, H. F. (1998). Sertraline treatment of children and adolescents with obsessive compulsive disorder or depression: Pharmacokinetics, tolerability, and efficacy. *Journal of the American Academy of Child and Adolescent Psychiatry, 37*, 386–394.

Alloy, L. B., Kelly, A. K., Mineka, S., & Clements, C. M. (1990). Comorbidity in anxiety and depressive disorders: A helplessness-hopelessness perspective. In J. D. Maser & C. R. Cloninger (Eds.), *Comorbidity of mood and anxiety disorders* (pp. 499–544). Washington, DC: American Psychiatric Press:.

Alpert-Gillis, L. J., Pedro-Carroll, J. L., & Cowen, E. L. (1989). The children of divorce intervention program: Development, implementation, and evaluation of a program for young urban children. *Journal of Consulting and Clinical Psychology, 57*, 583–589.

Amemori, K., Amemori, S., & Graybiel, A. M. (2015). Motivation and affective judgments differentially recruit neurons in the primate dorsolateral prefrontal and anterior cingulate cortex. *Journal of Neuroscience, 35*(5), 1939–1953.

American Psychiatric Association. (2004). Practice guideline for the treatment of patients with acute stress disorder and posttraumatic stress disorder. *American Journal of Psychiatry, 161* (Suppl 11), 1–31.

American Psychiatric Association. (2013). *Diagnostic and statistical manual of mental disorders* (5th ed.). Washington, DC: American Psychiatric Association.

Anderson, R. A., & Rees, C. S. (2007). Group versus individual cognitive-behavioural treatment for obsessive-compulsive disorder: A controlled trial. *Behaviour Research and Therapy, 45*(1), 123–137.

Andrykowski, M. A., & Cordova, M. J. (1998). Factors associated with PTSD symptoms following treatment for breast cancer: Test of the Andersen model. *Journal of Traumatic Stress, 11*, 189–203.

Anstendig, K. D. (1999). Is selective mutism an anxiety disorder? Rethinking its DSM-IV classification. *Journal of Anxiety Disorders, 13*, 417–434.

Apter, A., Ratzoni, G., King, R., Weizman, A., Doncy, I., Ginder, M., & Riddle, M. (1994). Fluvoxamine open-label treatment of adolescent inpatients with obsessive-compulsive disorder or depression. *Journal of the American Academy of Child and Adolescent Psychiatry, 33*, 342–348.

Arbelle, S., Benjamin, J., Galin, M., Kremer, I., Belmaker, R. H., & Ebstein, R. P. (2003). Relation of shyness in grade school children in the genotype for the long form of the serotonin transporter promoter region polymorphism. *American Journal of Psychiatry, 160*, 671–676.

Asbahr, F. R., Castillo, A. R., Ito, L. M., de Oliveira Latorre, M. R. D., Moreira, M. N., & Lotufo-Neto, F. (2005). Group cognitive-behavioral therapy versus sertraline for the treatment of children and adolescents with obsessive-compulsive disorder. *Journal of the American Academy of Child & Adolescent Psychiatry, 44*(11), 1128–1136.

Astin, M. C., Lawrence, K F. & Foy, D. W. (1993). Posttraumatic stress disorder among battered women: Risk and resiliency factors. *Violence & Victims, 8*, 17–28.

Bailey, K. A., Chavira, D. A., Stein, M. T., & Stein, M. B. (2006). Brief measures to screen for social phobia in primary care pediatrics. *Journal of Pediatric Psychology, 31*(5), 513–521.

Bakker, A., van Balkom, Anton J. L. M., & van Dyck, R. (2001). Comparing psychotherapy and pharmacotherapy. *American Journal of Psychiatry, 158*(7), 1164–1165.

Baldwin, D., Woods, R., Lawson, R., & Taylor, D. (2011). Efficacy of drug treatments for generalised anxiety disorder: Systematic review and meta-analysis. *BMJ,* 342.

Barlow, D. H. (1988). *Anxiety and its disorders: The nature and treatment of anxiety and panic.* New York: Guildford Press.

Barlow, D. H. (2001). *Anxiety and its disorders: The nature and treatment of anxiety and panic* (2nd ed.). New York: Guilford Press.

Barlow, D. H., & Craske, M. G. (1989). *Mastery of your anxiety and panic.* Albany, NY: Graywind Publications.

Barlow, D. H., & Craske, M. G. (2000). *Mastery of your anxiety and panic (MAP-3).* San Antonio, TX: Graywind Publications/The Psychological Corporation.

Barlow, D. H., Gorman, J. M., Shear, M. K. & Woods, S. W. (2000). Cognitive-behavioral therapy, imipramine, or their combination for panic disorder: A randomized controlled trial. *Journal of the American Medical Association, 283*, 2529–2536.

Barnas, M. V., Pollina, L. & Cummings, E. M. (1991). Life-span attachment: Relations between attachment and socioemotional functioning in adult women. *Genetic, Social, and General Psychology Monographs, 117*, 175–202.

Barrett, P. M. (1998). Evaluation of cognitive-behavioral group treatments for childhood anxiety disorders. *Journal of Clinical Child Psychology, 27*, 459–468.

Barrett, P. M., & Turner, C. (2001). Prevention of anxiety symptoms in primary school children: Preliminary results from a universal school-based trial. *British Journal of Clinical Psychology, 40*, 399–410.

Barrett, P. M., Dadds, M. R., & Rapee, R. M. (1996). Family treatment of childhood anxiety: A controlled trial. *Journal of Consulting and Clinical Psychology, 64*, 333–342.

Barrett, P. M., Farrell, L. J., Ollendick, T. H., & Dadds, M. (2006). Long-term outcomes of an Australian universal prevention trial of anxiety and depression symptoms in children and youth: An evaluation of the friends program. *Journal of Clinical Child and Adolescent Psychology, 35*(3), 403–411.

Barrett, P. M., Rapee, R. M., Dadds, M. M., & Ryan, S. M. (1996). Family enhancement of cognitive style in anxious and aggressive children. *Journal of Abnormal Child Psychology, 24*, 187–203.

Barrett, P., Farrell, L., Dadds, M., & Boulter, N., (2005). Cognitive-behavioral family treatment of childhood obsessive-compulsive disorder: Long-term follow-up and predictors of outcome. *Journal of the American Academy of Child and Adolescent Psychiatry, 44*, 1005–1014.

Barrett, P., Healy-Farrell, L., & March, J. S. (2004). Cognitive-behavioral family treatment of childhood obsessive-compulsive disorder: A controlled trial. *Journal of the American Academy of Child and Adolescent Psychiatry, 43*, 46–62.

Barrett, T. W., & Mizes, J. S. (1988). Combat level and social support in the development of posttraumatic stress disorder in Vietnam veterans. *Behavior Modification*, *12*, 100–115.

Basile, V. S, Masellis, M., Potkin, S. G., & Kennedy, J. L. (2002). Pharmacogenomics in schizophrenia: The quest for individualized therapy. *Human Molecular Genetics, 11*, 2517–2530.

Battaglia, M., Pesenti-Gritti, P., Medland, S. E., Ogliari, A., Tambs, K., & Spatola, C. A. (2009). A genetically informed study of the association between childhood separation anxiety, sensitivity to CO(2), panic disorder, and the effect of childhood parental loss. *Archives of General Psychiatry*, *66*(1), 64–71.

Baumeister, H., & Härter, M. (2007). Prevalence of mental disorders based on general population surveys. *Social Psychiatry and Psychiatric Epidemiology*, *42*(7), 537–546.

Beck, A. T. (1976). *Cognitive therapy and the emotional disorders*. Oxford: International Universities Press.

Beck, A. T., Emery, G., & Greenberg, R. L. (1985). *Anxiety disorders and phobias: A cognitive perspective*. New York: Basic Books.

Beidel, D. C., & Turner, S. M. (1988). Comorbidity of test anxiety and other anxiety disorders in children. *Journal of Abnormal Child Psychology*, *16*, 275–287.

Beidel, D. C., Turner, S. M. & Morris, T. L. (1999). Psychopathology of childhood social phobia. *Journal of the American Academy of Child and Adolescent Psychiatry*, *38*, 643–650.

Beidel, D. C., Turner, S. M., & Morris, T. L. (1995). A new inventory to assess childhood social anxiety and phobia: The Social Phobia and Anxiety Inventory for Children. *Psychological Assessment*, *7*, 73–79.

Beidel, D. C., Turner, S. M., & Morris, T. L. (2000). Behavioral treatment of childhood social phobia. *Journal of Consulting & Clinical Psychology*, *68*, 1072–1080.

Beidel, D. C., Turner, S. M., Hamlin, K., & Morris, T. L. (2000). The Social Phobia and Anxiety Inventory for Children (SPAI-C): External and discriminative validity. *Behavior Therapy*, *31*, 75–87.

Beidel, D. C., Turner, S. M., Sallee, F. R., Ammerman, R. T., Crosby, L. A., & Pathak, S. (2007). SET-C versus fluoxetine in the treatment of childhood social phobia. *Journal of the American Academy of Child & Adolescent Psychiatry*, *46*(12), 1622–1632.

Beidel, D. C., Turner, S. M., & Trager, K. N. (1994). Test anxiety and childhood anxiety disorders in African American and white school children. *Journal of Anxiety Disorders*, *8*, 169–174.

Bell-Dolan, D. J. (1995). Social cue interpretation of anxious children. *Journal of Clinical Child Psychology*, *24*, 1–10.

Belsky, J., & Rovine, M. (1987). Temperament and attachment security in the strange situation: An empirical rapprochement. *Child Development*, *58*, 787–795.

Bendor, S. J. (1990). Anxiety and isolation in siblings of pediatric cancer patients: The need for prevention. *Social Work in Health Care*, *14*, 17–35.

Benes, F. M. (1989). Myelination of cortical-hippocampal relays during late adolescence. *Schizophrenia Bulletin*, *15*, 585–593.

Bergman, R. L., Gonzalez, A., Piacentini, J., & Keller, M. L. (2013). Integrated behavior therapy for selective mutism: A randomized controlled pilot study. *Behaviour Research and Therapy*, *51*(10), 680–689.

Berman, S. L., Kurtines, W. M., Silverman, W. K., & Serafini, L. T. (1996). The impact of exposure to crime and violence on urban youth. *American Journal of Orthopsychiatry*, *66*, 329–336.

Berney, T. P., Bhate, S. R., Kolvin, I., Famuyiwa, O. O., Barrett, M. L., Fundudis, T., & Tyrer, P. S. (1991). The context of childhood depression: The Newcastle Childhood Depression Project. *British Journal of Psychiatry*, *159*, 28–35.

Berney, T., Kolvin, I., Bhate, S. R., Garside, R. F., Jeans, J., Kay, B., & Scarth, L. (1981). School phobia: A therapeutic trial with clomipramine and short-term outcome. *British Journal of Psychiatry*, *138*, 110–118.

Bernstein, G. A., Anderson, L. K., Hektner, J. M., & Realmuto, G. M. (2000). Imipramine compliance in adolescents. *Journal of the American Academy of Child and Adolescent Psychiatry*, *39*, 284–291.

Bernstein, G. A., Bernat, D. H., Davis, A. A., & Layne, A. E. (2008). Symptom presentation and classroom functioning in a nonclinical sample of children with social phobia. *Depression and Anxiety*, *25*(9), 752–760.

Bernstein, G. A., Garfinkel, B. D., & Borchardt, C. M. (1990). Comparative studies of pharmacotherapy for school refusal. *Journal of the American Academy of Child and Adolescent Psychiatry*, *29*, 773–781.

Biederman, J., Faraone, S. V., Hirshfeld-Becker, D. R., Friedman, D., Robin, J. A., & Rosenbaum, J. F. (2001). Patterns of psychopathology and dysfunction in high-risk children of parents with panic disorder and major depression. *American Journal of Psychiatry*, *158*, 49–57.

Biederman, J., Rosenbaum, J. R., Chaloff, J., & Kagan, J. (1995). Behavioral inhibition as a risk factor for anxiety disorders. In J. S. March (Ed.), *Anxiety disorders in children and adolescents*. New York: Guilford Press.

Bilder, R. M., Howe, A. G., & Sabb, F. W. (2013). Multilevel models from biology to psychology: Mission impossible? *Journal of Abnormal Psychology, 122*(3), 917–927.

Birmaher, B., Khetarpal, S., Brent, D., Cully, M., Balach, L., Kaufman, J., & Neer, S. M. (1997). The Screen for Child Anxiety Related Emotional Disorders (SCARED): Scale construction and psychometric characteristics. *Journal of the American Academy of Child and Adolescent Psychiatry, 36*, 545–553.

Birmaher, B., & Ollendick, T. H. (2004). Childhood onset panic disorder. In T. H. Ollendick & J. S. March (Eds.), *Phobic and anxiety disorders in children and adolescents: A clinician's guide to effective psychosocial and pharmacological interventions*. (pp. 306–333). New York: Oxford University Press.

Birmaher, B., Waterman, G. S., Ryan, N., Cully, M., Balach, L., Ingram, J., & Brodsky, M. (1994). Fluoxetine for childhood anxiety disorders. *Journal of the American Academy of Child and Adolescent Psychiatry, 33*, 993–999.

Bisson, J. I., & Shepherd, J. P. (1995). Psychological reactions of victims of violent crime. *British Journal of Psychiatry, 167*, 718–720.

Bisson, J. I., McFarlane, A. C., Susanna, R., Ruzek, J. I., & Watson, P. J. (2009). *Psychological debriefing for adults*. New York: Guilford Press.

Black, B. (1994). Separation anxiety disorder and panic disorder. In J. March (Ed.), *Anxiety disorders in children and adolescents*. New York: Guilford Press.

Black, M. C., Basile, K. C., Breidling, M. J., Smith, S. G., Walters, M. L., Merrick, M. T., Chen, J., & Stevens, M. R. (2011). The National Intimate Partner and Sexual Violence Survey (NISVS): 2010 Summary Report, Atlanta, GA: National Center for Injury Prevention and Control, Centers for Disease Control and Prevention.

Black, B., & Uhde, T. W. (1994). Treatment of elective mutism with fluoxetine: A double-blind, placebo-controlled study. *Journal of the American Academy of Child and Adolescent Psychiatry, 33*, 1000–1006.

Blackford, J. U., & Pine, D. S. (2012). Neural substrates of childhood anxiety disorders: A review of neuroimaging findings. *Child & Adolescent Psychiatric Clinics of North America, 21*(3), 501–525.

Blanco, C., Bragdon, L. B., Schneier, F. R., & Liebowitz, M. R. (2013). The evidence-based pharmacotherapy of social anxiety disorder. *International Journal of Neuropsychopharmacology, 16*(1), 235–249.

Boer, F. (1998). Anxiety disorders in the family: The contributions of heredity and family interactions. In D. A. Treffers (Ed.), *Emotionele Stoornissen en Somatoforme Stoornissen bij Kenderen en Adolescenten: de Stand van Zaken*, (pp. 109–114). Leiden: Boerhaave Commissie.

Bögels, S. M., Alden, L., Beidel, D. C., Clark, L. A., Pine, D. S., Stein, M. B., & Voncken, M. (2010). Social anxiety disorder: Questions and answers for the DSM-V. *Depression and Anxiety, 27*(2), 168–189.

Bögels, S., & Phares, V. (2008). Fathers' role in the etiology, prevention and treatment of child anxiety: A review and new model. *Clinical Psychology Review, 28*(4), 539–558.

Bolton, D., & Perrin, S. (2008). Evaluation of exposure with response-prevention for obsessive compulsive disorder in childhood and adolescence. *Journal of Behavior Therapy and Experimental Psychiatry, 39*, 11–22.

Bolton, D., Williams, T., Perrin, S., Atkinson, L., Gallop, C., Waite, P., & Salkovskis, P. (2011). Randomized controlled trial of full and brief cognitive-behaviour therapy and wait-list for paediatric obsessive-compulsive disorder. *Journal of Chld Psychology and Psychiatry, 52*, 1269–1278.

Bornas, X., Tortella-Feliu, M., & Llabrés, J. (2006). Do all treatments work for flight phobia? Computer-assisted exposure versus a brief multicomponent nonexposure treatment. *Psychotherapy Research, 16*(1), 41–50.

Boscarino, J. A. (1995). Post-traumatic stress and associated disorders among Vietnam veterans: The significance of combat exposure and social support. *Journal of Traumatic Stress, 8*, 317–336.

Bouton, M. E. (1994). Context, ambiguity, and classical conditioning. *Current Directions in Psychological Science, 3*(2), 49–53.

Bouton, M. E. (2000). A learning theory perspective on lapse, relapse, and the maintenance of behavior change. *Health Psychology, 19*(1), 57–63.

Bouwer, C., & Stein, D. J. (1997). Association of panic disorder with a history of traumatic suffocation. *American Journal of Psychiatry, 154*, 1566–1570.

Brady, E. U., & Kendall, P. C. (1992). Comorbidity of anxiety and depression in children and adolescents. *Psychological Bulletin, 11*, 244–255.

Bremner, J. D. (1999). Does stress damage the brain? *Biological Psychiatry, 45*, 797–805.

Bremner, J. D., Krystal, J. H., Charney, D. S. & Southwick, S, M. (1996). Neural mechanisms in dissociative amnesia for childhood abuse: Relevance to the current controversy surrounding the false memory syndrome. *American Journal of Psychiatry, 153*, 71–82.

Bremner, J. D., Staib, L. H., Kaloupek, D., Southwick, S. M., Soufer, R., & Charney, D. S. (1999). Neural correlates of exposure to traumatic pictures and sound in Vietnam combat veterans with and without posttraumatic stress disorder: A positron emission tomography study. *Biological Psychiatry, 45*, 806–816.

Breslau, N., Schultz, L., Peterson, E. (1995). Sex differences in depression: A role for preexisting anxiety. *Journal of Psychiatric Research, 58*, 1–12.

Britton, J. C., Grillon, C., Lissek, S., Norcross, M. A., Szuhany, K. L., Chen, G., ... Pine, D. S., (2013). Response to learned threat: An fMRI study in adolescent and adult anxiety. *American Journal of Psychiatry 170*(10), 1195–1204.

Britton, J. C., Lissek, S., Grillon, C., Norcross, M. A., & Pine, D. S. (2011). Development of anxiety: The role of threat appraisal and fear learning. *Depression and Anxiety 28*(1), 5–17.

Brooks-Gunn, J., Graber, J. A., & Paikoff, R. L. (1994). Studying links between hormones and negative affect: Models and measures. *Journal of Research on Adolescence, 4*, 469–486.

Brown, J. M., O'Keeffe, J., Sanders, S. H., & Baker, B. (1986). Developmental changes in children's cognition to stressful and painful situations. *Journal of Pediatric Psychology, 11*, 343–357.

Brownell, K. D., Marlatt, G. A., Lichtenstein, E., & Wilson, G. T. (1986). Understanding and preventing relapse. *American Psychologist, 41*, 765–782.

Bryant, R. A., Harvey, A. G., Sackville, T., Dang, S. T., & Basten, C. (1998). Treatment of acute stress disorder: A comparison between cognitive-behavioral therapy and supportive counseling. *Journal of Consulting and Clinical Psychology, 66*, 862–866.

Bryant, R. A., Mastrodomenico, J., Felmingham, K. L., Hopwood, S., Kenny, L., Kandris, E., ... Creamer, M. (2008). Treatment of acute stress disorder: A randomized controlled trial. *Archives of General Psychiatry, 2008*, 659–667.

Bryant, R. A., Moulds, M. L., Guthrie, R. M., & Nixon, R. D. V. (2005). The additive benefit of hypnosis and cognitive-behavioral therapy in treating acute stress disorder. *Journal of Consulting and Clinical Psychology, 73*, 334–340.

Bryant, R. A., Sackville, T., Dangh, S. T., Moulds, M., & Guthrie, R.(1999). Treating acute stress disorder: An evaluation of cognitive behavior therapy and supportive counseling techniques. *American Journal of Psychiatry, 156*, 1780–1786.

Buckley, T. C., Blanchard, E. B., & Hickling, E. J. (1996). A prospective examination of delayed onset PTSD secondary to motor vehicle accidents. *Journal of Abnormal Psychology, 105*, 617–625.

Carlbring, P., & Andersson, G. (2006). Internet and psychological treatment: How well can they be combined? *Computers in Human Behavior, 22*(3), 545–553.

Carlbring, P., Ekselius, L., & Andersson, G. (2003). Treatment of panic disorder via the Internet: A randomized trial of CBT versus applied relaxation. *Journal of Behavior Therapy and Experimental Psychiatry, 34*, 129–140.

Carlbring, P., Nilsson-Ihrfelt, E., Waara, J., Kollenstam, C., Buhrman, M., Kaldo, V, ... Andersson, G. (2006). Treatment of panic disorder: Live therapy versus self-help via Internet. *Behaviour Research and Therapy, 43*, 1321–1333.

Carrion, V. G., Garrett, A., Menon, V., Weems, C. F., & Reiss, A. L. (2008). Posttraumatic stress symptoms and brain function during a response-inhibition task: An fMRI study in youth. *Depression and Anxiety, 25*(6), 514–526.

Cartwright-Hatton, S. (2013). Treating anxiety in early life. *British Journal of Psychiatry, 203*(6), 401–402.

Casey, B. J., Duhoux, S., & Malter Cohen, M. (2010). Adolescence: What do transmission, transition, and translation have to do with it? *Neuron 67*(5), 749–760.

Casey, B. J., Giedd, J. N., & Thomas, K. M. (2000). Structural and functional brain development and its relation to cognitive development. *Biological Psychology, 54*, 241–257.

Casey, B. J., Jones, R. M., & Hare, T. A. (2008). The adolescent brain. *Annals of the New York Academy of Sciences, 1124*, 111–126.

Casey, B. J., Jones, R. M., Levita, L., Libby, V., Pattwell, S. S., Ruberry, E. J., ... Somerville, L. H. (2010). The storm and stress of adolescence: Insights from human imaging and mouse genetics. *Developmental Psychobiology, 52*(3), 225–235.

Casey, B. J., Pattwell, S. S., Glatt, C. E., & Lee, F. S. (2013). Treating the developing brain: Implications from human imaging and mouse genetics. *Annual Review of Medicine, 64*, 427–439.

Caspi, A., & Moffitt, T. E. (1991). Individual differences as accentuated during periods of social changes: The sample case of girls at puberty. *Journal of Personality and Social Psychology, 61*, 157–168.

Cassidy, J. (1995). Attachment and generalized anxiety disorder. In D. Cicchetti & S. Toth (Eds.), *Emotion, cognition, and representation: Rochester Symposium on Developmental Psychopathology VI* (pp. 343–370). Rochester, NY: University of Rochester Press.

Cassidy, J., & Berlin, L. J. (1994). The insecure/ambivalent pattern of attachment: Theory and research. *Child Development, 65*, 971–991.

Cavaiola, A. A., & Schiff, M. (1988). Behavioral sequelae of physical and/or sexual abuse in adolescents. *Child Abuse & Neglect, 12*, 181–188.

Chabane, N., Delorme, R., Millet, B., Mouren, M., Leboyer, M., & Pauls, D. (2005). Early-onset obsessive-compulsive disorder: A subgroup with a specific clinical and familial pattern? *Journal of Child Psychology and Psychiatry, 46*(8), 881–887.

Chambless, D. L., & Gillis, M. M. (1993). Cognitive therapy of anxiety disorders. *Journal of Consulting and Clinical Psychology, 61*(2), 248.

Chambless, D. L., & Hollon, S. D. (1998). Defining empirically supported therapies. *Journal of Consulting and Clinical Psychology, 66, 1*, 7–18.

Chambless, D. L., & Ollendick, T. H. (2001). Empirically supported psychological interventions: Controversies and evidence. *Annual Review of Psychology, 52*, 685–716.

Chambless, D. L., Goldstein, A. J., Gallagher, R., & Bright, P. (1986). Integrating behavior therapy and psychotherapy in the treatment of agoraphobia. *Psychotherapy: Theory, Research, Practice, Training, 23*(1), 150.

Charney, D. S., & Deutch, A. (1996). A functional neuroanatomy of anxiety and fear: Implications for the pathophysiology and treatment of anxiety disorders. *Critical Reviews in Neurobiology, 10*, 419–446.

Chemtob, C. M., Nakashima, J., & Carlson, J. G. (2002). Brief treatment for elementary school children with disaster-related posttraumatic stress disorder: A field study. *Journal of Clinical Psychology, 58, 1*, 99–112.

Chorpita, B. F., Albano, A. M., & Barlow, D. H. (1996). Cognitive processing in children: Relation to anxiety and family influences. *Journal of Clinical Child Psychology, 25*, 170–176.

Chorpita, B. F., Brown, T. A., & Barlow, D. H. (1998). Perceived control as a mediator of family environment in etiological models of childhood anxiety. *Behavior Therapy, 29*, 457–476.

Chronis-Tuscano, A., Degnan, A. M., Pine, D. S., Perez-Edgar, K., Henderson, H. A., Diaz, Y., ... & Fox, N. A. (2009). Stable early maternal report of behavioral inhibition predicts lifetime social anxiety disorder in adolescence. *Journal of the American Academy of Child and Adolescent Psychiatry, 48*, 928–935.

Chugani, H. T. (1996). Neuroimaging of developmental nonlinearity and developmental pathologies. In R. W. Thatcher, G. R. Lyon, J. Rumsey, & N. Krasnegor (Eds.), *Developmental neuroimaging: Mapping the development of brain and behavior* (pp. 187–195). San Diego: Academic Press.

Clark, D. M. (1986). A cognitive approach to panic. *Behaviour Research and Therapy, 24*(4), 461–470.

Clark, D. M. (1997). Panic disorder and social phobia. *Science and Practice of Cognitive Behaviour Therapy*, 119–153.

Clark, D. M., & Wells, A. (1995). A cognitive model of social phobia. In Heimberg, R. G., et al. (Eds.), *Social phobia: Diagnosis, assessment, and treatment* (pp. 69–93). New York: Guilford Press.

Claycomb, M. A., Charak, R., Kaplow, J., Layne, C. M., Pynoos, R., & Elhai, J. D. (2016). Persistent complex bereavement disorder symptom domains relate differentially to PTSD and depression: A study of war-exposed Bosnian adolescents. *Journal of Abnormal Child Psychology, 44*(7), 1361–1373.

Cobham, V. E., Dadds, M. R., & Spence, S. H. (1998). The role of parental anxiety in the treatment of childhood anxiety. *Journal of Consulting and Clinical Psychology, 66*, 893–905.

Cohen, J., Deblinger, E., Maedel, A. B., & Stauffer, L. B. (1999). Examining sex-related thoughts and feelings of sexually abused and nonabused children. *Journal of Interpersonal Violence, 14*(7), 701–712.

Cohen, J. A., Deblinger, E., Mannarino, A. P., & Steer, R. A. (2004). A multisite, randomized controlled trial for children with sexual abuse-related PTSD symptoms. *Journal of the American Academy of Child and Adolescent Psychiatry, 43*(4), 393–402.

Cohen, J. A., & Mannarino, A. P. (1996a). A treatment outcome study for sexually abused preschool children: Initial findings. *Journal of the American Academy of Child and Adolescent Psychiatry, 35*(1), 42–50.

Cohen, J. A., & Mannarino, A. P. (1996b). A treatment outcome study for sexually abused preschool children: Initial findings: Errata. *Journal of the American Academy of Child and Adolescent Psychiatry, 35*(6), 835.

Cohen, J. A., & Mannarino, A. P. (1998). Factors that mediate treatment outcome of sexually abused preschool children: Six- and 12-month follow-up. *Journal of the American Academy of Child & Adolescent Psychiatry, 37*(1), 44–51.

Cohen, J. A., Mannarino, A. P., Perel, J. M., & Stardon, V. (2007). A pilot randomized controlled trial of combined trauma-focused CBT and sertraline for childhood PTSD symptoms. *Journal of the American Academy of Child and Adolescent Psychiatry, 46*, 811–819.

Coldwell, S. E., Wilhelm, F. H., Milgrom, P., Prall, C. W., Getz, T., Spadafora, A., . . . Ramsay, D. (2007). Combining alprazolam with systematic desensitization therapy for dental injection phobia. *Journal of Anxiety Disorders, 21*(7), 871–887.

Collins, J. J., & Bailey, S. L. (1990). Traumatic stress disorder and violent behavior. *Journal of Traumatic Stress, 3*, 203–220.

Comeau, N., Stuart, S. H., & Loba, P. (2001). The relations of trait anxiety, anxiety sensitivity and sensation seeking to adolescents' motivations for alcohol, cigarette and marijuana use. *Addictive Behaviors, 26*, 803–825.

Compton, S. N., Peris, T. S., Almirall, D., Birmaher, B., Sherrill, J., Kendall, P. C., . . . Albano, A. M. (2014). Predictors and moderators of treatment response in childhood anxiety disorders: Results from the CAMS trial. *Journal of Consulting and Clinical Psychology, 82*(2), 212–224.

Compton, S. N., Walkup, J. T., Albano, A. M., Piacentini, J. C., Birmaher, B., Sherrill, J. T., . . . March, J. S. (2010). Child/Adolescent Anxiety Multimodal Study (CAMS): Rationale, design, and methods. *Child and Adolescent Psychiatry and Mental Health, 4*, 1.

Conners, C. K. (1997). *Conners Rating Scales: Revised technical manual*. Toronto: Multi-Health Systems.

Cooley-Strickland, M., Griffin, R. S., Darney, D., Otte, K., & Ko, J. (2011). Urban African American youth exposed to community violence: A school-based anxiety preventive intervention efficacy study. *Journal of Prevention & Intervention in the Community, 39*(2), 149–166.

Copeland, W. E., Angold, A., Shanahan, L., & Costello, E. J. (2014). Longitudinal patterns of anxiety from childhood to adulthood: The Great Smoky Mountains Study. *Journal of the American Academy of Child and Adolescent Psychiatry, 53*(1), 21–33.

Copeland, W. E., Shanahan, L., Costello, J., & Angold, A. (2009). Childhood and adolescent psychiatric disorders as predictors of young adult disorders. *Archives of General Psychiatry, 66*(7), 764–772.

Coplan, J. D., Moreau, D., Chaput, F., Martinez, J. M., Hoven, C. W., Mandell, D. J., . . . Pine, D. S. (2002). Salivary cortisol concentrations before and after carbon dioxide inhalations in children. *Biological Psychiatry, 51*(4), 326–333.

Coplan, J. D., Papp, L. A., Pine, D., Martinez, J., Cooper, T., Rosenblum, L. A., . . . Gorman, J. M. (1997). Clinical improvement with fluoxetine therapy and noradrenergic function in patients with panic disorder. *Archives of General Psychiatry, 54*, 643–648.

Cornelius, J. R., Kirisci, L., Reynolds, M., Clark, D. B., Hayes, J., & Tarter, R. (2010). PTSD contributes to teen and young adult cannabis use disorders. *Addictive Behaviors, 35*(2), 91–94.

Coryell, W., Fyer, A., Pine, D., Martinez, J., & Arndt, S. (2001). Aberrant respiratory sensitivity to CO(2) as a trait of familial panic disorder. *Biological Psychiatry, 49*, 582–587.

Costa, N. M., Weems, C. F., & Pina, A. A. (2009). Hurricane Katrina and youth anxiety: The role of perceived attachment beliefs and parenting behaviors. *Journal of Anxiety Disorders, 23*(7), 935–941.

Costello, E. J., & Angold, A. (1988). Scales to assess child and adolescent depression: Checklists, screens, and nets. *Journal of the American Academy of Child and Adolescent Psychiatry, 27*, 726–737.

Costello, E. J., & Angold, A. (1995). Epidemiology. In J. S. March (Ed.), *Anxiety disorders in children and adolescents* (pp. 109–124). New York: Guilford Press.

Costello, E. J., Burns, B. J., Angold, A., & Leaf, P. J. (1993). How can epidemiology improve mental health services for children and adolescents? *Journal of the American Academy of Child and Adolescent Psychiatry, 32*, 1106–1113.

Costello, E. J., Egger, H. L., & Angold, A. (2004). Developmental epidemiology of anxiety disorders. In T. H. Ollendick, & J. S. March (Eds.), *Phobic and anxiety disorders in children and adolescents: A clinician's guide to effective psychosocial and pharmacological interventions* (pp. 61–91). New York: Oxford University Press.

Costello, E. J., Erkanli, A, Federman, E., & Angold, A. (1999). Development of psychiatric comorbidity with substance abuse in adolescents: Effects of timing and sex. *Journal of Clinical Child Psychology, 28*, 298–311.

Costello, E. J., Mustillo, S., Erkanli, A., Keeler, G., & Angold, A. (2003). Prevalence and development of psychiatric disorders in childhood and adolescence. *Archives of General Psychiatry, 60*(8), 837–844.

Costello, E. J., Mustillo, S., Keeler, G., & Angold, A. (2004). Prevalence of psychiatric disorders in childhood and adolescence. In Levin, B. L., et al. (Eds.), *Mental health services: A public health perspective* (2nd ed., pp. 111–128). New York: Oxford University Press.

Cottreaux, J., Mollard, E., Bouvard, M., Marks, I., Sluys, M., Nury, A. M., ... & Cialdella, P. (1990). A controlled study of fluvoxamine and exposure in obsessive-compulsive disorder. *International Clinics in Psychopharmacology, 5*(1), 17–30.

Cottreaux, J., Note, I., Nan Yao, S., Lafont, S., Note, B., Mollard, E., . . . Dartigues, J. F. (2001). A randomized controlled trial of cognitive therapy versus intensive behavior therapy in obsessive–compulsive disorder. *Psychotherapy and Psychosomatics, 70*, 288–297.

Cowen, E. L., Wyman, P. A., Work, W. C. & Parker, G. R. (1990). The Rochester Child Resilience Project: Overview and summary of first year findings. *Development & Psychopathology, 2*, 193–212.

Craske, M. G., & Barlow, D. H. (2007). *Mastery of your anxiety and panic: Therapist guide*. New York: Oxford University Press.

Craske, M. G., Liao, B., Brown, L., & Vervliet, B. (2012). Role of inhibition in exposure therapy. *Journal of Experimental Psychopathology, 3*(3), 322–345.

Craske, M. G., Waters, A. M., Lindsey Bergman, R., Naliboff, B., Lipp, O. V., Negoro, H., & Ornitz, E. M. (2008). Is aversive learning a marker of risk for anxiety disorders in children? *Behaviour Research and Therapy, 46*(8), 954–967.

Craske, M. G., Waters, A. M., Nazarian, M., Mineka, S., Zinbarg, R. E., Griffith, J. W., . . . Ornitz, E. M. (2008). Does neuroticism in adolescents moderate contextual and explicit threat cue modulation of the startle reflex? *Biological Psychiatry, 65*(3), 220–226.

Craske, M. G., & Zucker, B. G. (2001). Prevention of anxiety disorders: A model for intervention. *Applied & Preventive Psychology, 10*, 155–175.

Crawley, S. A., Caporino, N. E., Birmaher, B., Ginsburg, G., Piacentini, J., Albano, A. M., . . . Kendall, P. C. (2014). Somatic complaints in anxious youth. *Child Psychiatry and Human Development, 45*(4), 398–407.

Crone, E. A., & Dahl, R. E. (2012). Understanding adolescence as a period of social-affective engagement and goal flexibility. *Nature Reviews Neuroscience, 13*(9), 636–650.

Crowe, R. (1985). The genetics of panic disorder and agoraphobia. *Psychiatric Developments, 3*(2), 171–185.

Crowell, J. A., O' Connor, E., Wollmers, G., & Sprafkin, J. (1991). Mothers' conceptualizations of parent-child relationships: Relation to mother-child interaction and child behavior problems. *Development and Psychopathology, 3*, 431–444.

Cuijpers, P., Sijbrandij, M., Koole, S., Huibers, M., Berking, M., & Andersson, G. (2014). Psychological treatment of generalized anxiety disorder: A meta-analysis. *Clinical Psychology Review, 34*(2), 130–140.

Cunningham, M. G., Bhattacharyya, S., & Benes, F. M. (2002). Amygdalo-cortical sprouting continues into early adulthood: Implications for the development of normal and abnormal function during adolescence. *Journal of Comparative Neurology, 453*, 116–130.

Dadds, M. R., Barrett, P. M., Rapee, R. M., & Ryan, S. (1996). Family process and child anxiety and aggression: An observational analysis. *Journal of Abnormal Child Psychology, 24*, 715–734.

Dadds, M. R., Holland, D. E., Laurens, K. R., Mullins, M., Barrett, P. M., & Spence, S. H. (1999). Early intervention and prevention of anxiety disorders in children: Results at 2-year follow-up. *Journal of Consulting and Clinical Psychology, 67*, 145–150.

Dadds, M. R., Spence, S. H., Holland, D. E., Barrett, P. M., & Laurens, K. R. (1997). Prevention and early intervention for anxiety disorders: A controlled trial. *Journal of Consulting and Clinical Psychology, 65*, 627–635.

Dalgleish, T., Taghavi, R., Neshat-Doost, H., Moradi, A., Canterbury, R., & Yule, W. (2003). Patterns of processing bias for emotional information across clinical disorders: A comparison of attention, memory, and prospective cognition in children and adolescents with depression, generalized anxiety, and posttraumatic stress disorder. *Journal of Clinical Child and Adolescent Psychology, 32*, 10–21.

Daniels, D., & Plomin, R. (1985). Origins of individual differences in infant shyness. *Developmental Psychology, 21*, 118–121.

Davidson, J. R. T., Foa, E. B., Huppert, J. D., Keefe, F. J., Franklin, M. E., Compton, J. S., ... Gadde, K. M. (2004). Fluoxetine, comprehensive cognitive behavioral therapy, and placebo in generalized social phobia. *Archives of General Psychiatry, 61*(10), 1005–1013.

Davidson, R. J., Abercrombie, H., Nitschke, J. B., & Putnam, K. (1999). Regional brain function, emotion and disorders of emotion. *Current Opinion in Neurobiology, 9*, 228–234.

Davis, M. (1992). The role of the amygdala in fear and anxiety. *Annual Review of Neuroscience, 15*, 353–375.

Davis, M. (1998). Are different parts of the extern al amygdala involved in fear versus anxiety? *Biological Psychiatry, 44*, 1239–1247.

Davis, M., & Whalen, P. J. (2001). The amygdala: Vigilance and emotion. *Molecular Psychiatry, 6*, 13–34.

Davis, M., Walker, D. L., Miles, L., & Grillon, C. (2010). Phasic vs. sustained fear in rats and humans: Role of the extended amygdala in fear vs anxiety. *Neuropsychopharmacology, 35*(1), 105–135.

Deacon, B., Kemp, J. J., Dixon, L. J., Sy, J. T., Farrell, N. R., & Zhang, A. R. (2013). Maximizing the efficacy of interoceptive exposure by optimizing inhibitory learning: A randomized controlled trial. *Behaviour Research and Therapy, 51*(9), 588–596.

De Bellis, M. D. (2001). Developmental traumatology: The psychobiological development of maltreated children and its implication for research, treatment, and policy. *Development and Psychopathology, 13*, 539–564.

De Bellis, M. D., Keshavan, M. S., Clark, D. B., Casey, B. J., Giedd, J. N., Boring, A. M., et al. (1999). A. E. Bennett Research Award. Developmental traumatology. Part II: Brain development. *Biological Psychiatry, 45*, 1271–1284.

De Bellis, M. D., Keshavan, M. S., Shifflett, H., Iyengar, S., Dahl, R. E., Axelson, D. A., et al. (2002). Superior temporal gyrus volumes in pediatric generalized anxiety disorder. *Biological Psychiatry, 51*, 553–562.

De Bellis, M. D., Keshavan, M. S., Spencer, S., & Hall, J. (2000). N-Acetylaspartate concentration in the anterior cingulate of maltreated children and adolescents with PTSD. *American Journal of Psychiatry, 157*, 1175–1177.

De Bellis, M. D., Spratt, E. G., & Hooper, S. R. (2011). Neurodevelopmental biology associated with childhood sexual abuse. *Journal of Child Sex Abuse, 20*(5), 548–587.

Deblinger, E., & Heflin, A. H. (1996). Treating sexually abused children and their nonoffending parents: A cognitive behavioral approach. *Interpersonal Violence: The Practice Series, 16*, 256.

Deblinger, E., Lippmann, J., & Steer, R. A. (1996). Sexually abused children suffering posttraumatic stress symptoms: Initial treatment outcome findings. *Child Maltreatment, 1*, 310–321.

Deblinger, E., Steer, R. A., & Lippmann, J. (1999a). Two-year follow-up study of cognitive behavioral therapy for sexually abused children suffering post-traumatic stress symptoms. *Child Abuse and Neglect, 23*(12), 1371–1378.

Deblinger, E., Steer, R. A., & Lippmann, J. (1999b). Maternal factors associated with sexually abused children's psychosocial adjustment. *Child Maltreatment, 4*(1), 13–20.

De Haan, E., Hoogduin, K. A., Buitelaar, J. K., & Keijsers, G. P. (1998). Behavior therapy versus clomipramine for the treatment of obsessive-compulsive disorder. *Journal of the American Academy of Child and Adolescent Psychiatry, 37*(10), 1022–1029.

Departments of Veterans Affairs and Defense. (2004). *VA/DoD clinical practice guideline for the management of post-traumatic stress.*

Derivois, D., Mérisier, G. G., Cénat, J., & Castelot, V. (2014). Symptoms of posttraumatic stress disorder and social support among children and adolescents after the 2010 Haitian earthquake. *Journal of Loss and Trauma, 19*(3), 202–212.

DeVeaugh-Geiss, J., Moroz, G., Biederman, J., et al. (1992). Clomipramine hydrochloride in childhood and adolescent obsessive-compulsive disorder—a multicenter trial. *Journal of the American Academy of Child and Adolescent Psychiatry, 31*, 45–49.

de Vries, A. P., Kassam-Adams, N., Cnaan, A., Sherman-Slate, E., Gallagher, P. R., & Winston, F. K. (1999). Looking beyond the physical injury: Posttraumatic stress disorder in children and parents after pediatric traffic injury. *Pediatrics, 104*(6), 1293–1299.

Deykin, E. Y., & Buka, S. L. (1997). Prevalence and risk factors for posttraumatic stress disorder among chemically dependent adolescents. *American Journal of Psychiatry, 154*, 752–757.

Dick-Niederhauser, A., & Silverman, W. K. (2003). *Courage and fearlessness: A positive approach to the etiology and treatment of anxiety disorders.* Paper submitted for publication.

Dierker, L. C., Albano, A. M., Clarke, G. N., Heimberg, R. G., et al. (2001). Screening for anxiety and depression in early adolescence. *Journal of the American Academy of Child and Adolescent Psychiatry, 40*, 929–936.

DiLalla, L. F., Kagan, J., & Reznick, J. S. (1994). Genetic etiology of behavioral inhibition among 2-year-old children. *Infant Behavior & Development, 17*, 405–412.

Doerfler, L. A., Connor, D. F., Volungis, A. M., & Toscano, P. F., Jr. (2007). Panic disorder in clinically referred children and adolescents. *Child Psychiatry and Human Development, 38*(1), 57–71.

Donovan, C. L., & Spence, S. H. (2000). Prevention of childhood anxiety disorders. *Clinical Psychology Review, 20*, 509–531.

Duckworth, A. L., Peterson, C., Matthews, M. D., & Kelly, D. R. (2007). Grit: Perseverance and passion for long-term goals. *Journal of Personality and Social Psychology, 92*(6), 1087–1101.

Duffy, M., Gillespie, K., & Clark, D. M. (2007). Post-traumatic stress disorder in the context of terrorism and other civil conflict in Northern Ireland: Randomised controlled trial. *BMJ, 334*, 1147–1150.

Dugas, M. J., Brillon, P., Savard, P., Turcotte, J., Gaudet, A., Ladouceur, R., . . . & Gervais, N. J. (2010). A randomized clinical trial of cognitive-behavioral therapy and applied relaxation for adults with generalized anxiety disorder. *Behavior Therapy, 41*(1), 46–58.

Dugas, M. J., Ladouceur, R., Léger, E., Freeston, M. H., Langolis, F., Provencher, M. D., & Boisvert, J. M. (2003). Group cognitive-behavioral therapy for generalized anxiety disorder: Treatment outcome and long-term follow-up. *Journal of Consulting and Clinical Psychology, 71*(4), 821.

D'Zurilla, T. J., & Nezu, A. M. (2001). Problem-solving therapies. In K. S. Dobson (Ed.), *Handbook of cognitive–behavioral therapies* (2nd ed., pp. 211–245). New York: Guilford Press.

Eaves, L. J., Eysenck, H. J., & Martin (1989). *Genes, culture and personality: An empirical approach.* New York: Academic Press.

Eaves, L. J., Silberg, J. L., et al. (1997). Genetics and developmental psychopathology: The main effects of genes and environment on behavioral problems in the Virginia Twin Study of adolescent behavior development. *Journal of Child Psychology and Psychiatry and Allied Disciplines, 38*(8), 965–980.

Ebata, A. T., & Moos, R. H. (1991). Coping and adjustment in distressed and healthy adolescents. *Journal of Applied Developmental Psychology, 12*, 33–54.

Ebesutani, C., Reise, S. P., Chorpita, B. F., Ale, C., Regan, J., Young, J., . . . Weisz, J. R. (2012). The Revised Child Anxiety and Depression Scale-Short Version: Scale reduction via exploratory bifactor modeling of the broad anxiety factor. *Psychological Assessment, 24*(4), 833–845.

Ehlers, A., Clark, D. M., Hackmann, A., McManus, F., Fennell, M., Herbert, C., & Mayou, R. (2003). A randomized controlled trial of cognitive therapy, a self-help booklet, and repeated assessments as early interventions for posttraumatic stress disorder. *Archives of General Psychiatry, 60*(10), 1024–1032.

Ehlers, A., Hackmann, A., Grey, N., Wild, J., Liness, S., Albert, I., . . . Clark, D. M. (2014). A randomized controlled trial of 7-day intensive and standard weekly cognitive therapy for PTSD and emotion-focused supportive therapy. *American Journal of Psychiatry, 171*(3), 294–304.

Eisen, A. R., & Silverman, W. K. (1998). Prescriptive treatment for generalized anxiety disorder in children. *Behavior Therapy, 29*, 105–121.

Eley, T. C., Rijsdijk, F. V., Perrin, S., O'Connor, T. G., & Bolton, D. (2008). A multivariate genetic analysis of specific phobia, separation anxiety, and social phobia in early childhood. *Journal of Abnormal Child Psychology, 36*, 839–848.

Epkins, C. C. (2002). A comparison of two self-report measures of children's social anxiety in clinical and community samples. *Journal of Clinical Child and Adolescent Psychology, 31*, 69–79.

Eriksson, P. S., Perfilieva, E., Björk-Eriksson, T., Alborn, A.-M., Nordborg, C., Peterson, D. A., et al. (1998). Neurogenesis in the adult human hippocampus. *Nature Medicine, 4*, 1313–1317.

Ernst, M., Pine, D. S., & Hardin, M. (2006). Triadic model of the neurobiology of motivated behavior in adolescence. *Psychology in Medicine, 36*(3), 299–312.

Essau, C.A., Conradt, J., & Petermann, F. (1999). Frequency of panic attacks and panic disorder in adolescents. *Depression & Anxiety, 9*, 19–26.

Essex, M. J., Klein, M. H., Cho, E., & Kalin, N. H. (2002). Maternal stress beginning in infancy may sensitize children to later stress exposure: Effects on cortisol and behavior. *Biological Psychiatry, 52*, 776–784.

Fairbanks, J. M., Pine, D. S., Tancer, N. K., Dummit, E. S., III, Kentgen, L. M., Asche, B. K., & Klein, R. G. (1997). Open fluoxetine treatment of mixed anxiety disorders in children and adolescents.

Journal of the American Academy of Child and Adolescent Psychiatry, 7, 17–29.

Farrell, A. D., & Bruce, S. E. (1997). Impact of exposure to community violence on violent behavior and emotional distress among urban adolescents. *Journal of Clinical Child Psychology, 26*, 2–14.

Farrell, L. J., & Barrett, P. M. (2007). Prevention of childhood emotional disorders: Reducing the burden of suffering associated with anxiety and depression. *Child and Adolescent Mental Health, 12*(2), 58–65.

Feigon, S., Waldman, I., et al. (2001). Genetic and environmental influences on separation anxiety disorder symptoms and their moderation by age and sex. *Behavior Genetics, 31*(5), 403–411.

Felner, R. D., & Adan, A. M. (1988). The School Transitional Environment Project: An ecological intervention and evaluation. In R. H. Price, E. L. Cowen, L. Emory, et al. (Eds.), *Fourteen ounces of prevention: A casebook for practitioners* (pp. 111–122). Washington, DC: American Psychological Association.

Feske, U., & Goldstein, A. J. (1997). Eye movement desensitization and reprocessing treatment for panic disorder: A controlled outcome and partial dismantling study. *Journal of Consulting and Clinical Psychology, 65*(6), 1026.

Festa, C. C., & Ginsburg, G. S. (2011). Parental and peer predictors of social anxiety in youth. *Child Psychiatry and Human Development, 42*(3), 291–306.

Field, A. P. (2006). Is conditioning a useful framework for understanding the development and treatment of phobias? *Clinical Psychology Review, 26*, 857–875.

Findling, R. L., Reed, M. D., Myers, C., et al (1999). Paroxetine pharmacokinetics in depressed children and adolescents. *Journal of the American Academy of Child and Adolescent Psychiatry, 38*, 952–959.

Fisak, B. J., Jr., Richard, D., & Mann, A. (2011). The prevention of child and adolescent anxiety: A meta-analytic review. *Prevention Science, 12*(3), 255–268.

Fisher, P. L. (2006). The efficacy of psychological treatments for generalised anxiety disorder. In G. C. L. Davey & A. Wells (Eds.), *Worry and its psychological disorders: Theory, assessment and treatment* (pp. 359–377). Chichester: John Wiley & Sons.

Fitzgerald, K. D., Stewart, C. M., Tawile, V., & Rosenberg, D. R. (1999). Risperidone augmentation of serotonin reuptake inhibitor treatment of pediatric obsessive compulsive disorder. *Journal of Child and Adolescent Psychopharmacology, 9*, 115–123.

Flament, M. F., Rapoport, J. L., Berg, C. J., et al. (1985). Clomipramine treatment of childhood obsessive-compulsive disorder. *Archives of General Psychiatry, 42*, 977–983.

Flannery-Schroeder, E. C. & Kendall, P. C. (2000). Group and individual cognitive-behavioral treatments for youth with anxiety disorders: A randomized clinical trial. *Cognitive Therapy & Research, 24*, 251–278.

Foa, E. B., Chrestman, K. R., & Gilboa-Schechtman, E. (2009). *Prolonged exposure therapy for adolescents with PTSD: Emotional processing of traumatic experiences: Therapist guide.* New York: Oxford University Press.

Foa, E. B., Dancu, C. V., Hembree, E. A., Jaycox, L. H., Meadows, E. A., & Street, G. P. (1999). A comparison of exposure therapy, stress inoculation training, and their combination for reducing posttraumatic stress disorder in female assault victims. *Journal of Consulting & Clinical Psychology, 67*, 194–200.

Foa, E. B., Feske, U., Murdock, T. B., Kozak, M. J., et al. (1991). Processing of threat-related information in rape victims. *Journal of Abnormal Psychology, 100*, 156–162.

Foa, E. B., Franklin, M. E., & Moser, J. (2002). Context in the clinic: How well do cognitive-behavioral therapies and medications work in combination? *Biological Psychiatry, 52*, 989–997.

Foa, E. B., Hearst-Ikeda, D., & Perry, K. J. (1995). Evaluation of a brief cognitive-behavioral program for the prevention of chronic PTSD in recent assault victims. *Journal of Consulting and Clinical Psychology, 63*, 948–955.

Foa, E. B., Hembree, E. A., Cahill, S. P., Rauch, S. A., Riggs, D. S., Feeny, N. C., & Yadin, E. (2005). Randomized trial of prolonged exposure for posttraumatic stress disorder with and without cognitive restructuring: outcome at academic and community clinics. *Journal of Consulting and Clinical Psychology, 73*(5), 953.

Foa, E. B., Johnson, K. M., Feeny, N. C., & Treadwell, K. R. H. (2001). The Child PTSD Symptom Scale (CPSS): A preliminary examination of its psychometric properties. *Journal of Clinical Child Psychology, 30*, 376–384.

Foa, E., Keane, T., & Friedman, M. (2000). *Effective treatments for PTSD: Practice guidelines from the International Society for Traumatic Stress Studies.* New York: Guilford Press.

Foa, E. B., & Kozak, M. J. (1985). Treatment of anxiety disorders: Implications for psychopathology.

In A. H. Tuma & J. D. Maser (Eds.), *Anxiety and the anxiety disorders*. Hillsdale, NJ: Lawrence Erlbaum Associates, Inc.

Foa, E. B., & Kozak, M. J. (1986). Emotional processing of fear: Exposure to corrective information. *Psychological Bulletin, 90*, 20–35.

Foa, E. B., & Kozak, M. J. (1996). Psychological treatment for obsessive-compulsive disorder. *Long-Term Treatments of Anxiety Disorders*, 285–309.

Foa, E. B., & Kozak, M. J. (1997a). Beyond the efficacy ceiling? Cognitive behavior therapy in search of theory. *Behavior Therapy, 28*, 601–611.

Foa, E. B., & Kozak, M. J. (1997b). *Mastery of obsessive-compulsive disorder: A cognitive-behavioral approach client workbook* (Vol. 2). New York: Oxford University Press.

Foa, E. B., Liebowitz, M. R., Kozak, M. J., Davies, S., Campeas, R., Franklin, M. E., . . . Tu, X. (2005). Randomized, placebo-controlled trial of exposure and ritual prevention, clomipramine, and their combination in the treatment of obsessive-compulsive disorder. *American Journal of Psychiatry, 162*(1), 151–161.

Foa, E. B., McLean, C. P., Capaldi, S., & Rosenfield, D. (2013). Prolonged exposure vs. supportive counseling for sexual abuse–related PTSD in adolescent girls: A randomized clinical trial. *Journal of the American Medical Association, 310*(24), 2650–2657.

Foa, E. B., Riggs, D. S., Dancu, C. V., & Rothbaum, B. O. (1993). Reliability and validity of a brief instrument for assessing post-traumatic stress disorder. *Journal of Traumatic Stress, 6*, 459–473.

Foa, E. B., & Rothbaum, B. O. (1998). *Treating the trauma of rape: Cognitive-behavioral treatment for PTSD*. New York: Guilford Press.

Foa, E. B., Yadin, E., & Lichner, T. K. (2012). *Exposure and response (ritual) prevention for obsessive-compulsive disorder: Therapist guide* (2nd ed.). New York: Oxford University Press.

Foa, E. B., Yusko, D. A., McLean, C. P., Suvak, M. K., Bux, D. A., Oslin, D., . . . Volpicelli, J. (2013). Concurrent naltrexone and prolonged exposure therapy for patients with comorbid alcohol dependence and PTSD: A randomized clinical trial. *Journal of the American Medical Association, 310*(5), 488–495.

Fontana, A., & Rosenheck, R. (1998a). Duty-related and sexual stress in the etiology of PTSD among women veterans who seek treatment. *Psychiatric Services. Special Issue: Women and Chronic Mental Illness, 49*, 658–662.

Fontana, A., & Rosenheck, R. (1998b). Effects of compensation-seeking on treatment outcomes among veterans with posttraumatic stress disorder. *Journal of Nervous & Mental Disease, 186*, 223–230.

Fontana, A., & Rosenheck, R. (1998c). Psychological benefits and liabilities of traumatic exposure in the war zone. *Journal of Traumatic Stress, 11*, 485–503.

Fontana, A., Schwartz, L. S., & Rosenheck, R. (1997). Posttraumatic stress disorder among female Vietnam veterans: A causal model of etiology. *American Journal of Public Health, 87*, 169–175.

Forbes, D., Lloyd, D., Nixon, R. D. V., Elliott, P., Varker, T., Perry, D., . . . Creamer, M. (2012). A multisite randomized controlled effectiveness trial of cognitive processing therapy for military-related posttraumatic stress disorder. *Journal of Anxiety Disorders, 26*(3), 442–452.

Ford, J. D., Steinberg, K. L., & Zhang, W. (2011). A randomized clinical trial comparing affect regulation and social problem-solving psychotherapies for mothers with victimization-related PTSD. *Behavior Therapy, 42*(4), 560–578.

Fox, N. A., & Bell, M. A. (1990). Electrophysiological indexes of frontal lobe development. *Annals of the New York Academy of Sciences, 608*, 677–698.

Fox, N. A., Henderson, H. A., Rabin, K. H., Caikins, S. D., & Schmidt, L. A. (2001). Continuity and discontinuity of behavioral inhibition and exuberance. *Child Development, 72*, 1–21.

Foy, D. W., Resnick, H. S., Sipprelle, R. C., & Carroll, E. M. (1987). Premilitary, military, and postmilitary factors in the development of combat-related posttraumatic stress disorder. *Behavior Therapist, 10*, 3–9.

Foy, D. W., Ritchie, I. K., & Conway, A. H. (2012). Trauma exposure, posttraumatic stress, and comorbidities in female adolescent offenders: Findings and implications from recent studies. *European Journal of Psychotraumatology* [E-pub before publication, May 31].

Franklin, M. E., & Foa, E. B. (2002). Cognitive behavioral treatments for obsessive compulsive disorder. In P. E. Nathan & J. M. Gormon (Eds.), *A guide to treatments that work* (2nd ed., pp. 367–386). London: Oxford University Press.

Franklin, M. E., Foa, E. B., & March, J. S. (2003). The Pediatric OCD Treatment Study (POTS): Rationale, design and methods. *Journal of Child and Adolescent Psychopharmacology, 13*(suppl. 1), 39–52.

Franklin, M. E., Kozak, M. J., et al. (1998). Cognitive-behavioral treatment of pediatric obsessive-compulsive disorder: An open clinical trial. *Journal of the American Academy of Child and Adolescent Psychiatry, 37*, 412–419.

Franklin, M. E., Sapyta, J., Freeman, J. B., Khanna, M., Compton, S., Almirall, D., ... March, J. S. (2011). Cognitive behavior therapy augmentation of pharmacotherapy in pediatric obsessive-compulsive disorder: The Pediatric OCD Treatment Study II (POTS II) randomized controlled trial. *Journal of the American Medical Association, 306*, 1224–1232.

Franklin, M. E., Tolin, D. F., March, J. S., & Foa, E. B. (2001). Treatment of pediatric obsessive-compulsive disorder: A case example of intensive cognitive-behavioral therapy involving exposure and ritual prevention. *Cognitive and Behavioral Practice, 8*(4), 297–304.

Frederick, C. J., Pynoos, R. S., & Nader, K. (1992). *Reaction Index to Psychic Trauma Form C (Child).* Unpublished manuscript, University of California at Los Angeles.

Freeman, J. B., Choate-Summers, M. L., Moore, P. S., Garcia, A. M., Sapyta, J. J., Leonard, H. L., & Franklin, M. E. (2007). Cognitive behavioral treatment of young children with obsessive compulsive disorder. *Biological Psychiatry, 61*, 337–343.

Freeman, J., Sapyta, J., Garcia, A., Compton, S., Khanna, M., Flessner, C., ... Franklin, M. (2014). Family-based treatment of early childhood obsessive-compulsive disorder: The Pediatric Obsessive Compulsive Disorder Treatment Study for Young Children (POTS Jr.) – A randomized clinical trial. *JAMA Psychiatry, 170*.

Gallo, K. P., Chan, P. T., Buzzella, B. A., Whitton, S. W., & Pincus, D. B. (2012). The impact of an 8-day intensive treatment for adolescent panic disorder and agoraphobia on comorbid diagnoses. *Behavior Therapy, 43*(1), 153–159.

Gar, N. S., Hudson, J. L., & Rapee, R. M. (2005). Family factors and the development of anxiety disorders. In J. L. Hudson & R. M. Rapee (Eds.), *Psychopathology and the family* (pp. 125–145). New York: Elsevier Science.

Garvey, M. A., Perlmutter, S. J., et al. (1999). A pilot study of penicillin prophylaxis for neuropsychiatric exacerbations triggered by streptococcal infections. *Biological Psychiatry, 45*, 1564–1571.

Geller, D. A., Biederman, J., Faraone, S. V., et al. (2001). Disentagling chronological age from age of onset in children and adolescents with obsessive-compulsive disorder. *International Journal of Neuropsycholopharmacology, 4*, 169–178.

Geller, D. A., Hoog, S. L., et al. (2001). Fluoxetine treatment for obsessive-compulsive disorder in children and adolescents: A placebo-controlled clinical trial. *Journal of the American Academy of Child and Adolescent Psychiatry, 40*, 773–779.

Gerlsma, C., Emmelkamp, P. M. G., & Arrindell, W. A. (1990). Anxiety, depression, and perception of early parenting: A meta-analysis. *Clinical Psychology Review, 10*, 251–277.

Giedd, J. N., Blumenthal, J., Jeffries, N. O., Castellanos, F. X., Liu, H., Zijdenbos, A., et al. (1999). Brain development during childhood and adolescence: A longitudinal MRI study. *Nature Neuroscience, 2*, 861–863.

Giedd, J. N., Castellanos, F. X., Rajapakse, J. C., Vaituzis, A. C., & Rapoport, J. L. (1997). Sexual dimorphism of the developing human brain. *Progress in Neuro-Psyphopharmacology & Biological Psychiatry, 21*, 1185–1201.

Giedd, J. N., Raznahan, A., Mills, K. L., & Lenroot, R. K. (2012). Review: Magnetic resonance imaging of male/female differences in human adolescent brain anatomy. *Biology of Sex Differentiation, 3*(1), 19.

Gilboa-Schechtman, E., Foa, E. B., Shafran, N., Aderka, I. M., Powers, M. B., Rachamim, L., ... Apter, A. (2010). Prolonged exposure versus dynamic therapy for adolescent PTSD: A pilot randomized controlled trial. *Journal of the American Academy of Child & Adolescent Psychiatry, 49*(10), 1034–1042.

Gillihan, S. J., Aderka, I. M., Conklin, P. H., Capaldi, S., & Foa, E. B. (2013). The child PTSD symptom scale: Psychometric properties in female adolescent sexual assault survivors. *Psychological Assessment, 25*(1), 23–31.

Ginsburg, G. S. (2009). The child anxiety prevention study: Intervention model and primary outcomes. *Journal of Consulting and Clinical Psychology, 77*(3), 580–587.

Ginsburg, G. S., & Scholossberg, M. C. (2002). Family-based treatment of childhood anxiety disorders. *International Review of Psychiatry. Special Issue: Anxiety Disorders in Children and Adolescents, 14*, 143–154.

Ginsburg, G. S., Becker, E. M., Keeton, C. P., Sakolsky, D., Piacentini, J., Albano, A. M., ... Kendall, P. C. (2014). Naturalistic follow-up of youths treated for pediatric anxiety disorders. *JAMA Psychiatry, 71*(3), 310–318.

Ginsburg, G. S., Silverman, W. K., & Kurtines, W. M. (1995). Family involvement in treating children with phobic and anxiety disorders: A look ahead. *Clinical Psychology Review, 15*, 457–473.

Gitlin, D. F., Schindler, B. A., Stern, T. A., Epstein, S. A., Lamdan, R. M., McCarty, T. A., ... Worley, L. L. (1996). Recommended guidelines for consultation-liaison psychiatric training in psychiatry residency programs: A report from the Academy of Psychosomatic Medicine Task Force on Psychiatric Resident Training in Consultation-Liaison Psychiatry. *Psychosomatics, 37*(1), 3–11.

Gittelman-Klein, R., & Klein, D. F. (1971). Controlled imipramine treatment of school phobia. *Archives of General Psychiatry, 2*, 204–207.

Gittelman-Klein, R., & Klein, D. F. (1973). School phobia: Diagnostic considerations in the light of imipramine effects. *Journal of Nervous & Mental Disease, 156*, 199–215.

Goddard, A. W., Brouette, T., Almai, A., Jetty, P., Woods, S. W., & Charney, D. (2001). Early coadministration of clonazepam with sertraline for panic disorder. *Archives of General Psychiatry, 58*, 681–686.

Goenjian, A. K., Karayan, I., Pynoos, R. S., Minassian, D., et al. (1997). Outcome of psychotherapy among early adolescents after trauma. *American Journal of Psychiatry, 154*, 536–542.

Goenjian, A., Stilwell, B. M., Steinberg, A. M., Fairbanks, L. A., Galvin, M. R., Karayan, I., & Pynoos, R. S. (1999). Moral development and psychopathological interference in conscience functioning among adolescents after trauma. *Journal of the American Academy of Child and Adolescent Psychiatry, 38*, 376–384.

Goldman-Rakic, P. S., Isseroff, A., Schwartz, M. L., & Bugbee, N. M. (1983). The neurobiology of cognitive development. In P. H. Mussen (Ed.), *Handbook of child psychology: Vol. II. Infancy and developmental psychobiology* (pp. 281–344). New York: Wiley.

Goldstein, A. J., de Beurs, E., Chambless, D. L., & Wilson, K. A. (2000). EMDR for panic disorder with agoraphobia: Comparison with waiting list and credible attention-placebo control conditions. *Journal of Consulting and Clinical Psychology, 68*(6), 947.

Gordon-Hollingsworth, A., Becker, E. M., Ginsburg, G. S., Keeton, C., Compton, S. N., Birmaher, B. B., ... March, J. S. (2015). Anxiety disorders in Caucasian and African American children: A comparison of clinical characteristics, treatment process variables, and treatment outcomes. *Child Psychiatry and Human Development, 46*(5), 643–655.

Gorman, J. M., & Sloan, R. P. (2000). Heart rate variability in depressive and anxiety disorders. *American Heart Journal, 140*, 77–83.

Gorwood, P., Feingold, J., et al. (1999). Genetic epidemiology and psychiatry: Scope and limitations of familial studies. Case of panic disorder. *Encephale, 25*(1), 21–29.

Gottesman, I. I., & Gould, T. D. (2003). The endophenotype concept in psychiatry: Etymology and strategic intentions. *American Journal of Psychiatry, 160*, 636–645.

Gould, R. A., Ott, M. W., & Pollack, M. H. (1995). A meta-analysis of treatment outcome for panic disorder. *Clinical Psychology Review, 15*(8), 819–844.

Graae, F., Milner, J., Rizzotto, L., et al. (1994). Clonazepam in childhood anxiety disorders. *Journal of the American Academy of Child and Adolescent Psychiatry, 33*, 372–376.

Graber, J. A., Brooks-Gunn, J., Paikoff, R. L., & Warren, M. P. (1994). Prediction of eating problems; an 8-year study of adolescent girls. *Developmental Psychology, 30*, 823–834.

Greaves-Lord, K., Tulen, J., Dietrich, A., Sondeijker, F., van Roon, A., Oldehinkel, A., ... Huizink, A. (2010). Reduced autonomic flexibility as a predictor for future anxiety in girls from the general population: The TRAILS study. *Psychiatry Research, 179*(2), 187–193.

Griffith, J. (1985). Social support providers: Who are they? Where are they met?—and the relationship of network characteristics to psychological distress. *Basic & Applied Social Psychology, 6*, 41–60.

Grillon, C., Dierker, L., & Merikangas, K. R. (1998). Fear-potentiated startle in adolescent offspring of parents with anxiety disorders. *Biological Psychiatry, 44*(10), 990–997.

Hadwin, J., Frost, S., French, C. C., & Richards, A. (1997). Cognitive processing and trait anxiety in typically developing children: Evidence for an interpretation bias. *Journal of Abnormal Psychology, 106*, 486–490.

Hagemann, D., Naumann, E., Thayer, J. F., & Bartussek, D., (2002). Does resting EEG asymmetry reflect a trait? *Journal of Personality and Social Psychology, 82*, 619–641.

Hagopian, L. P., & Ollendick, T. H. (1997). Anxiety disorders. In R. T. Ammerman, & M. Hersen (Eds.), *Handbook of prevention and treatment with children and adolescents: Intervention in the real world context* (pp. 431–454) Hoboken, NJ: John Wiley & Sons, Inc.

Hajcak, G., MacNamara, A., & Olvet, D. M. (2010). Event-related potentials, emotion, and emotion regulation: An integrative review. *Developmental Neuropsychology, 35*(2), 129–155.

Hanrahan, F., Field, A. P., Jones, F. W., & Davey, G. C. L. (2013). A meta-analysis of cognitive therapy for worry in generalized anxiety disorder. *Clinical Psychology Review, 33*(1), 120–132.

Hayes-Skelton, S. A., Roemer, L., & Orsillo, S. M. (2013). A randomized clinical trial comparing an acceptance-based behavior therapy to applied relaxation for generalized anxiety disorder. *Journal of Consulting and Clinical Psychology, 81*(5), 761.

Hayward, C., Killen, J. D., Kraemer, H. C., Blair-Greiner, A., Strachowski, D., Cunning, D., et al. (1997). Assessment and phenomenology of nonclinical panic attacks in adolescent girls. *Journal of Anxiety Disorders, 11*, 17–32.

Hayward, C., Killen, J. D., Wilson, D. M., & Hammer, L. D. (1997). Psychiatric risk associated with early puberty in adolescent girls. *Journal of the American Academy of Child and Adolescent Psychiatry, 36*, 255–262.

Hayward, C., Varady, S., Albano, A. M., Thienemann, M., Henderson, L., & Schatzberg, A. F. (2000). Cognitive-behavioral group therapy for social phobia in female adolescents: Results of a pilot study. *Journal of the American Academy of Child and Adolescent Psychiatry, 39*, 721–726.

Hedman, E., Andersson, G., Ljótsson, B., Andersson, E., Rück, C., Mörtberg, E., & Lindefors, N. (2011). Internet-based cognitive behavior therapy vs. cognitive behavioral group therapy for social anxiety disorder: A randomized controlled non-inferiority trial. *PLoS One, 6*(3), e18001.

Heim, C., & Nemeroff, C. B. (2002). Neurobiology of early life stress: Clinical studies. *Seminars in Clinical Neuropsychiatry, 7*, 147–159.

Heim, C., Owens, M. J., Plotsky, P. M., & Nemeroff, C. B. (1997). The role of early adverse life events in the etiology of depression and posttraumatic stress disorder. Focus on corticotropin-releasing factor. In R. Yehuda (Ed.), *Psychobiology of posttraumatic stress disorder* (pp. 194–207). New York: New York Academy of Sciences.

Herbert, J. D., Gaudiano, B. A., Rheingold, A. A., Moitra, E., Myers, V. H., Dalrymple, K. L., & Brandsma, L. L. (2009). Cognitive behavior therapy for generalized social anxiety disorder in adolescents: A randomized controlled trial. *Journal of Anxiety Disorders, 23*(2), 167–177.

Herman, J. L. (1992). Complex PTSD: A syndrome in survivors of prolonged and repeated trauma. *Journal of Traumatic Stress, 5*, 377–391.

Hettema, J., Neale, M. C., & Kendler, K. S. (2001). A review and meta-analysis of the genetic epidemiology of anxiety disorders. *American Journal of Psychiatry, 158*, 1568–1578.

Hettema, J. M., Prescott, C. A., & Kendler, K. S. (2001). A population-based twin study of generalized anxiety disorder in men and women. *Journal of Nervous and Mental Disease, 189*(7), 413–420.

Heyne, D., King, N. J., Tonge, B. J., Rollings, S., Young, D., Pritchard, M., et al. (2002). Evaluation of child therapy and caregiver training in the treatment of school refusal. *Journal of the American Academy of Child and Adolescent Psychiatry, 41*(6), 687–695.

Hightower, A. D., & Braden, J. (1991). Prevention. In T. R. Kratochwill & R. J. Morris (Eds.), *The practice of child therapy* (pp. 410–440). New York: Pergamon.

Hill, H. M., Levermore, M., Twaite, J., & Jones, L. P. (1996). Exposure to community violence and social support as predictors of anxiety and social and emotional behavior among African American children. *Journal of Child and Family Studies, 5*, 399–414.

Hirschmann, S., Dannon, P. N., Iancu, J., Dolberg, O. T., Zohar, J., & Grunhaus, L. (2000). Pindolol augmentation in patients with treatment-resistant panic disorder: A double-blind, placebo controlled trial. *Journal of Clinical Psychopharmacology, 20*(5), 556–559.

Hirshfeld-Becker, D. R., Dina, R., Petty, C., Micco, J. A., Henin, A., Park, J., . . . Biederman, J. (2008). Disruptive behavior disorders in offspring of parents with major depression: Associations with parental behavior disorders. *Journal of Affective Disorders, 111*, 176–184.

Hirshfeld-Becker, D., Masek, B., Henin, A., Blakely, L. R., Pollock-Wurman, R., McQuade, J., . . . Biederman, J. (2010). Cognitive behavioral therapy for 4- to 7-year-old children with anxiety disorders: A randomized clinical trial. *Journal of Consulting and Clinical Psychology, 78*(4), 498–510.

Hodges, K., Doucette-Gates, A., et al. (1999). The relationship between the Child and Adolescent Functional Assessment Scale (CAPAS) and indicators of functioning. *Journal of Child and Family Studies, 8*, 109–122.

Hodges, W. F. (1991). *Interventions for children of divorce*. New York: John Wiley & Sons.

Hofman, S. G., Bufka, L. F., & Barlow, D. H. (1999). Panic provocation procedures in the treatment of panic disorder: Early perspectives and case studies. *Behavior Therapy, 30*(2), 305–317.

Hoge, E. A., Bui, E., Marques, L., Metcalf, C. A., Morris, L. K., Robinaugh, D. J., . . . Simon, N. M. (2013). Randomized controlled trial of mindfulness meditation for generalized anxiety disorder: Effects on anxiety and stress reactivity. *Journal of Clinical Psychiatry, 74*(8), 786.

Hohagen, F., Winklemann, G., Rasche-Raeuchle, H., Hand, I., Koenig, A., Muenchau, N., et al. (1998). Combination of behaviour therapy with fluvoxamine in comparison with behaviour therapy and placebo: Results of a multicentre study. *British Journal of Psychiatry, 173*, 71–78.

Holmbeck, G. N., & Kendall, P. C. (2002). Introduction to the special section on clinical adolescent psychology: Developmental psychopathology and treatment. *Journal of Consulting and Clinical Psychology, 70*(1), 3–5.

Huang, F. F., Li, Z. J., Han, H. Y., Xiong, H. F., & Ma, Y. (2013). Cognitive behavioral therapy combined with pharmacotherapy for obsessive compulsive disorder: A meta-analysis. *Chinese Mental Health Journal, 27*(9), 643–649.

Hudson, J. L., Flannery-Schroeder, E., & Kendall, P. C. (2004). Primary prevention of anxiety disorders. In D. J. A. Dozois & K. S. Dobson (Eds.), *Primary prevention of anxiety disorders*. Washington, DC: American Psychological Association.

Hudson, J. L., & Rapee, R. M. (2002). Parent-child interactions in clinically anxious children and their siblings. *Journal of Clinical Child and Adolescent Psychology, 31*, 548–555.

Hughes, H. E., & Sparber, S. B. (1978). d-Amphetamine unmasks postnatal consequences of exposure to methylmercury in utero: Methods for studying behavioral teratogenesis. *Pharmacology, Biochemistry and Behavior, 8*, 365–375.

Hunot, V., Churchill, R., Silva de Lima, M., & Teixeira, V. (2007). Psychological therapies for generalised anxiety disorder. *Cochrane Database Systematic Reviews, 1*, CD001848.

Hunt, C., Andrews, G., Crino, R., Erskine, A., & Sakashita, C. (2009). Randomized controlled trial of an early intervention programme for adolescent anxiety disorders. *Australian and New Zealand Journal of Psychiatry, 43*(4), 300–304.

Huttenlocher, P. R. (1979). Synaptic density of human frontal cortex—developmental changes and effects of aging. *Brain Research, 163*, 195–205.

Ialongo, N., Edelsohn, G., Werthamer-Larsson, L., Crockett, L., & Kellam, S. (1993). Are self-reported depressive symptoms in first-grade children developmentally transient phenomena? A further look. *Development and Psychopathology, 5*, 433–452.

Ingul, J. M., Aune, T., & Nordahl, H. M. (2014). A randomized controlled trial of individual cognitive therapy, group cognitive behaviour therapy and attentional placebo adolescent social phobia. *Psychotherapy and Psychosomatics, 83*(1), 54–61.

Jaurrieta, N., Jimenez-Murcia, S., Menchón, J. M., Alonso, M. D. P., Segalas, C., Álvarez-Moya, E. M., . . . Vallejo, J. (2008). Individual versus group cognitive–behavioral treatment for obsessive–compulsive disorder: A controlled pilot study. *Psychotherapy Research, 18*(5), 604–614.

Jerremalm, A., Jansson, L., & Öst, L. (1986). Individual response patterns and the effects of different behavioral methods in the treatment of dental phobia. *Behaviour Research & Therapy, 24*, 587–596.

Johnson, J. G., Cohen, P., Pine, D. S., Kline, D. F., Kasen, S., & Book, J. S. (2000). Association between cigarette smoking and anxiety disorders during adolescence and early adulthood. *Journal of the American Medical Association, 284*, 2348–2351.

Jónsson, H., Hougaard, E., & Bennedsen, B. E. (2011). Randomized comparative study of group versus individual cognitive behavioural therapy for obsessive compulsive disorder. *Acta Psychiatrica Scandinavica, 123*(5), 387–397.

Jørstad-Stein, E. C., & Heimberg, R. G. (2009). Social phobia: An update on treatment. *Psychiatric Clinics of North America, 32*(3), 641–663.

Kagan, J. (1994a). *Galen's prophecy: Temperament in human nature*. New York: Basic Books.

Kagan, J. (1994b). Inhibited and uninhibited temperaments. In W. B. Carey & S. C. McDevitt (Eds.), *Prevention and early intervention: Individual differences as risk factors for the mental health of children: A festschrift for Stella Chess and Alexander Thomas* (pp. 35–41). Philadelphia, PA: Brunner/Mazel.

Kagan, J. (1994c). On the nature of emotion. *Monographs of the Society for Research in Child Development, 59*, 7–24, 250–283.

Kagan, J. (2002a). Childhood predictors of states of anxiety. *Dialogues in Clinical Neuroscience, 4*, 287–292.

Kagan, J. (2002b). *Surprise, uncertainty, and mental structures*. Cambridge, MA: Harvard University Press.

Kagan, J., Snidman, N., McManis, M., & Woodward, S. (2001). Temperamental contributions to the affect family of anxiety. *Psychiatric Clinics of North America, 24*, 677–688.

Kampman, M., Keijsers, G. P., Hoogduin, C. A., & Hendriks, G. J. (2002). A randomized, double-blind, placebo-controlled study of the effects of adjunctive paroxetine in panic disorder patients unsuccessfully treated with cognitive-behavioral therapy alone. *Journal of Clinical Psychiatry, 63*(9), 772–777.

Kaplan, M. L., Erensaft, M., Sanderson, W. C., Wetzler, S., Foote, B., & Asnis, G. M. (1998). Dissociative symptomatology and aggressive behavior. *Comprehensive Psychiatry, 39*(5), 271–276.

Kaplow, J. B., Curran, P. J., et al. (2001). The prospective relation between dimensions of anxiety and the initiation of adolescent alcohol use. *Journal of Clinical Child Psychology, 30*, 316–326.

Kaufman, J., Plotsky, P. M., Nemeroff, C. B., & Charney, D. S. (2000). Effects of early adverse experiences on brain structure and function: Clinical implications. *Biological Psychiatry, 48*, 778–790.

Kazak, A. E., Barakat, L. P, Meeske, K., Christakis, D., et al. (1997). Posttraumatic stress, family functioning, and social support in survivors of childhood leukemia and their mothers and fathers. *Journal of Consulting and Clinical Psychology, 65*, 120–129.

Kazdin, A. E. (1997). Parent management training: Evidence, outcomes, and issues. *Journal of the American Academy of Child and Adolescent Psychiatry, 36*(10), 1349–1356.

Kazdin, A. E., & Weisz, J. R. (1998). Identifying and developing empirically supported child and adolescent treatments. *Journal of Consulting and Clinical Psychology, 66, 1*, 19–36.

Keane, T. M., Fairbank, J. A., Caddell, J. M., & Zimmering, R. T. (1989). Implosive (flooding) therapy reduces symptoms of PTSD in Vietnam combat veterans. *Behavior Therapy, 20*, 245–260.

Keane, T. M., Fairbank, J. A., Caddell, J. M., Zimmering, R. T., et al. (1989). Clinical evaluation of a measure to assess combat exposure. *Psychological Assessment, 1*, 53–55.

Keane, T. M., Scott, W. O., Chavoya, G. A., Lamparski, D. M., & Fairbank, J. A. (1985). Social support in Vietnam veterans with posttraumatic stress disorder: A comparative analysis. *Journal of Consulting and Clinical Psychology, 53*, 95–102.

Keane, T. M., Zimering, R. T., & Caddell, J. M. (1985). A behavioral formulation of posttraumatic stress disorder in Vietnam veterans. *Behavior Therapist, 8*, 9–12.

Kearney, C. A. & Drake, K. L. (2002). Social phobia. In M. Hersen (Ed.), *Clinical behavior therapy: Adults and children*. New York: John Wiley & Sons, Inc.

Kearney, C. A., & Silverman, W. K. (1997). The evolution and reconciliation of taxonomic strategies for school refusal behavior. *Clinical Psychology: Science and Practice, 3*, 339–354.

Kearney, P. (2007). Cognitive assessment of game-based learning. *British Journal of Educational Technology, 38*(3), 529–531.

Kellogg, C. K. (1998). Early developmental modulation of GABA(A) receptor function: Influence on adaptive responses. *Perspectives on Developmental Neurobiology, 5*, 219–234.

Kemp, A., Green, B. L., Hovanitz, C., & Rawlings, E. I. (1995). Incidence and correlates of posttraumatic stress disorder in battered women: Shelter and community samples. *Journal of Interpersonal Violence, 10*, 43–55.

Kenardy, J. A., Dow, M. G. T., Johnston, D. W., Newman, M. G., Thomson, A., & Taylor, C. B. (2003). A comparison of delivery methods of cognitive-behavioral therapy for panic disorder: An international multicenter trial. *Journal of Consulting and Clinical Psychology, 71*(6), 1068–1075.

Kenardy, J., Robinson, S., & Dob, R. (2005). Cognitive behaviour therapy for panic disorder: Long-term follow-up. *Cognitive Behavior Therapy, 34*(2), 75–78.

Kendall, P. C. (1994). Treating anxiety disorders in youth: Results of a randomized clinical trial. *Journal of Consulting and Clinical Psychology, 62*, 100–110.

Kendall, P.C. (1989). The generalization and maintenance of behavior change: Comments, considerations and the "no-cure" criticism. *Behavior Therapy, 20*, 357–364.

Kendall, P. C. (2000a). *Cognitive-behavioral therapy for anxious children: Treatment manual* (2nd ed.). Ardmore, PA: Workbook Publishing.

Kendall, P. C. (2000b). *Coping Cat workbook*. Ardmore, PA: Workbook Publishing.

Kendall, P. C., Cantwell, D. P., & Kazdin, A. E. (1989). Depression in children and adolescents: Assessment issues and recommendations. *Cognitive Therapy and Research, 13*, 109–146.

Kendall, P. C., Chu, B., Gifford, A., Hayes, C., Nauta, M. (1998). Breathing life into a manual: Flexibility and creativity with manual-based treatments. *Cognitive and Behavioral Practice, 5*, 177–198.

Kendall, P. C., & Clarkin, J. F. (1992). Introduction to special section: Comorbidity and treatment implications. *Journal of Clinical and Consulting Psychology, 60*, 833–834.

Kendall, P. C., Compton, S. N., Walkup, J. T., Birmaher, B., Albano, A. M., Sherrill, J., . . . Piacentini, J. (2010). Clinical characteristics of anxiety disordered youth. *Journal of Anxiety Disorders, 24*(3), 360–365.

Kendall, P. C., Flannery-Schroeder, E., Panichelli-Mindel, S., Southam-Gerow, M. Henin, A., & Warman, M. (1997). Therapy for youth with anxiety disorders: A second randomized clinical trial. *Journal of Consulting & Clinical Psychology, 65*, 366–380.

Kendall, P. C., Hudson, J. L., Gosch, E., Flannery-Schroeder, E., & Suveg, C. (2008). Cognitive-behavioral therapy for anxiety disordered youth: A randomized clinical trial evaluating child and family modalities. *Journal of Consulting and Clinical Psychology, 76*(2), 282–297.

Kendall, P. C., Kortlander, E., et al. (1992). Comorbidity of anxiety and depression in youth: Treatment implications. *Journal of Consulting and Clinical Psychology, 60*(6), 869–880.

Kendall, P. C., Safford, S., Flannery-Schroeder, E., & Webb, A. (2004). Child anxiety treatment: Outcomes in adolescence and impact on substance use and depression at 7.4-year follow-up. *Journal of Consulting and Clinical Psychology, 72*(2), 276–287.

Kendall, P. C., & Southam-Gerow, M. A. (1995). Issues in the transportability of treatment: The case of anxiety disorders in youths. *Journal of Consulting & Clinical Psychology, 63*, 702–708.

Kendall, P. C., & Southam-Gerow, M. A. (1996). Long-term follow-up of a cognitive-behavioral therapy for anxiety-disordered youth. *Journal of Consulting & Clinical Psychology, 64*, 724–730.

Kendall, P. C., & Treadwell, K. R. H. (2007). The role of self-statements as a mediator in treatment for youth with anxiety disorders. *Journal of Consulting and Clinical Psychology, 75*(3), 380–389.

Kendler, K. S., Gardner, C. O., Annas, P., Neale, M. C., Eaves, L. J., & Lichtenstein, P. (2008). A longitudinal twin study of fears from middle childhood to early adulthood: Evidence for a developmentally dynamic genome. *Archives of General Psychiatry, 65*(4), 421–429.

Kendler, K. S., Neale, M. C., Kessler, R. C., Heath, A. C., & Eaves, L. J. (1992). A population-based twin study of major depression in women: The impact of varying definitions of illness. *Archives of General Psychiatry, 49*(4), 257–266.

Kerns, C. M., Read, K. L., Klugman, J., & Kendall, P. C. (2013). Cognitive behavioral therapy for youth with social anxiety: Differential short and long-term treatment outcomes. *Journal of Anxiety Disorders, 27*(2), 210–215.

Kessler, R. C., Berglund, P., Demler, O., Jin, R., Merikangas, K. R., & Walters, E. E. (2005). Lifetime prevalence and age-of-onset distributions of DSM-IV disorders in the National Comorbidity Survey Replication. *Archives of General Psychiatry, 62*, 593–602.

Kessler, R. C., Chiu, W. T., Demler, O., & Walters, E. E. (2005). Prevalence, severity, and comorbidity of 12-month DSM-IV disorders in the National Comorbidity Survey Replication. *Archives of General Psychiatry, 62*(6), 617–627.

Kessler, R. C., Sonnega, A., Bromet, E., Hughes, M., et al. (1995). Posttraumatic stress disorder in the National Comorbidity Survey. *Archives of General Psychiatry, 52*, 1048–1060.

Kilpatrick, D. G., Acierno, R., Resnick, H. S., Saunders, B. E., & Best, C. L. (1997). A 2-year longitudinal analysis of the relationships between violent assault and substance use in women. *Journal of Consulting and Clinical Psychology, 65*, 834–847.

Kilpatrick, D. G., Acierno, R., Saunders, B., Resnick, H. S., Best, C. L., & Schnurr, P. P. (2000). Risk factors for adolescent substance abuse and dependence: Data from a national sample. *Journal of Consulting and Clinical Psychology, 68*(1), 19–30.

Kilpatrick, D. G., Ruggerio, K. J., Acierno, R., Saunders, B. E., Resnick, H. S. & Best, C. L. (2003). Violence and risk of PTSD, major depression, substance abuse/dependence, and comorbidity: Results from the National Survey of Adolescents. *Journal of Consulting & Clinical Psychology, 71*, 692–700.

Kilpatrick, D. G., Saunders, B. E., Resnick, H. S., & Smith, D. W. (1995). *The National Survey of Adolescents: Preliminary findings on lifetime prevalence of traumatic events and mental health correlates*. Charleston: Medical University of South Carolina, National Crime Victims Research and Treatment Center.

Kindt, M., Bierman, D., & Brosschot, J. F. (1997). Cognitive bias in spider fear and control children: Assessment of emotional interference by a card format and a single-trial format of the Stroop task. *Journal of Experimental Child Psychology, 66*, 163–179.

Kindt, M., Brosschot, J. F., & Everaerd, W. (1997). Cognitive processing bias of children in a real-life stress situation and a neutral situation. *Journal of Experimental Child Psychology, 64*, 79–97.

Kindt, M., van den Hout, M., de Jong, P., & Hoekzema, B. (2000). Cognitive bias for pictorial and linguistic threat cues in children. *Journal of Psychopathology and Behavioral Assessment, 22*, 201–219.

King, N. J., Ollendick, T. H., Murphy, G. C., & Molloy, G. N. (1998). Utility of relaxation training with children in school settings: A plea for realistic goal setting and evaluation. *British Journal of Educational Psychology, 68*(1), 53–66.

King, R. A., Leonard, H., & March, J. (1998). Practice parameters for the assessment and treatment of children and adolescents with obsessive-compulsive disorder. *Journal of the American Academy of Child and Adolescent Psychiatry, 37*(10 Suppl.), 27S–45S.

King, R., Gaines, L. S., Lambert, E. W., Summerfelt, W. T., & Bickman, L. (2000). The co-occurence of psychiatric substance use diagnoses in adolescents in different service systems: Frequency, recognition, cost, and outcomes. *Journal of Behavioral Health Services & Research, 27*, 417–430.

Klein, B., Richards, J. C., & Austin, D. W. (2006). Efficacy of Internet therapy for panic disorder. *Journal of Behavior Therapy and Experimental Psychiatry, 37*(3), 213–238.

Klein, D. F. (1964). Delineation of two drug-responsive anxiety syndromes. *Psychopharmacologia (Berlin), 5*, 397.

Klein, D. F., & Fink, M. (1962). Behavioral reaction patterns with phenothiazines. *Archives of General Psychiatry, 7*, 449–459.

Klein, D. F., Mannuzza, S., Chapman, T. & Fyer, A. J. (1992). Child panic revisited. *Journal of the American Academy of Child & Adolescent Psychiatry, 31*, 112–114.

Klein, R. G. (1995). Is panic disorder associated with childhood separation anxiety disorder? *Clinical Neuropharmacology, 18*(Suppl 2), S7–S14.

Koch, E. I., Spates, C. R., & Himle, J. A. (2004). Comparison of behavioral and cognitive-behavioral one-session exposure treatments for small animal phobias. *Behaviour Research and Therapy, 42*(12), 1483–1504.

Koran, L. M., Hanna, G. L., Hollander, E., Nestadt, G., & Simpson, H. B. (2007). American Psychiatric Association practice guideline for the treatment of patients with obsessive-compulsive disorder. *American Journal of Psychiatry, 164*(7 Suppl), 5–53.

Kossowsky, J., Pfaltz, M. C., Schneider, S., Taeymans, J., Locher, C., & Gaab, J. (2013). The separation anxiety hypothesis of panic revisited: A meta-analysis. *American Journal of Psychiatry, 170*(7), 768–781.

Koszycki, D., Benger, M., Shlik, J., & Bradwejn, J. (2007). Randomized trial of a meditation-based stress reduction program and cognitive behavior therapy in generalized social anxiety disorder. *Behaviour Research and Therapy, 45*(10), 2518–2526.

La Bar, K. S., Gatenby, C., Gore, J. C., Le Doux, J. E., & Phelphs, E. A. (1998). Human amygdala activation during conditioned fear acquisition and extinction. *Neuron, 29*, 937–945.

La Greca, A. M., Lai, B. S., Joormann, J., Auslander, B. B., & Short, M. A. (2013). Children's risk and resilience following a natural disaster: Genetic vulnerability, posttraumatic stress, and depression. *Journal of Affective Disorders, 151*(3), 860–867.

La Greca, A. M., & Lopez, N. (1998). Social anxiety among adolescents: Linkages with peer relations and friendships. *Journal of Abnormal Child Psychology, 26*, 83–94.

La Greca, A. M., Silverman, W. K., Lai, B., & Jaccard, J. (2010). Hurricane-related exposure experiences and stressors, other life events, and social support: Concurrent and prospective impact on children's persistent posttraumatic stress symptoms. *Journal of Consulting and Clinical Psychology, 78*(6), 794–805.

La Greca, A. M., Silverman, W. K., Vernberg, E. M., & Prinstein, M. J. (1996). Symptoms of post-traumatic stress in children following Hurricane Andrew: A prospective study. *Journal of Consulting and Clinical Psychology, 105*, 712–723.

La Greca, A. M., & Stone, W. L. (1993). Social Anxiety Scale for Children—Revised: Factor structure and concurrent validity. *Journal of Clinical Child Psychology, 22*, 17–27.

Labellarte, M. J., Walkup, J. T., & Riddle, M. A. (1998). The new antidepressants: Selective serotonin reuptake inhibitors. *Pediatric Clinics of North America, 45*, 1137–1155.

Ladouceur, R., Dugas, M. J., Freeston, M. H., Léger, E., Gagnon, F., & Thibodeau, N. (2000). Efficacy of a cognitive–behavioral treatment for generalized anxiety disorder: Evaluation in a controlled clinical trial. *Journal of Consulting and Clinical Psychology, 68*(6), 957.

LaFreniere, P. J., & Capuano, F. (1997). Preventive intervention as means of clarifying direction of effects in socialization: Anxious-withdrawn preschoolers case. *Development & Psychopathology, 9*, 551–564.

Lang, P. J., (1977). Imagery in therapy: An information processing analysis of fear. *Behavior Therapy, 8*(5), 862–886.

Last, C. G., Hansen, C., & Franco, N. (1998). Cognitive-behavioral treatment of school phobia. *Journal of the American Academy of Child and Adolescent Psychiatry, 37*, 404–411.

Lavigne, J. V., Arend, R., et al. (1998). Psychiatric disorders with onset in the preschool years: I. Stability of diagnoses. *Journal of the American Academy of Child and Adolescent Psychiatry, 37*, 1246–1254.

Lavigne, J. V., Cicchetti, C., et al. (2001). Oppositional defiant disorder with onset in preschool years: Longitudinal stability and pathways to other disorders. *Journal of the American Academy of Child and Adolescent Psychiatry, 40*, 1393–1400.

Lavigne, J. V., Gibbons, R. D., et al. (1996). Prevalence rates and correlates of psychiatric disorders among preschool children. *Journal of the American Academy of Child and Adolescent Psychiatry, 35*,(2), 204–214.

Layne, C. M., Pynoos, R. S., & Cardenas, J. (2001). Wounded adolescence: School-based group psychotherapy for adolescents who sustained or witnessed violent injury. In M. Shafi & S. L. Shafi (Eds.), *School violence: Assessment, management, prevention* (pp. 163–186). Washington, DC: American Psychiatric Association.

Layne, C. M., Pynoos, R. S., Saltzman, W. R., Arslanagic, B., Black, M., Savjak, N., Popovic, T. et al. (2001). Trauma/grief-focused group psychotherapy: School-based postwar intervention with traumatized Bosnian adolescents. *Group Dynamics. Special Issue: Group-Based Interventions for Trauma Survivors, 5*, 277–290.

Leckman, J. F., & Mayes, L. C. (1998). Understanding developmental psychopathology: How useful are evolutionary accounts? *Journal of the American Academy of Child and Adolescent Psychiatry, 37*, 1011–1021.

Leckman, J. F., King, R. A., Gilbert, D. L., Coffey, B. J., Singer, H. S., Dure, L., ... Kaplan, E. L. (2011). Streptococcal upper respiratory tract infections and exacerbations of tic and obsessive-compulsive symptoms: A prospective longitudinal study. *Journal of the American Academy of Child and Adolescent Psychiatry, 50*(2), 108–118.

LeDoux, J. (1998). Fear and the brain: Where have we been, and where are we going? *Biological Psychiatry, 44*, 1229–1238.

LeDoux, J. (2012). Rethinking the emotional brain. *Neuron, 73*(4), 653–676.

LeDoux, J. E. (1996). *The emotional brain*. New York: Simon & Schuster.

LeDoux, J. E. (2000). Emotion circuits in the brain. *Annual Review of Neuroscience, 23*, 155–184.

LeDoux, J. E. (2013). The slippery slope of fear. *Trends in Cognitive Science, 17*(4), 155–156.

LeDoux, J. E. (2014). Coming to terms with fear. *Proceedings of the National Academy of Sciences, U S A, 111*(8), 2871–2878.

LeDoux, J. E., & Pine, D. S. (2016). Using neuroscience to help understand fear and anxiety: A two-system framework. *American Journal of Psychiatry, 173*(11), 1083–1093.

Leichsenring, F., Salzer, S., Beutel, M. E., Herpertz, S., Hiller, W., Hoyer, J., ... Leibing, E. (2013). Psychodynamic therapy and cognitive-behavioral therapy in social anxiety disorder: A multicenter randomized controlled trial. *American Journal of Psychiatry, 170*(7), 759–767.

Leonard, H. L, Topol, D., Bukstein, O., et al. (1994). Clonazepam as an augmenting agent in the treatment of childhood onset obsessive compulsive disorder. *Journal of the American Academy of Child and Adolescent Psychiatry, 33*, 792–794.

Leonard, H. L., & Swedo, S. E. (2001). Paediatric autoimmune neuropsychiatric disorders associated with streptococcal infection (PANDAS). *International Journal of Neuropsychopharmacology, 4*, 191–198.

Leonard, H. L., Swedo, S. E., Lenane, M. C., et al. (1991). A double-blind desipramine substitution during long-term clomipramine treatment in children and adolescents with obsessive compulsive disorder. *Archives of General Psychiatry, 48*, 922–926.

Leonard, H. L., Swedo, S., Rapoport, J. L., et al. (1989). Treatment of obsessive compulsive disorder with clomipramine and desipramine in children and adolescents: A double-blind crossover comparison. *Archives of General Psychiatry, 46*, 1088–1092.

Levisohn, L., Cronin-Golomb, A., & Schmahmann, J. D. (2000). Neuropsychological consequences of cerebellar tumour resection in children: Cerebellar cognition affective syndrome in a paediatric population. *Brain, 123*, 1041–1050.

Lewinsohn, P. M., Lewinsohn, M., et al. (1998). Gender differences in anxiety disorders and anxiety symptoms in adolescents. *Journal of Abnormal Psychology*, *107*, 109–117.

Lewinsohn, P., Zinbarg, J., et al. (1997). Lifetime comorbidity among anxiety disorders and between anxiety disorders and other mental disorders in adolescents. *Journal of Anxiety Disorders*, *14*(4), 377–394.

Lichtenstein, P., & Annas, P. (2000). Heritability and prevalence of specific fears and phobias in childhood. *Journal of Child Psychology and Psychiatry*, *41*(7), 927–937.

Liebowitz, M. R., Schneier, R., Campeas, R., Hollander, E., Hatterer, J., Fyer, A., et al. (1992). Phenelzine vs. atenolol in social phobia. *Archives of General Psychiatry*, *49*, 290–300.

Liebowitz, M. R., Turner, S. M., Piacentini, J., et al. (2002). Fluoxetine in children and adolescents with OCD: A placebo-controlled trial. *Journal of the American Academy of Child and Adolesc Psychiatry*, *41*, 1431–1438.

Lin, K. M. (2001). Biological differences in depression and anxiety across races and ethnic groups. *Journal of Clinical Psychiatry*, *62*(Suppl 13), 13–21.

Litz, B., Engel, C., Bryant, R., & Papa, A. (2007). A randomized, controlled proof-of-concept trial of an Internet-based, therapist-assisted self-management treatment for posttraumatic stress disorder. *American Journal of Psychiatry*, *164*(11), 1676–1684.

Loeber, R., Green, S. M., & Lahey, B. B. (1990). Mental health professionals' perception of the utility of children, mothers, and teachers as informants on childhood psychopathology. *Journal of Clinical Child Psychology*, *19*(2), 136–143.

Lovell, K., Cox, D., Haddock, G., Jones, C., Raines, D., Garvey, R., ... Hadley, S. (2006). Telephone-administered cognitive behaviour therapy for treatment of obsessive compulsive disorder: Randomised controlled non-inferiority trial. *BMJ*, *333*(7574), 883.

Lowry-Webster, H. M., Barrett, P. M. & Dadds, M. R. (2001). A universal prevention trial of anxiety and depressive symptomatology in childhood: Preliminary data from an Australian study. *Behaviour Change*, *18*, 36–50.

Lumpkin, P. W., Silverman, W. K, Weems, C. F., Markham, M. R., & Kurtines, W. M (2002). Treating a heterogeneous set of anxiety disorders in youths with group cognitive behavioral therapy: A partially nonconcurrent multiple-baseline evaluation. *Behavior Therapy*, *33*, 163–177.

Lutz, W. J., & Hock, E. (1995). Maternal separation anxiety: Relations to adult attachment representations in mothers of infants. *Journal of Genetic Psychology*, *156*, 57–72.

Ma, J. D., Wang, C. H., Li, H. F., Zhang, X. L., Zhang, Y. L., Hou, Y. H., ... Hu, X. Z. (2013). Cognitive-coping therapy for obsessive–compulsive disorder: A randomized controlled trial. *Journal of Psychiatric Research*, *47*(11), 1785–1790.

MacLeod, C., Mathews, A., & Tata, P. (1986). Attentional bias in emotional disorders. *Journal of Abnormal Psychology*, *95*, 15–20.

Madakasira, S., & O'Brien, K. F. (1987). Acute post-traumatic stress disorder in victims of a natural disaster. *Journal of Nervous & Mental Disease*, *175*, 286–290.

Main, M., & Goldwyn, R. (1991). Adult attachment classification system. In M. Main (Ed.), *Behavior and the development of representational models of attachment: Five methods of assessment*. Cambridge, UK: Cambridge University Press.

Main, M., & Solomon, J. (1990). Procedures for identifying infants as disorganized/disoriented during the Ainsworth Strange Situation. In M. T. Greenberg & D. Cicchetti (Eds.), *Attachment in the preschool years: Theory, research, and intervention* (pp. 121–160).The John D. and Catherine T. MacArthur Foundation Series on Mental Health and Development. Chicago: University of Chicago Press.

Malinosky-Rummell, R., & Hansen, D. J. (1993). Long-term consequences of childhood physical abuse. *Psychological Bulletin*, *114*, 68–79.

Manassis, K., & Bradley, S. J. (1994). The development of childhood anxiety disorders: Toward an integrated model. *Journal of Applied Developmental Psychology. Special Issue: Diversity and Development of Asian Americans*, *15*, 345–366.

Manassis, K., Bradley, S., Goldberg, S., Hood, J. & Swinson, R. P. (1994). Attachment in mothers with anxiety disorders and their children. *Journal of the American Academy of Child and Adolescent Psychiatry*, *33*, 1106–1113.

Manassis, K., Mendlowitz, S. L., Scapillato, D., Avery, D., Fiksenbaum, L., Freire, M., ... Owens, M. (2002). Group and individual cognitive-behavioral therapy for childhood anxiety disorders. A randomized trial. *Journal of the American Academy of Child and Adolescent Psychiatry*, *41*, 1423–1430.

Manicavasagar, V., Silove, D., et al. (2001). Parent-child concordance for separation anxiety: A clinical study. *Journal of Affective Disorders*, *65*(1), 81–84.

March, D., & Yonkers, K. A. (2001) Panic disorder. In K. Yonkers & B. Little (Eds.), *Management of psychiatric disorders in pregnancy* (pp. 134–148). New York: Oxford University Press.

March, J. S. (1995). Cognitive-behavioral psychotherapy for children and adolescents with OCD: A review and recommendations for treatment. *Journal of the American Academy of Child and Adolescent Psychiatry, 34*, 7–18.

March, J. (1999). Current status of pharmacotherapy for pediatric anxiety disorders. In D. Beidel (Ed.), *Treating anxiety disorders in youth: Current problems and future solutions* (ADAA/NIMH) (pp. 42–62). Washington, DC: Anxiety Disorders Association of America.

March, J. S., Amaya-Jackson, L., Murry, M. C., & Schulte, A. (1998). Cognitive-behavioral psychotherapy for children and adolescents with posttraumatic stress disorder after a single-incident stressor. *Journal of the American Academy of Child and Adolescent Psychiatry, 37*, 585–593.

March, J. S., Amaya-Jackson, L., Terry, R., & Costanzo, P. (1997). Post-traumatic stress symptomatology in children and adolescents after an industrial fire. *Journal of the American Academy of Child and Adolescent Psychiatry, 36*, 1080–1088.

March, J. S., Biederman, J., Wolkow, R., Safferman, A., Mardekian, J., Cook, E. H., ... Wagner, K. D. (1998). Sertraline in children and adolescents with obsessive-compulsive disorder: A multicenter randomized controlled trial. *Journal of the American Medical Association, 280*, 1752–1756.

March, J. S., Entusah, A. R., Rynn, M., Albano, A. M., & Tourian, K. A. (2007). A randomized controlled trial of venlafaxine ER versus placebo in pediatric social anxiety disorder. *Biological Psychiatry, 62*(10), 1149–1154.

March, J., Frances, A., Kahn, D., et al. (1997). Expert consensus guidelines: Treatment of obsessive-compulsive disorder. *Journal of Clinical Psychiatry, 58*, 1.

March, J. S., & Leonard, H. L. (1998). Obsessive-compulsive disorder in children and adolescents. In R. P. Swinson, M. M. Antony, et al. (Eds.), *Obsessive-compulsive disorder: Theory, research, and treatment*, New York: Guilford Press.

March, J., Mulle, K. & Herbel, B. (1994). Behavioral psychotherapy for children and adolescents with obsessive-compulsive disorder: An open trial of a new protocol driven treatment package. *Journal of the American Academy of Child and Adolescent Psychiatry, 33*, 333–341.

March, J. S., Parker, J. D. A., Sullivan, K., & Stallings, P. (1997). The Multidimensional Anxiety Scale for Children (MASC): Factor structure, reliability, and validity. *Journal of the American Academy of Child and Adolescent Psychiatry, 36*, 554–564.

Marchand, A., Beaulieu-Prévost, D., Guay, S., Bouchard, S., Drouin, M. S., & Germain, V. (2011). Relative efficacy of cognitive-behavioral therapy administered by videoconference for posttraumatic stress disorder: A six-month follow-up. *Journal of Aggression, Maltreatment & Trauma, 20*(3), 304–321.

Marchand, A., Roberge, P., Primiano, S., & Germain, V. (2009). A randomized, controlled clinical trial of standard, group and brief cognitive-behavioral therapy for panic disorder with agoraphobia: A two-year follow-up. *Journal of Anxiety Disorders, 23*(8), 1139–1147.

Marks, I. (1986). Genetics of fear and anxiety disorders (review). *British Journal of Psychiatry, 149*, 408–418.

Marks, I. M., Lelliott, P. T., Basoglu, M., Noshirvani, H., et al. (1988). Clomipramine, self-exposure and therapist-aided exposure for obsessive-compulsive rituals. *British Journal of Psychiatry, 152*, 522–534.

Marks, I. M., Swinson, R. P., Basoglu, M., Kuch, K., Noshirvani, H., O'Sullivan, G., ... Wickwire, K. (1993). Alprazolam and exposure alone and combined in panic disorder with agoraphobia: A controlled study in London and Toronto. *British Journal of Psychiatry, 162*, 776–787.

Marlatt, G. A., & Gordon, J. J. (1985). *Relapse prevention*. New York: Guilford Press.

Martenyi, F., Brown, E. B., Zhang, H., Koke, S. C., & Prakash, A. (2002a). Fluoxetine v. placebo in prevention of relapse in post-traumatic stress disorder. *British Journal of Psychiatry, 181*, 315–320.

Martenyi, F., Brown, E. B., Zhang, H., Prakash, A., & Koke, S. C. (2002b). Fluoxetine versus placebo in posttraumatic stress disorder. *Journal of Clinical Psychiatry, 63*, 199–206.

Martin, M., & Jones, G. V. (1995). Integral bias in the cognitive processing of emotionally linked pictures. *British Journal of Psychology, 86*(3), 419–435.

Martin, M., Horder, P., & Jones, G. V. (1992). Integral bias in naming of phobia-related words. *Cognition and Emotion, 6*(6), 479–486.

Masia, C. L., Klein, R. G., Storch, E. A., & Corda, B. (2001). School-based behavioral treatment for social anxiety disorder in adolescents: Results of a pilot study. *Journal of the American Academy of Child and Adolescent Psychiatry, 40*, 780–786.

Masia-Warner, C., Fisher, P. H., Shrout, P. E., Rathor, S., & Klein, R. G. (2007). Treating adolescents with social anxiety disorder in school: An attention control trial. *Journal of Child Psychology and Psychiatry, 48*(7), 676–686.

Masia-Warner, C., Klein, R. G., Dent, H. C., Fisher, P. H., Alvir, J., Albano, A. M., & Guardino, M. (2005). School-based intervention for adolescents with social anxiety disorder: Results of a controlled study. *Journal of Abnormal Child Psychology, 33*(6), 707–722.

Mathew, S. J., Coplan, J. D., & Gorman, J. M. (2001). Management of treatment-refractory panic disorder. *Psychopharmacology Bulletin, 35*, 97–110.

Mattis, S. G., & Ollendick, T. H. (2002). School refusal and separation anxiety. In M. Hersen (Ed.), *Clinical behavior therapy: Adults and children* (pp. 304–325). New York: John Wiley & Sons, Inc.

Mayou, R. A., Ehlers, A., & Bryant, B. (2002). Posttraumatic stress disorder after motor vehicle accidents: 3-year follow-up of a prospective longitudinal study. *Behaviour Research and Therapy, 40*, 665–675.

Mayou, R., Bryant, B., & Ehlers, A. (2001). Prediction of psychological outcomes one year after a motor vehicle accident. *American Journal of Psychiatry, 158*, 1231–1238.

McClure, E. B., Monk, C. S., Nelson, E. E., Parrish, J. M., Adler, A., Blair, R. J., . . . Pine, D. S. (2007). Abnormal attention modulation of fear circuit function in pediatric generalized anxiety disorder. *Archives of General Psychiatry, 64*(1), 97–106.

McCracken, J. T., Walkup, J. T., & Koplewicz, H. S. (2002). Childhood and early-onset anxiety: Treatment and biomarker studies. *Journal of Clinical Psychiatry, 63*, 8–11.

McDermott, J. M., Perez-Edgar, K., Henderson, H. A., Chronis-Tuscano, A., Pine, D. S., & Fox, N. A. (2009). A history of childhood behavioral inhibition and enhanced response monitoring in adolescence are linked to clinical anxiety. *Biological Psychiatry, 65*(5), 445–448.

McDermott, P. A., Watkins, M. W., Rovine, M. J., & Rikoon, S. H. (2013). Assessing changes in socioemotional adjustment across early school transitions—New national scales for children at risk. *Journal of School Psychology, 51*(1), 97–115.

McDougle, C. J., Epperson, C. N., Pelton, G. H., Wasylink, S., & Price, L. H. (2000). A double-blind, placebo-controlled study of risperidone addition in serotonin reuptake inhibitor-refractory obsessive-compulsive disorder. *Archives of General Psychiatry, 57*(8), 794–801.

McDougle, C. J., Goodman, W. K., & Price, L. H. (1994). Dopamine antagonists in tic-related and psychotic spectrum obsessive compulsive disorder. *Journal of Clinical Psychiatry, 55*(3), 24–31.

McLaughlin, K. A., Koenen, K. C., Hill, E. D., Petukhova, M., Sampson, N. A., Zaslavsky, A. M., & Kessler, R. C. (2013). Trauma exposure and posttraumatic stress disorder in a national sample of adolescents. *Journal of the American Academy of Child and Adolescent Psychiatry, 52*(8), 815–830.

McLean, C. P. & Foa, E. B. (2014). The use of prolonged exposure therapy to help patients with PTSD. *Clinical Practice, 11*(2), 233–241.

McManis, M. H., Kagan, J., Snidman, N. C., & Woodward, S. A. (2002). EEG asymmetry, power, and temperament in children. *Developmental Psychobiology, 41*, 169–177.

McNally, R. J. (1996). Cognitive bias in the anxiety disorders. *Nebraska Symposium on Motivation, 43*, 211–250.

McNally, R. J. (2001a). On Wakefield's harmful dysfunction analysis of mental disorder. *Behaviour Research and Therapy, 39*, 309–314.

McNally, R. J. (2001b). On the scientific status of cognitive appraisal models of anxiety disorder. *Behaviour Research and Therapy, 39*, 513–521.

McNally, R. J. (2011). *What is mental illness?* Cambridge, MA: Belknap Press of Harvard University Press.

Meaney, M. J. (2001). Nature, nurture, and the disunity of knowledge. *Annals of the New York Academy of Sciences, 935*, 50–61.

Meeske, K. A., Ruccione, K., Globe, D. R., & Stuber, M. L. (2001). Posttraumatic stress, quality of life, and psychological distress in young adult survivors of childhood cancer. *Oncology Nursing Forum, 28*, 481–489.

Menard, S. W. (2002). *Short and long-term consequences of adolescent victimization*. Washington, DC: US Department of Justice, Office of Justice Programs, Office of Juvenile Justice and Delinquency Prevention.

Mendlowitz, S., Manassis, Bradley, S., Scapillato, D., Miezitis, S., & Shaw, B. (1999). Cognitive-behavioral group treatments in childhood anxiety disorders: The role of parental involvement. *Journal of the American Academy of Child and Adolescent Psychiatry,* 38, 1223–1229.

Merikangas, K. R., & Avenevoli, S. (2002). Epidemiology of mood and anxiety disorders in children and adolescents. In M. T. Tsuang & M. Tohen (Eds.), *Textbook in psychiatric epidemiology* (2nd ed., pp. 657–704). New York: Wiley-Liss.

Merikangas, K. R., & Risch, N. (2003). Will the genomic revolution revolutionize psychiatry? *American Journal of Psychiatry, 160*, 625–635.

Merikangas, K. R., Avenevoli, S., Dierker, L., & Grillon, C. (1999). Vulnerability factors among children at risk for anxiety disorders. *Biological Psychiatry, 46*, 1523–1535.

Mills, K. L., Teesson, M., Back, S. E., Brady, K. T., Baker, A. L., Hopwood, S., . . . Ewer, P. L. (2012). Integrated exposure-based therapy for co-occurring posttraumatic stress disorder and substance dependence: A randomized controlled trial. *Journal of the American Medical Association, 308*(7), 690–699.

Minino, A. (2010). *Mortality among teenagers aged 12–19 years: United States, 1999-2006. NCHS Data Brief.* Centers for Disease Control and Prevention, National Center for Health Statistics.

Mitte, K. (2005). A meta-analysis of the efficacy of psycho-and pharmacotherapy in panic disorder with and without agoraphobia. *Journal of Affective Disorders, 88*(1), 27–45.

Moffitt, T. E., Caspi, A., Belsky, J., & Silva, P. A. (1992). Childhood experience and the onset of menarche: A test of a sociobiological model. *Child Development, 63*, 47–58.

Monk, C. S., Pine, D. S., & Charney, D. S. (2002). A developmental and neurobiological approach to early trauma research. *Seminars in Clinical Neuropsychiatry, 7*, 137–146.

Monson, C. M., Fredman, S. J., Adair, K. C., Stevens, S. P., Resick, P. A., Schnurr, P. P., ... & Macdonald, A. (2011). Cognitive–behavioral conjoint therapy for PTSD: Pilot results from a community sample. *Journal of Traumatic Stress, 24*(1), 97–101.

Mooney, P., Oakley, J., Ferriter, M., & Travers, R. (2004). Sertraline as a treatment for PTSD: A systematic review and meta-analysis. *Irish Journal of Psychological Medicine, 21*(3), 100–103.

Moreau, D. L., & Follet, C. (1993). Panic disorder in children and adolescents. *Child and Adolescent Psychiatric Clinics of North America, 2*, 581–602.

Moreau, D., & Weissman, M. M. (1992). Panic disorder in children and adolescents: A review. *American Journal of Psychiatry, 149*, 1306–1314.

Morris, T. L., & Masia, C. L. (1998). Psychometric evaluation of the Social Phobia and Anxiety Inventory for Children: Concurrent validity and normative data. *Journal of Clinical Child Psychology, 27*, 452–458.

Moss, H., & Damasio, A. R. (2001). Emotion, cognition, and the human brain. *Annals of the New York Academy of Sciences, 935*, 98–100.

Mrazek, P. J., & Haggerty, R. J. (1994). *Reducing risks for mental disorders: Frontiers for preventive intervention research.* Washington, DC: National Academy of Sciences, Institute of Medicine, Division of Biobehavioral Sciences & Mental Disorders, Committee on Prevention of Mental Disorders,.

Munoz, R. F., Mrazek, P. J., & Haggerty, R. J. (1996). Institute of Medicine report on prevention of mental disorders: Summary and commentary. *American Psychologist, 51*(11), 1116–1122.

Muris, P., Merckelbach, H., Ollendick, T., King, N., & Bogie, N. (2002). Three traditional and three new childhood anxiety questionnaires: Their reliability and validity in a normal adolescent sample. *Behaviour Research and Therapy, 40*(7), 753–772.

Muris, P., van Brakel, Anna M. L., Arntz, A., & Schouten, E. (2011). Behavioral inhibition as a risk factor for the development of childhood anxiety disorders: A longitudinal study. *Journal of Child and Family Studies, 20*(2), 157–170.

Murphy, G. M., Jr., Kremer, C., Rodrigues, H. E., & Schatzberg, A. F. (2003). Pharmacogenetics of antidepressant medication intolerance. *American Journal of Psychiatry, 160*, 1830–1835.

Murphy, M. L., & Pichichero, M. E. (2002). Prospective identification and treatment of children with pediatric autoimmune neuropsychiatric disorder associated with group A streptococcal infection (PANDAS). *Archives of Pediatric and Adolescent Medicine, 156*, 356–361.

Myers, H. F., & Durvasula, R. S. (1999). Psychiatric disorders in African American men and women living with HIV/AIDS. *Cultural Diversity & Ethnic Minority Psychology. Special Issue: HIV/AIDS and Ethnic Minority Women, Families, and Communities, 5*, 249–262.

Nader, P. R., Wexler, D. B., Patterson, T. L, McKusick, L., et al. (1989). Comparison of beliefs about AIDS among urban, suburban, incarcerated, and gay adolescents. *Journal of Adolescent Health Care, 10*, 413–418.

National Collaborating Centre for Mental Health. (2005). *Post-traumatic stress disorder (PTSD): The management of PTSD in adults and children in primary and secondary care.* Clinical Guideline 26. London: National Institute for Clinical Excellence.

National Institute for Health and Clinical Excellence. (2005). *Obsessive-compulsive disorder: Core interventions in the treatment of obsessive-compulsive disorder and body dysmorphic disorder*. NICE guideline 31. London: NIHCE. Accessed Aug. 1, 2014, at www.nice.org.uk/cg26.

National Institute for Health and Clinical Excellence. (2011). *Generalised anxiety disorder and panic disorder (with or without agoraphobia) in adults: Management in primary, secondary and community care*. NICE Clinical Guideline 113. Manchester: National Institute for Health and Clinical Excellence.

Nayak, N. H., Powers, M. B., & Foa, E. B. (2011). Empirically supported psychological treatments: Prolonged exposure. In G. J. Beck & D. M. Sloan (Eds.), *The Oxford handbook of traumatic stress disorders* (pp. 427–438). New York: Oxford University Press.

Nazari, H., Momeni, N., Jariani, M., & Tarrahi, M. J. (2011). Comparison of eye movement desensitization and reprocessing with citalopram in treatment of obsessive-compulsive disorder. *International Journal of Psychiatry in Clinical Practice*, *15*(4), 270–274.

Neil, A. L., & Christensen, H. (2009). Efficacy and effectiveness of school-based prevention and early intervention programs for anxiety. *Clinical Psychology Review*, *29*(3), 208–215.

Nelson, E. E., Shelton, S. E., & Kalin, N. H. (2003). Individual differences in the responses of naïve Rhesus monkeys to snakes. *Emotion*, *3*, 3–11.

Neuner, F., Schauer, M., Klaschik, C., Karunakara, U., & Elbert, T. (2004). A comparison of narrative exposure therapy, supportive counseling, and psychoeducation for treating posttraumatic stress disorder in an African refugee settlement. *Journal of Consulting and Clinical Psychology*, *72*(4), 579.

Newman, M. G., Castonguay, L. G., Borkovec, T. D., Fisher, A. J., Boswell, J. F., Szkodny, L. E., & Nordberg, S. S. (2011). A randomized controlled trial of cognitive-behavioral therapy for generalized anxiety disorder with integrated techniques from emotion-focused and interpersonal therapies. *Journal of Consulting and Clinical Psychology*, *79*(2), 171.

Nurse, S., & Lacaille, J.-C. (1999). Late maturation of GABA(B) synaptic transmission in area CA1 of the rat hippocampus. *Neuropharmacology*, *38*, 1733–1742.

Ollendick, T. H., & Cerny, J. A. (1981). *Clinical behavior therapy with children*. New York: Plenum.

Ollendick, T. H., & Francis, G. (1988). Behavioral assessment and treatment of childhood phobias. *Behavior Modification*, *12*(2), 165–204.

Ollendick, T. H., & King, N. J. (2000). Empirically supported treatments for children and adolescents. In P. C. Kendall (Ed.), *Child and adolescent therapy* (pp. 386–425). New York: Guilford.

Ollendick, T. H., & King, N.J. (1998). Empirically supported treatments for children with phobic and anxiety disorders: Current status. *Journal of Clinical Child Psychology. Special Issue: Empirically Supported Psychosocial Interventions for Children*, *27*, 156–167.

Ollendick, T. H., & March, J. S. (Eds.). (2004). *Phobic and anxiety disorders in children and adolescents: A clinician's guide to effective psychosocial and pharmacological interventions*. New York: Oxford University Press.

Ollendick, T. H., Halldorsdottir, T., Fraire, M. G., Austin, K. E., Noguchi, R. J. P., Lewis, K. M., ... Whitmore, M. J. (2015). Specific phobias in youth: A randomized controlled trial comparing one-session treatment to a parent-augmented one-session treatment. *Behavior Therapy*, *46*(2), 141–155.

Ollendick, T. H., King, N. J., & Muris, P. (2002). Fears and phobias in children: Phenomenology, epidemiology, and aetiology. *Child & Adolescent Mental Health*, *7*, 98–106.

Ollendick, T. H., Mattis, S. G., & King, N. J. (1994). Panic in children and adolescents: A review. *Journal of Child Psychology & Psychiatry & Allied Disciplines*, *35*, 113–134.

Ollendick, T. H., Öst, L., Reuterskiöld, L., Costa, N., Cederlund, R., Sirbu, C., ... Jarrett, M. A. (2009). One-session treatment of specific phobias in youth: A randomized clinical trial in the United States and Sweden. *Journal of Consulting and Clinical Psychology*, *77*(3), 504–516.

O'Neil, K. A., Brodman, D. M., Cohen, J. S., Edmunds, J. M., & Kendall, P. C. (2012). Childhood anxiety disorders: The coping cat program. In E. Szigethy, J. R. Weisz & R. L. Findling (Eds.), *Cognitive-behavior therapy for children and adolescents; cognitive-behavior therapy for children and adolescents* (pp. 227–261). Arlington, VA: American Psychiatric Publishing, Inc.

Orvaschel, H., Lewinsohn, P. M., et al. (1995). Continuity of psychopathology in a community sample of adolescents. *Journal of the American Academy of Child and Adolescent Psychiatry*, *34*(11), 1525–1535.

Öst, L. G. (1989). One-session treatment for specific phobias. *Behaviour Research and Therapy*, *27*(1), 1–7.

Öst, L. G., Ferebee, I., & Furmark, T. (1997). One-session group therapy of spider phobia: Direct versus indirect treatments. *Behaviour Research and Therapy, 35*(8), 721–732.

Öst, L. G., Salkovskis, P. M., & Hellström, K. (1991). One-session therapist-directed exposure vs. self-exposure in the treatment of spider phobia. *Behavior Therapy, 22*(3), 407–422.

Öst, L. G., Svensson, L., Hellstrom, K., & Lindwall, R. (2001). One-session treatment of specific phobias in youths: A randomized clinical trial. *Journal of Consulting and Clinical Psychology, 69*, 814–824.

Owley, T., Owley, S., Leventhal, B., & Cook, E. (2002). Case series: Adderall augmenation of serotonin reuptake inhibitors in childhood-onset obsessive compulsive disorder. *Journal of Child and Adolescent Psychopharmacology, 12*, 165–171.

Paget, K. D., & Reynolds, C. R. (1984). Dimensions, levels and reliabilities on the revised children's manifest anxiety scale with learning disabled children. *Journal of Learning Disabilities, 17*(3), 137–141.

Papp, L. A., Klein, D. F., Martinez, J., Schneier, F., Cole, R., Liebowitz, M. R., Hollander, E., et al. (1993). The diagnostic and substance specificity of carbon-dioxide-induced panic. *American Journal of Psychiatry, 150*, 250–257.

Papp, L. A., Martinez, J. M., Klein, D. F., Coplan, J., & Gorman, J. M. (1995). Rebreathing tests in panic disorder. *Biological Psychiatry, 38*, 240–245.

Paxling, B., Almlöv, J., Dahlin, M., Carlbring, P., Breitholtz, E., Eriksson, T., & Andersson, G. (2011). Guided Internet-delivered cognitive behavior therapy for generalized anxiety disorder: A randomized controlled trial. *Cognitive Behaviour Therapy, 40*(3), 159–173.

Pediatric OCD Treatment Study Team. (2004). Cognitive-behavioral therapy, sertraline, and their combination for children and adolescents with obsessive-compulsive disorder: The Pediatric OCD Treatment Study (POTS) randomized controlled trial. *Journal of the American Medical Association, 292*, 1969–1976.

Pedro-Carroll, J. L., & Cowen, E. L. (1985). The Children of Divorce Intervention Program: An investigation of the efficacy of a school-based prevention program. *Journal of Consulting & Clinical Psychology, 53*, 603–611.

Pelcovitz, D., Kaplan, S. J., DeRosa, R. R., Mandel, F. S., & Salzinger, S. (2000). Psychiatric disorders in adolescents exposed to violence and physical abuse. *American Journal of Orthopsychiatry, 70*, 360–369.

Perlmutter, S. J., Leitman, S. F., Garvey, M. A., et al. (1999). Therapeutic plasma exchange and intravenous immunoglobulin for OCD and tic disorders in children. *Lancet, 354*, 1153–1158.

Perry, B. D., & Pollard, R. (1998). Homeostasis, stress, trauma, and adaptation: A neurodevelopmental view of childhood trauma. *Child and Adolescent Psychiatric Clinics of North America, 7*(1), 33–51.

Peterson, L., & Shigetomi, C. (1981). The use of coping techniques to minimize anxiety in hospitalized children. *Behavioral Therapy, 12*, 1–14.

Petty, F., Brannan, S., Casada, J., Davis, L. L., Gajewski, V., Kramer, G. L., ... Young, K. A. (2001). Olanzapine treatment for post-traumatic stress disorder: An open-label study. *International Clinical Psychopharmacology, 16*(6), 331–337.

Piacentini, J., Bergman, R. L., Chang, S., Langley, A., Perls, T. S., Wood, J. J., & McCracken, J., (2011). Controlled comparison of family cognitive behavioral therapy and psychoeducation/relaxation training for child obsessive-compulsive disorder. *Journal of the American Academy of Child & Adolescent Psychiatry, 50*, 1149–1161.

Piacentini, J., Langley, A., & Roblek, T. (2007). *Cognitive-behavioral treatment of childhood OCD: It's only a false alarm, therapist guide*. New York: Oxford University Press.

Pickar, D. (2003). Pharmacogenomics of psychiatric drug treatment. *Psychiatric Clinics of North America, 26*, 303–321.

Pincus, D. B., May, J. E., Whitton, S. W., Mattis, S. G., & Barlow, D. H. (2010). Cognitive-behavioral treatment of panic disorder in adolescence. *Journal of Clinical Child and Adolescent Psychology, 39*(5), 638–649.

Pine, D. S. (1999). Pathophysiology of childhood anxiety disorders. *Biological Psychiatry, 46*, 1555–1566.

Pine, D. S. (2001). Affective neuroscience and the development of social anxiety disorder. *Psychiatric Clinics of North America, 24*, 689–705.

Pine, D. S. (2002). Brain development and the onset of mood disorders. *Seminars in Clinical Neuropsychiatry, 7*, 223–233.

Pine, D. S., & Grun, J. S. (1999). Childhood anxiety: Integrating developmental psychopathology and affective neuroscience. *Journal of Child and Adolescent Psychopharmacology, 9*, 1–12.

Pine, D. S., Cohen, P., & Brook, J. (2001). Adolescent fears as predictors of depression. *Biological Psychiatry, 50*, 721–724.

Pine, D. S., Cohen, P., Gurley, D., Brook, J., & Ma, Y. (1998). The risk for early-adulthood anxiety and depressive disorders in adolescents with anxiety and depressive disorders. *Archives of General Psychiatry, 55*, 56–64.

Pine, D. S., Fyer, A., Grun, J., Phelps, E. A., Szeszko, P. R., Koda, V., et al. (2001). Methods for developmental studies of fear conditioning circuitry. *Biological Psychiatry, 50*, 225–228.

Pine, D. S., Grun, J., Zarahn, E., Fyer, A., Koda, V., Li, W., et al. (2001). Cortical brain regions engaged by masked emotional faces in adolescents and adults: An fMRI study. *Emotion, 1*, 137–147.

Pine, D. S., Klein, R. G., Coplan, J. D., Papp, L. A., Hoven, C. W., Martinez, J., et al. (2000). Differential carbon dioxide sensitivity in childhood anxiety disorders and nonill comparison group. *Archives of General Psychiatry, 57*, 960–967.

Pine, D. S., Wasserman, G. A., & Workman, S. B. (1999). Memory and anxiety in prepubertal boys at risk for delinquency. *Journal of the American Academy of Child and Adolescent Psychiatry, 38*, 1024–1031.

Popper, C. W., & Ziminitzky, B. (1995). Sudden death putatively related to desipramine treatment in youth: A fifth case and a review of speculative mechanisms. *Journal of Child and Adolescent Psychopharmacology, 5*, 283–300.

Poulton, R., & Menzies, R. G. (2002). Non-associative fear acquisition: A review of the evidence from retrospective and longitudinal research. *Behaviour Research and Therapy, 40*, 127–149.

Prather, M. D., Lavenex, P., Mauldin-Jourdain, M. L., Mason, W. A., Capitanio, J. P., Mendoza, S. P., et al. (2001). Increased social fear and decreased fear of objects in monkeys with neonatal amygdala lesions. *Neuroscience, 106*, 653–658.

Prins, P. J. M., & Ollendick, T. H. (2003). Cognitive change and enhanced coping: Missing mediational links in cognitive behavior therapy with anxiety-disordered children. *Clinical Child and Family Psychology Review, 6*(2), 87–105.

Pynoos, R. S. (1992). Grief and trauma in children and adolescents. *Bereavement Care, 11*, 2–10.

Pynoos, R. S., Frederick, C., Nader, K., & Arroyo, W. (1987). Life threat and posttraumatic stress in school-age children. *Archives of General Psychiatry, 44*, 1057–1063.

Pynoos, R. S., Kinzie, J. D., & Gordon, M. (2001). Children, adolescents and families exposed to extreme trauma and torture. In E. Gerrity et al (Eds.), *Mental health consequences of torture and related violence and trauma* (pp. 211–225). New York: Plenum Publishing.

Pynoos, R. S., Steinberg, A. M., & Piacentini, J. C. (1999). A developmental psychopathology model of childhood traumatic stress and intersection with anxiety disorders. *Biological Psychiatry, 46*, 1542–1554.

Queen, A. H., Ehrenreich-May, J., & Hershorin, E. R. (2012). Preliminary validation of a screening tool for adolescent panic disorder in pediatric primary care clinics. *Child Psychiatry and Human Development, 43*(2), 171–183.

Rachman, S. (1977). The conditioning theory of fear acquisition: A critical examination. *Behaviour Research and Therapy, 15*, 375–387.

Radke-Yarrow, M., DeMulder, E., & Belmont, B. (1995). Attachment in the context of high-risk conditions. *Development and Psychopathology, 7*, 247–265.

Rakic, P., Bourgeois, J.-P., & Goldman-Rakic, P. S. (1994). Synaptic development of the cerebral cortex: Implications for learning, memory, and mental illness. In J. van Pelt, M. A. Corner, H. B. M. Uylings, & F. H. Lopes da Silva (Eds.), *Progress in brain research: Vol. 102. The self-organizing brain: From growth cones to functional networks* (pp. 227–243). Amsterdam: Elsevier.

Rapaport, M. H., Endicott, J., & Clary, C. M. (2002). Posttraumatic stress disorder and quality of life: results across 64 weeks of sertraline treatment. *Journal of Clinical Psychiatry, 63*(1), 59–65.

Rapee, R. M. (1997). Potential role of childrearing practices in the development of anxiety and depression. *Clinical Psychology Review, 17*, 47–67.

Rapee, R. M. (2002). The development and modification of temperamental risk for anxiety disorders: Prevention of a lifetime of anxiety. *Biological Psychiatry, 52*, 947–957.

Rapee, R. M. (2011). Treatments for childhood anxiety disorders: Integrating physiological and psychosocial interventions. *Expert Review of Neurotherapeutics, 11*(8), 1095–1097.

Rapee, R. M. (2013). The preventative effects of a brief, early intervention for preschool-aged children at risk for internalising: Follow-up into middle adolescence. *Journal of Child Psychology and Psychiatry, 54*(7), 780–788.

Rapee, R. M., & Heimberg, R. G. (1997). A cognitive-behavioral model of anxiety in social phobia. *Behaviour Research and Therapy, 35*(8), 741–756.

Rapee, R. M., Brown, T. A., Antony, M. M., & Barlow, D. H. (1992). Response to hyperventilation and inhalation of 5.5% carbon dioxide-enriched air across the DSM-III-R anxiety disorders. *Journal of Abnormal Psychology, 101*, 538–552.

Rapee, R. M., Kennedy, S. J., Ingram, M., Edwards, S. L., & Sweeney, L. (2010). Altering the trajectory of anxiety of at-risk young children. *American Journal of Psychiatry, 167*, 1518–1525.

Rapee, R. M., Kennedy, S., Ingram, M., Edwards, S., & Sweeney, L. (2005). Prevention and early intervention of anxiety disorders in inhibited preschool children. *Journal of Consulting and Clinical Psychology, 73*(3), 488–497.

Rauch, S. L., Savage, C. R., Alpert, N. M., Fischman, A. J., & Jenike, M. A. (1997). The functional neuroanatomy of anxiety: A study of three disorders using positron emission tomography and symptom provocation. *Biological Psychiatry, 42*, 446–452.

Rauch, S. L., Whalen, P. J., Shin, L. M., McInerney, S. C., Macklin, M. L., Lasko, N. B., et al. (2000). Exaggerated amygdala response to masked facial stimuli in posttraumatic stress disorder: A functional MRI study. *Biological Psychiatry, 47*, 769–776.

Raznahan, A., Lee, Y., Stidd, R., Long, R., Greenstein, D., Clasen, L., ... Giedd, J. N. (2010). Longitudinally mapping the influence of sex and androgen signaling on the dynamics of human cortical maturation in adolescence. *Proceedings of the National Academy of Sciences, U S A, 107*(39), 16988–16993.

Raznahan, A., Lerch, J. P., Lee, N., Greenstein, D., Wallace, G. L., Stockman, M., ... Giedd, J. N. (2011). Patterns of coordinated anatomical change in human cortical development: A longitudinal neuroimaging study of maturational coupling. *Neuron, 72*(5), 873–884.

Raznahan, A., Shaw, P. W., Lerch, J. P., Clasen, L. S., Greenstein, D., Berman, R., ... Giedd, J. N. (2014). Longitudinal four-dimensional mapping of subcortical anatomy in human development. *Proceedings of the National Academy of Sciences, U S A, 111*(4), 1592–1597.

Reiss, S., & Mc Nally, R. J. (1985). Expectancy model of fear. In S. Reiss & R. R. Bootzin (Eds.), *Theoretical issues in behavior therapy* (pp. 107–121). New York: Academic Press.

Renaud, J., Birmaher, B., Wassick, S. C., & Bridge, J. (1999). Use of selective serotonin reuptake inhibitors for the treatment of childhood panic disorder: A pilot study. *Journal of Child & Adolescent Psychopharmacology, 9*, 73–83.

Rescorla, R. A. (1988). Pavlovian conditioning: It's not what you think it is. *American Psychologist, 43*(3), 151–160.

Research Units of Pediatric Psychopharmacology (RUPP) Anxiety Group. (2001). Flovoxamine for the treatment of anxiety disorders in children and adolescents. *New England Journal of Medicine, 344*, 1279–1285.

Research Units on Pediatric Psychopharmacology Anxiety Study Group (RUPP). (2003). Searching for moderators and mediators of pharmacological treatment effects in children and adolescents with anxiety disorders. *Journal of the American Academy of Child and Adolescent Psychiatry, 42*, 13–21.

Resick, P. A. (1993). The psychological impact of rape. *Journal of Interpersonal Violence, 8*, 223–255.

Resick, P. A., Galovski, T. E., Uhlmansiek, M.O., et al. (2008). A randomized clinical trial to dismantle components of cognitive processing therapy for posttraumatic stress disorder in female victims of interpersonal violence. *Journal of Consulting and Clinical Psychology, 76*(2), 243–258.

Resick, P. A., Nishith, P., Weaver, T. L., Astin, M. C., & Feuer, C. A. (2002). A comparison of cognitive-processing therapy with prolonged exposure and a waiting condition for the treatment of chronic posttraumatic stress disorder in female rape victims. *Journal of Consulting and Clinical Psychology, 70*(4), 867–879.

Reynolds, C. R., & Richmond, B. O. (1978). What I think and feel: A revised measure of children's manifest anxiety. *Journal of Abnormal Child Psychology, 6*, 271–280.

Reynolds, C. R., & Richmond, B. O. (1979). Factor structure and construct validity of "what I think and feel": The revised children's manifest anxiety scale. *Journal of Personality Assessment, 43*(3), 281–283.

Richards, D. A., Lovell, K., & Marks, I. M. (1994). Post-traumatic stress disorder: Evaluation of a behavioral treatment program. *Journal of Traumatic Stress, 7*, 669–680.

Rickels, K., Case, W. G. & Diamond, L. R. (1980). Relapse after short-term drug therapy in neurotic outpatients. *International Pharmacopsychiatry, 15*(3), 186–192.

Rickels, K., Case, W. G., Downing, R. W., & Fridman, R. (1986). One-year follow-up of anxious patients treated with diazepam. *Journal of Clinical Psychopharmacology, 6*(1), 32–36.

Rickels, K., Schweizer, E., Case, W. G., & Greenblatt, D. J. (1990). Long-term therapeutic use of benzodiazepines, I. Effects of abrupt discontinuation. *Archives of General Psychiatry, 47*, 899–907.

Riddle, M. A., Geller, B., & Ryan, N. (1993). Case study: Another sudden death with a child treated with desipramine. *Journal of the American*

Academy of Child and Adolescent Psychiatry, 32, 792–797.

Riddle, M. A., Hardin, M. T., & King, R. A. (1990). Fluoxetine treatment of children and adolescents with Tourette's and obsessive compulsive disorders: Preliminary clinical experience. *Journal of the American Academy of Child and Adolescent Psychiatry, 29,* 45–48.

Riddle, M. A., King, R. A., Hardin, M. T., et al. (1991). Behavioral side effects of fluoxetine in children and adolescents. *Journal of Child and Adolescent Psychopharmacology, 1,* 193.

Riddle, M. A., Nelson, J. C., Kleinman, C. S., et al. (1991). Case study: Sudden death in children receiving norpramine: A review of three reported cases and commentary. *Journal of the American Academy of Child and Adolescent Psychiatry, 30,* 104–108.

Riddle, M., Reeve, E., Yaryura-Tobias, J., et al. (2001). Fluvoxamine for children and adolescents with obsessive compulsive disorder: A randomized controlled multicenter trial. *Journal of the American Academy of Child and Adolescent Psychiatry, 40,* 222–229.

Riggs, D. S., & Foa, E. B. (1993). Obsessive compulsive disorder. In D. H. Barlow (Ed.), *Clinical handbook of psychological disorders: A step-by-step treatment manual* (2nd ed.). New York: Guilford Press.

Riggs, D. S., Rothbaum, B. O. & Foa, E. B. (1995). A prospective examination of symptoms of posttraumatic stress disorder in vicitms of nonsexual assault. *Journal of Interpersonal Violence, 10,* 201–214.

Riggs, P. D., Baker, S., Mikulich, S. K., Young, S. E. et al. (1995). Depression in substance-dependent delinquents. *Journal of the American Academy of Child and Adolescent Psychiatry, 34,* 764–771.

Roberson-Nay, R., Eaves, L. J., Hettema, J. M., Kendler, K. S., & Silberg, J. L. (2012). Childhood separation anxiety disorder and adult onset panic attacks share a common genetic diathesis. *Depression and Anxiety, 29*(4), 320–327.

Roberson-Nay, R., Klein, D. F., Klein, R. G., Mannuzza, S., Moulton, J. L., Guardino, M., & Pine, D. S. (2010). Carbon dioxide hypersensitivity in separation-anxious offspring of parents with panic disorder. *Biological Psychiatry, 67*(12), 1171–1177.

Roberts, R. E., Lewinsohn, P. M., & Seeley, J. R. (1991). Screening for adolescent depression: A comparison of depression scales. *Journal of the American Academy of Child and Adolescent Psychiatry, 30,* 58–66.

Robinson, E., Titov, N., Andrews, G., McIntyre, K., Schwencke, G., & Solley, K. (2010). Internet treatment for generalized anxiety disorder: A randomized controlled trial comparing clinician vs. technician assistance. *PloS One, 5*(6), e10942.

Roemer, L., & Orsillo, S. M. (2009). *Mindfulness- and acceptance-based behavioral therapies in practice.* New York: Guilford Press.

Roemer, L., Orsillo, S. M., & Salters-Pedneault, K. (2008). Efficacy of an acceptance-based behavior therapy for generalized anxiety disorder: Evaluation in a randomized controlled trial. *Journal of Consulting and Clinical Psychology, 76,* 1083–1089.

Rohde, L. A., Roman, T., & Hutz, M. H. (2003). Attention-deficit/hyperactivity disorder: Current aspects on pharmacogenetics. *Pharmacogenomics Journal, 3,* 11–13.

Rosenberg, D. R., & Hanna, G. L. (2000). Genetic and imaging strategies in obsessive-compulsive disorder: Potential implications for treatment development. *Biological Psychiatry, 48,* 1210–1222.

Rosenberg, D. R., MacMillan, S. N., & Moore, G. J. (2001). Brain anatomy and chemistry may predict treatment response in pediatric obsessive-compulsive disorder. *International Journal of Neuropsychopharmacology, 4,* 179–190.

Rothbaum, B. O., Astin, M. C., & Marsteller, F. (2005). Prolonged exposure versus eye movement desensitization and reprocessing (EMDR) for PTSD rape victims. *Journal of Trauma Stress, 18,* 607–616.

Rothbaum, B. O., Foa, E. B., Riggs, D. S., Murdock, T., et al. (1992). A prospective examination of post-traumatic stress disorder in rape victims. *Journal of Traumatic Stress, 5,* 455–475.

Rothbaum, B. O., Kozack, M. J., Foa, B., & Whitaker, D. J. (2001). Posttraumatic stress disorder in rape victims: Autonomic habituation to auditory stimuli. *Journal of Traumatic Stress, 14*(2), 283–293.

Roy-Byrne, P. P., Craske, M. G., Stein, M. B., Sullivan, G., Bystritsky, A., Katon, W., . . . Sherbourne, C. D. (2005). A randomized effectiveness trial of cognitive-behavioral therapy and medication for primary care panic disorder. *Archives of General Psychiatry, 62*(3), 290–298.

Rutter, M., Bolton, P., Harrington, R., le Couteur, A., et al. (1990). Genetic factors in child psychiatric disorders: I. A review of research strategies. *Journal of Child Psychology & Psychiatry & Allied Disciplines, 31,* 3–37.

Rutter, M., Silberg, J., et al. (1999a). Genetics and child psychiatry, I: Advances in quantitative and molecular genetics. *Journal of Child Psychology and Psychiatry, 40,* 3–18.

Rutter, M., Silberg, T., et al. (1999b). Genetics and child psychiatry, II: Empirical research findings. *Journal of Child Psychology and Psychiatry, 40*(1), 19–56.

Rynn, M. A., Riddle, M. A., Yeung, P. P., & Kunz, N. R. (2007). Efficacy and safety of extended-release venlafaxine in the treatment of generalized anxiety disorder in children and adolescents: Two placebo-controlled trials. *American Journal of Psychiatry, 164*(2), 290–300.

Rynn, M. A., Siqueland, L., & Rickels, K. (2001). Placebo-controlled trial of sertraline in the treatment of children with generalized anxiety disorder. *American Journal of Psychiatry, 158,* 2008–2014.

Sacks, S., Chaple, M., Sacks, J. Y., McKendrick, K., & Cleland, C. M. (2012). Randomized trial of a reentry modified therapeutic community for offenders with co-occurring disorders: Crime outcomes. *Journal of Substance Abuse Treatment, 42*(3), 247–259.

Saigh, P. A., Mroueh, M., & Bremner, J. D. (1997). Scholastic impairments among traumatized adolescents. *Behaviour Research & Therapy, 35,* 429–436.

Salkovskis, P. M. (1985). Obsessional-compulsive problems: A cognitive-behavioral analysis. *Behaviour Research and Therapy, 23*(5), 571–583.

Sallee, F. R., & March, J. S. (2001). Neuropsychiatry of paediatric anxiety disorders. In W. K. Silverman & P. A. D. Treffers (Eds.), *Anxiety disorders in children and adolescents: Research, assessment and intervention* (pp. 90–125). New York: Cambridge University Press.

Sallee, F. R., Richman, H., Sethuraman, G., Dougherty, D., Sine, L., & Altman-Hamamdzic, S. (1998). Clonidine challenge in childhood anxiety disorder. *Journal of the American Academy of Child and Adolescent Psychiatry, 37,* 655–662.

Sallee, F. R., Sethuraman, G., Sine, L., & Liu, H. (2000). Yohimbine challenge in children with anxiety disorders. *American Journal of Psychiatry, 157,* 1236–1242.

Saltzman, W. R., Pynoos, R. S., Layne, C. M., Steinberg, A. M., & Aisenberg, E. (2001). Trauma- and grief-focused intervention for adolescents exposed to community violence: Results of a school-based screening and group treatment protocol. *Group Dynamics. Special Issue: Group-Based Interventions for Trauma Survivors, 5,* 291–303.

Sannibale, C., Teesson, M., Creamer, M., Sitharthan, T., Bryant, R. A., Sutherland, K., ... Peek-O'Leary, M. (2013). Randomized controlled trial of cognitive behaviour therapy for comorbid post-traumatic stress disorder and alcohol use disorders. *Addiction, 108*(8), 1397–1410.

Sanson, A., Pedlow, R., Cann, W., Prior, M., & Oberklaid, F. (1996). Shyness ratings: Stability and correlates in early childhood. *Journal of the American Academy of Child and Adolescent Psychiatry, 38,* 1008–1015.

Saranson, S., Davidson, K., Lighthall, F., & Waite, R. (1958). A test anxiety scale for children. *Child Development, 29,* 105–113.

Scahill, L., Riddle, M. A., McSwiggin-Hardin, M., Ort, S. I., King, R. A., Goodman, W. K., ... Leckman, J. F. (1997). Children's Yale-Brown obsessive compulsive scale: Reliability and validity. *Journal of the American Academy of Child & Adolescent Psychiatry, 36*(6), 844–852.

Scaini, S., Ogliari, A., Eley, T. C., Zavos, H. M., & Battaglia, M. (2012). Genetic and environmental contributions to separation anxiety: A meta-analytic approach to twin data. *Depression and Anxiety, 29*(9), 754–761.

Schlegel, A., & Barry, H., III. (1991) *Adolescence: An anthropological inquiry.* New York: The Free Press, Maxwell MacMillan International.

Schmahmann, J. D., & Sherman, J. C. (1998). The cerebellar cognitive affective syndrome. *Brain, 121,* 561–579.

Schmidt, N. B., Koselka, M., & Woolaway-Bickel, K. (2001). Combined treatments for phobic anxiety disorders. In M. T. Sammons & N. B. Schmidt (Eds.), *Combined treatment for mental disorders: A guide to psychological and pharmacological interventions* (pp. 81–110). Washington, DC: American Psychological Association.

Schmidt, N. B., Woolaway-Bickel, K. Trakowski, J., Santiago, H. Storey, J., Koselka, M., & Cook, J. (2000). Dismantling cognitive-behavioral treatment for panic disorder: Questioning the utility of breathing retraining. *Journal of Consulting & Clinical Psychology, 68,* 417–424.

Schneider, A. J., Mataix-Cols, D., Marks, I. M., & Bachofen, M. (2005). Internet-guided self-help with or without exposure therapy for phobic and panic disorders. *Psychotherapy and Psychosomatics, 74*(3), 154–164.

Schneider, S., Blatter-Meunier, J., Herren, C., Adornetto, C., In-Albon, T., & Lavallee, K.

(2011). Disorder-specific cognitive-behavioral therapy for separation anxiety disorder in young children: A randomized waiting-list-controlled trial. *Psychotherapy and Psychosomatics, 80*(4), 206–215.

Schneider, S., Blatter-Meunier, J., Herren, C., In-Albon, T., Adornetto, C., Meyer, A., & Lavallee, K. L. (2013). The efficacy of a family-based cognitive-behavioral treatment for separation anxiety disorder in children aged 8–13: A randomized comparison with a general anxiety program. *Journal of Consulting and Clinical Psychology, 81*(5), 932–940.

Schneier, F. R., Neria, Y., Pavlicova, M., Hembree, E., Suh, E. J., Amsel, L., & Marshall, M. R. D. (2012). Combined prolonged exposure therapy and paroxetine for posttraumatic stress disorder related to the World Trade Center attacks: A randomized controlled trial. *American Journal of Psychiatry, 169*(1), 80.

Schnurr, P. P., Friedman, M. J., Engel, C. C., et al. (2007). Cognitive behavioral therapy for posttraumatic stress disorder in women: A randomized controlled trial. *Journal of the American Medical Association, 297*, 820–830.

Schnurr, P. P., Friedman, M. J., Foy, D. W., Shea, M. T., Hsieh, F. Y., Lavori, P. W., ... Bernardy, N.C. (2003). A randomized trial of trauma-focused group therapy for posttraumatic stress disorder: Results from a Department of Veterans Affairs Cooperative Study. *Archives of General Psychiatry, 60*, 481–489.

Scholwinski, E., & Reynolds, C. R. (1985). Dimensions of anxiety among high IQ children. *Gifted Child Quarterly, 29*(3), 125–130.

Seligman, M. E. P. (2002). Positive psychology, positive prevention, and positive therapy. In C. R. Snyder & S. J. Lopez (Eds.), *Handbook of positive psychology* (pp. 3–9). New York: Oxford University Press.

Shaffer, D., Fisher, P., et al. (1996). The NIMH Diagnostic Interview Schedule for Children Version 2.3 (DISC 2.3): Description, acceptability, prevalence rates, and performance in the MECA study. *Journal of the American Academy of Child and Adolescent Psychiatry, 35*, 865–877.

Shaffer, D., Gould, M. S., et al. (1983). A Children's Global Assessment Scale (CGAS). *Archives of General Psychiatry, 40*, 1228–1231.

Shamir-Essakow, G., Ungerer, J. A., & Rapee, R. M. (2005). Attachment, behavioral inhibition, and anxiety in preschool children. *Journal of Abnormal Child Psychology, 33*(2), 131–143.

Sharf, A., Kimonis, E. R., & Howard, A. (2014). Negative life events and posttraumatic stress disorder among incarcerated boys with callous-unemotional traits. *Journal of Psychopathology and Behavioral Assessment, 36*(3), 401–414.

Sharp, D., Power, K. G., & Swanson, V. (2004). A comparison of the efficacy and acceptability of group versus individual cognitive behavioral therapy in the treatment of panic disorder and agoraphobia in primary care. *Clinical Psychology and Psychotherapy, 11*, 73–82.

Shear, M. K., Houck, P., Greeno, C., & Masters, S. (2001). Emotion-focused psychotherapy for patients with panic disorder. *American Journal of Psychiatry, 158*(12), 1993–1998.

Shear, M. K., & Oommen, M. (1995). Anxiety disorders in pregnant and postpartum women. *Psychopharmacology Bulletin, 31*, 693–703.

Shemesh, E., Lurie, S., Stuber, M. L., Emre, S., Patel, Y., Vohra, P., Aromando, M., & Shneider, B. L. (2000). A pilot study of posttraumatic stress and nonadherence in pediatric liver transplant recipients. *Pediatrics, 105*(2), E29.

Shemesh, E., Rudnick, A., Kaluski, E., Milovanov, O., Salah, A., Alon, D., et al. (2001). A prospective study of posttraumatic stress symptoms and nonadherence in survivors of a myocardial infarction (MI). *General Hospital Psychiatry, 23*, 215–222.

Short, J. L. (1998). Evaluation of a substance abuse prevention and mental health promotion program for children of divorce. *Journal of Divorce and Remarriage, 28*, 139–155.

Sickmund, M., Snyder, H. N., & Poe-Yamagata, E. (1997). Juvenile Offenders and Victims: 1997 Update on Violence. *Statistics Summary*.

Sijbrandij, M., Olff, M., Reitsma, J. B., Carlier, I. V. E., de Vries, M. H., & Gersons, B. P. R. (2007). Treatment of acute posttraumatic stress disorder with brief cognitive behavioral therapy: A randomized controlled trial. *American Journal of Psychiatry, 164*, 82–90.

Silberg, J. L., Rutter, M., & Eaves, L. (2001). Genetic and environmental influences on the temporal association between earlier anxiety and later depression in girls: Erratum. *Biological Psychiatry, 50*, 393.

Silberg, J., Neale, M., et al. (2001). Genetic moderation of environmental risk for depression and anxiety in adolescent girls. *British Journal of Psychiatry, 179*, 116–121.

Silberg, J., Rutter, M., et al. (2001). Genetic and environmental influences on the temporal association between earlier anxiety and later depression in girls. *Biological Psychiatry, 49*, 1040–1049.

Silberg, J., Rutter, M., Neale, M. & Eaves, L. (2001). Genetic moderation of environmental risk for depression and anxiety in adolescent girls. *British Journal of Psychiatry, 179*, 116–121

Silove, D., Manicavasagar, V., et al. (1996). Is early separation anxiety a risk factor for adult panic disorder? A critical review. *Comprehensive Psychiatry, 37*(3), 167–179.

Silver, R. C., Holman, E. A., McIntosh, D. N., Poulin, M., & Gil-Rivas, V. (2002). Nationwide longitudinal study of psychological responses to September 11. *Journal of the American Medical Association, 288*, 1235–1244.

Silverman, J. J., Singh, N. N., Carmanico, S. J., Lindstrom, K. A., Best, A. M., & Clearfield, S. (1999). Psychological distress and symptoms of posttraumatic stress disorder in Jewish adolescents following a brief exposure to concentration camps. *Journal of Child & Family Studies, 8*, 71–89.

Silverman, W. K., & Albano, A. M. (1996). *The Anxiety Disorders Interview Schedule for Children-IV (Child and Parent Versions)*. San Antonio, TX: Psychological Corporation.

Silverman, W. K., & Kurtines, W. M. (1996). Transfer of control: A psychosocial intervention model for internalizing disorders in youth. In E. D. Hibbs & P. S. Jensen (Eds.), *Psychosocial treatments for child and adolescent disorders: Empirically based strategies for clinical practice* (pp. 63–81). Washington, DC: American Psychological Association.

Silverman, W. K., & Weems, C. F. (1999). Anxiety sensitivity in children. In S. Taylor (Ed.), *Anxiety sensitivity: Theory, research, and treatment of the fear of anxiety* (pp. 239–268). Mahwah, NJ: Erlbaum.

Silverman, W. K., Cerny, J. A., Nelles, W. B., & Burke, A. E. (1988). Behavior problems in children of parents with anxiety disorders. *Journal of the American Academy of Child and Adolescent Psychiatry, 27*, 779–784.

Silverman, W. K., Fleisig, W., Rabian, B., & Peterson, R. A. (1991). Childhood anxiety sensitivity index. *Journal of Clinical Child Psychology, 20*, 162–168.

Silverman, W. K., Kurtines, W. M., Ginsburg, G. S., Weems, C. F., Lumpkin, P. W., & Carmichael, D. H. (1999). Treating anxiety disorders in children with group cognitive behavior therapy: A randomized clinical trial. *Journal of Consulting and Clinical Psychology, 67*, 995–1003.

Silverman, W. K., Kurtines, W. M., Ginsburg, G. S., Weems, C. F., Rabian, B. & Serafini, L. T. (1999). Contingency management, self-control, and education support in the treatment of childhood phobic disorders: A randomized clinical trial. *Journal of Consulting & Clinical Psychology, 67*, 675–687.

Silverman, W. K., La Greca, A. M., & Wasserstein, S. (1995). What do children worry about? Worries and their relation to anxiety. *Child Development, 66*, 671–686.

Simeon, J. G., Ferguson, H. B., Knott, V., Roberts, N., Gauthier, B., Dubois, C., et al. (1992). Clinical, cognitive, and neurophysiological effects of alprazolam in children and adolescents with overanxious and avoidant disorders. *Journal of the American Academy of Child and Adolescent Psychiatry, 31*, 29–33.

Simpson, H. B., Foa, E. B., Liebowitz, M. R., Huppert, J. D., Cahill, S., Maher, M. J., ... Campeas, R. (2013). Cognitive-behavioral therapy vs risperidone for augmenting serotonin reuptake inhibitors in obsessive-compulsive disorder: A randomized clinical trial. *JAMA Psychiatry, 70*(11), 1190–1198.

Simpson, H., Foa, E., Liebowitz, M., Ledley, D., Huppert, J., Cahill, S., ... Franklin, M. (2008). A randomized, controlled trial of cognitive-behavioral therapy for augmenting pharmacotherapy in obsessive-compulsive disorder. *American Journal of Psychiatry, 165*, 621–630.

Simpson, H. B., Liebowitz, M. R., Foa, E. B., Kozak, M. J., Schmidt, A. B., Rowan, V., ... Campeas, R. (2004). Post-treatment effects of exposure therapy and clomipramine in obsessive-compulsive disorder. *Depression and Anxiety, 19*(4), 225–233.

Siqueland, L., Kendall, P. C., & Steinberg, L. (1996). Anxiety in children: perceived family environments and observed family interaction. *Journal of Clinical Child Psychology, 25*, 225–237.

Skre, I., Onstad, S., et al. (1993). A twin study of DSM-III-R anxiety disorders. *Acta Psychiatrica Scandinavica, 88*(2), 85–92.

Slattery, M. J., Klein, D. F., Mannuzza, S., Moulton, J. L., III, Pine, D. S., & Klein, R. G. (2002). Relationship between separation anxiety disorder, parental panic disorder, and atopic disorders in children: A controlled high-risk study. *Journal of the American Academy of Child and Adolescent Psychiatry, 41*, 947–954.

Sloan, D. M., Marx, B. P., Bovin, M. J., Feinstein, B. A., & Gallagher, M. W. (2012). Written exposure as an intervention for PTSD: A randomized clinical trial with motor vehicle accident survivors. *Behaviour Research and Therapy, 50*(10), 627–635.

Smoller, J. W., Rosenbaum, J. F., Biederman, J., Kennedy, J., Dai, D., Racette, S. R., ... Slaugenhaupt, S. A. (2003). Association of a genetic marker at the corticotropin-releasing hormone locus with behavioral inhibition. *Biological Psychiatry, 54*, 1376–1381.

Snyder, H. N. (1999). Juvenile arrests, 1998. *Juvenile Justice Bulletin.*

Snyder, J., Bullard, L., Wagener, A., Leong, P. K., Snyder, J., & Jenkins, M. (2009). Childhood anxiety and depressive symptoms: Trajectories, relationship, and association with subsequent depression. *Journal of Clinical Child and Adolescent Psychology, 38*(6), 837–849.

Solomon, Z., Mikulincer, M., & Avitzur, E. (1988). Coping, locus of control, social support, and combat-related posttraumatic stress disorder: A prospective study. *Journal of Personality and Social Psychology, 55*, 279–285.

Sowell, E. R., Thompson, P. M., Holmes, C. J., Batth, R., Jernigan, T. L., & Toga, A. W. (1999a). Localizing age-related changes in brain structure between childhood and adolescence using statistical parametric mapping. *Neuroimage, 9*, 587–597.

Sowell, E. R., Thompson, P. M., Holmes, C. J., Jernigan, T. L., & Toga, A. W. (1999b). In vivo evidence for post-adolescent brain maturation in frontal and striatal regions. *Nature Neuroscience, 2*, 859–861.

Spear, L. P. (2000). The adolescent brain and age-related behavioral manifestations. *Neuroscience and Biobehavioral Reviews, 24*, 417–463.

Spence, J., Titov, N., Dear, B. F., Johnston, L., Solley, K., Lorian, C., ... Schwenke, G. (2011). Randomized controlled trial of Internet-delivered cognitive behavioral therapy for posttraumatic stress disorder. *Depression and Anxiety, 28*(7), 541–550.

Spence, S. H., Donovan, C. & Brechman-Toussaint, M. (2000). The treatment of childhood social phobia: The effectiveness of a social skills training-based, cognitive-behavioural intervention, with and without parental involvement. *Journal of Child Psychology & Psychiatry & Allied Disciplines, 41*, 713–726.

Stallard, P., Simpson, N., Anderson, S., & Goddard, M. (2008). The FRIENDS emotional health prevention programme: 12-month follow-up of a universal UK school-based trial. *European Child & Adolescent Psychiatry, 17*(5), 283–289.

Stangier, U., Schramm, E., Heidenreich, T., Berger, M., & Clark, D. M. (2011). Cognitive therapy vs interpersonal psychotherapy in social anxiety disorder: A randomized controlled trial. *Archives of General Psychiatry, 68*(7), 692–700.

Stein, D. J., Westenberg, H. G. M., Liebowitz, M. R. (2002). Social anxiety disorder and generalized anxiety disorder: Serotonergic and dopaminergic neurocircuitry. *Journal of Clinical Psychiatry, 63*, 12–19.

Stein, M. B., Chartier, M. J., Hazen, A. L., Kroft, C. D. L., Chale, R. A., Cote, D., et al. (1996). Paroxetine in the treatment of generalized social phobia: Open label and double-blind placebo-controlled discontinuation. *Journal of Clinical Psychopharmacology, 16*, 218–222.

Stein, M. B., Chavira, D. A., & Jang, K. L. (2001). Bringing up bashful baby: Developmental pathways to social phobia. *Psychiatric Clinics of North America, 24*, 661–675.

Steketee, G., & Foa, E. B. (1987). Rape victims: Post-traumatic stress responses and their treatment: A review of the literature. *Journal of Anxiety Disorders, 1*, 69–86.

Stenmark, H., Catani, C., Neuner, F., Elbert, T., & Holen, A. (2013). Treating PTSD in refugees and asylum seekers within the general health care system: A randomized controlled multicenter study. *Behaviour Research and Therapy, 51*(10), 641–647.

Stevens, S. J., Murphy, B. S., & McKnight, K. (2003). Traumatic stress and gender differences in relationship to substance abuse, mental health, physical health and HIV risk behavior in a sample of adolescents enrolled in drug treatment. *Child Maltreatment, 8*, 46–57.

Stevenson-Hinde, J., & Shouldice, A. (1990). Fear and attachment in 2.5-year-olds. *British Journal of Developmental Psychology, 8*, 319–333.

Storch, E. A., Caporino, N. E., Morgan, J. R., Lewin, A. B., Rojas, A., Brauer, L., ... Murphy, T. K. (2011). Preliminary investigation of web-camera delivered cognitive-behavioral therapy for youth with obsessive-compulsive disorder. *Psychiatry Research, 189*, 407–412.

Storch, E. A., Geffken, G. R., Merlo, L. J., Mann, G., Duke, D., Munson, M., et al. (2007). Family-based cognitive-behavioral therapy for pediatric obsessive-compulsive disorder: Comparison of intensive and weekly approaches. *Journal of the American Academy of Child and Adolescent Psychiatry, 46*, 469–478.

Storch, E. A., Murphy, T. K., Geffken, G. R., Mann, G., Adkins, J., Merlo, L. J., ... Goodman, W. K. (2006). Cognitive-behavioral therapy for PANDAS-related obsessive-compulsive disorder: Findings from a preliminary waitlist controlled open trial. *Journal of the American*

Academy of Child & Adolescent Psychiatry, 45(10), 1171–1178.

Stretch, R. H. (1985). Posttraumatic stress disorder among U.S. Army Reserve Vietnam and Vietnam-era veterans. *Journal of Consulting and Clinical Psychology, 53*, 935–936.

Suliman, S., Kaminer, D., Seedat, S., & Stein, D. J. (2005). Assessing post-traumatic stress disorder in South African adolescents: Using the Child and Adolescent Trauma Survey (CATS) as a screening tool. *Annals of General Psychiatry, 4*(1), 2.

Sullivan, G. M., Coplan, J. D., & Gorman, J. M. (1998). Psychoneuroendocrinology of anxiety disorders. *Psychiatric Clinics of North America, 21*, 397–412.

Sullivan, G. M., Coplan, J. D., Kent, J. M., & Gorman, J. M. (1999). The noradenergic system in pathological anxiety: A focus on panic with relevance to generalized anxiety and phobias. *Biological Psychiatry, 46*, 1205–1218.

Sutker, P. B., Davis, J. M., Uddo, M., & Ditta, S. R. (1995a). Assessment of psychological distress in Persian Gulf troops: Ethnicity and gender comparisons. *Journal of Personality Assessment, 64*, 415–427.

Sutker, P. B., Davis, J. M., Uddo, M., & Ditta, S. R. (1995b). War zone stress, personal resources, and PTSD in Persian Gulf War returnees. *Journal of Abnormal Psychology, 104*, 444–452.

Sutker, P. B., Vasterling, J. J., Brailey, K. Allain, A. N. et al. (1995). Memory, attention, and executive deficits in POW survivors: Contributing biological and psychological factors. *Neuropsychology, 9*, 118–125.

Swadi, H. (1999). Individual risk factors for adolescent substance abuse. *Drug and Alcohol Dependence, 55*, 209–224.

Swedo, S. E. (1994). Sydenham's chorea: A model for childhood autoimmune neuropsychiatric disorders. *Journal of the American Medical Association, 272*, 1788–1791.

Swedo, S. E. (2002). Pediatric autoimmune neuropsychiatric disorders associated with streptococcal infections. (PANDAS). *Molecular Psychiatry, 7*, S24–S25.

Swedo, S. E., Leonard, H. L., Garvey, M., et al (1998). Pediatric autoimmune neuropsychiatric disorders associated with streptococcal infections: Clinical description of the first 50 cases. *American Journal of Psychiatry, 155*, 264–271.

Swedo, S. E., Leonard, H. L., Mittleman, B. B., Allen, A. J., Rapoport, J. L., Dow, S. P., ... Zabriskie, J. (1997). Identification of children with pediatric autoimmune neuropsychiatric disorders associated with streptococcal infections by a marker associated with rheumatic fever. *American Journal of Psychiatry, 154*(1), 110–112.

Sweeney, M., & Pine, D. (2004). Etiology of fear and anxiety. In T. H. Ollendick & J. S. March (Eds.), *Phobic and anxiety disorders in children and adolescents: A clinician's guide to effective psychosocial and pharmacological interventions* (pp. 34–60). New York: Oxford University Press.

Swinson, R. P., Soulios, C., Cox, B. J. & Kuch, K. (1992). Brief treatment of emergency room patients with panic attacks. *American Journal of Psychiatry, 14*, 944–946.

Taghavi, M. R., Moradi, A. R., Neshat-Doost, H. T., Yule, W., & Dalgleish, T. (2000). Interpretation of ambiguous emotional information in clinically anxious children and adolescents. *Cognition and Emotion, 14*, 809–822.

Taghavi, M. R., Neshat-Doost, H. T., Moradi, A. R., Yule, W., & Dalgleish, T. (1999). Biases in visual attention in children and adolescents with clinical anxiety and mixed anxiety-depression. *Journal of Abnormal Child Psychology, 27*, 215–223.

Takahashi, L. K., & Goh, C. (1996). Presynaptic muscarinic cholinergic receptors in the dorsal hippocampus regulate behavioral inhibition of preweanling rats. *Brain Research, 731*(1-2), 230–235.

Teicher, M. H., & Andersen, S. L. (1999, October). *Limbic serotonin turnover plunges during puberty*. Poster session presented at the annual meeting of the Society for Neuroscience, Miami Beach, FL.

Teplin, L. A., Abram, K. M., McClelland, G. M., Dulcan, M. K., & Mericle, A. A. (2002). Psychiatric disorders in youth in juvenile detention. *Archives of General Psychiatry, 59*, 1133–1143.

Terasawa, E., & Timiras, P. S. (1968). Electrophysiological study of the limbic system in the rat at onset of puberty. *American Journal of Physiology, 215*, 1462–1467.

Teubert, D., & Pinquart, M. (2011). A meta-analytic review on the prevention of symptoms of anxiety in children and adolescents. *Journal of Anxiety Disorders, 25*(8), 1046–1059.

Thomas, K. M., Drevets, W. C., Dahl, R. E., Ryan, N. D., Birmaher, B., Eccard, C. H., et al. (2001a). Amygdala response to fearful faces in anxious and depressed children. *Archives of General Psychiatry, 58*, 1057–1063.

Thomas, K. M., Drevets, W. C., Whalen, P. J., Eccard, C. H., Dahl, R. E., Ryan, N. D., et al. (2001b). Amygdala response to facial expressions in children and adults. *Biological Psychiatry, 49,* 309–316.

Topolski, T., Hewitt, J., et al. (1997). Genetic and environmental influences on child reports of manifest anxiety and symptoms of separation anxiety and overanxious disorders: A community-based twin study. *Behavior Genetics, 27*(1), 15–28.

Tortella-Feliu, M., Botella, C., Llabrés, J., Bretón-López, J. M., del Amo, A. R., Baños, R. M., & Gelabert, J. M. (2011). Virtual reality versus computer-aided exposure treatments for fear of flying. *Behavior Modification, 35*(1), 3–30.

Treadwell, K. H., & Kendall, P. C. (1996). Self-talk in anxiety-disordered youth: States-of-mind, content specificity, and treatment outcome. *Journal of Consulting and Clinical Psychology, 64,* 941–950.

U.S. Department of Health and Human Services, Administration on Children, Youth and Families. (2003). *Child maltreatment 2001.* Washington, DC: U.S. Government Printing Office.

U.S. Department of Health & Human Services, Administration on Children, Youth, & Families. (2012). *Child maltreatment.* Washington, DC: Government Printing Office.

U.S. Department of Health & Human Services, Administration on Children, Youth, & Families. (2014). *Child maltreatment.* Washington, DC: Government Printing Office.

Upadhyaya, H., Deas, D., Brady, K., & Kruesi, M. (2002). Cigarette smoking and psychiatric comorbidity in children and adolescents. *Journal of the American Academy of Child and Adolescent Psychiatry, 41,* 1295–1303.

Vagi, K. J., Olsen, E. O. M., Basile, K. C., & Vivolo-Kantor, A. M. (2105). Teen dating violence (physical and sexual) among US high school students: Findings from the 2013 National Youth Risk Behavior Survey. *JAMA Pediatrics, 169(5),* 474–482.

van Balkom, A. J., Bakker, A., Spinhoven, P., Blaauw, B. M., Smeenk, S., & Ruesink, B. (1997). A meta-analysis of the treatment of panic disorder with or without agoraphobia: A comparison of psychopharmacological, cognitive-behavioral, and combination treatments. *Journal of Nervous and Mental Disease, 185*(8), 510–516.

van Balkom, A. J., de Haan, E., van Oppen, P., Spinhoven, P., Al Hoogduin, K. E. E. S., & van Dyck, R. (1998). Cognitive and behavioral therapies alone versus in combination with fluvoxamine in the treatment of obsessive compulsive disorder. *Journal of Nervous and Mental Disease, 186*(8), 492–499.

van Brakel, A. M., Muris, P., Bögels, S. M., & Thomassen, C. (2006). A multifactorial model for the etiology of anxiety in non-clinical adolescents: Main and interactive effects of behavioral inhibition, attachment, and parental rearing. *Journal of Child and Family Studies, 15*(5), 568–578.

van der Heiden, C., Muris, P., & van der Molen, H. T. (2012). Randomized controlled trial on the effectiveness of metacognitive therapy and intolerance-of-uncertainty therapy for generalized anxiety disorder. *Behaviour Research and Therapy, 50*(2), 100–109.

Varley, C. K., & McClellan, J. (1997). Case study: Two additional sudden deaths with tricyclic antidepressants. *American Journal of Child and Adolescent Psychiatry, 36,* 390–394.

Vasey, M. W., & MacLeod, C. (2001). Information-processing factors in childhood anxiety: A developmental perspective. In M. W. Vasey & M. R. Dadds (Eds.), *The developmental psychopathology of anxiety* (pp. 253–277). New York: Oxford University Press.

Vasey, M. W., Daleiden, E. L., Williams, L. L., & Brown. L. M. (1995). Biased attention in childhood anxiety disorders: A preliminary study. *Journal of Abnormal Child Psychology, 23,* 267–279.

Vasey, M. W., Dalgleish, T., & Silverman, W. K. (2003). Research on information-processing factors in child and adolescent psychopathology: A critical commentary. *Journal of Clinical Child and Adolescent Psychology, 32,* 81–93.

Vasey, M. W., El-Hag, N., & Daleiden, E. L. (1996). Anxiety and the processing of emotionally threatening stimuli: Distinctive patterns of selective attention among high- and low-test-anxious children. *Child Development, 67,* 1173–1185.

Vecchio, T. (1996). Predictive value of a single diagnostic test in unselected populations. *New England Journal of Medicine, 275,* 1171–1173.

Vernberg, E. M., La Greca, A. M., Silverman, W. K., Silverman, W. K., & Prinstein, M. J. (1996). Predictors of children's post-disaster functioning following Hurricane Andrew. *Journal of Abnormal Psychology, 105,* 237–248.

Viana, A. G., Beidel, D. C., & Rabian, B. (2009). Selective mutism: A review and integration of the last 15 years. *Clinical Psychology Review, 29*(1), 57–67.

Vika, M., Skaret, E., Raadal, M., Öst, L. G., & Kvale, G. (2009). One-vs. five-session treatment of intra-oral injection phobia: A randomized clinical study. *European Journal of Oral Sciences, 117*(3), 279–285.

Vos, S. P. F., Huibers, M. J. H., Diels, L., & Arntz, A. (2012). A randomized clinical trial of cognitive behavioral therapy and interpersonal psychotherapy for panic disorder with agoraphobia. *Psychological Medicine, 42*(12), 2661–2672.

Wagner, K. D., Berard, R., Stein, M. B., Wetherhold, E., Carpenter, D. J., Perera, P., ... Machin, A. (2004). A multicenter, randomized, double-blind, placebo-controlled trial of paroxetine in children and adolescents with social anxiety disorder. *Archives of General Psychiatry, 61*(11), 1153–1162.

Wakefield, J. C. (1992). The concept of mental disorder: On the boundary between biological facts and social values. *American Psychologist, 47*, 373–388.

Walker, J. R., Van Amerigen, M. A., Swinson, R., Bowen, R. C., Cokka, P. R., Goldner, E., ... Lane, R. M. (2000). Prevention of relapse in generalized social phobia: Results of a 24-week study in responders to 20 weeks of sertraline treatment. *Journal of Clinical Psychopharmacology, 20*(6), 636–643.

Walkup, J. T., Albano, A. M., Piacentini, J., Birmaher, B., Compton, S. N., Sherrill, J. T., ... Kendall, P. C. (2008). Cognitive behavioral therapy, sertraline, or a combination in childhood anxiety. *New England Journal of Medicine, 359*(26), 2753–2766.

Walkup, J. T., Labellarte, M. J., Riddle, M. A., Pine, D.S., Greenhill, L., Klein, R., ... Roper, M. (2001). Fluvoxamine for the treatment of anxiety disorders in children and adolescents. *New England Journal of Medicine, 344*, 1279–1285.

Warner, B. S., & Weist, M. D. (1996). Urban youth as witnesses to violence: Beginning assessment and treatment efforts. *Journal of Youth & Adolescence, 25*, 361–377.

Warren, S. L., Huston, L., Egeland, B., & Sroufe, L. A. (1997). Child and adolescent anxiety disorders and early attachment. *Journal of the American Academy of Child and Adolescent Psychiatry, 36*, 637–644.

Wasserman, G. A., McReynolds, L. S., Lucal, C. P., Fisher, P., & Santos, L. (2002). The Voice DISC-IV with incarcerated male youths: Prevalence of disorder, *Journal of the American Academy of Child and Adolescent Psychiatry, 41*, 314–321.

Waters, A. M., Craske, M. G., Bergman, R. L., Naliboff, B. D., Negoro, H., & Ornitz, E. M. (2008). Developmental changes in startle reactivity in school-age children at risk for and with actual anxiety disorder. *International Journal of Psychophysiology, 70*(3), 158–164.

Watts, B. V., Schnurr, P. P., Mayo, L., Young-Xu, Y., Weeks, W. B., & Friedman, M. J. (2013). Meta-analysis of the efficacy of treatments for posttraumatic stress disorder. *Journal of Clinical Psychiatry, 74*(6), 541–550.

Weems, C. F., Hayward, C., Killen, J., & Taylor, C. B. (2002). A longitudinal investigation of anxiety sensitivity in adolescence. *Journal of Abnormal Psychology, 111*, 471–477.

Weems, C. F., Silverman, W. K., & La Greca, A. M. (2000). What do youth referred for anxiety problems worry about? Worry and its relation to anxiety and anxiety disorders in children and adolescents. *Journal of Abnormal Child Psychology, 28*, 63–72.

Wegner, D. M. (1989). *White bears and other unwanted thoughts: Suppression, obsession, and the psychology of mental control.* New York: Penguin Books.

Weissberg, R. P., Kumpfer, K. L., & Seligman, M. E. P. (2003). Prevention that works for children and youth: An introduction. *American Psychologist. Special Issue: Prevention That Works for Children and Youth, 58*, 425–432.

Weissman, M. M. (1988). The epidemiology of anxiety disorders: Rates, risks and familial patterns. *Journal of Psychiatric Research, 22*, 99–114.

Weissman, M. M., Greenwald, S., Wichramarante, P., Bland, R. C., Newman, S. C., Canino, G. J., ... Wells, J. E. (1997). What happens to depressed men? Application of the Stirling County criteria. *Harvard Review of Psychiatry, 5*(1), 1–6.

Weissman, M. M., Wolk, S., Wichramaratne, P., Goldstein, R. B., Adams, P., Greenwald, S., ... Steinberg, D. (1999). Children with prepubertal-onset major depressive disorder and anxiety grown up. *Archives of General Psychiatry, 56*, 794–801.

Weizman, A., & Weizman, R. (2000). Serotonin transporter polymorphism and response to SSRIs in major depression and relevance to anxiety disorders and substance abuse. *Pharmacogenomics, 1*, 335–341.

Westen, D., & Morrison, K. (2001). A multidimensional meta-analysis of treatments for depression, panic, and generalized anxiety disorder: An empirical examination of the status of empirically supported therapies. *Journal of Consulting and Clinical Psychology, 69*(6), 875.

Wever, C., & Rey, J. M. (1997). Juvenile OCD. *Australian and New Zealand Journal of Psychiatry, 31*, 105–113.

White, K. S., Bruce, S. E., Farrell, A. D., & Kliewer, W. (1998). Impact of exposure to community violence on anxiety: A longitudinal study of family social support as a protective factor for urban children. *Journal of Child and Family Studies, 7*, 187–203.

Whittal, M. L., Thordarson, D. S., & McLean, P. D. (2005). Treatment of obsessive–compulsive disorder: Cognitive behavior therapy vs. exposure and response prevention. *Behaviour Research and Therapy, 43*(12), 1559–1576.

Wilhelm, F. H., & Roth, W. T. (1997). Acute and delayed effects of alprazolam on flight phobics during exposure. *Behavior Research and Therapy, 35*, 831–841.

Williams, J. M. G., Mathews, A., & MacLeod, C. (1996). The emotional Stroop task and psychopathology. *Psychological Bulletin, 120*, 3–24.

Williams, J. M. G., Watts, F. N., MacLeod, C., & Mathews, A. (1997). *Cognitive psychology and emotional disorders* (2nd ed.). Chichester, UK: Wiley.

Williams, T. I., Salkovskis, P. M., Forrester, L., Turner, S., White, H., & Allsopp, M. A. (2010). A randomised controlled trial of cognitive behavioural treatment for obsessive compulsive disorder in children and adolescents. *European Children and Adolescent Psychiatry, 19*, 449–456.

Wills, T. A., Vaccaro, D., & McNammar, G. (1992) The role of life events, family support and competence in adolescent substance abuse: A test of vulnerability and protective factors. *American Journal of Community Psychology, 20*, 349–374.

Wilson, F. A., & Rolls, E. T. (1993). The effect of stimulus novelty and familiarity on neuronal activity in the amygdala of monkeys performing recognition memory tasks. *Experimental Brain Research, 93*, 367–382.

Wims, E., Titov, N., Andrews, G., & Choi, I. (2010). Clinician-assisted Internet-based treatment is effective for panic: A randomized controlled trial. *Australian and New Zealand Journal of Psychiatry, 44*(7), 599–607.

Wittchen, H., Nelson, C. B., & Lachner, G. (1998). Prevalence of mental disorders and psychosocial impairments in adolescents and young adults. *Psychological Medicine, 28*, 109–126.

Wolfe, D. A., Scott, K., Reitzel-Jaffe, D., Wekerle, C. Grasley, C., & Straatman, A. (2001). Development and validation of the Conflict in Adolescent Dating Relationships Inventory. *Psychological Assessment, 13*, 277–293.

Wolfer, D. P., & Lipp, H.-P. (1995). Evidence for physiological growth of hippocampal mossy fiber collaterals in the guinea pig during puberty and adulthood. *Hippocampus, 5*, 329–340.

Wood, J., Foy, D., Layne, D., Pynoos, R., & James, C. B. (2002). An examination of the relationships among violence, posttraumatic stress symptomotology, and delinquent activity: An "ecological" model of delinquent behavior among incarcerated adolescents. *Journal of Aggression, Maltreatment and Trauma, 6*, 127–147.

Woods, S. W., & Charney, D. S. (1998). Applications of the pharmacologic challenge strategy in panic disorders research. *Journal of Anxiety Disorders, 2*, 31–49.

Yehuda, R. (2002). Post-traumatic stress disorder. *New England Journal of Medicine, 346*, 108–114.

Young, S. E., Smolen, A., Stallings, M. C., Corley, R. P., & Hewitt, J. K. (2003). Sibling-based association analyses of the serotonin transporter polymorphism and internalizing behavior problems in children. *Journal of Child Psychology and Psychiatry, 44*, 961–967.

Yurgelun-Todd, D. A., Killgore, W. D. S., & Cintron, C. B. (2003). Cognitive correlates of medial temporal lobe development across adolescence: A magnetic resonance imaging study. *Perceptual & Motor Skills, 96*, 3–17.

Zeller, M., Yuval, K., Nitzan-Assayag, Y., & Bernstein, A. (2015). Self-compassion in recovery following potentially traumatic stress: Longitudinal study of at-risk youth. *Journal of Abnormal Child Psychology, 43*(4), 645–653.

Zoellner, L. A., Foa, E. B., & Brigidi, B. D. (1999). Interpersonal friction and PTSD in female victims of sexual and nonsexual assault. *Journal of Traumatic Stress, 12*, 689–700.

Zubernis, L. S., Cassidy, K. W., Gillham, J. E., Reivich, K. J., & Jaycox, L. H. (1999). Prevention of depressive symptoms in preadolescent children of divorce. *Journal of Divorce and Remarriage, 30*, 11–36.

Zucker, B. G., Craske, M. G., Barrios, B., & Holguin, M. (2002). Thought action fusion: Can it be corrected? *Behaviour Research & Therapy, 40*, 652–664.

Zvolensky, M. J., & Bernstein, A. (2005). Cigarette smoking and panic psychopathology. *Current Directions in Psychological Science, 14*(6), 301–305.

Part IV: Eating Disorders

Abbassi, V. (1998). Growth and normal puberty. *Pediatrics, 102*, 507–511.

Abbott, D. W., de Zwaan, M., Mussell, M. P., Raymond, N. C., Seim, H. C., Crow, S. J., ...

Mitchell, J. E. (1998). Onset of binge eating and dieting in overweight women: Implications for etiology, associated features and treatment. *Journal of Psychosomatic Research, 44*, 367–374.

Abebe, D. S., Lien, L., Torgersen, L., & von Soest, T. (2012). Binge eating, purging and non-purging compensatory behaviours decrease from adolescence to adulthood: A population-based, longitudinal study. *BMC Public Health, 12*, 32.

Ackard, D. M., Fulkerson, J. A., & Neumark-Sztainer, D. (2007). Prevalence and utility of DSM-IV eating disorder diagnostic criteria among youth. *International Journal of Eating Disorders, 40*, 409–417.

Agras, W. S., Brandt, H., Bulik, C. M., Dolan-Sewell, R., Fairburn, C. G., Halmi, C. A., . . . Wilfley, D. (2004). Report of the National Health Institutes of Health Workshop on overcoming barriers to treatment research in anorexia nervosa. *International Journal of Eating Disorders, 35*, 509–521.

Agras, W. S., Lock, J., Brandt, H., Johnson, C., Halmi, K., Kaye, W., . . .Woodside, B. (2013, September). *A multisite study comparing two different family therapies for adolescent anorexia nervosa*. Paper presented at the annual Eating Disorders Research Society meeting, Bethesda, MD.

Agras, W. S., Walsh, B. T., Fairburn, C. G., Wilson, G. T., & Kraemer, H. C. (2000). A multicenter comparison of cognitive-behavioral therapy and interpersonal psychotherapy for bulimia nervosa. *Archives of General Psychiatry, 57*, 459–466.

Akkermann, K., Nordquist, N., Oreland, L., & Harro, J. (2010). Serotonin transporter gene promoter polymorphism affects the severity of binge eating in general population. *Progress in Neuro-psychopharmacology & Biological Psychiatry, 34*, 111–114.

Alegria, M., Woo, M., Cao, Z., Torres, M., Meng, X., & Striegel-Moore, R. (2007). Prevalence and correlates of eating disorders in Latinos in the United States. *International Journal of Eating Disorders, 40*, S15–S21.

Allan, R., Sharma, R., Sangani, B., Hugo, P. Frampton, I, Mason, H., & Lask, B. (2010). Predicting the weight gain required for recovery from anorexia nervosa with pelvic ultrasonography: An evidence-based approach. *European Eating Disorders Review, 18*, 43–48.

Almandil, N., Liu, Y., Murray, M., Besag, F., Aitchison, K., & Wong, I. (2013). Weight gain and other metabolic adverse effects associated with atypical antipsychotic treatment of children and adolescents: A systematic review and meta-analysis. *Pediatric Drugs, 15*, 139–150.

Altman, S. E., & Shankman, S. A. (2009). What is the association between obsessive-compulsive disorder and eating disorders? *Clinical Psychology Review, 29*, 638–645.

American Academy of Pediatrics Committee on Nutrition. (2014). Optimizing bone health in children and adolescents. *Pediatrics, 134*, e1229–1243.

American Dietetic Association. (2006). Position of the American Dietetic Association: Nutrition intervention in the treatment of anorexia nervosa, bulimia nervosa, and other eating disorders. *Journal of the American Dietetic Association, 106*, 2073–2082.

American Psychiatric Association. (2006). Treatment of patients with eating disorders, third edition. *American Journal of Psychiatry, 163*, 4–54.

American Psychiatric Association. (2013). *Diagnostic and statistical manual of mental disorders* (5th ed.). Washington, DC: American Psychiatric Association.

Anderluh, M., Tchanturia, K., Rabe-Hesketh, S., & Treasure, J. (2003). Childhood obsessive-compulsive personality traits in adult women with eating disorders: Defining a broader eating disorder phenotype. *American Journal of Psychiatry, 160*, 242–247.

Andersen, A. E., Bowers, W., & Evans, K. (1997). Inpatient treatment of anorexia nervosa. In D. M. Garner & P. E. Garfinkel (Eds.), *Handbook of treatment for eating disorders* (2nd ed., pp. 327–353). New York: Guilford Press.

Andersen, A. E., Watson, T., & Schlechte, J. (2000). Osteoporosis and osteopenia in men with eating disorders. *Lancet, 335*, 1967–1968.

Anderson, C. B., & Bulik, C. M. (2004). Gender differences in compensatory behaviors, weight and shape salience, and drive for thinness. *Eating Behaviors, 5*, 1–11.

Arden, M. R., Weiselberg, E. C., Nussbaum, M. P., Shenker, I. R., & Jacobson, M. S. (1990). Effect of weight restoration on the dyslipoproteinemia of anorexia nervosa. *Journal of Adolescent Health Care, 11*, 199–202.

Ata, R. N., Thompson, J. K., & Small, B. J. (2013). Effects of exposure to thin-ideal media images on body dissatisfaction: Testing the inclusion of a disclaimer versus warning label. *Body Image*. [epub before print]

Attia, E., Haiman, C., Walsh, B. T., & Flater, S. R. (1998). Does fluoxetine augment the inpatient treatment of anorexia nervosa? *American Journal of Psychiatry, 155*, 548–551.

Attia, E., Kaplan, A. S., Walsh, B. T., Gershkovich, M., Yilmaz, Z., Musante, D., & Wang, Y. (2011). Olanzapine versus placebo for outpatients with anorexia nervosa. *Psychological Medicine, 41*, 2177–2182.

Austin, S. B. (2012). A public health approach to eating disorders prevention: It's time for public health professionals to take a seat at the table. *BMC Public Health, 12*, 854.

Austin, S. B., Kim, J., Wiecha, J., Troped, P. J., Feldman H. A., & Peterson, K. E. (2007). School-based overweight preventive intervention lowers incidence of disordered weight-control behaviors in early adolescent girls. *Archives of Pediatric and Adolescent Medicine, 161*, 865–869.

Austin, S. B., Spadano-Gasbarro, J. L., Greaney, M. L., Blood, E. A., Hunt, A. T., Richmond, T. K., . . . Peterson, K. E. (2012). Effect of the Planet Health intervention on eating disorder symptoms in Massachusetts middle schools, 2005–2008. *Preventing Chronic Disease, 9*, E171.

Austin, S. B., Spadano-Gasbarro, J., Greaney, M. L., Richmond, T. K., Feldman, H. A., Osganian, S. K., . . . Peterson, K. E. (2011). Disordered weight control behaviors in early adolescent boys and girls of color: An under-recognized factor in the epidemic of childhood overweight. *Journal of Adolescent Health,* 48, 109–112.

Bacanu, S. A., Bulik, C. M., Klump, K. L., Fichter, M. M., Halmi, K. A., Keel, P., . . . Devlin, B. (2005). Linkage analysis of anorexia and bulimia nervosa cohorts using selected behavioral phenotypes as quantitative traits or covariates. *American Journal of Medical Genetics. Part B, Neuropsychiatric Genetics, 139B*, 61–68.

Bailer, U. F., & Kaye, W. H. (2011). Serotonin: Imaging findings in eating disorders. *Current Topics in Behavioral Neurosciences, 6*, 59–79.

Bair, C. E., Kelly, N. R., Serdar, K. L., & Mazzeo, S. E. (2012). Does the Internet function like magazines? An exploration of image-focused media, eating pathology, and body dissatisfaction. *Eating Behaviors, 13*, 398–401.

Bacaltchuk, J., & Hay, P. (2003). Antidepressants versus placebo for people with bulimia nervosa. *Cochrane Database of Systematic Reviews*, (4):CD003391.

Bacaltchuk, J., Hay, P., & Trefiglio, R. (2001). Antidepressants versus psychological treatments and their combination for bulimia nervosa. *Cochrane Database of Systematic Reviews*, (4):CD003385.

Bachrach, L. K., Guido, D., Katzman, D., Litt, I. F., & Marcus, R. (1990). Decreased bone density in adolescent girls with anorexia nervosa. *Pediatrics, 86*, 440–447.

Bachrach, L. K., Katzman, D. K., Litt, I. F., Guido, D., & Marcus, R. (1991). Recovery from osteopenia in adolescent girls with anorexia nervosa. *Journal of Clinical Endocrinology and Metabolism, 72*, 602–606.

Baker, J. H., Mazzeo, S. E., & Kendler, K. S. (2007). Association between broadly defined bulimia nervosa and drug use disorders: Common genetic and environmental influences. *International Journal of Eating Disorders, 40*, 673–678.

Ball, J., & Mitchell, P. (2004). A randomized controlled study of cognitive behavior therapy and behavioral family therapy for anorexia nervosa patients. *Eating Disorders, 12*, 303–314.

Baran, S. A., Weltzin, T. E., & Kaye, W. H. (1995). Low discharge weight and outcome in anorexia nervosa. *American Journal of Psychiatry, 152*, 1070–1072.

Barbarich, N. C., McConaha, C. W., Gaskill, J., La Via, M., Frank, G. K., Achenbach, S., . . . Kaye, W. H. (2004). An open trial of olanzapine in anorexia nervosa. *Journal of Clinical Psychiatry, 65*, 1480–1482.

Bardone-Cone, A. M., Abramson, L. Y., Vohs, K. D., Heatherton, T. F., & Joiner, T. E., Jr. (2006). Predicting bulimic symptoms: An interactive model of self-efficacy, perfectionism, and perceived weight status. *Behaviour Research and Therapy, 44*, 27–42.

Bardone-Cone, A. M., Harney, M. B., Maldonado, C. R., Lawson, M. A., Robinson, D. P., Smith, R., & Tosh, A. (2010). Defining recovery from an eating disorder: Conceptualization, validation, and examination of psychosocial functioning and psychiatric comorbidity. *Behaviour Research and Therapy, 48*, 194–202.

Bates, G. W., Bates, S. R., & Whitworth, N. S. (1982). Reproductive failure in women who practice weight control. *Fertility and Sterility, 37*, 373–378.

Bauer, S., Wolf, M., Haug, S., & Kordy, H. (2011). The effectiveness of Internet chat groups in relapse prevention after inpatient psychotherapy. *Psychotherapy Research, 21*, 219–226.

Becker, A. E. (1995). *Body, self, and society: The view from Fiji*. Philadelphia: University of Pennsylvania Press.

Becker, A. E., Arrindell, A. H., Perloe, A., Fay, K., & Striegel-Moore, R. H. (2010a). A qualitative study of perceived social barriers to care for eating disorders: Perspectives from ethnically diverse health care consumers. *International Journal of Eating Disorders, 43,* 633–647.

Becker, A. E., Burwell, R. A., Gilman, S. E., Herzog, D. B., & Hamburg, P. (2002). Eating behaviours and attitudes following prolonged television exposure among ethnic Fijian adolescent girls. *British Journal of Psychiatry, 180,* 509–514.

Becker, A. E., Fay, K., Agnew-Blais, J., Guarnaccia, P. M., Striegel-Moore, R. H., & Gilman, S. E. (2010b). Development of a measure of "acculturation" for ethnic Fijians: Methodologic and conceptual considerations for application to eating disorders research. *Transcultural Psychiatry, 47,* 754–788.

Becker, A. E., Fay, K., Agnew-Blais, J., Khan, A. N., Striegel-Moore, R. H., & Gilman, S. E. (2011). Social network media exposure and adolescent eating pathology in Fiji. *British Journal of Psychiatry, 198,* 43–50.

Becker, A. E., Franko, D., Speck, A., & Herzog, D. B. (2003). Ethnicity and differential access to care for eating disorder symptoms. *International Journal of Eating Disorders, 33,* 205–212.

Becker, A. E., Thomas, J. J., & Pike, K. M. (2009). Should non-fat-phobic anorexia nervosa be included in DSM-V? *International Journal of Eating Disorders, 42,* 620–635.

Becker, C. B., McDaniel, L., Bull, S., Powell, M., & McIntyre, K. (2012). Can we reduce eating disorder risk factors in female college athletes? A randomized exploratory investigation of two peer-led interventions. *Body Image, 9,* 31–42.

Beintner, A., Jacobi, C., & Taylor, C. B. (2012). Effects of an Internet-based prevention program for eating disorders in the U.S. and Germany: A meta-analytic review. *European Eating Disorders Review, 20,* 1–8.

Bello, N. T., & Hajnal, A. (2010). Dopamine and binge eating behaviors. *Pharmacology, Biochemistry, and Behavior, 97,* 25–33.

Bergen, A. W., Yeager, M., Welch, R. A., Haque, K., Ganjei, J. K., van den Bree, M. B., ... Kaye, W. H. (2005). Association of multiple DRD2 polymorphisms with anorexia nervosa. *Neuropsychopharmacology, 30,* 1703–1710.

Berger, U., Schaefer, J. M., Wick, K., Brix, C., Bormann, B., Sowa, M., ... Strauss, B. (2014). Effectiveness of reducing the risk of eating-related problems using the German school-based intervention program, "Torera", for preadolescent boys and girls. *Prevention Science, 15,* 557–569.

Berkman, N. D., Lohr, K. N., & Bulik, C. M. (2007). Outcomes of eating disorders: A systematic review of the literature. *International Journal of Eating Disorders, 40,* 293–309.

Berry, J. W., & Annis, R. C. (1974). Acculturative stress: The role of ecology, culture and differentiation. *Journal of Cross-Cultural Psychology, 5,* 382–406.

Bhugra, D., & Arya, P. (2005). Ethnic density, cultural congruity and mental illness in migrants. *International Review of Psychiatry, 17,* 133–137.

Bhugra, D., & Bhui, K. (2003). Eating disorders in teenagers in East London: A survey. *European Eating Disorders Review, 11,* 46–57.

Biederman, J., Herzog, D. B., Rivinus, T. M., Harper, G. P., Ferber, R. A., Rosenbaurm, J. F., ... Schildkraut, J. J. (1985). Amitriptyline in the treatment of anorexia nervosa: A double-blind placebo-controlled study. *Journal of Clinical Psychopharmacology, 5,* 10–16.

Birmingham, C. L., Goldmer, E. M., & Bakan, R. (1994). Controlled trial of zinc supplementation in anorexia nervosa. *International Journal of Eating Disorders, 15,* 251–255.

Bissada, H., Tasca, G. A., Barber, A. M., & Bradwejn, J. (2008). Olanzapine in the treatment of low body weight and obsessive thinking in women with anorexia nervosa: A randomized, double-blind, placebo-controlled trial. *American Journal of Psychiatry, 165,* 1281–1288.

Blinder, B. J., Cumella, E. J., & Sanathara, V. A. (2006). Psychiatric comorbidities of female inpatients with eating disorders. *Psychosomatic Medicine, 68,* 454–462.

Boachie, A., Goldfield, G. S., & Spettigue, W. (2003). Olanzapine use as an adjunctive treatment for hospitalized children with anorexia nervosa: Case reports. *International Journal of Eating Disorders, 33,* 98–103.

Bodell, L. P., & Keel, P. K. (2010). Current treatment for anorexia nervosa: Efficacy, safety and adherence. *Psychology Research and Behavior Management, 3,* 91–108.

Bodell, L. P., & Mayer, L. E. S. (2011). Percent body fat is a risk factor for relapse in anorexia nervosa: A replication study. *International Journal of Eating Disorders, 44,* 118–123.

Bohon, C., Stice, E., & Burton, E. (2009). Maintenance factors for persistence of bulimic pathology: A prospective natural history study. *International Journal of Eating Disorders, 42,* 173–178.

Boland, B., Beguin, C., Zech, F., Desager, J. P., & Lambert, M. (2001). Serum beta-carotene in anorexia nervosa patients: A case-control study.

International Journal of Eating Disorders, 30, 299–305.

Bonjour, J. P., Theintz, G., Buchs, B., Slosman, D., & Rizzoli, R. (1991). Critical years and stages of puberty for spinal and femoral bone mass accumulation during adolescence. *Journal of Clinical Endocrinology and Metabolism, 73,* 555–563.

Boraska, V., Davis, O. S., Cherkas, L. F., Helder, S. G., Harris, J., Krug, I., ... Zeggini, E. (2012). Genome-wide association analysis of eating disorder-related symptoms, behaviors, and personality traits. *American Journal of Medical Genetics. Part B, Neuropsychiatric Genetics, 159B,* 803–811.

Bosanac, P., Kurlender, S., Norman, T., Hallam, K., Wesnes, K., Manktelow, T., & Burrows, G. (2007). An open-label study of quetiapine in anorexia nervosa. *Human Psychopharmacology, 22,* 223–230.

Brambilla, F., Amianto, F., Grave, R. D., & Fassino, S. (2014). Lack of efficacy of psychological and pharmacological treatments of disorders of eating behavior: Neurobiological background. *BMC Psychiatry, 14,* 376. http://bmcpsychiatry.biomedcentral.com/articles/10.1186/s12888-014-0376-7

Brambilla, F., Garcia, C. S., Fassino, S., Daga, G. A., Favaro, A., Santonastaso, P., ... Monteleone, P. (2007). Olanzapine therapy in anorexia nervosa: Psychobiological effects. *International Clinical Psychopharmacology, 22,* 197–204.

Braun, D. L., Sunday, S. R., & Halmi, K. A. (1994). Psychiatric comorbidity in patients with eating disorders. *Psychological Medicine, 24,* 859–867.

Bravender, T., Bryant-Waugh, R., Herzog, D., Katzman, D., Kriepe, R. D., Lask, B., ... Zucker, N.; Workgroup for Classification of Eating Disorders in Children and Adolescents. (2010). Classification of eating disturbance in children and adolescents: Proposed changes for the DSM-V. *European Eating Disorders Review, 18,* 79–89.

Brewerton, T. D., Lydiard, R. B., Herzog, D. B., Brotman, A. W., O'Neil, P. M., & Ballenger, J. C. (1995). Comorbidity of Axis I psychiatric disorders in bulimia nervosa. *Journal of Clinical Psychiatry, 56,* 77–80.

Brietzke, E., Moreira, C. L., Toniolo, R. A., & Lafer, B. (2011). Clinical correlates of eating disorder comorbidity in women with bipolar disorder type I. *Journal of Affective Disorders, 130,* 162–165.

Broft, A. I., Spanos, A., Corwin, R.,L., Mayer, L., Steinglass, J., Devlin, M. J., ... Walsh, B. T. (2007). Baclofen for binge eating: An open-label trial. *International Journal of Eating Disorders, 40,* 687–691.

Brownell, K. (1991). Dieting and the search for the perfect body: Where physiology and culture collide. *Behavior Therapy, 22,* 1–12.

Brownell, K. D., Marlatt, G. A., Lichtenstein, E., & Wilson, G. T. (1986). Understanding and preventing relapse. *American Psychologist, 41,* 765–782.

Bruch, H. (1973). *Eating disorders.* New York: Basic Books.

Brumberg, J. J. (1988). *Fasting girls: The history of anorexia nervosa.* Cambridge, MA: Harvard University Press.

Bryant-Waugh, R., Markham, L., Kreipe, R. E., & Walsh, B. T. (2010). Feeding and eating disorders in childhood. *International Journal of Eating Disorders, 43,* 98–111.

Buchholz, A., Mack, H., McVey, G., Feder, S., & Barrowman, N. (2008). BodySense: An evaluation of a positive body image intervention on sport climate for female athletes. *Eating, 16,* 308–321.

Bulik, C. M. (2005). Exploring the gene-environment nexus in eating disorders. *Journal of Psychiatry & Neuroscience, 30,* 335–339.

Bulik, C. M., Berkman, N. D., Brownley, K. A., Sedway, J. A., & Lohr, K. N. (2007). Anorexia nervosa treatment: A systematic review of randomized controlled treatment trials. *International Journal of Eating Disorders, 40,* 310–320.

Bulik, C. M., Devlin, B., Bacanu, S. A., Thornton, L., Klump, K. L., Fichter, M. M., ... Kaye, W. H. (2003). Significant linkage on chromosome 10p in families with bulimia nervosa. *American Journal of Human Genetics, 72,* 200–207.

Bulik, C. M., Slof-Op't Landt, M. C., van Furth, E. F., & Sullivan, P. F. (2007). The genetics of anorexia nervosa. *Annual Review of Nutrition, 27,* 263–275.

Bulik, C. M., Sullivan, P. F., Fear, J. L., & Joyce, P. R. (1997). Eating disorders and antecedent anxiety disorders: A controlled study. *Acta Psychiatrica Scandinavica, 96,* 101–107.

Bulik, C., Sullivan, P., Fear, J., & Pickering, A. (2000). Outcome of anorexia nervosa: Eating attitudes, personality, and parental bonding. *International Journal of Eating Disorders, 28,* 139–147.

Bulik, C., Sullivan, P., Fear, J., Pickering, A., & Dawn, A. (1999). Fertility and reproduction in women with anorexia nervosa: A controlled study. *Journal of Clinical Psychiatry, 60,* 130–135.

Bulik, C. M., Sullivan, P. F., & Joyce, P. R. (1997). Eating disorders and antecedent anxiety disorders: A controlled study. *Acta Psychiatrica Scandanavia, 96,* 101–107.

Bulik, C. M., Sullivan, P. F., & Kendler, K. S. (2003). Genetic and environmental contributions to obesity and binge eating. *International Journal of Eating Disorders, 33,* 293–298.

Bulik, C. M., Sullivan, P. F., McKee, M., Weltzin, T. E., & Kaye, W. H. (1994). Characteristics of bulimic women with and without alcohol abuse. *American Journal of Drug and Alcohol Abuse, 20,* 273–283.

Bulik, C., Sullivan, P., Wade, T., & Kendler, K. (2000). Twin studies of eating disorders: A review. *International Journal of Eating Disorders, 27,* 1–20.

Bulik, C. M., Tozzi, F., Anderson, C., Mazzeo, S. E., Aggen, S., & Sullivan, P. F. (2003). The relation between eating disorders and components of perfectionism. *American Journal of Psychiatry, 160,* 366–368.

Bulik, C. M., Von Holle, A., Hamer, R., Knoph Berg, C., Torgersen, L., Magnus, P., ... Reichborn-Kjennerud, T. (2007). Patterns of remission, continuation and incidence of broadly defined eating disorders during early pregnancy in the Norwegian Mother and Child Cohort Study (MoBa). *Psychological Medicine, 37,* 1109–1118.

Bulik, C.M., Von Holle, A., Siega-Riz, A. M., Torgersen, L., Lie, K. K., Hamer, R. M., ... Reichborn-Kjennerud T. (2009). Birth outcomes in women with eating disorders in the Norwegian Mother and Child Cohort Study (MoBa). *International Journal of Eating Disorders, 42,* 9–18.

Burnet, P. W., Smith, K. A., Cowen, P. J., Fairburn, C. G., & Harrison, P. J. (1999). Allelic variation of the 5-HT2C receptor (HTR2C) in bulimia nervosa and binge eating disorder. *Psychiatric Genetics, 9,* 101–104.

Butryn, M. L., Juarascio, A., & Lowe, M. R. (2011). The relation of weight suppression and BMI to bulimic symptoms. *International Journal of Eating Disorders, 44,* 612–617.

Butryn, M. L., & Wadden, T. A. (2005). Treatment of overweight in children and adolescents: Does dieting increase the risk of eating disorders? *International Journal of Eating Disorders, 37,* 285–293.

Cadogan, J., Eastell, R., Jones, N., & Barker, M. E. (1997). Milk intake and bone mineral acquisition in adolescent girls: Randomised, controlled intervention trial. *British Medical Journal, 315,* 1255–1260.

Carrard, I., Norring, C., Fernandez-Aranda, F., Lam, T., Nevonen, L., Liwowsky, I., ... Van der Linden, M. (2011). Evaluation of a guided Internet self-treatment programme for bulimia nervosa in several European countries. *European Eating Disorders Review, 19,* 138–149.

Carretero-Garcia, A., Sanchez Planell, L., Doval, E., Rusinol Estragues, J., Raich Escursell, R. M., & Vanderlinden, J. (2012). Repeated traumatic experiences in eating disorders and their association with eating symptoms. *Eating and Weight Disorders, 17,* e267–e273.

Carter, J. C., Bewell, C., Blackmore, E., & Woodside, D. B. (2006). The impact of childhood sexual abuse in anorexia nervosa. *Child Abuse & Neglect, 30,* 257–269.

Carter, J. C., Blackmore, E., Sutandar-Pinnock, K., & Woodside, D. B. (2004). Relapse in anorexia nervosa: A survival analysis. *Psychological Medicine, 34,* 671–679.

Carter, J. C., McFarlane, T. L., Bewell, C., Olmsted, M. P., Woodside, D. B., Kaplan, A. S., & Crosby, R. D. (2009). Maintenance treatment for anorexia nervosa: A comparison of cognitive behavior therapy and treatment as usual. *International Journal of Eating Disorders, 42,* 202–207.

Carter, J. C., Stewart, D. A., Dunn, V. J., & Fairburn, C. G. (1997). Primary prevention of eating disorders: Might it do more harm than good? *International Journal of Eating Disorders, 22,* 167–172.

Casiero, D., & Frishman, W. H. (2006). Cardiovascular complications of eating disorders. *Cardiology in Review, 14,* 227–231.

Cassin, S. E., & von Ranson, K. M. (2005). Personality and eating disorders: A decade in review. *Clinical Psychology Review, 25,* 895–916.

Castellini, G., Lo Sauer, C., Mannucci, E., Ravaldi, C., Rotella, C. M., Faravelli, C., & Ricca, V. (2011). Diagnostic crossover and outcome predictors in eating disorders according to DSM-IV and DSM-5 proposed criteria: A 6-year follow-up study. *Psychosomatic Medicine, 73,* 270–279.

Castro-Fornieles, J., Díaz, R., Goti, J., Calvo, R., Gonzalez, L., Serrano, L., & Gual, A. (2010). Prevalence and factors related to substance use among adolescents with eating disorders. *European Addiction Research, 16,* 61–68.

Cattarin, J. A., & Thompson, J. K. (1994). A 3-year longitudinal study of body image, eating disturbance, and general psychological functioning in adolescent females. *Eating Disorders, 2,* 114–125.

Chao, Y. M., Pisetsky, E. M., Dierker, L. C., Dohm, F. A., Rosselli, F., May, A. M., & Striegel-Moore, R. H. (2008). Ethnic differences in weight control practices among U.S. adolescents from 1995 to 2005. *International Journal of Eating Disorders, 41*, 124–133.

Chisuwa, N., & O'Dea, J. A. (2010). Body image and eating disorders amongst Japanese adolescents: A review of the literature. *Appetite, 54*, 5–15.

Chumlea, W. C., Schubert, C. M., Roche, A. F., Kulin, H. E., Lee, P. A., Himes, J. H., & Sun S. S. (2003). Age at menarche and racial comparisons in US girls. *Pediatrics, 111*, 110–113.

Claes, L., & Vandereycken, W. (2007). Is there a link between traumatic experiences and self-injurious behaviors in eating-disordered patients? *Eating Disorders, 15*, 305–315.

Cnattingius, S., Hultman, C., Dahl, M., & Sparen, P. (1999). Very preterm birth, birth trauma, and the risk of anorexia nervosa among girls. *Archives of General Psychiatry, 56*, 634–638.

Collins, A. L., & Sullivan, P. F. (2013). Genome-wide association studies in psychiatry: What have we learned? *British Journal of Psychiatry, 202*, 1–4.

Cooley, E., & Toray, T. (2001). Body image and personality predictors of eating disorder symptoms during the college years. *International Journal of Eating Disorders, 30*, 28–36.

Cooper, P., Watkins, B., Bryant-Waugh, R., & Lask, B. (2002). The nosological status of early onset anorexia nervosa. *Psychological Medicine, 32*, 873–880.

Copeland, W. E., Bulik, C. M., Zucker, N., Wolke, D., Lereya, S. T., & Costello, E. J. (2015). Does childhood bullying predict eating disorder symptoms? A prospective, longitudinal analysis. *International Journal of Eating Disorders, 48*, 1141–1149.

Couturier, J., Kimber, M., & Szatmari, P. (2013). Efficacy of family-based treatment for adolescents with eating disorders: A systematic review and meta-analysis. *International Journal of Eating Disorders, 46*, 3–11.

Croll, J., Neumark-Sztainer, D., Story, M., & Ireland, M. (2002). Prevalence and risk and protective factors related to disordered eating behaviors among adolescents: Relationship to gender and ethnicity. *Journal of Adolescent Health, 31*, 166–175.

Crow, S. J., Mitchell, J. E., Roerig, J. D., & Steffen, K. (2009). What potential role is there for medication treatment in anorexia nervosa? *International Journal of Eating Disorders, 42*, 1–8.

Crow, S. J., Peterson, C. B., Swanson, S. A., Raymond, N. C., Specker, S., Eckert, E. D., & Mitchell, J. E. (2009). Increased mortality in bulimia nervosa and other eating disorders. *American Journal of Psychiatry, 166*, 1342–1346.

Currin, L., Schmidt, U., Treasure, J., & Jick, H. (2005). Time trends in eating disorder incidence. *British Journal of Psychiatry, 186*, 132–135.

Dalle Grave, R., Calugi, S., Doll, H. A., & Fairburn, C. G. (2013). Enhanced cognitive behaviour therapy for adolescents with anorexia nervosa: An alternative to family therapy? *Behavior Research and Therapy, 51*, 9–12.

Dalle Grave, R., Calugi, A., Ghoch, M., Conti, M., & Fairburn, C. (2014). Inpatient cognitive behavior therapy for adolescents with anorexia nervosa: Immediate and longer-term effects. *Frontiers in Psychiatry, 5*, 14.

Dansky, B. S., Brewerton, T. D., & Kilpatrick, D. G. (2000). Comorbidity of bulimia nervosa and alcohol use disorders: Results from the National Women's Study. *International Journal of Eating Disorders, 27*, 180–190.

Dare, C., Eisler, I., Russell, G., Treasure, J., & Dodge, L. (2001). Psychological therapies for adults with anorexia nervosa: Randomised controlled trial of outpatient treatments. *British Journal of Psychiatry, 178*, 216–221.

Davis, C., Levitan, R. D., Kaplan, A. S., Carter, J., Reid, C., Curtis, C., . . . Kennedy, J. L. (2008). Reward sensitivity and the D2 dopamine receptor gene: A case-control study of binge eating disorder. *Progress in Neuro-psychopharmacology & Biological Psychiatry, 32*, 620–628.

Day, J., Schmidt, U., Collier, D., Perkins, S., Van den Eynde, F., Treasure, J., . . . Eisler, I. (2011). Risk factors, correlates, and markers in early-onset bulimia nervosa and EDNOS. *International Journal of Eating Disorders, 44*, 287–294.

Decaluwé, V., & Braet, C. (2003). Prevalence of binge-eating disorder in obese children and adolescents seeking weight-loss treatment. *International Journal of Obesity and Related Metabolic Disorders, 27*, 404–409.

Decaluwé, V., Braet, C., & Fairburn, C. G. (2003). Binge eating in obese children and adolescents. *International Journal of Eating Disorders, 33*, 78–84.

De Caprio, C., Alfano, A., Senatore, I., Zarrella, L., Pasanisi, F., & Contaldo, F. (2006). Severe acute liver damage in anorexia nervosa: Two case reports. *Nutrition, 22*, 572–575.

Delgado, M. R., Nystrom, L. E., Fissell, C., Noll, D. C., & Fiez, J. A. (2000). Tracking the hemodynamic responses to reward and punishment in the striatum. *Journal of Neurophysiology, 84*, 3072–3077.

Dellava, J. E., Kendler, K. S., & Neale, M. C. (2011). Generalized anxiety disorder and anorexia nervosa: Evidence of shared genetic variation. *Depression and Anxiety*, *28*, 728–733.

Demyttenaere, K., Bruffaerts, R., Posada-Villa, J., Gasquet, I., Kovess, V., Lepine, J. P., ... Chatterji, S. (2004). Prevalence, severity, and unmet need for treatment of mental disorders in the World Health Organization World Mental Health Surveys. *Journal of the American Medical Association*, *291*, 2581–2590.

Dennis, K., Le Grange, D., & Bremer, J. (2006). Olanzapine use in adolescent anorexia nervosa. *Eating and Weight Disorders*, *11*, e53–e56.

DeSocio, J. E. (2013). The neurobiology of risk and pre-emptive interventions for anorexia nervosa. *Journal of Child and Adolescent Psychiatric Nursing*, *26*, 16–22.

Devlin, B., Bacanu, S. A., Klump, K. L., Bulik, C. M., Fichter, M. M., Halmi, K. A., ... Kaye, W. H. (2002). Linkage analysis of anorexia nervosa incorporating behavioral covariates. *Human Molecular Genetics*, *11*, 689–696.

de Zwaan, M., Mitchell, J. E., Seim, H. C., Specker, S. M., Pyle, R. L., Raymond, N. C., & Crosby, R. B. (1994). Eating related and general psychopathology in obese females with binge eating disorder. *International Journal of Eating Disorders*, *15*, 43–52.

DiVasta, A. D., Feldman, H. A., Quach, A. E., Balestrino, M., & Gordon, C. M. (2009). The effect of bed rest on bone turnover in young women hospitalized for anorexia nervosa: A pilot study. *Journal of Clinical Endocrinology and Metabolism*, *94*, 1650–1655.

Downey, C. A., & Chang, E. C. (2007). Perfectionism and symptoms of eating disturbances in female college students: Considering the role of negative affect and body dissatisfaction. *Eating Behaviors*, *8*, 497–503.

Eckert, E. D., Halmi, K. A., Marchi, P., Grove, W., & Crosby, R. (1995). Ten-year follow-up of anorexia nervosa: Clinical course and outcome. *Psychological Medicine*, *25*, 143–156.

Eddy, K. T., Keel, P. K., Dorer, D. J., Delinsky, S. S., Franko, D. L., & Herzog, D. B. (2002). Longitudinal comparison of anorexia nervosa subtypes. *International Journal of Eating Disorders*, *31*, 191–201.

Eisler, I. (2010, September). *A randomized controlled study of multi-family versus single-family therapy for adolescent anorexia nervosa*. Paper presented at the annual Eating Disorders Research Society meeting, Cambridge, MA.

Eisler, I., Dare, C., Hodes, M., Russell, G., Dodge, E., & Le Grange, D. (2000). Family therapy for adolescent anorexia nervosa: The results of a controlled comparison of two family interventions. *Journal of Child Psychology and Psychiatry*, *41*, 727–736.

Eisler, I., Dare, C., Russell, G. F., Szmukler, G., Le Grange, D., & Dodge, E. (1997). Family and individual therapy in anorexia nervosa: A 5-year follow-up. *Archives of General Psychiatry*, *54*, 1025–1030.

Eisler, I., Simic, M., Russell, G. F. M., & Dare, C. (2007). A randomized controlled treatment trial of two forms of family therapy in adolescent anorexia nervosa: A five-year follow-up. *Journal of Child Psychology and Psychiatry*, *48*, 552–560.

Enzmann, D. R., & Lane, B. (1977). Cranial computed tomography findings in anorexia nervosa. *Journal of Computer Assisted Tomography*, *1*, 410–414.

Espinoza, P., Penelo, E., & Raich, R. M. (2010). Disordered eating behaviors and body image in a longitudinal pilot study of adolescent girls: What happens 2 years later? *Body Image*, *7*, 70–73.

Fairburn, C. G. (2008). *Cognitive behavior therapy and eating disorders*. New York: Guilford Press.

Fairburn, C. G., Cooper, Z., Doll, H., Norman, P., & O'Connor, M. (2000). The natural course of bulimia nervosa and binge eating disorder in young women. *Archives of General Psychiatry*, *57*, 659–665.

Fairburn, C. G., Cooper, Z., Doll, H., & Welch, S. L. (1999). Risk factors for anorexia nervosa. *Archives of General Psychiatry*, *56*, 468–476.

Fairburn, C. G., Doll, H. A., Welch, S. L., Hay, P. J., Davies, B. A., & O'Connor, M. E. (1998). Risk factors for binge eating disorder: A community-based, case-control study. *Archives of General Psychiatry*, *55*, 425–432.

Fairburn, C. G., Marcus, M., & Wilson, G. T. (1993). Cognitive-behavioral therapy for binge eating and bulimia nervosa: A comprehensive treatment manual. In C. G. Fairburn & G. T. Wilson (Eds.), *Binge eating: Nature, assessment and treatment* (pp. 361–404). New York: Guilford Press.

Fairburn, C. G., Norman, P. A., Welch, S. L., O'Connor, M. E., Doll, H. A., & Peveler, R. C. (1995). A prospective study of outcome in bulimia nervosa and the long-term effects of three psychological treatments. *Archives of General Psychiatry*, *52*, 304–312.

Fairburn, C. G., Peveler, R. C., Jones, R., Hope, R. A., & Doll, H. A. (1993). Predictors of 12-month outcome in bulimia nervosa and the influence of attitudes to shape and weight. *Journal of Consulting and Clinical Psychology, 61*, 696–698.

Fairburn, C. G., Welch, S. L., Doll, H. A., Davies, B. A., & O'Connor, M. E. (1997). Risk factors for bulimia nervosa: A community-based case-control study. *Archives of General Psychiatry, 54*, 509–517.

Fallon, B. A., Sadik, C., Saoud, J. B., & Garfinkel, R. S. (1994). Childhood abuse, family environment, and outcome in bulimia nervosa. *Journal of Clinical Psychiatry, 55*, 424–428.

Faris, P. L., Kim, S. W., Meller, W. H., Goodale, R. L., Oakman, S. A., Hofbauer, R. D., ... Hartman, B. K. (2000). Effect of decreasing afferent vagal activity with ondansetron on symptoms of bulimia nervosa: A randomised, double-blind trial. *Lancet, 355*, 792–797.

Faulkner, R. A., Bailey, D. A., Drinkwater, D. T., McKay, H. A., Arnold, C., & Wilkinson, A. A. (1996). Bone densitometry in Canadian children 8–17 years of age. *Calcified Tissue International, 59*, 344–351.

Favaro, A., Caregaro, L., Tenconi, E., Bosello, R., & Santonastaso, P. (2009). Time trends in age at onset of anorexia nervosa and bulimia nervosa. *Journal of Clinical Psychiatry, 70*, 1715–1721.

Favaro, A., Tenconi, E., Bosello, R., Degortes, D., & Santonastaso, P. (2011). Perinatal complications in unaffected sisters of anorexia nervosa patients: Testing a covariation model between genetic and environmental factors. *European Archives of Psychiatry and Clinical Neuroscience, 261*, 391–396.

Favaro, A., Tenconi, E., & Santonastaso, P. (2006). Perinatal factors and the risk of developing anorexia nervosa and bulimia nervosa. *Archives of General Psychiatry, 63*, 82–88.

Fernández-Aranda, F., Nunez, A., Martinez, C., Krug, I., Cappozzo, M., Carrard, I., ... Lam, T. (2008). Internet-based cognitive-behavioral therapy for bulimia nervosa: A controlled study. *Cyberpsychology and Behavior, 12*, 37–41.

Fernandez-Aranda, F., Pinheiro, A. P., Tozzi, F., Thornton, L. M., Fichter, M. M., Halmi, K. A., ... Bulik, C. M. (2007). Symptom profile of major depressive disorder in women with eating disorders. *Australian and New Zealand Journal of Psychiatry, 41*, 24–31.

Fichter, M. M., Kruger, R., Rief, W., Holland, R., & Dohne, J. (1996). Fluvoxamine in prevention of relapse in bulimia nervosa: Effects on eating-specific psychopathology. *Journal of Clinical Psychopharmacology, 16*, 9–18.

Fichter, M., & Quadflieg, N. (1997) Six-year course of bulimia nervosa. *International Journal of Eating Disorders, 22*, 361–384.

Fichter, M. M., Quadflieg, N., Nisslmüller, K., Lindner, S., Osen, B., Huber, T., & Wünsch-Leiteritz, W. (2012). Does Internet-based prevention reduce the risk of relapse for anorexia nervosa? *Behaviour Research and Therapy, 50*, 180–190.

Field, A., Camargo, C., Taylor, C., Berkey, C., Frazier, A., Gillman, M., & Colditz, G. A. (1999). Overweight, weight concerns, and bulimic behaviors among girls and boys. *Journal of American Academy of Child Adolescent Psychiatry, 38*, 754–760.

Field, A. E., Camargo, C. A., Taylor, C. B., Berkey, C. S., Roberts, S. B., & Colditz, G. A. (2001). Peer, parent, and media influences on the development of weight concerns and frequent dieting among preadolescent and adolescent girls and boys. *Pediatrics, 107*, 54–60.

Field, A. E., Colditz, G. A., Herzog, D. B., & Heatherton, T. F. (1996). Disordered eating: Can women accurately recall their binging and purging behaviors 10 years later? *Obesity Research, 4*, 153–159.

Field, A. E., Javaras, K. M., Aneja, P., Kitos, N., Camargo, C. A., Jr., Taylor, C. B., & Laird, N. M. (2008). Family, peer, and media predictors of becoming eating disordered. *Archives of Pediatric and Adolescent Medicine, 162*, 574–579.

Field, A. E., Sonneville, K. R., Micali, N., Crosby, R. D., Swanson, S. A., Laird, N. M., ... Horton, N. J. (2012). Prospective association of common eating disorders and adverse outcomes. *Pediatrics, 130*, e289–e295.

Fischer, S., & Le Grange, D. (2007). Comorbidity and high-risk behaviors in treatment-seeking adolescents with bulimia nervosa. *International Journal of Eating Disorders, 40*, 751–753.

Fisher, C. A., Hetrick, S. E., & Rushford, N. (2010). Family therapy for anorexia nervosa. *Cochrane Database of Systematic Reviews*, (4):CD004780.

Fisher, M. M., Rosen, D. S., Ornstein, R. M., Mammel, K. A., Katzman, D. K., Rome, E. S., ... Walsh, B. T. (2014). Characteristics of avoidant/restrictive food intake disorder in children and adolescents: A "new disorder" in DSM-5. *Journal of Adolescent Health, 55*, 49–52.

Fisman, S., Steele, M., Short, J., Byrne, T., & Lavallee, C. (1996). Case study: Anorexia nervosa and autistic disorder in an adolescent girl. *Journal of the American Academy of Child and Adolescent Psychiatry, 35*, 937–940.

Fitzpatrick, K. K., Moye, A., Hoste, R., Lock, J., & Le Grange, D. (2010). Adolescent focused psychotherapy for adolescents with anorexia nervosa. *Journal of Contemporary Psychology, 40*, 31–39.

Fitzsimmons-Craft, E., Bardone-Cone, A., Bulik, C., Wonderlich, S., Crosby, R., & Engel, S. (2013). Examining an elaborated sociocultural model of disordered eating among college women: The roles of social comparison and body surveillance (under review).

Flament, M. F., Bissada, H., & Spettigue, W. (2012). Evidence-based pharmacotherapy of eating disorders. *International Journal of Neuropsychopharmacology, 15*, 189–207.

Foerde, K., Steinglass, J., Shohamy, D., & Walsh, B. T. (2015). Neural mechanisms supporting maladaptive food choices in anorexia nervosa. *Nature Neuroscience, 18*, 1571–1573.

Fornaro, M., Perugi, G., Gabrielli, F., Prestia, D., Mattei, C., Vinciguerra, V. & Fornaro, P. (2010). Lifetime co-morbidity with different subtypes of eating disorders in 148 females with bipolar disorders. *Journal of Affective Disorders, 121*, 147–151.

Foulon, C., Guilfi, J. D., Kipman, A., Adés, J., Romo, L., Houdeyer, K., ... Gorwood, P. (2007). Switching to the bingeing/purging subtype of anorexia nervosa is frequently associated with suicidal attempts. *European Psychiatry, 22*, 513–519.

Fowler, S., & Bulik, C. (1997). Family environment and psychiatric history in women with binge eating disorder and obese controls. *Behaviour Change, 14*, 106–112.

Frank, E., Prien, R., Jarnett, R., Keller, M. B., Kupfer, D., Lavori, P. W., ... Weissman, M. (1991). Conceptualization and rationale for consensus definitions of terms in major depressive disorders: Response, remission, recovery, relapse and recurrence. *Archives of General Psychiatry, 48*, 851–855.

Frank, G. K. (2012). Advances in the diagnosis of anorexia nervosa and bulimia nervosa using brain imaging. *Expert Opinion on Medical Diagnostics, 6*, 235–244.

Frank, G. K. (2016). Aripiprazole, a partial dopamine agonist to improve adolescent anorexia nervosa: A case series. *International Journal of Eating Disorders, 49*, 529–533.

Franko, D. L., Becker, A. E., Thomas, J. J., & Herzog, D. B. (2007). Cross-ethnic differences in eating disorder symptoms and related distress. *International Journal of Eating Disorders, 40*, 156–164.

Franko, D., Blais, M., Becker, A., Delinsky, S., Greenwood, D., Flores, A., ... Herzog, D. B. (2001). Pregnancy complications and neonatal outcomes in women with eating disorders. *American Journal of Psychiatry, 158*, 1461–1466.

Franko, D. L., Keshaviah, A., Eddy, K. T., Krishna, M., Davis, M. C., Keel, P. K., & Herzog, D. B. (2013). A longitudinal investigation of mortality in anorexia nervosa and bulimia nervosa. *American Journal of Psychiatry, 170*, 917–925.

French, S., Perry, C., Leon, G., & Fulkerson, J. (1995). Changes in psychological variables and health behaviors by dieting status over a three-year period in a cohort of adolescent females. *Journal of Adolescent Health, 16*, 438–447.

French, S., Story, M., Downes, B., Resnick, M., & Blum, R. (1995). Frequent dieting among adolescents: Psychosocial and health behavior correlates. *American Journal of Public Health, 85*, 695–701.

Friederich, H. C., Kumari, V., Uher, R., Riga, M., Schmidt, U., Campbell, I. C., ... Treasure, J. (2006). Differential motivational responses to food and pleasurable cues in anorexia and bulimia nervosa: A startle reflex paradigm. *Psychological Medicine, 36*, 1327–1335.

Furuta, S., Ozawa, Y., Maejima, K., Tashiro, H., Kitahora, T., Hasegawa, K., ... Ikuta, N. (1999). Anorexia nervosa with severe liver dysfunction and subsequent critical complications. *Internal Medicine, 38*, 575–579.

Gadalla, T., & Piran, N. (2007). Co-occurrence of eating disorders and alcohol use disorders in women: A meta-analysis. *Archives of Womens Mental Health, 10*, 133–140.

Galetta, F., Franzoni, F., Cupisti, A., Belliti, D., Prattichizzo, F., & Rolla, M. (2002). QT interval dispersion in young women with anorexia nervosa. *Journal of Pediatrics, 140*, 456–460.

Garber, A. K., Michihata, N., Hetnal, K., Shafer, M. A., & Moscicki, A. B. (2012). A prospective examination of weight gain in hospitalized adolescents with anorexia nervosa on a recommended refeeding protocol. *Journal of Adolescent Health, 50*, 24–29.

Garfinkel, P. E., & Garner, D. M. (1983). The multidetermined nature of anorexia nervosa. In P. L. Darby, P. E. Garfinkel, D. M. Garner, & D. V. Coscina (Eds.), *Anorexia nervosa: Recent developments in research* (pp. 3–14). New York: Alan R. Liss.

Garner, D. M., & Needleman, L. D. (1997). Sequencing and integration of treatments. In D. M. Garner & P. E. Garfinkel (Eds.), *Handbook of treatment for eating disorders* (2nd ed., pp. 50–66). New York: Guilford Press.

Garner, D. M., Vitousek, K. M., & Pike, K. M. (1997). Cognitive-behavioral therapy for anorexia nervosa. In D. M. Garner & P. E. Garfinkel (Eds.), *Handbook of treatment for eating disorders* (2nd ed., pp. 94–144). New York: Guilford Press.

Garnett, B. R., Buelow, R., Franko, D. L., Becker, C., Rodgers, R. F., & Austin, S. B. (2014). The importance of campaign saliency as a predictor of attitude and behavior change: A pilot evaluation of social marketing campaign Fat Talk Free Week®. *Health Communications, 29*, 984–995.

Geller, B., Reising, D., Leonard, H. L., Riddle, M. A., & Walsh, B. T. (1999). Critical review of tricyclic antidepressant use in children and adolescents. *Journal of the American Academy of Child and Adolescent Psychiatry, 38*, 513–516.

Gentile, M. G., Pastorelli, P., Ciceri, R., Manna, G. M., & Collimedaglia, S. (2010). Specialized refeeding treatment for anorexia nervosa patients suffering from extreme undernutrition. *Clinical Nutrition, 29*, 627–632.

Giovanni, A. D., Carla, G., Enrica, M., Federico, A., Maria, Z., & Secondo, F. (2011). Eating disorders and major depression: Role of anger and personality. *Depression Research and Treatment, 2011*, 194732.

Glastre, C., Braillon, P., David, L., Cochat, P., Meunier, P. J., & Delmas, P. D. (1990). Measurement of bone mineral content of the lumbar spine by dual energy x-ray absorptiometry in normal children: Correlations with growth parameters. *Journal of Clinical Endocrinology and Metabolism, 70*, 1330–1333.

Godart, N., Berthoz, S., Perdereau, F., & Jeammet, P. (2006). Comorbidity of anxiety with eating disorders and OCD. *American Journal of Psychiatry, 163*, 326.

Godart, N. T., Flament, M. F., Lecrubier, Y., & Jeammet, P. (2000). Anxiety disorders in anorexia nervosa and bulimia nervosa: Comorbidity and chronology of appearance. *European Psychiatry, 15*, 38–45.

Godart, N. T., Flament, M. F., Perdereau, F., & Jeammet, P. (2002). Comorbidity between eating disorders and anxiety disorders: A review. *International Journal of Eating Disorders, 32*, 253–270.

Goebel, G., Schweiger, U., Kruger, R., & Fichter, M. M. (1999). Predictors of bone mineral density in patients with eating disorders. *International Journal of Eating Disorders, 25*, 143–150.

Golden, N. H. (2010). Osteoporosis in anorexia nervosa. *Expert Reviews in Endocrinology and Metabolism, 5*, 723–732.

Golden, N. H., Ashtari, M., Kohn, M. R., Patel, M., Jacobson, M. S., Fletcher, A., & Shenker, I. R. (1996). Reversibility of cerebral ventricular enlargement in anorexia nervosa, demonstrated by quantitative magnetic resonance imaging. *Journal of Pediatrics, 128*, 296–301.

Golden, N. H., & Attia, E. (2011). Psychopharmacology of eating disorders in children and adolescents. *Pediatric Clinics of North America, 58*, 121–138.

Golden, N. H., Iglesias, E. A., Jacobson, M. S., Carey, D., Meyer, W., Schebendach, J., ... Shenker, I. R. (2005). Alendronate for the treatment of osteopenia in anorexia nervosa: A randomized, double-blind, placebo-controlled trial. *Journal of Clinical Endocrinology and Metabolism, 90*, 3179–3185.

Golden, N. H., Jacobson, M. S., Schebendach, J., Solanto, M. V., Hertz, S. M., & Shenker, I. R. (1997). Resumption of menses in anorexia nervosa. *Archives of Pediatrics and Adolescent Medicine, 151*, 16–21.

Golden, N. H., Katzman, D. K., Sawyer, S.M., Ornstein, R.M., Rome, E.S., Garber, A.K., ... Kreipe, R. E. (2015). Medical management of restrictive eating disorders in adolescents and young adults: A position paper of the Society for Adolescent Medicine. *Journal of Adolescent Health, 56*, 121–125.

Golden, N. H., Keane-Miller, C., Sainani, K. L., & Kapphahn, C. J. (2013). Higher caloric intake in hospitalized adolescents with anorexia nervosa is associated with reduced length of stay and no increased rate of refeeding syndrome. *Journal of Adolescent Health, 53*, 573–578.

Golden, N. H., Lanzkowsky, L., Schebendach, J., Palestro, C. J., Jacobson, M. S., & Shenker, I. R. (2002). The effect of estrogen-progestin treatment on bone mineral density in anorexia nervosa. *Journal of Pediatric and Adolescent Gynecology, 15*, 135–143.

Golden, N. H., & Shenker, I. R. (1992). Amenorrhrea in anorexia nervosa: Etiology and implications. In M. P. Nussbaum & J. T. Dwer (Eds.), *Adolescent nutrition and eating disorders* (3rd ed., pp. 503–518). Philadelphia: Hanley & Belfus, Inc.

Golden, N. H., Yang, W., Jacobson, M. S., Robinson, T., & Shaw, G. M. (2012). Expected body weight in adolescents: Comparison between weight-for-stature and BMI methods. *Pediatrics, 130*, e1607–e1613.

Goldschmidt, A. B., Wall, M., Loth, K. A., Le Grange, D., & Neumark-Sztainer, D. (2012). Which dieters are at risk for the onset of binge eating? A prospective study of adolescents and young adults. *Journal of Adolescent Health, 51*, 86–92.

Goodman, A., Heshmati, A., Malki, N., & Koupil, I. (2014). Associations between birth characteristics and eating disorders across the life course: Findings from 2 million males and females born in Sweden, 1975–1998. *American Journal of Epidemiology, 179*, 852–863.

Gordon, C. M., Goodman, E., Emans, S. J., Grace, E., Becker, K. A., Rosen, C. J., ... Leboff, M. S. (2002). Physiologic regulators of bone turnover in young women with anorexia nervosa. *Journal of Pediatrics, 141*, 64–70.

Gordon, C. M., Grace, E., Emans, S. J., Feldman, H. A., Goodman, E., Becker, K. A., ... LeBoff, M. S. (2002). Effects of oral dehydroepiandrosterone on bone density in young women with anorexia nervosa: A randomized trial. *Journal of Clinical Endocrinology and Metabolism, 87*, 4935–4941.

Gordon, C. M., Grace, E., Emans, S. J., Goodman, E., Crawford, M. H., & Leboff, M. S. (1999). Changes in bone turnover markers and menstrual function after short-term oral DHEA in young women with anorexia nervosa. *Journal of Bone Mineral Research, 14*, 136–145.

Gordon, I., Lask, B., Bryant-Waugh, R., Christie, D., & Timimi, S. (1997). Childhood-onset anorexia nervosa: Towards identifying a biological substrate. *International Journal of Eating Disorders, 22*, 159–165.

Gordon, K. H., Sitnikov, L., Castro, Y., & Holm-Denoma, J. M. (2010). Cultural body shape ideals and eating disorder symptoms among White, Latina, and Black college women. *Cultural Diversity & Ethnic Minority Psychology, 16*, 135–143.

Gowers, S. G., Clark, A., Roberts, C., Griffiths, A., Edwards, V., Bryan, C., ... Barrett, B. (2007). Clinical effectiveness of treatments for anorexia nervosa in adolescents. *British Journal of Psychiatry, 191*, 427–435.

Gowers, S., & Shore, A. (2001). Development of weight and shape concerns in the aetiology of eating disorders. *British Journal of Psychiatry, 179*, 236–242.

Graber, J., Brooks-Gunn, J., Paikoff, R., & Warren, M. (1994). Prediction of eating problems: An 8-year study of adolescent girls. *Developmental Psychology, 30*, 823–834.

Granillo, T., Jones-Rodriguez, G., Carvajal, S. C. (2005). Prevalence of eating disorders in Latina adolescents: Associations with substance use and other correlates. *Journal of Adolescent Health, 36*, 214–220.

Grice, D. E., Halmi, K. A., Fichter, M. M., Strober, M., Woodside, D. B., Treasure, J. T., ... Berrettini, W. H. (2002). Evidence for a susceptibility gene for anorexia nervosa on chromosome 1. *American Journal of Human Genetics, 70*, 787–792.

Grilo, C. M., & Masheb, R. M. (2000). Onset of dieting vs. binge eating in outpatients with binge eating disorder. *International Journal of Obesity and Related Metabolic Disorders, 24*, 404–409.

Grilo, C. M., Pagano, M. E., Stout, R. L., Markowitz, J. C., Ansell, E. B., Pinto, A., ... Skodol, A. E. (2012). Stressful life events predict eating disorder relapse following remission: Six-year prospective outcomes. *International Journal of Eating Disorders, 45*, 185–192.

Grilo, C. M., White, M. A., Barnes, R. D., & Masheb, R. M. (2012). Post-traumatic stress disorder in women with binge eating disorder in primary care. *Journal of Psychiatric Practice, 18*, 408–412.

Grilo, C. M., White, M. A., & Masheb, R. M. (2009). DSM-IV psychiatric disorder comorbidity and its correlates in binge eating disorder. *International Journal of Eating Disorders, 42*, 228–234.

Grinspoon, S., Baum, H., Lee, K., Anderson, E., Herzog, D., & Klibanski, A. (1996). Effects of short-term recombinant human insulin-like growth factor I administration on bone turnover in osteopenic women with anorexia nervosa. *Journal of Clinical Endocrinology and Metabolism, 81*, 3864–3870.

Grinspoon, S., Miller, K., Coyle, C., Krempin, J., Armstrong, C., Pitts, S., ... Klibanski, A. (1999). Severity of osteopenia in estrogen-deficient women with anorexia nervosa and hypothalamic amenorrhea. *Journal of Clinical Endocrinology and Metabolism, 84*, 2049–2055.

Grinspoon, S., Thomas, L., Miller, K., Herzog, D., & Klibanski, A. (2002). Effects of recombinant human IGF-I and oral contraceptive administration on bone density in anorexia nervosa. *Journal of Clinical Endocrinology and Metabolism, 87*, 2883–2891.

Grinspoon, S., Thomas, E., Pitts, S., Gross, E., Mickley, D., Miller, D., ... Klibanski, A. (2000). Prevalence and predictive factors for regional osteopenia in women with anorexia nervosa. *Annals of Internal Medicine, 133*, 790–794.

Groesz, L. M., Levine, M. P., & Murnen, S. K. (2002). The effects of experimental presentation of thin media images on body satisfaction: A meta-analytic review. *International Journal of Eating Disorders, 31*, 1–16.

Gross, H. A., Ebert, M. H., Faden, C. B., Goldberg, S. C., Nee, L. E., & Kaye, W. H. (1981). A double-blind controlled trial of lithium carbonate in primary anorexia nervosa. *Journal of Clinical Psychopharmacology, 1*, 376–381.

Gual, P., Perez-Gaspar, M., Martinez-Gonzalez, M., Lahortiga, F., de Irala-Estevez, J., & Cervera-Enguix, S. (2002). Self-esteem, personality, and eating disorders: Baseline assessment of a prospective population-based cohort. *International Journal of Eating Disorders, 31*, 261–273.

Gulec, H., Moessner, M., Mezei, A., Kohls, E., Tury, F., & Bauer, S. (2011). Internet-based maintenance treatment for patients with eating disorders. *Professional Psychology: Research and Practice, 42*, 479–486.

Hagman, J., Gralla, J., Sigel, E., Ellert, S., Dodge, M., . . . Wamboldt, M. Z. (2011). A double-blind, placebo-controlled study of risperidone for the treatment of adolescents and young adults with anorexia nervosa: A pilot study. *Journal of the American Academy of Child and Adolescent Psychiatry, 50*, 915–924.

Haines, J., Kleinman, K. P., Rifas-Shiman, S. L., Field, A. E., & Austin, S. B. (2010). Examination of shared risk and protective factors for overweight and disordered eating among adolescents. *Archives of Pediatric and Adolescent Medicine, 164*, 336–343.

Haines, J., Neumark-Sztainer, D., Eisenberg, M. E., & Hannan, P. J. (2006). Weight teasing and disordered eating behaviors in adolescents: Longitudinal findings from Project EAT (Eating Among Teens). *Pediatrics, 117*, e209–e215.

Halmi, K. A., Agras, W. S., Crow, S., Mitchell, J., Wilson, G. T., Bryson, S. W., & Kraemer, H. C. (2005). Predictors of treatment acceptance and completion in anorexia nervosa: Implications for future study designs. *Archives of General Psychiatry, 62*, 776–781.

Halmi, K. A., Agras, W. S., Mitchell, J., Wilson, G. T., Crow, S., Bryson, S. W., & Kraemer, H. (2002). Relapse predictors of patients with bulimia nervosa who achieved abstinence through cognitive behavioral therapy. *Archives of General Psychiatry, 59*, 1105–1109.

Halmi, K. A., Eckert, E., LaDu, T. J., & Cohen, J. (1986). Anorexia nervosa: Treatment efficacy of cyproheptadine and amitriptyline. *Archives of General Psychiatry, 43*, 177–181.

Halmi, K. A., Eckert, E., Marchi, P., Sampugnaro, V., Apple, R. & Cohen, J. (1991). Comorbidity of psychiatric diagnoses in anorexia nervosa. *Archives of General Psychiatry, 48*, 712–718.

Halmi, K. A., Struss, A., & Goldberg, S. C. (1978). An investigation of weights in the parents of anorexia nervosa patients. *Journal of Nervous and Mental Disease, 166*, 358–361.

Halmi, K., Tozzi, F., Thornton, L., Crow, S., Fichter, M., Kaplan, A., . . . Bulik, C. M. (2005). The relation among perfectionism, obsessive-compulsive personality disorder and obsessive-compulsive disorder in individuals with eating disorders. *International Journal of Eating Disorders, 38*, 371–374.

Hansen, L. (1999). Olanzapine in the treatment of anorexia nervosa. *British Journal of Psychiatry, 175*, 592.

Harper, K., Richter, N. L., & Gorey, K. M. (2009). Group work with female survivors of childhood sexual abuse: Evidence of poorer outcomes among those with eating disorders. *Eating Behaviors, 10*, 45–48.

Hartman, D., Crisp, A., Rooney, B., Rackow, C., Atkinson, R., & Patel, S. (2000). Bone density of women who have recovered from anorexia nervosa. *International Journal of Eating Disorders, 28*, 107–112.

Hay, P. (1998). The epidemiology of eating disorder behaviors: An Australian community-based survey. *International Journal of Eating Disorders, 23*, 371–382.

Hay, P. (2013). A systematic review of evidence for psychological treatments in eating disorders: 2005–2012. *International Journal of Eating Disorders, 46*, 462–469.

Hay, P. J., & Claudino, A. M. (2012). Clinical psychopharmacology of eating disorders: A research update. *International Journal of Neuropsychopharmacology, 15*, 209–222.

Hazell, P., O'Connell, D., Heathcote, D., Robertson, J., & Henry, D. (1995). Efficacy of tricyclic drugs in treatment child and adolescent depression: A meta-analysis. *British Medical Journal, 310*, 897–901.

Helverskov, J. L., Clausen, L., Mors, O., Frydenberg, M., Thomsen, P. H., & Rokkedal, K. (2010). Transdiagnostic outcome of eating disorders: A 30-month follow-up study of 629 patients. *European Eating Disorders Review, 18*, 453–463.

Henderson, N. K., Price, R. I., Cole, J. H., Gutteridge, D. H., & Bhagat, C. I. (1995). Bone density in young women is associated with body weight and muscle strength but not dietary intakes. *Journal of Bone and Mineral Research, 10*, 384–393.

Herpertz-Dahlmann, B. (2009). Adolescent eating disorders: Definitions, symptomatology, epidemiology and comorbidity. *Child and Adolescent Psychiatric Clinics of North America, 18*, 31–47.

Herpertz-Dahlmann, B., Müller, B., Herpertz, S., Heussen, N., Hebebrand, J., & Remschmidt, H. (2001). Prospective 10-year follow-up in adolescent anorexia nervosa: Course, outcome, psychiatric comorbidity, and psychosocial adaptation. *Journal of Child Psycholology and Psychiatry and Allied Disciplines, 42*, 103–162.

Herzog, D. B., Dorer, D. J., Keel, P. K., Selwyn, S. E., Ekeblad, E. R., Flores, A. T., ... Keller, M. B. (1999). Recovery and relapse in anorexia and bulimia nervosa: A 7.5-year follow-up study. *Journal of the American Academy of Child and Adolescent Psychiatry, 38*, 829–837.

Herzog, D. B., Keller, M. B., Sacks, N. R., Yeh, C. J., & Lavori, P. W. (1992). Psychiatric comorbidity in treatment-seeking anorexics and bulimics. *Journal of the American Academy of Child and Adolescent Psychiatry, 31*, 810–818.

Herzog, D. B., Nussbaum, K. M., & Marmor, A. K. (1996). Comorbidity and outcome in eating disorders. *Psychiatric Clinics of North America, 19*, 843–859.

Herzog, D. B., Staley, J. E., Carmody, S., Robbins, W. M., & van der Kolk, B. A. (1993). Childhood sexual abuse in anorexia nervosa and bulimia nervosa. *Journal of the American Academy of Child and Adolescent Psychiatry, 32*, 962–966.

Herzog, W., Minne, H., Deter, C., Leidig, G., Schellberg, D., Wuster, C. (1993). Outcome of bone mineral density in anorexia nervosa patients 11.7 years after first admission. *Journal of Bone Mineral Research, 8*, 597–605.

Hinney, A., Scherag, S., & Hebebrand, J. (2010). Genetic findings in anorexia and bulimia nervosa. *Progress in Molecular Biology and Translational Science, 94*, 241–270.

Hoek, H. W., van Harten, P. N., van Hoeken, D., & Susser, E. (1998). Lack of relation between culture and anorexia nervosa: Results of an incidence study on Curacao. *New England Journal of Medicine, 338*, 1231–1232.

Hoek, H., & van Hoeken, D. (2003). Review of prevalence and incidence of eating disorders. *International Journal of Eating Disorders, 34*, 383–396.

Holliday, J., Tchanturia, K., Landau, S., Collier, D., & Treasure, J. (2005). Is impaired set-shifting an endophenotype of anorexia nervosa? *American Journal of Psychiatry, 162*, 2269–2275.

Holt, K. E., & Ricciardelli, L. A. (2008). Weight concerns among elementary school children: A review of prevention programs. *Body Image, 5*, 233–243.

Holtkamp, K., Konrad, K., Kaiser, N., Ploenes, Y., Heussen, N., Grzella, I., & Herpertz-Dahlmann, B. (2005). A retrospective study of SSRI treatment in adolescent anorexia nervosa: Insufficient evidence for efficacy. *Journal of Psychiatric Research, 39*, 303–310.

Holtkamp, K., Muller, B., Heussen, N., Remschmidt, H., & Herpertz-Dahlmann, B. (2005). Depression, anxiety, and obsessionality in long-term recovered patients with adolescent-onset anorexia nervosa. *European Child & Adolescent Psychiatry, 14*, 106–110.

Hoopes, S. P., Reimherr, F. W., Hedges, D. W., Rosenthal, N. R., Kamin, M., Karim, R., ... Karvois, D. (2003) Treatment of bulimia nervosa with topiramate in a randomized, double-blind, placebo-controlled trial, part 1: Improvement in binge and purge measures. *Journal of Clinical Psychiatry, 64*, 1335–1341.

Horesh, N., Apter, A., Lepkifker, E., Ratzoni, G., Weizman, R., & Tyano, S. (1995). Life events and severe anorexia nervosa in adolescence. *Acta Psychiatrica Scandinavica, 91*, 5–9.

Hudson, J. I., Coit, C. E., Lalonde, J. K., & Pope, H. G. (2012). By how much will the proposed new DSM-5 criteria increase the prevalence of binge eating disorder? *International Journal of Eating Disorders, 45*, 139–141.

Hudson, J. I., Hiripi, E., Pope, H. G., Jr., & Kessler, R. C. (2007). The prevalence and correlates of eating disorders in the National Comorbidity Survey Replication. *Biological Psychiatry, 61*, 348–358.

Hudson, J., Lalonde, J., Pindyck, L., Bulik, C., Crow, S., McElroy, S., ... Pope, H. (2006). Familial aggregation of binge-eating disorder. *Archives of General Psychiatry, 63*, 313–319.

Hudson, J., Pope, H., Jonas, J., & Yurgelun-Todd, D. (1983). Family history study of anorexia and bulimia. *British Journal of Psychiatry, 142*, 133–138.

Hughes, P. L., Wells, L. A., & Cunningham, C. J. (1986). The dexamethasone suppression test in bulimia before and after successful treatment with desipramine. *Journal of Clinical Psychiatry, 47*, 515–517.

Hulley, A. J., & Hill, A. J. (2001). Eating disorders and health in elite women distance runners.

International Journal of Eating Disorders, 30, 312–317.

Iacovino, J. M., Gredysa, D. M., Altman, M., & Wilfley, D. E. (2012) Psychological treatments for binge eating disorder. *Current Psychiatry Reports, 14*, 432–446.

Insel, T., Cuthbert, B., Garvey, M., Heinssen, R., Pine, D. S., Quinn, K., ... Wang, P. (2010). Research domain criteria (RDoC): Toward a new classification framework for research on mental disorders. *American Journal of Psychiatry, 167*, 748–751.

Isnard, P., Michel, G., Frelut, M. L., Vila, G., Falissard, B., Naja, W., ... Mouren-Simeoni, M. C. (2003). Binge eating and psychopathology in severely obese adolescents. *International Journal of Eating Disorders, 34*, 235–243.

Isner, J. M., Roberts, W. C., Heymsfield, S. B., & Yager, J. (1985). Anorexia nervosa and sudden death. *Annals of Internal Medicine, 102*, 49–52.

Jacobi, C., Abascal, L., & Taylor, C. B. (2004). Screening for eating disorders and high risk behavior: Caution. *International Journal of Eating Disorders, 36*, 273–288.

Jacobi, C., Fittig, E., Bryson, S. W., Wilfley, D., Kraemer, H. C., & Taylor, C. B. (2011). Who is really at risk? Identifying risk factors for subthreshold and full syndrome eating disorders in a high-risk sample. *Psychological Medicine, 41*, 1939–1949.

Jacobi, C., Hayward, C., de Zwaan, M., Kraemer, H., & Agras, W. (2004). Coming to terms with risk factors for eating disorders: Application of risk terminology and suggestions for a general taxonomy. *Psychological Bulletin, 130*, 19–65.

Jacobi, C., Schmitz, G., & Agras, W. S. (2008). Interactions between disturbed eating and weight in children and their mothers. *Journal of Developmental and Behavioral Pediatrics, 29*, 360–366.

Jacobi, C., Volker, U., Trockel, M. T., & Taylor, C. B. (2012). Effects of an Internet-based intervention for subthreshold eating disorders: A randomized controlled trial. *Behavior Research and Therapy, 50*, 93–99.

Javaras, K. N., Laird, N. M., Reichborn-Kjennerud, T., Bulik, C. M., Pope, H. G., Jr., & Hudson, J. I. (2008). Familiality and heritability of binge eating disorder: Results of a case-control family study and a twin study. *International Journal of Eating Disorders, 41*, 174–179.

Jensen, V. S., & Mejlhede, A. (2000). Anorexia nervosa: Treatment with olanzapine. *British Journal of Psychiatry, 177*, 87.

Jeong, S. H., Cho, H., & Hwang, Y. (2012). Media literacy interventions: A meta-analytic review. *Journal of Communication, 62*, 454–472.

Jimerson, D. C., Lesem, M. D., Kaye, W. H., & Brewerton, T. D. (1992). Low serotonin and dopamine metabolite concentrations in cerebrospinal fluid from bulimic patients with frequent binge episodes. *Archives of General Psychiatry, 49*, 132–138.

John, U., Meyer, C., Rumpf, H. J., & Hapke, U. (2006). Psychiatric comorbidity including nicotine dependence among individuals with eating disorder criteria in an adult general population sample. *Psychiatry Research, 141*, 71–79.

Johnston, C. C., Jr., Miller, J. Z., Slemenda, C. W., Reister, T. K., Hui, S., Christian, J. C., & Peacock, M. (1992). Calcium supplementation and increases in bone mineral density in children. *New England Journal of Medicine, 327*, 82–87.

Jones, M., Volker, U., Lock, J., Taylor, C. B., & Jacobi, C. (2012). Family-based early intervention for anorexia nervosa. *European Eating Disorders Review, 20*, 137–143.

Judge, A. M., Thomas, J. J., & Becker, A.E. (2006) Ethnic disparities in overweight and obesity in the U.S.: A review of socio-cultural contributions. In L. F. Ditmier (Ed.), *New developments in obesity research* (pp. 85–119). New York: Nova Science Publishers.

Kafantaris, V., Leigh, E., Hertz, S., Berest, A., Schebendach, J., Sterling, W. M., ... Malhotra, A. K. (2011). A placebo-controlled pilot study of adjunctive olanzapine for adolescents with anorexia nervosa. *Journal of Child and Adolescent Psychopharmacology, 21*, 207–212.

Kaltiala-Heino, R., Rissanen, A., Rimpela, M., & Rantanen, P. (2003). Bulimia and impulsive behaviour in middle adolescence. *Psychotherapy and Psychosomatics, 72*, 26–33.

Kaplan, A. S., Walsh, B. T., Olmsted, M. P., Attia, E., Carter, J. C., Devlin, M. J., ... Parides, M. (2009). The slippery slope: Prediction of successful weight maintenance in anorexia nervosa. *Psychological Medicine, 39*, 1037–1045.

Karwautz, A., Rabe-Hesketh, S., Hu, X., Zhao, J., Sham, P., Collier, D. A., & Treasure, J. L. (2001). Individual-specific risk factors for anorexia nervosa: A pilot study using a discordant sister-pair design. *Psychological Medicine, 31*, 317–329.

Kassett, J. A., Gwirtsman, H. E., Kay, W. H., Brandt, H. A., & Jimerson, D. C. (1988). Pattern of onset of bulimic symptoms in anorexia nervosa. *American Journal of Psychiatry, 145*, 1287–1288.

Katz, R. L., Keen, C. L., Litt, I. F., Hurley, L. S., Kellams-Harrison, K. M., & Glader, L. J. (1987). Zinc deficiency in anorexia nervosa. *Journal of Adolescent Health Care*, *8*, 400–406.

Katzman, D. K., Bachrach, L. K., Carter, D. R., & Marcus, R. (1991). Clinical and anthropometric correlates of bone mineral acquisition in healthy adolescent girls. *Journal of Clinical Endocrinology and Metabolism*, *73*, 1332–1339.

Katzman, D. K., Lambe, E. K., Mikulis, D. J., Ridgley, J. N., Goldbloom, D. S., & Zipursky, R. B. (1996). Cerebral gray matter and white matter volume deficits in adolescent girls with anorexia nervosa. *Journal of Pediatrics*, *129*, 794–803.

Katzman, D., Peebles, R., Sawyer, S., Lock, J, & Le Grange, D. (2013). The role of the pediatrician in family-based treatment for adolescent eating disorders: Opportunities and challenges. *Journal of Adolescent Health*, *53*, 433–440.

Katzman, D. K., Zipursky, R. B., Lambe, E. K., & Mikulis, D. J. (1997). A longitudinal magnetic resonance imaging study of brain changes in adolescents with anorexia nervosa. *Archives of Pediatrics and Adolescent Medicine*, *151*, 793–797.

Katzman, M., Nasser, M., & Gordon, R. (2001). *Eating disorders and cultures in transition*. London: Routledge Press.

Kaye, W. (2008). Neurobiology of anorexia and bulimia nervosa. *Physiology & Behavior*, *94*, 121–135.

Kaye, W. H., Barbarich, N. C., Putnam, K., Gendall, K. A., Fernstrom, J., Fernstrom, M., . . . Kishore, A. (2003). Anxiolytic effects of acute tryptophan depletion in anorexia nervosa. *International Journal of Eating Disorders*, *33*, 257–267

Kaye, W. H., Bulik, C. M., Thornton, L., Barbarich, N., & Masters, K. (2004). Comorbidity of anxiety disorders with anorexia and bulimia nervosa. *American Journal of Psychiatry*, *161*, 2215–2221.

Kaye, W. H., Fudge, J. L., & Paulus, M. (2009). New insights into symptoms and neurocircuit function of anorexia nervosa. *Nature Reviews Neuroscience*, *10*, 573–584.

Kaye, W. H., Nagata, T., Weltzin, T. E., Hsu, L. K. G., Sokol, M. S., McConaha, C., . . . Deep, D. (2001). Double-blind placebo-controlled administration of fluoxetine in restricting- and restricting-purging type anorexia nervosa. *Biological Psychiatry*, *49*, 644–652.

Kaye, W. H., Wagner, A., Fudge, J. L., & Paulus, M. (2011). Neurocircuity of eating disorders. *Current Topics in Behavioral Neurosciences*, *6*, 37–57.

Kaye, W. H., Wierenga, C. E., Bailer, U. F., Simmons, A. N., & Bischoff-Grethe, A. (2013). Nothing tastes as good as skinny feels: The neurobiology of anorexia nervosa. *Trends in Neurosciences*, *36*, 110–120.

Keel, P. K., & Brown, T. A. (2010). Update on course and outcome in eating disorders. *International Journal of Eating Disorders*, *43*, 195–204.

Keel, P. K., Dorer, D. J., Franko, D. L., Jackson, S. C., & Herzog, D. B. (2005). Postremission predictors of relapse in women with eating disorders. *American Journal of Psychiatry*, *162*, 2263–2268.

Keel, P. K., & Forney, K. J. (2013). Psychosocial risk factors for eating disorders. *International Journal of Eating Disorders*, *46*, 433–439.

Keel, P. K., & Klump, K. L. (2003). Are eating disorders culture-bound syndromes? Implications for conceptualizing their etiology. *Psychological Bulletin*, *129*, 747–769.

Keel, P. K., & Mitchell, J. E. (1997). Outcome in bulimia nervosa. *American Journal of Psychiatry*, *154*, 313–321.

Keel, P. K., Mitchell, J. E., Miller, K. B., Davis, T. L., & Crow, S. J. (1999). Long-term outcome of bulimia nervosa. *Archives of General Psychiatry*, *56*, 63–69.

Kelly, N. R., Cotter, E. W., & Mazzeo, S. E. (2012). Eating Disorder Examination Question (EDE-Q): Norms for black women. *Eating Behaviors*, *13*, 429–432.

Kendler, K. S., Bulik, C. M., Silberg, J., Hettema, J. M., Myers, J., & Prescott, C. A. (2000). Childhood sexual abuse and adult psychiatric and substance use disorders in women: An epidemiological and cotwin control analysis. *Archives of General Psychiatry*, *57*, 953–959.

Kendler, K. S., Walters, E. E., Neale, M. C., Kessler, R. C., Heath, A. C., & Eaves, L. J. (1995). The structure of the genetic and environmental risk factors for six major psychiatric disorders in women: Phobia, generalized anxiety disorder, panic disorder, bulimia, major depression, and alcoholism. *Archives of General Psychiatry*, *52*, 374–383.

Keski-Rahkonen, A., Hoek, H. W., Linna, M. S., Raevuori, A., Sihvola, E., Bulik CM, . . . , Kaprio, J. (2009). Incidence and outcomes of bulimia nervosa: A nationwide population-based study. *Psychological Medicine*, *39*, 823–831.

Keski-Rahkonen, A., Hoek, H. W., Susser, E. S., Linna, M. S., Sihvola, E., Raevuori, A., . . . Rissanen, A. (2007). Epidemiology and course of anorexia nervosa in the community. *American Journal of Psychiatry*, *164*, 1259–1265.

Kessler, R. C., Berglund, P. A., Chiu, W. T., Deitz, A. C., Hudson, J. I., Shahly, V., . . . Xavier,

M. (2013). The prevalence and correlates of binge eating disorder in the World Health Organization World Mental Health Surveys. *Biological Psychiatry, 73,* 904–914.

Kessler, R. C., Berglund, P., Chiu, W. T., Demler, O., Heeringa, S., Hiripi, E., . . . Zheng, H. (2004). The US National Comorbidity Survey Replication (NCS-R): Design and field procedures. *International Journal of Methods in Psychiatric Research, 13,* 69–92.

Kessler, R. C., Chiu, W. T., Demler, O., Merikangas, K. R., & Walters, E. E. (2005). Prevalence, severity, and comorbidity of 12-month DSM-IV disorders in the National Comorbidity Survey Replication. *Archives of General Psychiatry, 62,* 617–627.

Key, A., Mason., Allan, R., & Lask, B. (2001). Restoration of ovarian and uterine maturity in adolescents with anorexia nervosa. *International Journal of Eating Disorders, 32,* 319–325.

Khan, K., Green, R., Saul, A., Bennell, K., Crichton, K., Hopper, J., & Wark, J. (1996). Retired elite female ballet dancers and nonathletic controls have similar bone mineral density at weightbearing sites. *Journal of Bone and Mineral Research, 11,* 1566–1574.

Killen, J., Taylor, C., Hayward, C., Wilson, D., Haydel, K., Hammer, L., . . . Kraemer, H. (1994). Pursuit of thinness and onset of eating disorder symptoms in a comunity sample of adolescent girls: A three-year prospective analysis. *International Journal of Eating Disorders, 16,* 227–238.

Kingston, K., Szmukler, G., Andrewes, D., Tress, B., & Desmond, P. (1996). Neuropsychological and structural brain changes in anorexia nervosa before and after refeeding. *Psychological Medicine, 26,* 15–28.

Kirkcaldy, B. D., Siefen, G. R., Kandel, I., & Merrick, J. (2007). A review on eating disorders and adolescence. *Minerva Pediatrics, 59,* 239–248.

Klibanski, A., Biller, B. M. K., Schoenfeld, D. A., Herzog, D. B., & Saxe, V. C. (1995). The effects of estrogen administration on trabecular bone loss in young women with anorexia nervosa. *Journal of Clinical Endocrinology and Metabolism, 80,* 898–903.

Klump, K., Ringham, R., Marcus, M., & Kaye, W. (2001). *A family history/family study approach to examining the nature of eating disorder risk in ballet dancers: Evidence for gene-environment combinations?* Paper presented at the Eating Disorder Research Society Annual Meeting, Albuquerque, NM.

Kohn, M. R., Golden, N. H., & Shenker, I. R. (1998). Cardiac arrest and delirium: Presentations of the refeeding syndrome in severely malnourished adolescents with anorexia nervosa. *Journal of Adolescent Health, 22,* 239–243.

Kohn, M. R., Madden, S., & Clarke, S. D. (2011). Refeeding in anorexia nervosa: Increased safety and efficiency through understanding the pathophysiology of protein calorie malnutrition. *Current Opinion in Pediatrics, 23,* 390–394.

Kordy, H., Kramer, B., Palmer, R. L., Papežová, H., Pellet, J., Richard, M., Treasure, J. (2002). Remission, recovery, relapse, and recurrence in eating disorders: Conceptualization and illustration of a validation strategy. *Journal of Clinical Psychology, 58,* 833–846.

Koschke, M., Boettger, M. K., & Macholdt, C. (2010). Increased QT variability in patients with anorexia nervosa: An indicator for increased cardiac mortality? *International Journal of Eating Disorders, 43,* 743–750.

Kotler, L., Cohen, P., Davies, M., Pine, D., & Walsh, B. (2001). Longitudinal relationships between childhood, adolescent, and adult eating disorders. *Journal of the American Academy of Child and Adolescent Psychiatry, 40,* 1434–1440.

Kotler, L. A., Devlin, M. J., Davies, M., & Walsh, B. T. (2003). An open trial of fluoxetine for adolescents with bulimia nervosa. *Journal of Child and Adolescent Psychopharmacology, 13,* 329–335.

Kotler, L. A., & Walsh, B. T. (2000). Eating disorders in children and adolescents: Pharmacological therapies. *European Child and Adolescent Psychiatry, 9,* 108–116.

Kurth, C. L., Krahn, D. D., Nairn, K., & Drewnowski, A. (1995). The severity of dieting and bingeing behaviors in college women: Interview validation of survey data. *Journal of Psychiatric Research, 29,* 211–225.

Lacey, J. H., & Crisp, A. H. (1980). Hunger, food intake and weight: The impact of clomipramine on a refeeding anorexia nervosa population. *Postgraduate Medical Journal, 56,* 79–85.

Lai, K. Y., De Bruyn, R., Lask, B., Bryant-Waugh, R., & Hankins, M. (1994). Use of pelvic ultrasound to monitor ovarian and uterine maturity in childhood-onset anorexia nervosa. *Archives of Disorders in Childhood, 71,* 228–231.

Langmesser, L., & Verscheure, S. (2009). Are eating disorder prevention programs effective? *Journal of Athletic Training, 44,* 304–305.

Lantzouni, E., Frank, G. R., Golden, N. H., & Shenker, R. I. (2002). Reversibility of growth stunting in early onset anorexia nervosa: A prospective study. *Journal of Adolescent Health, 31*, 162–165.

Lask, B., & Bryant-Waugh, R. (2000). *Anorexia nervosa and related eating disorders in children and adolescence*. Hove, East Sussex, UK: Psychology Press.

Lask, B., Fosson, A., Rolfe, U., & Thomas, S. (1993). Zinc deficiency and childhood-onset anorexia nervosa. *Journal of Clinical Psychiatry, 54*, 63–66.

La Via, M. C., Gray, N., & Kaye, W. H. (2000). Case reports of olanzapine treatment of anorexia nervosa. *International Journal of Eating Disorders, 27*, 363–366.

Lawrence, A. D., Dowson, J., Foxall, G. L., Summerfield, R., Robbins, T. W., & Sahakian, B. J. (2003). Impaired visual discrimination learning in anorexia nervosa. *Appetite, 40*, 85–89.

Lay, B., Jennen-Steinmetz, C., Reinhard, I., & Schmidt, M. H. (2002). Characteristics of inpatient weight gain in adolescent anorexia nervosa: Relation to speed of relapse and re-admission. *European Eating Disorders Review, 10*, 22–40.

Lee, S. (1991). Anorexia nervosa in Hong Kong: A Chinese perspective. *Psychological Medicine, 21*, 703–711.

Lee, S. (1995). Self-starvation in context: Towards a culturally sensitive understanding of anorexia nervosa. *Social Science & Medicine, 41*, 25–36.

Lee, S., Ng, L. K., Kwok, K., & Fung, C. (2010). The changing profile of eating disorders at a tertiary psychiatric clinic in Hong Kong (1987–2007). *International Journal of Eating Disorders, 43*, 307–314.

Lee, Y., Abbott, D., Seim, H., Crosby, R., Monson, N., Burgard, M., & Mitchell, J. (1999). Eating disorders and psychiatric disorders in the first-degree relatives of obese probands with binge eating disorder and obese non-binge eating disorder controls. *International Journal of Eating Disorders, 26*, 322–332.

Leggero, C., Masi, G., Brunori, E., Calderoni, S., Carissimo, R., Maestro, S., & Muratori, F. (2010). Low-dose olanzapine monotherapy in girls with anorexia nervosa, restricting subtype: Focus on hyperactivity. *Journal of Child and Adolescent Psychopharmacology, 20*, 127–113.

Le Grange, D., Crosby, R. D., Rathouz, P. J., & Leventhal, B. L. (2007). A randomized controlled comparison of family-based treatment and supportive psychotherapy for adolescent bulimia nervosa. *Archives of General Psychiatry, 64*, 1049–1056.

Le Grange, D., Eisler, I., Dare, C., & Hodes, M. (1992a). Family criticism and self-starvation: A study of expressed emotion. *Journal of Family Therapy, 14*, 177–192.

Le Grange, D., Eisler, I., Dare, C., & Russell, G. F. M. (1992b). Evaluation of family therapy in anorexia nervosa: A pilot study. *International Journal of Eating Disorders, 12*, 347–357.

Le Grange, D., Hughes, E. K., Court, A., Yeo, M., Crosby, R. D., & Sawyer, S. M. (2016). Randomized clinical trial of parent-focused treatment and family-based treatment for adolescent anorexia nervosa. *Journal of the American Academy of Child and Adolescent Psychiatry, 55*, 683–692.

Le Grange, D., & Lock, J. (2005). The dearth of psychological treatment studies for anorexia nervosa. *International Journal of Eating Disorders, 37*, 79–81.

Le Grange, D., & Lock, J. (2007). *Treating bulimia in adolescents: A family-based approach*. New York: Guilford Press.

Le Grange, D., Lock, J., Agras, W. S., Bryson, S. W., & Jo, B. (2015). Randomized clinical trial of family-based treatment and cognitive-behavioral therapy for adolescent bulimia nervosa. *Journal of the American Academy of Child and Adolescent Psychiatry, 54*, 886–894.

Le Grange, D., Lock, J., Agras, W. S., Moye, A., Bryson, S., Jo, B., & Kraemer, H. (2012). Moderators and mediators of remission in family-based treatment and adolescent focused therapy for anorexia nervosa. *Behaviour Research and Therapy, 50*, 85–92.

Leon, A. C. (2007). The revised warning for antidepressants and suicidality: Unveiling the black box of statistical analyses. *American Journal of Psychiatry, 164*, 1786–1789.

Lewinsohn, P. M., Seeley, J. R., Moerk, K. C., & Striegel-Moore, R. H. (2002). Gender differences in eating disorder symptoms in young adults. *International Journal of Eating Disorders, 32*, 426–440.

Lilenfeld, L. R., Kaye, W. H., Greeno, C. G., Merikangas, K. R., Plotnicov, K., Pollice, C., ... Nagy, L. (1998). A controlled family study of anorexia nervosa and bulimia nervosa: Psychiatric disorders in first-degree relatives and effects of proband comorbidity. *Archives of General Psychiatry, 55*, 603–610.

Lilenfeld, L. R., Ringham, R., Kalarchian, M. A., & Marcus, M. D. (2008). A family history study of binge-eating disorder. *Comprehensive Psychiatry, 49*, 247–254.

Lindenberg, K., Moessner, M., Harney, J., McLaughlin, O., & Bauer, S. (2011). E-health for individual prevention of eating disorders. *Clinical Practice and Epidemiology in Mental Health*, *7*, 74–83.

Lloyd, T., Andon, M. B., Rollings, N., Martel, J. K., Landis, J. R., Demers, L. M., ... Kulin, H. E. (1993). Calcium supplementation and bone mineral density in adolescent girls. *Journal of the American Medical Association*, *270*, 841–844.

Lock, J., Agras, W. S., Bryson, S., & Kraemer, H. (2005). A comparison of short-and long-term family therapy for adolescent anorexia nervosa. *Journal of the American Academy of Child and Adolescent Psychiatry*, *44*, 632–639.

Lock, J., Brandt, H., Woodside, B., Agras, W. S., Halmi, K., Johnson, C., ... Wilfley, D. (2012). Challenges in conducting a multi-site randomized clinical trial comparing treatments for adolescent anorexia nervosa. *International Journal of Eating Disorders*, *45*, 202–213.

Lock, J., Couturier, J., & Agras, W. S. (2006). Comparison of long-term outcomes in adolescents with anorexia nervosa treated with family therapy. *Journal of the American Academy of Child and Adolescent Psychiatry*, *45*, 666–672.

Lock, J., & Le Grange, D. (2001). Can family-based treatment of anorexia nervosa be manualized? *Journal of Psychotherapy Practice and Research*, *10*, 253–261.

Lock, J., & Le Grange, D. (2013). *Treatment manual for anorexia nervosa: A family-based approach* (2nd ed.). New York: Guilford Press.

Lock, J., Le Grange, D., Agras, W. S., & Dare, C. (2001). *Treatment manual for anorexia nervosa: A family-based approach.* New York: Guilford Press.

Lock, J., Le Grange, D., Agras, W. S., Moye, A., Bryson, S. W., & Jo, B. (2010). Randomized clinical trial comparing family-based treatment with adolescent-focused individual therapy for adolescents with anorexia nervosa. *Archives of General Psychiatry*, *67*, 1025–1032.

Loeb, K., Marcus, S., Striegel-Moore, R., Le Grange, D., Newcorn, J., Taylor, C. B., Lock, J., & Walsh, B. T. (2012, May). *Family-based treatment for prodromal anorexia nervosa: A hybrid efficacy-effectiveness trial.* Paper presented at the International Conference on Eating Disorders, Austin, TX.

Logue, C. M., Crowe, R. R., & Bean, J. A. (1989). A family study of anorexia nervosa and bulimia. *Comprehensive Psychiatry*, *30*, 179–188.

Löwe, B., Zipfel, S., Buchholz, C., Dupont, Y., Reas, D. L., & Herzog, W. (2001). Long-term outcome of anorexia nervosa in a prospective 21-year follow-up study. *Psychological Medicine*, *31*, 881–890.

Lucas, A. R., Beard, C. M., O'Fallon, W. M., & Kurland, L. T. (1988). Anorexia nervosa in Rochester, Minnesota: A 45-year study. *Mayo Clinic Proceedings*, *63*, 433–442.

Lucas, A. R., Beard, C. M., O'Fallon, W. M., & Kurland, L. T. (1991). 50-year trends in the incidence of anorexia nervosa in Rochester, Minn.: A population-based study. *American Journal of Psychiatry*, *148*, 917–922.

Lucas, A. R., Melton, L. J., Crowson, C. S., & O'Fallon, W. M. (1999). Long-term fracture risk among women with anorexia nervosa: A population-based cohort study. *Mayo Clinic Proceedings*, *74*, 972–977.

Luce, K. H., Osborne, M. I., Winzelberg, A. J., & Taylor, C. B. (2005). Application of an algorithm-driven protocol to simultaneously provide universal and targeted prevention programs. *International Journal of Eating Disorders*, *37*, 220–226.

Lunde, A. V., Fasmer, O. B., Akiskal, K. K., Akiskal, H. S., & Oedegaard, K. J. (2009). The relationship of bulimia and anorexia nervosa with bipolar disorder and its temperamental foundations. *Journal of Affective Disorders*, *115*, 309–314

Machado, P. P., Goncalves, S., & Hoek, H. W. (2013). DSM-5 reduces the proportion of EDNOS cases: Evidence from community samples. *International Journal of Eating Disorders*, *46*, 60–65.

Madden, S., Miskovic-Wheatley, J., Wallis, A., Kohn, M., Lock, J., Le Grange, D., ... Touyz, S. (under review). How much hospitalization is enough for anorexia nervosa? A randomized controlled trial of inpatient treatment in medically unstable adolescents. *JAMA Psychiatry.*

Mangweth-Matzek, B., Rupp, C. I., Hausmann, A., Kemmler, G., & Biebl, W. (2007). Menarche, puberty, and first sexual activities in eating-disordered patients as compared with a psychiatric and a nonpsychiatric control group. *International Journal of Eating Disorders*, *40*, 705–710.

Mann, T., Nolen-Hoeksema, S., Huang, K., Burgard, D., Wright, A., & Hanson, K. (1997). Are two interventions worse than none? Joint primary and secondary prevention of eating disorders in college females. *Health Psychology*, *16*, 1–11.

Manwaring, J. L., Hilbert, A., Wilfley, D. E., Pike, K. M., Fairburn, C. G., Dohm, F. A., & Striegel-Moore, R. H. (2006). Risk factors and patterns of onset in binge eating disorder. *International Journal of Eating Disorders, 39,* 101–107.

Marchi, M., & Cohen, P. (1990). Early childhood eating behaviors and adolescent eating disorders. *Journal of the American Academy of Child and Adolescent Psychiatry, 29,* 112–117.

Marcus, M. D., & Wildes, J. E. (2009). Obesity: Is it a mental disorder? *International Journal of Eating Disorders, 42,* 739–753.

Marino, D. D., & King, J. C. (1980). Nutritional concerns during adolescence. *Pediatric Clinics of North America, 27,* 125–139.

Marlatt, G. A., & Gordon, J. R. (Eds.). (1985). *Relapse prevention: Maintenance strategies in addictive behavior change.* New York: Guilford.

Marques, L., Alegria, M., Becker, A. E., Chen, C.-N., Fang, A., Chosak, A., & Diniz, J. B. (2011). Comparative prevalence, correlates of impairment, and service utilization for eating disorders across US ethnic groups: Implications for reducing ethnic disparities in health care access for eating disorders. *International Journal of Eating Disorders, 44,* 412–420.

Marrone, S., Mitchell, J. E., Crosby, R., Wonderlich, S., & Jollie-Trottier, T. (2009). Predictors of response to cognitive behavioral treatment for bulimia nervosa delivered via telemedicine versus face-to-face. *International Journal of Eating Disorders, 42,* 222–227.

Marzola, E., Desedime, N., Giovannone, C., Amianto, F., Fassino, S., & Abbate-Daga, G. (2015). Atypical antipsychotics as augmentation therapy in anorexia nervosa. *PLoS One, 10,* e0125569.

Mathes, W. F., Brownley, K. A., Mo, X., & Bulik, C. M. (2009). The biology of binge eating. *Appetite, 52,* 545–553.

Matusek, J. A., Wendt, S. J., & Wiseman, C. V. (2004). Dissonance thin-ideal and didactic healthy behavior eating disorder prevention programs: Results from a controlled trial. *International Journal of Eating Disorders, 36,* 376–388.

McElroy, S. L., Frye, M. A., Hellemann, G., Altshuler, L., Leverich, G. S., Suppes, T., ... Post, R. M. (2011). Prevalence and correlates of eating disorders in 875 patients with bipolar disorder. *Journal of Affective Disorders, 128,* 191–198.

McElroy, S. L., Hudson, J., Ferreira-Cornwell, M. C., Radewonuk, J., Whitaker, T., & Gasior, M. (2016). Lisdexamfetamine dimesylate for adults with moderate to severe binge eating disorder: Results of two pivotal phase 3 randomized controlled trials. *Neuropsychopharmacology, 41,* 1251–1260.

McFarlane, T., Olmsted, M. P., & Trottier, K. (2008). Timing and prediction of relapse in a transdiagnostic eating disorder sample. *International Journal of Eating Disorders, 41,* 587–593.

McIntosh, V. V. W., Jordan, J., Carter, F. A., Luty, S. E., McKenzie, J. M., Bulik, C. M., ... Joyce, P. R. (2005). Three psychotherapies for anorexia nervosa: A randomized, controlled trial. *American Journal of Psychiatry, 162,* 741–747.

McKay, H. A., Petit, M. A., Schutz, R. W., Prior, J. C., Barr, S. I., & Khan, K. M. (2000). Augmented trochanteric bone mineral density after modified physical education classes: A randomized school-based exercise intervention study in prepubescent and early pubescent children. *Journal of Pediatrics, 136,* 156–162.

McKnight, R. F., Park, R. J. (2010). Atypical antipsychotics and anorexia nervosa: A review. *European Eating Disorders Review, 18,* 10–21.

McVey, G., Gusella, J., Tweed, S., & Ferrari, M. A. (2009). A controlled evaluation of web-based training for teachers and public health practitioners on the prevention of eating disorders. *Eating Disorders, 17,* 1–26.

McVey, G., Tweed, S., & Blackmore, E. (2007). Healthy Schools, Healthy Kids: A controlled evaluation of a comprehensive universal eating disorder prevention program. *Body Image, 4,* 115–136.

Mecklenberg, R. S., Loriaux, D. L., Thompson, R. L., Andersen, A. E., & Lipsett, M. B. (1976). Hypothalamic dysfunction in patients with anorexia nervosa. *Medicine, 53,* 147–157.

Mehler, C., Wewetzer, C., Schulze, U., Warnke, A., Theisen, F., & Dittmann, R. W. (2001). Olanzapine in children and adolescents with chronic anorexia nervosa: A study of five cases. *European Child and Adolescent Psychiatry, 10,* 151–157.

Mehler, P. S., Lezotte, D., & Eckel, R. (1998). Lipid levels in anorexia nervosa. *International Journal of Eating Disorders, 24,* 217–221.

Mehler, P. S., Sabel, A. L., Watson, T., & Anderson, A. E. (2008). High risk of osteoporosis in male patients with eating disorders. *International Journal of Eating Disorders, 41,* 666–672.

Mehler-Wex, C., Romanos, M., Kirchheiner, J., & Schulze, U. M. (2008). Atypical antipsychotics in severe anorexia nervosa in children and adolescents—review and case reports. *European Eating Disorders Review, 16,* 100–108.

Merikangas, K. R., He, J. P., Burstein, M., Swendsen, J., Avenevoli, S., Case, B., ... Olfson, M. (2011).

Service utilization for lifetime mental disorders in U.S. adolescents: Results of the National Comorbidity Survey-Adolescent Supplement (NCS-A). *Journal of the American Academy of Child and Adolescent Psychiatry, 50*, 32–45.

Micali, N., De Stavola, B., dos-Santos-Silva, I., Steenweg-de Graaff, J., Jansen, P. W., Jaddoe, V. W., ... Tiemeier, H. (2012). Perinatal outcomes and gestational weight gain in women with eating disorders: A population-based cohort study. *British Journal of Obstetrics and Gynaecology, 119*, 1493–1502.

Micali, N., Simonoff, E., & Treasure, J. (2007). Risk of major adverse perinatal outcomes in women with eating disorders. *British Journal of Psychiatry, 190*, 255–259.

Mickley, D., Greenfeld, D., Quinlan, D. M., Roloff, P., & Zwas, F. (1996). Abnormal liver enzymes in outpatients with eating disorders. *International Journal of Eating Disorders, 20*, 325–329.

Milano, W., Petrella, C., Sabatino, C., & Capasso, A. (2004). Treatment of bulimia nervosa with sertraline: A randomized controlled trial. *Advances in Therapy, 21*, 232–237.

Milano, W., Siano, C., Putrella, C., & Capasso, A. (2005). Treatment of bulimia nervosa with fluvoxamine: A randomized controlled trial. *Advances in Therapy, 22*, 278–283.

Miller, K. K., Grieco, K. A., Mulder, J., Grinspoon, S., Mickley, D., Yehezkel, R., ... Klibanski, A. (2004). Effects of risedronate on bone density in anorexia nervosa. *Journal of Clinical Endocrinology and Metabolism, 89*, 3903–3906.

Miller, K. K., Meenaghan, E., Lawson, E. A., Misra, M., Gleysteen, S., Schoenfield, D., ... Klibanski, A. (2011). Effects of risedronate and low-dose transdermal testosterone on bone mineral density in women with anorexia nervosa: A randomized, placebo-controlled study. *Journal of Clinical Endocrinology and Metabolism, 96*, 2081–2088.

Mischoulon, D., Eddy, K. T., Keshaviah, A., Dinescu, D., Ross, S. L., Kass, A. E., ... Herzog, D. B. (2011). Depression and eating disorders: Treatment and course. *Journal of Affective Disorders, 130*, 470–477.

Misra, M., Aggarwal, A., Miller, K. K., Almazan, C., Worley, M., & Soyka, L.A. (2004). Effects of anorexia nervosa on clinical, hematologic, biochemical, and bone density parameters in community-dwelling adolescent girls. *Pediatrics, 114*, 1574–1583.

Misra, M., Katzman, D. K., Cord, J., Manning, S. J., Mendes, N., Herzog, D. B., ... Klibanski, A. (2008). Bone metabolism in adolescent boys with anorexia nervosa. *Journal of Clinical Endocrinology and Metabolism, 93*, 3029–3036.

Misra, M., Prabhakaran, R., Miller, K. K., Goldstein, M. A., Mickley, D., Clauss, L., ... Klibanski, A. (2008). Weight gain and restoration of menses as predictors of bone mineral density change in adolescent girls with anorexia nervosa. *Journal of Clinical Endocrinology and Metabolism, 93*, 1231–1237.

Mitchell, J. E., Specker, S. M., & de Zwaan, M. (1991). Comorbidity and medical complications of bulimia nervosa. *Journal of Clinical Psychiatry, 52*, 13–20.

Mitchell, K. S., Mazzeo, S. E., Schlesinger, M. R., Brewerton, T. D., & Smith, B. N. (2012). Comorbidity of partial and subthreshold ptsd among men and women with eating disorders in the National Comorbidity Survey-Replication Study. *International Journal of Eating Disorders, 45*, 307–315.

Mitchell, K. S., Neale, M. C., Bulik, C. M., Aggen, S. H., Kendler, K. S., & Mazzeo, S. E. (2010). Binge eating disorder: A symptom-level investigation of genetic and environmental influences on liability. *Psychological Medicine, 40*, 1899–1906.

Modan-Moses, D., Yaroslavsky, A., Novikov, I., Segev, S., Toledano, A., Miterany, E., & Stein, D. (2003). Stunting of growth as a major feature of anorexia nervosa in male adolescents. *Pediatrics, 111*, 270–276.

Mondraty, N., Birmingham, C. L., Touyz, S., Sundakov, V., Chapman, L., & Beumont, P. (2005). Randomized controlled trial of olanzapine in the treatment of cognitions in anorexia nervosa. *Australasian Psychiatry, 13*, 72–75.

Mont, L., Castro, J., Herreros, B., Pare, C., Azqueta, M., Magrina, J., ... Brugada, J. (2003). Reversibility of cardiac abnormalities in adolescents with anorexia nervosa after weight recovery. *Journal of the American Academy of Child and Adolescent Psychiatry, 42*, 808–813.

Montague, P. R., Hyman, S. E., & Cohen, J. D. (2004). Computational roles for dopamine in behavioural control. *Nature, 431*, 760–767.

Monteleone, P., Brambilla, F., Bortolotti, F., Ferraro, C., & Maj, M. (1998). Plasma prolactin response to D-fenfluramine is blunted in bulimic patients with frequent binge episodes. *Psychological Medicine, 28*, 975–983.

Moodie, D. S., & Salcedo, E. (1983). Cardiac function in adolescents and young adults with anorexia nervosa. *Journal of Adolescent Health Care, 4*, 9–14.

Morgan, H. G., Purgold, J., & Welbourne, J. (1983). Management and outcome in anorexia nervosa: A standardized prognostic study. *British Journal of Psychiatry, 143*, 282–287.

Munsch, S., Biedert, E., Meyer, A. H., Herpertz, S., & Beglinger, C. (2009). CCK, ghrelin, and PYY responses in individuals with binge eating disorder before and after a cognitive behavioral treatment. *Physiology & Behavior, 97*, 14–20.

Murphy, F., Troop, N., & Treasure, J. (2000). Differential environmental factors in anorexia nervosa: A sibling pair study. *British Journal of Clinical Psychology, 39*, 193–203.

Murray, C. J. L., Vos, T., Lozano, R., Naghavi, M., Abraham, D., Flaxman, A. D. . . . Lopez, A.D. (2012). Global Burden of Disease Study Diseases and Injuries Group. Disability-adjusted life years (DALYs) for 291 diseases and injuries in 21 regions, 1990–2010: A systematic analysis for the Global Burden of Disease Study 2010. *Lancet, 380*, 2197–2223.

Mussell, M. P., Mitchell, J. E., Weller, C. L., Raymond, N. C., Crow, S. J., & Crosby, R. D. (1995). Onset of binge eating, dieting, obesity, and mood disorders among subjects seeking treatment for binge eating disorder. *International Journal of Eating Disorders, 17*, 395–401.

Naessen, S., Carlstrom, K., Glant, R., Jacobsson, H., & Hirshberg, A. I. (2006). Bone mineral density in bulimic women: Influence of endocrine factors and previous anorexia. *European Journal of Endocrinology, 155*, 245–251.

Nakabayashi, K., Komaki, G., Tajima, A., Ando, T., Ishikawa, M., Nomoto, J., . . . Shirasawa, S. (2009). Identification of novel candidate loci for anorexia nervosa at 1q41 and 11q22 in Japanese by a genome-wide association analysis with microsatellite markers. *Journal of Human Genetics, 54*, 531–537.

Nakash-Eisikovits, O., Dierberger, A., & Westen, D. (2002). A multidimensional meta-analysis of pharmacotherapy for bulimia nervosa: Summarizing the range of outcomes in controlled clinical trials. *Harvard Review of Psychiatry, 10*, 193–211.

Nakazato, M., Hashimoto, K., Schmidt, U., Tchanturia, K., Campbell, I. C., Collier, D. A., . . . Treasure, J. (2010). Serum glutamine, set-shifting ability and anorexia nervosa. *Annals of General Psychiatry, 9*, 29.

Narayanan, V., Gaudiani, J. L., Harris, R. H., & Mehler, P. S. (2010). Liver function test abnormalities in anorexia nervosa: Cause or effect. *International Journal of Eating Disorders, 43*, 378–381.

Nascimento, A. L., Luna, J. V., & Fontenelle, L. F. (2012). Body dysmorphic disorder and eating disorders in elite professional female ballet dancers. *Annals of Clinical Psychiatry, 24*, 191–194.

Nasser, M., Katzman, M. A., & Gordon, R. A. (2001). *Eating disorders and cultures in transition.* East Sussex, UK: Brunner-Routledge.

National Task Force on the Prevention and Treatment of Obesity. (2000). Dieting and the development of eating disorders in overweight and obese adults. *Archives of Internal Medicine, 160*, 2581–2589.

Nazar, B. P., Pinna, C. M., Coutinho, G., Segenreich, D., Duchesne, M., Appolinario, J. C., & Mattos, P. (2008). Review of literature of attention-deficit/hyperactivity disorder with comorbid eating disorders. *Revista Brasileira de Psiquiatria, 30*, 384–389.

Nemeroff, C. B., Kalali, A., Keller, M. B., Charney, D. S., Lenderts, S. E., Cascade, E. F., . . . Schatzberg, A. F. (2007). Impact of publicity concerning pediatric suicidality data on physician practice patterns in the United States. *Archives of General Psychiatry, 64*, 466–472.

Neumark-Sztainer, D. (1996). School-based programs for preventing eating disturbances. *Journal of School Health, 66*, 64–71.

Neumark-Sztainer, D. (2012). Integrating messages from the eating disorders field into obesity prevention. *Adolescent Medicine: State of the Art Reviews, 23*, 529–543.

Neumark-Sztainer, D., Butler, R., & Palti, H. (1995). Eating disturbances among adolescent girls: Evaluation of a school-based primary prevention program. *Journal of Nutrition Education, 27*, 24–30.

Neumark-Sztainer, D., Falkner, N., Story, M., Perry, C., Hannan, P. J., & Mulert, S. (2002). Weight-teasing among adolescents: Correlations with weight status and disordered eating behaviors. *International Journal of Obesity and Related Metabolic Disorders, 26*, 123–131.

Neumark-Sztainer D., Sherwood N., Coller T., & Hannan, P. J. (2000). Primary prevention of disordered eating among pre-adolescent girls: Feasibility and short-term impact of a community-based intervention. *Journal of the American Dietetic Association*, 100, 1466–1473.

Neumark-Sztainer, D., Wall, M., Guo, J., Story, M., Haines, J., & Eisenberg, M. (2006). Obesity, disordered eating, and eating disorders in a longitudinal study of adolescents: How do dieters fare 5 years later? *Journal of the American Dietetic Association, 106*, 559–568.

Neumark-Sztainer, D. R., Wall, M. M., Haines, J. I., Story, M. T., Sherwood, N. E., & van den Berg, P. A. (2007). Shared risk and protective factors for overweight and disordered eating in adolescents. *American Journal of Preventive Medicine, 33*, 359–369.

Neumark-Sztainer, D., Wall, M. M., Larson, N., Story, M., Fulkerson, J. A., Eisenberg, M. E., & Hannan, P. J. (2012). Secular trends in weight status and weight-related attitudes and behaviors in adolescents from 1999 to 2010. *Preventive Medicine, 54*, 77–81.

Newman-Toker, J. (2000). Risperidone in anorexia nervosa. *Journal of the American Academy of Child and Adolescent Psychiatry, 39*, 941–942.

Nicholls, D. E., Lynn, R., & Viner, R. M. (2011). Childhood eating disorders: British national surveillance study. *British Journal of Psychiatry, 198*, 295–301.

Nickel, C., Tritt, K., Muehlbacher, M., Pedrosa Gil, F., Mitterlehner, F. O., Kaplan, P., ... Nickel, M. K. (2005). Topiramate treatment in bulimia nervosa patients: A randomized, double-blind, placebo-controlled trial. *International Journal of Eating Disorders, 38*, 295–300.

Noordenbos, G. (2011) Which criteria for recovery are relevant according to eating disorder patients and therapists. *Eating Disorders, 19*, 441–451.

Norris, M. L., & Katzman, D. K. (2015). Change is never easy, but it is possible: Reflections on avoidant/restrictive food intake disorder two years after its introduction in the DSM-5. *Journal of Adolescent Health, 57*, 8–9.

Norris, M. L., Spettigue, W., Buchholz, A., & Henderson, K. A. (2007). Challenges associated with controlled psychopharmacological research trials in adolescents with eating disorders. *Journal of the Canadian Academy of Child and Adolescent Psychiatry, 16*, 167–172.

Nouri, M., Hill, L. G., & Orrell-Valente, J. K. (2011). Media exposure, internalization of the thin ideal, and body dissatisfaction: Comparing Asian American and European American college females. *Body Image, 8*, 366–372.

Nudel, D. B., Gootman, N., Nussbaum, M. P., & Shenker, I. R., (1984). Altered exercise performance and abnormal sympathetic responses to exercise in patients with anorexia nervosa. *Journal of Pediatrics, 105*, 34–37.

Nussbaum, M., Baird, D., Sonnenblick, M., Cowan, K., & Shenker, I. R. (1985). Short stature in anorexia nervosa patients. *Journal of Adolescent Health Care, 6*, 453–455.

Nussbaum, M., Shenker, I. R., Marc, J., & Klein, M. (1980). Cerebral atrophy in anorexia nervosa. *Journal of Pediatrics, 96*, 867–869.

Ogren, F. P., Huerter, J. V., Pearson, P. H., Antonson, C. W., & Moore, G. F. (1987). Transient salivary gland hypertrophy in bulimics. *Laryngoscope, 97*, 951–953.

Ohlmer, R., Jacobi, C., & Taylor, C. B. (2013). Preventing symptom progression in women at risk of anorexia: A pilot study. *European Eating Disorders Review, 21*, 323–329

Olfson, M., Marcus, S. C., & Druss, B. G. (2008). Effects of Food and Drug Administration warnings on antidepressant use in a national sample. *Archives of General Psychiatry, 65*, 94–101.

Olmsted, M. P., Daneman, D., Rydall, A. C., Lawson, M. L., & Rodin, G. M. (2002). The effects of psychoeducation on disturbed eating attitudes and behavior in young women with Type 1 diabetes mellitus. *International Journal of Eating Disorders, 32*, 230–239.

Olmsted, M. P., Kaplan, A. S., & Rockert, W. (1994). Rate and prediction of relapse in bulimia nervosa. *American Journal of Psychiatry, 151*, 738–743.

Olmsted, M. P., Kaplan, A. S., & Rockert, W. (2005). Defining remission and relapse in bulimia nervosa. *International Journal of Eating Disorders, 38*, 1–6.

Ornstein, R. M., Golden, N. H., Jacobson, M. S., & Shenker, I. R. (2003). Hypophosphatemia during nutritional rehabilitation in anorexia nervosa: Implications for refeeding and monitoring. *Journal of Adolescent Health, 32*, 83–88.

Ornstein, R. M., Rosen, D. S., Mammel, K. A., Callahan, S. T., Forman, S., Jay, M. S., ... Walsh, B. T. (2013). Distribution of eating disorders in children and adolescents using the proposed DSM-5 criteria for feeding and eating disorders. *Journal of Adolescent Health, 53*, 303–305.

Oswalt, S. B., & Wyatt, T. J. (2007). Mirror, mirror, help me like my body: Examining a body image media campaign. *Californian Journal of Health Promotion, 5*, 135–147.

Palla, B., & Litt, I. F. (1988). Medical complications of eating disorders in adolescents. *Pediatrics, 81*, 613–623.

Papadopoulos, F. C., Ekbom, A., Brandt, L., & Ekselius, L. (2009). Excess mortality, causes of death and prognostic factors in anorexia nervosa. *British Journal of Psychiatry, 194*, 10–17.

Paxton, S. J. (1993). A prevention program for disturbed eating and body dissatisfaction in adolescent girls: A 1-year follow-up. *Health Education Research: Theory & Practice, 8,* 43–51.

Peat, C., Mitchell, J. E., Hoek, H. W., & Wonderlich, S. A. (2009). Validity and utility of subtyping anorexia nervosa. *International Journal of Eating Disorders, 42,* 590–594.

Peebles, R., Hardy, K. K., Wilson, J. L., & Lock, J. D. (2010). Are diagnostic criteria for eating disorders markers of medical severity? *Pediatrics, 125,* e1193–e1201.

Peñas-Lledó, E., Vaz, F. J., Ramos, M. I., & Waller, G. (2002). Impulsive behaviors in bulimic patients: Relation to general psychopathology. *International Journal of Eating Disorders, 32,* 98–102.

Penniment, K. J., & Egan, S. J. (2012). Perfectionism and learning experiences in dance class as risk factors for eating disorders in dancers. *European Eating Disorders Review, 20,* 13–22.

Perez, M., Becker, C. B., & Ramirez, A. (2010). Transportability of an empirically supported dissonance-based prevention program for eating disorders. *Body Image, 7,* 179–186.

Pike, K. M., & Borovoy, A. (2004). The rise of eating disorders in Japan: Issues of culture and limitations of the model of "westernization." *Culture, Medicine, and Psychiatry, 28,* 493–531.

Pike, K. M., Carter, J. C., & Olmsted, M. P. (2009). Cognitive-behavioral therapy for anorexia nervosa. In C. M. Grilos & J. E. Mitchell (Eds.), *The treatment of eating disorders: A clinical handbook* (pp. 83–107). New York: Guilford Press.

Pike, K. M., Devlin, M. J., & Loeb, K. L. (2003). Cognitive-behavioral therapy in the treatment of anorexia nervosa, bulimia nervosa, and binge eating disorder. In J. K. Thompson (Ed.), *Handbook of eating disorders and obesity* (pp. 130–162). Hoboken, NJ: John Wiley & Sons.

Pike, K. M., Hilbert, A., Wilfley, D. E., Fairburn, C. G., Dohm, F. A., Walsh, B. T., & Striegel-Moore, R. (2008). Toward an understanding of risk factors for anorexia nervosa: A case-control study. *Psychological Medicine, 38,* 1443–1453.

Pike, K. M., Walsh, B. T., Vitousek, K., Wilson, G. T., & Bauer, J. (2003). Cognitive behavior therapy in the post-hospitalization treatment of anorexia nervosa. *American Journal of Psychiatry, 160,* 2046–2049.

Pinhas, L., Morris, A., Crosby, R. D., & Katzman, D. K. (2011). Incidence and age-specific presentation of restrictive eating disorders in children: A Canadian paediatric surveillance program study. *Archives of Pediatric and Adolescent Medicine, 165,* 895–899.

Piran, N. (1999). Eating disorders: A trial of prevention in a high risk school setting. *Journal of Primary Prevention, 20,* 75–90.

Polivy, J., & Herman, C. P. (1985). Dieting and binging: A causal analysis. *American Psychologist, 40,* 193–201.

Powers, P. S. (1982). Heart failure during treatment of anorexia nervosa. *American Journal of Psychiatry, 139,* 1167–1170.

Powers, P. S., Bannon, Y. S., Eubanks, R., & McCormick, T. (2007). Quetiapine in anorexia nervosa patients: An open label outpatient pilot study. *International Journal of Eating Disorders, 40,* 21–26.

Powers, P. S., Santana, C. A., & Bannon, Y. S. (2002). Olanzapine in the treatment of anorexia nervosa: An open label trial. *International Journal of Eating Disorders, 32,* 146–154.

Powers, P., Schocken, D., & Boyd, F. (1998). Comparison of habitual runners and anorexia nervosa patients. *International Journal of Eating Disorders, 23,* 133–143.

Presnell, K., Stice, E., & Tristan, J. (2008). Experimental investigation of the effects of naturalistic dieting on bulimic symptoms: Moderating effects of depressive symptoms. *Appetite, 50,* 91–101.

Preti, A., Girolamo, G., Vilagut, G., Alonso, J., Graaf, R., Bruffaerts, R., ... Morosini, P. (2009). The epidemiology of eating disorders in six European countries: Results of the ESEMeD-WMH project. *Journal of Psychiatric Research, 43,* 1125–1132.

Pyle, R. L., Mitchell, J. E., Ecker, E. D., Hatsukami, D., Pomeroy, C., & Zimmerman, R. (1990). Maintenance treatment and 6-month outcome for bulimic patients who respond to initial treatment. *American Journal of Psychiatry, 147,* 871–875.

Raj, K. S., Keane-Miller, C., & Golden, N. H. (2012). Hypomagnesemia in adolescents with eating disorders hospitalized for medical instability. *Nutrition and Clinical Practice, 27,* 689–694.

Ramacciotti, C. E., Coli, E., Biadi, O., & Dell'Osso, L. (2003). Silent pericardial effusion in a sample of anorexic patients. *Eating and Weight Disorders, 8,* 6871.

Raney, T. J., Thornton, L. M., Berrettini, W., Brandt, H., Crawford, S., Fichter, M. M., ... Bulik, C. M. (2008). Influence of overanxious disorder of childhood on the expression of anorexia nervosa. *International Journal of Eating Disorders, 41,* 326–332.

Rautou, P. E., Cazals-Hatem, D., Moreau, R., Francoz, C., Feldmann, G., Lebrec, D., ...

Durand, F. (2008). Acute liver cell damage in patients with anorexia nervosa: A possible role of starvation-induced hepatocyte autophagy. *Gastroenterology, 135*, 840–848.

Reagan, P., & Hersch, J. (2005). Influence of race, gender, and socioeconomic status on binge eating frequency in a population-based sample. *International Journal of Eating Disorders, 38*, 252–256.

Reichborn-Kjennerud, T., Bulik, C. M., Tambs, K., & Harris, J. R. (2004). Genetic and environmental influences on binge eating in the absence of compensatory behaviors: A population-based twin study. *International Journal of Eating Disorders, 36*, 307–314.

Reid, I. R., Ames, R. W., Evans, M. C., Gamble, G. D., & Sharpe, S. J. (1995). Long-term effects of calcium supplementation on bone loss and fractures in postmenopausal women: A randomized controlled trial. *American Journal of Medicine, 98*, 331–335.

Richard, M., Bauer, S., & Kordy, H. (2005). Relapse in anorexia and bulimia nervosa: A 2.5-year follow-up study. *European Eating Disorders Review, 13*, 180–190.

Richardson, S. M., & Paxton, S. J. (2010). An evaluation of a body image intervention based on risk factors for body dissatisfaction: A controlled study with adolescent girls. *International Journal of Eating Disorders, 43*, 112–122.

Richardson, S. M., Paxton, S. J., & Thomson, J. S. (2009). Is BodyThink an efficacious body image and self-esteem program? A controlled evaluation with adolescents. *Body Image, 6*, 75–82.

Rierdan, J., Koff, E., & Stubbs, M. L. (1989). A longitudinal analysis of body image as a predictor of the onset and persistence of adolescent girls' depression. *Journal of Early Adolescence, 9*, 454–466.

Rigotti, N. A., Neer, R. M., Skates, S. J., Herzog, D. B., & Nussbaum, S. R. (1991). The clinical course of osteoporosis in anorexia nervosa: A longitudinal study of cortical bone mass. *Journal of the American Medical Association, 265*, 1133–1138.

Rivinus, T., Biederman, J., Herzog, D., Kemper, K., Harper, G., Harmatz, J., & Houseworth, S. (1984). Anorexia nervosa and affective disorders: A controlled family history study. *American Journal of Psychiatry, 141*, 1414–1418.

Rohde, P., Auslander, B. A., Shaw, H., Raineri, K. M., Gau, J. M., & Stice, E. (2014). Dissonance-based prevention of eating disorder risk factors in middle school girls: Results from two pilot trials. *International Journal of Eating Disorders, 47*, 483–494.

Roberts, M. E., Tchanturia, K., Stahl, D., Southgate, L., & Treasure, J. (2007). A systematic review and meta-analysis of set-shifting ability in eating disorders. *Psychological Medicine, 37*, 1075–1084.

Roberts, M. E., Tchanturia, K., & Treasure, J. L. (2010). Exploring the neurocognitive signature of poor set-shifting in anorexia and bulimia nervosa. *Journal of Psychiatric Research, 44*, 964–970.

Robin, A. L., & Le Grange, D. (2010). Treating adolescents with anorexia nervosa using behavioral family systems therapy. In J. R. Weisz & A. E. Kazdin (Eds.), *Evidence-based psychotherapies for children and adolescents* (2nd ed., pp. 345–358). New York: Guilford Press.

Robin, A., Siegel, P., Gilroy, M., Dennis, A., Sikand, A. (1999). A controlled comparison of family versus individual therapy for adolescents with anorexia nervosa. *Journal of the American Academy of Child and Adolescent Psychiatry, 38*, 1482–1489.

Robinson, E., Bachrach, L. K., & Katzman, D. K. (2000). Use of hormone replacement therapy to reduce the risk of osteopenia in adolescent girls with anorexia nervosa. *Journal of Adolescent Health, 26*, 343–348.

Rodin, J., Silberstein, L., & Streigel-Moore, R. (1985). Women and weight: A normative discontent. In T. Sonderegger (Ed.), *Psychology and gender: Nebraska Symposium on Motivation* (pp. 267–307). Lincoln: University of Nebraska Press.

Rogers Wood, N. A., & Petrie, T. A. (2010). Body dissatisfaction, ethnic identity, and disordered eating among African American women. *Journal of Counseling Psychology, 57*, 141–153.

Romano, S. J., Halmi, K. A., Sarkar, N. P., Koke, S. C., & Lee, J. S. (2002). A placebo-controlled study of fluoxetine in continued treatment of bulimia nervosa after successful acute fluoxetine treatment. *American Journal of Psychiatry, 159*, 96–102.

Romans, S., Martin, J., & Mullen, P. (1994). Child sexual abuse (CSA) and later eating disorders: A New Zealand epidemiological study. *Neuropsychopharmacology, 10*, 92S.

Root, A. W., & Powers, P. S. (1983). Anorexia nervosa presenting as growth retardation in adolescents. *Journal of Adolescent Health Care, 4*, 25–30.

Root, T. L., Pinheiro, A. P., Thornton, L., Strober, M., Fernandez-Aranda, F., Brandt, H., ... Bulik CM. (2010). Substance use disorders in women with anorexia nervosa. *International Journal of Eating Disorders, 43*, 14–21.

Root, T. L., Pisetsky, E. M., Thornton, L., Lichtenstein, P., Pedersen, N. L., & Bulik, C. M. (2010). Patterns of co-morbidity of eating disorders and substance use in Swedish females. *Psychological Medicine, 40*, 105–115.

Rosval, L., Steiger, H., Bruce, K., Israel, M., Richardson, J., & Aubut, M. (2006). Impulsivity in women with eating disorders: Problem of response inhibition, planning, or attention? *International Journal of Eating Disorders, 39*, 590–593.

Rubin, L. R., Fitts, M. L., & Becker, A. E. (2003). 'Whatever feels good in my soul': Body ethics and aesthetics among African American and Latina women. *Culture, Medicine and Psychiatry, 27*, 49–75.

Rubinstein, T. B., McGinn, A. P., Wildman, R. P., & Wylie-Rosett, J. (2010). Disordered eating in adulthood is associated with reported weight loss attempts in childhood. *International Journal of Eating Disorders, 43*, 663–666.

Russell, G. F. (1985). Premenarchal anorexia nervosa and its sequelae. *Journal of Psychiatric Research, 19*, 363–369.

Russell, G. F. M., Szmukler, G. I., Dare, C., & Eisler, I. (1987). An evaluation of family therapy in anorexia nervosa and bulimia nervosa. *Archives of General Psychiatry, 44*, 1047–1056.

Ruuska, J., Kaltiala-Heino, R., Koivisto, A. M., & Rantanen, P. (2003). Puberty, sexual development and eating disorders in adolescent outpatients. *European Child & Adolescent Psychiatry, 12*, 214–220.

Sánchez-Carracedo, D., Neumark-Sztainer, D., & López-Guimerà, G. (2012). Integrated prevention of obesity and eating disorders: Barriers, developments and opportunities. *Public Health Nutrition, 15*, 2295–2309.

Sánchez-Ortiz, V. C., Munro, C., Stahl, D., House, J., Startup, H., Treasure, J., ... Schmidt, U. (2011). A randomized controlled trial of internet-based cognitive-behavioral therapy for bulimia nervosa or related disorders in a student population. *Psychological Medicine, 41*, 407–417.

Sanci, L., Coffey, C., Olsson, C., Reid, S., Carlin, J. B., & Patton, G. (2008). Childhood sexual abuse and eating disorders in females: Findings from the Victorian Adolescent Health Cohort Study. *Archives of Pediatrics & Adolescent Medicine, 162*, 261–267.

Sands, R., Tricker, J., Sherman, C., Armatas, C., & Maschette, W. (1997). Disordered eating patterns, body image, self-esteem, and physical activity in preadolescent school children. *International Journal of Eating Disorders, 21*, 159–166.

Schebendach, J., Golden, N. H., Jacobson, M. S., Arden, M., Pettei, M., Hardoff, D., ... Hertz, S. (1995). Indirect calorimetry in the nutritional management of eating disorders. *International Journal of Eating Disorders, 17*, 59–66.

Schebendach, J. E., Golden, N. H., Jacobson, M. S., Hertz, S., & Shenker, I. R. (1997). The metabolic responses to starvation and refeeding in adolescents with anorexia nervosa. *Annals of the New York Academy of Sciences, 817*, 110–119.

Schebendach, J. E., Mayer, L. E., Devlin, M. J., Attia, E., Contento, I. R., Wolf, R. L., & Walsh, B. T. (2008). Dietary energy density and diet variety as predictors of outcome in anorexia nervosa. *American Journal of Clinical Nutrition, 87*, 810–816.

Schebendach, J. E., Mayer, L. E. S., Devlin, M. J., Attia, E., & Walsh, B. T. (2012). Dietary energy density and diet variety as risk factor for relapse in anorexia nervosa: A replication. *International Journal of Eating Disorders, 45*, 79–84.

Schiff, R. J., Wurzel, C. L., Brunson, S. C., Kasloff, I., Nussbaum, M. P., & Frank, S. D. (1986). Death due to chronic syrup of ipecac use in a patient with bulimia. *Pediatrics, 78*, 412–416.

Schizophrenia Working Group of the Psychiatric Genomics Consortium. (2014). Biological insights from 108 schizophrenia-associated genetic loci. *Nature, 511*, 421–427.

Schmidt, U., Andiappan, M., Grover, M., Robinson, S., Perkins, S., Dugmore, O., ... Williams, C. (2008). A randomized controlled trial of the effectiveness of a CD-ROM-based cognitive-behavioral self-care intervention for bulimia nervosa. *British Journal of Psychiatry, 193*, 493–500.

Schmidt, U., Cooper, P. J., Essers, H., Freeman, C. P., Holland, R. L., Palmer, R. L., ... Webster J. (2004). Fluvoxamine and graded psychotherapy in the treatment of bulimia nervosa: A randomized, double-blind, placebo-controlled, multicenter study of short-term and long-term pharmacotherapy combined with a stepped care approach to psychotherapy. *Journal of Clinical Psychopharmacology, 24*, 549–552.

Schmidt, U., Lee, S., Beecham, J., Perkins, S., Treasure, J., Yi, I., ... Eisler I. (2007). A randomized controlled trial of family therapy and cognitive behavior therapy guided self-care for adolescents with bulimia nervosa and related disorders. *American Journal of Psychiatry, 164*, 591–598.

Schmidt, U., Tiller, J., Blanchard, M., Andrews, B., & Treasure, J. (1997). Is there a specific trauma precipitating anorexia nervosa? *Psychological Medicine*, *27*, 523–530.

Schultz, W. (2004). Neural coding of basic reward terms of animal learning theory, game theory, microeconomics and behavioural ecology. *Current Opinion in Neurobiology*, *14*, 139–147.

Serfaty, M. A., Trukington, D., Heap, M., Ledsham, L., & Jolley, E. (1999). Cognitive therapy versus dietary counselling in the outpatient treatment of anorexia nervosa: Effects of the treatment phase. *European Eating Disorders Review*, *7*, 334–350.

Shamim, T., Golden, N. H., Arden, M., Filiberto, L., & Shenker, I. R. (2003). Resolution of vital sign instability: An objective measure of medical stability in anorexia nervosa. *Journal of Adolescent Health*, *32*, 73–77.

Shapiro, J. R., Reba-Harrelson, L., Dymek-Valentine, M., Woolson, S. L., Hamer, R. M., & Bulik, C. M. (2007). Feasability and acceptability of CD-ROM-based cognitive-behavioral treatment for binge-eating disorder. *European Eating Disorders Review*, *15*, 175–184.

Sharp, C. W., & Freeman, C. P. (1993). The medical complications of anorexia nervosa. *British Journal of Psychiatry*, *162*, 452–462.

Shaw, H., Ramirez, L., Trost, A., Randall, P., & Stice, E. (2004). Body image and eating disturbances across ethnic groups: More similarities than differences. *Psychology of Addictive Behaviors*, *18*, 12–18.

Shaw, H. E., Stice, E., & Springer, D. W. (2004). Perfectionism, body dissatisfaction, and self-esteem in predicting bulimic symptomatology: Lack of replication. *International Journal of Eating Disorders*, *36*, 41–47.

Sherman, P., Leslie, K., Goldberg, E., Rybczynski, J., & St. Louis, P. (1994). Hypercarotenemia and transaminitis in female adolescents with eating disorders: A prospective, controlled study. *Journal of Adolescent Health*, *15*, 205–209.

Shoebridge, P., & Gowers, S. (2000). Parental high concern and adolescent-onset anorexia nervosa. *British Journal of Psychiatry*, *176*, 132–137.

Shomaker, L. B., Tanofsky-Kraff, M., Savastano, D. M., Kozlosky, M., Columbo, K. M., Wolkoff, L. E., . . .Yanovski, J. A. (2010). Puberty and observed energy intake: Boy, can they eat! *American Journal of Clinical Nutrition*, *92*, 123–129.

Silberg, J. L., & Bulik, C. M. (2005). The developmental association between eating disorders symptoms and symptoms of depression and anxiety in juvenile twin girls. *Journal of Child Psychology and Psychiatry, and Allied Disciplines*, *46*, 1317–1326.

Silverman, J. A., & Krongrad, E. (1983). Anorexia nervosa: A cause of pericardial effusion? *Pediatric Cardiology*, *4*, 125–127.

Silvetti, M. S., Magnani, M., Santilli, A., Di Liso, G., Diamanti, A., Pompei, E., . . . Ragonese, P. (1998). The heart of anorexic adolescents. *Giornale Italiano di Cardiologia*, *28*, 131–139.

Sinton, M., & Taylor, C. B. (2010). Prevention: Current status and underlying theory. In W. S. Agras (Ed.), *Oxford handbook of eating disorders* (pp. 307–331). Oxford: Oxford University Press.

Slof-Op 't Landt, M. C., van Furth, E. F., Meulenbelt, I., Slagboom, P. E., Bartels, M., Boomsma, D. I., & Bulik, C. M. (2005). Eating disorders: From twin studies to candidate genes and beyond. *Twin Research and Human Genetics*, *8*, 467–482.

Snow-Harter, C., Bouxsein, M. L., Lewis, B. T., Carter, D. R., & Marcus, R. (1992). Effects of resistance and endurance exercise on bone mineral status of young women: A randomized exercise intervention trial. *Journal of Bone and Mineral Research*, *7*, 761–769.

Sobanski, E., Hiltmann, W. D., Blanz, B., Klein, M., Schmidt, M. H. (1997). Pelvic ultrasound scanning of the ovaries in adolescent anorectic patients at low weight and after weight recovery. *European Child & Adolescent Psychiatry*, *6*, 207–211.

Solanto, M. V., Jacobson, M. S., Heller, L., Golden, N. H., & Hertz, S. (1994). Rate of weight gain of inpatients with anorexia nervosa under two behavioral contracts. *Pediatrics*, *93*, 989–991.

Sollid, C. P., Wisborg, K., Hjort, J., & Secher, N. J. (2004). Eating disorder that was diagnosed before pregnancy and pregnancy outcome. *American Journal of Obstetrics and Gyncecology*, *190*, 206–210.

Sonneville, K.R., Calzo, J. P., Horton, N. J., Haines, J., Austin, S. B., & Field, A. E. (2012). Body satisfaction, weight gain and binge eating among overweight adolescent girls. *International Journal of Obesity*, *36*, 944–949.

Sonneville, K. R., Horton, N. J., Micali, N., Crosby, R. D., Swanson, S. A., Solmi, F., & Field, A. E. (2013). Longitudinal associations between binge eating and overeating and adverse outcomes among adolescents and young adults: Does loss of control matter? *JAMA Pediatrics*, *167*, 149–155.

Southard, R. N., Morris, J. D., Mahan, J. D., Hayes, J. R., Torch, M. A., Sommer, A., & Zipf, W. B. (1991). Bone mass in healthy children: Measurement with quantitative DXA. *Radiology, 179*, 735–738.

Soyka, L. A., Misra, M., Frenchman, A., Miller, K. K., Grinspoon, S., Schoenfeld, D. A., & Kilbanski, A. (2002). Abnormal bone mineral accrual in adolescent girls with anorexia nervosa. *Journal of Clinical Endocrinology and Metabolism, 87*, 4177–4185.

Spettigue, W., Buchholz, A., Henderson, K., Feder, S., Moher, D., Kourad, K., . . . Ledoux S. (2008). Evaluation of the efficacy and safety of olanzapine as an adjunctive treatment for anorexia nervosa in adolescent females: A randomized, double-blind, placebo-controlled trial. *BMC Pediatrics, 8*, 4.

Spindler, A., & Milos, G. (2007). Links between eating disorder symptom severity and psychiatric comorbidity. *Eating Behaviors, 8*, 364–373.

Spurrell, E. B., Wilfley, D. E., Tanofsky, M. B., & Brownell, K. D. (1997). Age of onset for binge eating: Are there different pathways to binge eating? *International Journal of Eating Disorders, 21*, 55–65.

Stahl, S. M. (2008). *Stahl's essential psychopharmacology: Neuroscientific basis and practical applications* (3rd ed.). New York: Cambridge University Press.

Steele, A., Corsini, N., & Wade, T. D. (2007). The interaction of perfectionism, perceived weight status, and self-esteem to predict bulimic symptoms: The role of "benign" perfectionism. *Behaviour Research and Therapy, 45*, 1647–1655.

Steinglass, J., & Walsh, B. T. (2006). Habit learning and anorexia nervosa: A cognitive neuroscience hypothesis. *International Journal of Eating Disorders, 39*, 267–275.

Steinhausen, H. C. (1997). Outcome of anorexia nervosa in the younger patient. *Journal of Child Psychology and Psychiatry and Allied Disciplines, 38*, 271–276.

Steinhausen, H. C. (2002). The outcome of anorexia nervosa in the 20th century *American Journal of Psychiatry, 159*, 1284–1293.

Steinhausen, H. C. (2009). Outcome of eating disorders. *Child and Adolescent Psychiatric Clinics of North America, 18*, 225–242.

Steinhausen, H. C., & Weber, S. (2009). The outcome of bulimia nervosa: Findings from one-quarter century of research. *American Journal of Psychiatry, 166*, 1331–1341.

Stice, E. (1994). Review of the evidence for a sociocultural model of bulimia nervosa and exploration of mechanisms of action. *Clinical Psychology Review, 14*, 633–661.

Stice, E. (2001). A prospective test of the dual-pathway model of bulimic pathology: Mediating effects of dieting and negative affect. *Journal of Abnormal Psychology, 110*, 124–135.

Stice, E., Agras, W., & Hammer, L. (1999). Risk factors for the emergence of childhood eating disturbances: A five-year prospective study. *International Journal of Eating Disorders, 25*, 375–387.

Stice, E., & Bearman, S. K. (2001). Body image and eating disturbances prospectively predict growth in depressive symptoms in adolescent girls: A growth curve analysis. *Developmental Psychology, 37*, 597–607.

Stice, E., Becker, C. B., & Yokum, S. (2013). Eating disorder prevention: Current evidence-base and future directions. *International Journal of Eating Disorders, 46*, 478–485.

Stice, E., Cameron, R. P., Killen, J. D., Hayward, C., & Taylor, C. B. (1999). Naturalistic weight-reduction efforts prospectively predict growth in relative weight and onset of obesity among female adolescents. *Journal of Consulting and Clinical Psychology, 67*, 967–974.

Stice, E., Durant, S., Burger, K. S., & Schoeller, D. A. (2011). Weight suppression and risk of future increases in body mass: Effects of suppressed resting metabolic rate and energy expenditure. *American Journal of Clinical Nutrition, 94*, 7–11.

Stice, E., Durant, S., Rohde, P., & Shaw, H. (2014). Effects of a prototype Internet dissonance-based eating disorder prevention program at 1- and 2-year follow-up. *Health Psychology, 33*, 1558–1567.

Stice, E., Marti, C. N., & Rohde, P. (2013). Prevalence, incidence, impairment, and course of the proposed DSM-5 eating disorder diagnoses in an 8-year prospective community study of young women. *Journal of Abnormal Psychology, 122*, 445–457.

Stice, E., Marti, C. N., Spoor, S., Presnell, K., & Shaw, H. (2008). Dissonance and healthy weight eating disorder prevention programs: Long-term effects from a randomized efficacy trial. *Journal of Consulting and Clinical Psychology, 76*, 329–340.

Stice, E., Presnell, K., & Bearman, S. K. (2001). Relation of early menarche to depression, eating disorders, substance abuse, and comorbid psychopathology among adolescent girls. *Developmental Psychology, 37*, 608–619.

Stice, E., Presnell, K., & Spangler, D. (2002). Risk factors for binge eating onset in adolescent girls: A 2-year prospective investigation. *Health Psychology, 21*, 131–138.

Stice, E., Rohde, P., Butryn, M. L., Shaw, H., & Marti, C. N. (2015). Effectiveness trial of a selective dissonance-based eating disorder prevention program with female college students: Effects at 2- and 3-year follow-up. *Behaviour Research and Therapy*, *71*, 20–26.

Stice, E., Rohde, P., Gau, J., & Shaw, H. (2009). An effectiveness trial of a dissonance-based eating disorder prevention program for high-risk adolescent girls. *Journal of Consulting and Clinical Psychology*, *77*, 825–834.

Stice, E., Rohde, P., & Shaw, H. (2013). *The Body Project: A dissonance-based eating disorder prevention intervention (Programs That Work)*. Oxford: Oxford University Press.

Stice, E., Rohde, P., Shaw, H., & Marti, C. N. (2013). An efficacy trial of a selective prevention program targeting both eating disorders and obesity among female college students: 1- and 2-year follow-up effects. *Journal of Consulting and Clinical Psychology*, *81*, 183–189.

Stice, E., & Shaw, H. E. (2002). Role of body dissatisfaction in the onset and maintenance of eating pathology: A synthesis of research findings. *Journal of Psychosomatic Research*, *53*, 985–993.

Stice, E., & Shaw, H. (2004). Eating disorder prevention programs: A meta-analytic review. *Psychological Bulletin*, *130*, 206–227.

Stice, E., Shaw, H., & Marti, C. N. (2007). A meta-analytic review of eating disorder prevention programs: Encouraging findings. *Annual Review of Clinical Psychology*, *3*, 207–231.

Stice, E., Spoor, S., Bohon, C., & Small, D. M. (2008). Relation between obesity and blunted striatal response to food is moderated by TaqIA A1 allele. *Science*, *322*, 449–452.

Stice, E., & Whitenton, K. (2002). Risk factors for body dissatisfaction in adolescent girls: A longitudinal investigation. *Developmental Psychology*, *38*, 669–678.

Stock, S. L., Goldberg, E., Corbett, S., & Katzman, D. K. (2002). Substance use in female adolescents with eating disorders. *Journal of Adolescent Health*, *31*, 176–182.

Stormer, S. M., & Thompson, J. K. (1996). Explanations of body image disturbance: A test of maturational status, negative verbal commentary, social comparison, and sociocultural hypotheses. *International Journal of Eating Disorders*, *19*, 193–202.

Striegel-Moore, R. H., & Bulik, C. M. (2007). Risk factors for eating disorders. *American Psychologist*, *62*, 181–198.

Striegel-Moore, R. H., Dohm, F. A., Kraemer, H. C., Schreiber, G. B., Crawford, P. B., & Daniels, S. R. (2005). Health services use in women with a history of bulimia nervosa or binge eating disorder. *International Journal of Eating Disorders*, *37*, 11–18.

Striegel-Moore, R., Dohm, F., Kraemer, H., Taylor, C., Daniels, S., Crawford, P., & Schreiber, G. (2003). Eating disorders in white and black women. *American Journal of Psychiatry*, *160*, 1326–1331.

Striegel-Moore, R. H., Fairburn, C. G., Wilfley, D. E., Pike, K. M., Dohm, F. A., & Kraemer, H. C. (2005). Toward an understanding of risk factors for binge-eating disorder in black and white women: A community-based case-control study. *Psychological Medicine*, *35*, 907–917.

Striegel-Moore, R. H., Franko, D. L., Thompson, D., Barton, B., Schreiber, G. B., & Daniels, S. R. (2004). Changes in weight and body image over time in women with eating disorders. *International Journal of Eating Disorders*, *36*, 315–327.

Striegel-Moore, R. H., Leslie, D., Petrill, S. A., Garvin, V., & Rosenheck, R.A. (2000). One-year use and cost of inpatient and outpatient services among female and male patients with an eating disorder: Evidence from a national database of health insurance claims. *International Journal of Eating Disorders*, *27*, 381–389.

Striegel-Moore, R. H., Schrieber, G. B., Lo, A., Crawford, P., Obarzanek, E., & Rodin, J. (2000). Eating disorder symptoms in a cohort of 11- to 16-year-old black and white girls: The NHLBI Growth and Health Study. *International Journal of Eating Disorders*, *27*, 49–66.

Strober, M., Freeman, R., Lampert, C., & Diamond, J. (2007). The association of anxiety disorders and obsessive compulsive personality disorder with anorexia nervosa: Evidence from a family study with discussion of nosological and neurodevelopmental implications. *International Journal of Eating Disorders*, *40*, 46–51.

Strober, M., Freeman, R., Lampert, C., Diamond, J., & Kaye, W. (2000). Controlled family study of anorexia nervosa and bulimia nervosa: Evidence of shared liability and transmission of partial syndromes. *American Journal of Psychiatry*, *157*, 393–401.

Strober, M., Freeman, R., & Morrell, W. (1997). The long-term course of severe anorexia nervosa in adolescents: Survival analysis of recovery, relapse, and outcome predictors over

10–15 years in a prospective study. *International Journal of Eating Disorders*, *22*, 339–360.

Strober, M., Lampert, C., Morrell, W., Burroughs, J., & Jacobs, C. (1990). A controlled family study of anorexia nervosa: Evidence of familial aggregation and lack of shared transmission with affective disorders. *International Journal of Eating Disorders*, *9*, 239–253.

Strokosch, G. R., Friedman, A. J., Wu, S. C., & Kamin, M. (2006). Effects of an oral contraceptive (norgestimate/ethinyl estradiol) on bone mineral density in adolescent females with anorexia nervosa: A double-blind, placebo-controlled study. *Journal of Adolescent Health*, *39*, 819–827.

Sudi, K., Ottl, K., Payerl, D., Baumgartl, P., Tauschmann, K., & Muller, W. (2004). Anorexia athletica. *Nutrition*, *20*, 657–661.

Sullivan, P. F. (1995). Mortality in anorexia nervosa. *American Journal of Psychiatry*, *152*, 1073–1074.

Sundblad, C., Landén, M., Eriksson, T., Bergman, L., & Eriksson, E. (2005). Effects of the androgen antagonist flutamide and the serotonin reuptake inhibitor citalopram in bulimia nervosa: A placebo-controlled pilot study. *Journal of Clinical Psychopharmacology*, *25*, 85–88.

Sundgot-Borgen, J., & Torstveit, M. K. (2004). Prevalence of eating disorders in elite athletes is higher than in the general population. *Clinical Journal of Sport Medicine*, *14*, 25–32.

Sundgot-Borgen, J., & Torstveit, M. K. (2010). Aspects of disordered eating continuum in elite high-intensity sports. *Scandinavian Journal of Medicine & Science in Sports*, *20*, 112–121.

Swanson, S. A., Crow, S. J., Le Grange, D., Swendsen, J., & Merikangas, K. R. (2011). Prevalence and correlates of eating disorders in adolescents. Results from the National Comorbidity Survey Replication Adolescent Supplement. *Archives of General Psychiatry*, *68*, 714–723.

Swinbourne, J., Hunt, C., Abbott, M., Russell, J., St Clare, T., & Touyz, S. (2012). The comorbidity between eating disorders and anxiety disorders: Prevalence in an eating disorder sample and anxiety disorder sample. *Australian and New Zealand Journal of Psychiatry*, *46*, 118–131.

Swinbourne, J. M., & Touyz, S. W. (2007). The comorbidity of eating disorders and anxiety disorders: A review. *European Eating Disorders Review*, *15*, 253–274.

Sysko, R., Roberto, C. A., Barnes, R., Grilo, C. M., Attia, E., & Walsh, B. T. (2012). Test-retest reliability of the proposed DSM-5 eating disorder diagnostic criteria. *Psychiatry Research*, *196*, 302–308.

Sysko, R., Sha, N., Wang, Y., Duan, N., & Walsh, B. T. (2010). Early response to antidepressant treatment in bulimia nervosa. *Psychological Medicine*, *49*, 999–1006.

Tanofsky-Kraff, M., Bulik, C. M., Marcus, M. D., Striegel, R. H., Wilfley, D. E., Wonderlich, S. A., & Hudson, J. I. (2013). Binge eating disorder: The next generation of research. *International Journal of Eating Disorders*, *46*, 193–207.

Tanofsky-Kraff, M., Cohen, M. L., Yanovski, S. Z., Cox, C., Theim, K. R., Keil, M., . . . Yanovski, J. A. (2006). A prospective study of psychological predictors of body fat gain among children at high risk for adult obesity. *Pediatrics*, *117*, 1203–1209.

Tanofsky-Kraff, M., Shomaker, L. B., Olsen, C., Roza, C. A., Wolkoff, L. E., Columbo, K. M., . . . Yanovski, J. A. (2011). A prospective study of pediatric loss of control eating and psychological outcomes. *Journal of Abnormal Psychology*, *120*, 108–118.

Tanofsky-Kraff, M., Shomaker, L. B., Stern, E. A., Miller, R., Sebring, N., Dellavalle, D., Yanovski, S. Z., . . . Yanovski, J. A. (2012). Children's binge eating and development of metabolic syndrome. *International Journal of Obesity*, *36*, 956–962.

Tanofsky-Kraff, M., Yanovski, S. Z., Schvey, N. A., Olsen, C. H., Gustafson, J., & Yanovski, J. A. (2009). A prospective study of loss of control eating for body weight gain in children at high risk for adult obesity. *International Journal of Eating Disorders*, *42*, 26–30.

Taylor, C. B., Bryson, S., Luce, K. H., Cunning, D., Celio, A., Abascal, L. B., . . . Wilfley, D. E. (2006). Prevention of eating disorders in at-risk college-age women. *Archives of General Psychiatry*, *63*, 831–838.

Taylor, C. B., Franko, D. L., Neumark-Sztainer, D., Paxton, S. J., & Shapiro, J. R. (2007). Public-health approach to eating disorders. *Lancet*, *9*, 369.

Taylor, C. B., Kass, A. E., Trockel, M., Cunning, D., Weisman, H., Bailey, J., . . . Wilfley, D. E. (2016). Reducing eating disorder onset in a very high risk sample with significant comorbid depression: A randomized controlled trial. *Journal of Consulting and Clinical Psychology*, *84*, 402–414.

Taylor, C. B., Taylor, K., Jones, M., Shorter, A., Yee, M., Genkin, B., . . . Wilfley, D. E. (2012). Obesity prevention in defined (high school) populations. *International Journal of Obesity Supplements*, *2*, S30–S32.

Taylor, J. Y., Caldwell, C. H., Baser, R. E., Faison, N., & Jackson, J. S. (2007). Prevalence of eating disorders among Blacks in the National Survey of American Life. *International Journal of Eating Disorders, 40*, S10–S14.

Taylor, J. Y., Caldwell, C. H., Baser, R. E., Matusko, N., Faison, N., & Jackson, J. S. (2013). Classification and correlates of eating disorders among blacks: Findings from the National Survey of American Life. *Journal of Health Care for the Poor and Underserved, 24*, 289–310.

Tchanturia, K., Davies, H., Roberts, M., Harrison, A., Nakazato, M., Schmidt, U., ... Morris, R. (2012). Poor cognitive flexibility in eating disorders: Examining the evidence using the Wisconsin Card Sorting Task. *PloS One, 7*, e28331.

Tchanturia, K., Morris, R. G., Anderluh, M. B., Collier, D. A., Nikolaou, V., & Treasure, J. (2004). Set shifting in anorexia nervosa: An examination before and after weight gain, in full recovery and relationship to childhood and adult OCPD traits. *Journal of Psychiatric Research, 38*, 545–552.

Tenconi, E., Santonastaso, P., Degortes, D., Bosello, R., Titton, F., Mapelli, D., & Favaro, A. (2010). Set-shifting abilities, central coherence, and handedness in anorexia nervosa patients, their unaffected siblings and healthy controls: Exploring putative endophenotypes. *World Journal of Biological Psychiatry, 11*, 813–823.

Theintz, G., Buchs, B., Rizzoli, R., Slosman, D., Clavien, H., Sizonenko, P. C., & Bonjour, J. P. (1992). Longitudinal monitoring of bone mass accumulation in healthy adolescents: Evidence for a marked reduction after 16 years of age at the levels of lumbar spine and femoral neck in female subjects. *Journal of Clinical Endocrinology and Metabolism, 75*, 1060–1065.

Thomas, J. J., Crosby, R. D., Wonderlich, S. A., Striegel-Moore, R. H., Becker, A. E. (2011). A latent profile analysis of the typology of bulimic symptoms in an indigenous Pacific population: Evidence of cross-cultural variation in phenomenology. *Psychological Medicine, 41*, 195–206.

Thomas, J. J., Eddy, K. T., Murray, H. B., Tromp, M. D., Hartmann, A. S., Stone, M. T., ... Becker, A. E. (2015). The impact of revised DSM-5 criteria on the relative distribution and inter-rater reliability of eating disorder diagnoses in a residential treatment setting. *Psychiatry Research, 229*, 517–523.

Thomas, J. J., Keel, P. K., & Heatherton, T. F. (2011). Disordered eating and injuries among adolescent ballet dancers. *Eating and Weight Disorders, 16*, e216–e222.

Thompson, J. K., & Shroff, H. (2006). The tripartite influence model of body image and eating disturbance: A replication with adolescent girls. *Body Image, 3*, 17–23.

Thornton, L., Watson, H., Jangmo, A., Welch, E., Wiklund, C., von Hausswolff-Juhlin, Y., ... Bulik, C. M. (2017). Binge-eating disorder in the Swedish National Registers: Somatic comorbidity. *International Journal of Eating Disorders, 50*, 58–65.

Tiggemann, M., Slater, A., Bury, B., Hawkins, K., & Firth, B. (2013). Disclaimer labels on fashion magazine advertisements: Effects on social comparison and body dissatisfaction. *Body Image, 10*, 45–53.

Touchette, E., Henegar, A., Codart, N. T., Pryor, L., Falissard, B., Tremblay, R. E., & Côté, S. M. (2011). Subclinical eating disorders and their comorbidity with mood and anxiety disorders in adolescent girls. *Psychiatry Research, 185*, 185–192.

Trace, S. E., Thornton, L. M., Root, T. L., Mazzeo, S. E., Lichtenstein, P., Pedersen, N. L., & Bulik, C. M. (2012). Effects of reducing the frequency and duration criteria for binge eating on lifetime prevalence of bulimia nervosa and binge eating disorder: Implications for DSM-5. *International Journal of Eating Disorders, 45*, 531–536.

Treasure, J. L., Wheeler, M., King, E. A., Gordon, P. A., & Russell, G. F. M. (1988). Weight gain and reproductive function: Ultrasonographic and endocrine features in anorexia nervosa. *Clinical Endocrinology, 29*, 607–616.

Trunko, M. E., Schwartz, T. A., Duvvuri, V., & Kaye, W. H. (2011). Aripiprazole in anorexia nervosa and low-weight bulimia nervosa: Case reports. *International Journal of Eating Disorders, 44*, 269–275.

Uher, R., Murphy, T., Brammer, M. J., Dalgleish, T., Phillips, M. L., Ng, V. W., ... Treasure, J. (2004). Medial prefrontal cortex activity associated with symptom provocation in eating disorders. *American Journal of Psychiatry, 161*, 1238–1246.

U.S. Food and Drug Administration. (2004). *Labeling change request letter for antidepressant medications*. Rockville, MD.

Vandereycken, W. (1984). Neuroleptics in the short-term treatment of anorexia nervosa: A double-blind placebo-controlled study with sulpiride. *British Journal of Psychiatry, 144*, 288–292.

Vandereycken, W., & Pierloot, R. (1982). Pimozide combined with behavior therapy in the short-term treatment of anorexia nervosa. *Acta Psychiatrica Scandinavica, 66*, 445–450.

Van Durme, K., Goossens, L., & Braet, C. (2012). Adolescent aesthetic athletes: A group at risk for eating pathology? *Eating Behaviors, 13*, 119–122.

Van Hoeken, D., Veling, W., Smink, F. R. E., & Hoek, H. (2010). The incidence of anorexia nervosa in Netherlands Antilles immigrants in the Netherlands. *European Eating Disorders Review, 18*, 399–403.

van Son, G. E., van Hoeken, D., Bartelds, A. I., van Furth, E. F., & Hoek, H. W. (2006a). Time trends in the incidence of eating disorders: A primary care study in the Netherlands. *International Journal of Eating Disorders, 39*, 565–569.

van Son, G. E., van Hoeken, D., Bartelds, A. I., van Furth, E. F., & Hoek, H. W. (2006b). Urbanisation and the incidence of eating disorders. *British Journal of Psychiatry, 189*, 562–563.

Vaughn, C., & Leff, J. (1976). The measurement of expressed emotion in the families of psychiatric patients. *British Journal of Social and Clinical Psychiatry, 15*, 157–165.

Vestergaard, P., Emborg, C., Stoving, R. K., Hagen, C., Mosekilde, L., & Brixen, K. (2002). Fractures in patients with anorexia nervosa, bulimia nervosa, and other eating disorders: A nationwide register study. *International Journal of Eating Disorders, 32*, 301–308.

Viljakainen, H.T., Natri, A.M., Karkkainen, M., Huttunen, M.M., Palssa, A., Jakobsen, J., . . . Lamberg-Allardt, C. (2006). A positive dose-response effect of vitamin D supplementation on site-specific bone mineral augmentation in adolescent girls: A double-blinded randomized placebo-controlled 1-year intervention. *Journal of Bone Mineral Research, 21*, 836–844.

Villarejo, C., Fernández-Aranda, F., Jiménez-Murcia, S., Peñas-Lledó, E., Granero, R., Penelo, E., . . . Menchón, J. M. (2012). Lifetime obesity in patients with eating disorders: Increasing prevalence, clinical and personality correlates. *European Eating Disorders Review, 20*, 250–254.

Vohs, K. D., Bardone, A. M., Joiner, T. E., Jr., Abramson, L. Y., & Heatherton, T. F. (1999). Perfectionism, perceived weight status, and self-esteem interact to predict bulimic symptoms: A model of bulimic symptom development. *Journal of Abnormal Psychology, 108*, 695–700.

von Lojewski, A., Boyd, D., Abraham, S., & Russell, J. (2012). Lifetime and recent DSM and ICD psychiatric comorbidity of inpatients engaging in different eating disorder behaviors. *Eating and Weight Disorders, 17*, 185–193.

von Ranson, K. M., Kaye, W. H., Weltzin, T. E., Rao, R., & Matsunaga, H. (1999). Obsessive-compulsive disorder symptoms before and after recovery from bulimia nervosa. *American Journal of Psychiatry, 156*, 1703–1708.

Wade, T. D., Bergin, J. L., Tiggemann, M., Bulik, C. M., & Fairburn, C. G. (2006). Prevalence and long-term course of lifetime eating disorders in an adult Australian twin cohort. *Australia and New Zealand Journal of Psychiatry, 40*, 121–128.

Wade, T. D., Bulik, C. M., Neale, M., & Kendler, K. S. (2000). Anorexia nervosa and major depression: Shared genetic and environmental risk factors. *American Journal of Psychiatry, 157*, 469–471.

Wade, T. D., Tiggemann, M., Bulik, C. M., Fairburn, C. G., Wray, N. R., & Martin, N. G. (2008). Shared temperament risk factors for anorexia nervosa: A twin study. *Psychosomatic Medicine, 70*, 239–244.

Wadsworth. (2003). *Dietary reference intakes*. Belmont, CA: Thomson-Wadsworth.

Waller, G., Halek, C., & Crisp, A. (1993). Sexual abuse as a factor in anorexia nervosa: Evidence from two separate case series. *Journal of Psychosomatic Research, 37*, 873–879.

Walsh, B. T., Hadigan, C. M., Devlin, M. J., Gladis, M., & Roose, S. P. (1991). Long-term outcome of antidepressant treatment for bulimia nervosa. *American Journal of Psychiatry, 148*, 1206–1212.

Walsh, B. T., Kaplan, A. S., Attia, E., Olmsted, M., Parides, M., Carter, J. C., et al. (2006). Fluoxetine after weight restoration in anorexia nervosa: A randomized controlled trial. *Journal of the American Medical Association, 295*, 2605–2612.

Walsh, B. T., Wilson, G. T., Loeb, K. L., Devlin, M. J., Pike, K. M., Roose, S. P., . . . Waternaux, C. (1997). Medication and psychotherapy in the treatment of bulimia nervosa. *American Journal of Psychiatry, 154*, 523–531.

Walters, E. E., & Kendler, K. S. (1995). Anorexia nervosa and anorexic-like syndromes in a population-based female twin sample. *American Journal of Psychiatry, 152*, 64–71.

Wang, K., Zhang, H., Bloss, C. S., Duvvuri, V., Kaye, W., Schork, N. J., . . . Hakonarson, H. (2011). A genome-wide association study on common

SNPs and rare CNVs in anorexia nervosa. *Molecular Psychiatry, 16*, 949–959.

Wang, M. L., Walls, C. E., Peterson, K. E., Richmond, T. K., Spadano-Gasbarro, J., Greaney, M. L., ... Bryn Austin, S. (2013). Dietary and physical activity factors related to eating disorder symptoms among middle school youth. *Journal of School Health, 83*, 14–20.

Ward, A., Brown, N., Lightman, S., Campbell, I. C., & Treasure, J. (1998). Neuroendocrine, appetitive and behavioural responses to d-fenfluramine in women recovered from anorexia nervosa. *British Journal of Psychiatry, 172*, 351–358.

Ward, A., Brown, N., & Treasure, J. (1997). Persistent osteopenia after recovery from anorexia nervosa. *International Journal of Eating Disorders, 22*, 71–75.

Watson, H., Jangmo, A., Munn-Chernoff, M., Thornton, L. M., Welch, E., Wiklund, C., ... Bulik, C. M. (2016). A register-based case-control study of prescription medication utilization in binge-eating disorder. *The Primary Care Companion for CNS Disorders, 18*.

Watson, H. J., Steele, A. L., Bergin, J. L., Fursland, A., & Wade, T. D. (2011). Bulimic symptomatology: The role of adaptive perfectionism, shape and weight concern, and self-esteem. *Behaviour Research and Therapy, 49*, 565–572.

Watson, K. K., Werling, D. M., Zucker, N. L., & Platt, M. L. (2010). Altered social reward and attention in anorexia nervosa. *Frontiers in Psychology, 1*, 36.

Welch, E., Jangmo, A., Thornton, L., Herman, B., Pawaskar, M., Larsson H, ... Bulik, C. M. (2016). Treatment-seeking patients with binge-eating disorder in the Swedish national registers: Clinical course and psychiatric comorbidity. *BMC Psychiatry, 16*, 163.

Wentz, E., Gillberg, C., Gillberg, I. C., & Rastam, M. (2001). Ten-year follow-up of adolescent-onset anorexia nervosa: Psychiatric disorders and overall functioning scales. *Journal of Child Psychology and Psychiatry and Allied Disciplines, 42*, 613–622.

Wertheim, E. H., Koerner, J., & Paxton, S. (2001). Longitudinal predictors of restrictive eating and bulimic tendencies in three different age groups of adolescent girls. *Journal of Youth and Adolescence, 30*, 69–81.

Whisenhunt, B. L., Williamson, D. A., Drab-Hudson, D. L., & Walden, H. (2008). Intervening with coaches to promote awareness and prevention of weight pressures in cheerleaders. *Eating and Weight Disorders, 13*, 102–110.

Whitelaw, M., Gilbertson, H., Lam, P. Y., & Sawyer, S. M. (2010). Does aggressive refeeding in hospitalized adolescents with anorexia nervosa result in increased hypophosphatemia? *Journal of Adolescent Health, 46*, 577–582.

Wildes, J. E., & Marcus, M. D. (2013). Incorporating dimensions into the classification of eating disorders: Three models and their implications for research and clinical practice. *International Journal of Eating Disorders, 46*, 396–403.

Wildes, J. E., Marcus, M. D., Kalarchian, M. A., Levine, M. D., Houck, P. R., & Cheng, Y. (2010). Self-reported binge eating in severe pediatric obesity: Impact on weight change in a randomized controlled trial of family-based treatment. *International Journal of Obesity, 34*, 1143–1148.

Wilfley, D., Agras, W. S., & Taylor, C. B. (2013). Reducing the burden of eating disorders: A model for population-based prevention and treatment for university and college campuses. *International Journal of Eating Disorders, 46*, 529–532.

Wilksch, S. M., Paxton, S. J., Byrne, S. M., Austin, S. B., McLean, S. A., Thompson, K. M., ... Wade, T. D. (2015). Prevention across the spectrum: A randomized controlled trial of three programs to reduce risk factors for both eating disorders and obesity. *Psychological Medicine, 45*, 1811–1823.

Wilksch, S. M., & Wade, T. D. (2009). Reduction of shape and weight concern in young adolescents: A 30-month controlled evaluation of a media literacy program. *Journal of the American Academy of Child and Adolescent Psychiatry, 48*, 652–661.

Wilksch, S. M., & Wade, T. D. (2013). Life Smart: A pilot study of a school-based program to reduce the risk of both eating disorders and obesity in young adolescent girls and boys. *Journal of Pediatric Psychology, 38*, 1021–1029.

Williams, S. E., Watts, T. K., & Wade, T. D. (2012). A review of the definitions of outcome used in the treatment of bulimia nervosa. *Clinical Psychology Review, 32*, 292–300.

Wilson, G. T., Grilo, C. M., & Vitousek, K. M. (2007). Psychological treatment of eating disorders. *American Psychologist, 62*, 199–216.

Wilson, G. T., Vitousek, K. M., & Loeb, K. L. (2000). Stepped care treatment for eating disorders. *Journal of Consulting and Clinical Psychology, 68*, 564–572.

Wilson, G. T., Wilfley, D. E., Agras, W. S., & Bryson, S. W. (2010). Psychological treatments for binge eating disorder. *Archives of General Psychiatry, 67*, 94–101.

Wilson, G. T., & Zandberg, L. J. (2012). Cognitive-behavioral guided self-help for eating disorders: Effectiveness and scalability. *Clinical Psychology Review, 32*, 343–357.

Wittchen, H. U., Nelson, C. B., & Lachner, G. (1998). Prevalence of mental disorders and psychosocial impairments in adolescents and young adults. *Psychological Medicine, 28*, 109–126.

Wonderlich, S. A., Brewerton, T. D., Jocic, Z., Dansky, B. S., & Abbott, D. W. (1997). Relationship of childhood sexual abuse and eating disorders. *Journal of the American Academy of Child and Adolescent Psychiatry, 36*, 1107–1115.

Wonderlich, S. A., & Mitchell, J. E. (1997). Eating disorders and comorbidity: Empirical, conceptual, and clinical implications. *Psychopharmacology Bulletin, 33*, 381–390.

Woodside, D. B., Garfinkel, P. E., Lin, E., Goering, P., Kaplan, A. S., Goldbloom, D. S., & Kennedy, S. H. (2001). Comparisons of men with full or partial eating disorders, men without eating disorders, and women with eating disorders in the community. *American Journal of Psychiatry, 158*, 570–574.

World Health Organization. (2003). *Caring for children and adolescents with mental disorders: Setting WHO directions*. Geneva, Switzerland: World Health Organization.

Xanthopoulos, M. S., Borradaile, K. E., Hayes, S., Sherman, S., Vander Veur, S., Grundy, K. M., . . . Foster, G. D. (2011). The impact of weight, sex, and race/ethnicity on body dissatisfaction among urban children. *Body Image, 8*, 385–389.

Yager, J., Anderson, A., & Devlin, M. (2000). American Psychiatric Association Practice Guideline for the Treatment of Patients with Eating Disorders. *American Journal of Psychiatry, 157*, 1–39.

Yates, W. R., Lund, B. C., Johnson, C., Mitchell, J., & McKee, P. (2009). Attention-deficit hyperactivity symptoms and disorder in eating disorder inpatients. *International Journal of Eating Disorders, 42*, 375–378.

Young, J. K. (2010). Anorexia nervosa and estrogen: Current status of the hypothesis. *Neuroscience and Biobehavioral Reviews, 34*, 1195–1200.

Zerwas, S., Lund, B. C., Von Holle, A., Thornton, L. M., Berrettini, W. H., Brandt, H., . . . Bulik, C. M. (2013). Factors associated with recovery from anorexia nervosa. *Journal of Psychiatric Research, 47*, 972–979.

Zucker, N. L., Losh, M., Bulik, C. M., LaBar, K. S., Piven, J., & Pelphrey, K. A. (2007). Anorexia nervosa and autism spectrum disorders: Guided investigation of social cognitive endophenotypes. *Psychological Bulletin, 133*, 976–1006.

Part V: Substance Use Disorders

Abdalla, R. R., Madruga, C. S., Ribeiro, M., Pinsky, I., Caetano, R., & Laranjeira, R. (2014). Prevalence of cocaine use in Brazil: Data from the II Brazilian National Alcohol and Drugs Survey (BNADS). *Addictive Behaviors, 39*, 297–301.

Abraham, H. D., Aldridge, A. M., & Gogia, P. (1996). The psychopharmacology of hallucinogens. *Neuropsychopharmacology, 14*, 285–298.

Abraham, H., McCann, U., & Ricaurte, G. (2002). Psychedelic drugs. In K. Davis, D. Charney, J. Coyle, & C. Nemeroff (Eds.), *Neuropsychopharmacology, the fifth generation of progress,* (pp. 1545–1556) New York: Lippincott Williams & Wilkins.

Abreu-Villaca, Y., Seidler, F. J., Qiao, D., Tate, C. A., Cousins, M. M., Thillai, I., et al. (2003). Shortterm adolescent nicotine exposure has immediate and persistent effects on cholinergic systems: Critical periods, patterns of exposure, dose thresholds. *Neuropsychopharmacology, 28*(11), 1935–1949.

Addolorato, G., Caputo, F., Capristo, E., Colombo, G., Gessa, G. L., & Gasbarrini, G. (2000). Ability of baclofen in reducing alcohol craving and intake: II—Preliminary clinical evidence. *Alcoholism, Clinical and Experimental Research, 24*, 67–71.

Adelman, H. S., & Taylor, L. (2003). On sustainability of project innovations as systemic change. *Journal of Educational and Psychological Consultation,* 14(1): 1–25.

Agabio, R., & Colombo, G. (2014). GABAB receptor ligands for the treatment of alcohol use disorder: Preclinical and clinical evidence. *Frontiers in Neuroscience, 8*, 140.

Aghajanian, G. K., & Marek, G. J. (1999). Serotonin and hallucinogens. *Neuropsychopharmacology, 21*(2 Suppl), 16S–23S.

Ahmed, S. H., & Koob, G. F. (1998). Transition from moderate to excessive drug intake: Change in hedonic set point. *Science, 282*, 298–300.

Aigner, T. G., & Balster, R. L. (1978). Choice behavior in rhesus monkeys: Cocaine versus food. *Science, 201*, 534–535.

Akhondzadeh, S., Ahmadi-Abhari, S. A., Assadi, S. M., Shabestari, O. L., Kashani, A. R., &

Farzanehgan, Z. M. (2000). Double-blind randomized controlled trial of baclofen vs. clonidine in the treatment of opiates withdrawal. *Journal of Clinical Pharmacy and Therapeutics, 25*, 347–353.

Alper, K. R. (2001). Ibogaine: A review. *The Alkaloids, Chemistry & Biology, 56*, 1–38.

Alshaarawy, O., & Anthony, J. C. (2015). Cannabis smoking and diabetes mellitus: Results from meta-analysis with eight independent replication samples. *Epidemiology, 26*(4), 597–600.

Altman, D. G. (1995). Sustaining interventions in community systems: On the relationship between researchers and communities. *Health Psychology, 14*(6), 526–536.

Alvarado, A., Kendell, K., Beesley, S., & LeeCavaness, C. (2000). *Strengthening American families: Model family programs for substance abuse and delinquency prevention*. Salt Lake City, UT: University of Utah, Department of Health Promotion and Education.

American Legacy Foundation. (2002). Media tracking survey (unpublished data).

American Psychiatric Association. (1994). *Diagnostic and statistical manual of mental disorders* (4th ed.). Washington, DC: Author.

American Psychiatric Association. (2013). *Diagnostic and statistical manual of mental disorders* (5th ed.). Washington, DC: American Psychiatric Association.

American Society of Addiction Medicine. (2001). *Patient placement criteria for the treatment of substance-related disorders* (2nd ed., rev.; ASAM PPC-2R). Available at http://www.asam.org/PatientPlacementCriteria.html.

Amitai, N., Liu, J., & Schulteis G. (2006). Discrete cues paired with naloxone-precipitated withdrawal from acute morphine dependence elicit conditioned withdrawal responses. *Behavioural Pharmacology, 17*(3), 213–222.

Anderson, C. E., & Loomis, G. A. (2003). Recognition and prevention of inhalant abuse. *American Family Physician, 68*, 869–874.

Anonymous. (2003). Inhalant abuse treatment and prevention. *Public Health Reports, 118*, 276.

Anthony, J. C., Barondess, D. A., Radovanovic, M., & Lopez-Quintero, C. (2016). Polydrug use: Research topics and issues. In K. J. Sher (Ed.), *The Oxford handbook of substance use and substance use disorders* (Vol. 2, pp. 29–59). New York: Oxford University Press.

Anthony, J. C.. Warner, L. A.. & Kessler, R. C. (1994). Comparative epidemiology of dependence on tobacco, alcohol, controlled substances, and inhalants: Basic findings from the National Comorbidity Survey. *Experimental and Clinical Psychopharmacology, 2*(3), 244–268.

Arnold, M. E., & Hughes, J. N. (1999). First do no harm: Adverse effects of grouping deviant youth for skills training. *Journal of School Psychology, 37*, 99–115.

Arrazola, R. A., Singh, T., Corey, C. G., Husten, C. G., Neff, L., Apelberg, B. J., et al. (2015). Tobacco use among middle and high school students—United States, 2011–2014. *Morbidity and Mortality Weekly Report, 64*(14), 381–385.

Arthur, M. W., Ayers, C. D., Graham, K. A., & Hawkins, J. D. (2003). Mobilizing communities to reduce risks for drug abuse: A comparison of two strategies. In Z. Sloboda & W. J. Bukoski (Eds.), *Handbook of drug abuse prevention: Theory, science and practice* (pp. 129–144). New York: Plenum Press.

Asensio, S., Romero, M. J., Romero, F. J., Wong, C., Alia-Klein, N., Tomasi, D., . . . Goldstein, R. Z. (2010). Striatal dopamine D2 receptor availability predicts the thalamic and medial prefrontal responses to reward in cocaine abusers three years later. *Synapse, 64*(5), 397–402.

Asmaro, D., Jaspers-Fayer, F., Sramko, V., Taake, I., Carolan, P., & Liotti, M. (2012) Spatiotemporal dynamics of the hedonic processing of chocolate images in individuals with and without trait chocolate craving. *Appetite, 58*(3), 790–799.

Audrain-McGovern, J., & Tercyak, K. P. (2011). Genes, environment, and adolescent smoking: Implications for prevention. In K. S. Kendler, S. R. Jaffee, & D. Romer (Eds.), *The dynamic genome and mental health: The role of genes and environments in youth development* (pp. 294–321). New York: Oxford University Press.

Audrain-McGovern, J., Al Koudsi, N., Rodriguez, D., Wileyto, E. P., Shields, P. G., & Tyndale, R. F. (2007). The role of CYP2A6 in the emergence of nicotine dependence in adolescents. *Pediatrics, 119*(1), e264–274.

Audrain-McGovern, J., Rodriguez, D., Epstein, L. H., Cuevas, J., Rodgers, K., & Wileyto, E. P. (2009). Does delay discounting play an etiological role in smoking or is it a consequence of smoking? *Drug and Alcohol Dependence, 103*(3), 99–106.

Audrain-McGovern, J., Rodriguez, D., & Moss, H. B. (2003). Smoking progression and physical activity. *Cancer Epidemiology, Biomarkers & Prevention, 12*(11 Pt 1), 1121–1129.

Aydin, K., Sencer, S., Demir, T., Ogel, K., Tunaci, A., & Minareci, O. (2002). Cranial MR findings in chronic toluene abuse by inhalation. *American Journal of Neuroradiology, 23*, 1173–1179.

Azrin, N. H., Donohue, B., & Besalel, V. A. (1994). Youth drug abuse treatment: A controlled outcome study. *Journal of Child and Adolescent Substance Abuse, 3*, 1–16.

Bachman, J. G., Johnston, L. D., & O'Malley, P. M. (1990). Explaining the recent decline in cocaine use among young adults: Further evidence that perceived risks and disapproval lead to reduced drug use. *Journal of Health and Social Behavior, 31*, 173–184.

Bachman, J. G., Johnston, L. D., & O'Malley, P. M. (1998). Explaining the recent increases in students' marijuana use: The impacts of perceived risks and disapproval from 1976 through 1996. *American Journal of Public Health, 88*, 887–892.

Bachman, R., & Peralta, R. L. (2002). The relationship between drinking and violence in an adolescent population: Does gender matter? *Deviant Behavior, 23*, 1–19.

Baer, J. S., & Carney, M. M. (1993). Biases in the perceptions of the consequences of alcohol use among college students. *Journal of Studies on Alcohol, 54*(1), 54–60.

Baker, T. B., Mermelstein, R., Collins, L. M., Piper, M.E., Jorenby, D. E., Smith, S. S., . . . Fiore, M. C. (2011). New methods for tobacco dependence treatment research. *Annals of Behavioral Medicine, 41*, 192–207.

Balster, R. L. (1987). Abuse potential evaluation of inhalants. *Drug and Alcohol Dependence, 19*, 7–15.

Barrickman, L. L., Perry, P. J., Allen, A. J., Kuperman, S., Arndt, S. V., Herrmann, K. J., et al. (1995). Bupropion versus methylphenidate in the treatment of attention-deficit hyperactivity disorder. *Journal of the American Academy of Child and Adolescent Psychiatry, 34*, 649–657.

Barry, A. E., King, J., Sears, C., Harville, C., Bondoc, I., & Joseph, K. (2016). Prioritizing alcohol prevention: Establishing alcohol as the gateway drug and linking age of first drink with illicit drug use. *Journal of School Health, 86*(1), 31–38.

Beauvais, F., Wayman, J. C., Jumper-Thurman, P., Plested, B., & Helm, H. (2002). Inhalant abuse among American Indian, Mexican American, and non-Latino white adolescents. *American Journal of Drug and Alcohol Abuse, 28*, 171–187.

Becker, S. J., & Curry, J. F. (2008). Outpatient interventions for adolescent substance abuse: A quality of evidence review. *Journal of Consulting and Clinical Psychology, 76*(4), 531–543.

Belin, D., Mar, A. C., Dalley, J. W., Robbins, T. W., & Everitt. (2008). High impulsivity predicts the switch to compulsive cocaine-taking. *Science, 320*(5881), 1352–1355.

Benjet, C., Borges, G., Méndez, E., Casanova, L., & Medina-Mora, M. E. (2014). Adolescent alcohol use and alcohol use disorders in Mexico City. *Drug and Alcohol Dependence, 136*, 43–50.

Benowitz, N. L. (1990). Pharmacokinetic considerations in understanding nicotine dependence. In G. Block & J. Marsh (Eds.), *The biology of nicotine dependence* (Vol. Ciba Foundation Symposium 152, pp. 186–209). Chichester: John Wiley & Sons.

Benowitz, N. L., & Jacob, P., III. (1999). Pharmacokinetics and metabolism of nicotine and related alkaloids. In S. P. Arneric & J. D. Brioni (Eds.), *Neuronal nicotinic receptors* (pp. 213–234). New York: Wiley-Liss.

Benowitz, N. L., Perez-Stable, E. J., Herrera, B., & Jacob, P., 3rd. (2002). Slower metabolism and reduced intake of nicotine from cigarette smoking in Chinese-Americans. *Journal of the National Cancer Institute, 94*, 108–115.

Benson, P. L., Leffert, W., Scates, P. C., & Blyth, D. A. (1998). Beyond the "village" rhetoric: Creating healthy communities for children and adolescents. *Applied Developmental Science, 2*, 138–159.

Bergamini, E., Demidenko, E., & Sargent, J. D. (2013). Trends in tobacco and alcohol brand placements in popular US movies, 1996 through 2009. *JAMA Pediatrics, 167*(7), 634–639.

Bergen, A. W., Korczak, J. F., Weissbecker K. A., Goldstein, A. M., et al. (1999). A genome-wide search for loci contribution to smoking and alcoholism. *Genetic Epidemiology, 17*, S55–60.

Berrettini, W. H., Alexander, R., Ferraro, T. N., & Vogel, W. H. (1994). A study of oral morphine preference in inbred mouse strains. *Psychiatric Genetics, 4*, 81–86.

Berrettini, W. H., & Doyle, G. A. (2012). The CHRNA5-A3-B4 gene cluster in nicotine addiction. *Molecular Psychiatry, 17*(9), 856–866.

Bevilacqua, L., & Goldman, D. (2013). Genetics of impulsive behavior. *Philosophical Transactions of the Royal Society B, 368*, 20120380.

Bickel, W. K., Jarmolowicz, D. P., Mueller, E. T., Koffarnus, M. N., & Gatchalian, K. M. (2012). Excessive discounting of delayed reinforcers as a trans-disease process contributing to addiction and other disease-related vulnerabilities: Emerging evidence. *Pharmacology & Therapeutics, 134*, 287–297.

Bickel, W. K., Yi, R., Landes, R. D., Hill, P. F., & Baxter, C. (2011). Remember the future: Working memory training decreases delay discounting among stimulant addicts. *Biological Psychiatry*, *69*, 260–265.

Biederman, J., Wilens, T., Mick, E., Faraone, S. V, Weber, W., Curtis, S., ... Soriano, J. (1997). Is ADHD a risk factor for psychoactive substance use disorders? Findings from a four-year prospective follow-up study. *Journal of the American Academy of Child and Adolescent Psychiatry*, *36*(1), 21–29.

Biederman, J., Wilens, T., Mick, E., Spencer, T., & Faraone, S. V. (1999). Pharmacotherapy of attention-deficit/hyperactivity disorder reduces risk for substance use disorder. *Pediatrics*, *104*, e20.

Bierut, L. J., Saccone, N. L., Rice, J. P., Goate, A., Foroud, T., Edenberg, H., et al. (2002). Defining alcohol-related phenotypes in humans. The Collaborative Study on the Genetics of Alcoholism. *Alcohol Research and Health*, *26*, 208–213.

Bieurt, L., Rice, J., Edenberg, H., Goate, A., Foroud, T., & Cloninger, C. (2000). Family-based study of the association of the dopamine D2 receptor gene (DRD2) with habitual smoking. *American Journal of Medical Genetics*, *90*, 299–302.

Bigelow, G. E., Stitzer, M. L., & Liebson, I. A. (1984). The role of behavioral contingency management in drug abuse treatment. In J. Grabowski, M. L. Stitzer, & J. E. Henningfield (Eds.) *Behavioral intervention techniques in drug abuse treatment* (pp. 36–52). Rockville, MD: National Institute on Drug Abuse.

Blaho, K., Merigian, K., Winbery, S., Geraci, S. A., & Smartt, C. (1997). Clinical pharmacology of lysergic acid diethylamide: Case reports and review of the treatment of intoxication. *American Journal of Therapeutics*, *4*, 211–221.

Blum, K., Noble, E. P., Sheridan, P. J., Mongomery, A., Ritchie, T., Jagadeeswaran, P., et al. (1990). Allelic association of human dopamine D2 receptor gene in alcoholism. *Journal of the American Medical Association*, *263*, 2055–2060.

Bolos, A. M., Dean, M., Lucas-Derse, S., Ramsburg, M., Brown, G. L., & Goldman, D. (1990). Population and pedigree studies reveal a lack of association between the dopamine D2 receptor gene and alcoholism. *Journal of the American Medical Association*, *264*, 3156–3160.

Bonnie, R. J., & O'Connell, M. E. (2004). *Reducing underage drinking: A collective responsibility.* United States National Research Council and United States Institute of Medicine Committee on Developing a Strategy to Reduce and Prevent Underage Drinking. Washington, DC: National Academies Press.

Bonson, K. R., Grant, S. J., Contoreggi, C. S., Links, J. M., Metcalfe, J., Weyl, H. L., ... London, E. D. (2002). Neural systems and cue-induced cocaine craving. *Neuropsychopharmacology*, *26*, 376–386.

Borduin, C. M., Mann, B. J., Cone, L. T., Henggeler, S. W., Fucci, B. R., Blaske, D. M., et al. (1995). Multisystemic treatment of serious juvenile offenders: Long-term prevention of criminality and violence. *Journal of Consulting and Clinical Psychology*, *63*, 569–578.

Borras, E., Coutelle, C., Rosell, A., Fernandez-Muixi, F., Broch., M., Crosas, B., et al. (2000). Genetic polymorphism of alcohol dehydrogenase in Europeans: The ADH2*2 allele decreases the risk for alcoholism and is associated with ADH3*1. *Hepatology*, *31*, 984–989.

Botvin, G. J., Baker, E., Dusenbury, L., Botvin, E. M., & Diaz, T. (1995). Long-term follow-up results of a randomized drug abuse prevention trial in a white middle-class population. *Journal of the American Medical Association*, *273*(14), 1106–1112.

Brebner, K., Childress, A. R., & Roberts, D. C. (2002). A potential role for GABA(B) agonists in the treatment of psychostimulant addiction. *Alcohol and Alcoholism*, *37*, 478–484.

Brebner, K., Froestl, W., & Roberts, D. C. S. (2002). The GABA(B) antagonist CGP56433A attenuates the effect of baclofen on cocaine but not heroin self-administration in the rat. *Psychopharmacology*, *160*(1), 49–55.

Brehm, J. W. (1966). *A theory of psychological reactance*. New York: Academy Press.

Brehm, S. S., & Brehm, J. W. (1981). *Psychological reactance*. New York: John Wiley & Sons.

Brenhouse, H. C., & Stellar, J. R. (2006). c-Fos and deltaFosB expression are differentially altered in distinct subregions of the nucleus accumbens shell in cocaine-sensitized rats. *Neuroscience*, *137*(3), 773–780.

Bresleau, N. (1995). Psychiatric comorbidity of smoking and nicotine dependence. *Behavioral Genetics*, *25*, 95–101.

Brinn, M. P., Carson, K. V., Esterman, A. J., Chang, A. B., & Smith, B. J. (2010). Mass media interventions for preventing smoking in young people. *Cochrane Database of Systemic Reviews*, *11*(CD001006), 1–57.

Brody, A. L., Mandelkern, M. A., London, E. D., Childress, A. R., Lee, G. S., Bota, R. G., ... Jarvik, M. E. (2002). Brain metabolic changes during cigarette craving. *Archives of General Psychiatry*, *59*(12), 1162–1172.

Brody, G. H., Chen, Y.-F., Kogan, S. M., Yu, T., Molgaard, V. K., DiClemente, R. J., & Wingood, G. M. (2012). Family-centered program deters substance use, conduct problems, and depressive symptoms in black adolescents. *Pediatrics, 129*(1), 108–115.

Brody, G. H., Yu, T., & Beach, S. R. H. (2015). A differential susceptibility analysis reveals the "who and how" about adolescents' responses to preventive interventions: Tests of firstand second-generation gene times environment hypotheses. *Development and Psychopathology, 27*, 37–49.

Brouette, T., & Anton, R. (2001). Clinical review of inhalants. *American Journal on Addictions, 10*, 79– 94.

Brown, R. A., Ramsey, S. E., Strong, D. R., Myers, M. G., Kahler, C. W., Lejuez, C. W., ... Abrams, D. B. (2003). Effects of Motivational Interviewing on smoking cessation in adolescents with psychiatric disorders. *Tobacco Control, 12*(Suppl. 4), IV3–10.

Brown, S. (1993). Recovery patterns in adolescent substance abuse. In J. S. Baer, G. A. Marlott, & McMahon, R. J. (Eds.), *Addictive behaviors across the life span: Prevention, treatment, and policy issues* (pp. 161–183). Newbury Park, CA: Sage Publications.

Brown, S. A., Brumback, T., Tomlinson, K., Cummins, K., Thompson, W. K., Nagel, B. J., ... Tapert, S. F. (2015). The National Consortium on Alcohol and NeuroDevelopment in Adolescence (NCANDA): A multisite study of adolescent eevelopment and substance use. *Journal of Studies on Alcohol and Drugs, 76*(6), 895–908.

Buchan, B. J., Dennis, M. L., Tims, F. M., & Diamond, G. S. (2002). Cannabis use: Consistency and validity of self-report, on-site urine testing, and laboratory testing. *Addiction, 97* (Suppl. 1), 98–108.

Buchert, R., Obrocki, J., Thomasius, R., Vaterlein, O., Petersen, K., Jenicke, L., et al. (2001). Longterm effects of "ecstasy" abuse on the human brain studied by FDG PET. *Nuclear Medicine Communications, 22*, 889–897.

Budney, A. J., & Higgins, S. T. (1998). A Community Reinforcement Plus Vouchers Approach: Treating Cocaine Addiction. Rockville, MD: NIDA.

Budney, A. J., & Moore, B. A. (2002). Development and consequences of cannabis dependence. *Journal of Clinical Pharmacology, 42* (11 Suppl), 28S–33S.

Budney, A. J., Higgins, S. T., Radonovich, K. J., & Novy, P. L. (2000). Adding voucher-based incentives to coping skills and motivational enhancement improves outcomes during treatment for marijuana dependence. *Journal of Consulting and Clinical Psychology, 68*, 1051–1061.

Budney, A. J., Roffman, R., Stephens, R. S., & Walker, D. (2007). Marijuana dependence and its treatment. *Addiction Science and Clinical Practice, 4*(1), 4–16.

Bukstein, O. G., Bernet, W., Arnold, V., Beitchman, J., Shaw, J., Benson, R. S., ... Ptakowski, K. K. (2005). Work Group on Quality Issues. Practice parameter for the assessment and treatment of children and adolescents with substance use disorders. *Journal of the American Academy of Child and Adolescent Psychiatry, 44*(6), 609–621.

Bukstein, O. G., Glancy, L. J., & Kaminer, Y. (1992). Patterns of affective comorbidity in a clinical population of dually diagnosed adolescent substance abusers. *Journal of the American Academy of Child and Adolescent Psychiatry, 31*, 1041–1045.

Burke, B. L., Arkowitz, H., & Menchola, M. (2003). The efficacy of motivational interviewing: A meta-analysis of controlled clinical trials. *Journal of Consulting and Clinical Psychology, 71*, 843–861.

Cadoret, R. J., Troughton, E., O'Gorman, T. W., & Heywood, E. (1986). An adoption study of genetic and environmental factors in drug abuse. *Archives of General Psychiatry, 43*(12), 1131–1136.

Caetano, R., & Babor, T. F. (2006). Diagnosis of alcohol dependence in epidemiological surveys: An epidemic of youthful alcohol dependence or a case of measurement error? *Addiction, 101*(S1), 111–114.

Cahill, L., & McGaugh, J. L. (1998). Mechanisms of emotional arousal and lasting declarative memory. *Trends in Neurosciences, 21*, 294–299.

Caldwell, B. M., Harenski, C. L., Harenski, K. A., Fede, S. J., Steele, V. R., Koenigs, M. R., & Kiehl, K. A. (2015). Abnormal frontostriatal activity in recently abstinent cocaine users during implicit moral processing. *Frontiers in Human Neuroscience, 16*(9), 565.

California Department of Public Health. (2015). *California Tobacco Facts and Figures 2015: 25 years of tobacco control in California*. Sacramento: California Tobacco Control Program. Retrieved from http://www.cdph.ca.gov/programs/tobacco/Documents/

Resources/Fact%20Sheets/2015FactsFigures-web2.pdf.

Carpenter, C. S., & Stehr, M. (2008). The effects of mandatory seatbelt laws on seatbelt use, motor vehicle fatalities, and crash-related injuries among youths. *Journal of Health Economics, 27*, 642–661.

Carroll, K. M. (1996). Relapse prevention as a psychosocial treatment approach: A review of controlled clinical trials. *Experimental and Clinical Psychopharmacology, 4*, 46–54.

Carroll, K. M., Ball, S. A., & Martino, S. (2004). Cognitive, behavioral and motivational therapies. In M. Galanter & H. D. Kleber (Eds.), *The American Psychiatric Publishing textbook of substance abuse treatment* (3rd ed., pp. 365–376). Washington, DC: American Psychiatric Association Press.

Carroll, K. M., Nich, C., Ball, S. A., McCance-Katz, E., & Rounsaville, B. J. (1998). Treatment of cocaine and alcohol dependence with psychotherapy and disulfiram. *Addiction, 93*, 713–728.

Carroll, K. M., Rounsaville, B. J., Gordon, L. T., Nich, C., Jatlow, P. M., Bisighini, R. M., et al. (1994). Psychotherapy and pharmacotherapy for ambulatory cocaine abusers. *Archives of General Psychiatry, 51*, 177–197.

Carroll, K. M., Rounsaville, B. J., Nich, C., Gordon, T., Wirtz, P. W., & Gawin, F. H. (1994). One-year follow-up of psychotherapy and pharmacotherapy for cocaine dependence: Delayed emergence of psychotherapy effects. *Archives of General Psychiatry, 51*, 989–997.

Catalano, R. F., Berglund, M. L., Ryan, J.A.M., Lonczak, H. S., & Hawkins, J. D. (2004). Positive youth development in the United States: Research findings on evaluations of positive youth development programs. *Annals of the American Academy of Political and Social Science, 591*, 98–124.

Catalano, R. F., Haggerty, K., Gainey, R., & Hoppe, M. J. (1997). Reducing parental risk factors for children's substance misuse: Preliminary outcomes with opiate-addicted parents. *Substance Use and Misuse, 32*, 699–721.

Catalano, R., Gainey, R., Fleming, C., Haggerty, K., & Johnson, N. (1999). An experimental intervention with families of substance abusers: One-year follow-up of the focus on families project. *Addiction, 94*, 241–254.

Caulkins, J. P., Hawken, A., Kilmer, B., & Kleiman, M. (2012). *Marijuana legalization: What everyone needs to know* (1st ed.). New York: Oxford University Press.

Center for Substance Abuse Treatment (CSAT). (1999). Adolescents and young adults in treatment. In www.health.org/nties/young/yung text.htm

Center for the Study and Prevention of Violence. (2003). Blueprints Model Programs. Boulder: Center for the Study and Prevention of Violence, Institute of Behavioral Science, University of Colorado at Boulder. http//colorado.edu.cspv/blueprints/

Centers for Disease Control and Prevention. (1998). Youth risk behavior surveillance—United States, 1997. *Morbidity and Mortality Weekly Report, 47*(SS-3), 1–89.

Centers for Disease Control and Prevention (CDC). (2002a). Adolescent and school health. Atlanta: National Center for Chronic Disease Prevention and Health Promotion.

Centers for Disease Control and Prevention (CDC). (2002b). Trends and cigarette smoking among high school students—United States, 1991–2001. *Morbidity and Mortality Weekly Report, 51*, 409–412.

Centers for Disease Control and Prevention. (2015). *Results from the school health policies and practices study, 2014*. Atlanta, GA: U.S. Department of Health and Human Services, Centers for Disease Control and Prevention. http://www.cdc.gov/healthyyouth/data/shpps/pdf/shpps-508-final_101315.pdf

Chambers, R. A., Taylor, J. R., & Potenza, M. N. (2003). Developmental neurocircuitry of motivation in adolescence: A critical period of addiction vulnerability. *American Journal of Psychiatry, 160*, 1041–1052.

Chambless, D. L., & Hollon, S. D. (1998). Defining empirically supported therapies. *Journal of Consulting and Clinical Psychology, 66*, 7–18.

Chang, Y. C., Li, T. K., et al. (1999). Interaction between the functional polymorphisms of the alcohol-metabolism genes in protection against alcoholism. *American Journal of Human Genetics, 65*, 795–807.

Chen, C. C., Lu, R. B., Chen, Y. C., Wang, M. F., Chang, Y. C., Li, T. K., et al. (1999). Interaction between the functional polymorphisms of the alcohol-metabolism genes in protection against alcoholism. *American Journal of Human Genetics, 65*, 795–807.

Chen, C. Y., & Anthony, J. C. (2004). Epidemiological estimates of risk to become dependent upon cocaine: Cocaine hydrochloride powder vs. crack coccaine. *Psychopharmacology, 172*, 78–86.

Chen, C. Y., Storr, C. L., & Anthony, J. C. (2009). Early-onset drug use and risk for drug dependence problems. *Addictive Behavior, 34*(3), 319–322.

Cheng, H. G., & Anthony, J. C. (2016). Does our legal minimum drinking age modulate risk of first heavy drinking episode soon after drinking onset? Epidemiological evidence for the United States, 2006–2014. *Peer Journal, 4*, e2153.

Cheng, H. G., & Anthony, J. C. Age-specific risk of first heavy episodic drinking soon after drinking onset in young people: United States, 2006–2014. Under review.

Cheng, H. G., Cantave, M. D., & Anthony, J. C. (2016). Alcohol experiences viewed mutoscopically: Newly incident drinking of 12- to 25-year-olds in the United States, 2002–2013. *Journal of Studies on Alcohol and Drugs, 77*(3), 405–412.

Cheng, H. G., Cantave, M. D., & Anthony, J. C. (2016). Taking the first full drink: Epidemiological evidence on male–female differences in the United States. *Alcoholism: Clinical & Experimental Research, 40*(4), 816–825.

Cheng, H. G., Chandra, M., Alcover, K. C., & Anthony, J. C. (2016). Rapid transition from drinking to alcohol dependence among adolescent and young-adult newly incident drinkers in the United States, 2002–2013. *Drug and Alcohol Dependence, 168*, 61–68.

Cheng, H. G., Chen, S., McBride, O., & Phillips, M. R. (2016). Prospective relationship of depressive symptoms, drinking, and tobacco smoking among middle-aged and elderly community-dwelling adults: Results from the China Health and Retirement Longitudinal Study (CHARLS). *Journal of Affective Disorders, 195*(195), 136–143.

Cheng, H. G., Deng, F., Xiong, W., & Phillips, M. R. (2015) Prevalence of alcohol use disorders in mainland China: A systematic review. *Addiction, 110*(5), 761–774.

Cheng, H. G., Wetherington, C. L., & Anthony, J. C. (under review). Male-female differences in the onset of heavy episodic drinking soon after first full drink in contemporary United States: From early adolescence to young adulthood.

Chick, C. F. (2015). Reward processing in the adolescent brain: Individual differences and relation to risk taking. *Journal of Neuroscience, 35*(40), 13539–13541.

Chilcoat, H. D., Dishion, T. J., & Anthony, J. C. (1995). Parent monitoring and the incidence of drug sampling in urban elementary school children. *American Journal of Epidemiology, 14*, 25–31.

Childress, A. R., Franklin, T., Listerud, J., Acton, P., & O'Brien, C. P. (2002). Neuroimaging of cocaine craving states: Cessation, stimulant administration, and drug cue paradigms. In K. L. Davis, D. Charney, J. Coyle, & C. Nemeroff (Eds.), *Neuropsychopharmacology: The fifth generation of progress* (pp. 1575–1590). New York: Lippincott Williams & Wilkins.

Childress, A. R., McElgin, W., Franklin, T., Acton, P., & O'Brien, C. P. (1999). Impact of GABAergics on brain activity during cue-induced cocaine craving. *Society for Neuroscience* Abstracts Annual meeting. Abstract Book Vol. 328.14, 25(1), 815.

Childress, A. R., McElgin, W., & Mozley, P. D. (1999). Limbic activation during cue-induced craving for cocaine and for natural rewards. *Biological Psychiatry, 45*, 53S.

Childress, A. R., McLellan, A. T., Ehrman, R., & O'Brien, C. P. (1988). Classifically conditioned responses in opioid and cocaine dependence: A role in relapse? In B. A. Ray (Ed.), *Learning factors in substance abuse* (NIDA Research Monograph, pp. 25–43). Rockville, MD: National Institute on Drug Abuse.

Childress, A. R., Mozley, P. D., McElgin, W., Fitzgerald, J., Reivich, M., & O'Brien, C. P. (1999). Limbic activation during cue-induced cocaine craving. *American Journal of Psychiatry, 156*, 11– 18.

Choi, W. S., Gilpin, E. A., Farkas, A. J., & Pierce, J. P. (2001). Determining the probability of future smoking among adolescents. *Addiction, 96*(2), 313–323.

Choi, W. S., Pierce, J. P., Gilpin, E. A., Farkas, A. J., & Berry, C. C. (1997). Which adolescent experimenters progress to established smoking in the United States. *American Journal of Preventive Medicine, 13*(5), 385–391.

Chung, T., Cornelius, J. R., Martin, C. S., Ferrell, R., Maisto, S. A., & Clark, D. B. (2014). Serotonin transporter genotype linked to adolescent substance use treatment outcome through externalizing behavior. *Frontiers in Pediatrics, 2*, 71.

Chung, T., Martin, C. S., Armstrong, T. D., & Labouvie, E. W. (2002). Prevalence of DSM-IV alcohol diagnoses and symptoms in adolescent community and clinical samples. *Journal of the American Academy of Child and Adolescent Psychiatry, 41*(5), 546–554.

Clark, D. B. (2012). Pharmacotherapy for adolescent alcohol use disorder. *CNS Drugs, 26*(7), 559–569.

Clark, D. B., Bukstein, O., & Cornelius, J. (2002). Alcohol use disorders in adolescents: Epidemiology, diagnosis, psychosocial interventions, and pharmacological treatment. *Paediatric Drugs, 4*, 493–502.

Clark, D. B., Cornelius, J., Wood, D. S., & Vanyukov, M. (2004). Psychopathology risk transmission in children of parents with substance use disorders. *American Journal of Psychiatry, 161*(4), 685–691.

Clark, D. B., Pollock, N., Bukstein, O. G., Mezzich, C., Bromberger, J. T., & Donovan, J. E. (1997). Gender and comorbid psychopathology in adolescents with alcohol dependence. *Journal of the American Academy of Child and Adolescent Psychiatry, 36*, 1195–1203.

Clark, D. B., Vanyukov, M., & Cornelius, J. (2002). Childhood antisocial behavior and adolescent alcohol use disorders. *Alcohol Research and Health, 26*, 109–115.

Clayton, R. R., Cattarello, A. M., & Johnstone, B. M. (1996). The effectiveness of Drug Abuse Resistance Education (Project DARE): 5-year follow-up results. *Preventive Medicine, 25*(3), 307–318.

Coatsworth, J. D., Santisteban, P. A., McBride, K., Szapocznik, J. (2001). Brief strategic family therapy versus community control: Engagement, retention, and an exploration of the moderating role of adolescent symptom severity. *Family Process, 40*, 313–332.

Colby, S. M., Tiffany, S. T., Shiffman, S., & Niaura, R. S. (2000a). Are adolescent smokers dependent on nicotine? A review of the evidence. *Drug and Alcohol Dependence, 59* (Suppl 1), S83–95.

Colby, S. M., Tiffany, S. T., Shiffman, S., & Niaura, R. S. (2000b). Measuring nicotine dependence among youth: A review of available approaches and instruments. *Drug and Alcohol Dependence, 59* (Suppl 1), S23–39.

Cole, J. C., & Sumnall, H. R. (2003). Altered states: The clinical effects of Ecstasy. *Pharmacology Therapeutics, 98*, 35–58.

Cole, J. C., Bailey, M., Sumnall, H. R., Wagstaff, G. F., & King, L. A. (2002). The content of ecstasy tablets: Implications for the study of their long-term effects. *Addiction, 97*, 1531–1536.

Collins, L. M., Baker, T. B., Mermelstein, R. J., Piper, M. E., Jorenby, D. F., Smith, S. S., . . . Fiore, M. C. (2011). The multiphase optimization strategy for engineering effective tobacco use interventions. *Annals of Behavioral Medicine, 41*, 208–226.

Comer, J. S., Olfson, M., & Mojtabai, R. (2010). National trends in child and adolescent psychotropic polypharmacy in office-based practice, 1996–2007. *Journal of the American Academy of Child and Adolescent Psychiatry, 49*(10), 1001–1010.

Comings, D., Ferry, L., Bradshaw-Robinson, S., Burchette, R., Chiu, C., & Muhleman, D. (1996). The dopamine D2 receptor (DRD2) gene: A genetic risk factor in smoking. *Pharmacogenetics, 6*, 73–79.

Comings, D. E., Wu, S., Gonzalez, N., Iacono, W. G., McGue, M., Peters, W. W., & MacMurray, J. P. (2001). Cholecystokinin (CCK) gene as a possible risk factor for smoking: A replication in two independent samples. *Molecular Genetics & Metabolism, 73*, 349–353.

Compton, R. P., & Berning, A. (2015, February). Drug and alcohol crash risk. *Traffic Safety Facts Research Note.*

Conrad, K. M., Flay, B. R., & Hill, D. (1992). Why children start smoking cigarettes: Predictors of onset. *British Journal of Addiction, 87*, 1711–1724.

Corby, E. A., Roll, J. M., Ledgerwood, D. M., & Schuster, C. R. (2000). Contingency management interventions for treating the substance abuse of adolescents: A feasibility study. *Experimental and Clinical Psychopharmacology, 8*, 371.

Cornelius, J. R., Bukstein, O. G., Douaihy, A. B., Clark, D. B., Chung, T. A., Daley, D. C., . . . Brown, S. J. (2010). Double-blind fluoxetine trial in comorbid MDD-CUD youth and young adults. *Drug and Alcohol Dependence, 112*(1–2), 39–45.

Cornelius, J. R., Bukstein, O. G., Wood, D. S., Kirisci, L., Douaihy, A., & Clark, D. B. (2009). Double-blind placebo-controlled trial of fluoxetine in adolescents with comorbid major depression and an alcohol use disorder. *Addictive Behaviors, 34*(10), 905–909.

Cornelius, J. R., Douaihy, A., Bukstein, O. G., Daley, D. C., Wood, S. D., Kelly, T. M., & Salloum, I. M. (2011). Evaluation of cognitive behavioral therapy/motivational enhancement therapy (CBT/MET) in a treatment trial of comorbid MDD/AUD adolescents. *Addictive Behaviors, 36*(8), 843–848.

Cornelius, J. R., Salloum, I. M., Ferrell, R., Douaihy, A. B., Hayes, J., Kirisci, L., . . . Daley, D. C. (2012). Treatment trial and long-term follow-up evaluation among comorbid youth with major depression and a cannabis use disorder. *International Journal of Medical and Biological Frontiers, 18*(6), 399–411.

Corrigall, W. A., Zack, M., Eissenberg, T., Belsito, L., & Scher, R. (2001). Acute subjective and physiological responses to smoking in adolescents. *Addiction, 96*, 1409–1417.

Cottler, L. B., Schuckit, M. A., Helzer, J. E., Crowley, T., Woody, G., Nathan, P., et al. (1995). The DSMIV field trial for substance use disorders: Major results. *Drug and Alcohol Dependence, 38*, 59–69; discussion 71–83.

Cottrell, D., & Boston, P. (2000). Practitioner review: The effectiveness of systemic family therapy for children and adolescents. *Journal of Child Psychology and Psychiatry, 43*, 573–586.

Craig, A. R., Maxfield, A. D., & Stein, J. S. (2014). Do the adjusting-delay and increasing-delay tasks measure the same construct: Delay discounting? *Behavioural Pharmacology, 25*, 306–315.

Craig, E. L., Zhao, B., Cui, J. Z., Novalen, M., Miksys, S., & Tyndale, R. F. (2014). Nicotine pharmacokinetics in rats is altered as a function of age, impacting the interpretation of animal model data. *Drug Metabolism and Disposition, 42*(9), 1447–1455.

Crews, F., He, J., & Hodge, C. (2007). Adolescent cortical development: A critical period of vulnerability for addiction. *Pharmacology Biochemisty and Behavior, 86*(2), 189–199.

Crits-Christoph, P., Siqueland, L., Blaine, J. D., Frank, A., Luborsky, L., Onken, L. S., et al. (1999). Psychosocial treatments for cocaine dependence: Results of the National Institute on Drug Abuse Collaborative Cocaine Study. *Archives of General Psychiatry, 56*, 495–502.

Crome, I. B., Christian, J., & Green, C. (1998). Tip of the national iceberg? Profile of adolescent subjects prescribed methadone in an innovative community drug service. *Drugs: Education, Prevention and Policy, 5*, 195–197.

Crowley, J. J., Oslin, D. W., Patkar, A. A., Gottheil, E., DeMaria, P. A., Jr., O'Brien, C. P., et al. (2003). A genetic association study of the mu opioid receptor and severe opioid dependence. *Psychiatric Genetics, 13*, 169–173.

Crowley, T. J., & Riggs, P. D. (1995). Adolescent substance use disorder with conduct disorder and comorbid conditions. In D. Czechowicz (Ed.), *NIDA research monograph 156: Adolescent drug abuse: Clinical assessment and therapeutic interventions* (Vol. 156, pp. 49–111). Rockville, MD: National Institute on Drug Abuse.

Czoty, P. W., Gage, H. D., & Nader, M. A. (2010). Differences in D2 dopamine receptor availability and reaction to novelty in socially housed male monkeys during abstinence from cocaine. *Psychopharmacology (Berlin), 208*(4), 585–592.

Dackis, C. A., & Gold, M. S. (1992). Psychiatric hospitals for treatment of dual diagnosis. In J. H. Lowinson (Ed.), *Substance abuse, a comprehensive textbook* (2nd ed., pp. 467–485). Baltimore: Williams & Wilkins.

Dackis, C. A., Lynch, K. G., Yu, E., Samaha, F. F., Kampman, K. M., Cornish, J. W., et al. (2003). Modafinil and cocaine: A double-blind, placebocontrolled drug interaction study. *Drug and Alcohol Dependence, 70*, 29–37.

Dackis, C. A., & O'Brien, C. P. (2001). Cocaine dependence: A disease of the brain's reward centers. *Journal of Substance Abuse Treatment, 21*, 111–117.

Dackis, C. A., & O'Brien, C. P. (2002). Cocaine dependence: The challenge for pharmacotherapy. *Current Opinion in Psychiatry, 15*, 261–267.

Dackis, C., & O'Brien, C. (2003). Glutamatergic agents for cocaine dependence. *Annals of the New York Academy of Sciences, 1003*, 328–345.

Dackis, C., Yu, E., Samaha, F., Kampman, K., Cornish, J., Rowan, A., et al. (2001). Modafinil—Cocaine safety study; a double-blind, placebo-controlled drug interaction study. College on Problems of Drug Dependence, Presented at the Annual Meeting at San Juan, Puerto Rico.

Daglish, M., Weinstein, A., Malizia, A. L., Wilson, S., Melichar, J. K., Britten, S., ... Nutt, D. J. (2001). Changes in regional cerebral blood flow elicited by craving memories in abstinent opiate-dependent subjects. *American Journal of Psychiatry, 158*, 1680–1686.

Daumann, J., Schnitker, R., Weidemann, J., Schnell, K., Thron, A., & Gouzoulis-Mayfrank, E. (2003). Neural correlates of working memory in pure and polyvalent ecstasy (MDMA) users. *Neuroreport, 14*, 1983–1987.

Davies, R., Gabbert, S., & Riggs, P. D. (2001). Anxiety disorders in neurologic illness. *Current Treatment Options in Neurology, 3*, 333–346.

Daviss, W. B., Bentivoglio, P., Racusin, R., Brown, K. M., Bostic, J. Q., & Wiley, L. (2001). Bupropion sustained release in adolescents with comorbid attention-deficit/hyperactivity disorder and depression. *Journal of the American Academy of Child and Adolescent Psychiatry, 40*, 307–314.

Dawson, D. A., Goldstein, R. B., Chou, S. P., Ruan, W. J., & Grant, B. F. (2008). Age at first drink and the first incidence of adult-onset DSM-IV alcohol use disorders. *Alcoholism: Clinical and Experimental Research, 32*(12), 2149–2160.

Deandrea, D. C., Troost, J. P., & Anthony, J. C. (2013). Toward primary prevention of extra-medical OxyContin® use among young people. *Preventive Medicine, 57*(3), 244–246.

Deas, D., Riggs, P., Langenbucher, J., Goldman, M., & Brown, S. (2000). Adolescents are not adults: Developmental considerations in alcohol users. *Alcoholism, Clinical and Experimental Research, 24*, 232–237.

Deas, D., & Thomas, S. E. (2001). An overview of controlled studies of adolescent substance abuse treatment. *American Journal on Addictions, 10*, 178–189.

Deas, D., & Thomas, S. (2002). Comorbid psychiatric factors contributing to adolescent alcohol and other drug use. *Alcohol Research & Health, 26*(2), 116–121.

Deas-Nesmith, D., Brady, K., & Campbell, S. (1998). Comorbid substance use and anxiety disorders in adolescents. *Journal of Psychopathology and Behavioral Assessment, 20*, 139–148.

Deas-Nesmith, D., Campbell, S., & Brady, K. T. (1998). Substance use disorders in an adolescent inpatient psychiatric population. *Journal of the National Medical Association, 90*, 233–238.

DeJong, W., & Blanchette, J. (2014). Case closed: Research evidence on the positive public health impact of the age 21 minimum legal drinking age in the United States. *Journal of Studies on Alcohol and Drugs, S17*, 108–115.

De Jong, W. J., Cleveringa, A. M., Greijdanus, B., Meyer, P., Heineman, E., & Hulscher, J. B. (2015). The effect of acute alcohol intoxication on gut wall integrity in healthy male volunteers; a randomized controlled trial. *Alcohol, 49*(1), 65–70.

Dennis, M., Babor, T. F., Roebuck, M. C., & Donaldson, J. (2002). Changing the focus: The case for recognizing and treating cannabis use disorders. *Addiction, 97* (Suppl 1), 4–15.

Dennis, M., Godley, S. H., Diamond, G., Tims, F. M., Babor, T., Donaldson, J., ... Funk R. (2004). The Cannabis Youth Treatment (CYT) Study: Main findings from two randomized trials. *Journal of Substance Abuse Treatment, 27*(3), 197–213.

Dennis, M., Titus, J. C., Diamond, G., Donaldson, J., Godley, S. H., Tims, F. M., et al. (2002). The Cannabis Youth Treatment (CYT) experiment: Rationale, study design and analysis plans. *Addiction 97*, 16–34.

Dennis, M. L., & White, M. K. (2003). The effectiveness of adolescent substance abuse treatment: A brief summary of studies through 2001. Bloomington, IL: Chestnut Health Systems.

Denoth, F., Siciliano, V., Iozzo, P., Fortunato, L., & Molinaro, S. (2011). The association between overweight and illegal drug consumption in adolescents: Is there an underlying influence of the sociocultural environment? *PLoS One, 6*(11), 1–8.

DeRubeis, R. J., & Crits-Christoph, P. (1998). Empirically supported individual and group psychological treatments for adult mental disorders. *Journal of Consulting and Clinical Psychology, 66*, 37–52.

Developmental Research and Programs. (2000). In *Communities that care: A comprehensive prevention program*. Seattle, WA.

De Win, M. M., Reneman, L., Reitsma, J. B., Den Heeten, G. J., Booij, J., & Van Den Brink, W. (2004). Mood disorders and serotonin transporter density in ecstasy users—the influence of long-term abstention, dose, and gender. *Psychopharmacology (Berlin)*, 173, 376–382.

DeWit, D. J., Adlaf, E. M., Offord, D. R., & Ogborne, A. C. (2000). Age at first alcohol use: A risk factor for the development of alcohol disorders. [Comment]. *American Journal of Psychiatry, 157*, 745–750.

Di Chiara, G. (1999). Drug addiction as dopamine-dependent associative learning disorder. *European Journal of Pharmacology, 375*, 13–30.

Di Chiara, G., Acquas, E., Tanda, G., & Cadoni, C. (1993). Drugs of abuse: Biochemical surrogates of specific aspects of natural reward? *Biochemical Society Symposium, 59*, 65–81.

Di Chiara, G., Bassareo, V., Fenu, S., De Luca, M. A., Spina, L., Cadoni, C., ... Lecca, D. (2004) Dopamine and drug addiction: The nucleus accumbens shell connection. *Neuropharmacology, 47*(Suppl 1), 227–241.

Di Ciano, P., & Everitt, B. J. (2003). The GABA(B) receptor agonist baclofen attenuates cocaine and heroin-seeking behavior by rats. *Neuropsychopharmacology, 28*(3), 510–518.

Diamond, A. (2013). Executive functions. *Annual Review of Psychology, 64*,135–168.

Diamond, G. M., Izzard, M. C., Kedar, T., Hutlzer, A., & Mell, H. J. (2005). Psychological symptoms and drug use severity among Israeli adolescents presenting for outpatient drug abuse treatment. *Journal of Adolescence, 28*(4), 495–505.

Diamond, G. S., & Liddle, H. A. (1996). Resolving a therapeutic impasse between parents and adolescents in multidimensional family therapy. *Journal of Consulting and Clinical Psychology, 64*, 481–488.

Diamond, G. S., Liddle, H. A., Wintersteen, M. B., Dennis, M. L., Godley, S. H., & Tims, F. (2006). Early therapeutic alliance as a predictor of treatment outcome for adolescent cannabis users in outpatient treatment. *American Journal of Addiction, 15*(Suppl 1), 26–33.

Diamond, G., Godley, S. H., Liddle, H. A., Sampl, S., Webb, C., Tims, F. M., & Meyers R. (2002).

Five outpatient treatment models for adolescent marijuana use: A description of the Cannabis Youth Treatment Interventions. *Addiction, 97*(Suppl. 1), 70–83.

Diamond, G., Panichelli-Mindel, S. M., Shera, D., Tims, F., Ungemack, J. (in press). Psychiatric distress in adolescents presenting for outpatient treatment for marijuana abuse and dependency: Prevalence and diagnostic algorithms. *Journal of Child and Adolescent Substance Abuse Treatment.*

Dick, D. (2011). The dynamic nature of genetic and environmental influences on alcohol use and dependence. In K. S. Kendler, S. R. Jaffee, & D. Romer (Eds.), *The dynamic genome and mental health: The role of genes and environments in youth development*. New York: Oxford University Press.

Dick, D., Viken, R., Purcell, S., Kaprio, J., Pulkkinen, L., & Rose, R. J. (2007). Parental monitoring moderates the importance of genetic and environmental influences on adolescent smoking. *Journal of Abnormal Psychology, 116*(1), 213–218.

Dickson, S. L., Egecioglu, E., Landgren, S., Skibicka, K., Engel, J., & Jerlhag, E. (2011). The role of the central ghrelin system in reward from food and chemical drugs. *Molecular and Cellular Endocrinology, 340*(1), 80–87.

DiFranza, J. R., Rigotti, N. A., McNeill, A. D., Ockene, J. K., Savageau, J. A., St Cyr, D., et al. (2000). Initial symptoms of nicotine dependence in adolescents. *Tobacco Control, 9*, 313–319.

DiFranza, J. R., Savageau, J. A., Rigotti, N. A., Fletcher, K., Ockene, J. K., McNeill, A. D., et al. (2002). Development of symptoms of tobacco dependence in youths: 30-month follow-up data from the DANDY study. *Tobacco Control, 11*, 228–235.

Dillon, P., Copeland, J., & Jansen, K. (2003). Patterns of use and harms associated with nonmedical ketamine use. *Drug and Alcohol Dependence, 69*, 23–28.

Dishion, T. J., & Dodge, K. A. (2005). Peer contagion in interventions for children and adolescents: Moving towards an understanding of the ecology and dynamics of change. *Journal of Abnormal Child Psychology, 33*(3), 395–400.

Dishion, T., & Kavanagh, K. (2000). A multilevel approach to family-centered prevention in schools: Process and outcome. *Addictive Behaviors, 25*(6), 899–911.

Dishion, T. J., McCord, J., & Poulin, F. (1999). When interventions harm: Peer groups and problem behavior. *American Psychologist, 54*, 755–764.

Dishion, T., Patterson, G., Stoolmiller, M., & Skinner, M. (1991). Family, school and behavioral antecedents to early adolescent involvement with antisocial peers. *Developmental Psychology, 27*(1), 172–180.

Dishion, T., Véronneau, M-H, Stormshak, E. A., & Kavanagh, K. (2015). Family-centered prevention of adolescent drug abuse: Translational research in a public health framework. In L. M. Scheier (Ed.), *Handbook of adolescent drug use prevention: Research, intervention strategies, and practice* (pp. 293–309). Washington, DC: American Psychological Association.

Donohew, L., Lorch, E., & Palmgreen, P. (1991). Sensation seeking and targeting of televised antidrug PSAs. In L. Donohew, H. E. Sypher, & W. J. Bukoski (Eds.), *Persuasive communication and drug abuse prevention* (pp. 209–226). Hillsdale, NJ: Lawrence Erlbaum.

Drake, R. E., Mchugo, G. J., & Noordsy, D. L. (1993). Treatment of alcoholism among schizophrenic outpatients: 4-year outcomes. *American Journal of Psychiatry, 150*, 328–329.

Drake, R. E., Mercer-McFadden, C., Muesser, K. T., McHugo, G. J., & Bond, G. R. (1998). A review of integrated mental health and substance abuse treatment for patients with dual disorders. *Schizophrenia Bulletin, 24*, 589–608.

Drug Strategies. (2003). In *Making the grade: A guide to school drug prevention programs*. Washington, D.C.

Duggirala, R., Almasy, L., & Blangero, J. (1999). Smoking behavior is under the influence of a major quantitative trait locus on human chromosome 5q. *Genetic Epidemiology, 17*, S139–144.

Dunn, C., Deroo, I., & Rivara, F. P. (2001). The use of brief interventions adapted from motivational interviewing across behavioral domains: A systematic review. *Addiction, 96*, 1725–1742.

Dunne, E. M., Hearn, L. E., Rose, J. J., & Latimer, W. W. (2014). ADHD as a risk factor for early onset and heightened adult problem severity of illicit substance use: An accelerated gateway model. *Addictive Behaviors, 39*(12), 1755–1758.

DuRant, R. H., Getts, A., Cadenhead, C., Emans, S. J., & Woods, E. R. (1995). Exposure to violence and victimization and depression, hopelessness, and purpose in life among adolescents living in and around public housing. *Journal of Developmental and Behavioral Pediatrics, 16*, 233–237.

DuRant, R. H. (1995). Adolescent health research as we proceed into the twenty-first century. *Journal of Adolescent Health, 17*, 199–203.

Dwyer, J. B., & Leslie, F. M. (2016). Adolescent maturation of dopamine D1 and D2 receptor function and interactions in rodents. *PLoS One, 11*(1), e0146966.

Eccles, J., & Gootman, J. A. (2002). *Community programs to promote youth development* (National Research Council and Institute of Medicine). Washington, DC: National Academy Press.

Eddy, N. B., Halbach, H., Isbell, H., & Seevers, M. H. (1965). Drug dependence: Its significance and characteristics. *Bulletin of the World Health Organization, 32*, 721–733.

Eggert, L. L., Thompson, E. A., Herting, J. R., & Nicholas, L. J. (1995). Reducing suicide potential among high-risk youth: Tests of school-based prevention program. *Suicide and Life Threatening Behavior, 25*(2), 276–296.

Eggert, L. L., Thompson, E. A., Herting, J. R., Nicholas, L. J., & Dicker, B. G. (1994). Preventing adolescent drug abuse and high school dropout through an intensive school-based social network development program. *American Journal of Health Promotion, 8*(3), 202–215.

Eissenberg, T., & Balster, R. (2000). Initial tobacco use episodes in children and adolescent: Current knowledge, future direction (review). *Drug and Alcohol Dependence, 59*(Suppl. 51), S41–60.

Elkins, I., McGue, M., & Iacono, W. G. (2007). Prospective effects of attention-deficit/hyperactivity disorder, conduct disorder, and sex on adolescent substance use and abuse. *Archives of General Psychiatry, 64*, 1145–1152.

Ellickson, P. L., Tucker, J. S., & Klein, D. J. (2003). Ten-year prospective study of public health problems associated with early drinking. *Pediatrics, 111*(5), 949–956.

Elliott, R., Newman, J. L., Longe, O. A., & Deakin, J. F. W. (2003) Differential response patterns in the striatum and orbitofrontal cortex to financial reward in humans: A parametric functional magnetic resonance imaging study. *Journal of Neuroscience, 23*, 303–307.

Emslie, G. J., Rush, A. J., Weinberg, W. A., Kowatch, R. A., Hughes, C. W., Carmody, T., et al. (1997). A double-blind, randomized, placebo-controlled trial of fluoxetine in children and adolescents with depression. *Archives of General Psychiatry, 54*, 1031–1037.

Ercan, E. S., Coskunol, H., Varan, A., & Toksoz, K. (2003). Childhood attention deficit/hyperactivity disorder and alcohol dependence: A 1-year follow-up. *Alcohol and Alcoholism, 38*, 352–356.

Ercan, E. S., Uysal, T., Ercan, E., Ardıc, U. A., Niederhofer, H., & Staffen, W. (2012). Aripiprazole in children and adolescents with conduct disorder: A single-center, open-label study. *Pharmacopsychiatry, 45*(1), 13–19.

Erol, A., & Karpyak, V. M. (2015). Sex and gender-related differences in alcohol use and its consequences: Contemporary knowledge and future research considerations. *Drug and Alcohol Dependence, 156*, 1–13.

Escobedo, L. G., Kirch, D. G., & Anda, R. F. (1996). Depression and smoking initiation among US Latinos. *Addiction, 91*, 113–119.

Escobedo, L. G., Marcus, S. E., Holtzman, D., & Giovino, G. A. (1993). Sports participation, age at smoking initiation, and the risk of smoking among US high school students. *Journal of the American Medical Association, 269*, 1391–1395.

Everitt, B. J., & Robbins, T. W. (2016). Drug addiction: Updating actions to habits to compulsions ten years on. *Annual Review of Psychology, 67*, 23–50.

Faessel, H., Ravva, P., & Williams, K. (2009). Pharmacokinetics, safety, and tolerability of varenicline in healthy adolescent smokers: A multicenter, randomized, double-blind, placebo-controlled, parallel-group study. *Clinical Therapeutics*, 31, 177–189. doi: 10.1016/j.clinthera.2009.01.003.

Faggiano, F., Vigna-Taglinati, F. D., Versino, E., Zambon, A., Borraccino, A., Lemma, P., ... EU-Dap Study Group. (2008). School-based prevention for illicit drugs use: A systematic review. *Drug and Alcohol Dependence, 46*, 385–396.

Fahim, R. E., Kessler, P. D., Fuller, S. A., & Kalnik, M. W. (2011). Nicotine vaccines. *CNS and Neurological Disorders Drug Targets*, 10, 905–915.

Faraone, S. V., Biederman, J., Spencer, T. J., & Aleardi, M. (2006). Comparing the efficacy of medications for ADHD using meta-analysis. *Medscape General Medicine, 8*(4), 4.

Farkas, A. J., Gilpin, E. A., White, M. M., & Pierce, J. P. (2000). Association between household and workplace smoking restrictions and adolescent smoking. *Journal of the American Medical Association, 284*, 717–722.

Farre, M., De La Torre, R., O Marthuna, B., Roset, P. N., Peiro, A. M., Torrens, M., ... Cami, J. (2004). Repeated doses administration of MDMA in humans: Pharmacological effects and pharmacokinetics. *Psychopharmacology (Berlin), 173*, 364–375.

Feinberg, M. E., Greenberg, M. T., Osgood, D. W., Anderson, A., & Babinski, L. (2002). The effects of training community leaders in prevention science: Communities that Care in Pennsylvania. *Evaluation and Program Planning, 25*(3), 245–259.

Feldman, E. A. (2013). Shots for tots? *Hastings Center Report*, 43(3), 34–35.

Ferri, M., Allara, E., Gasparrini, A., & Faggiano, F. (2013). Media campaigns for the prevention of illicit drug use in young people. *Cochrane Database of Systemic Reviews, 6*(CD009287), 1–107.

Fishman, M. J., Winstanley, E. L., Curran, E., Garrett, S., & Subramaniam, G. (2010). Treatment of opioid dependence in adolescents and young adults with extended release naltrexone: Preliminary case-series and feasibility. *Addiction, 105*(9), 1669–1676.

Flachmeier, C., Kidd, K. K., et al. (2000). Sequence variability and candidate gene analysis in complex disease: Association of mu opioid receptor gene variation with substance dependence. *Human Molecular Genetics, 9*, 2895–2908.

Flay, B. R. (2002). Positive youth development requires comprehensive health promotion programs. *American Journal of Health Behavior, 26*(6), 407–424.

Flay, B. R., d'Avernas, J., Best, J., Kersell, M., & Ryan, K. (1983). Cigarette smoking: Why young people do it and ways of preventing it. In P. J. McGrath & P. Firestone (Eds.), *Pediatric and adolescent behavioral medicine* (pp. 132–183). New York: Springer-Verlag.

Fletcher, J. M., Deb, P., & Sindelar, J. L. (2009). *Tobacco use, taxation and self control in adolescence* (Working Paper No. 15130). Cambridge, MA: National Bureau of Economic Research. Retrieved from www.nber.org/papers/w15130.

Flynn, A. B., Falco, M., & Hocini, S. (2015). Independent evaluation of middle school-based drug prevention curricula: A systematic review. *JAMA Pediatrics, 169*(11), 1046–1052.

Fone, K. C., Beckett, S. R., Topham, I. A., Swettenham, J., Ball, M., & Maddocks, L. (2002). Long-term changes in social interaction and reward following repeated MDMA administration to adolescent rats without accompanying serotonergic neurotoxicity. *Psychopharmacology (Berlin), 159*, 437–444.

Forrester, M. B. (2012). Adolescent synthetic cannabinoid exposures reported to Texas poison centers. *Pediatric Emergency Care, 28*(10), 985–989.

Fosco, G. M., Frank, J. L., Stormshak, E. A., & Dishion, T. J. (2013). Opening the "Black Box": Family check-up intervention effects on self-regulation that prevents growth in problem behavior and substance use. *Journal of School Psychology, 51*(4), 455–468.

Foster, S. E., Vaughan, R. D., Foster, W. H., & Califano, J. A., Jr. (2003). Alcohol consumption and expenditures for underage drinking and adult excessive drinking. *Journal of the American Medical Association, 289*(8), 989–995. [Erratum in *Journal of the American Medical Association* April 9, 2003, vol. 289, issue 14, p. 1782.]

Foxcroft, D. R., & Tsertsvadze, A. (2012). Universal alcohol misuse prevention programmes for chidren and adolescents: Cochrane systematic reviews. *Perspectives in Public Health, 132*(3), 128–134.

Foxcroft, D. R., Coombes, L., Wood, S., Allen, D., & Almeida Santimano, N. M. (2014). Motivational Interviewing for alcohol misuse in young adults. *Cochrane Database of Systematic Reviews, 8*, CD007025.

Freese, T. E., Miotto, K., & Reback, C. J. (2002). The effects and consequences of selected club drugs. *Journal of Substance Abuse Treatment, 23*, 151–156.

French, S. A., Perry, C. L., Leon, G. R., & Fulkerson, J. A. (1994). Food preferences, eating patterns, and physical activity among adolescents: Correlates of eating disorders symptoms. *Journal of Adolescent Health, 15*, 286–294.

Frenois, F., Le Moine, C., & Cador, M. (2005) The motivational component of withdrawal in opiate addiction: Role of associative learning and aversive memory in opiate addiction from a behavioral, anatomical and functional perspective. *Reviews in the Neurosciences, 16*(3), 255–276.

Friedman, A. (1989). Family therapy vs. parent groups: Effects on adolescent drug abusers. *American Journal of Family Therapy, 17*, 335–347.

Friedman, L., Lichtenstein, E., & Biglan, A. (1985). Smoking onset among teens: An empirical analysis of initial situation. *Addictive Behaviors, 10*, 1–13.

Galloway, G. P., Frederick-Osborne, S. L., Seymour, R., Contini, S. E., & Smith, D. E. (2000). Abuse and therapeutic potential of gamma-hydroxybutyric acid. *Alcohol, 20*, 263–269.

Garavan, H., Pankiewicz, H. J., Bloom, A., Cho, J.-K., Sperry, L., Ross, T. J., et al. (2000).

Cue-induced cocaine craving: Neuroanatomical specificity for drug-users and drug stimuli. *American Journal of Psychiatry, 157*, 1789–1798.

Garner, B. G., Godley, S. H., Funk, R. R., Dennis, M. L., Smith, J. E., & Godley, M. D. (2009). Exposure to Adolescent Community Reinforcement Approach (A-CRA) treatment procedures as a mediator of the relationship between adolescent substance abuse treatment retention and outcome. *Journal of Substance Abuse Treatment, 36*(3), 252–264.

Gautam, P., Lebel, C., Narr, K. L., Mattson, S. N., May, P. A., Adnams, C. M., ... Sowell, E. R. (2015). Volume changes and brain-behavior relationships in white matter and subcortical gray matter in children with prenatal alcohol exposure. *Human Brain Mapping, 36*(6), 2318–2329.

Gelernter, J., Kranzler, H., & Cubells, J. (1999). Genetics of two mu opioid receptor gene (OPRM1) exon 1 polymorphisms: Population studies, and allele frequencies in alcoholand drugdependent subjects. *Molecular Psychiatry, 4*, 476–483.

Geller, B., Cooper, T. B., Sun, K., Zimerman, B., Frazier, J., Williams, M., et al. (1998). Double-blind and placebo-controlled study of lithium for adolescent bipolar disorders with secondary substance dependency. [see comment]. *Journal of the American Academy of Child and Adolescent Psychiatry, 37*, 171–178.

Gerra, G., Zaimovic, A., Ferri, M., Zambelli, U., Timpano, M., Neri, E., et al. (2000). Long-lasting effects of (+/−)3,4-methylenedioxymethamphetamine (ecstasy) on serotonin system function in humans. *Biological Psychiatry, 47*, 127– 136.

Gerstein, D. R., & Johnson, R. A. (1999). Adolescents and young adults in the National Treatment Improvement Evaluation Study. Retrieved from http//www.ilpsr.umich.edu/SAMHDA/ NTIES/ebm-summaries.html

Giesbrecht, H., Krempulec, L., & West, P. (1993). Community-based prevention research to reduce alcohol-related problems. *Alcohol Health and Research World, 28*(3), 309–321.

Gilbert, D., & Gilbert, B. (1995). Personality, psychopathology and nicotine responses as mediators of the genetics of smoking. *Behavior Genetics, 25*, 133–147.

Gilpin, R. (2009). The use of Theravada Buddhist practices and perspectives in mindfulness-based cognitive therapy. *Contemporary Buddhism, 9*, 227–251.

Gilvarry, E. (2000). Substance abuse in young people. *Journal of Child Psychology and Psychiatry, and Allied Disciplines, 41*(1), 55–80.

Glasser, A. M., Collins, L., Pearson, J. L., Abudayyeh, H., Niaura, R. S., Abrams, D. B., & Villanti, A. C. (2017). Overview of electronic nicotine delivery systems: A systematic review. *American Journal of Preventive Medicine*, 52(2), e33–e66. Epub 2016 Nov 30.

Godley, M. D., Godley, S. H., Dennis, M. L., Funk, R. R., & Passetti, L. L. (2007). The effect of assertive continuing care on continuing care linkage, adherence and abstinence following residential treatment for adolescents with substance use disorders. *Addiction, 102*(1), 81–93.

Godley, M., Godley, S., Karvinen, T., Slown, L., & Wright, K. (2006). *The assertive continuing care protocol: A clinician's manual for working with adolescents after treatment of alcohol and other substance abuse disorders*. Center for Substance Abuse Treatment.

Godley, S. H. (1994). A treatment system for persons with mental illness and substance abuse: The Illinois ME/SA Project. Springfield, IL: Illinois Department of Mental Health and Developmental Disabilities.

Godley, S. H., Garner, B. R., Passetti, L. L., Funk, R. R., Dennis, M. L., & Godley, M. D. (2010). Adolescent outpatient treatment and continuing care: Main findings from a randomized clinical trial. *Drug and Alcohol Dependence, 110*(1–2), 44–54.

Godley, S. H., Meyers, R. J., Smith, J. E., Godley, M. D., Titus, J. C., Karvinen, T., ... Kelberg P. (2001). *Cannabis Youth Treatment Series Volume 4: The Adolescent Community Reinforcement Approach.* Rockville, MD: Center for Substance Abuse Treatment, Substance Abuse and Mental Health Services Administration. DHHS Publication No (SMA) 01-3489.

Gold, M. S., Dackis, C. A., & Washton, A. M. (1984). The sequential use of clonidine and naltrexone in the treatment of opiate addicts. *Advances in Alcohol and Substance Abuse, 3*, 19–39.

Goldberg, L., Elliot, D. L., MacKinnon, D. P., Moe, E. L., Kuehl, K. S., Yoon, M., & Williams, J. (2007). Outcomes of a prospective trial of student-athlete drug testing: The Student Athlete Testing Using Notification (SATURN) study. *Journal of Adolescent Health, 41*, 421–429.

Goldberg, S. R., & Schuster, C. R. (1967). Conditioned suppression by a stimulus associated with nalorphine in morphine-dependent monkeys. *Journal of the Experimental Analysis of Behavior, 10*, 235–242.

Goniewicz, M. L., Knysak, J., Gawron, M., Kosmider, L., Sobczak, A., Kurek, J., . . . Benowitz, N. (2014). Levels of selected carcinogens and toxicants in vapour from electronic cigarettes. *Tobacco Control, 23*(2), 133–139.

Gonzalez, G., Oliveto, A., & Kosten, T. R. (2002). Treatment of heroin (Diamorphine) addiction: Current approaches and future prospects. *Drugs, 62*, 1331–1343.

Gonzalez, R., Carey, C., & Grant, I. (2002). Nonacute (residual) neuropsychological effects of cannabis use: A qualitative analysis and systematic review. *Journal of Clinical Pharmacology, 42* (11 Suppl.), 48S–57S.

Goodman, R. M. (2000). Bridging the gap in effective program implementation: From concept to application. *Journal of Community Psychology, 28*(3), 309–321.

Goodwin, R. D., Wall, M. M., Choo, T., Galea, S., Horowitz, J., Nomura, Y., . . . Hasin, D. S. (2014). Changes in the prevalence of mood and anxiety disorders among male and female current smokers in the United States: 1990–2001. *Annals of Epidemiology, 24*(7), 493–497.

Gottfredson, D., & Wilson, D. B. (2003). Characteristics of effective school-based substance abuse prevention. *Prevention Science, 4*(1), 27–38.

Gowing, L. R., Henry-Edwards, S. M., Irvine, R. J., & Ali, R. L. (2002). The health effects of ecstasy: A literature review. *Drug and Alcohol Review, 21*, 53–63.

Grant, B. F., & Dawson, D. A. (1997). Age at onset of alcohol use and its association with DSM-IV alcohol abuse and dependence: Results from the National Longitudinal Alcohol Epidemiologic Survey. *Journal of Substance Abuse, 9*, 103–110.

Grant, S., London, E. D., Newlin, D. B., Villemagne, V. L., Liu, X., Contoreggi, C., . . . Margolin A. (1996). Activation of memory circuits during cue-elicited cocaine craving. *Proceedings of the National Academy of Sciences of the United States of America, 93*(21), 12040–12045.

Gray, K. M., Carpenter, M. J., Baker, N. L., Hartwell, K. J., Lewis, A. L., Hiott, D. W., . . . Upadhyaya, H. P. (2011). Bupropion SR and contingency management for adolescent smoking cessation. *Journal of Substance Abuse Treatment*, 40, 77–86. Epub 2010 Oct 8.

Gray, K. M., Carpenter, M. J., Lewis, A. L., Klintworth, E. M., & Upadhyaya, H. P. (2012). Varenicline versus bupropion XL for smoking cessation in older adolescents: A randomized, double-blind pilot trial. *Nicotine and Tobacco Research*, 14, 234–239. Epub 2011 Jul 20.

Green, A. R., Mechan, A. O., Elliott, J. M., O'Shea, E., & Colado, M. I. (2003). The pharmacology and clinical pharmacology of 3,4-methylenedioxymethamphetamine (MDMA, "ecstasy"). *Pharmacological Reviews, 55*, 463–508.

Green, B., Kavanagh, D., & Young, R. (2003). Being stoned: A review of self-reported cannabis effects. *Drug and Alcohol Review, 22*, 453–460.

Greenberg, M. T., Domitrovich, C., & Bumbarger, B. (2000). Preventing mental disorders in schoolaged children: A review of the effectiveness of prevention programs. *Prevention & Treatment.* Washington, DC: American Psychological Association.

Grella, C. E., Hser, Y. I., Joshi, V., & Rounds-Bryant, J. (2001). Drug treatment outcomes for adolescents with comorbid mental and substance use disorders. *Journal of Nervous and Mental Disease, 189*(6), 384–392.

Griffith, J. D., Rowan-Szal, G. A., Roark, R. R., & Simpson, D. D. (2000). Contingency management in outpatient methadone treatment: A meta-analysis. *Drug and Alcohol Dependence, 58*, 55–66.

Gross, S. R., Barrett, S. P., Shestowsky, J. S., & Pihl, R. O. (2002). Ecstasy and drug consumption patterns: A Canadian rave population study. *Canadian Journal of Psychiatry, 47*, 546–551.

Grunbaum, J. A, Kann, L., Kinchen, S. A., Williams, B., Ross, J. G., Lowry, R., et al. (2002). Youth Risk Behavior Surveillance—United States, 2001. *Morbidity and Mortality Weekly Review Surveillance Summaries, 51*(No.SS-4).

Haggerty, R. J., & Mrazek, P. J. (1994). *Reducing the risk of mental disorders.* Washington, DC: National Academies Press.

Hall, W., & Solowij, N. (1998). Adverse effects of cannabis. *Lancet, 352*(9140), 1611–1616.

Hallfors, D. (2001, April). Diffusion of federal policy to promote effective school-based prevention: State and local perspectives. Paper presented at the Drug Abuse Prevention Summit, Snowbird, UT.

Hallikainen, T., Saito, T., Lachman, H. M., Volavka, J., Pohjalainen, T., Ryynanen, O. P., et al. (1999). Association between low activity serotonin transporter promoter genotype and early onset alcoholism with habitual impulsive violent behavior. *Molecular Psychiatry, 4*, 385–388.

Halpern, J. H., & Pope, H. G. (2003). Hallucinogen persisting perception disorder: What do we know after 50 years? *Drug and Alcohol Dependence, 69*, 109–119.

Halpern, J. H., & Pope, H. G., Jr. (1999). Do hallucinogens cause residual neuropsychological toxicity? *Drug and Alcohol Dependence*, 53, 247–256.

Handelsman, L., Aronson, M. J., Ness, R., Cochrane, K. J., & Kanof, P. D. (1992). The dysphoria of heroin addiction. *American Journal of Drug and Alcohol Abuse, 18*, 275–287.

Hanewinkel, R., Sargent, J. D., Hunt, K., Sweeting, H., Engels, R. C., Scholte, R. H., ... Morgenstern M. (2014). Portrayal of alcohol consumption in movies and drinking initiation in low-risk adolescents. *Pediatrics. 133*(6), 973–982.

Hansen, W. B. (1992). School-based substance abuse prevention: A review of the state of the art in curriculum, 1980–1990. *Health Education Research: Theory and Practice, 7*, 403–430.

Harrison, L. (2001). Understanding the differences in youth drug prevalence rates produced by the MTF, NHSDA, and YRBS studies. *Journal of Drug Issues, 31*, 665–694.

Hasin, D. S., O'Brien, C. P., Auriacombe, M., Borges, G., Bucholz, K., Budney, A., ... Grant, B. F. (2013). DSM-5 criteria for substance use disorders: Recommendations and rationale. *American Journal of Psychiatry, 170*(8), 834–851.

Hasin, D. S., Stinson, F. S., Ogburn, E., & Grant, B. F. (2007). Prevalence, correlates, disability, and comorbidity of DSM-IV alcohol abuse and dependence in the United States: Results from the National Epidemiologic Survey on Alcohol and Related Conditions. *Archives of General Psychiatry, 64*(7), 830–842.

Hatsukami, D. K., & Fischman, M. W. (1996). Crack cocaine and cocaine hydrochloride: Are the differences myth or reality? *Journal of the American Medical Association, 276*, 1580–1588.

Hawkins, J. D., Catalano, R. F., & Miller, J. Y. (1992). Risk and protective factors for alcohol and other drug problems in adolescence and early adulthood: Implications for substance abuse prevention. *Psychological Bulletin 112*, 64–105.

Heath, A. C., Madden, P. A., Grant, J. D., McLaughlin, T. L., Todorov, A. A., & Bucholz, K. K. (1999). Resiliency factors protecting against teenage alcohol use and smoking, influences of religion, religious involvement and values and ethnicity in the Missouri Adolescent Female Twin Study. *Twin Research, 2*, 145–155.

Heath, A. C., & Martin, N. (1988). Teenage alcohol use in the Australian twin register; genetic and social determinants of starting to drink. *Alcoholism, Clinical and Experimental Research, 12*, 735–741.

Heath, A. C., & Martin, N. G. (1993). Genetic models for the natural history of smoking: Evidence for a genetic influence on smoking persistence. *Addictive Behaviors, 18*, 19–34.

Hecht, M. L., Marsiglia, F. F., Elek, E., Wagstaff, D. A., Kulis, S., Dustman, P., & Miller-Day, M. (2003). Culturally grounded substance use prevention: An evaluation of the Keepin' it R.E.A.L. curriculum. *Prevention Science, 4*(4), 233–248.

Hedlund, J. H., Ulmer, R. G., & Preusser, D. F. (2001). *Determine why there are fewer young alcohol-impaired drivers*. Washington, DC: National Highway Traffic Safety Administration (publication no. DOT-HS-809-348).

Heeten, G. J., Booij, J., & Van Den Brink, W. (2004). Mood disorders and serotonin transporter density in ecstasy users—the influence of long-term abstention, dose, and gender. *Psychopharmacology (Berlin)*, 173, 376–382.

Heimer, L., & Alheid, G. (1991) Piecing together the puzzle of basal forebrain anatomy. In T. C. Napier, P. W. Kalivas & I. Hanin (Eds.), *The basal forebrain: Anatomy to function*, series title: Advances in experimental medicine and biology (Vol. 295, pp. 1–42). New York: Plenum Press.

Heimer, L., & Alheid, G. (1991). Piecing together the puzzle of basal forebrain anatomy. In T. C. Napier, P. W. Kalivas, & I. Hanin (Eds.), The basal forebrain: Anatomy to function (series title: *Advances in Experimental Medicine and Biology*, Vol. 295, pp. 1–42). New York: Plenum Press.

Heinz, A., Goldman, D., Jones, D. W., Palmour, R., Hommer, D., Gorey, J, G., et al. (2000). Genotype influences in vivo dopamine transporter availability in human striatum. *Neuropsychopharmacology, 22*, 133–139.

Hellerstein, D. J., Rosenthal, R. N., & Miner, C. R. (2001). Integrating services for schizophrenia and substance abuse. *Psychiatric Quarterly, 72*, 291–306.

Henderson, C. E., Dakof, G. A., Greenbaum, P. E., & Liddle, H. A. (2010). Effectiveness of multidimensional family therapy with higher severity substance-abusing adolescents: Report from two randomized controlled trials. *Journal of Consulting and Clinical Psychology, 78*(6), 885–897.

Hendriks, V., van der Schee, E., & Blanken P. (2012). Matching adolescents with a cannabis use disorder to multidimensional family therapy or cognitive behavioral therapy: Treatment effect moderators in a randomized controlled trial. *Drug and Alcohol Dependence, 125*(1–2), 119–126.

Hendriks, V., van der Schee, E., & Blanken, P. (2011). Treatment of adolescents with a cannabis use disorder: Main findings of a randomized controlled trial comparing multidimensional family therapy and cognitive behavioral therapy in The Netherlands. *Drug and Alcohol Dependence, 119*(1–2), 64–71.

Henggeler, S. W., & Borduin, C. M. (1990). *Family therapy and beyond: A multisystemic approach to treating the behavior problems of children and adolescents.* Pacific Grove, CA: Brooks/Cole.

Henggeler, S. W., Clingempeel, W. G., Brondino, M. J., & Pickrel, S. G. (2002). Four-year follow-up of multisystemic therapy with substance-abusing and substance-dependent juvenile offenders. *Journal of the American Academy of Child and Adolescent Psychiatry, 41*(7), 868–874.

Henggeler, S. W., Melton, G. B., Brondino, M. J., Scherer, D. G., & Hanley, J. H. (1997). Multisystemic therapy with violent and chronic juvenile offenders and their families: The role of treatment fidelity. *Journal of Consulting and Clinical Psychology, 65*, 821–833.

Henggeler, S. W., Pickrel, S. G., Brondino, M. J., & Crouch, J. L. (1996). Eliminating (almost) treatment dropout of substance abusing or dependent delinquents through home-based multisystemic therapy. *American Journal of Psychiatry, 153*, 427–428.

Henggeler, S. W., Schoenwald, S. K., Borduin, M., Rowland, M. D., & Cunningham, P. B. (1998). *Multisystemic treatment of antisocial behavior in children and adolescents.* New York: Guilford Press.

Hennessy, E. A., & Tanner-Smith, E. E. (2015). Effectiveness of brief school-based interventions for adolescents: A meta-analysis of alcohol use prevention programs. *Prevention Science, 16*, 463–474.

Hersh, J., Curry, J. F., & Kaminer, Y. (2014). What is the impact of comorbid depression on adolescent substance abuse treatment? *Substance Abuse, 35*(4), 364–375.

Hibell, B., Andersson, B., Ahlstrom, S., Balakireva, O., Bjarnason, T., Kokkevi, A., et al. (2000). *The 1999 ESPAD report on alcohol and other drug use among students in 30 European countries.* Paper presented at the Information on Alcohol and Other Drugs, Stockholm, Sweden.

Hicks, B. M., Blonigen, D. M., Kramer, M. D., Kreuger, R. F., Patrick, C. J., et al. (2007). Gender differences and developmental changes in externalizing disorders from late adolescence to early adulthood: A longitudinal twin study. *Journal of Abnormal Psychology, 116*, 433–447.

Higgins, S. T. (1999). We've come a long way: Comments on cocaine treatment outcome research. *Archives of General Psychiatry, 56*, 516–518.

Hill, S. Y., Locke, J., Zezza, N., Kaplan, B., Neiswanger, K., Steinhauer, S. R., et al. (1998). Genetic association between reduced P300 amplitude and the DRD2 dopamine receptor A1 allele in children at high risk for alcoholism. *Biological Psychiatry, 43*, 40–51.

Hill, S. Y., Zezza, N., Wipprecht, G., Locke, J., & Neiswanger, K. (1999). Personality traits and dopamine receptors (D2 and D4): Linkage studies in families of alcoholics. *American Journal of Medical Genetics 88*, 634–641.

Himelstein, S., Saul, S., Garcia-Romeu, A., & Pinedo, D. (2014). Mindfulness training as an intervention for substance user incarcerated adolescents: A pilot grounded theory study. *Substance Use and Misuse, 49*(5):560–570.

Himmelsbach, C. K. (1943). Can the euphoric, analgetic, and physical dependence effects of drugs be separated? IV With reference to physical dependence. *Federation Proceedings, 2*, 201–203.

Hingson, R. W., Heeren, T., Zakocs, R. C., Kopstein, A., & Wechsler, H. (2002). Magnitude of alcohol-related mortality and morbidity among U. S. college students ages 18–24. *Journal of Studies on Alcohol, 63*(2), 136–144.

Hingson, R., Zha, W., & Weitzman, E. R. (2009). Magnitude of and trends in alcohol-related mortality and morbidity among US college students ages 18–24, 1998–2005. *Journal of Studies in Alcohol and Drugs Supplement, 16*, 12–20.

Hoehe, M. R., Kopke, K., Wendel, B., Rohde, K., Hofmann, A. (1994). History of the discovery of LSD. In A. Pletscher & D. Ladewig (Eds.), *Fifty years of LSD: Current status and prospectives of hallucinogens.* Parthenon, NY: Parthenon Publishing Group.

Hogue, A., Henderson, C. E., Ozechowski, T. J., & Robbins, M. S. (2014.). Evidence base on outpatient behavioral treatments for adolescent substance use: Updates and recommendations 2007–2013. *Journal of Clinical Child and Adolescent Psychology, 43*(5), 695–720.

Holder, H. D. (2001). Prevention of alcohol problems in the 21st century. *American Journal of the Addictions, 10*, 1–15.

Holder, H. D. (2002). Prevention of alcohol and drug "abuse" problems at the community level: What research tells us. *Substance Use and Misuse, 37*, 901–921.

Hollister, L. E. (1968). *Chemical psychoses: LSD and related drugs*. Springfield, IL: C. C. Thomas.

Hopfer, C., Salomonsen-Sautel, S., Mikulich-Gilbertson, S., Min, S. J., McQueen, M., Crowley, T., ... Hewitt, J. (2013). Conduct disorder and initiation of substance use: a prospective longitudinal study. *Journal of the Academy of Child and Adolescent Psychiatry, 52*(5), 511–518.

Horner, B. R., & Scheibe, K. E. (1997). Prevalence and implications of attention-deficit hyperactivity disorder among adolescents in treatment for substance abuse. *Journal of the American Academy of Child and Adolescent Psychiatry, 36*, 30–36.

Hornik, R. (2003). Alcohol, tobacco, and marijuana use among youth: Same-time and lagged and simultaneous-change associations in a nationally representative sample of 9- to 18-year-olds. In D. Romer (Ed.), *Reducing adolescent risk: Toward an integrated approach* (pp. 335–344). Thousand Oaks, CA: Sage Publications.

Hornik, R., Jacobsohn, L., Orwin, R., Piesse, A., & Kalton, G. (2008). Effects of the National Youth Anti-Drug Media Campaign on youths. *American Journal of Public Health, 98*(12), 2229–2236.

Hornik, R., Maklan, D., Cadell, D., Barmada, C., Jacobsohn, L., Prado, A., et al. (2002). *Evaluation of the National Youth Anti-Drug Media Campaign: Fifth semi-annual report of findings*. Washington, DC: Campaign Publications.

Hser, Y., Hoffman, V., Grella, C. E., & Anglin, M. D. (2001). A 33-year follow-up of narcotics addicts. *Archives of General Psychiatry, 58*, 503–508.

Hu, S., Brody, C., Fisher, C., Gunzerath, L., Nelson, M., Sabol, S., et al. (2000). Interaction between the serotonin transporter gene and neuroticism in cigarette smoking behavior. *Molecular Psychiatry, 5*, 181–188.

Huang, J., & Chaloupka, F. L. (2012). *The impact of the 2009 federal tobacco excise tax increase on youth tobacco use* (Working Paper No. 18026). Cambridge, MA: National Bureau of Economic Research. Retrieved from www.nber.org/papers/w18026.

Hubbard, R. L., Rachal, J. V., Craddock, S. G., & Cavanaugh, E. R. (1984). Treatment Outcome Prospective Study (TOPS): client characteristics and behaviors before, during, and after treatment. *NIDA Research Monographs, 51*, 42–68.

Hublet, A., Bendtsen, P., de Looze, M. E., Fotiou, A., Donnelly, P., Vilhjalmsson, R., ... ter Bogt, T. F. (2015). Trends in the co-occurrence of tobacco and cannabis use in 15-year-olds from 2002 to 2010 in 28 countries of Europe and North America. *European Journal of Public Health, 25*(Suppl 2), 73–75.

Hughes, A., Williams, M. R., Lipari, R. N., Bose, J., Copello, E., A., P., & Kroutil, L. A. (2016). *Prescription drug use and misuse in the United States: Results from the 2015 National Survey on Drug Use and Health*. National Survey on Drug Use and Health Data Review. Rockville, MD: U.S. Substance Abuse and Mental Health Services Administration. Retrieved Sept. 23, 2016, from http://www.samhsa.gov/data/sites/default/files/NSDUH-FFR2-2015/NSDUH-FFR2-2015.htm

Hyman, S. E., & Malenka, R. C. (2001). Addiction and the brain: The neurobiology of compulsion and its persistence. *Nature Reviews Neuroscience, 2*, 695–703.

Iacono, W. G., Malone, S. M., & McGue, M. (2008). Behavioral disinhibition and the development of early-onset addiction: Common and specific influences. *Annual Review of Clinical Psychology, 4*, 325–348.

Irons, D. E., McGue, M., Iacono, W. G., & Oetting, W. (2007). Mendellian randomization: A novel test of the gateway hypothesis and models of gene-environment interplay. *Development and Psychopathology, 19*, 1181–1195.

Ishiguro, H., Saito, T., Akazawa, S., Mitushio, H., Tada. K., Enomoto, M., et al. (1999). Association between drinking-related antisocial behavior and a polymorphism in the serotonin transporter gene in a Japanese population. *Alcoholism, Clinical and Experimental Research, 23*, 1281– 1284.

Iversen, L. (2003). Cannabis and the brain. *Brain, 126* (Pt 6), 1252–1270.

Jacobson, K. C., Prescott, C. A., & Kendler, K. S. (2002). Sex differences in the genetic and environmental influences on the development of antisocial behavior. *Development and Psychopathology, 14*, 395–416.

Jaffe, S. L., & Simkin, D. R. (2002). Alcohol and drug abuse in children and adolescents. In M. Lewis (Ed.), *Child and adolescent psychiatry: A comprehensive textbook* (3rd ed., pp. 895–911). New Haven, CT: Lippincott Williams and Wilkins.

James-Burdumy, S., Goesling, B., Deke, J., & Einspruch, E. (2012). The effectiveness of mandatory-random student drug testing: A cluster randomized trial. *Journal of Adolescent Health, 50*, 172–178.

Jamieson, P., & Romer, D. (2001). What do young people think they know about the risks of smoking. In P. Slovic (Ed.), *Smoking risks, perception and policy,* (pp. 51–63). Philadelphia: Sage Publications.

Jansen, K. L., & Darracot-Cankovic, R. (2001). The nonmedical use of ketamine, part two: A review of problem use and dependence. *Journal of Psychoactive Drugs, 33*, 151–158.

Jasinska, A. J., Stein, E. A., Kaiser, J., Naumer, M. J., & Yalachkov, Y. (2014). Factors modulating neural reactivity to drug cues in addiction: A survey of human neuroimaging studies. *Neuroscience and Biobehavioral Reviews, 38*, 1–16.

Jentsch, J. D., Olausson, P., De La Garza, R., 2nd, & Taylor, J. R. (2002). Impairments of reversal learning and response perseveration after repeated, intermittent cocaine administrations to monkeys. *Neuropsychopharmacology, 26*, 183–190.

Jernigan, D. H., Ostroff, J., Ross, C., & O'Hara, J. A., 3rd. (2004). Sex differences in adolescent exposure to alcohol advertising in magazines. *Archives of Pediatric and Adolescent Medicine, 158*(7), 629–634.

Jerrell, J. M., & Ridgely, M. S. (1995). Comparative effectiveness of three approaches to serving people with severe mental illness and substance abuse disorders. *Journal of Nervous and Mental Disease, 183*, 566–576.

Jessor, R. (1991). Risk behavior in adolescence: A psychosocial framework for understanding and action. *Journal of Adolescent Health, 12*, 597–605.

Jessor, R., & Jessor, S. (1977). *Problem behavior and psychosocial development.* New York: Academic Press.

Joanning, H., Thomas, F., & Quinn, W. (1992). Treating adolescent drug abuse: A comparison of family systems therapy, group therapy, and family drug education. *Journal of Marital and Family Therapy, 18*, 345–356.

Johnston, L. D. (1973). *Drugs and American youth.* Paper presented at the Institute for Social Research, Ann Arbor, MI.

Johnston, L. D. (1991). Toward a theory of drug epidemics. In L. Donohew, H. Syper & W. Bukoski (Eds.), *Persuasive communication and drug abuse prevention* (pp. 93–131). Hillsdale, NJ: Lawrence Erlbaum.

Johnston, L. D. (2003). Alcohol and illicit drugs: The role of risk perceptions. In D. Romer (Ed.), *Reducing adolescent risk: Toward an integrated approach* (pp. 56–74). Thousand Oaks, CA: Sage Publications.

Johnston, L. D., O'Malley, P. M., & Bachman, J. G. (1998). *National survey results on drug use from the Monitoring the Future Study 1995–1997. Volume 1: Secondary school students.* Rockville, MD: National Institute on Drug Abuse.

Johnston, L. D., O'Malley, P. M., & Bachman, J. G. (2000). *National survey results on drug use from the Monitoring the Future Study, 1975–1999. Volume I: Secondary school students* (NIH publication no. 00-4802). Bethesda, MD: National Institute on Drug Abuse. 480 pp.

Johnston, L. D., O'Malley, P. M., & Bachman, J. G. (2002a). *National survey results on drug use from the Monitoring the Future Study, 1975–2001. Volume I: Secondary school students* (NIH Publication No. 02-5106). Bethesda, MD: National Institute on Drug Abuse.

Johnston, L., O'Malley, P., & Bachman, J. (2002b). Overview of key findings of the Monitoring the Future study on drug use, national survey results 2001. Bethesda, MD: National Institute on Drug Abuse.

Johnston, L. D., O'Malley, P. M., & Bachman, J. G. (2003a). Demographic subgroup trends for various licit and illicit drugs, 1975–2002. (Monitoring the Future Occasional Paper #58) Ann Arbor, MI: Institute for Social Research 25pp.

Johnston, L. D., O'Malley, P. M., & Bachman, J. G. (2003b). *National survey results on drug use from the Monitoring the Future Study, 1975–2002: Volume I: Secondary school students* (NIH publication no. 03-5375). Bethesda, MD: National Institute on Drug Abuse.

Johnston, L. D., O'Malley, P. M., & Bachman, J. G. (2003c). *National survey results on drug use from the Monitoring the Future study, 1975–2002. Volume II: College students and adults ages 19–40* (NIH Publication No. 03-5376). Bethesda, MD: National Institute on Drug Abuse.

Johnston, L. D., O'Malley, P. M., Bachman, J. G., & Schulenberg, J. E. (2013). *Monitoring the Future national survey results on drug use, 1975–2012. Volume I: Secondary school students.* Ann Arbor: Institute for Social Research, The University of Michigan.

Johnston, L. D., O'Malley, P. M., Bachman, J. G., Schulenberg, J. E., & Miech, R. A. (2014). *Monitoring the Future national survey results on drug use, 1975–2013: Volume I, Secondary school students.* Ann Arbor: Institute for Social Research, The University of Michigan.

Johnston, L. D., O'Malley, P. M., Miech, R. A., Bachman, J. G., & Schulenberg, J. E. (2015). *Monitoring the Future national results on drug use: 1975–2014: Overview, key findings on adolescent drug use*. Ann Arbor, MI: Institute for Social Research, University of Michigan.

Johnston, L. D., O'Malley, P. M., Miech, R. A., Bachman, J. G., & Schulenberg, J. E. (2016a). *Monitoring the Future: National survey results on drug use, 1975–2015: Overview, key findings on adolescent drug use*. Ann Arbor, MI: Institute for Social Research, University of Michigan.

Johnston, L. D., O'Malley, P. M., Miech, R. A., Bachman, J. G., & Schulenberg, J. E. (2016b). *Demographic subgroup trends among adolescents in the use of various licit and illicit drugs, 1975–2015*. Monitoring the Future Occasional Paper No. 86. Ann Arbor: Institute for Social Research, University of Michigan.

Jones, C. M., Logan, J., Gladden, R. M., & Bohm, M. K. (2015). Vital signs: Demographic and substance use trends among heroin users—United States, 2002–2013. *Morbidity and Mortality Weekly Reports*, *64*(26), 719–725.

Jonkman, S., & Kenny, P. J. (2013). Molecular, cellular, and structural mechanisms of cocaine addiction: A key role for microRNAs. *Neuropsychopharmacology*, *38*(1), 198–211.

Jorm, A., Henderson, A., Jacomb, P., Christensen, H., Korten, A., Rodgers, B., et al. (2000). Association of smoking and personality with a polymorphism of the dopamine transpoter gene: Results from a community survey. *American Journal of Medical Genetics*, *96*, 331–334.

Jupp, B., & Dalley, J. W. (2014). Behavioral endophenotypes of drug addiction: Etiological insights from neuroimaging studies. *Neuropharmacology*, *76*, 487–497.

Jureidini, J., Tonkin, A., & Jureidini, E. (2013). Combination pharmacotherapy for psychiatric disorders in children and adolescents: Prevalence, efficacy, risks and research needs. *Paediatric Drugs*, *15*(5), 377–391.

Kaminer, Y., Burleson, J. A., Burke, R., & Litt, M. D. (2014). The efficacy of contingency management for adolescent cannabis use disorder: A controlled study. *Substance Abuse*, *35*(4), 391–398.

Kampman, K. M. (2010). What's new in the treatment of cocaine addiction? *Current Psychiatry Reports*, *12*(5), 441–447.

Kandel, D. B. (1975). Stages in adolescent involvement in drug use. *Science*, *190*, 912–914.

Kandel, D. B. (Eds). (2002). *Stages and pathways of drug involvement: Examining the gateway hypothesis*. Cambridge, UK: Cambridge University Press.

Kandel, D. B., & Jessor, R. (2002). The gateway hypothesis revisited. In D. B. Kandel (Ed.), *Stages and pathways of drug involvement: Examining the gateway hypothesis*. (pp. 365–372). Cambridge, UK: Cambridge University Press.

Kandel, D. B., & Logan, J. A. (1984). Patterns of drug use from adolescence to young adulthood: I. Periods of risk for initiation, continued use, and discontinuation. *American Journal of Public Health*, *74*(7), 660–666.

Kandel, D., & Yamaguchi, K. (1993). From beer to crack: Developmental patterns of drug involvement. *American Journal of Public Health*, *83*, 851– 855.

Kann, I., & Solevåg, A. (2014). Economic and health consequences of non-invasive respiratory support in newborn infants: A difference-in-difference analysis using data from the Norwegian patient registry. *BMC Health Services Research*, *14*(1), 494.

Kann, L. (2002). The Youth Risk Behavior Surveillance System: Measuring health-risk behaviors. *American Journal of Health Behavior 2001*, *25*, 272–277.

Karama, S., Lecours, A. R., Leroux, J. M., Bourgouin, P., Beaudoin, G., Joubert, S., & Beauregard, M. (2002). Areas of brain activation in males and females during viewing of erotic film excerpts. *Human Brain Mapping*, *16*, 1–13.

Kazdin, A. E. (1991). Effectiveness of psychotherapy with children and adolescents. *Journal of Consulting and Clinical Psychology*, *59*, 785–798.

Kazdin, A. E. (1993). Treatment of conduct disorder: Progress and directions in psychotherapy research. *Development and Psychopathology*, *5*, 277–310.

Kellam, S. G., Reid, J., & Balster, R. L. (2008). Universal classroom behavior program in first and second grades on young adult outcomes. *Drug and Alcohol Dependence*, *95*(Suppl 1), S5–S28.

Kendler, K. S. (2001). Twin studies of psychiatric illness an update. *Archives of General Psychiatry*, *58*, 1005–1014.

Kendler, K. S., Gardner, C. O., & Gardner, C.O.J. (1998). Twin studies of adult psychiatric and substance dependence disorders: Are they biased by differences in the environmental experiences of monozygotic and dizygotic twins in childhood and adolescence? *Psychological Medicine*, *28*, 625–633.

Kendler, K. S., Jaffee, S. R., & Romer, D. (Eds.). (2011). *The dynamic genome and mental health: The role of genes and environments in youth development*. New York: Oxford University Press.

Kendler, K. S., Prescott, C. A., Myers, J., & Neale, M. C. (2003). The structure of genetic and environmental risk factors for common psychiatric and substance use disorders in men and women. *Archives of General Psychiatry, 60,* 929–937.

Kessler, R. C. (1994). The National Comorbidy Survey of the United States. *International Review of Psychiatry, 6,* 365–376.

Kessler, R. C., Aguilar-Gaxiola, S., Andrade, L., Bijl, R., Borges, G., Caraveo-Anduaga, J. J., et al. (2001). Mental–substance comorbidities in the ICPE surveys. *Psychiatria Fennica, 32* (Suppl. 2), 62–80.

Kessler, R. C., McGonagle, K. A., Zhao, S., Nelson, C. B., Hughes, M., Eshleman, S., et al. (1994). Lifetime and 12-month prevalence of DSM-III-R psychiatric disorders in the United States: Results from the National Comorbidity Survey. *Archives of General Psychiatry, 51,* 8–19.

Keyes, K. M., Wall, M., Cerdá, M., Schulenberg, J., O'Malley, P. M., Galea, S., ... Hasin, D. S. (2016). How does state marijuana policy affect US youth? Medical marijuana laws, marijuana use and perceived harmfulness: 1991–2014. *Addiction, 111*(12), 2187–2195.

Khokhar, J. Y., Ferguson, C. S., Zhu, A. Z., & Tyndale, R. F. (2010). Pharmacogenetics of drug dependence: Role of gene variations in susceptibility and treatment. *Annual Review of Pharmacology and Toxicology, 50,* 39–61.

Khurana, A., Romer, D., Betancourt, L. M., & Hurt, H. (2017). Working memory ability and early drug use progression as predictors of substance use disorders. *Addiction.* [Epub before press].

Khurana, A., Romer, D., Betancourt, L. M., Brodsky, N. L., Giannetta, J. M., & Hurt, H. (2013). Working memory ability predicts trajectories of early alcohol use in adolescents: The mediational role of impulsivity. *Addiction, 108*(3), 506–515.

Khurana, A., Romer, D., Betancourt, L. M., Brodsky, N. L., Giannetta, J. M., & Hurt, H. (2015). Experimentation versus progression in adolescent drug use: A test of an emerging neurobehavioral imbalance model. *Development and Psychopathology, 27*(3), 901–913.

Kilpatrick, D. G., Acierno, R., Saunders, B., Resnick, H. S., Best, C. L., & Schnurr, P. P. (2000). Risk factors for adolescent substance abuse and dependence: Data from a national sample. *Journal of Consulting and Clinical Psychology, 68*(1), 19–30.

Kilts, C. D., Schweitzer, J. B., Quinn, C. K., Gross, R. E., Faber, T. L., Muhammad, F., ... Drexler, K. P. G. (2001). Neural activity related to drug craving in cocaine addiction. *Archives of General Psychiatry, 58*(4), 334–341.

Kinnunen, J. M., Ollila, H., El-Amin, S.-T., Pere, L. A., Lindfors, P. L., & Rimpelä, A. H. (2015). Awareness and determinants of electronic cigarette use among Finnish adolescents in 2013: A population-based study. *Tobacco Control,* 24, e264–270. Epub 2014 May 14.

Kirby, K. C., Marlowe, D. B., Festinger, D. S., Lamb, R. J., & Platt, J. J. (1998). Schedule of voucher delivery influences initiation of cocaine abstinence. *Journal of Consulting and Clinical Psychology, 66,* 761–767.

Kirby, T., & Barry, A. E. (2012). Alcohol as a gateway drug: A study of US 12th graders. *Journal of School Health, 82*(8), 371–379.

Klassen, L. J., Bilkey, T. S., Katzman, M. A., & Chokka, P. (2012). Comorbid attention deficit/hyperactivity disorder and substance use disorder: Treatment considerations. *Current Drug Abuse Reviews, 5*(3), 190–198.

Klein-Schwartz, W., & McGrath, J. (2003). Poison centers' experience with methylphenidate abuse in pre-teens and adolescents. *Journal of the American Academy of Child and Adolescent Psychiatry, 42,* 288–294.

Koesters, S. C., Rogers, P. D., & Rajasingham, C. R. (2002). MDMA ("Ecstasy") and other "club drugs." The new epidemic. *Pediatric Clinics of North America, 49,* 415–433.

Kohler, S., & Hofmann, A. (2015). Can motivational interviewing in emergency care reduce alcohol consumption in young people? A systematic review and meta-analysis. *Alcohol and Alcoholism, 50*(2), 107–117.

Kollath-Cattano, C., Abad-Vivero, E. N., Mejia, R., Perez-Hernandez, R., Sargent, J. D., & Thrasher, J. F. (2016). Portrayals of character smoking and drinking in Argentine-, Mexican- and US-produced films. *Preventive Medicine, 90,* 143–147.

Kollins, S. H. (2008). A qualitative review of issues arising in the use of psycho-stimulant medications in patients with ADHD and co-morbid substance use disorders. *Current Medical Research and Opinion, 24*(5), 1345–1357.

Koob, G. F. (1992). Drugs of abuse: Anatomy, pharmacology, and function of reward pathways. *Trends in Pharmacological Sciences, 13,* 177–184.

Koob, G. F. (2006). The neurobiology of addiction: A neuroadaptational view relevant for diagnosis. *Addiction, 101,* 23–30.

Koob, G. F. (2009). Neurobiological substrates for the dark side of compulsivity in addiction. *Neuropharmacology, 56*(1), 18–31.

Koob, G. F. (2013). Theoretical frameworks and mechanistic aspects of alcohol addiction: Alcohol addiction as a reward deficit disorder. *Current Topics Behavioral Neuroscience, 13*, 3–30.

Koob, G. F. (2015). The dark side of emotion: The addiction perspective. *European Journal of Pharmacology, 753*, 73–87.

Koob, G. F., Buck, C. L., Cohen, A., Edwards, S., Park, P. E., Schlosburg, J. E., . . George, O. (2014). Addiction as a stress surfeit disorder. *Neuropharmacology, 76*(Pt B), 370–382.

Koob, G. F., & Heinricks, S. C. (1999). A role for corticotropin-releasing factors and urocortin in behavioral responses to stressors. *Brain Research, 848*, 141–152.

Koob, G. F., & Le Moal, M. (1997). Drug abuse: Hedonic homeostatic dysregulation. *Science, 278*, 52–58.

Koob, G. F., & Le Moal, M. (2001). Drug addiction, dysregulation of reward, and allostasis. *Neuropsychopharmacology, 24*, 97–129.

Koob, G. F., & Nestler, E. J. (1997). The neurobiology of drug addiction. *Journal of Neuropsychiatry and Clinical Neuroscience, 9*, 482–497.

Koob, G. F., Sanna, P. P., & Bloom, F. E. (1998). Neuroscience of addiction. *Neuron, 21*, 467–476.

Koob, G. F., & Volkow, N. D. (2010). Neurocircuitry of addiction. *Neuropsychopharmacology, 35*(1), 217–238.

Kosten, T. R. (in press). Cocaine and psychostimulants. In H. R. Kranzler & D. A. Ciraulo (Eds.), *Clinical manual of addiction psychopharmacology.* Washington, DC: APPI Press.

Kosten, T. R., & Biegel, D. (2002). Therapeutic vaccines for substance dependence. *Expert Review of Vaccines, 1*, 363–371.

Kosten, T. R., & O'Connor, P. G. (2003). Current concepts—Management of drug withdrawal. *New England Journal of Medicine, 348*, 1786–1795.

Kreuger, R. F., & Markon, K. E. (2006). Reinterpreting comorbidity: A model-based approach to understanding and classifying psychopathology. *Annual Review of Clinical Psychology, 2*, 111–133.

Kreuger, R. F., Hicks, B. M., Patrick, C. J., Carlson, S. R., Iacono, W. G., & McGue, M. (2002). Etiologic connections among substance dependence, antisocial behavior, and personality: Modeling the externalizing spectrum. *Journal of Abnormal Psychology, 111*, 411–424.

Kruesi, M. J., Rapoport, J. L., Hamburger, S., Hibbs, E., Potter, W. Z., Lenane, M., et al. (1990). Cerebrospinal fluid monoamine metabolites, aggression, and impulsivity in disrsuptive behavior disorders of children and adolescents. *Archives of General Psychiatry, 47*, 419–426.

Kulis, S., Nieri, T., Yabiku, S., Stromwall, L. K., & Marsiglia, F. F. (2007). Promoting reduced and discontinued substance use among adolescent substance users: Effectiveness of a universal prevention program. *Prevention Science, 8*, 35–49.

Kumar, R., O'Malley, P. M., Johnston, L. D., & Laetz, V. B. (2013). Alcohol, tobacco, and other drug use prevention in U.S. schools: A descriptive summary. *Prevention Science, 14*, 581–592.

Kumpfer, K. L. (2014). Family-based interventions for the prevention of substance abuse and other impulse control disorders in girls. *ISRN Addiction, 2014*, 308789.

Kumpfer, K., & Alvardo, R. (1995). Strengthening families to prevent drug use in multi-ethnic youth. In G. Botvin, S. Schinke, & M. Orlandi (Eds.), *Drug abuse prevention with multi-ethnic youth* (pp. 253–292). Newbury Park, CA: Sage Publications.

Kumpfer, K. L., Alvarado, R., & Whiteside, H. O. (2003). Family-based interventions for substance use and misuse prevention. *Substance Use and Misuse, 38*(11–13), 1759–1789.

Kumpfer, K., Molgaard, V., & Spoth, R. (1996). The Strengthening Families Program for the prevention of delinquency and drug use. In R. D. Peters & R. J. McMahon (Eds.), *Preventing childhood disorders, substance abuse, and delinquency* (pp. 241–267). Thousand Oaks, CA: Sage Publications.

Kuo, M., Adlaf, E. M., Lee, H., Glicksman, L., Demers, A., & Wechsler, H. (2002). More Canadian students drink but American students drink more: Comparing college alcohol use in two countries. *Addiction, 97*(12), 1583–1592.

Kuperman, S., Calarge, C., Kolar, A., Holman, T., Barnett, M., & Perry, P. (2011). An open-label trial of aripiprazole in the treatment of aggression in male adolescents diagnosed with conduct disorder. *Annals of Clinical Psychiatry, 23*(4), 270–276.

Kuperman, S., Schlosser, S. S., Kramer, J. R., Bucholz, K., Hesselbrock, V., Reich, T., et al. (2001). Developmental sequence from disruptive behavior diagnosis to adolescent alcohol dependence. *American Journal of Psychiatry, 158*, 2022–2026.

Kurtzman, T. L., Otsuka, K. N., & Wahl, R. A. (2001). Inhalant abuse by adolescents. *Journal of Adolescent Health, 28*, 170–180.

Lam, S. C., Wang, Z., Li, Y. Franklin, T., O'Brien, C., Magland, J., & Childress, A. R. (2013). Wavelet-transformed temporal cerebral blood flow signals during attempted inhibition of cue-induced cocaine craving distinguish prognostic phenotypes. *Drug and Alcohol Dependence, 128*(1–2), 140–147.

Langenbucher, J., Martin, C. S., Labouvie, E., Sanjuan, P. M., Bavly, L., & Pollock, N. K. (2000). Toward the DSM-V: The withdrawal-gate model versus the DSM-IV in the diagnosis of alcohol abuse and dependence. *Journal of Consulting and Clinical Psychology, 68*(5), 799–809.

Langleben, D. D., Loughead, J. W., Ruparel, K., Hakun, J. G., Bush-Winokur, S., Holloway, M. B., Strasser, A. A., ... Lerman, C. (2009). Reduced prefrontal and temporal processing and recall of high "sensation value" ads. *Neuroimage, 46*, 219–225.

Lasagna, L., von Felsinger, J. M., & Beecher, H. K. (1955). Drug-induced mood changes in man: Observations on healthy subjects, chronically ill patients, and "postaddicts." *Journal of the American Medical Association, 157*(12), 1006–1020.

Lee, S. S., Humphreys, K. L., Flory, K., Liu, R., & Glass, K. (2011). Prospective association of childhood attention-deficit/hyperactivity disorder (ADHD) and substance use and abuse/dependence: A meta-analytic review. *Clinical Psychology Reviews, 31*(3), 328–341.

Lerman, C., Caporaso, N. E., Audrain, J., Main, D., Boyd, N. R., & Shields, P. G. (2000). Interacting effects of the serotonin transporter gene and neuroticism in smoking practices and nicotine dependence. *Molecular Psychiatry, 5*, 189–192.

Lerman, C., Caporaso, N., Bush, A., Zheng, Y., Audrian, J., Main, D., et al. (2001). Tryptophan hydroxylase gene variant and smoking behavior. *American Journal of Medical Genetics, 105*, 518– 520.

Lerman, C., Gold, K., Audrain, J., Lin, T. H., Boyd, N. R., Orleans, C. T., et al. (1997). Incorporating biomarkers of exposure and genetic susceptibility into smoking cessation treatment: Effects on smoking-related cognitions, emotions and behavior change. *Health Psychology, 16*, 87–99.

Lerman, C., Patterson, F., & Shields, P. (2003). *Genetic basis of substance use and dependence: Implication for prevention in high-risk youth.* Philadelphia: Sage Publications.

Lerman, C., Shields, P., Audrain, J., Main, D., Cobb, B., Boyd, N., et al. (1998). The role of the serotonin transporter gene in cigarette smoking. *Cancer Epidemiology, Biomarkers, and Prevention, 7*, 253–255.

Lerner, R. (1995). *America's youth in crisis: Challenges and options for programs and policies*. Thousand Oaks, CA: Sage Publications.

Lerner, R. (2001). Promoting promotion in the development of prevention science. *Applied Developmental Science, 5*, 254–257.

Lesch, K. P., & Merschdorf, U. (2000). Impulsivity, aggression, and serotonin: A molecular psychobiological perspective. *Behavioral Science Law, 18*, 581–604.

Levin, E. D., Rezvani, A. H., Montoya, D., Rose, J. E., & Swartzwelder, H. S. (2003). Adolescent-onset nicotine self-administration modeled in female rats. *Psychopharmacology (Berl), 169*, 141–149.

Lewinsohn, P. M., Rohde, P., & Seeley, J. R. (1996). Adolescent suicidal ideation and attempts: Prevalence, risk factors, and clinical implications. *Clinical Psychology: Science and Practice, 3*(1), 25–46.

Lichtermann, D., Hranoiovic, D., Trixler, M., Franke, P., Jernej, B., Delmo, C. D., et al. (2000). Support for allelic association of a polymorphic site in the promoter region of the serotonin transporter gene with risk for alcohol dependence. *American Journal of Psychiatry, 159*, 2045– 2047.

Liddle, H. A., & Dakof, G. (1995). Efficacy of family therapy for drug abuse: Promising but not definitive. *Journal of Marital and Family Therapy, 21*, 511–543.

Liddle, H. A., & Dakof, G. A. (2002). *A family-based, intensive outpatient alternative to residential drug treatment for co-morbid adolescent substance abusers: Preliminary finding of a controlled trial*. Santa Fe, NM: Society for Psychotherapy Research.

Liddle, H. A., & Rowe, C. L. (in press). Advances in family therapy research: Bridging gaps and expanding frontiers. In M. Nichols & Schwartz (Eds.), *Family therapy: Concepts and methods*. Boston: Allyn & Bacon.

Liddle, H. A., Dakof, G. A., Parker, K., Diamond, S., Barrett, K., & Tejeda, M. (2001). Multidimensional family therapy for adolescent drug abuse: Results of a randomized clinical trial. *American Journal of Drug and Alcohol Abuse, 27*, 651–688.

Liddle, H. A., Dakof, G. A., Turner, R. M., Henderson, C. E., & Greenbaum, P. E. (2008). Treating adolescent drug abuse: A randomized trial comparing multidimensional family therapy and cognitive behavior therapy. *Addiction, 103*(10), 1660–1670.

Liddle, H. A., Rowe, C. L., Dakof, G. A., Henderson, C. E., & Greenbaum, P. E. (2009). Multidimensional family therapy for young adolescent substance abuse: Twelve-month outcomes of a randomized controlled trial. *Journal of Consulting and Clinical Psychology, 77*(1), 12–25.

Lieber, S. R., & Millum, J. (2013). Preventing sin: The ethics of vaccines against smoking. *Hastings Center Report*, 43(3), 23–33.

Liepman, M. R., Calles, J. L., Kizilbash, L., Nazeer, A., & Sheikh, S. (2002). Genetic and nongenetic factors influencing substance use by adolescents. *Adolescent Medicine State of the Art Reviews, 13*(2), 375–401.

Lifrak, P. D., Alterman, A. E., O'Brien, C. P., & Volpicelli, J. R. (1997). Naltrexone for alcoholic adolescents [Letter]. *American Journal of Psychiatry, 153*, 439–441.

Ling, W., Shoptaw, S., & Majewska, D. (1998). Baclofen as a cocaine anti-craving medication: A preliminary clinical study. *Neuropsychopharmacology, 18*, 403–404.

Lingford-Hughes, A. R., Acton, P. D., Gacinovic, S., Suckling, J., Busatto, G. F., Boddington, S. J., et al. (1998). Reduced levels of GABA-benzodiazepine receptor in alcohol dependency in the absence of grey matter atrophy. *British Journal of Psychiatry, 173*, 116–22.

Lipari, R. N. (2015, Aug. 27). *Monthly variation in substance use initiation among full-time college students. The CBHSQ Report*. Rockville, MD: U.S. Substance Abuse and Mental Health Services Administration, Center for Behavioral Health Statistics and Quality. Retrieved October 3, 2016, from http://www.samhsa.gov/data/sites/default/files/report_2049/ShortReport-2049.pdf

Lipari, R. N., & Hughes, A. (2015). *Trends in heroin use in the United States: 2002 to 2013. The CBHSQ Report*. Rockville, MD: U.S. Substance Abuse and Mental Health Services Administration: Rockville, MD. Retrieved Sept. 23, 2016, from http://www.samhsa.gov/data/sites/default/files/report_1943/ShortReport-1943.html

Liu, H. Y., Potter, M. P., Woodworth, K. Y., Yorks, D. M., Petty, C. R., Wozniak, J. R., ... Biederman, J. (2011). Pharmacologic treatments for pediatric bipolar disorder: A review and meta-analysis. *Journal of the American Academy of Child and Adolescent Psychiatry, 50*(8), 749–762.

Lohman, M., Riggs, P. D., Hall, S. K., Mikulich, K., & Klein, C. A. (2002). *Perceived motivations for treatment in depressed, substance-dependent adolescents with conduct disorder*. Paper presented at the College on Problems of Drug Dependence: 64th Annual Scientific Meeting, Quebec, Canada, June 2004.

London, S. J., Idle, J. R., Daly, A. K., & Coetzee, G. A. (1999). Genetic variation of CYP2A6, smoking, and risk of cancer. *Lancet, 353*, 898– 899.

Lopez-Quintero, C., & Anthony, J. C. (2015). Drug use disorders in the polydrug context: New epidemiological evidence from a foodborne outbreak approach. *Annals of the New York Academy of Science, 1349*, 119–126.

Lopez-Quintero, C., Pérez de los Cobos J, Hasin, D. S., Okuda, M., Wang, S., Grant, B. F., & Blanco, C. (2011). Probability and predictors of transition from first use to dependence on nicotine, alcohol, cannabis, and cocaine: Results of the National Epidemiologic Survey on Alcohol and Related Conditions (NESARC). *Drug and Alcohol Dependence, 115*(1–2), 120–130.

Lorenc, J. D. (2003). Inhalant abuse in the pediatric population: A persistent challenge. *Current Opinion in Pediatrics, 15*, 204–209.

Loy, J. H., Merry, S. N., & Stasiak, K. (2012). Atypical antipsychotics for disruptive behaviour disorders in children and youths. *Cochrane Database of Systematic Reviews, 9*, CD008559.

Lueders, K. K., Hu, S., McHugh, L., Myakishev, M. V., Sirota, L. A., & Hamer, D. H. (2002). Genetic and functional analysis of single nucleotide polymorphisms in the beta2-neuronal nicotinic acetylcholine receptor gene (CHRNB2). *Nicotine and Tobacco Research, 4*, 115–125.

Luo, X., Kranzler, H. R., Zhao, H., & Gelernter, J. (2003). Haplotypes at the OPRM1 locus are associated with susceptibility to substance dependence in European-Americans. *American Journal of Medical Genetics, 120B(1)*, 97–108.

Lynam, D. R., Milich, R., Zimmerman, R., Novak, S. P., Logan, T. K., Martin, C., et al. (1999). Project DARE: No effects at 10-year follow-up. *Journal of Consulting and Clinical Psychology, 67*(4), 292–296.

Maas, L. C., Lukas, S. E., Kaufman, M. J., Weiss, R. C., Daniels, S. L., Rogers, V. W., et al. (1996). *Functional MRI of human brain activation during cue-induced cocaine craving*. Paper presented at the Proceedings on College on Problems of Drug Dependence 1996, Nashville, TN.

MacKillop, K., Obasi, E., Amlung, M. T., McGeary, J. E., & Knopik, V. S. (2010). The role of genetics in nicotine dependence: Mapping the pathways from genome to syndrome. *Current Cardiovascular Risk Reports, 4*(6), 446–453.

Madden, P. A., Heath, A., Pederson, N., Kaprio, J., Koskenvuo, M., & Martin, N. (1999). The genetics of smoking persistence in men and women: A multicultural study. *Behavior Genetics, 29*, 423– 431.

Magno Zito, J., Safer, D. J., dosReis, S., Gardner, J. F., Magder, L., Soeken, K., et al. (2003). Psychotropic practice patterns of youth: A 10-year perspective. *Archives of Pediatrics and Adolescent Medicine, 157*, 17–25.

Malik, S. A., Khan, C., Jabbar, A., & Iqbal, A. (1992). Heroin addiction and sex hormones in males. *Journal of the Pakistan Medical Association, 42*, 210–212.

Mannuzza, S., Klein, R. G., Truong, N. L., Moulton, J. L., 3rd, Roizen, E. R., Howell, K. H., & Castellanos, F. X. (2008). Age of methylphenidate treatment initiation in children with ADHD and later substance abuse: Prospective follow-up into adulthood. *American Journal of Psychiatry, 165*(5), 604–609.

Markou, A., Kosten, T. R., & Koob, G. F. (1998). Neurobiological similarities in depression and drug dependence: A self-medication hypothesis. *Neuropsychopharmacology, 18*, 135–174.

Marsch, L. A., Bickel, W. K., Badger, G. J., Stothart, M. E., Quesnel, K. J., Stanger, C., & Brooklyn, J. (2005). Comparison of pharmacological treatments for opioid-dependent adolescents: A randomized controlled trial. *Archives of General Psychiatry, 62*(10), 1157–1164

Marteau, J., & Lerman, C. (2001). Genetic risk and behavioral change. *BMJ, 322*, 1056–1059.

Martin, C. S., & Winters, K. C. (1998). Diagnosis and assessment of alcohol use disorders among adolescents. *Alcohol Health and Research World, 22*, 95–105.

Martin, C. S., Kaczynski, N., Maisto, S., Bukstein, O. M., & Moss, H. B. (1995). Patterns of DSM-IV alcohol abuse and dependence symptoms in adolescent drinkers. *Journal of Studies on Alcohol, 56*(6), 672–680.

Mason, P. E., & Kerns, W. P., 2nd. (2002). Gamma hydroxybutyric acid (GHB) intoxication. *Academic Emergency Medicine, 9*, 730–739.

Masse, L., & Tremblay, R. (1997). Behavior of boys in kindergarten and the onset of substance use during adolescence. *Archives of General Psychiatry, 54*, 62–68.

Matsushita, S., Yoshino, A., Murayama, M., Kimura, M., Muramatsu, T., & Higuchi, S. (2001). Association study of serotonin transporter gene regulatory region polymorphism and alcoholism. *Behavior Genetics, 31*, 231–239.

Maxwell, J. C. (2015). The pain reliever and heroin epidemic in the United States: Shifting winds in the perfect storm. *Journal of Addictive Diseases, 34*(2–3), 127–140.

McAfee, T., Davis, K. C., Alexander, R. L., Pechacek, T. F., & Bunnell, R. (2013). Effect of the first federally funded US antismoking national media campaign. *Lancet, 382*, 2003–2011.

McCabe, S. E., West, B. T., Schepis, T. S., & Teter, C. J. (2015). Simultaneous co-ingestion of prescription stimulants, alcohol and other drugs: A multi-cohort national study of US adolescents. *Human Psychopharmacology, 30*(1),42–51.

McCabe, S. E., West, B. T., Teter, C. J., & Boyd, C. J. (2014). Trends in medical use, diversion, and nonmedical use of prescription medications among college students from 2003 to 2013: Connecting the dots. *Addictive Behaviors, 39*(7), 1176–1182.

McCabe, S. E., West, B. T., Teter, C. J., Ross-Durow, P., Young, A., & Boyd, C. J. (2011). Characteristics associated with the diversion of controlled medications among adolescents. *Drug and Alcohol Dependence, 118*(2–3), 452–458.

McCambridge, J., & Strang, J. (2004). The efficacy of single-session motivational interviewing in reducing drug consumption and perceptions of drug-related risk and harm among young people. *Addiction, 99*, 39–52.

McCance, E. F., & Kosten, T. R. (1998). Psychopharmacological treatments. In R. Frances & S. Miller (Eds.), *Clinical textbook of addictive disorders* (2nd ed., Section V, pp. 596–624). New York: Guilford Publications.

McGue, M., & Iacono, W. G. (2005). The association of early adolescent problem behavior with adult psychopathology. *American Journal of Psychiatry, 162*, 1118–1124.

McGue, M., Pickens, R. W., & Svikis, D. S. (1992). Sex and age effects on the inheritance of alcohol problems: A twin study. *Journal of Abnormal Psychology, 101*, 3–17.

McKance-Katz, E. F., Kosten, T. R., & Jatlow, P. (1998). Concurrent use of cocaine and alcohol is more potent and potentially more toxic than use of either alone—A multiple-dose study. *Biological Psychiatry, 44*, 250–259.

McKay, J. R., Alterman, A. I., Cacciola, J. S., Rutherford, M. J., O'Brien, C. P., & Koppenhaver, J. (1997). Group counseling versus individualized relapse prevention aftercare following intensive outpatient treatment for cocaine dependence. *Journal of Consulting and Clinical Psychology, 65*, 778–788.

McLellan, A. T., Lewis, D. C., O'Brien, C. P., & Kleber, H. D. (2000). Drug dependence, a chronic medical illness: Implications for treatment, insurance, and outcomes evaluation. *Journal of the American Medical Association, 284*, 1689–1695.

Merikangas, K. R., He, J. P., Rapoport, J. Vitiello, B., & Olfson, M. (2013). Medication use in US youth with mental disorders. *JAMA Pediatrics, 167*(2), 141–148.

Merikangas, K. R., Stolar, M., Stevens, D. E., Goulet, J., Preisig, M. A., Fenton, B., et al. (1998). Familial transmission of substance use disorders. *Archives of General Psychiatry, 55*, 973–979.

Mermelstein, R. (2003). Teen smoking cessation. *Tobacco Control,* 12(Suppl. 1), 125–134.

Metzler, C. W., Biglan, A., Rusby, J. C., & Sprague, J. R. (2001). Evaluation of a comprehensive behavior management program to improve school-wide positive behavior support. *Education and Treatment of Children, 24*, 448–479.

Meyers, J. L., & Dick, D. (2010). Genetic and environmental risk factors for adolescent-onset substance use disorders. *Child and Adolescent Psychiatric Clinics of North America, 19*(3), 465–477.

Meyers, J. L., Salvatore, J. E., Vuoksimaa, E., Korhonen, T., Pulkkinen, L., Rose, R. J., ... Dick, D. M. (2014). Genetic influences on alcohol use behaviors have diverging developmental trajectories: A prospective study among male and female twins. *Alcoholism: Clinical and Experimental Research, 38*(11), 2869–2877.

Michelson, D., Allen, A. J., Busner, J., Casat, C., Dunn, D., Kratochvil, C., et al. (2002). Once-daily atomoxetine treatment for children and adolescents with attention deficit hyperactivity disorder: A randomized, placebo-controlled study. *American Journal of Psychiatry, 159*, 1896– 1901.

Miech, R. A., Johnston, L. D., O'Malley, P. M., Bachman, J. G., & Schulenberg, J. E. (2015a). *Teen cigarette smoking drops to historic low in 2015.* Ann Arbor: University of Michigan News Service. Retrieved May 5, 2016, from http://www.monitoringthefuture.org

Miech, R. A., Johnston, L. D., O'Malley, P. M., Bachman, J. G., & Schulenberg, J. E. (2015b). *Cigarillo use increases estimates of teen smoking rates by half.* Ann Arbor: University of Michigan News Service. Retrieved May 5, 2016, from http://www.monitoringthefuture.org

Miech, R. A., Johnston, L. D., O'Malley, P. M., Bachman, J. G., & Schulenberg, J. E. (2015c). *Most youth use e-cigarettes for novelty, flavors—not to quit smoking.* Ann Arbor: University of Michigan News Service. Retrieved May 5, 2016, from http://www.monitoringthefuture.org

Milberger, S., Biederman, J., Faraone, S. V., Chen, L., & Jones, J. (1997). ADHD is associated with early initiation of cigarette smoking in children and adolescents. *Journal of the American Academy of Child and Adolescent Psychiatry, 36*, 37–44.

Miliano, C., Serpelloni, G., Rimondo, C., Mereu, M., Marti, M., & De Luca, M. A. (2016). Neuropharmacology of new psychoactive substances (NPS): Focus on the rewarding and reinforcing properties of cannabimimetics and amphetamine-like stimulants. *Frontiers in Neuroscience, 10*, 153.

Miller, W. R., & DelBoca, F. K. (1994). Measurement of drinking behavior using the Form 90 family of instruments. *Journal of Studies on Alcohol, 12* (Suppl.), 112–117.

Miller, W. R., & Rollnick, S. (1991). *Motivational interviewing: Preparing people to change addictive behavior.* New York: Guilford Press.

Miller, W. R., & Rollnick, S. (2002). *Motivational interviewing: Preparing people for change* (2nd ed). New York: Guilford Press.

Miller, W. R., & Wilbourne, P. L. (2002). Mesa Grande: A methodological analysis of clinical trials of treatments for alcohol use disorders. *Addiction, 97*, 265–277.

Minkoff, K., & Drake, R. E. (1991). Dual diagnosis of serious mental illness and substance disorder. San Francisco: Jossey-Bass.

Minozzi, S., Amato, L., Bellisario, C., & Davoli, M. (2014a). Detoxification treatments for opiate-dependent adolescents. *Cochrane Database of Systematic Reviews, 4*, CD006749.

Minozzi, S., Amato, L., Bellisario, C., & Davoli, M. (2014b). Maintenance treatments for opiate-dependent adolescents. *Cochrane Database of Systematic Reviews, 6*, CD007210.

Minozzi, S., Cinquini, M., Amato, L., Davoli, M., Farrell, M. F., Pani, P. P., & Vecchi, S. (2015). Anticonvulsants for cocaine dependence. *Cochrane Database Systematic Reviews, 4*, CD006754.

Miotto, K., Darakjian, J., Basch, J., Murray, S., Zogg, J., & Rawson, R. (2001). Gamma-hydroxybutyric acid: Patterns of use, effects and withdrawal. *American Journal of Addiction, 10*, 232–241.

Miranda, R., Ray, L., Blanchard, A., Reynolds, E. K., Monti, P. M., Chun, T., ... Ramirez J. (2014). Effects of naltrexone on adolescent alcohol cue reactivity and sensitivity: An initial randomized trial. *Addiction Biology, 19*(5), 941–954.

Moffitt, T. E., Arseneault, L., Belsky, D., Dickson, N., Hancox, R. J., Harrington, H., et al. (2011). A gradient of childhood self-control predicts health, wealth, and public safety. *Proceedings of the National Academy of Sciences, U S A, 108*(7), 2693–2698.

Molgaard, V., & Kumpfer, K. (1995). *The Strengthening Families program for families with pre- and early teens: Leader guide*. Ames, IA: Iowa State University Extension.

Molina, B. S., Hinshaw, S. P., Eugene Arnold, L., Swanson, J. M., Pelham, W. E., Hechtman, L., ... Marcus, S. (2013). Adolescent substance use in the Multimodal Treatment Study of Attention-Deficit/Hyperactivity Disorder as a function of childhood ADHD, random assignment to childhood treatments, and subsequent medication. *Journal of the American Academy of Child and Adolescent Psychiatry, 52*(3), 250–263.

Monterosso, J., Ehrman, J., Franklin, T., Napier, K., O'Brien, C. P., & Childress, A. R. (2001). *Decision-making task performance in cocainedependent patients*. Paper presented at the Drug and Alcohol Dependence: Abstracts for the 63rd Annual Meeting of the College on Problems of Drug Dependence, Phoenix, AZ, June 2001.

Monti, P. M., Colby, S. M., Barnett, N. P., Spirito, A., Rohsenow, D. J., Myers, M. G., et al. (1999). Brief intervention for harm reduction with alcohol-positive older adolescents in a hospital emergency department. *Journal of Consulting and Clinical Psychology, 67*, 989–994.

Moolchan, E. T., Ernst, M., & Henningfield, J. E. (2000). A review of tobacco smoking in adolescents: Treatment implications. *Journal of the American Academy of Child and Adolescent Psychiatry, 39*, 682–693.

Morel, C., Fattore, L., Pons, S., Hay, Y. A., Marti, F., Lambolez, B., ... Faure, P. (2014). Nicotine consumption is regulated by a human polymorphism in dopamine neurons. *Molecular Psychiatry, 19*(8), 930–936.

Morgan, C., & Kosten, T. R. (1990). Potential toxicity of high dose naltrexone in patients with appetitive disorders. In L. Ried (Ed.), *Opioids, bulimia, and alcohol abuse and alcoholism* (pp. 261– 274). New York: Springer-Verlag.

Morgan, D., Grant, K. A., Gage, H. D., Mach, R. H., Kaplan, J. R., Prioleau, O., et al. (2002). Social dominance in monkeys: dopamine D2 receptors and cocaine self-administration [Comment]. *Nature Neuroscience, 5*, 169–174.

Morgenstern, J., & Longabaugh, R. (2000). Cognitive-behavioral treatment for alcohol dependence: A review of the evidence for its hypothesized mechanisms of action. *Addiction, 95*, 1475–1490.

Morley-Fletcher, S., Bianchi, M., Gerra, G., & Laviola, G. (2002). Acute and carryover effects in mice of MDMA ("ecstasy") administration during periadolescence. *European Journal of Pharmacology, 448*, 31–38.

Morral, A. R., McCaffrey, D. F., & Paddock, S. M. (2002). Reassessing the marijuana gateway effect. *Addiction, 97*(12), 1493–1504.

Morrisey, E., Wandersmand, A., Seybolt, D., Nation, M., Crusto, C., & Davino, K. (1997). Toward a framework for bridging the gap between science and practice in prevention: A focus on evaluator and practitioner perspectives. *Evaluation and Program Planning, 20*, 367–377.

Moss, H. B., & Lynch, K. G. (2001). Comorbid disruptive behavior disorder symptoms and their relationship to adolescent alcohol use disorders. *Drug and Alcohol Dependence, 64*(1), 75–83.

Mrazek, P. J., & Haggerty, K. (1994). Reducing Risks for Mental Disorders: Frontiers for Preventive Intervention Research. Washington, DC.: National Academy Press.

Munafò, M. R., Timpson, N. J., David, S. P., Ebrahim, S., & Lawlor, D. A. (2009). Association of the DRD2 gene Taq1A polymorphism and smoking behavior: A meta-analysis and new data. *Nicotine and Tobacco Research 11*(1), 64–76.

Muramoto, M. L., Leischow, S. J., Sherrill, D., Matthews, E., & Strayer, L. J. (2007). Randomized, double-blind, placebo-controlled trial of 2 dosages of sustained-release bupropion for adolescent smoking cessation. *Archives of Pediatrics and Adolescent Medicine*, 161, 1068–1074.

Mwenifumbo, J. C., & Tyndale, R. F. (2007). Genetic variability in CYP2A6 and the pharmacokinetics of nicotine. *Pharmacogenomics, 8*(10), 1385–1402.

Myers, M. G., Stewart, D. G., & Brown, S. A. (1998). Progression from conduct disorder to antisocial personality disorder following treatment for adolescent substance abuse. *American Journal of Psychiatry, 155*, 479–485.

Nader, M. A., Nader, S. H., Czoty, P. W., Riddick, N. V., Gage, H. D., Gould, R. W., ... Reboussin, B. A. (2012). Social dominance in female monkeys: Dopamine receptor function and cocaine reinforcement. *Biological Psychiatry, 72*(5), 414–421.

Naimi, T. S., Stockwell, T., Zhao, J., Xuan, Z., Dangardt, F., Saitz, R., ... Chikritzhs T. (2017). Selection biases in observational studies affect associations between "moderate" alcohol consumption and mortality. *Addiction, 112*(2), 207–214.

National Cancer Institute. (2008). *The role of the media in promoting and reducing tobacco use* (Tobacco Control Monograph No. 19 No. NIH Pub No. 07-6242). Bethesda, MD: National Institutes of Health.

National Center on Alcohol and Substance Abuse (CASA). (2003). *Teen tipplers: America's underage drinking epidemic.* The National Center on Addiction and Substance Abuse at Columbia University. New York: Columbia University.

National Commission on Marihuana (1972). *Marihuana: A signal of misunderstanding.* Washington, DC: Government Printing Office.

National Highway Traffic Safety Administration. (2016). Alcohol-Impaired Driving 2015 data. Retrieved from https://crashstats.nhtsa.dot.gov/Api/Public/ViewPublication/812350

National Institute on Alcohol Abuse and Alcoholism (NIAAA). (2003). *Alcohol alert, underage drinking: A major public health challenge* (Vol. 59). From http//www.niaaa.gov/publications/a/alerts.htm

National Institute on Drug Abuse. (2000). *Principles of drug abuse treatment: A research-based guide.* Bethesda, Maryland: NIDA.

National Research Council. (2004). *Reducing underage drinking: A collective responsibility.* Washington, DC: National Academies Press.

Negus, S. S., & Miller, L. L. (2014). Intracranial self-stimulation to evaluate abuse potential of drugs. *Pharmacology Reviews, 66*(3), 869–917.

Nestler, E. J., Kelz, M. B., & Chen, J. (1999). Delta Fos B: A molecular mediator of long-term neural and behavioral plasticity. *Brain Research, 835,* 10–17.

Nestor, L. J., Ghahremani, D. G., Monterosso, J., & London, E. D. (2011). Prefrontal hypoactivation during cognitive control in early abstinent methamphetamine-dependent subjects. *Psychiatry Research, 194*(3), 287–295.

Neta, G., Glasgow, R. E., Carpenter, C. R., Grimshaw, J. M., Rabin, B. A., Femandez, M. E., & Brownson, R. C. (2015). A framework for enhancing the value of research for dissemination and implementation. *American Journal of Public Health, 105,* 49–57.

Newcomb, M. D. (1997). Psychosocial predictors and consequences of drug use: A developmental perspective within a prospective study. *Journal of Addictive Diseases, 16*(1), 51–89.

Nicholson, K. L., & Balster, R. L. (2001). GHB: A new and novel drug of abuse. *Drug and Alcohol Dependence, 63,* 1–22.

Niederhofer, H., & Staffen, W. (2003a). Comparison of disulfiram and placebo in treatment of alcohol dependence of adolescents. *Drug and Alcohol Reviews, 22*(3), 295–297.

Niederhofer, H., & Staffen, W. (2003b). Acamprosate and its efficacy in treating alcohol dependent adolescents. *European Child and Adolescent Psychiatry, 12*(3), 144–148.

Nielsen, D. A., Virkkunen, M., Lappalainen, J., Eggert, M., Brown, G. L., Long, J. C., et al. (1998). A tryptophan hydroxylase gene marker for suicidality and alcoholism. *Archives of General Psychiatry, 55,* 593–602.

Noble, E. P. (1993). The D2 dopamine receptor gene: A review of association studies in alcoholism. *Behavior Genetics, 23,* 119–129.

Noble, E., Ozkaragoz, T., Ritchie, T., Zhang, X., Belin, T., & Sparkes, R. (1998). D2 and D4 dopamine receptor polymorphisms and personality. *American Journal of Medical Genetics, 81,* 257–267.

Noble, E., St Jeor, S. T., Ritchie, T., Syndulko, K., St Jeor, S. C., Fitch, R., & Brunner, R. L. (1994). D2 dopamine receptor gene and cigarette smoking: A reward gene? *Medical Hypotheses, 42,* 257.

O'Brien, C. (2001). Drug addiction and drug abuse. In J. G. Hardman & C. L. Lee (Eds.), *Goodman & Gilman's the pharmacological basis of therapeutics* (10th ed., pp. 621–642). New York: McGrawHill.

O'Brien, C. P. (2008). Evidence-based treatments of addiction. *Philosophical Transactions of the Royal Society B: Biological Sciences, 363*(1507), 3277–3286.

O'Brien, C. P., Childress, A. R., Ehrman, R., & Robbins, S. J. (1998). Conditioning factors in drug abuse: Can they explain compulsion? *Journal of Psychopharmacology, 12,* 15–22.

O'Brien, C. P., Childress, A. R., McLellan, A. T., & Ehrman, R. (1992). Classical conditioning in drug-dependent humans. *Annals of the New York Academy of Science, 654,* 400–415.

O'Brien, C. P., Testa, T., O'Brien, T. J., Brady, J. P., & Wells, B. (1977). Conditioning narcotic withdrawal in humans. *Science, 195,* 1000–1002.

O'Loughlin, J., Tarasuk, J., DiFranza, J., & Paradis, G. (2002). Reliability of selected measures of nicotine dependence among adolescents. *Annals of Epidemiology, 12,* 353–362.

Obrocki, J., Schmoldt, A., Buchert, R., Andresen, B., Petersen, K., & Thomasius, R. (2002). Specific neurotoxicity of chronic use of ecstasy. *Toxicology Letters, 127*, 285–297.

Olfson, M., King, M., & Schoenbaum, M. (2015). Treatment of young people with antipsychotic medications in the United States. *JAMA Psychiatry, 72*(9), 867–874.

Osgood, D. W., Johnston, L. D., O'Malley, P. M., & Bachman, J. G. (1988). The generality of deviance in late adolescence and early adulthood. *American Sociological Review, 53*, 81–93.

Osher, F. C., & Drake, R. E. (1996). Reversing a history of unmet needs: Approaches to care for persons with co-occurring addictive and mental disorders. *American Journal of Orthopsychiatry, 66*, 4–11.

Padhy, R., Saxena, K., Remsing, L., Huemer, J., Plattner, B., & Steiner, H. (2011). Symptomatic response to divalproex in subtypes of conduct disorder. *Child Psychiatry and Human Development, 42*(5), 584–593.

Pal, H. R., Berry, N., Kumar, R., & Ray, R. (2002). Ketamine dependence. *Anaesthesia and Intensive Care, 30*, 382–384.

Pandey, S. C., Zhang, H., & Roy, A. (2003). Effect of PKA activator infusion into the central amygdala on anxiety and on NPY expression during ethanol withdrawal. *Alcoholism: Clinical and Experimental Research, 27* (5 Suppl.), 188A.

Park, M. S., Sohn, J. H., Suk, J. A., Kim, S. H., Sohn, S., & Sparacio, R. (2007). Brain substrates of craving to alcohol cues in subjects with alcohol use disorder. *Alcohol and Alcoholism, 42*(5), 417–422.

Parker, M. A., & Anthony, J C. (2014). Should anyone be riding to glory on the now-descending limb of the crack-cocaine epidemic curve in the United States? *Drug and Alcohol Dependence, 138*, 225–228.

Parker, M. A., & Anthony, J. C. (2015). Epidemiological evidence on extra-medical use of prescription pain relievers: Transitions from newly incident use to dependence among 12–21 year olds in the United States using meta-analysis, 2002–13. *Peer Journal, 20*(3), e1340.

Parrott, A. C. (2001). Human psychopharmacology of Ecstasy (MDMA): A review of 15 years of empirical research. *Human Psychopharmacology, 16*, 557–577.

Parrott, A. C. (2002). Recreational ecstasy/MDMA, the serotonin syndrome, and serotonergic neurotoxicity. *Pharmacology, Biochemistry, and Behavior, 71*, 837–844.

Parrott, A. C., Buchanan, T., Scholey, A. B., Heffernan, T., Ling, J., & Rodgers, J. (2002). Ecstasy/MDMA-attributed problems reported by novice, moderate and heavy recreational users. *Human Psychopharmacology, 17*, 309–312.

Parsian, A., Chakraverty, S., Fishler, L., & Cloninger, C. R. (1997). No association between polymorphisms in the human dopamine D3 and D4 receptor genes and alcoholism. *American Journal of Medical Genetics, 74*, 281–285.

Pas, E. T., & Bradshaw, C. P. (2015). Dissemination of evidence-based prevention programs: The broad picture. In L. M. Scheier (Ed.), *Handbook of adolescent drug use prevention: Research, intervention strategies, and practice* (pp. 527–540). Washington, DC: American Psychological Association.

Patrick, M. E., & Schulenberg, J. E. (2010). Alcohol use and heavy episodic drinking prevalence and predictors among national samples of American eighth- and tenth-grade students. *Journal of Studies on Alcohol and Drugs, 71*(1), 41–45.

Patterson, G., DeBaryshe, B., & Ramsey, E. (1989). A developmental perspective on antisocial behavior. *American Psychologist, 44*, 329–335.

Patton, G. C., Carlin, J. B., Coffey, C., Wolfe, R., Hibbert, M., & Bowers, G. (1998). The course of early smoking: A population-based cohort study over three years. *Addiction, 93*, 1251–1260.

Pbert, L., Moolchan, E. T., Muramoto, M., Winickoff, J. P., Curry, S., Lando, H., et al. (2003). The state of office-based interventions for youth tobacco use. *Pediatrics, 111*(6 Pt. 1), e650–660.

Pedroni, A., Koeneke, S., Velickaite, A., & Jäncke, L. (2011). Differential magnitude coding of gains and omitted rewards in the ventral striatum. *Brain Research, 1411*, 76–86.

Peeters, M., Monshouwer, K., van de Schoot, R., Janssen, T., Vollebergh, W. A., & Wiers, R. W. (2014). Personality and the prediction of high-risk trajectories of alcohol use during adolescence. *Journal of Studies in Alcohol and Drugs, 75*(5), 790–798.

Pentz, M. A., Dwyer, J. H., MacKinnon, D. P., Flay, B. R., Hansen, W. B., Wang, E. Y., et al. (1989). A multicommunity trial for primary prevention of adolescent drug abuse: Effects on drug use prevalence. *Journal of the American Medical Association, 261*(22), 3259–3266.

Perry, C. L., Komro, K. A., Veblen-Mortenson, S., Bosma, L. M., Farbakhsh, K., Munson, K. A., et al. (2003). A randomized controlled trial of the middle and junior high school D.A.R.E. and

D.A.R.E. Plus programs. *Archives of Pediatrics and Adolescent Medicine, 157*(2), 178–184.

Petrakis, I. L., Gonzalez, G., Rosenheck, R., & Krystal, J. H. (2002). Comorbidity of alcoholism and psychiatric disorders: An overview. *Alcohol Research and Health, 26*, 81–90.

Petry, N. M. (2001). Substance abuse pathological gambling, and impulsiveness. *Drug and Alcohol Dependence 63*, 29–38.

Petry, N. M., Martin, B., Cooney, J. L., & Kranzler, H. R. (2000). Give them prizes and they will come: Contingency management treatment of alcohol dependence. *Journal of Consulting and Clinical Psychology, 68*, 250–257.

Pianca, T. G., Rohde, L. A., Rosa, R. L., Begnis, A. P. A., Ferronatto, P. B., Jensen, M... . Szobot, C. M. (2016). Crack-cocaine in adolescents: Clinical characteristics and predictors of early initiation. *Journal of Clinical Psychiatry, 77*(10), e1205–e1210.

Pianezza, M., Sellers, E., & Tyndale, R. (1998). Nicotine metabolism defect reduces smoking. *Nature, 393*, 750.

Pickens, R. W., & Svikis, D. S. (1991). Genetic influences in human substance abuse. *Journal of Addictive Diseases, 10*, 205–213.

Pickens, R. W., Svikis, D. S., McGue, M., & LaBuda, M. C. (1995). Common genetic mechanisms in alcohol, drug, and mental disorder comorbidity. *Drug and Alcohol Dependence, 39*, 129–138.

Pierce, J. P., Choi, W. S., Gilpin, E. A., Farkas, A. J., & Berry, C. C. (1998). Tobacco industry promotion of cigarettes and adolescent smoking. *Journal of the American Medical Association, 279*, 511– 515.

Pierce, J. P., White, M. M., & Gilpin, E. A. (2005). Adolescent smoking decline during California's Tobacco Control program. *Tobacco Control, 14*(3), 207–212.

Pittman, K., Irby, M., & Ferber, T. (2000). Unfinished business: Further reflections on a decade of promoting youth development. In Public/Private Ventures, *Youth development: Issues, challenges, and directions* (pp. 17–64). Philadelphia, PA: Public/Private Ventures.

Pliszka, S. R., Crismon, M. L., Hughes, C. W., Corners, C. K., Emslie, G. J., Jensen, P. S., et al. (2006). The Texas Children's Medication Algorithm Project: Revision of the algorithm for pharmacotherapy of attention-deficit/hyperactivity disorder. *Journal of the American Academy of Child and Adolescent Psychiatry, 45*, 642–657.

Pollock, N. K., & Martin, C. S. (1999). Diagnostic orphans: Adolescents with alcohol symptoms who do not qualify for DSM-IV abuse or dependence diagnoses. *American Journal of Psychiatry, 156*(6), 897–901.

Pomerleau, O. F., & Pomerleau, C. S. (1984). Neuroregulators and the reinforcement of smoking: Towards a biobehavioral explanation. *Neuroscience and Biobehavioral Reviews, 8*, 503–513.

Pomerleau, O. F., Pomerleau, C. S., & Namenek, R. J. (1998). Early experiences with tobacco among women smokers, ex-smokers and never-smokers. *Addiction, 93*, 595–599.

Ponomarev, I., & Crabbe, J. C. (2002). A novel method to assess initial sensitivity and acute functional tolerance to hypnotic effects of ethanol. *Journal of Pharmacology and Experimental Therapeutics, 302*, 257–263.

Porath-Waller, A. J., Beasley, E., & Beirness, D. J. (2010). A meta-analytic review of school-based prevention for cannabis use. *Health Education & Behavior, 37*(5), 709–723.

Prescott, C. A., & Kendler, K. S. (1999). Genetic and environmental contributions to alcohol abuse and dependence in a population-based sample of male twins. *American Journal of Psychiatry, 156*, 34–40.

Price, R. H., & Behrens, T. (2003). Working Pasteur's quadrant: Harnessing science and action for community change. *American Journal of Community Psychology, 31*, 219–223.

Project MATCH Research Group. (1997). Matching alcohol treatments to client heterogeneity: Project MATCH posttreatment drinking outcomes. *Journal of Studies on Alcohol, 58*, 7–29.

Pulvirenti, L., Balducci, C., Piercy, M., & Koob, G. F. (1998). Characterization of the effects of the partial dopamine agonist terguride on cocaine selfadministration in the rat. *Journal of Pharmacology and Therapeutics, 286*, 1231–1238.

Rawson, R. A., Huber, A., McCann, M. J., Shoptaw, S., Farabee, D., Reiber, C., et al. (2002). A comparison of contingency management and cognitive-behavioral approaches during methadone maintenance for cocaine dependence. *Archives of General Psychiatry, 59*, 817–824.

Reboussin, B. A., & Anthony, J. C. (2006). Is there epidemiological evidence to support the idea that a cocaine dependence syndrome emerges soon after onset of cocaine use? *Neuropsychopharmacology, 31*(9), 2055–2064.

Rennie, L. J., Bazillier-Bruneau, C., & Rouëssé, J. (2016). Harm reduction or harm introduction? Prevalence and correlates of e-cigarette use among French adolescents. *Journal of Adolescent Health*, 58, 440–445. Epub 2016 Feb 3.

Rey, J. M., Bella-Awusah, T. T., & Liu, J. (2015). Depression in children and adolescents. In *IACAPAP Textbook of Child and Adolescent Mental Health*. Geneva: International Association for Child and Adolescent Psychiatry and Allied Professions, 2015.

Richardson, M. A., Craig, T. J., and Haughland, G. (1985). Treatment patterns of young chronic schizophrenic patients in the era of deinstitutionalization. *Psychiatric Quarterly*, *57*, 243–249.

Ridenour, T. A., Reynolds, M., Ahlqvist, O., Zhai, Z. W., Kirisci, L., Vanyukov, M. M., & Tarter, R. E. (2013). High and low neurobehavior disinhibition clusters within locales: Implications for community efforts to prevent substance use disorder. *American Journal of Drug and Alcohol Abuse*, *39*(3), 194–203.

Ridgely, M. S., & Lambert D., et al., (1999). Interagency collaboration in services for people with co-occurring mental illness and substance use disorders. *Psychiatric Services*, *49*, 236–238.

Ridgely, M. S., Goldman, H. H., & Willenbring, M. (1990). Barriers to the care of persons with dual diagnoses: Organizational and financing issues. *Schizophrenia Bulletin*, *16*, 123–132.

Riggs, P. D., Leon, S. L., Mikulich, S. K., & Pottle, L. C. (1998). An open trial of bupropion for ADHD in adolescents with substance use disorders and conduct disorder. *Journal of the American Academy of Child and Adolescent Psychiatry*, *37*, 1271–1278.

Riggs, P. D., Mikulich, S. K., & Hall, S. (2001). Effects of pemoline on ADHD, antisocial behaviors, and substance use in adolescents with conduct disorder and substance use disorder. Paper presented at the College on Problems of Drug Dependence, 63rd Annual Scientific Meeting, Scottsdale, AZ, June

Riggs, P. D., Mikulich, S. K., Coffman, L. M., & Crowley, T. J. (1997). Fluoxetine in drug-dependent delinquents with major depression: An open trial. *Journal of Child and Adolescent Psychopharmacology*, *7*, 87–95.

Riggs, P. D., Mikulich-Gilbertson, S. K., Davies, R. D., Lohman, M., Klein, C., & Stover, S. K. (2007). A randomized controlled trial of fluoxetine and cognitive behavioral therapy in adolescents with major depression, behavior problems, and substance use disorders. *Archives of Pediatric and Adolescent Medicine*, *161*(11), 1026–1034.

Riggs, P. D., Thompson, L. L., Mikulich, S. K., Whitmore, E. A., & Crowley, T. J. (1996). An open trial of pemoline in drug-dependent delinquents with attention-deficit hyperactivity disorder. *Journal of the American Academy of Child and Adolescent Psychiatry*, *35*, 1018–1024.

Riggs, P. D., & Whitmore, E. A. (1999). Substance use disorders and disruptive behavior disorders. In R. L. Hendren (Ed.), *Disruptive behavior disorders in children and adolescents* (pp. 133–173). Washington, DC: American Psychiatric Association Press.

Riggs, P. D., Winhusen, T., Davies, R. D., Leimberger, J. D., Mikulich-Gilbertson, S., Klein, C., ... Liu, D. (2011). Randomized controlled trial of osmotic-release methylphenidate with CBT in adolescents with ADHD and substance use disorders. *Journal of the American Academy of Child and Adolescent Psychiatry*, *50*(9), 903–914.

Ringwalt, C., Vincus, A. A., Hanley, S., Ennett, S. T., Bowling, J. M., & Haws, S. (2011). Prevalence of evidence-based drug use prevention curricula in U.S. middle schools in 2008. *Prevention Science*, *12*, 63–69.

Robbins, M. S., Feaster, D. J., Horigian, V. E., Rohrbaugh, M., Shoham, V., Bachrach, K., ... Szapocznik, J. (2011). Brief strategic family therapy versus treatment as usual: Results of a multisite randomized trial for substance using adolescents. *Journal of Consulting and Clinical Psychology*, *79*(6), 713–727.

Roberts, D. C. (2005). Preclinical evidence for GABAB agonists as a pharmacotherapy for cocaine addiction. *Physiology and Behavior*, *86*(1–2), 18–20.

Roberts, D. C. S., Andrews, M. M., & Vickers, G. J. (1996). Baclofen attenuates the reinforcing effects of cocaine in rats. *Neuropsychopharmacology*, *15*(4), 417–423.

Roberts, D. C. S., & Ranaldi, R. (1995). Effect of dopaminergic drugs on cocaine reinforcement. *Clinical Neuropharmacology*, *18*, S84–S95.

Robins, L., & Regier, D. (1991). *Psychiatric disorders in America; the Epidemiological Catchment Area Study*. New York: The Free Press.

Robinson, J. M., Ladd, B. O., & Anderson, K. G. (2014). When you see it, let it be: Urgency, mindfulness and adolescent substance use. *Addictive Behaviors*, *39*(6), 1038–1041.

Rodriguez, S., Cook, D. G., Gaunt, T. R., Nightingale, C. M., Whincup, P. H., & Day, I. N. (2011). Combined analysis of CHRNA5, CHRNA3 and CYP2A6 in relation to adolescent smoking behaviour. *Journal of Psychopharmacology*, *25*, 915–923.

Rohde, P., Lewinsohn, P. M., & Seeley, J. R. (1996). Psychiatric comorbidity with problematic alcohol use in high school students. *Journal of the American Academy of Child and Adolescent Psychiatry*, *35*(1), 101–109.

Romer, D., Betancourt, L. M., Brodsky, N. L., Giannetta, J. M., Yang, W., & Hurt, H. (2011). Does adolescent risk taking imply weak executive function? A prospective study of relations between working memory performance, impulsivity, and risk taking in early adolescence. *Developmental Science*, *14*(5), 1119–1133.

Romer, D., Betancourt, L., Giannetta, J. M., Brodsky, N. L., Farah, M. J., & Hurt, H. (2009). Executive cognitive functions and impulsivity as correlates of risk taking and problem behavior in preadolescents. *Neuropsychologia*, *47*(13), 2916–2926.

Roozendaal, B., Barsegyan, A., & Lee, S. (2008). Adrenal stress hormones, amygdala activation, and memory for emotionally arousing experiences. *Progress in Brain Research*, *167*, 79–97.

Rose, R. J., Dick, D., Viken, R., & Kaprio, J. (2001). Gene-environment interaction in patterns of adolescent drinking: Regional residency moderates longitudinal influences on alcohol use. *Alcoholism: Clinical and Experimental Research*, *25*, 637–643.

Rosenberg, H. (2009). Clinical and laboratory assessment of the subjective experience of drug craving. *Clinical Psychology Reviews*, *29*(6), 519–534.

Roth, J. L., & Brooks-Gunn, J. (2002). Youth development programs and healthy development: Next steps. In D. Romer (Ed.), *Reducing adolescent risk: Toward an integrated approach*. Thousand Oaks, CA.: Sage Publications.

Roth, J., Brooks-Gunn, J., Murray, L., & Foster, W. (1998). Promoting healthy adolescents: Synthesis of youth development program evaluations. *Journal of Research on Adolescence*, *8*, 423–459.

Roy, A., & Pandey, S. C. (2002). The decreased cellular expression of neuropeptide Y protein in rat brain structures during ethanol withdrawal after chronic ethanol exposure. *Alcoholism; Clinical and Experimental Research*, *26*, 796–803.

Rutledge, P. C., Park, A., & Sher, K. J. (2008). 21st birthday drinking: Extremely extreme. *Journal of Consulting and Clinical Psychology*, *76*(3), 511–516.

Rutter, M., Giller, H., & Hagell, A. (1998). *Antisocial behavior by young people*. Cambridge, UK: Cambridge University Press.

Scherphof, C. S., van den Eijnden, R. J., Engels, R. C., & Vollebergh, W. A. (2014b). Long-term efficacy of nicotine replacement therapy for smoking cessation in adolescents: A randomized controlled trial. *Drug and Alcohol Dependence*, *140*, 217–220.

Schneider, F., Habel, U., Wagner, M., Franke, P., Salloum, J. B., Hah, N. J., Toni, I., ... Zilles, K. (2001). Subcortical correlates of craving in recently abstinent alcoholic patients. *American Journal of Psychiatry*, *158*, 1075–1089.

Schneider, S., & Diehl, K. (2016). Vaping as a catalyst for smoking? An initial model on the initiation of electronic cigarette use and the transition to tobacco smoking among adolescents. *Nicotine and Tobacco Research*, 18, 647–653. Epub 2015 Sep 18.

Schoenwald, S. K., Ward, D. M., Henggeler, S. W., Pickerl, S. G., & Patel, H. (1996). Multisystemic therapy treatment of substance abusing or dependent adolescent offenders: Cost of reducing incarceration, inpatient and residential placement. *Journal of Child and Family Studies*, *5*, 431– 444.

Schreiber, L., Odlaug, B. L., & Grant, J. E. (2011). Impulse control disorders: Updated review of clinical characteristics and pharmacological management. *Frontiers in Psychiatry*, *2*, 1.

Schuckit, M. A. (2000). Genetics of the risk for alcoholism. *American Journal on Addictions*, *9*, 103– 112.

Schulenberg, J. E., & Maggs, J. L. (2002). A developmental perspective on alcohol use and heavy drinking during adolescence and the transition to young adulthood. *Journal of Studies on Alcohol Supplement*, *14*, 54–70.

Schulenberg, J., O'Malley, P. M., Bachman, J. G., Wadsworth, K. N., & Johnston, L. D. (1996). Getting drunk and growing up: Trajectories of frequent binge drinking during the transition to young adulthood. *Journal of Studies on Alcohol*, *57*, 289–304.

Schulteis, G., Ahmed, S. H., Morse, A. C., Koob, G. F., & Everitt, B. J. (2000). Conditioning and opiate withdrawal: The amygdala links neutral stimuli with the agony of overcoming drug addiction. *Nature*, *405*, 1013–1014.

Schulteis, G., & Koob, G. F. (1996). Reinforcement processes in opiate addiction: A homeostatic model. *Neurochemical Research*, *21*, 1437–1454.

Schultz, W. (2002). Getting formal with dopamine and reward. *Neuron*, *36*, 241–263.

Schwartz, R. H., Milteer, R., & LeBeau, M. A. (2000). Drug-facilitated sexual assault ("date rape"). *Southern Medical Journal*, *93*, 558–561.

Seedall, R. B., & Anthony, J. C. (2015). Monitoring by parents and hypothesized male/female differences in evidence from a nationally representative cohort re-sampled from age 12 to 17 years: An exploratory study using a "mutoscope" approach. *Prevention Science, 16*(5), 696–706.

Sees, K. L., Delucchi, K. L., Masson, C., Rosen, A., Clark, H. W., Robillard, H., et al. (2000). Methadone maintenance vs 180-day psychosocially enriched detoxification for treatment of opioid dependence: A randomized controlled trial [see comments]. *Journal of the American Medical Association, 283*, 1303–1310.

Self, D. W., & Nestler, E. J. (1995). Molecular mechanisms of drug reinforcement and addiction. *Annual Review of Neuroscience, 18*, 463–495.

Sell, L. A., Morris, J, Bearn, J., Frackowiak, R. S. J., Friston, K. J., & Dolan, R. J., (1999). Activation of reward circuitry in human opiate addicts. *European Journal of Neuroscience, 11*, 1042–1048.

Sell, L. A., Morris, J., Bearn, J., Frackowiak, R. S., Friston, K. J., & Dolan, R. J. (1999). Activation of reward circuitry in human opiate addicts. *European Journal of Neuroscience, 11*, 1042–1048.

Sellers, E. M., Tyndale, R. F., & Fernandes, L. C. (2003). Decreasing smoking behavior and risk through CYP2A6 inhibition. *Drug Discovery Today, 8*, 487–493.

Shamosh, N. A., Deyoung, C. G., Green, A. E., Reis, D. L., Johnson, M. R., Conway, A. R., . . . Gray, J. R. (2008). Individual differences in delay discounting: Relation to intelligence, working memory, and anterior prefrontal cortex. *Psychological Science, 19*(9), 904–111.

Shane, P., Diamond, G. S., Mensinger, J. L., Shera, D., & Wintersteen, M. B. (2006). Impact of victimization on substance abuse treatment outcomes for adolescents in outpatient and residential substance abuse treatment. *American Journal of Addiction, 15*(Suppl 1), 34–42.

Shea, S. H. Wall, T. L., Carr, L. G., & Li, T. K. (2001). ADH2 and alcohol-treated phenotypes in Ashkenazic Jewish American college students. *Behavior Genetics, 31*, 231–239.

Sheffler, D. J., & Roth, B. L. (2003). Salvinorin A: The "magic mint" hallucinogen finds a molecular target in the kappa opioid receptor. *Trends in Pharmacological Science, 24*, 107–109.

Shillington, A. M., Woodruff, S. I., Clapp, J. D., Reed, M. B., & Lemus, H. (2012). Self-reported age of onset and telescoping for cigarettes, alcohol, and marijuana across eight years of the National Longitudinal Survey of Youth. *Journal of Child and Adolescent Substance Abuse, 21*(4), 333–348.

Shimada, S., Kitayama, S., Lin, C. L., Patel, A., Nanthakumar, E., Gregor, P., et al. (1991). Cloning and expression of a cocaine-sensitive dopamine transporter complementary DNA [published erratum appears in *Science* 1992 Mar 6;255(5049); 1195]. *Science, 254* (5031), 576–578.

Shytle, R. D., Silver, A. A., Lukas, R. J., Newman, M. B., Sheehan, D. V., & Sanberg, P. R. (2002). Nicotinic acetylcholine receptors as targets for antidepressants. *Molecular Psychiatry, 7*(6), 525–535.

Siegel, M., DeJong, W., Naimi, T. S., Fortunato, E. K., Albers, A. B., & Heeren, T. (2013). Brand-specific consumption of alcohol among underage youth in the United States. *Alcoholism: Clinical and Experimental Research, 37*(7), 1195–1203.

Siegel, S. (1975). Evidence from rats that morphine tolerance is a learned response. *Journal of Comparative and Physiological Psychology, 89*, 498–506.

Silverman, K., Higgins, S. T., Brooner, R. K., Montoya, I. D., Cone, E. J., Schuster, C. R., et al. (1996). Sustained cocaine abstinence in methadone maintenance patients through voucherbased reinforcement therapy. *Archives of General Psychiatry, 53*, 409–415.

Silverman, M., Neale, M., Sullivan, P., Harris-Kerr, C., Wormley, B., & Sadek, H. (2001). Haplotypes of four novel single nucleotide polymorphisms in the nicotine acetylcholine receptor □-subunit (CHRNB2) gene show no association smoking initiation or nicotine dependence. *American Journal of Medical Genetics, 96*, 646–653.

Simkin, D. R., & Black, N. B. (2014). Meditation and mindfulness in clinical practice. *Child and Adolescent Psychiatric Clinics of North America, 23*, 487–534.

Simmons, M. M., & Cupp, M. J. (1998). Use and abuse of flunitrazepam. *Annals of Pharmacotherapy, 32*, 117–119.

Simpson, D. D., Savage, L. J., & Sells, S. B. (1978). Data book on drug treatment outcomes: Follow-up study of the 1969–71 admission to the Drug Abuse Report Program. Fort Worth, TX: Texas Christian University.

Singh, T., Marynak, K., Arrazola, R. A., Cox, S., Rolle, I. V., & King, B. A. (2016). Vital signs: Exposure to electronic cigarette advertising among middle and high school students—United States, 2014. *Morbidity and Mortality Weekly Reports, 64*(52), 1403–1408.

Slaughter, L. (2000). Involvement of drugs in sexual assault. *Journal of Reproductive Medicine, 45*, 425–430.

Slutske, W. S., True, W. R., Scherrer, J. F., Heath, A. C., Bucholz, K. K., Eisen, S. A., et al. (1999). The heritability of alcoholism symptoms: Indicators of genetic and environmental influence in alcohol-dependent individuals: Revisited. *Alcoholism, Clinical and Experimental Research, 23*, 757–758.

Small, D. M., Zatorre, R. J., Dagher, A., Evans, A. C., & Jones-Gotman, M. (2001). Changes in brain activity related to eating chocolate: From pleasure to aversion. *Brain, 124*(Pt 9), 1720–1733.

Smith, D. C., Ureche, D. J., Davis, J. P., & Walters, S. T. (2015). Motivational Interviewing with and without normative feedback for adolescents with substance use problems: A preliminary study. *Substance Abuse, 36*(3), 350–358.

Smith, K. M., Larive, L. L., & Romanelli, F. (2002). Club drugs: Methylenedioxymethamphetamine, flunitrazepam, ketamine hydrochloride, and gamma-hydroxybutyrate. *American Journal of Health-System Pharmacy, 59*, 1067–1076.

Smith, T. A., House, R. F., Jr., Croghan, I. T., Gauvin, T. R., Colligan, R. C., Offord, K. P., et al. (1996). Nicotine patch therapy in adolescent smokers. *Pediatrics, 98* (4 Pt. 1), 659–667.

Smyth, B. P., Fagan, J., & Kernan, K. (2012). Outcome of heroin-dependent adolescents presenting for opiate substitution treatment. *Journal of Substance Abuse Treatment, 42*(1), 35–44.

Solhkhah, R., & Wilens, T. E. (1998). Pharmacotherapy of adolescent AOD use disorders. *Alcohol Health and Research World, 22*, 122–126.

Solomon, R. L., & Corbit, J. D. (1974). An opponent-process theory of motivation: 1. Temporal dynamics of affect. *Psychological Reviews, 81*, 119–145.

Spano, M. S., Fattore, L., Fratta, W., & Fadda, P. (2007). The GABAB receptor agonist baclofen prevents heroin-induced reinstatement of heroin-seeking behavior in rats. *Neuropharmacology, 52*(7), 1555–1562.

Spear, L. P. (2002) Alcohol's effects on adolescents. *Alcohol Research & Health, 26*, 287–291.

Spear, L. P. (2002). The adolescent brain and the college drinker: Biological basis of propensity to use and misuse alcohol. *Journal of Studies on Alcohol Supplement, 14*, 71–81.

Spear, L. P., & Varlinskaya, E. I. (2010). Sensitivity to ethanol and other hedonic stimuli in an animal model of adolescence: Implications for prevention science? *Developmental Psychobiology, 52*(3), 236–243.

Spencer, T., Heiligenstein, J. H., Biederman, J., Faries, D. E., Kratochvil, C. J., Conners, C. K., et al. (2002). Results from 2 proof-of-concept, placebo-controlled studies of atomoxetine in children with attention-deficit/hyperactivity disorder. *Journal of Clinical Psychiatry, 63*, 1140– 1147.

Spielman, A. I., Najai, H., Sunavala, G., Dasso., M., Breer, H., Boekhoff, I., et al. (1996). Rapid kinetics of second messenger production in bitter taste. *American Journal of Physiology, 270*(3 pt 1), C926–931.

Spitz, M., Shi, H., Yang, F., Hudmon, K., Jiang, H., & Chanberlain, R. (1998). Case–control study of the D2 dopamine receptor gene and smoking status in lung cancer patients. *Journal of the National Cancer Institute, 90*, 358–363.

Spoth, R. (2008). Translating family-focused prevention science into effective practice: Toward a translational impact paradigm. *Current Directions in Psychological Science, 17*(6), 415–421.

Spoth, R. L., & Greenberg, M. T. (in press). Toward a comprehensive strategy for effective practitioner-scientist partnerships and larger-scale community benefits. *American Journal of Community Psychology.*

Spoth, R., Greenberg, M., & Turisi, R. (2009). Overview of preventive interventions addressing underage drinking. *Alcohol Research & Health, 32*(1), 53–66.

Spoth, R., Guyll, M., Chao, W., & Molgaard, V. (2003). Exploratory study of a preventive intervention with general population African American families. *Journal of Early Adolescence, 23*, 435–468.

Spoth, R., Guyll, M., & Day, S. X. (2002). Universal family-focused interventions in alcohol-use disorder prevention: Cost-effectiveness and cost-benefit analyses of two interventions. *Journal of Studies on Alcohol and Drugs, 63*(2), 219–228.

Spoth, R., Redmond, C., Clair, S., Shin, C., Greenberg, M. T., & Feinberg, M. (2011). Preventing substance misuse through community-university partnerships: Randomized controlled trial outcomes 4-1/2 years past baseline. *American Journal of Preventive Medicine, 40*(4), 440–447.

Spoth, R., Redmond, C., Mason, W. A., Schainker, L., & Borduin, L. (2015). Research on the strengthening families program for parents and youth ages 10–14: Long-term effects, mechanisms, translation to public health, prosper partnership scale up. In L. M. Scheier (Ed.), *Handbook of adolescent drug use prevention: Research, intervention strategies, and practice* (pp. 267–292). Washington, DC: American Psychological Association.

Spoth, R., Redmond, C., & Shin, C. (2000). Reducing adolescents' aggressive and hostile behaviors: Randomized trail effects of a brief family intervention four years past baseline. *Archives of Pediatrics and Adolescent Medicine, 154*, 1248–1257.

Spoth, R., Redmond, C., & Shin, C. (2001). Randomized trial of brief family interventions for general populations: Adolescent substance use outcomes four years following baseline. *Journal of Consulting and Clinical Psychology, 69*, 627– 642.

Spoth, R., Redmond, C., Shin, C., Greenberg, M., Feinberg, M., & Schainker, L. (2013). PROSPER community-university partnership delivery system effects on substance misuse through 6 1/2 years past baseline from a cluster randomized controlled intervention trial. *Preventive Medicine, 56*, 190–196.

Spoth, R., Reyes, M. L., Redmond, C., & Shin, C. (1999). Assessing the public health approach to delay onset and progression of adolescent substance use: Latent transition and loglinear analyses of longitudinal family preventive intervention outcomes. *Journal of Consulting and Clinical Psychology, 67*, 619–630.

Spoth, R., Trudeau, L., Guyll, C., & Redmond, C. (2009). Universal intervention effects on substance use among young adults mediated by delayed adolescent substance initiation. *Journal of Consulting and Clinical Psychology, 77*(4), 620–632.

Spoth, R. L., Trudeau, L., Guyll, M., & Shin, C. (2012). Benefits of universal intervention effects on a youth protective shield 10 years after baseline. *Journal of Adolescent Health, 50*, 414–417.

Stalnaker, T. A., Takahashi, Y., Roesch, M. R., & Schoenbaum, G. (2009). Neural substrates of cognitive inflexibility after chronic cocaine exposure. *Neuropharmacology, 56*(Suppl 1), 63–72.

Stanger, C., & Budney, A. J. (2010). Contingency management approaches for adolescent substance use disorders. *Child & Adolescent Psychiatric Clinics of North America, 19*(3), 547–562.

Stanger, C., Budney, A. J., Kamon, J. L., & Thostensen, J. (2009). A randomized trial of contingency management for adolescent marijuana abuse and dependence. *Drug and Alcohol Dependence, 105*(3), 240–247.

Stanger, C., Ryan, S. R., Scherer, E. A., Norton, G. E., & Budney, A. J. (2015). Clinic- and home-based contingency management plus parent training for adolescent cannabis use disorders. *Journal of the American Academy of Child and Adolescent Psychiatry, 54*(6), 445–453.

Stanton, A., & Grimshaw, G. (2013). Tobacco cessation interventions for young people. *Cochrane Database of Systematic Reviews, 8*, CD003289.

Stanton, M. D., & Shadish, W. R. (1997). Outcome, attrition, and family-couples treatment for drug abuse: A meta-analysis and review of the controlled, comparative studies. *Psychological Bulletin, 122*, 170–191.

Stanton, W. R. (1995). DSM-III-R tobacco dependence and quitting during late adolescence. *Addictive Behaviors, 29*, 595–603.

Steiner, H., Petersen, M. L., Saxena, K., Ford, S., & Matthews, Z. (2003). Divalproex sodium for the treatment of conduct disorder: A randomized controlled clinical trial. *Journal of Clinical Psychiatry, 64*(10), 1183–1191.

Stephens, P. C., Sloboda, Z., Stephens, R. C., Teasdale, B., Grey, S. F., Hawthorne, R. D., & Williams, J. (2009). Universal school-based substance abuse prevention programs: Modeling targeted mediators and outcomes for adolescent cigarette, alcohol and marijuana use. *Drug and Alcohol Dependence, 102*, 19–29.

Stephens, R., Roffman, R. A., & Curtin, L. (2000). Comparison of extended versus brief treatments for marijuana use. *Journal of Consulting and Clinical Psychology, 68*, 898–908.

Sterling, R. C., Dean, J., Weinstein, S. P., Murphy, J., & Gottheil, E. (2004). Gender differences in cue exposure reactivity and 9-month outcome. *Journal of Substance Abuse Treatment, 27*(1), 39–44.

Stitzer, M. L., & Bigelow, G. E. (1978). Contingency management in a methadone maintenance program: Availability of reinforcers. *International Journal of the Addictions, 13*, 737–746.

Stitzer, M. L., Iguchi, M. Y., & Felch, L. J. (1992). Contingent take-home incentive: Effects on drug use of methadone maintenance patients. *Journal of Consulting and Clinical Psychology, 60*, 927–934.

Stitzer, M. L., Iguchi, M. Y., Kidorf, M., & Bigelow, G. E. (1993). Contingency management in methadone treatment: The case for positive incentives. In L. S. Onken, J. D. Blaine, & J. J. Boren (Eds.), *Behavioral treatments for drug abuse and dependence* (pp. 19–36). Rockville, MD: National Institute on Drug Abuse.

Stoléru, S., Fonteille, V., Cornélis, C., Joyal, C., & Moulier, V. (2012). Functional neuroimaging studies of sexual arousal and orgasm in healthy men and women: A review and meta-analysis. *Neuroscience and Biobehavioral Reviews, 36*(6), 1481–1509.

Stolzenberg, L., D'Alessio, S. J., & Dariano, D. (2016). The effect of medical cannabis laws on juvenile cannabis use. *International Journal of Drug Policy, 27*, 82–88.

Strassman, R. J. (1984). Adverse reactions to psychedelic drugs: A review of the literature. *Journal of Nervous and Mental Disease, 172*, 577–595.

Strengthening America's Families. (1999). In *Effective family programs for the prevention of delinquency*. Maintained by the University of Utah, with funding by the Office of Juvenile Justice and Delinquency Prevention.

Stucky, B. D., Edelen, M. O., Vaughan, C. A., Tucker, J. S., & Butler, J. (2014). The psychometric development and initial validation of the DCI-A short form for adolescent therapeutic community treatment process. *Journal of Substance Abuse Treatment, 46*(4), 516–521.

Substance Abuse and Mental Health Administration (SAMHSA). (1997). *Preliminary results from the 1996 National Household Survey on Drug Abuse*. Rockville, MD: U.S. Department of Health and Human Services.

Substance Abuse and Mental Health Administration (SAMHSA). (2000). *National Household Survey on Drug Use and Health*. Rockville, MD: U.S. Department of Health and Human Services.

Substance Abuse and Mental Health Services Administration (SAMHSA). (2002a). *Results from the 2001 National Household Survey on Drug Abuse: Volume 1. Summary of national findings* (Office of Applied Studies, NHSDA Series H-17, DHHS Publication No. SMA 02-3758). Rockville, MD:

Substance Abuse and Mental Health Services Administration (SAMHSA). (2002b). *Emergency department trends from the Drug Abuse Warning Network, Final estimates 1994–2000* (Office of Applied Statistics, DAWN Series D-21, DHHS Publication No. SMA 02-3635. Rockville, MD: U.S. Department of Health and Human Services.

Substance Abuse and Mental Health Services Administration. (2009). *The NSDUH report: Children living with substance-dependent or substance-abusing parents: 2002 to 2007*. Rockville, MD: Substance Abuse and Mental Health Services Administration.

Substance Abuse and Mental Health Services Administration. (2013). *Drug Abuse Warning Network, 2011: Selected tables of national estimates of drug-related emergency department visits*. HHS Publication No. (SMA) 13-4760. DAWN Series D-39. Rockville, MD: Center for Behavioral Health Statistics and Quality, Substance Abuse and Mental Health Services Administration.

Substance Abuse and Mental Health Services Administration. (2014). *Results from the 2013 National Survey on Drug Use and Health: Summary of national findings*. NSDUH Series H-48, HHS Publication SMA 14-4863. Rockville, MD: Substance Abuse and Mental Health Services Administration.

Substance Abuse and Mental Health Services Administration. (2015). *Behavioral health barometer: United States, 2015* (No. SMA-16-2015) (p. 21). Rockville, MD: Substance Abuse and Mental Health Services Administration. Retrieved from http://store.samhsa.gov/shin/content//SMA16-BARO-2015/SMA16-BARO-2015.pdf

Sullivan, P. F., Jiang, Y., Neal, M. C., Kendler, K. S., & Straud, R. E. (2001). Association of the tryptophan hydroxylase gene with smoking initiation but not progression to nicotine dependence. *American Journal of Medical Genetics, 105*(5), 479–484.

Sullivan, P., & Kendler, K. (1999). The genetic epidemiology of smoking. *Nicotine and Tobacco Research, 1*(S), 51–57.

Sung, M., Erkanli, A., & Costello, E. J. (2012). Estimating the causal effect of conduct disorder on the time from first substance use to substance use disorders using g-estimation. *Substance Abuse, 35*(2), 141–146.

Swan, G. E., Carmelli, D., & Cardon, L. R. (1996). The consumption of tobacco, alcohol and coffee in Caucasian male twins: A multivariate genetic analysis. *Journal of Substance Abuse, 8*, 19–31.

Szapocznik, J., & Hervis, O. (2003). *Brief strategic family therapy*. Rockville, MD: National Institute on Drug Abuse. (NIH Pub. No. 03-4751).

Szapocznik, J., Kurtines, W. M., Foote, F. H., PerezVidal, A., & Hervis, O. (1986). Conjoint versus one person family therapy: Some evidence for the effectiveness of conducting family therapy through one person. *Journal of Consulting and Clinical Psychology, 54*, 395–397.

Szapocznik, J., Perez-Vidal, A., Brickman, A. L., Foote, F. H., Santisteban, D. A., Hervis, O., et al. (1988). Engaging adolescent drug abusers and their families in treatment: A strategic structural systems approach. *Journal of Consulting and Clinical Psychology, 56*, 552–557.

Szapocznik, J., Schwartz, S. J., Muir, J. A., & Brown, C. H. (2012). Brief strategic family therapy: An intervention to reduce adolescent risk behavior. *Couple & Family Psychology, 1*(2), 134–145.

Sznitman, S., Dunlop, S., Nalkur, P., & Romer, D. (2012). Student drug testing in the context of positive and negative school climates: Results from a national survey. *Journal of Youth and Adolescence, 41*, 146–155.

Sznitman, S., & Romer, D. (2014). Student drug testing and positive school climates: Testing the effects of two school characteristics on drug use behavior in a national longitudinal study. *Journal of Studies on Alcohol and Drugs, 75*, 1–9.

Szobot, C. M., Rohde, L. A., Bukstein, O., Molina, B. S., Martins, C., Ruaro, P., & Pechansky, F. Is attention-deficit/hyperactivity disorder associated with illicit substance use disorders in male adolescents? A community-based case-control study. *Addiction, 102*(7), 1122–1130.

Szobot, C. M., Rohde, L. A., Katz, B., Ruaro, P., Schaefer, T., Walcher, M., ... Pechansky, F. (2008). A randomized crossover clinical study showing that methylphenidate-SODAS improves attention-deficit/hyperactivity disorder symptoms in adolescents with substance use disorder. *Brazilian Journal of Medical and Biological Research, 41*(3), 250–257.

Takahashi, H. (2013) PET neuroimaging of extrastriatal dopamine receptors and prefrontal cortex functions. *Journal of Physiology Paris, 107*(6), 503–509.

Tamm, L., Trello-Rishel, K. Riggs, P., Nakonezny, P. A., Acosta, M., Bailey, G., & Winhusen, T. (2013). Predictors of treatment response in adolescents with comorbid substance use disorder and attention-deficit/hyperactivity disorder. *Journal of Substance Abuse Treatment, 44*(2), 224–230.

Tapert, S. F. Cheung, E. H., Brown, G. G., Frank, L. R., Paulus, M., Schweinsburg, A. D., Meloy, M. J., & Brown, S. A. (2003). Neural response to alcohol stimuli in adolescents with alcohol use disorder. *Archives of General Psychiatry*, 60(7), 727–735.

Tarter, R. E. (2002). Etiology of adolescent substance abuse: A developmental perspective. *American Journal on Addictions, 11*, 171–191.

Taylor, B., Irving, H. M., Kanteres, F., Room, R., Borges, G., Cherpitel, C., ... Rehm, J. (2010). The more you drink, the harder you fall: A systematic review and meta-analysis of how acute alcohol consumption and injury or collision risk increase together. *Drug and Alcohol Dependence, 110*, 108–116.

Tellier, P. P. (2002). Club drugs: Is it all ecstasy? *Pediatric Annals, 31*, 550–556.

Terry-McElrath, Y. M., O'Malley, P. M., & Johnston, L. D. (2013). Middle and high school drug testing and student illicit drug use: A national study 1998–2011. *Journal of Adolescent Health, 52*, 707–715.

Terry-McElrath, Y. M., O'Malley, P. M., & Johnston, L. D. (2014). Alcohol and marijuana use patterns associated with unsafe driving among U. S. high school seniors: High use frequency, concurrent use, and simultaneous use. *Journal of Studies on Alcohol and Drugs, 75*, 378–389.

Teter, C. J., & Guthrie, S. K. (2001). A comprehensive review of MDMA and GHB: Two common club drugs. *Pharmacotherapy, 21*, 1486–1513.

Thompson, T., & Pickens, R. W. (1971). *Stimulus properties of drugs*. New York: Appleton-CenturyCrofts.

Thorlindsson, T., & Vihjalmsson, R. (1991). Factors related to cigarette smoking and alcohol use among adolescents. *Adolescence, 26*, 399–418.

Thrasher, J. F., Niederdeppe, J., Farrelly, M. C., Davis, K. C., Ribisl, K. M., & Haviland, M. L. (2004). The impact of anti-tobacco industry prevention messages in tobacco producing regions: Evidence from the US Truth campaign. *Tobacco Control, 13*(3), 283–288.

Thurstone, C., Riggs, P. D., Salomonsen-Sautel, S., & Mikulich-Gilbertson, S. K. (2010). Randomized, controlled trial of atomoxetine for attention-deficit/hyperactivity disorder in adolescents with substance use disorder. *Journal of the American Academy of Child and Adolescent Psychiatry, 49*(6), 573–582.

Tims, F. M., Dennis, M. L., Hamilton, N., Buchanan, J. B., Diamond, G., Funk, R., & Brantley, B. (2002). Characteristics and problems of 600 adolescent cannabis abusers in outpatient treatment. *Addiction, 97*(Suppl 1), 46–57.

Tobacco Advisory Group Royal College of Physicians. (2000). *Nicotine addiction in Britain: A report of the Tobacco Advisory Group of the Royal College of Physicians*. London: Royal College of Physicians.

Toumbourou, J. W., Stockwell, T., Neighbors, C., Marlatt, G. A., Sturge, J., & Rehm, J. (2007). Interventions to reduce harm associated with adolescent substance use. *Lancet, 369*, 1391–1401.

Tripodi, S. J. (2009). A comprehensive review: Methodological rigor of studies on residential treatment centers for substance-abusing adolescents. *Journal of Evidence-Based Social Work*, *6*(3), 288–299.

Trudeau, L., Spoth, R., Randall, G. K., & Azevedo, K. (2007). Longitudinal effects of a universal family-focused intervention on growth patterns of adolescent internalizing symptoms and polysubstance use: Gender comparisons. *Journal of Youth and Adolescence*, *36*, 725–740.

True, W. R., Xian, H., Scherrer, J. F., Madden, P., Bucholz, K. K., Heath, A. C., et al. (1999). Common genetic vulnerability for nicotine and alcohol dependence in men. *Archives of General Psychiatry*, *56*, 655–661.

Uhl, G., Blum, K., Noble, E., & Smith, S. (1993). Substance abuse vulnerability and D2 receptor genes. *Trends in Neuroscience*, *16*, 83–86.

Vandenbergh, D. J., Rodriguez, L. A., Miller, I. T., Uhl, G. R., & Lachman, H. M. (1997). High-activity catechol-*O*-methyltransferase allele is more prevalent in polysubstance abusers. *American Journal of Medical Genetics*, *74*, 439–442.

Vandenbergh, D., Bennett, C., Grant, M., Strasser, A., O'Connor, R., Stauffer, R., Vogler, G. P., & Kozlowski, L. T. (2002). Smoking status and the human dopamine transporting variable number of tandem repeats (VNTR) polymorphism: Failure to replicate and finding that never-smokers may be different. *Nicotine and Tobacco Research* 4, 333–340.

Volkow, N. D., Wang, G.-J., Fischman, M. W., Foltin, R. W., Fowler, J. S., Abumrad, N. N., et al. (1997). Relationship between subjective effects of cocaine and dopamine transporter occupancy. *Nature*, *386*(6627), 827–830.

Volkow, N. D., Wang, G. J., Fowler, J. S., & Ding, Y. S. (2005). Imaging the effects of methylphenidate on brain dopamine: New model on its therapeutic actions for attention-deficit/hyperactivity disorder. *Biological Psychiatry*, *57*, 1410–1415.

Zuckerman, M., & Kuhlman, D. M. (2000). Personality and risk-taking: common biosocial factors. *Journal of Personality*, *68*(6), 999–1029.

Part VI: Youth Suicide

American Academy of Pediatrics. (2000). Firearm-related injuries affecting the pediatric population. *Pediatrics*, *105*, 888–895.

American College Health Association. (2016). American College Health Association—National College Health Assessment (ACHA-NCHA) Executive Summary. Available at http://www.acha-ncha.org/docs/NCHA-II%20SPRING%202016%20US%20REFERENCE%20GROUP%20EXECUTIVE%20SUMMARY.pdf

American Foundation for Suicide Prevention and Suicide Prevention Resource Center. (2011). *After a Suicide: A Toolkit for Schools*. Newton, MA.

Apter, A., Plutchik, R., & van Praag, H.M. (1993). Anxiety, impulsivity and depressed mood in relation to suicidal and violent behavior. *Acta Psychiatrica Scandinavica*, *87*, 1–5.

Arango, V., Ernsberger, P., Marzuk, P. M., Chen, J. S., Tierney, H., Stanley, M., et al. (1990). Autoradiographic demonstration of increased serotonin 5HT2 and β-adrenergic receptor binding sites in the brain of suicide victims. *Archives of General Psychiatry*, *47*, 1038–1046.

Arensman, E., Townsend, E., Hawton, K., Bremner, S., Feldman, E., Goldney, R., ... Traskman-Bendz, L. (2001). Psychosocial and pharmacological treatment of patients following deliberate self-harm: The methodological issues involved in evaluating effectiveness. *Suicide & Life-Threatening Behavior*, *31*(2), 169–180.

Arreola, S., Neilands, T., Pollack, L., et al. (2008). Childhood sexual experiences and adult health sequelae among gay and bisexual men: Defining childhood sexual abuse. *Journal of Sex Research*, *45*, 246–252.

Asarnow, J. R., Baraf, L. J., Berk, M., Grob, C.S., Devich-Navaro, M., Suddath, R., ... Tang, L. (2011). An emergency department intervention linking pediatric suicidal patients to follow-up mental health treatment. *Psychiatric Services*, *62*(11), 1303–1309

Åsberg, M., Traksman, L., & Thoren, P. (1976). 5-HIAA in the cerebrospinal fluid. A biochemical suicide predictor? *Archives of General Psychiatry*, *33*, 1193–1197

Aseltine, R., Jacobs, D., Kopans, B., & Bloom, A. (2003, June). *Evaluation of the SOS suicide prevention program.* Presented at the Annenberg Center for Communications and the American Foundation for Suicide Prevention's Youth Suicide Prevention Workshop, New York.

Aseltine, R., James, A., Schilling, E., & Glanovsky, J. (2007). Evaluation of the SOS suicide prevention program: A replication and extension. *BMC Public Health*, *7*, 161–168.

Askland, K. D., Sonnenfeld, N., & Crosby, A. (2003). A public health response to a cluster of suicidal behaviors: Clinical psychiatry, prevention, and community health. *Journal of Psychiatric Practice*, *9*, 219–227.

Azrael, D. (2001). *Risk factors for suicide by children: What can we learn from Child Fatality Review*

Team data? Unpublished doctoral dissertation, Harvard University.

Azrael, D., Miller, M., & Hemenway, D. (2000). Are household firearms stored safely? It depends on whom you ask. *Pediatrics, 10*, E31.

Bailly, D. (2008). Benefits and risks of using antidepressants in children and adolescents. *Expert Opinions Drug Safety, 7*, 9–27

Barbui, C., Campomori, A., D'Avanzo, B., Negri, E., & Garattini, S. (1999). Antidepressant drug use in Italy since the introduction of SSRIs: National trends, regional differences, and impact on suicide rates. *Social Psychiatry and Psychiatric Epidemiology, 34*, 152–156.

Barrish, H. H., Saunders, M., & Wolf, M. M. (1969). Good Behavior Game: Effects of individual contingencies for group consequences on disruptive behavior in classroom 1. *Journal of Applied Behavior Analysis, 2*(2), 119–124.

Battle, A. O., Battle, M. V. & Tolley, E. A. (1993). Potential for suicide and aggression in delinquents at juvenile court in a Southern city. *Suicide and Life-Threatening Behavior, 23*(3), 230–244.

Beautrais, A. L. (2001). Child and young adolescent suicide in New Zealand. *Australian New Zealand Journal of Psychiatry, 35*, 647–653.

Beautrais, A. L. (2004). Further suicidal behavior among medically serious suicide attempters. *Suicide and Life-Threatening Behavior, 34*(1), 1–11.

Beautrais, A. L., Joyce, P. R., & Mulder, R. T. (1996). Risk factors for serious suicide attempts among youths aged 13 through 24 years. *Journal of the American Academy of Child and Adolescent Psychiatry, 35*(9), 1174–1182.

Beautrais, A. L., Joyce, P. R., & Mulder, R. T. (1997). Precipitating factors and life events in serious suicide attempts among youths aged 13 through 24 years. *Journal of the American Academy of Child and Adolescent Psychiatry, 36*(11), 1543–1551.

Benchmark Research and Safety Inc. (2009). Idaho Suicide Prevention Research Project. http://www.healthandwelfare.idaho.gov/Portals/0/Families/Suicide%20Prevention/Suicide%20Prevention%20Programs/CAST_Coping_And_Support_Training.pdf

Best Practice Registry for Suicide Prevention. (n.d.). Suicide Prevention Resource Center. Retrieved August 30, 2013, from http://www.sprc.org/bpr/using-bpr

Birckmayer, J., & Hemenway, D. (2001). Suicide and firearm prevalence: Are youth disproportionately affected? *Suicide and Life-Threatening Behavior, 31*, 303–310.

Bodfish, J. W., Symons, F. J., Parker, D. E., & Lewis, M. H. (2000). Varieties of repetitive behavior in autism: Comparison to mental retardation. *Journal of Autism and Developmental Disorders, 30*, 237–243.

Bongiovi-Garcia, M. E., Merville, J., Almeida, M. G., Burke, A., Ellis, S., Stanley, B. H., & Oquendo, M. A. (2009). Comparison of clinical and research assessments of diagnosis, suicide attempt history and suicidal ideation in major depression. *Journal of Affective Disorders, 115*(1), 183–188.

Brady, S. (2008) The impact of sexual abuse on sexual identity formation in gay men. *Journal of Child Sexual Abuse, 17*, 359–376.

Brain & Behavior Research Foundation. Retrieved Oct. 8, 2014, from https://bbrfoundation.org/brain-matters-discoveries/computerized-screening-tool-for-youth-suicide-risk-coming-soon?utm_source=eNews+List&utm_campaign=cb799b2292-eNews_10_7_2014&utm_medium=email&utm_term=0_fb7d503c0e-cb799b2292-159660645

Brand, E. F., King, C. A., Olson, E., Ghaziuddin, N., & Naylor, M. (1996). Depressed adolescents with a history of sexual abuse: Diagnostic comorbidity and suicidality. *Journal of Child & Adolescent Psychiatry. 35*, 34–41.

Brent, D. A., Baugher, M., Birmaher, B., Kolko, D. J., & Bridge, J. (2000). Compliance with recommendations to remove firearms in families participating in a clinical trial for adolescent depression. *Journal of the American Academy of Child and Adolescent Psychiatry, 39*, 1220–1226.

Brent, D. A., Baugher, M., Bridge, J., Chen, T., & Chiappetta, L. (1999). Age- and sex-related risk factors for adolescent suicide. *Journal of American Academy of Child and Adolescent Psychiatry, 38*, 1497–1505.

Brent, D. A., & Bridge, J. (2003). Firearms availability and suicide. *American Behavioral Scientist, 46*, 1192–1210.

Brent, D. A., Bridge, J., Johnson, B. A., & Connolly, J. (1996). Suicidal behavior runs in families: A controlled family study of adolescent suicide victims. *Archives of General Psychiatry, 53*, 1145–1152.

Brent, D. A., Greenhill, L. L., Compton, S., Emsleie, G., Wells, K., Walkup, J. T., et al. (2009). The Treatment of Adolescent Suicide Attempters study (TASA): Predictors of suicidal events in an open treatment style. *Journal of the American Academy of Child and Adolescent Psychiatry, 48*, 987–996.

Brent, D. A., Holder, D., Kolko, D., Birmaher, B., Baugher, M., Roth, C., et al. (1997). A clinical psychotherapy trial for adolescent depression comparing cognitive, family and supportive therapy. *Archives of General Psychiatry, 54*, 877–885.

Brent, D. A., Johnson, B. A., Perper, J., Connolly, J., Bridge, J., Bartle, S., et al. (1994). Personality disorder, personality traits, impulsive violence, and completed suicide in adolescents. *Journal of American Academy of Child and Adolescent Psychiatry, 33*, 1080–1086.

Brent, D. A., Oquendo, M., Birmaher, B., Greenhill, L., Kolko, D., Stanley, B., et al. (2002). Familial pathways to early-onset suicide attempt: Risk for suicidal behavior in offspring of mood-disordered suicide attempters. *Archives of General Psychiatry, 59*, 801–807.

Brent, D. A., Oquendo, M., Birmaher, B., Greenhill, L., Kolko, D., Stanley, B., et al. (2003). Peripubertal suicide attempts in offspring of suicide attempters with siblings concordant for suicidal behavior. *American Journal of Psychiatry, 160*, 1486–1493.

Brent, D. A., Perper, J. A., Goldstein, C. E., Kolko, D. J., Allan, M. J., Allman, C. J., et al. (1988). Risk factors for adolescent suicide: A comparison of adolescent suicide victims with suicidal inpatients. *Archives of General Psychiatry, 45*(6), 581–588.

Brent, D. A., Perper, J. A., Moritz, G., Allman, C., Friend, A., Roth, C., et al. (1993a). Psychiatric risk factors for adolescent suicide: A case-control study. *Journal of the American Academy of Child and Adolescent Psychiatry*, 32, 521–529.

Brent, D. A., Perper, J. A., Moritz, G., Baugher, M., Roth, C., Balach, L., et al. (1993b). Stressful life events, psychopathology and adolescent suicide: A case control study. *Suicide and Life-Threatening Behavior, 23*, 179–187.

Brent, D. A., Perper, J. A., Mortiz, G. M., Allman, C., Schweers, C., & Roth, C. (1993c). Psychiatric sequale to the loss of an adolescent peer to suicide. *Journal of the American Academy of Child and Adolescent Psychiatry. 32*, 509–517.

Brent, D. A., Perper, J. A., Moritz, G. M., Baugher, M., Schweers, J., & Ross, C. (1993d). Firearms and adolescent suicide: A community case control study. *American Journal of Diseases of Children, 147*, 1066–1071.

Brent, D. A., Perper, J. A., Moritz, G. M., Friend, A., Schweers, J., Allman, C., . . . Balach, L. (1993e). Adolescent witness to a peer suicide. *Journal of the American Academy of Child and Adolescent Psychiatry, 32*, 1184–1188.

Brent, D. A., Perper, J. A., Moritz, G. M., Liotus, L., Schweers, J., Balach, L. et al. (1994). Familial risk factors for adolescent suicide: A case-control study. *Acta Psychiatrica Scandinavica, 89*, 52–58.

Bridge, J. A., Goldstein, T. R., & Brent, D. A. (2006). Adolescent suicide and suicidal behavior. *Journal of Child Psychology and Psychiatry, 47*(3-4), 372–394.

Bridge, J. A., Iyengar, S., Salary, C. B., Barbe, R. P., Birmaher, B., et al. (2007). Clinical response and risk for reported suicidal ideation and suicide attempts in pediatric antidepressant treatment: A meta-analysis of randomized controlled trials. *Journal of the American Medical Association, 297*, 1683–1696.

Brown, M. M., & Grumet, J. G. (2009). School-based suicide prevention with African American youth in an urban setting. *Professional Psychology: Research and Practice, 40*(2), 111.

Byford, S., Harrington, R., Torgerson, D., Kerfoot, M., Dyer, E., Harrington, V., et al. (1999). Cost-effectiveness analysis of a home-based social work intervention for children and adolescents who have deliberately poisoned themselves: Results of a randomized control trial. *British Journal of Psychiatry, 174*, 56–62.

Carlsten, A., Wearen, M., Ekedahl, A., & Ranstam, J. (2001). Antidepressant medication and suicide in Sweden. *Pharmacoepidemiology and Drug Safety, 10*, 525–530.

Centers for Disease Control and Prevention. (1988). CDC recommendations for a postvention and containment of suicide clusters. *Morbidity and Mortality Weekly Report, 37*, 1–12.

Centers for Disease Control and Prevention. *1991–2013 High School Youth Risk Behavior Survey Data*. Accessed June 18, 2014, at http://nccd.cdc.gov/youthonline/

Centers for Disease Control and Prevention. (2013, August). Youth Risk Behavior Survey, System Overview. http://www.cdc.gov/healthyyouth/yrbs/pdf/ system_overview_yrbs.pdf

Centers for Disease Control and Prevention. (2013, August). National Violent Death Reporting System. http://www.cdc.gov/injury/wisqars/fatal_injury_reports.html

Centers for Disease Control and Prevention, National Center for Health Statistics. (2013, August). http://www.nchs.gov

Centers for Disease Control and Prevention, National Center for Injury Prevention and Control. (2014). *Web-based Injury Statistics*

Query and Reporting System (WISQARS). http://webappa.cdc.gov/cgi-bin/broker.exe

Cohen-Sandler, R., Berman, A. L., & King, R. A. (1982). A follow-up study of hospitalized suicidal children. *Journal of the American Academy of Child and Adolescent Psychiatry, 20*, 398–403.

Cornelius, J. R. (2003). *Medication trials with depressed suicidal adolescent substance abusers*. Presented at the Annenberg Center for Communications and the American Foundation for Suicide Prevention's Youth Suicide Prevention Workshop, New York.

Cornelius, J. R., Bukstein, O. G., Birmaher, B., Salloum, I. M., Lynch, K., Pollack, N. K., et al. (2001). Flouxotine in adolescents with major depression and an alcohol use disorder: An open-label trial. *Addictive Behaviors, 26*, 735–739.

Cornelius, J. R., Salloum, I. M., Lynch, K., Clark, D. B., & Mann, J. J. (2001). Treating the substance abusing suicidal patient. In H. Hendin & J. J. Mann (Eds.), *The clinical science of suicide prevention* (pp. 78–93). New York: New York Academy of Sciences.

Courtney, D. B. (2004). Selective serotonin reuptake inhibitor and venlafaxine use in children and adolescents with major depressive disorder: A systematic review of published randomized controlled trials. *Canadian Journal of Psychiatry, 49*, 557–563

Coyne-Beasley, T., McGee, K. S., Johnson, M. R., & Bordley, W. C. (2002). The association of hand-gun ownership and storage practices with safety consciousness. *Archives of Pediatric and Adolescent Medicine, 156*, 763–768.

Coyne-Beasley, T., Schoenbach, V. J., & Johnson, R. M. (2001). Love our kids, lock your guns: A community firearm safety counseling and gun lock distribution program. *Archives of Pediatric and Adolescent Medicine, 155*, 659–664.

Crepeau-Hobson, M. F., & Leech, N. L. (2014). The impact of peer suicidal self-directed violence on youth suicidal behavior: A critical review of the literature. *Suicide & Life-Threatening Behavior, 44*(1), 58–77.

Cummings, P., Grossman, D. C., Rivara, F. P., & Koepsell, T. D. (1997). State gun safe storage laws and child mortality due to firearms. *Journal of the American Medical Association, 278*, 1084–1086.

Currier, G. W., Fisher, S. G., & Caine, E. D. (2010). Mobile crisis team intervention to enhance linkage of discharged suicidal emergency department patients to outpatient psychiatric services: A randomized controlled trial. *Academic Emergency Medicine, 17*(1), 36–43.

Cutler, D. M., Glaeser, E. L. & Norberg, K. E. (2001). Explaining the rise in youth suicide. In J. Gruber (Ed.), *Risky behavior among youths: An economic analysis* (pp. 219–269). Chicago: University of Chicago Press.

D'Augelli, A. R., Grossman, A. H., Salter, N. P., Vasey, J. J., Starks, M. T., & Sinclair, K. O. (2005). Predicting the suicide attempts of lesbian, gay, and bisexual youth. *Suicide and Life-Threatening Behavior, 35*(6), 646–660.

D'Augelli, A. R., Hershberger, S. L., & Pilkington, N. W. (2001). Suicidality patterns and sexual orientation-related factors among lesbian, gay, and bisexual youths. *Suicide and Life-Threatening Behavior, 31*(3), 250–264.

De Leo, D., Dwyer, J., Firman, D., & Neulinger, K. (2003). Trends in hanging and firearm suicide rates in Australia: Substitution of method? *Suicide and Life-Threatening Behavior, 33*, 151–164.

Diamond, G. M., Diamond, G. S., Levy, S., Closs, C., Ladipo, T., & Siqueland, L. (2012). Attachment-based family therapy for suicidal lesbian, gay, and bisexual adolescents: A treatment development study and open trial with preliminary findings. *Psychotherapy, 49*, 62–71.

Diamond, G. S., Reis, B. F., Diamond, G. M., Siqueland, L., & Isaacs, L. (2002). Attachment-based family therapy for depressed adolescents: A treatment development study. *Journal of the American Academy of Child and Adolescent Psychiatry, 41*, 1190–1196.

Diamond, G. S., Wintersteen, M. B., Brown, G. K., Diamond, G. M., Gallop, R., Shelef, K., & Levy, S. (2010). Attachment-based family therapy for adolescents with suicidal ideation: A randomized controlled trial. *Journal of the American Academy of Child and Adolescent Psychiatry, 49*, 122–131.

Dinh-Zarr, T., Diguiseppi, C., Heitman, E., & Roberts, I. (1999). Preventing injuries through interventions for problem drinking: A systematic review of randomized controlled trials. *Alcohol and Alcoholism, 34*, 609–621.

Eggert, L. L., Krakovsky, P. P., & Pike, K. C. (1999). *Washington state youth suicide prevention program: Pathways to enhancing community capacity in preventing youth suicidal behavior, final report*. Seattle: University of Washington School of Nursing.

Eggert, L. L., Thompson, E. A., Herting, J. R., & Nicholas, L. J. (1994). A prevention research program: Reconnecting at-risk youth. *Issues of Mental Heath Nursing, 15*, 107–135.

Eggert, L. L., Thompson, E. A., Herting, J. R., & Nicholas, L. J. (1995). Reducing suicide potential among high-risk youth: Tests of a school-based prevention program. *Suicide and Life-Threatening Behavior, 25*(2), 276–296.

Eisenberg, D., Gollust, S. E., Golberstein, E., & Hefner, J. L. (2007). Prevalence and correlates of depression, anxiety, and suicidality among university students. *American Journal of Orthopsychiatry, 77*(4), 534–542.

Emslie, G. J., Mayes, T., Porta, G., Vitiello, B., Clarke, G., Wagner, K. D., ... Brent D. (2010). Treatment of Resistant Depression in Adolescents (TORDIA): week 24 outcomes. *American Journal of Psychiatry, 167*(7), 782–791.

Emslie, G. J., Waslick, B., Weller, E. B., Kloos, A., Weller, R., & Kratochvil, C. J. (2007). Antidepressant management in context of suicidal ideation. *Journal of the American Academy of Child and Adolescent Psychiatry, 46*, 1222–1225.

Epstein, N. B., Baldin, L. M., & Bishop, D. S. (1983). Family Assessment Device (FAD). George Warren Brown School of Social Work at Washington University in St. Louis. Center for Mental Health Services Research.

Espelage, D. L., & Holt, M. K. (2013). Suicidal ideation and school bullying experiences after controlling for depression and delinquency. *Journal of Adolescent Health, 53*(1), S27–S31.

Farand, L., Chagnon, F., Renaud, J., & Rivard, M. (2004). Completed suicides among Quebec adolescents involved with juvenile justice and child welfare services. *Suicide and Life-Threatening Behavior, 34*(1), 24–35.

Feigelman, W., & Gorman, B. S. (2008). Assessing the effects of peer suicide on youth suicide. *Suicide and Life-Threatening Behavior, 38*(2),181–194.

Fergusson, D. M., Horwood, L. J., & Beautrais, A. L. (1999). Is sexual orientation related to mental health problems and suicidality in young people? *Archives of General Psychiatry, 56*, 876–880.

Fergusson, D. M., Horwood, L. J., & Lynskey, M. T. (1996). Childhood sexual abuse and psychiatric disorder in young adulthood, II. Psychiatric outcomes of childhood sexual abuse. *Journal of the American Academy of Child and Adolescent Psychiatry, 35*, 1365–1374.

Fergusson, D. M., Woodward, L. J., & Horwood, L. J. (2000). Risk factors and life processes associated with the onset of suicidal behavior during adolescence and early adulthood. *Psychological Medicine, 30*, 23–39.

Fleischhaker, C., Böhme, R., Sixt, B., Brück, C., Schneider, C., & Schulz, E. (2011). Dialectical Behavioral Therapy for Adolescents (DBT-A): A clinical trial for patients with suicidal and self-injurious behavior and borderline symptoms with a one-year follow-up. *Child and Adolescent Psychiatry and Mental Health, 5*, 3, http://www.capmh.com/content/5/1/3

Friedman, M. S., Marshal, M. P., Guadamuz, T. E., Wei, C., Wong, C. F., Saewyc, E. M., & Stall, R. (2011). A meta-analysis of disparities in childhood sexual abuse, parental physical abuse, and peer victimization among sexual minority and sexual nonminority individuals. *American Journal of Public Health, 101*, 1481–1494.

Garland, A. F., & Zigler, E. (1993). Adolescent suicide prevention: Current research and social policy implications. *American Psychologist, 48*, 169–182.

Garlow, S. J., Rosenberg, J., Moore, J. D., Haas, A. P., Koestner, B., Hendin, H., & Nemeroff, C. B. (2008). Depression, desperation, and suicidal ideation in college students: Results from the American Foundation for Suicide Prevention College Screening Project at Emory University. *Depression and Anxiety, 25*(6), 482–488.

George, M., Taylor, L., Schmidt, S. C., & Weist, M. D. (2013). A Review of school mental health programs in SAMHSA's national registry of evidence-based programs and practices. *Psychiatric Services, 64*(5), 483–486.

Gibbons, R. D., Brown, C. H., Hur, K., Davis, J. M., & Mann, J. J. (2012). Suicidal thoughts and behavior with antidepressant treatment: Reanalysis of the randomized placebo-controlled studies of fluoxetine and venlafaxine. *Archives of General Psychiatry, 69*, 580–587.

Glowinski, A. L., Bucholz, K. K., Nelson, E. C., Fu, Q., Madden, P. A., Reich, W., & Heath, A. C. (2001). Suicide attempts in an adolescent female twin sample. *Journal of the American Academy of Child & Adolescent Psychiatry, 40*(11), 1300–1307.

Gogtay, N., & Rapoport, J., (2008). Clozapine use in children and adolescents. *Expert Opinion Pharmacotherapy, 9*, 459–465.

Goldsmith, S. K., Pellmar, T. C., Kleinman, A. M, & Bunney, W. E.; National Research Council. (2002). *Reducing suicide: A national imperative*. Washington, DC: National Academies Press.

Goldstein, T. R, Birmaher, B., Axelson, D., Ryan, N. D., Strober, M. A, Gill, M. K., ... Keller M. (2005). History of suicide attempts in pediatric bipolar disorder: Factors associated with increased risk. *Bipolar Disorders, 7*(6), 525–535.

Gonzalez, V. M. (2012). Association of solitary binge drinking and suicidal behavior among emerging adult college students. *Psychology of Addictive Behaviors, 26*(3), 609.

Goode, E. (2003). British warning on antidepressant use for youth. *New York Times*. Retrieved December 11, 2003, from http://www.nytimes.com.

Gould, M. S., Fisher, P., Parides, M., Flory, M., & Shaffer, D. (1996). Psychosocial risk factors of child and adolescent completed suicide. *Archives of General Psychiatry, 53*, 1155–1162.

Gould, M. S., Greenberg, T. E. D., Velting, D. M., & Shaffer, D. (2003). Youth suicide risk and preventive interventions: A review of the past 10 years. *Journal of the American Academy of Child and Adolescent Psychiatry, 42*(4), 386–405.

Gould, M., Jamieson, P., & Romer, D. (2003). Media contagion and suicide among the young. *American Behavioral Scientist, 46*(9), 1269–1284.

Gould, M. S., King, R., Greenwald, S., et al. (1998). Psychopathology associated with suicidal ideation and attempts among children and adolescents. *Journal of the American Academy of Child and Adolescent Psychiatry, 37*, 915–923.

Gould, M. S., Kleinman, M. H., Lake, A. M., Forman, J, & Midle, J. B. (2014). Newspaper coverage of suicide and initiation of suicide clusters in teenagers in the USA, 1988–96: A retrospective, population-based case-control study. *Lancet Psychiatry, 1*(1), 34–43.

Gould, M. S., & Kramer, R. A. (2001). Youth suicide prevention. *Suicide and Life-Threatening Behavior, 31*(Supp. 1), 6–31.

Gould, M. S., Petrie, K., Kleinman, M., & Wallenstein, S. (1994). Clustering of attempted suicide: New Zealand national data. *International Journal of Epidemiology, 23*, 1185–1189.

Gould, M. S., Wallenstein, S., & Davidson, L. (1989). Suicide clusters: A critical review. *Suicide and Life-Threatening Behavior, 19*, 17–27.

Gould, M. S., Wallenstein, S., & Kleinman, M. (1990). Time-space clustering of teenage suicide. *American Journal of Epidemiology, 131*(1), 71–78.

Gould, M. S., Wallenstein, S., Kleinman, M. H., O'Carroll, P., & Mercy, J. (1990). Suicide clusters: An examination of age-specific effects. *American Journal of Public Health, 80*(2), 211–212.

Greenfield, B., Larson, C., Hetchman, L., Rousseau, C., & Platt, R. (2002) A rapid-response outpatient model for reducing hospitalization rates among suicidal adolescents. *Psychiatric Services, 53*, 1574–1579.

Grøholt, B., Ekeberg, Ø., Wichstrom, L., & Haldorsen, T. (1997). Youth suicide in Norway, 1990–1992: A comparison between children and adolescents completing suicide and age- and gender-matched controls. *Suicide and Life-Threatening Behavior, 27*(3), 250–263.

Grøholt, B., Ekeberg, Ø., Wichstrøm, L., & Haldorsen, T. (1998). Suicide among children and younger and older adolescents in Norway: A comparative study. *Journal of the American Academy of Child & Adolescent Psychiatry, 37*(5), 473–481.

Grossman, D. C., Cummings, P., Koepsell, T. D., Marshall, J., D'Ambrosio, L., Thompson, R. S., & Mack, C. (2000). Firearm safety counseling in primary care pediatrics: A randomized controlled trial. *Pediatrics, 106*(1 Pt 1), 22–26.

Grossman, D. C., Mueller, B. A., Riedy, C., Dowd, M. D., Villaveces, A., Prodzinski, J., Nakagawara, J., et al. (2005). Gun storage practices and risk of youth suicide and unintentional firearms injuries. *Journal of the American Medical Association, 293*, 707–714.

Grunbaum, J. A., Kann, I., Kinchen, S. A., Williams, B., Ross, J. G., Lowry, R., et al. (2002). Youth suicide risk behavior surveillance—United States, 2001. *Morbidity and Mortality Weekly Report Surveillance Summary, 51*, 1–64.

Gunnel, D., Middleton, N., Whitley, E., Dorling, D., & Frankel, S. (2003). Why are suicide rates rising in young men but falling in the elderly? A time series analysis of trends in England and Wales, 1959–1998. *Social Science and Medicine, 57*, 595–611.

Guttormsen T., Hoifodt T., Silvola K., & Burkeland O. (2003). Applied suicide intervention: An evaluation. *Tidsskr Nor Laegeforen, 123*(16), 2284–2286.

Haas, A. P., Eliason, M., Mays, V. M., Mathy, R. M., Cochran, S. D., D'Augelli, et al. (2011). Suicide and suicide risk in lesbian, gay, bisexual, and transgender populations: Review and recommendations. *Journal of Homosexuality, 58*(1), 10–51.

Haas, A. P., Hendin, H. M., & Mann, J. J. (2003). Suicide in college students. *American Behavioral Scientist, 46*, 1224–1240.

Haas, A. P., Koestner, B., Rosenberg, J., Moore, D., Garlow, S. J., Sedway, J., ... Nemeroff, C. B. (2008). An interactive web-based method of outreach to college students at risk for suicide. *Journal of American College Health, 57*(1), 15–22.

Hacker, K., Collins, J., Gross-Young, L., Almeida, S., & Burke, N. (2008). Coping with youth suicide and overdose: One community's efforts to investigate, intervene, and prevent suicide contagion. *Crisis, 29*, 86–95.

Hammand, T. A. (2004). Results of analysis of suicidality in pediatric trials of newer antidepressants. Presented at the FDA Center Evaluation and Research (CDER), Bethesda, MD. Retrieved January 5, 2005, from http://www.fda.gov/ohrms/dockets/ac/cder04.html#PsychopharmacologidDrugs

Harrington, R., Kerfoot, M., Dyer, E., McNiven, F., Gill, J., Harrington, V., et al. (1998). Randomized trial of a home-based family intervention for children who have deliberately poisoned themselves. *Journal of the American Academy of Child and Adolescent Psychiatry, 37*, 512–518.

Harrington, R., Kerfoot, M., Dyer, E., McNiven, F., Gill, J., Harrington, V., et al., (2000). Deliberate self-poisoning in adolescence: Why does a brief family intervention work in some cases and not in others? *Journal of Adolescence, 23*, 13–20.

Hatzenbuehler, M. L. (2011). The social environment and suicide attempts in lesbian, gay, and bisexual youth. *Pediatrics, 127*(5), 896–903.

Haw, C., Hawton, K., Niedzwiedz, C., & Platt, S. (2013). Suicide clusters: A review of risk factors and mechanisms. *Suicide & Life-Threatening Behavior, 43*(1), 97–108.

Hawton, K., & Sinclair, J. (2003). The challenge of evaluating the effectiveness of treatments for deliberate self-harm. *Psychological Medicine, 33*, 955–958.

Hayes, L. (2004). *Juvenile suicides in confinement: A national survey* (NCJ 206354). Washington, DC: U.S. Department of Justice, Office of Juvenile Justice and Delinquency Prevention.

Hazell, P., & Lewin, T. (1993). An evaluation of postvention following adolescent suicide. *Suicide and Life-Threatening Behavior, 23*, 101–109.

Hazell, P. L., Martin, G., McGill, K., Kay, T., Wood, A., Trainor, G., & Harrington, R. (2009). Group therapy for repeated deliberate self-harm in adolescents: Failure of replication of a randomized trial. *Journal of the American Academy of Child & Adolescent Psychiatry, 48*, 662–670.

Hjern, A., Vinnerljung, B., & Lindblad, F. (2004). Avoidable mortality among child welfare recipients and intercountry adoptees: A national cohort study. *Journal of Epidemiology and Community Health, 58*(5), 412–417.

Horowitz, J. L., Garber, J., Ciesla, J. A., Young, J. F., & Mufson, L. (2007). Prevention of depressive symptoms in adolescents: A randomized trial of cognitive-behavioral and interpersonal prevention programs. *Journal of Consulting & Clinical Psychology, 75*(5), 693–706.

Hunt, J., & Eisenberg, D. (2010). Mental health problems and help-seeking behavior among college students. *Journal of Adolescent Health, 46*, 3–10.

Husky, M. M., Kaplan, A., McGuire, L., et al. (2011). Identifying adolescents at risk through voluntary school-based mental health screening. *Journal of Adolescence, 34*(3), 505–511.

Insel, B. J., & Gould, M.S. (2008). Impact of modeling on adolescent suicidal behavior. *Psychiatric Clinics of North America, 31*(2), 293–316.

Isacsson, G. (2000). Suicide prevention—a medical breakthrough. *Acta Psychiatrica Scandinavica, 102*, 113–117.

Jessor, R. (1991). Risk behavior in adolescence: A psychosocial framework for understanding and action. *Journal of Adolescent Health, 12*, 597–605.

Joffe, P. (2003). *An empirically supported program to prevent suicide among a college population.* Paper presented at Stetson College of Law, Clearwater Beach, FL.

Joffe, P. (2008). An empirically supported program to prevent suicide in a college student population. *Suicide and Life-Threatening Behavior, 38*, 87–103.

Johnson, B. A., Brent, D. A., Bridge, J., & Connolly, J. (1998). The familial aggregation of adolescent suicide attempts. *Acta Psychiatrica Scandinavica, 97*(1), 18–24.

Johnson, J. G., Cohen, P., Brown, J., Smailes, E. M., & Bernstein, D. P. (1999). Childhood maltreatment increases risk for personality disorders during early adulthood. *Archives of General Psychiatry, 56*(7), 600–606.

Johnson, J. G., Cohen, P., Gould, M. S., Kasen, S., Brown, J., & Brook, J. S. (2002). Childhood adversities, interpersonal difficulties, and risk for suicide attempts during late adolescence and early adulthood. *Archives of General Psychiatry, 59*(8), 741.

Joiner, T. E., Voelz, Z. R., & Rudd, M. D. (2001). For suicidal young adults with comorbid depressive and anxiety disorders, problem-solving treatment may be better than treatment as usual. *Professional Psychology: Research and Practice, 32*(3), 278–282.

Kalafat, J. (2003). Adolescents' views of seeking help from school-based adults. *Prevention Researcher, 10*(4), 10–12.

Kalafat, J., & Elias, M. J. (1995). Suicide prevention in an educational context: Broad and narrow foci. *Suicide and Life-Threatening Behavior, 25*(1), 123–133.

Kalafat, J., Madden, M., Haley, D., & O'Halloran, S. (2007). *Evaluation of Lifelines classes: A component of the school-community based Maine Youth Suicide Prevention Project*. Report for NREPP. Unpublished manuscript.

Kalafat, J., & Ryerson, D. M. (1999). The implementation and institutionalization of a school-based youth suicide prevention program. *Journal of Primary Prevention, 19*, 157–175.

Kaminski, J. W., Puddy, R. W., Hall, D. M., Cashman, S. Y., Crosby, A. E., & Ortega, L. A. (2010). The relative influence of different domains of social connectedness on self-directed violence in adolescence. *Journal of Youth and Adolescence, 39*(5), 460–473.

Kann, L., Olsen, E. O., McManus, T., Harris, W. A., Shanklin, S. L., Flint, K. H., ... Zaza, S. (2016). Sexual identity, sex of sexual contacts, and health-related behaviors among students in grades 9–12—United States and Selected Sites, 2015. *Morbidity and Mortality Weekly Report Surveillance Summary, 65*(9), 1–202.

Karch, D. L., Logan, J., McDaniel, D. D., Floyd, C. F., & Vagi, K. J. (2013) Precipitating circumstances of suicide among youth aged 10–17 years by sex: Data from the National Violent Death Reporting System, 16 states, 2005–2008. *Journal of Adolescent Health, 53*, S51–53.

Katz, L. Y., Cox, B. J., Gunasekara, S., & Miller, A. L. (2004). Feasibility of dialectical behavior therapy for suicidal adolescent inpatients. *Journal of the American Academy of Child and Adolescent Psychiatry, 43*, 276–282.

Kellermann, A. L., Rivara, F. P., Somes, G., Reay, D. T., Francisco, J., Banton, J. G., ... Hackman, B. B. (1992). Suicide in the home in relation to gun ownership. *New England Journal of Medicine, 327*(7), 467–472.

Kerfoot, M. (1988). Deliberate self-poisoning in childhood and early adolescence. *Journal of Child Psychology and Psychiatry, 29*, 335–345.

Kerfoot, M., Dyer, E., Harrington, V., Woodham, A., & Harrington, R. C. (1996). Correlates and short-term course of self-poisoning in adolescents. *British Journal of Psychiatry, 168*, 38–42.

Kerr, M. M., Brent, D. A., & McKain, B. W. (1997). *Postvention standards guidelines: A guide for a school's response in the aftermath of a sudden death* (3rd ed.). Pittsburgh, PA: STAR Center Outreach.

Kessler, R. C., Borges, G., & Walters, E. E. (1999). Prevalence of risk factors for lifetime suicide attempts in the National Comorbidity Survey. *Archives of General Psychiatry, 56*, 617–626.

Kim, Y. S., & Leventhal, B. (2008). Bullying and suicide: A review. *International Journal of Adolescent Medicine and Health, 20*(2), 133–154.

King, C. A. (2003). *Post-hospitalization support program for suicide survivors*. Presented at the Annenberg Center for Communications and the American Foundation of Suicide Prevention's Youth Suicide Prevention Workshop, New York.

King, C. A., Hoevey, J. D., Brand, E., Wilson, R., & Ghaziuddin, N. (1997). Suicidal adolescents after hospitalization: Parent and family impacts on treatment follow-through. *Journal of the American Academy of Child and Adolescent Psychiatry, 36*, 85–93.

King, C. A., Preuss, L., & Krammer, A. (2001). *Youth-Nominated Support Team (YST) for suicidal adolescents*. Poster session presented at the 49th Annual Meeting of the American Academy of Child and Adolescent Psychiatry, Honolulu, HI.

King, M., Semlyen, J., Tai, S. S., Killaspy, H., Osborn, D., Popelyuk, D., & Nazareth, I. (2008). A systematic review of mental disorder, suicide, and deliberate self-harm in lesbian, gay and bisexual people. *BMC Psychiatry, 8*(1), 70.

Klomek, A. B., Sourander, A., & Gould, M. S. (2011). Bullying and suicide. *Psychiatric Times, 28*(2), 27–31.

Kochel, K. P., Ladd, G. W., & Rudolph, K. D. (2012). Longitudinal associations among youth depressive symptoms, peer victimization, and low peer acceptance: An interpersonal process perspective. *Child Development, 83*(2), 637–650.

Kreipe, R. E. (2013). Public health approaches to adolescent health beyond disease and illness. In W. T. O'Donohue, L. T. Benuto, & L. Woodward Tolle (Eds.), *Handbook of adolescent health psychology* (pp. 61–75). New York: Springer.

Kruessi, J. M., Grossman, J., Pennington, J. M., Woodward, P. J., Duda, D., & Hirsch, J. G. (1999). Suicide and violence prevention: Parent education in the emergency department. *Journal of the American Academy of Child and Adolescent Psychiatry, 38*, 250–255.

LaFramboise, T. D., & Howard-Pitney, B. (1995). The Zuni Life Skills Development curriculum: Description and evaluation of a suicide prevention program. *Journal of Counseling Psychology, 42*, 479–486.

LaFromboise, T. D., & Lewis, H. A. (2008). The Zuni Life Skills Development program: A school/community-based suicide prevention intervention. *Suicide and Life-Threatening Behavior, 38*, 343–353.

Lake, A., & Gould, M. (2011). School-based strategies for youth suicide prevention. In R. C. O'Connor, S. Platt, & J. Gordon (Eds)., *International handbook of suicide prevention: Research, policy and practice* (1st ed., pp. 507–529). West Sussex, UK: John Wiley & Sons.

Lake, A. M., & Gould, M.S. (2014) Suicide clusters and suicide contagion. In S. Koslow, P. Ruiz, & C. Nemeroff (Eds.), *A concise guide to understanding suicide: Epidemiology, pathophysiology and prevention* (pp. 52–61). Cambridge, UK: Cambridge University Press.

Lamis, D. A., & Bagge, C. L. (2011). Alcohol involvement and suicidality in college students. In D. A. Lamis & D. Lester (Eds.), *Understanding and preventing college student suicide* (pp. 119–133). Springfield, IL: Charles C. Thomas Publishers.

Lewinsohn, P. M., Rhode, P., & Seeley, J. R. (1993). Psychological characteristics of adolescents with a history of suicide attempts. *Journal of the American Academy of Child and Adolescent Psychiatry*, *32*, 60–68.

Lewinsohn, P. M., Rohde, P., & Seeley, J. R. (1994). Psychosocial risk factors for future adolescent suicide attempts. *Journal of Consulting and Clinical Psychology*, *62*(2), 297.

Lewinsohn, P. M., Rohde, P., & Seeley, J. R. (1996). Adolescent suicidal ideation and attempts: Prevalence, risk factors, and clinical implications. *Clinical Psychology: Science and Practice*, *3*(1), 25–46.

Linehan, M. M., Armstrong, H. E., Suarez, A., Allmon, D., & Heard, H. L. (1991). Cognitive-behavioral treatment of chronically parasuicidal borderline patients. *Archives of General Psychiatry*, *50*, 971–974.

Lubin, G., Werbeloff, N., Halperin, D., Shmushkevitch, M., Weiser, M., & Knobler, H. Y. (2010). Decrease in suicide rates after a change of policy reducing access to firearms in adolescents: A naturalistic epidemiological study. *Suicide and Life-Threatening Behavior*, *40*, 421–424.

Malone, R. P., Delaney, M. A., Leubbert, J. F., Cater, J., & Campbell, M. (2000). A double-blind placebo-controlled study of lithium in hospitalized aggressive children and adolescents with conduct disorder. *Archives of General Psychiatry*, *57*, 649–654

Mandoki, M. W., Tapia, M. R., Tapia, M A., Sumner, G. S., & Parker, J. L. (1997). Venlafaxine in treatment of children and adolescents with major depression. *Psychopharmacology Bulletin*, *33*, 149–154.

Mann, J. J. (2003). Neurobiology of suicidal behavior. *Nature Reviews Neuroscience*, *4*, 819–828.

Mann, J. J., Stanley, M., McBride, P. A., & McEwen, B. S. (1986). Increased serotonin and beta-adrenergic receptor binding in the frontal cortices of suicide victims. *Archives of General Psychiatry*, *43*(10), 954.

March, J., Silva, S., Petrycki, S., Curry, J., Wells, K., Fairbank, J., et al. (2004). Fluoxetine, cognitive behavioral therapy, and their combination for adolescents with depression: Treatment of Adolescents with Depression Study (TADS) randomized controlled trial. *Journal of the American Medical Association*, *292*, 807–820.

Marion, M. S., & Range, L. M. (2003). African American college women's suicide buffers. *Suicide and Life-Threatening Behavior*, *33*(1), 33–43.

Marshal, M. P., Dietz, L. J., Friedman, M. S., Stall, R., Smith, H. A., McGinley, J., ... Brent, D. A. (2011). Suicidality and depression disparities between sexual minority and heterosexual youth: A meta-analytic review. *Journal of Adolescent Health*, *49*(2), 115–123.

Marttunen, M. J., Aro, H. M., Henriksson, M. M., & Lönnqvist, J. K. (1991). Mental disorders in adolescent suicide: DSM-III-R axes I and II diagnoses in suicides among 13- to 19-year-olds in Finland. *Archives of General Psychiatry*, *48*, 834–839.

Marttunen, M. J., Aro, H. M., Henriksson, M. M., & Lönnqvist, J. K. (1994). Psychosocial stressors more common in adolescent suicides with alcohol abuse compared with depressive adolescent suicides. *Journal of the American Academy of Child and Adolescent Psychiatry*, *33*(4), 490–497.

Marttunen, M. J., Aro, H. M., & Lönnqvist, J. K. (1993). Precipitant stressors in adolescent suicide. *Journal of the American Academy of Child and Adolescent Psychiatry*, *32*(6), 1178–1183.

May, P. A., & Van Winkle, N. (1994). Indian adolescent suicide: The epidemiological picture in new Mexico. In C. W. Duclos & M. Manson (Eds.), *Calling from the rim: Suicide behavior among American Indian and Alaska Native adolescents* (pp. 2–23). Boulder: University of Colorado Press.

Mayes, S. D., Gorman, A. A., Hillwig-Garcia, J., & Syed, E. (2013). Suicide ideation and attempts in children with autism. *Research in Autism Spectrum Disorders*, *7*(1), 109–119.

McKeown, R. E., Garrison, C. Z., Cuffe, S. P., Waller, J. L., Jackson, K. L., & Addy, C. L. (1998). Incidence and predictors of suicidal behaviors in a longitudinal sample of young adolescents. *Journal of the American Academy of Child and Adolescent Psychiatry, 37*(6), 612–619.

Middlebrook, D. L., LeMaster, P. L., Beals, J., Novins, D. K., & Manson, S. M. (2001). Suicide prevention in American Indian and Alaska Native communities: A critical review of programs. *Suicide and Life-Threatening Behavior, 31*(Suppl.), 132–149.

Miller, A. L., Rathus, J. H., Linehan, M. M., Wetzler, S., & Leigh, E. (1997). Dialectical behavioral therapy adapted for suicidal adolescents. *Journal of Practical Psychiatry and Behavioral Health, 3*, 78–86.

Miller, D. N., Eckert, T. L., DuPaul, G. J., & White, G. P. (1999). Adolescent suicide prevention: Acceptability of school-based programs among secondary school principals. *Suicide and Life-Threatening Behavior, 29*, 72–85.

Miller, D. N., Eckert, T. L., & Mazza, J. J. (2009). Suicide prevention programs in the schools: A review and public health perspective. *School Psychology Review, 38*(2), 168.

Miller, M., Barber, C., White, R. A., & Azrael, D. (2013). Firearms and suicide in the United States: Is risk independent of underlying suicidal behavior? *American Journal of Epidemiology, 178*(6), 946–955.

Miller, M., Lippmann, S. J., Azrael, D., & Hemenway, D. (2007). Household firearm ownership and rates of suicide across the 50 United States. *Journal of Trauma and Acute Care Surgery, 62*(4), 1029–1035.

Moffit, L.B., Garcia-Williams, A., Berg, J. P., Calderon, M. E., Haas, A. P., & Kaslow, N. J. (2014). Reaching graduate students at risk for suicidal behavior through the interactive screening program, *Journal of College Student Psychotherapy, 28*(1), 23–34.

Moreno, C., Laje, G., Blanco, C., Jiang, H., Schmidt, A. B., & Olfson, M. (2007). National trends in the outpatient diagnosis and treatment of bipolar disorder in youth. *Archives of General Psychiatry*, 64, 1032–1039.

Moskos, M. A., Halbem, S. R., Alder, S., Kim, H., & Gray, D. (2007). Utah Youth Suicide Study: Evidence-based suicide prevention for juvenile offenders. *Journal of Law & Family Studies, 10*, 127–139.

Moutier, C., Norcross, W., Jong, P., Norman, M., Kirby, B., McGuire, T., & Zisook, S. (2012). The Suicide Prevention and Depression Awareness Program at the University of California, San Diego School of Medicine. *Journal of Academic Medicine, 87*(3), 320–326.

Mufson, L., Dorta, K. P., Wickramaratne, P., Nomura, Y., Olfson, M., & Weissman, M. M. (2004). A randomized effectiveness trial of interpersonal psychotherapy for depressed adolescents. *Archives of General Psychiatry, 61*(6), 577–584.

Mustanski, B., & Liu, R. T. (2013). A longitudinal study of predictors of suicide attempts among lesbian, gay, bisexual, and transgender youth. *Archives of Sexual Behavior, 42*(3), 437–448.

National Commission on Correctional Health Care. (2009). Position Statement: Prevention of juvenile suicide in correctional settings. *Journal of Correctional Health Care, 15*, 227–231.

Nemeroff, C. B., Compton, M. T., & Berger, J. (2001). The depressed suicidal patient: Assessment and treatment. *Annals of the New York Academy of Science, 932*, 1–19.

NIMH (Online). Antidepressant medications for children and adolescents: Information for parents and caregivers.

Nock, M. K., Joiner, T. E., Jr, Gordon, K. H., Lloyd-Richardson, E., & Prinstein, M. J. (2006). Non-suicidal self-injury among adolescents: Diagnostic correlates and relation to suicide attempts. *Psychiatry Research, 144*(1), 65–72.

Nock, M. K., & Kessler, R. C. (2006). Prevalence of and risk factors for suicide attempts versus suicide gestures: Analysis of the National Comorbidity Survey. *Journal of Abnormal Psychology, 115*(3), 616.

Nordstrom, P., & Asberg, M. (1992). Suicide risk and serotonin. *International Clinical Psychopharmacology, 6*, 12–21.

Oatis, P. J., Fenn Buderer, N. M., Cummings, P., & Fleitz, R. (1999). Pediatric practice based evaluation of the Steps to Prevent Firearm Injury program. *Injury Prevention, 5*, 48–52.

Olfson, M., Shaffer, D., Marcus, S. C., & Greenberg, T. (2003). Relationship between antidepressant medication treatment and suicide in adolescents. *Archives of General Psychiatry, 60*, 978–982.

Oquendo, M. A., & Mann, J. J. (2000). The biology of impulsivity and suicidality. *Psychiatric Clinics of North America, 23*(1), 11–25.

Oquendo, M. A., Melone, K. M., & Mann, J. J. (1997). Suicide: Risk factors and prevention in refractory major depression. *Depression and Anxiety, 5*, 202–211.

Ostroff, R. B., & Nelson, C. (1999). Risperidone augmentation of selective serotonin reuptake inhibitors in major depression. *Journal of Clinical Psychiatry, 60*, 256–259.

Overholser, J. C., Hemstreet, A., Spirito, A., & Vyse, S. (1989). Suicide awareness programs in the schools: Effects of gender and personal experience. *Journal of the American Academy of Child and Adolescent Psychiatry, 28*, 925–930.

Pandey, G. N. (2002). Higher expression of serotonin 5-ht(2a) receptors in the postmortem brains of teenage suicide victims. *American Journal of Psychiatry, 159*(3), 419–429.

Pandey, G. N., Rizavi, H. S., Ren, X., Dwivedi, Y., & Palkovits, M. (2013). Region-specific alterations in glucocorticoid receptor expression in the postmortem brain of teenage suicide victims. *Psychoneuroendocrinology, 38*(11), 2628–2639.

Papanikolau, K., Richardson, C., Pehlivanidis, A., & Papadopoulou-Diafoti, Z. (2006). Efficacy in antidepressants in child and adolescent depression: A meta-analytic study. *Journal of Neural Transmission, 113*, 399–415.

Pathak, S., Johns, E. S., & Kowatch, R. A. (2005). Adjunctive quetiapine for treatment-resistant adolescent major depressive disorder: A case series. *Journal of Child and Adolescent Psychopharmacology, 4*, 696–702.

Patrick, D. L., Bell, J. F., Huang, J. Y., Lazarakis, N. C., & Edwards, T. C. (2013). Bullying and quality of life in youths perceived as gay, lesbian, or bisexual in Washington State, 2010. *American Journal of Public Health, 103*(7), 1255–1261.

Pearce, C. M., & Martin, G. (1994). Predicting suicide attempts among adolescents. *Acta Psychiatrica Scandinavica, 90*, 324–328.

Pilowsky, D. J., & Wu, L. T. (2006). Psychiatric symptoms and substance use disorders in a nationally representative sample of American adolescents involved with foster care. *Journal of Adolescent Health, 38*(4), 351–358.

Pineda, J., & Dadds, M. R. (2013). Family intervention for adolescents with suicidal behavior: A randomized controlled trial and medication analysis. *Journal of the American Academy of Child and Adolescent Psychiatry, 52*, 851–862.

Pirkis, J., & Blood, R. W. (2001a). Suicide and the media: Part I. Reportage in nonfictional media. *Journal of Crisis Intervention and Suicide Prevention, 22*, 146–154.

Pirkis, J., & Blood, R. W. (2001b). Suicide and the media: Part II. Reportage in fictional media. *Journal of Crisis Intervention and Suicide Prevention, 22*, 152–162.

Ploderal, M., Wagermakers, E. J., Tremblay, P., Ramsay, R., Kravolec, K., et al. (2013). Suicide risk and sexual orientation: A critical review. *Archives of Sexual Behavior, 42*(5), 715–727.

Poijula, S., Wahlberg, K. E., & Dyregrov, A. (2001). Adolescent suicide and suicide contagion in three secondary schools. *International Journal of Emergency Mental Health, 3*(3), 163–168.

Pössel, P., & Hauzinger, M. (2006). Effekte pharmakilogischer und psychotherapeutischer interventionen auf depressionen bei kindern und jugendlichen. *Z Kinder Jugendpsychiatr Psychother 34*, 243–255

Ramsay, R., Cooke, M., & Lang, W. (1990). Alberta's suicide prevention training programs: A retrospective comparison with Rothman's developmental research model. *Suicide and Life-Threatening Behavior, 20*, 335–351.

Randell, B. P (1999). *Promoting CARE: Counselors and parents prevent youth suicide risk*. Bethesda, MD: National Institute of Health, National Institute for Nursing Research.

Randell, B. P., Eggert, L. L., & Pike, K. C. (2001). Immediate post intervention effects of two brief youth suicide prevention interventions. *Suicide & Life-Threatening Behavior, 31*(1), 41–61.

Rathus, J. H., & Miller, A. L. (2002). Dialectical behavior therapy adapted for suicidal adolescents. *Suicide and Life-Threatening Behavior, 32*, 146–157.

Ray, N. (2006). *Lesbian, gay bisexual and transgender youth: An epidemic of homelessness*. New York: National Gay and Lesbian Task Force Policy Institute and the National Coalition for the Homeless.

Remafedi, G., Farrow, J. A., & Deisher, R. W. (1991). Risk factors for attempted suicide in gay and bisexual youth. *Pediatrics, 87*(6), 869–875.

Renaud, J., Berlim, M. T., & Turecki, G. (2010). Sexual orientation and suicide: A comment on Renaud et al response. *Canadian Journal of Psychiatry, 55*(11), 747–747.

Resnick, M. D., Bearman, P. S., Blum, W. R., Bauman, K. E., Harris, K. M., Jones, J., et al. (1997). Protecting adolescents from harm: Findings from the National Longitudinal Study on adolescent health. *Journal of the American Medical Association, 278*, 823–832.

Rew, L., Taylor-Seehafer, M., & Fitzgerald, L. (2001). Sexual abuse, alcohol and other drug use, and suicidal behaviors in homeless adolescents.

Issues in Comprehensive Pediatric Nursing, 24(4), 225–240.

Robinson, J., Cox, G., Malone, A., Williamson, M., Baldwin, G., Fletcher, K., & O'Brien, M. (2013). A systematic review of school-based interventions aimed at preventing, treating, and responding to suicide-related behavior in young people. *Crisis: The Journal of Crisis Intervention and Suicide Prevention, 34*(3), 164.

Rossouw, T. I., & Fonagy, P. (2012). Mentalization-based treatment for self-harm in adolescents: A randomized controlled trial. *Journal of the American Academy of Child and Adolescent Psychiatry, 51*, 1304–1313.

Rotheram-Borus, M. J., Piacentini, J., Cantwell, C., Belin, T. R., & Song, J. (2000). The 18-month impact of an emergency room intervention for adolescent female suicide attempters. *Journal of Consulting and Clinical Psychology, 68*, 1081–1093.

Rotheram-Borus, M. J., Piacentini, J., Van Rossem, R., Graaw, F., Cantwell, C., Castro-Blanco, D., et al. (1996). Enhancing treatment adherence with a specialized emergency room program for adolescent suicide attempters. *Journal of the American Academy of Child and Adolescent Psychiatry, 35*, 654–663

Rotheram-Borus, M. J., & Trautman, P. D. (1988). Hopelessness, depression, and suicidal intent among adolescent suicide attempters. *Journal of the American Academy of Child and Adolescent Psychiatry, 27*(6), 700–704.

Rotheram-Borus, M. J., Trautman, P. D., Dopkins, S. C., & Shrout, P. E. (1990). Cognitive style and pleasant activities among female adolescent suicide attempters. *Journal of Consulting and Clinical Psychology, 58*(5), 554.

Rothman, J. (1980). *Social R & D: Research development in the human services.* Englewood Cliffs, NJ: Prentice-Hall.

Rubenstein, J. L., Halton, A., Kasten, L., Rubin, C., & Stechler, G. (1998). Suicidal behavior in adolescents. *American Journal of Orthopsychiatry, 68*(2), 274–284.

Rubenstein, J. L., Heeren, T., Housman, D., Rubin, C., & Stechler, G. (1989). Suicidal behavior in "normal" adolescents: Risk and protective factors. *American Journal of Orthopsychiatry, 59*(1), 59–71.

Rudd, M. D., Rajab, M. H., Orman, D. T., Stulman, D. A., Joiner, T., & Dixon, W. (1996). Effectiveness of an outpatient intervention targeting suicidal young adults: Preliminary results. *Journal of Consulting and Clinical Psychology, 64*, 179–190.

Russell, S. T., Van Campen, K. S., Hoefle, J. M., & Boor, J. K. (2011). Suicide risk and lesbian, gay, bisexual, and transgender college students. In D. A. Lamis & D. Lester (Eds.), *Understanding and preventing college student suicide* (pp. 146–156). Springfield, IL: Charles C. Thomas.

Ryan, C., Huebner, D., Diaz, R. M., & Sanchez, J. (2009). Family rejection as a predictor of negative health outcomes in white and Latino lesbian, gay, and bisexual young adults. *Pediatrics, 123*(1), 346–352.

Ryan, C., Russell, S. T., Huebner, D., Diaz, R., & Sanchez, J. (2010). Family acceptance in adolescence and the health of LGBT young adults. *Journal of Child and Adolescent Psychiatric Nursing, 23*(4), 205–213.

Saewyc, E., Konishi, C., Rose, H., & Homma, Y. (2014). School-based strategies to reduce suicidal ideation, suicide attempts, and discrimination among sexual minority and heterosexual adolescents in western Canada. *International Journal of Child, Youth & Family Studies, 5*(1), 89–112.

Sakinofsky, I. (2002). Repetition of suicidal behavior. In K. Hawton & K. Van Heering (Eds.), *The international handbook of suicide and attempted suicide* (pp. 385–404). New York: John Wiley & Sons.

Sarchiapone, M., Mandelli, L., Iosue, M., Andrisano, C., & Roy, A. (2011). Controlling access to suicide means. *International Journal of Environmental Research and Public Health, 8*, 4550–4562.

Schmidtke, A., & Schaller, S. (2000). The role of mass media in suicide prevention. In K. Hawton & K. Van Heering (Eds.), *The international handbook of suicide and attempted suicide* (pp. 675–697). New York: John Wiley & Sons.

Schuster, M. A., Franke, T., Bastian, A., Sor, S., & Halfon, N. (2000). Firearm storage patterns in US homes with children. *American Journal of Public Health, 90*, 588–594.

Schwartz, A. J. (2006). College student suicide in the United States: 1990–1991 through 2003–2004. *Journal of American College Health, 54*(6), 341–352.

Schwartz, A. J. (2011). Rate, relative risk, and method of suicide by students at 4-year colleges and universities in the United States, 2004–2005 through 2008–2009. *Suicide and Life-Threatening Behavior, 41*(4), 353–371.

Scott, M. A., Wilcox, H. C., & Schonfeld, I. S. (2009). School-based screening to identify at-risk students not already known to school professionals: The Columbia suicide screen. *American Journal of Public Health, 99*(2), 334–339.

Senturia, Y. D., Christoffeln, K. K., & Donovan, M. (1994). Children's household exposure to guns: A pediatric practice-based survey. *Pediatrics, 93*, 469–475.

Shaffer, D., Fisher, P., Hiscks, R., Pardes, H., & Gould, M. (1995). Sexual orientation in adolescents who commit suicide. *Suicide and Life-Threatening Behavior, 25*, 64–70.

Shaffer, D., Fisher, P., Lucas, C. P., Dulcan, M. K., & Schwab-Stone, M. E. (2000). NIMH Diagnostic Interview Schedule for Children Version IV (NIMH DISC-IV): Description, differences from previous versions, and reliability of some common diagnoses. *Journal of the American Academy of Child and Adolescent Psychiatry, 39*, 28–38.

Shaffer, D., Gould, M.S., Fisher, P., Trautman, P., Moreau, D., Kleinman, M., et al. (1996). Psychiatric diagnosis in child and adolescent suicide. *Archives of General Psychiatry, 53*, 339–348.

Shaffer, D., Scott, M., Wilcox, H. (2004). The Columbia Suicide Screen: Validity and reliability of a screen for youth suicide and depression. *Journal of the American Academy of Child and Adolescent Psychiatry, 43*(1), 71–79.

Shah, S., Hoffman, R. E., Wake, L., & Marine, W. M. (2000). Adolescent suicide and household access to firearms in Colorado: Results of a case-control study. *Journal of Adolescent Health, 26*(3), 157–163.

Sharma, V. (2003). Atypical antipsychotics and suicide in mood and anxiety disorders. *Bipolar Disorders, 5*, 48–52.

Shpigel, M. S., Diamond, G. M., & Diamond, G. S. (2012). Changes in parenting behaviors, attachment, depressive symptoms and suicidal ideation in Attachment-Based Family Therapy for depressive and suicidal adolescents. *Journal of Marital and Family Therapy, 38*, 271–283.

Silverman, A. B., Reinherz, H. Z., & Giaconia, R. M. (1996). The long-term sequelae of child and adolescent abuse: A longitudinal community study. *Child Abuse & Neglect, 20*(8), 709–723.

Silverman, M. M., Meyer, P. M., Sloane, F., Raffel, M., & Pratt, D. M. (1997). The Big Ten Student Suicide Study: A 10-year study of suicides on Midwestern university campuses. *Suicide and Life-Threatening Behavior*, 27(3), 285–303.

Smith, A. R., Silva, C., Covington, D. W., & Joiner, T. E., Jr. (2014). An assessment of suicide-related knowledge and skills smong health professionals. *Health Psychology, 33*(2), 110–119.

Sourander, A., Helstelä, L., Haavisto, A., & Bergroth, L. (2001). Suicidal thoughts and attempts among adolescents: A longitudinal 8-year follow-up study. *Journal of Affective Disorders, 63*(1), 59–66.

Spirito, A. (2003). *Suicide attempters identified in emergency rooms*. Presented at the Annenberg Center for Communications and the American Foundation of Suicide Prevention's Youth Suicide Prevention workshop, New York.

Spirito, A., Boergers, J., Donaldson, D., Bishop, B., & Lewander, W. (2002). An intervention trial to improve adherence to community treatment by adolescents after a suicide attempt. *Journal of the American Academy of Child and Adolescent Psychiatry, 41*, 435–442.

Spirito, A., Brown, L., Overholser, J., & Fritz, G. (1989). Attempted suicide in adolescence: A review and critique of the literature. *Clinical Psychology Review, 9*, 335–363.

Spirito, A., Overholser, J., Ashworth, S., Morgan, J., & Benedict-Drew, C. (1988). Evaluation of a suicide awareness curriculum for high school students. *Journal of the American Academy of Child and Adolescent Psychiatry, 27*, 705–711.

Spirito, A., Plummer, B., Gispert, M., Levy, S., Kurkjian, J., Lewander, W., et al. (1992). Adolescent suicide attempts: Overcomes at follow-up. *American Journal of Orthopsychiatry, 62*, 464–468.

Spitzer, R. L., Kroenke, K., Williams, J. B. L., & the Patient Health Questionnaire Study Group. (1999). Validity and utility of a self-report version of PRIME-MD: The PHQ Primary Care Study. *Journal of the American Medical Association, 282*, 1737–1744.

Spitzer, R. L., Williams, J. B., Kroenke, K., Hornyak, R., McMurray, J., Heartwell, S. F., et al. (2000). Validity and utility of the Patient Health Questionnaire in assessment of 3000 obstetric-gynecology patients: The PRIME-MD Patient Health Questionnaire Obstetric-Gynecology Study. *American Journal of Obstetrics and Gynecology, 183*, 759–769.

Sporn, A. L., Vermani, A., Greenstein, D. K., Bobb, A. J., Spencer, E. P., Clasen, L. S., . . . Gogtay N. (2007). Clozapine treatment of childhood-onset schizophrenia: Evaluation of effectiveness, adverse effects, and long-term outcome. *Journal of the American Academy of Child and Adolescent Psychiatry, 46*, 1349–1356.

Stack, S. (2000). Media impacts on suicide: A quantitative review of 293 findings. *Social Science Quarterly, 81*, 957–971.

Stack, S. (2005). Suicide in the media: A quantitative review of studies based on nonfictional stories. *Suicide & Life-Threatening Behavior, 35*, 121–133.

Stanley, B., Brown, G., Brent, D. A., Wells, K., Poling, K., Curry, J., ... Hughes, J. (2009). Cognitive-Behavioral Therapy for Suicide Prevention (CBT-SP): Treatment model, feasibility, and acceptability. *Journal of the American Academy of Child and Adolescent Psychiatry, 48*, 1005–1013.

Stanley, B., Molcho, A., Stanley, M., Winchel, R., Gameroff, M. J., Parsons, B., & Mann, J. J. (2000). Association of aggressive behavior with altered serotonergic function in patients who are not suicidal. *American Journal of Psychiatry, 157*, 609–614.

Stennies, G., Ikeda, R., Leadbetter, S., Houston, B., & Sacks, J. (1999). Firearm storage practices and children in the home, United States. *Archives of Pediatrics & Adolescent Medicine, 153*, 586–590.

Stewart, S. E., Mansion, I. G., Davidson, S., & Cloutier, P. (2001). Suicidal youth and adolescents with first emergency room presentations: Prediction of six-month outcome. *Journal of American Academy of Child and Adolescent Psychiatry, 40*, 580–587.

Stone, D. M., Luo, F., Ouyang, L., Lippy, C., Hertz, M. F., & Crosby, A. E. (2014). Sexual orientation and suicide ideation, plans, attempts, and medically serious attempts: Evidence from local Youth Risk Behavior Surveys, 2001–2009. *American Journal of Public Health, 104*(2), 262–271.

Substance Abuse and Mental Health Services Administration. (2012). *Preventing suicide: A toolkit for high schools*. HHS Publication No. SMA-12-4669. Rockville, MD: Center for Mental Health Services, Substance Abuse and Mental Health Services Administration, 2012. Development Center, Inc.

Suicide Prevention Resource Center (SPRC) celebrates tenth anniversary. (2012). http://www.sprc.org/directorsblog/suicide-prevention-resource-center-celebrates-tenth-anniversary

Swanson, S. A., & Coleman, I. (2013). Association between exposure to suicide and suicidality outcomes in youth. *Canadian Medical Association Journal,185*(10), 870–877.

Szalacha, L. A. (2003) Safer sexual diversity climates: Lessons learned from an evaluation of Massachusetts' Safe Schools Program for Gay and Lesbian Students. *American Journal of Education* 110, 58–88.

Taurines, R., Gerlach, M., Warnke, A., Thome, J., & Wewetzer, C. (2011). Pharmacotherapy in depressed children and adolescents. *World Journal of Biological Psychiatry 12*, 11–15.

Taylor, L. M. W., Oldershaw, A., Richards, C., Davidson, K., Schmidt, U., & Simic, M. (2011). Development and pilot evaluation of a manualized cognitive-behavioural treatment package for adolescent self-harm. *Behavioural and Cognitive Psychotherapy, 39*, 619–625.

Thompson, E. A. (2003). *Washington state program.* Presented at the Annenberg Center for Communications and The American Foundation for Suicide Prevention's Youth Suicide Prevention Workshop, New York.

Thompson, E. A., & Eggert, L. L. (1999). Using the suicide risk screen to identify suicidal adolescents among potential high school dropouts. *Journal of the American Academy of Child and Adolescent Psychiatry, 38*(12), 1506–1514.

Thompson, E. A., Eggert, L. L., & Herting, J. R. (2000). Mediating effects of an indicated prevention program for reducing youth depression and suicide risk behaviors. *Suicide and Life-Threatening Behavior, 30*(3), 252–271.

Thompson, E. A., Eggert, L. L., Randell, B. P., & Pike, K. C. (2001). Evaluation of indicated suicide risk prevention approaches for potential high school dropouts. *American Journal of Public Health, 91*(5), 742.

Tidemalm, D., Långström, N., Lichtenstein, P., & Runeson, B. (2008). Risk of suicide after suicide attempt according to coexisting psychiatric disorder: Swedish cohort study with long term follow-up. *BMJ, 337*, a2205.

Tierney, R. J. (1994). Suicide intervention training evaluation: A preliminary report. *Crisis, 15*, 70–76.

Tondo, L., Jamison, K. R., & Baldessarini, R. J. (1997). Effect of lithium maintenance on suicidal behavior in major mood disorders. *Annals of the New York Academy of Sciences: Neurobiology of Suicide, 836*, 339–351

Trautman, P., Stewart, M., & Morishima, A. (1993). Are adolescent suicide attempters noncompliant with outcome care? *Journal of American Academy of Child and Adolescent Psychiatry, 32*, 89–94.

Turley, B., & Tanney, B. (1998). *Evaluation report on suicide intervention field trial Australia.* Deakin, Australia: Lifeline Australia, Inc. and LivingWorks Education., Inc.

U.S. Department of Health and Human Services. (2001). *National strategy for suicide prevention: Goals and objectives for action*. Rockville, MD: Public Health Services.

U.S. Department of Health and Human Services, Office of the Surgeon General and National Action Alliance for Suicide Prevention. (2012). *National strategy for suicide prevention: Goals and objectives for action*. Rockville, MD: Public Health Services.

Vitiello, B., Brent, D., Greenhill, L. L., et al. (2009). Depressive symptoms and clinical status during the Treatment of Adolescent Suicide Attempters study (TASA). *Journal of the American Academy of Child and Adolescent Psychiatry, 48*, 997–1004.

Wagner, B. M. (1997). Family risk factors for child and adolescent suicidal behavior. *Psychological Bulletin, 121*, 246–298.

Wagner, B. M., Silverman, M. A., & Martin, C. E. (2003). Family factors in youth suicidal behaviors. *American Behavioral Scientist, 46*, 1171–1191.

Wagner, K. D. (2005). Pharamacotherapy for major depression in children and adolescents. *Progress in Neuropsychopharmacology and Biological Psychiatry, 29*, 819–826.

Walsh, M., & Perry, C. (2000). *Youth Based Suicide Prevention Strategies in a Rural Community, Quesnel, BC: A Community Suicide Prevention Study*. Quesnel, BC.

Walter, G. (2009). *Nessun dorma* ("none shall sleep") ... at least not before we digest Treatment of Adolescent Suicide Attempters (TASA). *Journal of the American Academy of Child and Adolescent Psychiatry, 48*, 977–978.

Wasserman, G. A., & McReynolds, L. S. (2006). Suicide risk at juvenile justice intake. *Suicide and Life-Threatening Behavior, 36*(2), 239–249.

Webster, D. W., Vernick, J. S., Zeoli, A. M., & Manganello, J. A. (2004). Association between youth-focused firearm laws and youth suicides. *Journal of the American Medical Association, 292*(5), 594–601.

Westefeld, J. S., Button, C., Haley, J. T., Kettmann, J. J., MacConnell, J., Sandil, R., & Tallman, B. (2006). College student suicide: A call to action. *Death Studies, 30*, 931–956.

Wichstrøm, L. (2000). Predictors of adolescent suicide attempts: A nationally representative longitudinal study of Norwegian adolescents. *Journal of the American Academy of Child and Adolescent Psychiatry, 39*(5), 603–610.

Wilcox, H. C., Sheppard, K. G., Brown, C. H., Poducka, J., Ialongo, N. S., Wang, W., & Anthony, J. C. (2008). The impact of two universal randomized first- and second-grade classroom interventions on young adult suicide ideation and attempt. *Drug and Alcohol Dependency, 95*(1), 60–73.

Wong, S. S., Zhou, B., Goebert, D., & Hishinuma, E. S. (2013). The risk of adolescent suicide across patterns of drug use: A nationally representative study of high school students in the United States from 1999 to 2009. *Social Psychiatry and Psychiatric Epidemiology, 48*(10), 1611–1620.

Wood, A., Harrington, R., & Moore, A. (1996). Controlled trial of brief cognitive-behavioral intervention in adolescent patients with depressive disorders. *Journal of Child Psychology and Psychiatry, 37*, 737–746

Wood, A., Trainor, G., Rothwell, J., Moore, A., & Harrington, R. (2001). Randomized trial of group therapy of repeated deliberate self-harm adolescents. *Journal of the American Academy of Child and Adolescent Psychiatry, 40*, 1246–1253.

Wunderlich, U., Bronisch, T., & Wittchen, H. U. (1998). Comorbidity patterns in adolescents and young adults with suicide attempts. *European Archives of Psychiatry and Clinical Neuroscience, 248*(2), 87–95.

Wyman, P. A., Brown, C. H., Inman, J., Cross, W., Schmeelk-Cone, K., Guo, J., & Pena, J. B. (2008). Randomized trial of a gatekeeper program for suicide prevention: 1-year impact on secondary school staff. *Journal of Consulting and Clinical Psychology, 76*(1), 104.

Wyman, P. A., Brown, C. H., LoMurray, M., Schmeelk-Cone, K., Petrova, M., Yu, Q., & Wang, W. (2010). An outcome evaluation of the Sources of Strength suicide prevention program delivered by adolescent peer leaders in high schools. *American Journal of Public Health, 100*(9), 1653–1661.

Yoder, K. A., Hoyt, D. R., & Whitbeck, L. B. (1998). Suicidal behavior among homeless and runaway adolescents. *Journal of Youth and Adolescence, 27*(6), 753–771.

Zenere, F. J., III, & Lazarus, P. J. (1997). The decline of youth suicidal behavior in an urban, multicultural public school system following the introduction of a suicide prevention and intervention program. *Suicide and Life-Threatening Behavior, 27*, 387–403.

Zenere, F. J., & Lazarus, P. J. (2009). The sustained reduction of youth suicidal behaviour in an urban, multicultural school district. *School Psychology Review, 38*, 189–199.

Zhang, J., & Jin, S. (1996). Determinants of suicide ideation: A comparison of Chinese and American college students. *Adolescence, 31*, 451–467.

Part VII: Beyond Disorder

Agans, J. P., Champine, R. B., DeSouza, L. M., Mueller, M. K., Johnson, S. K., & Lerner, R. M. (2014). Activity involvement as an ecological asset: Profiles of participation and youth outcomes. *Journal of Youth and Adolescence, 43*, 919–932.

Ainsworth, M. S., Blehar, M. C., Waters, E., & Wall, S. (1978). *Patterns of attachment: A psychological study of the strange situation.* Potomac, MD: Lawrence Erlbaum.

Aknin, L., Barrington-Leigh, C., Dunn, E., Helliwell, J., Biswas-Diener, R., Kemeza, I., ... Norton, M. (2012). Prosocial spending and well-being: Cross-cultural evidence for a psychological universal. *Journal of Personality and Social Psychology, 104*, 635–652.

Albee, G. W. (1982). Preventing psychopathology and promoting human potential. *American Psychologist, 37*, 1043–1050.

Allen, J. P., Porter, M., McFarland, C., McElhaney, K. B., & March, P. (2007). The relation of attachment security to adolescents' paternal and peer relationships, depression, and externalizing behavior. *Child Development, 78*, 1222–1239.

Allen, K., Kern, M. L., Vella-Brodrick, D., Hattie, J., & Waters, L. (in press). What schools need to know about fostering school belonging: A meta-analysis. *Educational Psychology Review.*

Anderson, I. M., Ferrier, I. N., Baldwin, R. C., Cowen, P. J., Howard, L., Lewis, G., ... Tylee, A. (2008). Evidence-based guidelines for treating depressive disorders with antidepressants: A revision of the 2000 British Association for Psychopharmacology guidelines. *Journal of Psychopharmacology, 22*, 343–396.

Appleton, J. J., Christenson, S. L., & Furlong, M. L. (2008). Student engagement with school: Critical conceptual and methodological issues of the construct. *Psychology in the Schools, 45*, 369–386.

Arbeit, M. R., Johnson, S. K., Champine, R. B., Greenman, K. N., Lerner, J. V., & Lerner, R. M. (2014). Profiles of problematic behaviors across adolescence: Covariations with indicators of positive youth development. *Journal of Youth and Adolescence, 43*, 971–990.

Bandura, A. (1989). Human agency in social cognitive theory. *American Psychologist, 14*, 175–184.

Bandura, A. (1993). Perceived self-efficacy in cognitive development and functioning. *Educational Psychologist, 28*, 117–148.

Barasch, M. (1994). Innovative approaches in a community based educational/treatment unit for mentally ill adolescents. *International Journal of Adolescent Medicine and Health, 7*, 11–26.

Baumeister, R. F., Vohs, K. D., Aaker, J. L., & Garbinsky, E. N. (2013). Some key differences between a happy life and a meaningful life. *The Journal of Positive Psychology, 8*, 505–516.

Baumrind, D. (1998). Reflections on character and competence. In A. Colby, J. James, & D. Hart (Eds.), *Competence and character through life* (pp. 1–28). Chicago: University of Chicago Press.

Benard, B. (1991). *Fostering resiliency in kids: Protective factors in the family, school and community.* Western Regional Center for Drug Free Schools and Communities, Far West Laboratory, San Francisco, CA.

Benson, P. (1997). *All kids are our kids.* San Francisco: Jossey-Bass.

Benson, P. L., & Scales, P. C. (2009). The definition and preliminary measurement of thriving in adolescence. *The Journal of Positive Psychology, 4*, 85–104.

Berkowitz, M. W., & Bier, M. C. (2007). What works in character education. *Journal of Research in Character Education, 5*, 29–48.

Birmaher, B., Arbelaez, C., & Brent, D. (2002). Course and outcome of child and adolescent major depressive disorder. *Child and Adolescent Psychiatric Clinics of North America, 111*, 619–638.

Biswas-Diener, R. (2015). A brief history of eudemonia in positive psychology. *Positive Acorn.* Retrieved from https://www.positiveacorn.com/Brief_History_Eudemonia.pdf?

Bond, L. A., & Hauf, A. M. C. (2004). Taking stock and putting stock in primary prevention: Characteristics of effective programs. *Journal of Primary Prevention, 24*, 199–221.

Botvin, G. J. (1998). Preventing adolescent drug abuse through life skills training: Theory, evidence of effectiveness, and implementation issues. In J. Crane (Ed.), *Social programs that work* (pp. 225–257). New York: Russell Sage Foundation.

Botvin, G. J. (2000). Preventing drug abuse in schools: Social and competence enhancement approaches targeting individual-level etiologic factors. *Addictive Behaviors, 25*, 887–897.

Botvin, G. J., Baker, E., Dusenbury, L., Botvin, E. M., & Diaz, T. (1995). Long-term follow-up results of a randomized drug abuse prevention trial in a white middle-class population. *Journal of the American Medical Association, 273*, 1106–1112.

Bowers, E. P., Geldhof, G., Schmid, K. L., Napolitano, C. M., Minor, K., & Lerner, J. V.

(2012). Relationships with important nonparental adults and positive youth development: An examination of youth self-regulatory strengths as mediators. *Research in Human Development, 9,* 298–316.

Bowers, E. P., Johnson, S. K., Buckingham, M. H., Gasca, S., Warren, D. J. A., Lerner, J. V., & Lerner, R. M. (2014). Important non-parental adults and positive youth development across mid to late adolescence: The moderating effect of parenting profiles. *Journal of Youth and Adolescence, 43,* 897–918.

Bowlby, J. (1969). *Attachment and loss, Vol. I. Attachment.* New York: Basic Books.

Bowlby, J. (1973). *Attachment and loss, Vol. II. Separation: Anxiety and anger.* New York: Basic Books.

Bowlby, J. (1980). *Attachment and loss, Vol. III. Loss, sadness, and depression.* New York: Basic Books.

Boyle, P. A., Barnes, L. L., Buchman, A. S., & Bennett, D. A. (2009). Purpose in life is associated with mortality among community-dwelling older persons. *Psychosomatic Medicine, 71,* 574–579.

Brandstädter, J. (1998). Action perspectives on human development. In W. Damon (Series Ed.) & R. Lerner (Vol. Ed.), *Handbook of child psychology: Vol. 1. Theoretical models of human development* (pp. 1029–1144). New York: Wiley.

Bronfenbrenner, U. (1977). Toward an experimental ecology of human development. *American Psychologist, 32,* 513–531.

Bronfenbrenner, U. (1979). *The ecology of human development: Experiments by nature and design.* Cambridge, MA: Harvard University Press.

Bronfenbrenner, U. (1986). Ecology of the family as a context for human development: Research perspectives. *Developmental Psychology, 22,* 723–742.

Bronfenbrenner, U., & Ceci, S. J. (1994). Nature-nurture reconceptualized: A bio-ecological model. *Psychological Review, 101,* 568–586.

Bronk, K. C., Hill, P. L., Lapsley, D. K., Talib, N., & Finch, H. (2009). Purpose, hope, and life satisfaction in three age groups. *The Journal of Positive Psychology, 4,* 500–510.

Brook, J. S., Brook, D. W., Gordon, A. S., Whiteman, M., & Cohen, P. (1990). The psychosocial etiology of adolescent drug use: A family interactional approach. *Genetic, Social, and General Psychology Monographs, 116,* 111–267.

Brophy, J. (1988). Research linking teacher behavior to student achievement: Potential implications for instruction of Chapter 1 students. *Educational Psychologist, 23,* 235–286.

Brophy, J., & Good, T. L. (1986). Teacher behavior and student achievement. In M. C. Wittrock (Ed.), *Handbook of research on teaching* (pp. 328–375). New York: MacMillan.

Burrow, A. L., O'Dell, A. C., & Hill, P. L. (2010). Profiles of a developmental asset: Youth purpose as a context for hope and well-being. *Journal of Youth and Adolescence, 39,* 1265–1273.

Byalin, K., Smith, A., Chatkin, M., & Wilmot, J. (1987). A bridge over troubled waters: An innovative day-treatment program for older adolescents. *International Journal of Partial Hospitalization, 4,* 217–226.

Cacioppo, J. T., Hawley, L. C., & Berntson, G. G. (2003). The anatomy of loneliness. *Current Directions in Psychological Science, 12,* 71–74.

Cameron, K. S., & Caza, A. (2004). Introduction: Contributions to the discipline of positive organizational scholarship. *American Behavioral Scientist, 47,* 731–739.

Cameron, K. S., Dutton, J. E., & Quinn, R. E. (2003). *Positive organizational scholarship: Foundations of a new discipline.* San Francisco: Berrett-Koehler.

Cannon, T. D., Huttunen, M. O., Dahlstrom, M., Larmo, I., Rasanen, P., & Juriloo, A. (2002). Antipsychotic drug treatment in the prodromal phase of schizophrenia. *American Journal of Psychiatry, 159,* 1230–1232.

Caplan, M., Weissberg, R. P., Grober, J. S., Sivo, P. J., Grady, K., & Jacoby, C. (1992). Social competence promotion with inner-city and suburban young adolescents: Effects on social adjustment and alcohol use. *Journal of Consulting and Clinical Psychology, 60,* 56–63.

Carver, C. S., Scheier, M. F., & Segerstrom, S. C. (2010). Optimism. *Clinical Psychology Review, 30,* 879–889.

Casacalenda, N., Perry, C., & Looper, K. (2002). Remission in major depressive disorder: A comparison of pharmacotherapy, psychotherapy, and control conditions. *American Journal of Psychiatry, 159,* 1354–1360.

Catalano, R. F., Berglund, M. L., Ryan, J. A. M., Lonczak, H. S., & Hawkins, J. D. (1999). *Positive youth development in the United States. Research findings on evaluations of the positive youth development programs.* New York: Carnegie Corporation of New York.

Catalano, R. F., Berglund, M. L., Ryan, J. A. M., Lonczak, H. S., & Hawkins, J. D. (2004). Positive youth development in the United States: Research findings on evaluations of positive youth development programs. *Annals of the American Academy of Political and Social Science, 591,* 98–124.

Catalano, R. F., Fagan, A. A., Gavin, L. E., Greenberg, M. T., Irwin, C. E., Jr., Ross, D. A., & Shek, D. T. (2012). Worldwide application of prevention science in adolescent health. *Lancet, 379*(9826), 1653–1664.

Clarke, G. N., Hornbrook, M., Lynch, F., Polen, M., Gale, J., Beardslee, W. R., O'Connor, E., & Seeley, J. (2001). A randomized trial of a group cognitive intervention for preventing depression in adolescent offspring of depressed parents. *Archives of General Psychiatry, 58*, 1127–1134.

Clonan, S. M., Chafouleas, S. M., McDougal, J. L., & Riley-Tillman, T. C. (2004). Positive psychology goes to school: Are we there yet? *Psychology in the Schools, 51*, 101–110.

Cohen, J. (2006) Social, emotional, ethical, and academic education: Creating a climate for learning, participation in democracy, and well-being. *Harvard Educational Review, 76*, 201–237.

Collaborative for Academic, Social, and Emotional Learning (CASEL). (2003). *Safe and sound: An educational leader's guide to social and emotional learning programs*. Chicago, IL: Author. Retrieved from http://casel.org/publications/safe-and-sound-an-educational-leaders-guide-to-evidence-based-sel-programs/

Connell, J. P., Gambone, M. A., & Smith, T. J. (2000). Youth development in community settings: Challenges to our field and our approach. In N. Jaffe (Ed.), *Youth development: Issues, challenges, and directions* (pp. 281–300). Philadelphia: Public/Private Ventures.

Connell, J. P., & Wellborn, J. G. (1991). Competence, autonomy, and relatedness: A motivational analysis of self-system processes. In M. R. Gunnar & L. A. Sroufe (Eds.), *Self processes and development* (Vol. 23, pp. 43–77). Hillsdale, NJ: Lawrence Erlbaum.

Cowen, E. L. (1994). The enhancement of psychological wellness: Challenges and opportunities. *American Journal of Community Psychology, 22*, 149–179.

Csikszentmihalyi, M. (1990). *Flow: The psychology of optimal experience*. New York: HarperCollins.

Dadds, M. R. Holland, D. E., Laurens, K. R. Mullins, M., Barrett, P. M., & Spence, S. H. (1999). Early intervention and prevention of anxiety disorders in children: Results at 2-year follow-up. *Journal of Consulting and Clinical Psychology, 67*, 145–150.

Damon, W. (2004). What is positive youth development? *Annals of the American Academy of Political and Social Science, 591*, 13–24.

Damon, W. (2008). *The path to purpose: Helping our children find their calling in life*. New York: Simon and Schuster.

Davis, C. G., Nolen-Hoeksema, S., & Larson, J. (1998). Making sense of loss and benefiting from the experience: Two construals of meaning. *Journal of Personality and Social Psychology, 75*, 561–574.

Deci, E. L., & Ryan, R. M. (2000). The "what" and "why" of goal pursuits: Human needs and the self-determination of behavior. *Psychological Inquiry, 11*, 227–268.

Deci, E. L., & Ryan, R. M. (2008). Hedonia, eudaimonia, and well-being: An introduction. *Journal of Happiness Studies, 9*, 1–11.

Deci, E. L., & Ryan, R. M. (2011). Levels of analysis, regnant causes of behavior and well-being: The role of psychological needs. *Psychological Inquiry, 22*, 17–22.

deVries, M. W. (Ed.). (1992). *The experience of psychopathology: Investigating mental disorders in their natural settings*. New York: Cambridge University Press.

Diener, E. (1984). Subjective well-being. *Psychological Bulletin, 95*, 542–575.

Diener, E., & Chan, M. Y. (2011). Happy people live longer: Subjective well-being contributes to health and longevity. *Applied Psychology: Health and Well-being, 3*, 1–43.

Diener, E., Emmons, R. A., Larsen, R. J., & Griffin, S. (1985). The satisfaction with life scale. *Journal of Personality Assessment, 49*, 71–75.

Diener, E., Inglehart, R., & Tay, L. (2012). Theory and validity of life satisfaction scales. *Social Indicators Research, 112*, 497–527.

Diener, E., Wirtz, D., Tov, W., Kim-Prieto, C., Choi, D-W., Oishi, S., & Biswas-Diener, R. (2010). New well-being measures: Short scales to assess flourishing and positive and negative feelings. *Social Indicators Research, 97*, 143–156.

Dolan, L., Kellam, S., & Brown, C. H. (1989). *Short-term impact of a mastery learning preventive intervention on early risk behaviors*. Baltimore: Johns Hopkins University.

Dryfoos, J. G. (1990). *Adolescents at risk: Prevalence and prevention*. New York: Oxford University Press.

Duckworth, A. L., Gendler, T. S., & Gross, J. J. (2014). Self-control in school-age children. *Educational Psychologist, 49*, 199–217.

Duckworth, A., & Gross, J. J. (2014). Self-control and grit: Related but separable determinants of success. *Current Directions in Psychological Science, 23*, 319–325.

Duckworth, A. L., & Kern, M. L. (2011). A meta-analysis of the convergent validity of self-control measures. *Journal of Research in Personality, 45*, 259–268.

Duckworth, A. L., Peterson, C., Matthews, M. D., & Kelly, D. R. (2007). Grit: Perseverance and passion for long-term goals. *Journal of Personality and Social Psychology, 92*, 1087–1101.

Duckworth, A. L., & Seligman, M. E. P. (2005). Self-discipline outdoes IQ in predicting academic performance of adolescents. *Psychological Science, 16*, 939–944.

Duke, N. N., Skay, C. L., Pettingell, S. L., & Borowsky, I. W. (2009). From adolescent connections to social capital: Predictors of civic engagement in young adulthood. *Journal of Adolescent Health, 44*, 161–168.

Durlak, J. A. (1997). *Successful prevention programs for children and adolescents*. New York: Plenum.

Durlak, J. A., Weissberg, R. P., Dymnicki, A. B., Taylor, R. D., & Schellinger, K. B. (2011). The impact of enhancing students' social and emotional learning: A meta-analysis of school-based universal interventions. *Child Development, 82*, 405–432.

Durlak, J. A., Weissberg, R. P., & Pachan, M. (2010). A meta-analysis of after-school programs that seek to promote personal and social skills in children and adolescents. *American Journal of Community Psychology, 45*, 294–309.

Dusenbury, L., & Falco, M. (1995). Eleven components of effective drug abuse prevention curricula. *Journal of School Health, 65*, 420–425.

Dweck, C. S. (2006). *Mindset: The new psychology of success*. New York: Ballantine Books.

Dweck, C. S., Walton, G. M., & Cohen, G. L. (2014). *Academic tenacity: Mindsets and skills that promote long-term learning*. Bill & Melinda Gates Foundation. Retrieved from https://web.stanford.edu/~gwalton/home/Welcome_files/DweckWaltonCohen_2014.pdf

Eccles, J. S., & Gootman, J. A. (Eds.). (2002). *Community programs to promote youth development*. Washington, DC: National Academy Press.

Eisenberg, N., Huerta, S., & Edwards, A. (2012). Relation of empathy-related responding to children's and adolescents' social competence. In J. Decety (Ed.), *Empathy: From bench to bedside* (pp. 148–163). Cambridge, MA: MIT Press.

Erickson, J. B. (1999). *Directory of American youth organizations: A guide to 500 clubs, groups, troops, teams, societies, lodges, and more for young people, 1998-1999* (7th ed.). Minneapolis, MN: Free Spirit.

Erickson, L. D., McDonald, S., & Elder, G. H. (2009). Informal mentors and education: Complementary or compensatory resources? *Sociology of Education, 82*(4), 344–367.

Felsman, J. K., & Vaillant, G. E. (1987). Resilient children as adults: A forty-year study. In E. J. Anthony & B. J. Cohler (Eds.), *Invulnerable child* (pp. 289–314). New York: Guilford Press.

Feshbach, N. D., & Feshbach, S. (2009). Empathy and education. In J. Decey & W. Ickes (Eds.), *The social neuroscience of empathy* (pp. 85–98). Cambridge, MA: MIT Press.

Flay, B. R., & Allred, C. G. (2010). The Positive Action program: Improving academics, behavior and character by teaching comprehensive skills for successful learning and living. In T. Lovat & R. Toomey (Eds.), *International handbook on values education and student well-being* (pp. 471–501). Dordrecht: Springer.

Forgeard, M. J. C., Jayawickreme, E., Kern, M. L., & Seligman, M. E. P. (2011). Doing the right thing: Measuring well-being for public policy. *International Journal of Well-Being, 1*, 79–106.

Fox, J. (2008). *Your child's strengths: Discover them, develop them, use them*. New York: Viking.

Fox Eades, J. M. (2008). *Celebrating strengths: Building strengths-based schools*. Coventry: CAPP Press.

Fredrickson, B. L. (2001). The role of positive emotions in positive psychology: The broaden-and-build theory of positive emotions. *American Psychologist, 56*, 218–226.

Fredrickson, B. L. (2013a). Positive emotions broaden and build. In P. Devine & A. Plant (Eds.), *Advances in experimental social psychology* (Vol. 47, pp. 1–54). San Diego, CA: Academic Press.

Fredrickson, B. L. (2013b). *Love 2.0: Creating happiness and health in moments of connection*. New York: Hudson Street Press.

Fredrickson, B. L. (2013c). Updated thinking on positivity ratios. *American Psychologist, 68*, 814–822.

Friedman, H. S. (2000). *The self-healing personality: Why some people achieve health and others succumb to illness*. Lincoln, NE: iUniverse.

Friedman, H. S., & Kern, M. L. (2014). Personality, well-being, and health. *Annual Review of Psychology, 65*, 719–742.

Friedman, H. S., & Martin, L. R. (2011). *The Longevity Project: Surprising discoveries for health and long life from the landmark eight-decade study*. New York: Hudson Street Press.

Froh, J., Yurkewicz, C., & Kashdan, T. (2009). Gratitude and subjective well-being in early adolescence: Examining mechanisms and gender differences. *Journal of Adolescence, 32*, 633–650.

Fruedenberger, H. J., & Carbone, J. (1984). The reentry process of adolescents. *Journal of Psychoactive Drugs, 16*, 95–99.

Gable, S. L., & Haidt, J. (2005). What (and why) is positive psychology. *Review of General Psychology, 9*, 103–110.

Gambone, M. A. (1997). *Launching a resident-driven initiative: Community Change for Youth Development (CCYD) from site-selection to early implementation.* Philadelphia: Public/Private Ventures.

Gardner, H. (1983). *Frames of mind: The theory of multiple intelligences.* New York: Basic Books.

Gavin, L. E., Catalano, R. F., David-Ferdon, C., Gloppen, K. M., & Markham, C. M. (2010). A review of positive youth development programs that promote adolescent sexual and reproductive health. *Journal of Adolescent Health, 46*, S75–S91.

Geldhof, G. J., Bowers, E. P., Mueller, M. K., Napolitano, C. M., Callina, K. S., & Lerner, R. M. (2014). Longitudinal analysis of a very short measures of positive youth development. *Journal of Youth and Adolescence, 43*, 933–949.

Gilham, J. E., Abenavoli, R. M., Brunwasser, S. M., Linkins, M., Reivich, K. J., & Seligman, M. E. P. (2013). Resilience education. In I. Boniwell, S. A. David, & A. C. Ayers (Eds.), *Oxford handbook of happiness*. New York: Oxford University Press.

Gillham, J. E., Jaycox, L. H., Reivich, K. J., Seligman, M. E. P., & Silver, T. (1990). *The Penn Resiliency Program.* Unpublished manual, University of Pennsylvania, Philadelphia.

Gillham, J. E., & Reivich, K. J. (2004). Cultivating optimism in childhood and adolescence. *Annals of the American Academy of Political and Social Science, 591*, 146–163.

Gilligan, C. (1982). *In a different voice: Psychological theory and women's development.* Cambridge, MA: Harvard University Press.

Gilman, R., & Huebner, S. (2003). A review of life satisfaction research with children and adolescents. *School Psychology Quarterly, 18*, 192–205.

Green, S., Oades, L., & Robinson, P. (2011, April). Positive education: Creating flourishing students, staff and schools. *InPsych.* Retrieved from http://www.psychology.org.au/publications/inpsych/2011/april/green

Greenberg, M., Domitrovich, C., & Bumbarger, B. (1999). *Preventing mental disorders in school-age children.* Washington, DC: Center for Mental Health Services, U.S. Department of Health and Human Services.

Greenberg, M. T. & Kusche, C. A. (1998). *Promoting alternative thinking strategies. Blueprint for violence prevention* (Book 10). Institute of Behavioral Sciences, University of Colorado.

Greenberger, E., Chen, C., & Beam, M. R. (1998). The role of "very important" nonparental adults in adolescent development. *Journal of Youth and Adolescence, 27*(3), 321–343.

Guerra, N. G., & Bradshaw, C. P. (2008). Linking the prevention of problem behaviors and positive youth development: Core competencies for positive youth development and risk prevention. In N. G. Guerra & C. P. Bradshaw (Eds.), *Core competencies to prevent problem behaviors and promote positive youth development: New directions for child and adolescent development, 122*, 1–17. Jossey-Bass.

Hahn, A., Leavitt, T., & Aaron, P. (1994). *Evaluation of the Quantum Opportunity Program (QOP): Did the program work?* Waltham, MA: Brandeis University, Heller Graduate School.

Halpern, R., Barker, G., & Mollard, W. (2000). Youth programs as alternatives spaces to be: A study of neighborhood youth programs in Chicago's West Town. *Youth and Society, 31*, 469–506.

Harms, P. D., Herian, M. N., Krasikova, D. V., Vanhove, A., & Lester, P. B. (2013). The Comprehensive Soldier and Family Fitness Program evaluation report #4: Evaluation of resilience training and mental and behavioral health outcomes. U.S. Army Research Facilitation Team. Retrieved from http://www.ppc.sas.upenn.edu/csftechreport4mrt.pdf

Harrigan, S. M., McGorry, P. D., & Krstev, H. (2003). Does treatment delay in first-episode psychosis really matter? *Psychological Medicine, 33*, 97–110.

Hattie, J. M., Neill, J. T., & Richards, G. E. (1997). Adventure education and Outward Bound: Out-of-class experiences that make a lasting difference. *Review of Educational Research, 67*, 43–87.

Hawkins, J. D., Brown, E. C., Oesterle, S., Artuhur, M. W., Abbott, R. D., & Catalano, R.F. (2007). Early effects of Communities That Care on targeted risks and initiation of delinquent behavior and substance use. *Journal of Adolescent Health, 43*, 15–22.

Hawkins, J. D., Catalano, R. F., Kosterman, R., Abbott, R., & Hill, K. G. (1999). Preventing adolescent health-risk behaviors by strengthening protection during childhood. *Archives of Pediatric Adolescent Medicine, 153*, 226–234.

Hawkins, J. D., Catalano, R. F., & Miller, J. Y. (1992). Risk and protective factors for alcohol and other drug problems in adolescence and early adulthood: Implications for substance-abuse prevention. *Psychological Bulletin, 112*, 64–105.

Hawkins, J. D., Catalano, R. F., Morrison, D. M., O'Donnell, J., Abbott, R. D., & Day, L. E. (1992). The Seattle Social Development Project: Effects of the first four years on protective factors and problem behaviors. In J. McCord & R. E. Tremblay (Eds.), *Preventing antisocial behavior: Interventions from birth through adolescence* (pp. 139–161). New York: Guilford Press.

Hawkins, J. D., Kosterman, R., Catalano, R. F., Hill, K. G., & Abbott, R. D. (2008). Effects of social development intervention in childhood fifteen years later. *Archives of Pediatrics & Adolescent Medicine, 162*(12), 1133–1141.

Hawkley, L. C., & Cacioppo, J. T. (2010). Loneliness matters: A theoretical and empirical review of consequences and mechanisms. *Annals of Behavioral Medicine, 40*, 218–227.

Hill, P. L., Burrow, A. L., O'Dell, A. C., & Thornton, M. A. (2011). Classifying adolescents' conceptions of purpose in life. *The Journal of Positive Psychology, 5*, 466–473.

Hill, P. L., & Turiano, N. A. (2014). Purpose in life as a predictor of mortality across adulthood. *Psychological Science,* 25, 1482–1486.

Hoffman, M. L. (1981). Is altruism part of human nature? *Journal of Personality and Social Psychology, 40*, 121–137.

Hogan, M. J. (2008). Modest systems psychology: A neutral complement to positive psychological thinking. *Systems Research & Behavioral Science, 25*, 717–732.

Howell, R., Kern, M. L, & Lyubomirsky, S. (2007). Health benefits: Meta-analytically determining the impact of well-being on objective health outcomes. *Journal of Health Psychology, 13*, 1092–1104.

Hoyt, L. T., Chase-Lansdale, P. L., McDade, T. W., & Adam, E. K. (2012). Positive youth, healthy adults: Does positive well-being in adolescence predict better perceived health and fewer risky behaviors in young adulthood? *Journal of Adolescent Health, 50*, 66–73.

Huebner, E. S. (2004). Research on assessment of life satisfaction of children and adolescents. *Social Indicators Research, 66*, 3–33.

Huebner, E. S., Funk, B. A., I. I. I., & Gilman, R. (2000). Cross-sectional and longitudinal psychosocial correlates of adolescent life satisfaction reports. *Canadian Journal of School Psychology, 16*, 53–64.

Huppert, F. A., & So, T. T. C. (2013). Flourishing across Europe: Application of a new conceptual framework for defining well-being. *Social Indicators Research, 110*, 837–861.

Jensen-Campbell, L. A., Knack, J. M., & Gomez, H. L. (2010). The psychology of nice people. *Social and Personality Psychology Compass, 4*, 1042–1056.

Jessor, R., & Jessor, S. L. (1977). *Problem behavior and psychosocial development: A longitudinal study of youth.* New York: Academic Press.

Joiner, T. J. (2000). Depression's vicious scree: Self-propagating and erosive processes in depression chronicity. *Clinical Psychology: Science and Practice, 72*, 203–218.

Joseph, S., & Linley, P. A. (2005). Positive adjustment to threatening events: An organismic valuing theory of growth through adversity. *Review of General Psychology, 9*, 262–280.

Kern, M. L., Adler, A., Waters, L. E., & White, M. (2015. Measuring whole-school well-being in students and staff. In M. White & S. Murray (Eds.), *Evidence-based approaches in positive education.* Heidelberg: Springer.

Kern, M. L., Duckworth, A. L., Urzue, S. S., Loeber, R., Stouthamer-Loeber, M., & Lynam, D. R. (2013). "Do as you're told": Facets of agreeableness and early outcomes for inner-city boys. *Journal of Research in Personality, 47*, 795–599.

Kern, M. L., & Friedman, H. S. (2008). Do conscientious individuals live longer? A quantitative review. *Health Psychology, 27*, 505–512.

Keyes, C. L. M. (2002). The mental health continuum: From languishing to flourishing in life. *Journal of Health and Social Behavior, 43*, 207–222.

Kohlberg, L. (1963). The development of children's orientations toward a moral order: I. Sequence in the development of moral thought. *Vita Humana, 6*, 11–33.

Kohlberg, L. (1969). Stage and sequence: The cognitive-developmental approach. In D. A. Goslin (Ed.), *Handbook of socialization theory and research* (pp. 347–480). Chicago: Rand McNally.

Kornberg, M. S., & Caplan, G. (1980). Risk factors and preventive intervention in child psychotherapy: A review. *Journal of Primary Prevention, 1*, 71–133.

Kristjánsson, K. (2012). Positive psychology and positive education: Old wine in new bottles? *Educational Psychologist, 47*, 86–105.

Larson, R. W. (2000). Toward a psychology of positive youth development. *American Psychologist, 55*, 170–183.

LaRusso, M., Romer, D., & Selman, R. L. (2007). Teachers as builders of respectful school climates: Implications for adolescent drug use norms and depressive symptoms in high school. *Journal of Youth and Adolescence, 37*, 386–398.

LaRusso, M. D., & Selman, R. L. (2003) The influence of school atmosphere and development on adolescents' perceptions of risks and prevention: Cynicism versus skepticism. In D. Romer (Ed.), *Reducing adolescent risk: Toward an integrated approach* (pp. 113–122). San Francisco: Sage Publications.

Layous, K., & Lyubomirsky, S. (2014). The how, who, what, when, and why of happiness: Mechanisms underlying the success of positive interventions. In J. Gruber & J. Moskowitz (Eds.), *Positive emotion: Integrating the light sides and dark sides* (pp. 473–495). Oxford: Oxford University Press.

Leffert, N., Benson, P. L., Scales, P. C., Sharma, A. R., Drake, D. R., & Blyth, D. A. (1998). Developmental assets: Measurement and prediction of risk behaviors among adolescents. *Applied Developmental Science, 2*, 209–230.

Lerner, J. V., Bowers, E. P., Minor, K., Boyd, M. J., Mueller, M. K., Schmid, K. L., ... Lerner, R. M. (2013). Positive youth development: Processes, philosophies, and programs. In R. M. Lerner, M. A. Easterbrooks, & J. Mistry (Eds.); I. B. Weiner (Editor-in-Chief). *Handbook of psychology: Developmental psychology* (Vol. 6, pp. 365–392). Hoboken, NJ: Wiley.

Lerner, J. V., Phelps, E., Forman, Y., & Bowers, E. P. (2009). Positive youth development. In R. M. Lerner, L. Steinberg, R. M. Lerner, & L. Steinberg (Eds.), *Handbook of adolescent psychology, Vol. 1: Individual bases of adolescent development* (3rd ed., pp. 524–558). Hoboken, NJ: Wiley.

Lerner, R. M., Fisher, C. B., & Weinberg, R. A. (2000). Toward a science for and of the people: Promoting civil society through the application of developmental science. *Child Development, 71*, 11–20.

Lerner, R. M., & Kauffman, M. B. (1985). The concept of development in contextualism. *Developmental Review, 5*, 309–333.

Lerner, R. M., Lerner, J. V., Almerigi, J. Theokas, C., Naudeau, S., Gestsdottir, S., ... von Eye, A. (2005). Positive youth development, participation in community youth development programs, and community contributions of fifth grade adolescents: Findings from the first wave of the 4-H study of positive youth development. *Journal of Early Adolescence, 25*(1), 17–71.

Lerner, R. M., & Steinberg, L. (2009). The scientific study of adolescent development: Historical and contemporary perspectives. In R. M. Lerner & L. Steinberg (Eds.), *Handbook of adolescent psychology* (pp. 3–14). Hoboken, NJ: John Wiley & Sons.

Lerner, R. M., von Eye, A., Lerner, J. V., Lewin-Bizan, S., & Bowers, E. P. (Eds.). (2010). The meaning and measurement of thriving in adolescence: Findings from the 4-H study of positive youth development [Special Issue]. *Journal of Youth and Adolescence, 39*(7), 113–143.

Levitt, A. J., Hogan, T. P., & Bucosky, C. M. (1990). Quality of life in chronically mentally ill patients in day treatment. *Psychological Medicine, 20*, 703–710.

Lewinsohn, P. M., Pettit, J. W., Joiner, T. E., & Seeley, J. R. (2003). The symptomatic expression of major depressive disorder in adolescents and young adults. *Journal of Abnormal Psychology, 112*, 244–252.

Linley, P. A., & Joseph, S. (2004). Positive change following trauma and adversity: A review. *Journal of Traumatic Stress, 17*, 11–21.

Lippman, L. H., Moore, K. A., & McIntosh, H. (2011). Positive indicators of child well-being: A conceptual framework, measures, and methodological issues. *Applied Research in Quality of Life, 6*, 425–449.

Luthar, S. S. (2006). Resilience in development: A synthesis of research across five decades. In D. Cicchetti & D. J. Cohen (Eds.), *Developmental psychopathology: Vol. 3. Risk, disorder, and adaptation* (pp. 739–795). Hoboken, NJ: John Wiley & Sons, Inc.

Luthar, S. S., Cicchetti, D., & Becker, B. (2000). The construct of resilience: A critical evaluation and guidelines for future work. *Child Development, 71*, 543–562.

Lyubomirsky, S., King, L. A., & Diener, E. (2005). The benefits of frequent positive affect: Does happiness lead to success? *Psychological Bulletin, 131*, 803–855

Lyubomirsky, S., Sheldon, K. M., & Schkade, D. (2005). Pursuing happiness: The architecture of sustainable change. *Review of General Psychology, 9*, 111–131

Mariano, J. M., & Going, J. (2011). Youth purpose and positive youth development. *Advances in Child Development and Behavior, 41*, 39–68.

Maslow, A. H. (1970). *Motivation and personality* (2nd ed.). New York: Harper & Row.

Masten, A. S. (2001). Ordinary magic: Resilience processes in development. *American Psychologist, 56*, 227–238.

Masten, A. S. (2011). Resilience in children threatened by extreme adversity: Frameworks for research, practice, and translational synergy. *Development and Psychopathology, 23*, 141–154.

Masten, A. S. (2014). Global perspectives on resilience in children and youth. *Child Development, 85*, 6–20.

Maton, K. I., Schellenbach, C. J., Leadbetter, B. J., & Solarz, A. L. (Eds.) (2003). *Investing in children, youth, families, and communities: Strengths-based research and policy*. Washington, DC: American Psychological Association.

McGorry, P. D., Yung, A. R., Phillips, L. J., Yuen, H. P., Francey, S., Cosgrave, E. M., ... Jackson, H. (2002). Randomized controlled trial of interventions designed to reduce the risk of progression to first-episode psychosis in a clinical sample with subthreshold symptoms. *Archives of General Psychiatry, 59*, 921–928.

McGrath, H., & Noble, T. (2011). *BounceBack! A wellbeing and resilience program* (2nd ed.). Sydney, Australia: Pearson Education.

McGrath, R. E. (2015a). Character strengths in 75 nations: An update. *The Journal of Positive Psychology, 10*, 41–52.

McGrath, R. E. (2015b). Integrating psychological and cultural perspectives on virtue: The hierarchical structure of character strengths. *The Journal of Positive Psychology, 10*(5), 407–424.

Mikulincer, M., & Shaver, P. R. (2012). An attachment perspective on psychopathology. *World Psychiatry, 11*, 11–15.

Mishna, F., Michalski, J., & Cummings, R. (2001). Camps as social work interventions: Returning to our roots. *Social Work with Groups, 24*, 153–171.

Moffitt, T. E., Poulton, R., & Caspi, A. (2013). Lifelong impact of early self-control: Childhood self-discipline predicts adult quality of life. *American Scientist, 101*, 352–359.

Moore, K. A., Lippman, L., & Brown, B. (2004). Indicators of child well-being: The promise for positive youth development. *Annals of the American Academy of Political and Social Science, 591*, 125–145.

Morgan, B., Gulliford, L., & Kristjánsson, K. (2016). A new approach to measuring moral virtues: the multi-component gratitude measure. *Personality and Individual Differences, 107*, 179–189.

Nakamura, J., & Csikszentmihalyi, M. (2009). Flow theory and research. In C. R. Snyder & S. J. Lopez (Eds.), *Oxford handbook of positive psychology* (2nd ed., pp. 195–206). New York: Oxford University Press.

Nation, M., Crusto, C., Wandersman, A., Kumpfer, K. L., Seybolt, D., Morrisey-Kane, E., & Davino, K. (2003). What works in prevention: Principles of effective prevention programs. *American Psychologist, 58*, 449–456.

Neill, A. S. (1960). *Summerhill: A radical approach to child rearing*. New York: Hart.

Nelson, G., Westhues, A., & Macleod, J. (2004). A meta-analysis of longitudinal research on preschool intervention programs for children. *Prevention and Treatment, 6*(31). Retrieved from http://journals.apa.org/prevention/volume6/pre0060031a.html

Newman, R. P., Smith, S. M., & Murphy, R. (2000). A matter of money: The cost and financing of youth development. In N. Jaffe (Ed.), *Youth development: Issues, challenges, and directions* (pp. 81–142). Philadelphia: Public/Private Ventures.

Niemiec, R. (2014). What the research says about character strengths. VIA Institute on Character. Retrieved from https://www.viacharacter.org/www/Research/Character-Strengths-Research-Findings-Summary

Noddings, N. (2003). *Happiness and education*. New York: Cambridge University Press.

Norrish, J. M., Williams, P., O'Connor, M., & Robinson, J. (2013). An applied framework for positive education. *International Journal of Wellbeing, 3*, 147–161.

Park, N. (2004). The role of subjective well-being in positive youth development. *Annals of the American Academy of Political and Social Science, 591*, 25–39.

Park, N., & Peterson, C. (2003). Virtues and organizations. In K. S. Cameron, J. E. Dutton, & R. E. Quinn (Eds.), *Positive organizational scholarship: Foundations of a new discipline* (pp. 33–47). San Francisco: Berrett-Koehler.

Park, N., & Peterson, C. (2004). Early intervention from the perspective of positive psychology. *Prevention and Treatment, 6*(35). Retrieved from http://journals.apa.org/prevention/volume6/pre0060035c.html

Park, N., & Peterson, C. (2006). Moral competence and character strengths among adolescents: The development and validation of the Values in Action Inventory of Strengths for youth. *Journal of Adolescence, 29*, 891–909.

Park, N., & Peterson, C. (2009). Strengths of character in schools. In R. Gilman, E. S. Huebner, & M. J. Furlong (Eds.), *Handbook of positive psychology in the schools: Promoting wellness in children and youth* (pp. 65–76). Mahwah, NJ: Erlbaum.

Parks, A. C., & Biswas-Diener, R. (2013). Positive interventions: Past, present and future. In T. Kashdan & J. Ciarrochi (Eds.), *Mindfulness, acceptance and positive psychology: The seven foundations of well-being*. Oakland, CA: Context Press.

Peterson, C. (2006). *Primer in positive psychology*. New York: Oxford University Press.

Peterson, C., Park, N., & Seligman, M. E. (2006). Greater strengths of character and recovery from illness. *The Journal of Positive Psychology, 1*, 17–26.

Peterson, C., & Seligman, M. E. P. (2004). *Character strengths and virtues: A handbook and classification*. New York: Oxford University Press/Washington, DC: American Psychological Association.

Phelps, E., Balsano, A. B., Fay, K., Peltz, J. S., Zimmerman, S. M., Lerner, R. M., & Lerner, J. V. (2007). Nuances in early adolescent developmental trajectories of positive and problematic/risk behaviors: Findings from the 4-H study of positive youth development. *Child and Adolescent Psychiatric Clinics of North America, 16*, 473–496.

Phillips, L. J., Yung, A. R., Yuen, H. P., Pantelis, C., & McGorry, P. D. (2002). Prediction and prevention of transition to psychosis in young people at incipient risk for schizophrenia. *American Journal of Medical Genetics, 114*, 929–937.

Piaget, J. (1965). *The moral judgment of the child*. New York: Free Press.

Pittman, K. J. (1991). *Promoting youth development: Strengthening the role of youth-serving and community organizations*. Washington, DC: U. S. Department of Agriculture Extension Services.

Pittman, K. J. (2000, May 2). *What youth need: Services, supports, and opportunities, the ingredients for youth*. Paper prepared for presentation at the White House Conference on Teenagers, Washington, DC.

Pittman, K., Irby, M., & Ferber, T. (2001). Unfinished business: Further reflections on a decade of promoting youth development. In P. L. Benson & K. J. Pittman (Eds.), *Trends in youth development: Visions, realities and challenges* (pp. 4–50). Norwell, MA: Kluwer.

Pollard, J. A., Hawkins, J. D., & Arthur, M. W. (1999). Risk and protection: Are both necessary to understand diverse behavioral outcomes in adolescence? *Social Work Research, 23*, 145–158.

Poortinga, W. (2012). Community resilience and health: The role of bonding, bridging, and linking aspects of social capital. *Health & Place, 18*, 286–295.

Pressman, S. D., & Cohen, S. (2005). Does positive affect influence health? *Psychological Bulletin, 131*, 925–971.

Proctor, C., Tsukayama, E., Wood, A., M., Maltby, J., Fox Eades, J., & Linley, P. A. (2011). Strengths Gym: The impact of a character strengths-based intervention on the life satisfaction and well-being of adolescents. *The Journal of Positive Psychology, 6* (5), 377–388.

Ranson, K. E., & Urichuk, L. J. (2008). The effect of parent-child attachment relationships on child biopsychosocial outcomes: A review. *Early Child Development and Care, 178*, 129–152.

Rashid, T. (2015). Positive psychotherapy: A strength-based approach. *The Journal of Positive Psychology, 10*, 25–40.

Rathunde, K. R., & Csikszentmihalyi, M. (1993). Undivided interest and the growth of talent: A longitudinal study of adolescents. *Journal of Youth and Adolescence, 22*, 385–405.

Reivich, K. J., Seligman, M. E. P., & McBride, S. (2011). Master resilience training in the U.S. Army. *American Psychologist, 66*, 25–34.

Rey, R. A., Valero, A. P. B., Paniello, S. H., & Monge, M del M. S. (2012). *The "Happy Classrooms" programme: Positive psychology applied to education*. Zaragosa, Spain: SATI.

Rhodes, J. E. (2014). Invited commentary: Improving the human condition through rigorous, applied developmental research. *Journal of Youth and Adolescence, 43*, 1025–1026.

Rhodes, J. E., Ebert, L., & Fischer, K. (1992). Natural mentors: An overlooked resource in the social networks of young, African American mothers. *American Journal of Community Psychology, 20*(4), 445–461.

Roberts, B. W., Kuncel, N., Shiner, R. N., Caspi, A., & Goldberg, L. R. (2007). The power of personality: The comparative validity of personality traits, socio-economic status, and cognitive ability for predicting important life outcomes. *Perspectives in Psychological Science, 2*, 313–345.

Roberts, B. W., Lejuez, C., Krueger, R. F., Richards, J. M., & Hill, P. L. (2014). What is conscientiousness and how can it be assessed? *Developmental Psychology, 50*, 1315–1330.

Rogers, C. R. (1951). *Client-centered therapy: Its current practice, implications, and theory*. Boston: Houghton Mifflin.

Romer, D. (2003). *Reducing adolescent risk: Toward an integrated approach*. Thousand Oaks, CA: Sage Publications.

Roth, J., & Brooks-Gunn, J. (2003). Youth development programs: Risk, prevention, and policy. *Journal of Adolescent Health*, *32*, 170–182.

Roth, J., Brooks-Gunn, J., Murray, L., & Foster, W. (1998). Promoting healthy adolescents: Synthesis of youth development program evaluations. *Journal of Research on Adolescence*, *8*, 423–459.

Roth, J. L., Malone, L. M., & Brooks-Gunn, J. (2010). Does the amount of participation in afterschool programs relate to developmental outcomes? A review of the literature. *American Journal of Community Psychology*, *45*, 310–324.

Rothbart, M. K., & Posner, M. I. (2006). Temperament, attention, and developmental psychopathology. In D. Cicchetti & D. Cohen (Eds.), *Developmental psychopathology: Vol. 2. Developmental neuroscience* (2nd ed., pp. 465–501). New York: Wiley.

Rund, B. R., Moe, L., Sollien, T., Fjell, A., Borchgrevink, T., Hallert, M., & Naess, P. O. (1994). The Psychosis Project: Outcome and cost-effectiveness of a psychoeducational treatment program for schizophrenic adolescents. *Acta Psychiatrica Scandinavica*, *89*, 211–218.

Rusk, R. D., & Waters, L. E. (2013). Tracing the size, reach, impact, and breadth of positive psychology. *The Journal of Positive Psychology*, *8*, 207–221.

Ryff, C. D., & Keyes, C. L. M. (1995). The structure of psychological well-being revisited. *Journal of Personality and Social Psychology*, *69*, 719–727.

Scales, C., Benson, P. L., Leffert, N., & Blyth, D. A. (2000). Contribution of developmental assets to the prediction of thriving among adolescents. *Applied Developmental Science*, *4*, 27–46.

Schneider, B. H., Atkinson, L., & Tardif, C. (2001). Child-parent attachment and children's peer relations: A quantitative review. *Developmental Psychology*, *37*, 86–100.

Seivewright, H., Tyrer, P., & Johnson, T. (1998). Prediction of outcome in neurotic disorder: A 5-year prospective study. *Psychological Medicine*, *28*, 1149–1157.

Seligman, M. E. P. (2011). *Flourish*. New York: Simon & Schuster.

Seligman, M. E. P., & Csikszentmihalyi, M. (2000). Positive psychology: An introduction. *American Psychologist*, *55*, 5–14.

Seligman, M. E. P., Ernst, R. M., Gillham, J., Reivich, K., & Linkins, M. (2009). Positive education: Positive psychology and classroom interventions. *Oxford Review of Education*, *35*, 293–311.

Seligman, M. E. P., Rashid, T., & Parks, A. C. (2006). Positive psychotherapy. *American Psychologist*, *61*, 774–788.

Seligman, M. E. P., Steen, T. A., Park, N., & Peterson, C. (2005). Positive psychology progress: Empirical validation of interventions. *American Psychologist*, *60*, 410–421.

Shih, M. (2004). Positive stigma: Examining resilience and empowerment in overcoming stigma. *Annals of the American Academy of Political and Social Science*, *591*, 175–185.

Shoshani, A., & Slone, M. (2013). Middle school transition from the strengths perspective: Young adolescents' character strengths, subjective well-being, and school adjustment. *Journal of Happiness Studies*, *14*, 1163–1181.

Sin, N. L., & Lyubomirsky, S. (2009). Enhancing well-being and alleviating depressive symptoms with positive psychology interventions: A practice-friendly meta-analysis. *Journal of Clinical Psychology*, *65*, 467–487.

Snyder, C. R. (1994). *The psychology of hope: You can get there from here*. New York: Free Press.

Snyder, H., & Sickmund, M. (1999). *Juvenile offenders and victims: 1999 national report*. Washington, DC: Office Juvenile Justice and Delinquency Prevention.

Snyder, M., Schactman, L., & Young, S. (2015). Three dimensions of recovery within a recovery model oriented therapeutic community. *Psychiatric Quarterly*, *86*, 123–136.

Social and Character Development Research Consortium. (2010). *Efficacy of schoolwide programs to promote social and character development and reduce problem behavior in elementary school children* (NCER 2011–2001). Washington, DC: National Center for Education Research, Institute of Education Sciences, U.S. Department of Education.

Solomon, D., Battistich, V., Watson, M., Schaps, E., & Lewis, C. (2000). A six-district study of educational change: Direct and mediated effects of the Child Development Project. *Social Psychology of Education*, *4*, 3–51.

Spooner, C., Mattick, R. P., & Noffs, (2001). Outcomes of a comprehensive treatment program for adolescents with a substance-use disorder. *Journal of Substance Abuse Treatment*, *20*, 205–213.

Sroufe, L. A. (1997). Psychopathology as an outcome of development. *Development & Psychopathology*, *9*, 251–268.

Steger, M. F. (2012). Making meaning in life. *Psychological Inquiry*, *23*, 381–385.

Steger, M. F., Oishi, S., & Kashdan, T. B. (2009). Meaning in life across the life span: Levels and correlates of meaning in life from emerging adulthood to older adulthood. *The Journal of Positive Psychology, 4*, 43–52.

Steinbrueck, S. M., Maxwell, S. E., & Howard, G. S. (1983). A meta-analysis of psychotherapy and drug therapy in the treatment of unipolar depression with adults. *Journal of Consulting and Clinical Psychology, 51*, 856–863.

Sternberg, R. J. (1985). *Beyond IQ: A triarchic theory of human intelligence*. Cambridge: Cambridge University Press.

Stice, E., & Shaw, H. (2004). Eating disorder prevention programs: A meta-analytic review. *Psychological Bulletin, 130*, 206–227.

Taylor, S. E. (2011). Social support: A review. In H. S. Friedman (Ed.), *Oxford handbook of health psychology*. (pp. 189–214). New York: Oxford University Press.

Theokas, C., & Lerner, R. M. (2006). Promoting positive development in adolescence: The role of ecological assets in families, schools, and neighborhoods. *Applied Developmental Science, 10*, 61–74.

Tierney, J. P., & Grossman, J. B. (2000). *Making a difference: An impact study of Big Brothers/Big Sisters*. Philadelphia: Public/Private Ventures.

Toner, E., Haslam, N., Robinson, J., & Williams, P. (2012). Character strengths and wellbeing in adolescence: Structure and correlates of the Values in Action Inventory of Strengths for Children. *Personality and Individual Differences, 52*(5), 637–642.

Torney-Purta, J., Richardson, W. K., & Barber, C. H. (2004). *Trust in government-related institutions and civic engagement among adolescents: Analysis of five countries from the IEA Civic Education Study*. College Park, MD: Center for Information & Research on Civic Learning & Engagement (CIRCLE).

Tugade, M. M., Fredrickson, B. L., & Feldman Barrett, L. (2004). Psychological resilience and positive emotional granularity: Examining the benefits of positive emotions on coping and health. *Journal of Personality, 72*, 1161–1190.

Vaillant, G. E. (2012). *Triumphs of experience: The men of the Harvard Grant Study*. Cambridge, MA: Belknap.

Valle, M. F., Huebner, E. S., & Suldo, S. M. (2006). An analysis of hope as a psychological strength. *Journal of School Psychology, 44*, 393–406.

Walker, G. (2001). *The policy climate for early adolescent initiatives. P/PV Briefs*. Philadelphia, PA: Public/Private Ventures.

Wang, M.-T. (2009). School climate support for behavioral and psychological adjustment: Testing the mediating effect of social competence. *School Psychology Quarterly, 24*, 240–251.

Waters, L. E. (2011). A review of school-based positive psychology interventions. *Australian Educational and Developmental Psychologist, 28*, 75–90.

Waters, L., & White, M. (2015). Case study of a school wellbeing initative: Using appreciative inquiry to support positive change. *International Journal of Wellbeing, 5*, 19–32.

Weber, M., & Ruch, W. (2012). The role of a good character in 12-year-old school children: Do character strengths matter in the classroom? *Child Indicators Research, 5* (2), 317–334.

Weissberg, R. P., Caplan, M. Z., & Sivo, P. J. (1989). A new conceptual framework for establishing school-based social competence promotion programs. In L. A. Bond & B. E. Compas (Eds.), *Primary prevention and promotion in the schools* (pp. 255–296). Newbury Park, CA: Sage.

Weissberg, R. P., & Greenberg, M. T. (1997). School and community competence-enhancement and prevention programs. In W. Damon (Ed.), *Handbook of child psychology* (pp. 877–954). New York: John Wiley & Sons.

Weissman, M. M. (1994). Psychotherapy in the maintenance treatment of depression. *British Journal of Psychiatry, 51*, 42–50.

Weissman, M. M., Wolk, S., Goldstein, R. B., Moreau, D., Adams, P., Greenwald, S., ... Wickramaratne, P. (1999). Depressed adolescents grown up. *Journal of the American Medical Association, 281*, 1707–1713.

Werner, E. E. (1982). *Vulnerable but invincible: A longitudinal study of resilient children and youth*. New York: McGraw-Hill.

Werner, E., & Smith, R. (2001). *Journeys from childhood to midlife. Risk, resilience, and recovery*. Ithaca, NY: Cornell University Press.

White, M. A., & Waters, L. E. (2015). A case study of "the good school": Examples of the use of Peterson's strengths-based approach with students. *The Journal of Positive Psychology, 10*(1), 69–76.

Winner, E. (2000). The origins and ends of giftedness. *American Psychologist, 55*, 159–169.

Wood, A. M., Froh, J. J., & Garaghty, A. W. A. (2010). Gratitude and well-being: A review and theoretical integration. *Clinical Psychology Review, 30*, 890–905.

World Health Organization. (1946). *Preamble to the Constitution of the World Health Organization as adopted by the International Health Conference.* New York, June 19–22, 1946.

Yeager, J. M., Fisher, S. W., & Shearon, D. N. (2011). *SMART strengths. Building character, resilience and relationships in youth.* New York: Kravis Publishing.

Zigler, E., & Berman, W. (1983). Discerning the future of early childhood intervention. *American Psychologist, 38*, 894–906.

Zimmerman, M. A., Bingenheimer, J. B., & Notaro, P. C. (2002). Natural mentors and adolescent resiliency: A study with urban youth. *American Journal of Community Psychology, 30*(2), 221–243.

Part VIII: Other Behavioral Disorders

Abbott, M. W., & Volberg, R. A. (2000). *Taking the pulse on gambling and problem gambling in New Zealand: Phase One of the 1999 National Prevalence Study. Report Number Three of the New Zealand Gaming Survey.* Wellington: Department of Internal Affairs.

Abbott, M. W., & Volberg, R. A., Bellringer, M., & Reith, G. (2004). *A review of research on aspects of problem gambling: Final report.* Prepared for the Responsibility in Gambling Trust, London.

Ariyabuddhiphongs, V. (2013). Problem gambling prevention: Before, during, and after measures. *International Journal of Mental Health and Addiction, 11*(5), 568–582.

Arndt, S., & Palmer, J. (2013). *Iowa youth gambling using the 2012 Iowa Youth Survey: Who, what, where and what else?* Iowa City: Iowa Consortium for Substance Abuse Research and Evaluation.

Beard, K. W. (2005). Internet addiction: A review of current assessment techniques and potential assessment questions. *CyberPsychology & Behavior, 8*(1), 7–14.

Beard, K. W., & Wolf, E. M. (2001). Modification in the proposed diagnostic criteria for Internet addiction. *CyberPsychology & Behavior, 4*(3), 377–383.

Bergevin, T., Gupta, R., Derevensky, J., & Kaufman, F. (2006). Adolescent gambling: Understanding the role of stress and coping. *Journal of Gambling Studies, 22*(2), 195–208.

Billieux, J., Deleuze, J., Griffiths, M. D., & Kuss, D. J. (2015). Internet gaming addiction: The case of massively multiplayer online role-playing games. In N. el-Guebaly, G. Carrà, & M. Galanter (Eds.), *Textbook of addiction treatment: International perspectives* (pp. 1515–1525). Milan: Springer.

Blaszczynski, A. P., & McConaghy, N. (1993). A two- to nine-year treatment follow-up study of pathological gambling. In W. Eadington & J. A. Cornelius (Eds.), *Gambling behavior and problem gambling.* Reno, NV: Institute for the Study of Gambling and Commercial Gambling.

Blaszczynski, A. P., & Nower, L. (2013). Cognitive behavioral therapy: Translating research into clinical practice. In D. Richard, A. Blaszczynski & L. Nower (Eds.), *The Wiley-Blackwell handbook of disordered gambling* (pp. 204–224). West Sussex: John Wiley and Sons.

Blaszczynski, A. P., Winter, S., & McConaghy, N. (1986). Plasma endorphin levels in pathological gambling. *Journal of Gambling Behavior, 2*(1), 3–14.

Bleakley, A., Ellithorpe, M., & Romer, D. (2016). The role of parents in problematic internet use among US adolescents. *Media and Communication, 4*(3).

Bleakley, A., Vaala, S. E., Jordan, A., & Romer, D. (2014). The Annenberg Media Environment Survey: Media access and use in U.S. homes with children and adolescents. In A. Jordan & D. Romer (Eds.), *Media and the well-being of children and adolescents* (pp. 1–19). New York: Oxford University Press.

Blinn-Pike, L., Worthy, S. L., & Jonkman, J. (2010). Adolescent gambling: A review of an emerging field of research. *Journal of Adolescent Health, 47*(3), 223–236.

Block, J. (2008). Issues for DSM-V: Internet addiction. *American Journal of Psychiatry, 165*(3), 306–307.

Brand, M., Young, K. S., & Laier, C. (2014). Prefrontal control and Internet addiction: A theoretical model and review of neuropsychological and neuroimaging findings. *Frontiers in Human Neuroscience, 8*, 375.

Brown, R. I. (1986). Dropouts and continuers in Gamblers Anonymous: Life context and other factors. *Journal of Gambling Behavior, 2*, 130–140.

Brown, R. I. (1987). Dropouts and continuers in Gamblers Anonymous: IV. Evaluation and summary. *Journal of Gambling Behavior, 3*, 202–210.

Bujold, A., Ladouceur, R., Sylvain, C., & Boisvert, J. M. (1994). Treatment of pathological gamblers: An experimental study. *Journal of Behavioral Therapy and Experimental Psychiatry, 25*, 275–282.

Cain, N., & Gradisar, M. (2010). Electronic media use and sleep in school-aged children and adolescents: A review. *Sleep Medicine, 11*(8), 735–742.

Campbell, C., Derevensky, J., Meerkamper, E., & Cutajar, J. (2011). Parents' perceptions of adolescent gambling: A Canadian national study. *Journal of Gambling Issues, 25*, 36–53.

Cao, F., Su, L., Liu, T., & Gao, X. (2007). The relationship between impulsivity and Internet addiction in a sample of Chinese adolescents. *European Psychiatry, 22*(7), 466–471.

Caplan, S. E. (2010). Theory and measurement of generalized problematic Internet use: A two-step approach. *Computers in Human Behavior, 26*, 1089–1097.

Cheng, C., & Li, A. Y.-L. (2014). Internet addiction prevalence and quality of (real) life: A meta-analysis of 31 nations across seven world regions. *Cyberpsychology, Behavior, and Social Networking, 17*(12), 755–760.

Chng, G. S., Li, D., Liau, A. K., & Khoo, A. (2015). Moderating effects of the family environment for parental mediation and pathological Internet use in youths. *Cyberpsychology, Behavior, and Social Networking, 18*(1), 30–36.

Davis, R. A. (2001). A cognitive-behavioral model of pathological Internet use. *Computers in Human Behavior, 17*(2), 187–195.

DeCaria, C., Hollander, E., & Wong, C. (1997, August). *Neuropsychiatric functioning in pathological gamblers.* Paper presented at the National Conference on Problem Gambling, New Orleans.

Delfabbro, P., & Thrupp, L. (2003). The social determinants of youth gambling in South Australian adolescents. *Journal of Adolescence, 26*(3), 313–330.

Derevensky, J. (2012). *Teen gambling: Understanding a growing epidemic.* New York: Rowman & Littlefield Publishing.

Derevensky, J., & Gainsbury, S. (2016). Social casino gaming and adolescents: Should we be concerned and is regulation in sight? *International Journal of Law and Psychiatry, 44*, 1–6.

Derevensky, J., & Gupta, R. (1999). Youth gambling problems: A new issue for school psychologists. *Nova Scotia Psychologist, 12* (11), 8–11.

Derevensky, J., & Gupta, R. (2001). Le probleme de jeu touche aussi les jeunes. *Psychologie Quebec, 18*(6), 23–27.

Derevensky, J., & Gupta, R. (2004). Adolescents with gambling problems: A synopsis of our current knowledge. *eGambling: The Electronic Journal of Gambling Issues, 10*. Available at http://www.camh.net/egambling

Derevensky, J., & Gupta, R. (2007). Internet gambling amongst adolescents: A growing concern. *International Journal of Mental Health and Addiction, 5*(2), 93–101.

Derevensky, J., & Gupta, R. (2011). Youth gambling prevention initiatives: A decade of research. In J. Derevensky, D. Shek, & J. Merrick (Eds.), *Youth gambling problems: The hidden addiction* (pp. 213–230). Berlin: De Gruyter.

Derevensky, J., Gupta, R., & Della-Cioppa, G. (1996). A developmental perspective of gambling behavior in children and adolescents. *Journal of Gambling Studies, 12*, 49–66.

Derevensky, J., Pratt, L., Hardoon, K., & Gupta, R. (2007). Gambling problems and features of attention deficit hyperactivity disorder among children and adolescents. *Journal of Addiction Medicine, 1*(3), 165–172.

Derevensky, J., Shek, D. & Merrick, J. (Eds.). (2011). *Youth gambling problems: The hidden addiction.* Berlin: De Gruyter.

Derevensky, J., St-Pierre, R., Temcheff, C., & Gupta, R. (2014). Teacher awareness and attitudes regarding adolescent risky behaviors: Is adolescent gambling perceived to be a problem? *Journal of Gambling Studies, 30*, 435–451.

Derevensky, J., Temcheff, C., & Gupta, R. (2011). Treatment of adolescent gambling problems: More art than science. In J. Derevensky, D. Shek, & J. Merrick (Eds.), *Youth gambling problems: The hidden addiction* (pp. 168–187). Berlin: De Gruyter.

Dickson, L., Derevensky, J., & Gupta, R. (2002). The prevention of youth gambling problems: A conceptual model. *Journal of Gambling Studies, 18*(2), 97–159.

Dickson, L., Derevensky, J., & Gupta, R. (2004). Youth gambling problems: A harm reduction prevention model. *Addiction Research and Theory, 12*(4), 305–316.

Dickson, L., Derevensky, J., & Gupta, R. (2008). Youth gambling problems: Examining risk and protective factors. *International Gambling Studies, 8*(1), 25–47.

Dickson-Gillespie, L., Rugle, L., Rosenthal, R., & Fong, T. (2008). Preventing the incidence and harm of gambling problems. *Journal of Primary Prevention, 29*(1), 37–55.

Douglas, A. C., Mills, J. E., Niang, M., Stepchenkova, S., Byun, S., Ruffini, C., ... Atallah, M. (2008). Internet addiction: Meta-synthesis of qualitative research for the decade 1996–2006. *Computers in Human Behavior, 24*(6), 3027–3044.

Dowling, N. A. (2013). The cognitive-behavioral treatment of female problem gambling. In D. Richard, A. Blaszczynski, & L. Nower (Eds.), *The Wiley-Blackwell handbook of disordered gambling* (pp. 225–250). West Sussex: John Wiley and Sons.

Durkee, T., Kaess, M., Carli, V., Parzer, P., Wasserman, C., Floderus, B., . . . Bobes, J. (2012). Prevalence of pathological internet use among adolescents in Europe: Demographic and social factors. *Addiction, 107*(12), 2210–2222.

el-Guebaly, N., Casey, D. M., Currie, S. R., Hodgins, D. C., Schopflocher, D. P., Smith, G. J., & Williams, R. J. (2015). *The Leisure, Lifestyle, & Lifecycle Project (LLLP): A longitudinal study of gambling in Alberta.* Final Report for the Alberta Gambling Research Institute, February 2015.

Ellenbogen, S., Gupta, R., & Derevensky, J. L. (2007). A cross-cultural study of gambling behavior among adolescents. *Journal of Gambling Studies, 23*(1), 25–39.

Felsher, J., Derevensky, J., & Gupta, R. (2010). Young adults with gambling problems: The impact of childhood maltreatment. *International Journal of Mental Health and Addiction, 8*(4), 545–556.

Ferentzy, P., Skinner, W., & Antze, P. (2013). Understanding Gamblers Anonymous: A practitioner's guide. In D. Richard, A. Blaszczynski, & L. Nower (Eds.), *The Wiley-Blackwell handbook of disordered gambling* (pp. 251–262). West Sussex: John Wiley and Sons.

Fisher, S. (1992). Measuring pathological gambling in children: The case of fruit machines in the U.K. *Journal of Gambling Studies, 8*, 263–285.

Fisher, S. (2000). Developing the DSM-IV-MR-J criteria to identify adolescent problem gambling in non-clinical populations. *Journal of Gambling Studies, 16*(2/3), 253–273.

Garmez-Guadix, M. (2014). Depressive symptoms and problematic Internet use among adolescents: Analysis of the longitudinal relationships from the cognitive-behavioral model. *Cyberpsychology, Behavior, and Social Networks, 17*(11), 714–719.

Gentile, D. A., Choo, H., Liau, A., Sim, T., Li, D., Fung, D., & Khoo, A. (2011). Pathological video game use among youths: A two-year longitudinal study. *Pediatrics, 127*, e319–e329.

Gerrits, R. S., van der Zanden, R. A. P., Visscher, R. F. M., & Conijn, B. P. (2007). Master your mood online: A preventive chat group intervention for adolescents. *Advances in Mental Health, 6*(3), 152–162.

Gillespie, M., Gupta, R., Derevensky, J., Pratt, L., & Vallerand, R. (2005). *Adolescent problem gambling: Evaluating perceived risks and benefits (Le jeu problématique chez les adolescents: Perceptions des risques et des bénéfices).* Report prepared for the Fonds de recherché en santé du Québec (FRSQ), Québec.

Grant, J., Chambers, R., & Potenza, M. (2004). Adolescent problem gambling: Neurodevelopment and pharmacological treatment. In J. Derevensky & R. Gupta (Eds.), *Gambling problems in youth: Theoretical and applied perspectives* (pp. 81–98). New York: Kluwer Academic/Plenum Publishers.

Grant, J., Kim, S., & Potenza, M. (2003). Advances in the pharmacological treatment of pathological gambling. *Journal of Gambling Studies, 19*, 85–109.

Grant, J., & Potenza, M. (Eds.). (2011). *Understanding impulse control disorders.* New York: Oxford University Press.

Griffiths, M. (1999). Internet addiction: Internet fuels other addictions. *Student British Medical Journal, 7*, 428–429.

Griffiths, M. (2000). Does Internet and computer "addiction" exist? Some case study evidence. *CyberPsychology and Behavior, 3*(2), 211–218.

Griffiths, M. (2005). A "components" model of addiction within a biopsychosocial framework. *Journal of Substance Use, 10*(4), 191–197.

Griffiths, M. (2010). Internet abuse and Internet addiction in the workplace. *Journal of Workplace Learning, 22*(7), 463–472.

Griffiths, M. (2012). Facebook addiction: Concerns, criticism, and recommendations—a response to Andreassen and colleagues 1. *Psychological Reports, 110*(2), 518–520.

Griffiths, M., King, D., & Delfabbro, P. (2009). Adolescent gambling-like experiences: Are they a cause for concern? *Education and Health, 27*(2), 27–30.

Griffiths, M., & Parke, J. (2010). Adolescent gambling on the Internet: A review. *International Journal of Adolescent Medicine and Health, 22*(1), 59–75.

Griffiths, M., & Pontes, H. M. (2014). Internet addiction disorder and Internet gaming disorder are not the same. *Journal of Addiction Research & Therapy, 5*(4), e124–e125.

Griffiths, M., & Wood, R. (2007). Adolescent Internet gambling: Preliminary results of a national survey. *Education and Health, 25*(2), 23–26.

Gupta, R., & Derevensky, J. L. (1997). Familial and social influences on juvenile gambling behavior. *Journal of Gambling Studies, 13*, 179–192.

Gupta, R., & Derevensky, J. (1998a). Adolescent gambling behavior: A prevalence study and examination of the correlates associated with excessive gambling. *Journal of Gambling Studies, 14*, 319–345.

Gupta, R., & Derevensky, J. (1998b). An empirical examination of Jacobs' general theory of addictions: Do adolescent gamblers fit the theory? *Journal of Gambling Studies, 14*, 17–49.

Gupta, R., & Derevensky, J. (2000). Adolescents with gambling problems: From research to treatment. *Journal of Gambling Studies, 16*, 315–342.

Gupta, R., & Derevensky, J. (2004). A treatment approach for adolescents with gambling problems. In J. Derevensky & R. Gupta (Eds.), *Gambling problems in youth: Theoretical and applied perspectives* (pp. 165–188). New York: Kluwer Academic/ Plenum Publishers.

Gupta, R., & Derevensky, J. (2011). Defining and assessing binge gambling. In J. Derevensky, D. Shek, & J. Merricks (Eds.), *Youth gambling problems: The hidden addiction* (pp. 79–97). Berlin: De Gruyter.

Gupta, R., Derevensky, J., & Ellenbogen, S. (2006). Personality characteristics and risk-taking tendencies among adolescent gamblers. *Canadian Journal of Behavioural Science, 38*(3), 201.

Gupta, R., Nower, L., Derevensky, J., Blaszczynski, A., Faregh, N., & Temcheff, C. (2013). Problem gambling in adolescents: An examination of the pathways model. *Journal of Gambling Studies, 29*(3), 575–588.

Haagsma, M. C., Caplan, S. E., Peters, O., & Pieterse, M. E. (2013). A cognitive-behavioral model of problematic online gaming in adolescents aged 12–22 years. *Computers in Human Behavior, 29*, 202–209.

Haller, R., & Hinterhuber, H. (1994). Treatment of pathological gambling with carbamazepine. *Pharmacopsychiatry, 27*, 129.

Hammond, C., Pilver, C., Rugle, L., Steinberg, M., Mayes, L., Malison, R., Krishnan-Sarin, S., Desai, R. & Potenza, M. (2014). An exploratory examination of marijuana use, problem-gambling severity, and health correlates among adolescents. *Journal of Behavioral Addictions, 3*(2), 90–101.

Han, D. H., Lee, Y. S., Na, C., Ahn, J. Y., Chung, U. S., Daniels, M. A., . . . Renshaw, P. F. (2009). The effect of methylphenidate on Internet video game play in children with attention-deficit/ hyperactivity disorder. *Comprehensive Psychiatry, 50*(3), 251–256.

Hanss, D., Rune, A., Mentzoni, R., Delfabbro, P., Myrseth, H., & Pallesen, S. (2014). Attitudes toward gambling among adolescents. *International Gambling Studies, 14*(3), 505–519.

Hardoon, K., Derevensky, J., & Gupta, R. (2002). *An examination of the influence of familial, emotional, conduct and cognitive problems, and hyperactivity upon youth risk-taking and adolescent gambling problems.* Report prepared for the Ontario Problem Gambling Research Centre, Ontario.

Hardoon, K., Derevensky, J., & Gupta, R. (2003). Empirical vs. perceived measures of gambling severity: Why adolescents don't present themselves for treatment. *Addictive Behaviors, 28*, 933–946.

Hardoon, K., Gupta, R., & Derevensky, J. (2004). Psychosocial variables associated with adolescent gambling: A model for problem gambling. *Psychology of Addictive Behaviors, 18*(2), 170–179.

Hayer, T., Griffiths, M., & Meyer, G. (2005). Gambling. In T. P. Gullotta & G. R. Adams (Eds.), *Handbook of adolescent behavioral problems* (1st ed., pp. 467–486). New York: Springer.

Herodotou, C., Kambouri, M., & Winters, N. (2014). Dispelling the myth of the socio-emotionally dissatisfied gamer. *Computers in Human Behavior, 32*, 23–31.

Ho, R. C., Zhang, M. W., Tsang, T. Y., Toh, A. H., Pan, F., Lu, Y., . . . Watanabe, H. (2014). The association between Internet addiction and psychiatric co-morbidity: A meta-analysis. *BMC Psychiatry, 14*(1), 183.

Hodgins, D. (2014). *Finding the 10%.* Presentation at the Responsible Gambling Council of Ontario annual conference, Toronto.

Hodgins, D., Stea, J., & Grant, J. (2011). Gambling disorders. *Lancet, 378*(9806), 1874–1884.

Hollander, E., Frenkel, M., DeCaria, C., Trungold, S., & Stein, D. (1992). Treatment of pathological gambling with chlomipramine. *American Journal of Psychiatry, 149*, 710–711.

Hollander, E., Sood, E., Pallanti, S., Baldini-Rossi, N., & Baker, B. (2005). Pharmacological treatments of pathological gamblers. *Journal of Gambling Studies, 21*, 101–110.

Huang, X. Q., Li, M. C., & Tao, R. (2010). Treatment of Internet addiction. *Current Psychiatry Reports, 12*(5), 462–470.

Insel, T. R., & Cuthbert, B. N. (2015). Brain disorders? Precisely. *Science, 348*(6234), 499–500.

Ipsos MORI. (2014). *The prevalence of underage gambling: A research study among 11 to 16 year olds on behalf of the Gambling Commission.* Young People Omnibus, 2014.

Jackson, A., Dowling, N., Thomas, S., Bond, L., & Patton, G. (2008). Adolescent gambling behaviour and attitudes: A prevalence study and correlates in an Australian population. *International Journal of Mental Health and Addiction, 6*(3), 325–352.

Jacobs, D. (2000). Juvenile gambling in North America: An analysis of long-term trends and future prospects. *Journal of Gambling Studies, 16*, 119–152.

Jacobs, D. (2004). Youth gambling in North America: An analysis of long-term trends and future prospects. In J. Derevensky & R. Gupta (Eds.), *Gambling problems in youth: Theoretical and applied perspectives* (pp. 1–26). New York: Kluwer Academic/Plenum Publishers.

Jacobs, D., Marston, A., Singer, R., Widaman, K., Little, T., & Veizades, J. (1989). Children of problem gamblers. *Journal of Gambling Behavior, 5*, 261–267.

Jessor, R. (Ed.). (1998). *New perspectives on adolescent risk behavior.* Cambridge, UK: Cambridge University Press.

Johansson, A., & Götestam, K. G. (2004). Internet addiction: Characteristics of a questionnaire and prevalence in Norwegian youth (12–18 years). *Scandinavian Journal of Psychology, 45*(3), 223–229.

Khurana, A., Bleakley, A., Jordan, A. B., & Romer, D. (2015). The protective effects of parental monitoring and Internet restriction on adolescents' risk of online harassment. *Journal of Youth and Adolescence, 44*(5), 1039–1047.

King, D. L., & Delfabbro, P. H. (2014). The cognitive psychology of Internet gaming disorder. *Clinical Psychology Review, 34*(4), 298–308.

King, S., Abrams, K., & Wilkinson, T. (2010). Personality, gender, and family history in the prediction of college gambling. *Journal of Gambling Studies, 26*(3), 347–359.

Király, O., Griffiths, M. D., Urbán, R., Farkas, J., Kökönyei, G., Elekes, Z., ... Demetrovics, Z. (2014). Problematic Internet use and problematic online gaming are not the same: Findings from a large nationally representative adolescent sample. *Cyberpsychology, Behavior, and Social Networking, 17*(12), 749–754.

Ko, C. H., Yen, J. Y., Yen, C. F., Lin, H. C., & Yang, M. J. (2007). Factors predictive for incidence and remission of Internet addiction in young adolescents: A prospective study. *CyberPsychology & Behavior, 10*(4), 545–551.

Kong, G., Tsai, J., Krishnan-Sarin, S., Cavallo, D., Hoff, R., Steinberg, M., Rugle, L. & Potenza, M. (2014). A latent class analysis of pathological-gambling criteria among high school students: Associations with gambling, risk and health/functioning characteristics. *Journal of Addiction Medicine, 8*(6), 421–430.

Kundu, P., Pilver, C., Desai, R., Steinberg, M., Rugle, L., Krishnan-Sarin, S., & Potenza, M. N. (2013). Gambling-related attitudes and behaviors in adolescents having received instant (scratch) lottery tickets as gifts. *Journal of Adolescent Health, 52*(4), 456–464.

Kuss, D. J., & Griffiths, M. D. (2012). Internet gaming addiction: A systematic review of empirical research. *International Journal of Mental Health and Addiction, 10*(2), 278–296.

Kuss, D. J., Griffiths, M. D., & Binder, J. F. (2013). Internet addiction in students: Prevalence and risk factors. *Computers in Human Behavior, 29*(3), 959–966.

Kuss, D., Shorter, G., van Rooij, A., Griffiths, M., & Schoenmakers, T. (2014). Assessing Internet addiction using the parsimonious Internet addiction components model—a preliminary study. *International Journal of Mental Health and Addiction, 12*(3), 351–366.

Ladouceur, R., Boisvert, J.-M., & Dumont, J. (1994). Cognitive behavioral treatment for adolescent pathological gamblers. *Behavior Modification, 18*, 230–242.

Ladouceur, R., Goulet, A., & Vitaro, F. (2013). Prevention programmes for youth gambling: A review of the empirical evidence. *International Gambling Studies, 13*(2), 141–159.

Ladouceur, R., & Shaffer, H. (2005). Treating problem gamblers: Working towards empirically supported treatments. *Journal of Gambling Studies, 21*, 1–4.

Ladouceur, R., & Walker, M. (1998). Cognitive approach to understanding and treating pathological gambling. In A. S. Bellack & M. Hersen (Eds.), *Comprehensive clinical psychology.* New York: Pergamon, 587–601.

Lam, L. T. (2014). Internet gaming addiction, problematic use of the Internet, and sleep problems: A systematic review. *Current Psychiatry Reports, 16*(4), 1–9.

Lam, L. T., & Peng, Z. W. (2010). Effect of pathological use of the internet on adolescent mental health: A prospective study. *Archives of Pediatrics & Adolescent Medicine, 164*(10), 901–906.

LaPlante, D., & Shaffer, H. (2007). Understanding the influence of gambling opportunities: Expanding exposure models to include adaptation. *American Journal of Orthopsychiatry, 77*(4), 616–623.

Ledgerwood, D., Loree, A. & Lundahl, L. (2013). Predictors of treatment outcome in disordered gambling. In D. Richard, A. Blaszczynski, & L. Nower (Eds.), *The Wiley-Blackwell handbook of disordered gambling* (pp. 283–305). West Sussex: John Wiley and Sons.

Leeman, R., Hoff, R., Krishnan-Sarin, S., Patock-Peckham, J., & Potenza, M. (2014). Impulsivity, sensation-seeking, and part-time job status in relation to substance use and gambling in adolescents. *Journal of Adolescent Health, 54*(4), 460–466.

Lesieur, H. (1990). Working with and understanding Gamblers Anonymous. In *Working with self-help*. Homewood, IL: Dorsey.

Lesieur, H., & Blume, S. (1991). Evaluation of patients treated for pathological gambling in a combined alcohol, substance abuse, and pathological gambling treatment unit using the Addiction Severity Index. *British Journal of Addictions, 86*, 1017–1028.

Lesieur, H., & Rothschild, J. (1989). Children of Gamblers Anonymous members. *Journal of Gambling Behavior, 5*, 269–281.

Lin, M.-P., Ko, H.-C., & Wu, J. Y.-W. (2011). Prevalence and psychosocial risk factors associated with Internet addiction in a nationally representative sample of college students in Taiwan. *Cyberpsychology, Behavior, and Social Networking, 14*(12), 741–746.

Liu, L., Yip, S. W., Khang, J-T., Wang, L-J., Shen, Z-J., Liu, B., Ma, S-S., ... Fang, X-Y. (2016). Activation of the ventral and dorsal striatum during cue reactivity in Internet gaming disorder. *Addiction Biology*, Jan. 5 [E-pub ahead of print].

Liu, Q. X., Fang, X. Y., Deng, L. Y., Zhang, J. T. (2012). Parent-adolescent communication, parental Internet use and Internet-specific norms and pathological Internet use among Chinese adolescents. *Computers in Human Behavior, 28*, 1269–1275.

Lortie, C. L., & Guitton, M. J. (2013). Internet addiction assessment tools: Dimensional structure and methodological status. *Addiction, 108*(7), 1207–1216.

Lupu, I. R., & Lupu, V. (2013). Gambling prevention program for teenagers. *Journal of Cognitive & Behavioral Psychotherapies, 13*(2a), 575–584.

Lussier, I., Derevensky, J., & Gupta, R. (2004, August). *Youth gambling behaviour: An examination of resilience*. Paper presented at the 5th National Child Welfare Symposium, Ottawa.

Lussier, I., Derevensky, J. L., Gupta, R., Bergevin, T., & Ellenbogen, S. (2007). Youth gambling behaviors: An examination of the role of resilience. *Psychology of Addictive Behaviors, 21*(2), 165–173.

Lussier, I., Derevensky, J., Gupta, R. & Vitaro, F. (2014). Risk, compensatory, protective, and vulnerability processes influencing youth gambling problems and other high-risk behaviours. *Psychology of Addictive Behaviors, 28*, 404–413.

Madden, M., Lenhart, A., Duggan, M., Cortesi, S., & Gasser, U. (2013). *Teens and technology 2013*. Pew Internet & American Life Project.

Mak, K. K., Lai, C. M., Watanabe, H., Kim, D. I., Bahar, N., Ramos, M., ... Cheng, C. (2014). Epidemiology of internet behaviors and addiction among adolescents in six Asian countries. *Cyberpsychology, Behavior, and Social Networking, 17*(11), 720–728.

Masten, A. S., Best, K. M., & Garmezy, N. (1990). Resilience and development: Contributions from the study of children who overcome adversity. *Development and Psychopathology*, 2(04), 425–444.

Messerlian, C., & Derevensky, J. (2005). Youth gambling: A public health perspective. *Journal of Gambling Issues, 14*, 97–116.

Messerlian, C., Derevensky, J. & Gupta, R. (2005). Youth gambling problems: A public health framework. *Health Promotion International, 20*, 69–79.

Mitchell, P. (2000). Internet addiction: Genuine diagnosis or not? *Lancet, 355*(9204), 632.

Moreno, M. A., Jelenchick, L., Cox, E., Young, H., & Christakis, D. A. (2011). Problematic Internet use among US youth: A systematic review. *Archives of Pediatrics & Adolescent Medicine, 165*(9), 797–805.

National Research Council. (1999). *Pathological gambling: A critical review*. Washington, DC: National Academy Press.

Nower, L., & Blaszczynski, A. (2004). A pathways approach to treating youth gamblers. In J. Derevensky & R. Gupta (Eds.), *Gambling problems in youth: Theoretical and applied perspectives* (pp. 189–210). New York: Kluwer Academic/Plenum Publishers.

Nower, L., Derevensky, J., & Gupta, R. (2004). The relationship of impulsivity, sensation seeking, coping and substance use in youth gamblers. *Psychology of Addictive Behaviors, 18*, 49–55.

Nower, L., Gupta, R., Blaszczynski, A., & Derevensky, J. (2004). Suicidality ideation and depression among youth gamblers: A preliminary examination of three studies. *International Gambling Studies*, *4*(1), 69–80.

Petry, N. (2005). *Pathological gambling: Etiology, comorbidity, and treatment.* Washington, DC: American Psychological Association Press.

Petry, N. M., & O'Brien, C. P. (2013). Internet gaming disorder and the DSM-5. *Addiction*, *108*(7), 1186–1187.

Petry, N. M., Rehbein, F., Gentile, D. A., Lemmens, J. S., Rumpf, H.-J., Mößle, T., ... O'Brien, C. P. (2014). An international consensus for assessing internet gaming disorder using the new DSM-5 approach. *Addiction*, *109*(9), 1399–1406.

Petry, N. M., Rehbein, F., Ko, C.-K., & O'Brien (2015). Internet gaming disorder in the DSM-5. *Current Psychiatry Reports*, *17*, 72.

Petry, N., & Roll, J. (2001). A behavioral approach to understanding and treating pathological gambling. *Seminars in Clinical Neuropsychiatry*, *6*, 177–183.

Pies, R. (2009). Should DSM-5 designate "Internet addiction" a mental disorder? *Psychiatry (Edgmont)*, *6*(2), 31–37.

Potenza, M. N. (2006). Should addictive disorders include non-substance-related conditions? *Addiction*, *101*, 142–151.

Prizant-Passal, S., Shechner, T., & Aderka, I. M, (2016). Social anxiety and internet use: A meta-analysis: What do we know? What are we missing? *Computers in Human Behavior*, *62*, 221–229.

Productivity Commission. (1999). *Australia's gambling industries*. Report No. 10. Canberra: AusInfo. Available at http://www.pc.gov.au/

Productivity Commission. (2010). *Gambling Productivity Commission Inquiry Report*. Australian Government.

Przepiorka, A. M., Blachnio, A., Miziak, B., & Czuczwar, S. J. (2014). Clinical approaches to treatment of Internet addiction. *Pharmacological Reports*, *66*(2), 187–191.

Rahman, A., Pilver, C., Desai, R., Steinberg, M., Rugle, L., Krishnan-Sarin, S., & Potenza, M. (2012). The relationship between age of gambling onset and adolescent problematic gambling severity. *Journal of Psychiatric Research*, *46*(5), 675–683.

Raylu, N., & Oei, T. (2002). Pathological gambling: A comprehensive review. *Clinical Psychology Review*, *22*, 1009–1061.

Richard, D. Blaszczynski, A., & Nower, L. (Eds.) (2013) *The Wiley-Blackwell handbook of disordered gambling*. West Sussex: John Wiley and Sons.

Rideout, V. J., Foehr, U. G., & Roberts, D. F. (2010). *Generation M2: Media in the lives of 8- to 18-year-olds*. Henry J. Kaiser Family Foundation.

Roberts, D. F., & Foehr, U. G. (2004). *Kids and the media in America*. New York: Cambridge University Press.

Romer, D., Bagdasarov, Z., & More, E. (2013). Older versus newer media and the well-being of United States youth: Results from a national longitudinal panel. *Journal of Adolescent Health*, *52*(5), 613–619.

Romer, D., & Rich, M. (2016). Afterword to the issue "Adolescents in the Digital Age: Effects on Health and Development." *Media and Communication*, *4*(3), 90–94.

Rosenthal, R. (1987). The psychodynamics of pathological gambling: A review of the literature. In T. Galski (Ed.), *The handbook of pathological gambling*. Springfield, IL: Charles C. Thomas.

Rugle, L., & Rosenthal, R. (1994). Transference and countertransference in the psychotherapy of pathological gamblers. *Journal of Gambling Studies*, *10*, 43–65.

Schüll, N. (2012). *Addiction by design: Machine gambling in Las Vegas*. Princeton, NJ: Princeton University Press.

Shaffer, H., LaBrie, R., Scanlan, K., & Cummings, T. (1994). Pathological gambling among adolescents: Massachusetts Gambling Screen. *Journal of Gambling Studies*, *10*, 339–362.

Shaffer, H. J., LaPlante, D. A., LaBrie, R. A., Kidman, R. C., Donato, A. N., & Stanton, M. V. (2004). Toward a syndrome model of addiction: Multiple expressions, common etiology. *Harvard Review of Psychiatry*, *12*, 367–374.

Shapira, N. A., Goldsmith, T. D., Keck, P. E., Jr., Khosla, U. M., & McElroy, S. L. (2000). Psychiatric features of individuals with problematic Internet use. *Journal of Affective Disorders*, *57*(1), 267–272.

Shapira, N. A., Lessig, M. C., Goldsmith, T. D., Szabo, S. T., Lazoritz, M., Gold, M. S., & Stein, D. J. (2003). Problematic Internet use: Proposed classification and diagnostic criteria. *Depression and Anxiety*, *17*(4), 207–216.

Shead, N., Derevensky, J., & Gupta, R. (2010). Risk and protective factors associated with youth problem gambling. *International Journal of Adolescent Medicine and Health*, *22*(1), 39.

Siomos, K., Floros, G., Fisoun, V., Evaggelia, D., Farkonas, N., Sergentani, E., ... Geroukalis, D. (2012). Evolution of Internet addiction in Greek adolescent students over a two-year period: The impact of parental bonding. *European Child & Adolescent Psychiatry*, *21*(4), 211–219.

Slutske, W., Blaszczynski, A., & Martin, N. (2009). Sex differences in the rates of recovery, treatment-seeking, and natural recovery in pathological gambling: Results from an Australian community-based twin survey. *Twin Research and Human Genetics*, *12*(5), 425–432.

Smith, A. (2014). African Americans and technology use: A demographic portrait. http://www.pewinternet.org/files/2014/01/African-Americans-and-Technology-Use.pdf

Ste-Marie, C., Gupta, R., & Derevensky, J. (2002). Anxiety and social stress related to adolescent gambling behavior. *International Gambling Studies, 2(1),* 123–141.

Ste-Marie, C., Gupta, R., & Derevensky, J. (2006). Anxiety and social stress related to adolescent gambling behavior and substance use. *Journal of Child & Adolescent Substance Abuse*, *15*(4), 55–74.

Stinchfield, R. (2000). Gambling and correlates of gambling among Minnesota public school students. *Journal of Gambling Studies*, *16*, 153–173.

Stinchfield, R. (2010). A critical review of adolescent problem gambling assessment instruments. *International Journal of Adolescent Medicine and Health*, *22*(1), 77–93.

St-Pierre, R., Walker, D., Derevensky, J., & Gupta, R. (2014). How availability and accessibility of gambling venues influence problem gambling: A review of the literature. *Gaming Law Review and Economics*, *18*(2), 150–172.

Suurvali, H., Hodgins, D., & Cunningham, J. (2010). Motivators for resolving or seeking help for gambling problems: A review of the empirical literature. *Journal of Gambling Studies*, *26*(1), 1–33.

Temcheff, C., Derevensky, J., St-Pierre, R, Gupta, R., & Martin, I. (2014). Beliefs and attitudes of mental health professionals with respect to gambling and other high-risk behaviors in schools. *International Journal of Mental Health and Addiction*, *12*, 716–729.

Tokunaga, R. S., & Rains, S. A. (2016). A review and meta-analysis examining conceptual and operational definitions of problematic Internet use. *Human Communication Research*, *42*, 165–199.

Toneatto, T., & Sobell, L. (1990). Pathological gambling treated with cognitive behavior therapy: A case report. *Addictive Behaviors*, *15*, 497–501.

Tsitsika, A., Janikian, M., Schoenmakers, T. M., Tzavela, E. C., Ólafsson, K., Wójcik, S., ... Richardson, C. (2014). Internet addictive behavior in adolescence: A cross-cectional study in seven European countries. *Cyberpsychology, Behavior, and Social Networking*, *17*(8), 528–535.

Turner, N., Macdonald, J., & Somerset, M. (2008). Life skills, mathematical reasoning and critical thinking: A curriculum for the prevention of problem gambling. *Journal of Gambling Studies*, *24*(3), 367–380.

van Rooij, A. J., Schoenmakers, T. M., Van de Eijnden, R. J., & van de Mheen, D. (2010). Compulsive Internet use: The role of online gaming and other Internet applications. *Journal of Adolescent Health*, *47*(1), 51–57.

Vitaro, F., Brendgen, M., Ladouceur, R., & Tremblay, R. (2001). Gambling, delinquency, and drug use during adolescence: Mutual influences and common risk factors. *Journal of Gambling Studies*, *17*(3), 171–190.

Vitaro, F., Ferland, F., Jacques, C., & Ladouceur, R. (1998). Gambling, substance use, and impulsivity during adolescence. *Psychology of Addictive Behaviors*, *12*, 185–194.

Vitaro, F. Wanner, B., Ladouceur, R., Brendgen, M., & Tremblay, R. E. (2004). Trajectories of gambling during adolescence. *Journal of Gambling Studies*, *20*, 47–69.

Volberg, R., Gupta, R., Griffiths, M. D., Olason, D. T., & Delfabbro, P. (2010). An international perspective on youth gambling prevalence studies. In J. Derevensky, D. Shek, & J. Merrick (Eds.), *Youth gambling problems: The hidden addiction* (pp. 21–56). Berlin: De Gruyter.

Walker, M. (1993). Treatment strategies for problem gambling: A review of effectiveness. In W. R. Eadington & J. A. Cornelius (Eds.), *Gambling behavior and problem gambling* (pp. 533–566). Reno: University of Nevada.

Wardle, H., Moody, A., Spence, S., Orford, J., Volberg, R. Jotangia, D., ... Dobbie, F. (2011). *British gambling prevalence survey*. Report to the UK Gambling Commission. London: National Centre for Social Research.

Welte, J., Barnes, G., Tidwell, M., & Hoffman, J. (2008). The prevalence of problem gambling among US adolescents and young adults: Results from a national survey. *Journal of Gambling Studies*, *24*(2), 119–133.

Widyanto, L., & Griffiths, M. (2006). "Internet addiction": A critical review. *International Journal of Mental Health and Addiction*, *4*(1), 31–51.

Widyanto, L., & McMurran, M. (2004). The psychometric properties of the Internet Addiction Test. *CyberPsychology & Behavior*, *7*(4), 443–450.

Wiebe, J., Wynne, H., Stinchfield, R., & Tremblay, J. (2005). *Measuring problem gambling in adolescent populations*. Canadian Consortium for Gambling Research.

Wiebe, J., Wynne, H., Stinchfield, R., & Tremblay, J. (2007). *The Canadian Adolescent Gambling Inventory (CAGI): Phase II final report*. Canadian Centre on Substance Abuse.

Williams, R., Hann, R., Schopflocher, D., West, B., McLaughlin, P., White, N., ... Flexhaug, T. (2015). *Quinte longitudinal study of gambling and problem gambling*. Report prepared for the Ontario Problem Gambling Research Centre.

Williams, R., Volberg, R., & Stevens, R. (2012). *The population prevalence of problem gambling: Methodological influences, standardized rates, jurisdictional differences, and worldwide trends*. Report Prepared for the Ontario Problem Gambling Research Centre & the Ontario Ministry of Health and Long Term Care.

Williams, R., West, B., & Simpson, R. (2012). *Prevention of problem gambling: A comprehensive review of the evidence, and identified best practices*. Report prepared for the Ontario Problem Gambling Research Centre and the Ontario Ministry of Health and Long Term Care.

Wilson, D., & Ross, N. (2011). Place, gender and the appeal of video lottery terminal gambling: Unpacking a focus group study of Montreal youth. *GeoJournal, 76*(2), 123–138.

Winkler, A., Dörsing, B., Rief, W., Shen, Y., & Glombiewski, J. A. (2013). Treatment of internet addiction: A meta-analysis. *Clinical Psychology Review, 33*(2), 317–329.

Winters, K., & Anderson, N. (2000). Gambling involvement and drug use among adolescents. *Journal of Gambling Studies, 16*, 175–198.

Winters, K., Stinchfield, R., & Fulkerson, J. (1993). Toward the development of an adolescent gambling problem severity scale. *Journal of Gambling Studies, 9*, 371–386.

Wynne, H., Smith, G., & Jacobs, D. (1996). *Adolescent gambling and problem gambling in Alberta*. Alberta, Canada: Alberta Alcohol and Drug Abuse Commission.

Yellowlees, P. M., & Marks, S. (2007). Problematic Internet use or Internet addiction? *Computers in Human Behavior, 23*(3), 1447–1453.

Young, K. S. (1996). *Internet addiction: The emergence of a new clinical disorder*. Paper presented at the 104th annual meeting of the American Psychological Association, Toronto.

Young, K. S. (1998). Internet addiction: The emergence of a new clinical disorder. *CyberPsychology & Behavior, 1*(3), 237–244.

Young, K. S. (2007). Cognitive behavior therapy with Internet addicts: Treatment outcomes and implications. *CyberPsychology & Behavior, 10*(5), 671–679.

Zuckerman, M. (1994). *Behavioral expressions and biosocial bases of sensation seeking*. New York: Cambridge University Press.

Part IX: Conclusions, Recommendations, Priorities

AAP Council on Community Pediatrics. (2016). Poverty and child health in the United States. *Pediatrics, 137*(4), e20160339.

Aarons, G., Hurlburt, M., & Horwitz, S. (2011). Advancing a conceptual model of evidence-based practice implementation in public service sectors. *Administration and Policy in Mental Health and Mental Health Services Research, 38*(1), 4–23.

Abeles, P., Verduyn, C., Robinson, A., Smith, P., Yule, W., & Proudfoot, J. (2009). Computerized CBT for adolescent depression ("Stressbusters") and its initial evaluation through an extended case series. *Behavioural and Cognitive Psychotherapy, 37*(2), 151–165.

Administration for Children and Families. (2013). *Trends in foster care and adoption: FY2002-2012 (based on data submitted by states as of July 19, 2013)*. Washington, DC: Administration for Children and Families.

Allen, S. (2010). Medicaid and pediatric Accountable Care Organizations: A case study. *Accountable Care News, 1*(5), 1–4. http://www.network-health.org/uploadedFiles/About_Us/Newsroom/In_the_News/Accountable%20Care%20News%20-%20December%202010%281%29.pdf

American Academy of Pediatrics. Bright Futures. Retrieved Sept. 18, 2013, from http://brightfutures.aap.org/.

American Academy of Pediatrics, Division of Child Health Research. (1998). Research update: 45% of Fellows routinely screen for alcohol use. *AAP News, 14*(10), 1–12.

American Psychiatric Association. (2013). *Diagnostic and statistical manual of mental disorders* (5th ed.). Washington, DC: American Psychiatric Association.

American Recovery and Reinvestment Act of 2009, Pub. L. No. 111-5, 123 Stat. (2009).

Angermeyer, M. C., & Schulze, B. (2001). Reinforcing stereotypes: How the focus on forensic cases in news reporting may influence public attitudes towards the mentally ill. *International Journal of Law and Psychiatry, 24*, 469–486.

Appelbaum, P. (2013). Public safety, mental disorders, and guns, *JAMA Psychiatry*, *70*, 565–566.

Asarnow, J. R., Rozenman, M., Wiblin, J. & Zeltzer, L. (2015). Integrated medical-behavioral care compared with usual primary care for child and adolescent behavioral health; a meta-analysis. *JAMA Pediatrics*, *169*(10), 929–937.

Ashwood, J. S., Briscombe, B., Collins, R. L., Wong, E. C., Eberhart, N. K., Cerully, J. L., . . . Burnam, A. (2016). *Investment in social marketing campaign to reduce stigma and discrimination associated with mental illness yields positive economic benefits to California*. Santa Monica, CA: RAND Corporation.

Baum, R. A., Epstein, J. N., & Kelleher, K. (2013). Healthcare reform, quality, and technology: ADHD as a case study. *Current Psychiatry Reports*, *15*(7), 1–7.

Berenson, R. A., Pronovost, P. J., & Krumholz, H. M. (2013). Achieving the potential of health care performance measures: Timely analysis of immediate health policy issues. *Research and Publications*. http://www.rwjf.org/en/research-publications/find-rwjf-research/2013/05/achieving-the-potential-of-health-care-performance-measures.html.

Bernstein, J., Heeren, T., Edward, E., Dorfman, D., Bliss, C., Winter, M., & Bernstein, E. (2010). A brief motivational interview in a pediatric emergency department, plus 10-day telephone follow-up, increases attempts to quit drinking among youth and young adults who screen positive for problematic drinking. *Academic Emergency Medicine*, *17*, 890–902.

Bethell, C., Klein, J., & Peck, C. (2001). Assessing health system provision of adolescent preventive services: The Young Adult Health Care Survey. *Medical Care*, *39*(5), 478–490.

Bickman, L., Kelley, S. D., Breda, C., de Andrade, A. R., & Riemer, M. (2011). Effects of routine feedback to clinicians on youth mental health outcomes: A randomized cluster design. *Psychiatric Services*, *62*(12), 1423–1429.

Blau, G. B., Caldwell, B., Fisher, S., Kuppinger, A., Levinson-Johnson, J., & Lieberman, R. (2010). The Building Bridges initiative: Residential and community-based providers, families, and youth coming together to improve outcomes. *Child Welfare*, *89*(2), 21–38.

Brannigan, R., Schackman, B. R., Falco, M., & Millman, R. B. (2004). The quality of highly regarded adolescent substance abuse treatment programs: Results of an in-depth national survey. *Archives of Pediatrics & Adolescent Medicine*, *158*, 904–909.

Brewer, M. B. (1981). Perceptions of the elderly: Stereotypes as prototypes. *Journal of Personality and Social Psychology*, *41*(4), 656–670.

Brockington, I., Hall, P., Levings, J., & Murphy, C. (1993). The community's tolerance of the mentally ill. *British Journal of Psychiatry*, *162*, 93–99.

Brown, J. D., & Witherspoon, E. M. (2001). The mass media and the health of adolescents in the United States. In Y. R. Kamalipour & K. R. Rampal (Eds.), *Media, sex, violence, and drugs in the global village* (pp. 77–96). New York: Rowman & Littlefield.

Brown, S. A., & Tapert, S. F. (2004). Adolescence and the trajectory of alcohol use: Basic to clinical studies. *Annals of the New York Academy of Sciences*, *1021*, 234–244.

Brown, S. A., Vik, P. W., & Creamer, V. A. (1989). Characteristics of relapse following adolescent substance abuse treatment. *Addictive Behaviors*, *14*(3), 291–300.

Bruns, E. J., & Hoagwood, K. E. (2008). State implementation of evidence-based practice for youths, Part I: Responses to the state of the evidence. *Journal of the American Academy of Child and Adolescent Psychiatry*, *47*(4), 369–373.

Buck, D., Baker, G. A., Chadwick, D. W., & Jacoby, A. (1997). Factors influencing compliance with antiepileptic drug regimes. *Seizure*, *6*, 87–93.

Bushman, B. J., & Anderson, C. A. (2001). Media violence and the American public: Scientific fact versus media misinformation. *American Psychologist*, *56*, 477–489.

Bushman, B. J., Newman, K., Calvert, S. L., Downey, G., Dredze, M., Gottfredson, M., . . . Webster, D. W. (2016). Youth violence: What we know and what we need to know. *American Psychologist*, 71(1), 17–39.

Cacciola, J., Camilleri, A., Kolwicz, T., Brooks, A., & Alterman, A. (2012). *Does clinical monitoring impact treatment outcomes?* Poster presentation at the 74th Annual Meeting of the College on Problems of Drug Dependence, Palm Springs, CA.

Cacciola, J. S., Meyers, K., Ward, S., Rosenwasser, B., Arria, A., & McLellan, A. T. (2015). Assessing adolescent substance abuse programs with updated quality indicators: The development of a consumer guide for adolescent treatment. *Journal of Child & Adolescent Substance Abuse*, *24*(3), 142–154.

California Evidence-based Clearinghouse. (2013). Information and resources for child welfare professional. Retrieved November 5, 2013, from http://www.cebc4cw.org.

Campbell, F., Conti, G., Heckman, J. J., Moon, S.H., Pinto, R., Pungello, E., & Pan, Y. (2014). Early childhood investments substantially boost adult health. *Science, 343*(6178), 1478–1485.

Campbell-Heider, N., Finnell, D. S., Feigenbaum, J. C., Feeley, T. H., Rejman, K. S., Austin-Ketch, T., ... Schmitt, A. (2009). Survey on addictions: Toward curricular change for family nurse practitioners. *International Journal of Nursing Education Scholarship*, *6*(1), Article 4.

CASA. (2011). Adolescent substance use: America's #1 public health problem. New York: National Center on Addiction and Substance Abuse.

Center for Behavioral Health Statistics and Quality. (2015). Behavioral health trends in the United States: Results from the 2014 National Survey on Drug Use and Health (HHS Publication No. SMA 15-4927, NSDUH Series H-50). Retrieved from http://www.samhsa.gov/data/

Center for Health Care Strategies Inc. (2012). Medicaid financing for family and youth peer support: A scan of state programs. Retrieved September 13, 2013, from http://www.chcs.org/usr_doc/FYPS_Matrix.pdf

Center for Medicare & Medicaid Services. (2013). The Affordable Care Act: Helping providers help patients—A menu of options of improving care. Accountable Care Organizations (ACO). Retrieved September 13, 2013, from http://www.cms.gov/Medicare/Medicare-Fee-for-Service-Payment/ACO/Downloads/ACO-Menu-Of-Options.pdf

Center for Substance Abuse Research. (2012). 60% of high school students report drugs are used, kept, or sold in their schools *CESAR FAX*. College Park: University of Maryland.

Centers for Disease Control and Prevention. (2007). Use of niacin in attempts to defeat urine drug testing—Five states, January–September 2006. *MMWR. Morbidity and Mortality Weekly Report*, *56*(15), 365–366.

Chaffin, M., Hecht, D., Bard, D., Silovsky, J. F., & Beasley, W. H. (2012). A statewide trial of the SafeCare home-based services model with parents in Child Protective Services. *Pediatrics*, *129*(3), 509–515.

Chaloupka, F. J., & Laixuthal, A. (2002). Controversial drug testing yields mixed results. *Drug Policy News*, from http://www.dpj.org/news/12_30_02testing.cfm.

Chamberlain, P., Brown, C. H., & Saldana, L. (2011). Observational measure of implementation progress in community based settings: The Stages of Implementation Completion (SIC). *Implementation Science*, *6*, 116.

Chambers, D. (2010). *Overview of NIH dissemination and implementation funding opportunities*. Paper presented at the 3rd Annual NIH Conference on the Science of Dissemination and Implementation: Methods and Measurement, Bethesda, MD.

Chambers, D. (2012). *NIH dissemination and implementation research at the crossroads*. Paper presented at the 5th Annual NIH Conference on the Science of Dissemination and Implementation: Research at the Crossroads, Bethesda, MD.

Chaplin, R. (2000). Psychiatrists can cause stigma too. *British Journal of Psychiatry*, *177*, 467.

Cheng, T. L., Savageau, J. A., Sattler, A. L., & DeWitt, T. G. (1993). Confidentiality in health care: A survey of knowledge, perceptions, and attitudes among high school students. *Journal of the American Medical Association*, *269*(11), 1404–1407.

Children's Health Insurance Program Reauthorization Act of 2009 Pub. L. No. 111-3, 123 Stat. (2009).

Choe, D. E., Olson, S. L., & Sameroff, A. J. (2013). Effects of early maternal distress and parenting on the development of children's self-regulation and externalizing behavior. *Development and Psychopathology*, *25*, 437–453.

Chorpita, B. F., Bernstein, A., & Daleiden, E. L. (2011). Empirically guided coordination of multiple evidence-based treatments: An illustration of relevance mapping in children's mental health services. *Journal of Consulting and Clinical Psychology*, *79*(4), 470–480.

Chorpita, B. F., Daleiden, E. L., Ebesutani, C., Young, J., Becker, K. D., Nakamura, B. J., ... Starace, N. (2011). Evidence-based treatments for children and adolescents: An updated review of indicators of efficacy and effectiveness. *Clinical Psychology: Science and Practice*, *18*(2), 154–172.

Chorpita, B. F., & Weisz, J. R. (2009). *MATCH-ADTC: Modular Approach to Therapy for Children (MATCH) with anxiety, depression, trauma, or conduct problems* Satellite Beach, FL: PracticeWise.

Clark, W., Welch, S. H., Berry, S. H., Collentine, A. M., Collins, R. L., Lebron, D., & Shearer, A. L. (2013). California's historic effort to reduce the stigma of mental illness: The Mental Health

Services Act. *American Journal of Public Health, 103*(5), 786–794.

Clayton, S., Chin, T., Blackburn, S., & Echeverria, C. (2010). Different setting, different care: Integrating prevention and clinical care in school-based health centers. *American Journal of Public Health, 100*, 1592–1596.

Clement, S., Schauman, O., Graham, T., Maggioni, F., Evans-Lacko, S., Bezborodovs, N., ... Thornicroft, G. (2015). What is the impact of mental health-related stigma on help-seeking? A systematic review of quantitative studies. *Psychological Medicine, 45*, 11–27.

Clinic Technical Assistance Center. (2013). Training and Resources. Retrieved November 8, 2013, from http://www.ctacny.com.

Co, J. P. T., Johnson, S. A., Poon, E. G., Fiskio, J., Rao, S. R., Van Cleave, J., ... Ferris, T. G. (2010). Electronic health record decision support and quality of care for children with ADHD. *Pediatrics, 126*(2), 239–246.

Comer, J. S., & Barlow, D. H. (2013). The occasional case against broad dissemination and implementation: Retaining a role for specialty care in the delivery of psychological treatments. *American Psychologist* [E-pub August 5].

Conrad, P., & Schneider, J. (1992). *Deviance and medicalization* (expanded ed.) Philadelphia, PA: Temple University Press.

Copeland, W., & Costello, E. J. (2010). Parents' incomes and children's outcomes: A quasi-experiment. *American Economic Journal of Applied Economics, 2*(1), 86–115.

Cornelius, J. R., Maisto, S. A., Martin, C. S., Bukstein, O. G., Salloum, I. M., Daley, D. C., ... Clark, D. B. (2004). Major depression associated with earlier alcohol relapse in treated teens with AUD. *Addictive Behaviors, 29*(5), 1035–1038.

Cornelius, J. R., Maisto, S. A., Pollock, N. K., Martin, C. S., Salloum, I. M., Lynch, K. G., & Clark, D. B. (2003). Rapid relapse generally follows treatment for substance use disorders among adolescents. *Addictive Behaviors, 28*(2), 381–386.

Cornelius, J. R., Pringle, J., Jernigan, J., Kirisci, L., & Clark, D. B. (2001). Correlates of mental health service utilization and unmet need among a sample of male adolescents. *Addictive Behaviors, 26*(1), 11–19.

Corrigan, P. W. (2000). Mental health stigma as social attribution: Implications for research methods and attitude change. *Clinical Psychology: Science and Practice, 7*, 48–67.

Corrigan, P. W. (2002). Testing social cognitive models of mental illness stigma: The Prairie State stigma studies. *Psychiatric Rehabilitation Skills, 6*, 232–254.

Corrigan, P. W. (2004). How stigma interferes with mental health care. *American Psychologist, 59*, 614–625.

Corrigan, P. W., Michaels, B., & Morris, S. (2014). Do the effects of antistigma programs persist over time? Findings from a meta-analysis. *Psychiatric Services*. 66, 543–546. Available at http://wx3zg9re3e.scholar.serialssolutions.com/?sid=googleandauinit=Pandaulast=Corriganand atitle=Do+the+effects+of+antistigma+programs+persist+over+time%3F+Findings+from+a+meta-analysisandid=doi:10.1176/appi.ps.201400291. Accessed March 31, 2016.

Corrigan, P. W., Morris, S. B., Michaels, P. J., Rafacz, J. D., & Rüsch, N. (2012). Challenging the public stigma of mental illness: A meta-analysis of outcome studies. *Psychiatric Services, 63*, 963–973. Available at http://dx.doi.org/10.1176/appi.ps.201100529. Accessed March 25, 2016.

Couture, S., & Penn, D. L. (2003). Contact and the stigma of mental illness: A review of the literature. *Journal of Mental Health, 12*, 291–305.

Cullen, E., & Salganicoff, A. (2011). *Adolescent health: Coverage and access to care.* Issue brief: An update on women's health policy. Publication #8236: The Henry J. Kaiser Family Foundation.

Cummings, J. R., Lucas, S. M., & Druss, B. G. (2013). Addressing public stigma and disparities among persons with mental illness: The role of federal policy. *American Journal of Public Health, 103*(5), 781–785.

Curran, G. M., Bauer, M., Mittman, B., Pyne, J. M., & Stetler, C. (2012). Effectiveness-implementation hybrid designs: Combining elements of clinical effectiveness and implementation research to enhance public health impact. *Medical Care, 50*(3), 217–226.

Curtin, S. C., Warner, M., & Hedegaard, H. (2016). *Increase in suicide in the United States, 1999–2014.* NCHS data brief, no 241. Hyattsville, MD: National Center for Health Statistics.

Curtis, B. L., McLellan, A. T., & Gabellini, B. N. (2014). Translating SBIRT to public school settings: An initial test of feasibility. *Journal of Substance Abuse Treatment, 46*(1), 15–21.

Damschroder, L. J., Aron, D. C., Keith, R. E., Kirsh, S. R., Alexander, J. A., & Lowery, J. C. (2009). Fostering implementation of health services research findings into practice: A consolidated framework for advancing implementation science. *Implementation Science, 4*, 50.

Deas, D., Riggs, P., Langenbucher, M., Goldman, M., & Brown, S. (2000). Adolescents are not adults: Developmental considerations in alcohol users. *Alcoholism: Clinical and Experimental Research, 24,* 232–237.

Deegan, P. E. (1993). Recovering our sense of value after being labeled mentally ill. *Journal of Psychosocial Nursing and Mental Health Services, 31*(4), 7–9.

DeNavas-Walt, C., & Proctor, B. D. (2015). *Income and poverty in the United States: 2014.* U.S. Census Bureau, Current Population Reports, P60-252. Washington, DC: U.S. Government Printing Office.

Dennis, M. L. (2009). *Understanding and managing addiction as a chronic condition.* Paper presented at the Congressional Addiction, Treatment, and Recovery Caucus Briefing, "Reducing Health Care Costs: Chronic Disease Management for Alcohol & Drug Problems," Washington, DC.

Desai, R. A., Goulet, J. L., Robbins, J., Chapman, J. F., Migdole, S. J., & Hoge, M. A. (2006). Mental health care in juvenile detention facilities: A review. *Journal of the American Academy of Psychiatry and the Law Online, 34*(2), 204–214.

Diefenbach, D. (1997). The portrayal of mental illness on prime-time television. *Journal of Community Psychology, 25,* 289–302.

Doherty, M. K., Meyers, K., Williams, L., Bonner, R., Reed, D., Tomlinson, A., & Hurtig, L. (2011). *Considerations for a child/adolescent oriented system of substance use care in Philadelphia.* Philadelphia, PA: Office of Addiction Services Advisory Board.

Donovan, C. L., Spence, S. H., & March, S. (2013). Using new technologies to deliver cognitive behaviour therpay with children and adolescents. In P. Graham & S. Reynolds (Eds.), *Cognitive behavior therapy for children and families* (pp. 351–370). New York: Cambridge University Press.

Ducharme, L. J., Mello, H. L., Roman, P. M., Knudsen, H. K., & Johnson, J. A. (2007). Service delivery in substance abuse treatment: Reexamining "comprehensive" care. *Journal of Behavioral Health Services & Research, 34*(2), 121–136.

Dudley, J. R. (2000). Confronting stigma within the services system. *Social Work, 45,* 449–455.

Durlak, J. A., & DuPre, E. P. (2008). Implementation matters: A review of research on the influence of implementation on program outcomes and the factors affecting implementation. *American Journal of Community Psychology, 41*(3-4), 327–350.

English, A., Gold, R. B., Nash, E., & Levine, J. (2012). *Confidentiality for individuals insured as dependents: A review of state laws and policies.* New York: Guttmacher Institute.

Esters, I. G., Cooker, P. G., & Ittenbach, R. F. (1998). Effects of a unit of instruction in mental health on rural adolescents' conceptions of mental illness and attitudes about seeking help. *Adolescence, 33,* 469–476.

Estroff, S. E., Penn, D. L., & Toporek, J. R. (2004). From stigma to discrimination: An analysis of community efforts to reduce the negative consequences of having a psychiatric disorder and label. *Schizophrenia Bulletin.* 30(3), 493–509.

Evans-Lacko, S., Corker, E., Williams, P., Henderson, C., & Thornicroft, G. (2014). Effect of the Time to Change anti-stigma campaign on trends in mental-illness-related public stigma among the English population in 2003–13: An analysis of survey data. *Lancet Psychiatry, 1*(2), 121–128.

Farina, A. & Felner, R. D. (1973). Employment interviewer reactions to former mental patients. *Journal of Abnormal Psychology, 82,* 268–272.

Farmer, E. M. Z., Mustillo, S. A., Wagner, H. R., Burns, B. J., Kolko, D. J., Barth, R. P., & Leslie, L. K. (2010). Service use and multi-sector use for mental health problems by youth in contact with child welfare. *Children and Youth Services Review, 32*(6), 815–821.

Feldstein, A. C., & Glasgow, R. E. (2008). A practical, robust implementation and sustainability model (PRISM) for integrating research findings into practice. *Joint Commission Journal on Quality and Patient Safety, 34*(4), 228–243.

Fiks, A. G., Grundmeier, R. W., Mayne, S., Song, L., Feemster, K., Karavite, D., . . . Bell, L. M. (2013). Effectiveness of decision support for families, clinicians, or both on HPV vaccine receipt. *Pediatrics, 131*(6), 1114–1124.

Finnell, D. S., Garbin, M., & Scarborough, J. (2004). Advanced practice addictions nursing specialty certification. *Journal of Addictions Nursing, 15,* 37–40.

Fixsen, D., Blase, K., Metz, A., & van Dyke, M. (2013). Statewide implementation of evidence-based programs. *Exceptional Children, 79*(2), 213–230.

Fixsen, D. L., Naoom, S. F., Blase, K. A., Friedman, R. M., & Wallace, F. (2005). *Implementation research: A synthesis of the literature.* Tampa, FL: University of South Florida, Louis de la Parte

Florida Mental Health Institute, The National Implementation Research Network.

Ford, C. A., Millstein, S. G., Halpern-Felsher, B. L., & Irwin, C. E. (1997). Influence of physician confidentiality assurances on adolescents' willingness to disclose information and seek future health care: A randomized controlled trial. *Journal of the American Medical Association, 278*(12), 1029–1034.

Ford, J., Green, C., Hoffman, K., Wisdom, J., Riley, K., Bergman, L., & T., M. (2008). Process improvement needs in substance abuse treatment: Admissions walk-through results. *Journal of Substance Abuse & Treatment, 33*(4), 379–389.

Freeborn, D. K., Polen, M. R., & Mullooly, J. P. (1995). Adolescent drug misuse treatment and use of medical care services. *Substance Use & Misuse, 30*(7), 795–822.

Gabel, S. (2010). The integration of mental health into pediatric practice: Pediatricians and child and adolescent psychiatrists working together in new models of care. *Journal of Pediatrics, 157*(5), 848–851.

Garner, B. R., Godley, S. H., Funk, R. R., Dennis, M. L., Smith, J. E., & Godley, M. D. (2009). Exposure to Adolescent Community Reinforcement Approach treatment procedures as a mediator of the relationship between adolescent substance abuse treatment retention and outcome. *Journal of Substance Abuse Treatment, 36*(3), 252–264.

Gewirtz, A., & Gossart-Walker, S. (2000). Home-based treatment for children and families affected by HIV and AIDS. Dealing with stigma, secrecy, disclosure, and loss. *Child and Adolescent Psychiatric Clinics of North America, 9*(2), 313–330.

Giesbers, J., Verdonck-de Leeuw, I. M., van Zuuren, F. J., Kleverlaan, N., & van der Linden, M. H. (2010). Coping with parental cancer: Web-based peer support in children. *Psycho-Oncology, 19*(8), 887–892.

Glasgow, R. E., Lichtenstein, E., & Marcus, A. C. (2003). Why don't we see more translation of health promotion research to practice? Rethinking the efficacy-to-effectiveness transition. *American Journal of Public Health, 93*(8), 1261–1267.

Gleacher, A. A., Nadeem, E., Moy, A. J., Whited, A. L., Albano, A. M., Radigan, M., . . . Eaton Hoagwood, K. (2011). Statewide CBT training for clinicians and supervisors treating youth: The New York State Evidence Based Treatment Dissemination Center. *Journal of Emotional and Behavioral Disorders, 19*(3), 182–192.

Glisson, C. (2007). Assessing and changing organizational culture and climate for effective services. *Research on Social Work Practice, 17*(6), 736–747.

Glisson, C., Hemmelgarn, A., Green, P., Dukes, D., Atkinson, S., & Williams, N. J. (2012). Randomized trial of the Availability, Responsiveness, and Continuity (ARC) organizational intervention with community-based mental health programs and clinicians serving youth. *Journal of the American Academy of Child & Adolescent Psychiatry, 51*(8), 780–787.

Glisson, C., & Schoenwald, S. K. (2005). The ARC organizational and community intervention strategy for implementing evidence-based children's mental health treatments. *Administration and Policy in Mental Health and Mental Health Services Research, 7*(4), 243–259.

Godley, M. D., & Godley, S. H. (2011). Assertive Continuing Care for adolescents. In J. Kelly & W. White (Eds.), *Addiction recovery management: Theory, science, and practice* (pp. 103–126). New York: Springer Publishing.

Godley, M. D., & Godley, S. H. (2012). Continuing care following residential treatment: History, current practice, critical issues, and emerging approaches. In N. Jainchill (Ed.), *Understanding and treating adolescent substance use disorders: Assessment, treatment, juvenile justice responses*. Kingston, NJ: Civic Research Institute, Inc.

Godley, M. D., Godley, S. H., Dennis, M. L., Funk, R., & Passetti, L. L. (2002). Preliminary outcomes from the assertive continuing care experiment for adolescents discharged from residential treatment. *Journal of Substance Abuse Treatment, 23*(1), 21–32.

Godley, S. H., Meyers, R. J., Smith, J. E., Godley, M. D., Titus, J. C., Karvinen, T., . . . Kelberg, P. (2001). The Adolescent Community Reinforcement Approach (ACRA) for adolescent cannabis users. *Cannabis Youth Treatment (CYT) Manual Series* (Vol. 4). Rockville, MD: Center for Substance Abuse Treatment, Substance Abuse and Mental Health Services Administration.

Gomory, T. (2013). The limits of evidence-based medicine and its application to mental health evidence-based practice: Part 1. *Ethical Human Psychology and Psychiatry, 15*(1), 18–34.

Gonzales, R., Anderer, T., McCulloch, C. E., Maselli, J. H., Bloom, F. J., Graf, T. R., . . . Metlay, J. P. (2013). A cluster randomized trial of decision support strategies for reducing antibiotic use in acute bronchitis. *JAMA Internal Medicine, 173*(4), 267–273.

Gonzales, R., Ang, A., Murphy, D. A., Glik, D. C., & Anglin, M. D. (2014). Substance use recovery outcomes among a cohort of youth participating in a mobile-based texting aftercare pilot program. *Journal of Substance Abuse Treatment, 47*(1), 20–26.

Granello, D., & Pauley, P. S. (2000). Television viewing habits and their relationship to tolerance toward people with mental illness. *Journal of Mental Health Counseling, 22*, 162–175.

Granello, D., Pauley, P. S., & Carmichael, A. (1999). Relationship of the media to attitudes toward people with mental illness. *Journal of Humanistic Counseling, Education, and Development, 38*, 98–110.

Gray, S. H., Pasternak, R. H., Gooding, H. C., Woodward, K., Hawkins, K., Sawyer, S., & Anoshiravani, A. (2014). Recommendations for electronic health record use for delivery of adolescent health care. *Journal of Adolescent Health, 54*(4), 487–490.

Green, L. W. (2001). From research to best practices in other settings and populations. *American Journal of Health Behavior, 25*(3), 165–178.

Green, L. W. (2007). *PRECEDE-PROCEED & RE-AIM as Frameworks for Practice-Based Planning and Evaluation: If We Want More Evidence-Based Practice, We Need More Practice-Based Evidence.* Paper presented at the CDC Oral Health Workshop, Atlanta, GA.

Groesz, L. M., Levine, M. P., & Murnen S. K. (2002). The effect of experimental presentation of thin media images on body satisfaction: A meta-analytic review. *International Journal of Eating Disorders, 31*, 1–16.

Gulliver, A., Griffiths, K. M., & Christensen, H. (2010). Perceived barriers and facilitators to mental health-seeking in young people: A systematic review. *BMC Psychiatry, 10*, 13.

Gustafson, D. H., McTavish, F. M., Chih, M.-Y., Atwood, A. K., Johnson, R. A., Boyle, M. G., ... Dillenburg, L. (2014). A smartphone application to support recovery from alcoholism: A randomized clinical trial. *JAMA Psychiatry, 71*(5), 566–572.

Hardesty, C. (2014). *Five things to know about opioid overdose.* Office of Drug Control Policy, from http://whitehouse.gov/blog/2014/02/10/5-things-know-about-opioid-overdoses

Harrell, E., Langton, L., Berzofsky, M., Couzens, L., & Smiley-McDonald, H. (2014). *Household poverty and nonfatal violent victimization, 2008–2012.* Report No. 248384. Washington, DC: U.S. Dept. of Justice, Bureau of Justice Statistics.

Hasui, C., Sakamoto, S., Sugiura, T., & Kitamua, T. (2000). Stigmatization of mental illness in Japan: Images and frequency of encounters with diagnostic categories of mental illness among medical and non-medical university students. *Journal of Psychiatry and Law, 28*, 253–266.

Henault, C. (2001). Zero tolerance in schools. *Journal of Law & Education, 30*, 547.

Henderson, C., Corker, E., Lewis-Holmes, E., Hamilton, S., Flach, C., Rose, D. & Thornicroft, G. (2012). England's Time to Change anti-stigma campaign: One-year outcomes of service user-rated experiences of discrimination. *Psychiatric Services*, 63, 451–457.

Hibbard, J. H., Stockard, J., & Tusler, M. (2005). Hospital performance reports: Impact on quality, market share, and reputation. *Health Affairs, 24*(4), 1150–1160.

Hilt, R., McDonell, M. G., Rockhill, C., Golombek, A., & Thompson, J. (2009). The Partnership Access Line: Establishing an empirically based child psychiatry consultation program for Washington State. *Report on Emotional and Behavioral Disorder in Youth, 9*(1), 3–7.

Hingson, R. W., Heeren, T., & Winter, M. R. (2006). Age at drinking onset and alcohol dependence: Age at onset, duration, and severity. *Archives of Pediatrics & Adolescent Medicine, 160*(7), 739–746.

Hingson, R. W., Heeren, T., Winter, M. R., & Wechsler, H. (2003). Early age of first drunkenness as a factor in college students' unplanned and unprotected sex attributable to drinking. *Pediatrics, 111*(1), 34–41.

Hingson, R. W., & Zha, W. (2009). Age of drinking onset, alcohol use disorders, frequent heavy drinking, and unintentionally injuring oneself and others after drinking. *Pediatrics, 123*(6), 1477–1484.

Hingson, R. W., Zha, W., & Weitzman, E. R. (2009). Magnitude of and trends in alcohol-related mortality and morbidity among U.S. college students ages 18–24, 1998–2005. *Journal of Studies on Alcohol and Drugs, Supplement No. 16*, 12–20.

Hirth, R. A. (1999). Consumer information and competition between nonprofit and for-profit nursing homes. *Journal of Health Economics, 18*(2), 219–240.

Hoagwood, K. E. (2013). Don't mourn: Organize. Reviving mental health services research for healthcare quality improvement. *Clinical Psychology: Science and Practice, 20*(1), 120–126.

Hoagwood, K. E., Burns, B. J., & Weisz, J. R. (2002). A profitable conjunction: From science to service in children's mental health. In B. J. Burns & K. E. Hoagwood (Eds.), *Community treatment for youth: Evidence-based interventions for severe emotional and behavioral disorders* (pp. 327–338). Oxford, UK: Oxford University Press.

Hoagwood, K. E., Cavaleri, M. A., Olin, S. S., Burns, B. J., Slaton, E., Gruttadaro, D., & Hughes, R. (2010). Family support in children's mental health: A review and synthesis. *Clinical Child and Family Psychology Review*, *13*(1), 1–45.

Hoagwood, K. E., Green, E., Kelleher, K., Schoenwald, S. K., Rolls-Reutz, J., Landsverk, J., . . . Mayberg, S. (2008). Family advocacy, support and education in children's mental health: Results of a national survey. *Administration and Policy in Mental Health and Mental Health Services Research*, *35*(1), 73–83.

Hoagwood, K., Olin, S., & Cleek, A. (2013). Beyond context to the skyline: Thinking in 3D. *Administration and Policy in Mental Health and Mental Health Services Research*, *40*(1), 23–28.

Hoagwood, K. E., Olin, S. S., Horwitz, S. M., McKay, M. M., Cleek, A. F., Gleacher, A., . . . Hogan, M. (2014). Scaling up evidence-based practices for children and families in New York State: Towards evidence-based policies on implementation for state mental health systems. *Journal of Clinical Child & Adolescent Psychology*, *43*(2), 145–157.

Horwitz, S. M., Kelleher, K. J., Stein, R. E., Storfer-Isser, A., Youngstrom, E. A., Park, E. R., . . . Hoagwood, K. E. (2007). Barriers to the identification and management of psychosocial issues in children and maternal depression. *Pediatrics*, *119*(1), e208–e218.

Hutchings, G. P., & King, K. (2009). *Ensuring U.S. health reform includes prevention and treatment of mental and substance use disorders—A framework for discussion: Core consensus principles for reform from the mental health and substance abuse community*. Rockville, MD: Substance Abuse and Mental Health Services Administration.

Hyler, S. E., Gabbard, G. O., & Schneider, I. (1991). Homicidal maniacs and narcissistic parasites: Stigmatization of mentally ill persons in the movies. *Hospital and Community Psychiatry*, *42*, 1044–1048.

IMDB. (2016). Box office for *A beautiful mind*. Available at http://www.imdb.com/title/tt0268978/business. Retrieved May 4, 2016.

Insel, T. (2013). Transforming diagnosis. *About NIMH: Director's blog*. Retrieved September 13, 2013, from http://www.nimh.nih.gov/about/director/2013/transforming-diagnosis.shtml

Institute of Medicine. (1989). *Report of a study on research on children and adolescents with mental, behavioral, and developmental disorders*. Division of Mental Health and Behavioral Medicine. Washington, DC: National Academies Press.

Institute of Medicine. (2001). *Crossing the quality chasm: A new health system for the 21st century*. Washington, DC: National Academies Press.

Institute of Medicine. (2006). *Improving the quality of health care for mental and substance-use conditions: Quality chasm series*. Washington, DC: National Academies Press.

Institute of Medicine. (2009). *On being a scientist: A guide to responsible conduct in research* (3rd ed.). Washington, DC: National Academies Press.

Institute of Medicine & National Research Council. (2011). *Child and adolescent health and health care quality: Measuring what matters*. Washington, DC: National Academies Press.

Ippolito, R. A. (1992). Consumer reaction to measures of poor quality. *Journal of Law and Economics*, *35*, 45–67.

Jackson, J. W. (1993). Contact theory of intergroup hostility: A review and evaluation of the theoretical and empirical literature. *International Journal of Group Tensions*, *23*, 43–65.

Jainchill, N. (2012). *Understanding and treating adolescent substance use disorders: Assessment, treatment, juvenile justice responses*. Kingston, NJ: Civic Research Institute, Inc.

Jamieson, P. E., Romer, D., &and Jamieson, K. H. (2006). Do films about mentally disturbed characters promote ineffective coping in vulnerable youth? *Journal of Adolescence*, *29*(5), 749–760.

Johnstone, L., & Hewstone, M. (1992). Cognitive models of stereotype change: 3. Subtyping and the perceived typicality of disconfirming group members. *Journal of Experimental Social Psychology*, *28*, 360–386.

Kaminer, Y. (1994). *Adolescent substance abuse: A comprehensive guide to theory and practice*. New York: Plenum.

Kaminer, Y., Burleson, J. A., & Burke, R. H. (2008). Efficacy of outpatient aftercare for adolescents with alcohol use disorders: A randomized controlled study. *Journal of the American Academy of Child and Adolescent Psychiatry*, *47*(12), 1405–1412.

Kandel, D. B., Yamaguchi, K., & Chen, K. (1992). Stages of progression in drug involvement from adolescence to adulthood: Further evidence for the gateway theory. *Journal of Studies on Alcohol and Drugs, 53*(5), 447.

Katon, W. J., & Unützer, J. (2013). Health reform and the Affordable Care Act: The importance of mental health treatment to achieving the triple aim. *Journal of Psychosomatic Research, 74*(6), 533–537.

Kauer, S. D., Reid, S. C., Crooke, A. H., Khor, A., Hearps, S. J., Jorm, A. F., ... Patton, G. (2012). Self-monitoring using mobile phones in the early stages of adolescent depression: Randomized controlled trial. *Journal of Medical Internet Research, 14*(3), e67.

Kazak, A. E., Hoagwood, K., Weisz, J. R., Hood, K., Kratochwill, T. R., Vargas, L. A., & Banez, G. A. (2010). A meta-systems approach to evidence-based practice for children and adolescents. *American Psychologist, 65*(2), 85–97.

Kazdin, A. E. (2013). Evidence-based treatment and usual care: Cautions and qualifications. *JAMA Psychiatry, 70*(7), 666–667.

Kazdin, A. E., & Rabbitt, S. M. (2013). Novel models for delivering mental health services and reducing the burdens of mental illness. *Clinical Psychological Science, 1*(2), 170–191.

Kealey, E., Scholle, S. H., Byron, S. C., Hoagwood, K. E., Leckman-Westin, E., Kelleher, K., & Finnerty, M. (2014). *Quality concerns in antipsychotic prescribing for youth: A review of treatment guidelines. Academic Pediatrics, 14*(5), S68–S75.

Kelleher, K. (2010). Organizational capacity to deliver effective treatments for children and adolescents. *Administration and Policy in Mental Health and Mental Health Services Research, 37*(1-2), 89–94.

Kendall, P. C., Khanna, M. S., Edson, A., Cummings, C., & Harris, M. S. (2011). Computers and psychosocial treatment for child anxiety: Recent advances and ongoing efforts. *Depression and Anxiety, 28*(1), 58–66.

Khanna, M. S., & Kendall, P. C. (2010). Computer-assisted cognitive behavioral therapy for child anxiety: Results of a randomized clinical trial. *Journal of Consulting and Clinical Psychology, 78*(5), 737–745.

Kim, H., & Eaton, N. R. (2015). The hierarchical structure of common mental disorders: Connecting multiple levels of comorbidity, bifactor models, and predictive validity. *Journal of Abnormal Psychology, 124*(4), 1064–1078.

Kim, H. S., Munson, M. R., & McKay, M. M. (2012). Engagement in mental health treatment among adolescents and young adults: A systematic review. *Child and Adolescent Social Work Journal, 29*(3), 241–266.

Klin, A., & Lemish, D. (2008). Mental disorders stigma in the media: Review of studies on production, content, and influences. *Journal of Health Communication: International Perspectives, 13*(5), 434–449.

Knaak, S., Modgill, G., & Patten, S. B. (2014). Key ingredients of anti-stigma programs for health care providers: A data synthesis of evaluative studies. *Canadian Journal of Psychiatry, 59* (10 Suppl 1), S19–S26.

Knight, J. R., Sherritt, L., Van Hook, S., Gates, E. C., Levy, S., & Chang, G. (2005). Motivational interviewing for adolescent substance use: A pilot study. *Journal of Adolescent Health, 37*, 167–169.

Knudsen, H. K. (2009). Adolescent-only substance abuse treatment: Availability and adoption of components of quality. *Journal of Substance Abuse Treatment, 36*, 195–204.

Kolko, D. (2015). The effectiveness of integrated care on pediatric behavioral health; outcomes and opportunities. *JAMA Pediatrics, 169*(10), 894–896.

Kolodziej, M. E., & Johnson, B. T. (1996). Interpersonal contact and acceptance of persons with psychiatric disorders: A research synthesis. *Journal of Consulting and Clinical Psychology, 64*, 1387–1396.

Kutash, K., Acri, M., Pollock, M., Armusewicz, K., Serene Olin, S.-C., & Hoagwood, K. E. (2014). Quality indicators for multidisciplinary team functioning in community-based children's mental health services. *Administration and Policy in Mental Health and Mental Health Services Research*, 41(1), 55–68.

Kutash, K., Duchnowski, A. J., Green, A. L., & Ferron, J. M. (2011). Supporting parents who have youth with emotional disturbances through a parent-to-parent support program: A proof of concept study using random assignment. *Administration and Policy in Mental Health and Mental Health Services Research, 38*(5), 412–427.

Lagnado, L. (2013). U.S. probes use of antipsychotic drugs on children. *Wall Street Journal*. Available at http://online.wsj.com/article/SB10001424127887323477604578654130865747470.html

Lahey, B. B., Rathouz, P. J., Keenan, K., Stepp, S. D., Loeber, R., & Hipwell, A. E. (2015). Criterion validity of the general factor of psychopathology in a prospective study of girls. *Journal of Child Psychology and Psychiatry, 56*(4), 415–422.

Landon, B. E., Onnela, J. P., Keating, N. L., Barnett, M. L., Paul, S., O'Malley, A. J., ... Christakis, N. A. (2013). Using administrative data to identify naturally occurring networks of physicians. *Medical Care, 51*(8), 715–721.

Langley, A., Nadeem, E., Kataoka, S., Stein, B., & Jaycox, L. (2010). Evidence-based mental health programs in schools: Barriers and facilitators of successful implementation. *School Mental Health, 2*(3), 105–113.

Lawrie, S. M. (1999). Stigmatisation of psychiatric disorder. *Psychiatric Bulletin, 23*, 129–131.

Lear, J. G. (2002). Schools and adolescent health: Strengthening services and improving outcomes. *Journal of Adolescent Health, 31*, 310–320.

Levey, S., & Howells, K. (1995). Dangerousness, unpredictability, and the fear of people with schizophrenia. *Journal of Forensic Psychiatry, 6*, 19–39.

Levy, S. J., & Kokotailo, P. K. (2011). Substance use screening, brief intervention, and referral to treatment for pediatricians. *Pediatrics, 128*, e1330-e1340.

Levy, S., Schizer, M., Ammerman, S. D., Gonzalez, P. K., Ryan, S. A., Siqueira, L. M., & Smith, V. C. (2015). Adolescent drug testing policies in schools. *Pediatrics, 135*(4), e1107–e1112.

Lewandowski, R. E., Acri, M. C., Hoagwood, K. E., Olfson, M., Clarke, G., Gardner, W., ... Horwitz, S. M. (2013). Evidence for the management of adolescent depression. *Pediatrics, 132*(4), e996–e1009.

Lewis, V. A., & Fisher, E. S. (2012). Social networks in health care: So much to learn. *Journal of the American Medical Association, 308*(3), 294–296.

Lieberman, J. A., Perkins, D., Belger, A., Chakos, M., Jarskog, F., Boteva, K., & Gilmore, J. (2001). The early stages of schizophrenia: Speculations on pathogenesis, pathophysiology, and therapeutic approaches. *Biological Psychiatry, 50*(11), 884–897.

Link, B. G., Cullen, F. T., Struening, E., Shrout, P. E., & Dohrenwend, B. P. (1989). A modified labeling theory approach to mental disorders: An empirical assessment. *American Sociological Review, 54*(3), 400–423.

Link, B. G., Mirotznik, J., & Cullen, F. T. (1991). The effectiveness of stigma coping orientations: Can negative consequences of mental illness be avoided? *Journal of Health and Social Behavior, 32*, 302–320.

Link, B. G., & Phelan, J. C. (1999). The labeling theory of mental disorder (II): The consequences of labeling. In A. V. Horwitz & T. L. Scheid (Eds.), *A handbook for the study of mental health: Social contexts, theories, and systems* (pp. 361–376). New York: Cambridge University Press.

Link, B. G., & Phelan, J. C. (2001). Conceptualizing stigma. *Annual Review of Sociology, 27*, 363–385.

Link, B. G., Struening, E. L., Neese-Todd, S., Asmussen, S., & Phelan, J. (2001). Stigma as a barrier to recovery: The consequences of stigma for the self-esteem of people with mental illness. *Psychiatric Services, 52*, 1621–1626.

Lipsey, M. W., Tanner-Smith, E. E., & Wilson, S. J. (2010). *Comparative effectiveness of adolescent substance abuse treatment: Three meta-analyses with implications for practice*. Peabody Research Institute: Vanderbilt University.

Livingston, J. D., & Boyd, J. E. (2010). Correlates and consequences of internalized stigma for people living with mental illness: A systematic review and meta-analysis. *Social Science and Medicine, 71*(12), 2150–2161.

Lofink, H., Kuebler, J., Juszczak, L., Schlitt, J., Even, M., Rosenberg, J., & White, I. (2013). *2010-2011 School-Based Health Alliance Census Report*. Washington, DC: School-Based Health Alliance.

Luxton, D. D., McCann, R. A., Bush, N. E., Mishkind, M. C., & Reger, G. M. (2011). mHealth for mental health: Integrating smartphone technology in behavioral healthcare. *Professional Psychology: Research and Practice, 42*(6), 505–512.

Ma, Z. (2017). How the media cover mental illness; a review. *Health Education, 117*(1), 90–109.

Madras, B. K., Compton, W. M., Avula, D., Stegbauer, T., Stein, J. B., & Clark, H. W. (2009). Screening, brief interventions, referral to treatment (SBIRT) for illicit drug and alcohol use at multiple healthcare sites: Comparison at intake and 6 months later. *Drug and Alcohol Dependence, 99*(1), 280–295.

Mann, J. J., & Michel, C. A. (2016). Prevention of firearm suicide in the United States: What works and what is possible. *American Journal of Psychiatry, 173*(10), 969–979.

March, S., Spence, S. H., & Donovan, C. L. (2009). The efficacy of an Internet-based cognitive-behavioral therapy intervention for child anxiety disorders. *Journal of Pediatric Psychology, 34*(5), 474–487.

Mark, T. L., Song, X., Vandivort, R., Duffy, S., Butler, J., Coffey, R., & Schabert, V. F. (2006). Characterizing substance abuse programs that treat adolescents. *Journal of Substance Abuse Treatment, 31*, 59–65.

Markowitz, F. E. (1998). The effects of stigma on the psychological well-being and life satisfaction of persons with mental illness. *Journal of Health and Social Behavior, 39*, 335–347.

Martin, C. S., & Winters, K. C. (1998). Diagnosis and assessment of alcohol use disorders among adolescents. *Alcohol Health and Research World, 22*(2), 95–105.

Martin, W. M. (2000). Does zero mean zero? Balancing policy with procedure in the fight against weapons at school. *American School Board Journal, 187*(3), 39–41.

McAndrews, T. (2001). Zero tolerance policies. *ERIC Digest Number 146*.

McCarty, D., Gustafson, D. H., Wisdom, J. P., Ford, J., Choi, D., Molfenter, T., . . . Cotter, F. (2007). The Network for the Improvement of Addiction Treatment (NIATx): Enhancing access and retention. *Drug and Alcohol Dependence, 88*(2), 138–145.

McGinty, E. E., Goldman, H. H., Pescosolido, B., & Barry, C. L. (2015). Portraying mental illness and drug addiction as treatable health conditions: Effects of a randomized experiment on stigma and discrimination. *Social Science and Medicine, 126*, 73–85.

McGorry, P. D., Yung, A., & Phillips, L. (2001). Ethics and early intervention in psychosis: Keeping the pace and staying in step. *Schizophrenia Research, 51*, 17–29.

McHugh, R. K., & Barlow, D. H. (2010). The dissemination and implementation of evidence-based psychological treatments. *American Psychologist, 65*(2), 73–84.

McKay, J. R., Lynch, K. G., Shepard, D. S., & Pettinati, H. M. (2005). The effectiveness of telephone-based continuing care for alcohol and cocaine dependence: 24-month outcomes. *Archives of General Psychiatry, 62*(2), 199–207.

McKay, J. R., Lynch, K. G., Shepard, D. S., Ratichek, S., Morrison, R., Koppenhaver, J., & Pettinati, H. M. (2004). The effectiveness of telephone-based continuing care in the clinical management of alcohol and cocaine use disorders: 12-month outcomes. *Journal of Consulting and Clinical Psychology, 72*(6), 967.

McKay, M. M., Gopalan, G., Franco, L., Dean-Assael, K., Chacko, A., Jackson, J. M., & Fuss, A. (2011). A collaboratively designed child mental health service model: Multiple Family Groups for urban children with conduct difficulties. *Research on Social Work Practice, 21*(6), 664–674.

McLellan, A. T., Curtis, B. L., Nordstrom, B., & Skrajewski, J. (2014). *Web-based medical school education on substance use disorders*. Poster presented at the annual conference of the Committee on Drug Dependence, Puerto Rico.

McLellan, A. T., Lewis, D. C., O'Brien, C. P., & Kleber, H. D. (2000). Drug dependence, a chronic medical illness: Implications for treatment, insurance, and outcomes evaluation. *Journal of the American Medical Association, 284*(13), 1689–1695.

McLellan, A. T., & Meyers, K. (2004). Contemporary addiction treatment: A review of systems problems for adults and adolescents. *Biological Psychiatry, 56*(10), 764–770.

Mechanic, D., McAlpine, D. D., & Rochefort, D. A. (2014). *Mental health and social policy: Beyond managed care* (6th ed.). Upper Saddle River, NJ: Pearson Education, Inc.

Mechanic, D., McAlpine, D., Rosenfield, S., & Davis, D. (1994). Effects of illness attribution and depression on the quality of life among persons with serious mental illness. *Social Science and Medicine, 39*, 155–164.

Medical University of South Carolina. (2013). *TF-CBTWeb: A web-based learning course for trauma-focused cognitive-behavioral therapy*. Retrieved November 8, 2013, from http://tfcbt.musc.edu

Mee-Lee, D., Shulman, G. D., Fishman, M. J., Gastfriend, D. R., & Miller, M. M. (2013). *The ASAM criteria: Treatment criteria for addictive, substance-related, and co-occurring conditions*. Carson Ciy, NV: The Change Companies.

Mellor, C. (2014). School-based interventions targeting stigma of mental illness: Systematic review. *Psychiatric Bulletin, 38*, 164–171.

Melnick, G., De Leon, G., Hawke, J., Jainchill, N., & Kressel, D. (1997). Motivation and readiness for therapeutic community treatment among adolescents and adult substance abusers. *American Journal of Drug and Alcohol Abuse, 23*(4), 485–506.

Meltzer, H., Bebbington, P., Brugha, T., Farrell, M., Jenkins, R., & Lewis, G. (2003). The reluctance to seek treatment for neurotic disorders. *International Review of Psychiatry, 15*, 123–128.

Mental Health Commission of Canada. (2015). *Opening Minds Program*. Available at http://www.mentalhealthcommission.ca/English/system/files/private/document/opening_minds_interim_report.pdf

Mericle, A. A., Arria, A. M., Meyers, K., Cacciola, J., Winters, K. C., & Kirby, K. (2015). National trends in adolescent substance use disorders and treatment availability: 2003–2010. *Journal of Child & Adolescent Substance Abuse, 24*(5), 255–263.

Merikangas, K. R., He, J.-P., Brody, D., Fisher, P. W., Bourdon, K., & Koretz, D. S. (2010). Prevalence and treatment of mental disorders among US children in the 2001–2004 NHANES. *Pediatrics, 125*(1), 75–81.

Merikangas, K. R., He, J.-P., Burstein, M., Swanson, S. A., Avenevoli, S., Cui, L., ... Swendsen, J. (2010). Lifetime prevalence of mental disorders in U.S. adolescents: Results from the National Comorbidity Survey Replication–Adolescent Supplement (NCS-A). *Journal of the American Academy of Child and Adolescent Psychiatry, 49*(10), 980–989.

Merikangas, K. R., He, J.-P., Burstein, M., Swendsen, J., Avenevoli, S., Case, B., ... Olfson, M. (2011). Service utilization for lifetime mental disorders in U.S. adolescents: Results of the National Comorbidity Survey–Adolescent Supplement (NCS-A). *Journal of the American Academy of Child and Adolescent Psychiatry, 50*(1), 32–45.

Merikangas, K. R., He, J. P., Rapoport, J., Vitiello, B., & Olfson, M. (2013). Medication use in US youth with mental disorders. *JAMA Pediatrics, 167*(2), 141–148.

Mermelstein, R., & Turner, L. (2006). Web-based support as an adjunct to group-based smoking cessation for adolescents. *Nicotine & Tobacco Research, 8*(Suppl 1), S69–S76.

Meyers, K., Cacciola, J., Ward, S., Kaynak, O., & Woodworth, A. (2014). *Paving the way to change: Advancing quality interventions for adolescents who use, abuse or are dependent upon alcohol and other drugs*. Philadelphia, PA: Treatment Research Institute.

Meyers, K., & McLellan, A. T. (2005a). The American treatment system for adolescent substance abuse: Formidable challenges, fundamental revisions and mechanisms for improvements. In M. E. P. Seligman & D. Evans (Eds.), *Adolescent health care*. New York: Oxford University Press.

Meyers, K., & McLellan, A. T. (2005b). The American treatment system for adolescent substance abuse: Formidable challenges, fundamental revisions, and mechanisms for improvements. In D. Evans, E. Foa, R. Gur, H. Hendin, C. O'Brien, M. Seligman, & T. Walsh (Eds.), *Treating and preventing adolescent mental health disorders* (1st ed., pp. 561–578). New York: Oxford University Press.

Miller, J. W., Naimi, T. S., Brewer, R. D., & Jones, S. E. (2007). Binge drinking and associated health risk behaviors among high school students. *Pediatrics, 119*(1), 76–85.

Miller, N., Shepard, L. M., & Magen, J. (2001). Barriers to improving education and training in addiction medicine. *Psychiatric Annals, 31*, 649–656.

Minkoff, K. (1987). Resistance of mental health professionals to working with the chronically mentally ill. In A. T. Meyerson (Ed.), *Barriers to treating the chronic mentally ill* (pp. 3–20). New Directions in Mental Health Services, 33. San Francisco, CA: Jossey-Bass.

Missouri Therapy Network. (2013). Resources for therapists. Retrieved November 8, 2013, from https://motherapynetwork.wustl.edu

Mitchell, S. G., Gryczynski, J., O'Grady, K. E., & Schwartz, R. P. (2013). SBIRT for adolescent drug and alcohol use: Current status and future directions. *Journal of Substance Abuse Treatment, 44*(5), 463–472.

Mitchell, S. G., Schwartz, R. P., Kirk, A. S., Dusek, K., Oros, M., Hosler, C., ... Brown, B. S. (2016). SBIRT implementation for adolescents in urban federally qualified health centers. *Journal of Substance Abuse treatment, 60*, 81–90.

Mittal, D., Sullivan, G., Chekuri, L., Allee, E., & Corrigan, P. W. (2012). Empirical studies of self-stigma reduction strategies: A critical review of the literature. *Psychiatric Services, 63*(10), 974–981.

Moberg, D. P., & Finch, A. J. (2008). Recovery high schools: A descriptive study of school programs and students. *Journal of Groups in Addiction & Recovery, 2*(2-4), 128–161.

Mohr, D. C., Cheung, K., Schueller, S. M., Brown, C. H., & Duan, N. (2013). Continuous evaluation of evolving behavioral intervention technologies. *American Journal of Preventive Medicine, 45*(4), 517–523.

Monahan, J. (1992). Mental disorder and violent behavior: Perceptions and evidence. *American Psychologist, 47*(4), 511.

Monti, P. M., Colby, S. M., Barnett, N. P., Spirito, A., Rohsenow, D. J., Myers, M., ... Lewander, W. (1999). Brief intervention for harm reduction with alcohol-positive older adolescents in a hospital emergency department. *Journal of Consulting and Clinical Psychology, 67*, 989–994.

Morrison, C., & Bailey, C. (2011). The Alternative Peer Group: A recovery model for teens and young adults Retrieved Sept. 20, 2013, from http://www.recoverytoday.net/2011/50-march/286-the-alternative-peer-group-a-recovery-model-for-teens-and-young-adults?format=pdf.

Muck, R., Zempolich, K. A., Titus, J. C., Fishman, M., Godley, M. D., & Schwebel, R. (2001). An overview of the effectiveness of adolescent substance abuse treatment models. *Youth & Society, 33*(2), 143–168.

Muennig, P. (2015). Can universal pre-kindergarten programs improve population health and longevity? Mechanisms, evidence, and policy implications. *Social Science & Medicine, 127,* 116–123.

Mueser, K. T., & Bellack, A. S. (1998). Social skills and social functioning. In K. T. Mueser & N. Tarrier (Eds.), *Handbook of social functioning in schizophrenia* (pp. 79–96). Needham Heights, MA: Allyn & Bacon.

Mukherjee, R., Fialho, A., Wijetunge, A., Checinski, K., & Surgenor, T. (2002). The stigmatization of psychiatric illness: The attitudes of medical students and doctors in a London teaching hospital. *Psychiatric Bulletin, 26,* 178–181.

Mutter, R., Ali, M. M., Smith, K., & Strashny, A. (2015). Factors associated with substance use treatment completion in residential facilities. *Drug and Alcohol Dependence, 154,* 291–295.

Myers, M. G., Brown, S. A., & Mott, M. A. (1995). Preadolescent conduct disorder behaviors predict relapse and progression of addiction for adolescent alcohol and drug abusers. *Alcoholism: Clinical and Experimental Research, 19*(6), 1528–1536.

Nairn, R., Coverdale, J., & Claasen, D. (2001). From source material to news story in New Zealand print media: A prospective study of the stigmatizing processes depicting mental illness. *Australian and New Zealand Journal of Pyschiatry, 35,* 654–659.

Nakamura, M. M., Harper, M. B., & Jha, A. K. (2013). Change in adoption of electronic health records by US children's hospitals. *Pediatrics, 131*(5), e1563–e1575.

NASADAD. (1998). *Improving the dialogue in co-occurring mental health and substance abuse disorders.* Washington, DC.

NASADAD. (2002). *Identification and description of multiple alcohol and other drug treatment systems.* Final report for SAMHSA/CSAT Health Care Reform Technical Assistance and Knowledge Development, Synthesis and Dissemination Project.

National Academies of Sciences, Engineering, and Medicine. (2016). *Ending discrimination against people with mental and substance use disorders: The evidence for stigma change.* Washington, DC: National Academies Press. Available at http://www.nap.edu/23442. Retrieved April 27, 2016.

National Alliance for the Mentally Ill (2002). NAMI honors *A beautiful mind* for year's most outstanding contribution to public understanding of mental illness. Available at https://www.nami.org/Press-Media/Press-Releases/2002/Nami-Honors-A-Beautiful-Mind-For-Year-s-Most-Outst. Retrieved April 26, 2016.

National Association of School Nurses. (2015). *Naloxone use in the school setting: The role of the school nurse (Position Statement).* Silver Spring, MD.

National Cancer Institute. (2013). *Grid-enabled measure database.* Retrieved September 2, 2013, from https://www.gem-beta.org/public/Home.aspx?cat=0.

National Child Traumatic Stress Network. (2013). *Empirically supported treatments and promising practices.* Retrieved November 5, 2013, from http://www.nctsn.org/resources/topics/treatments-that-work/promising-practices

National Institute of Health. (2012). *NIH awards $100 million for Autism Centers of Excellence Program.* News & Events. Retrieved November 2, 2013, from http://www.nih.gov/news/health/sep2012/nichd-04.htm

National Institute of Mental Health. (2001). *Blueprint for change: Research on child and adolescent mental health.* The National Advisory Mental Health Council Workgroup on Child and Adolescent Mental Health Intervention Deployment and Development. Bethesda, MD: Office of Communications and Public Liaison, Information Resources and Inquiries Branch.

National Institute of Mental Health. (2013). *Advances in global mental health research and research capacity building.* Research Priorities/Scientific Meetings. Retrieved November 2, 2013, from http://www.nimh.nih.gov/research-priorities/scientific-meetings/2013/advances-in-global-mental-health-research-and-research-capacity-building.shtml

Newacheck, P. W., Brindis, C. D., Cart, C. U., Marchi, K., & Irwin, C. E. (1999). Adolescent health insurance coverage: recent changes and access to care. *Pediatrics, 104*(2), 195–202.

New Freedom Commission on Mental Health. (2003). *Achieving the promise: Transforming mental health care in America. Final Report.* DHHS Pub. No. SMA-03-3832. Rockville, MD.

New York State Department of Health. (2011). *Redesigning New York's Medicaid program.* Retrieved November 5, 2013, from www.health.ny.gov/health_care/medicaid/redesign/

New York State Office of Mental Health. (2012). *Behavioral health organizations implementation.*

Retrieved September 13, 2013, from http://www.omh.ny.gov/omhweb/bho/.

Norman, R. M. G., & Malla, A. (2001). Duration of untreated psychosis: A critical examination of the concept and its importance. *Psychological Medicine, 31*, 381–400.

Office of Juvenile Justice and Delinquency Prevention. (2009). *Juvenile court statistics 2009*. Washington, DC: Office of Juvenile Justice and Delinquency Prevention.

Office of Juvenile Justice and Deliquency Prevention. (2013). *Model program guide*. Retrieved November 5, 2013, from http://www.ojjdp.gov/MPG/Default.aspx

O'Kearney, R., Gibson, M., Christensen, H., & Griffiths, K. M. (2006). Effects of a cognitive-behavioural internet program on depression, vulnerability to depression and stigma in adolescent males: A school-based controlled trial. *Cognitive Behaviour Therapy, 35*(1), 43–54.

Olin, S. S., Kutash, K., Pollock, M., Burns, B. J., Kuppinger, A., Craig, N., ... Hoagwood, K. E. (2014). Developing quality indicators for family support services in community team-based mental health care. *Administration and Policy in Mental Health and Mental Health Services Research, 41*(1), 7–20.

Olin, S. S., Williams, N., Pollock, M., Armusewicz, K., Kutash, K., Glisson, C., & Hoagwood, K. E. (2014). Quality indicators for family support services and their relationship to organizational social context. *Administration and Policy in Mental Health and Mental Health Services Research, 41*(1), 43–54.

Oxford English Dictionary Online (2016). Stigma. Retrieved May 6, 2016, from http://www.oed.com/view/Entry/190242?redirectedFrom=stigma

Page, S. (1995). Effects of the mental illness label in 1993: Acceptance and rejection in the community. *Journal of Health and Social Policy, 7*, 61–68.

Patient-Centered Outcomes Research Institute (PCORI). (2013). *Pilot projects*. Funding Opportunities. Retrieved September 13, 2013, from http://www.pcori.org/pilot-projects

Patient Protection and Affordable Care Act of 2010, Pub. L. No. 111-148, 124 Stat. 119-1205 (2010).

Paul Wellstone and Pete Domenici Mental Health Parity and Addiction Equity Act of 2008, 3765, Pub. L. No. 110-343 § 511, 122 Stat. (2008).

Penn, D. L., Judge, A., Jamieson, P., Garczynski, J., Hennessy, M., & Romer, D. (2005). Stigma. In D. L. Evans, E. B. Foa, R. E. Gur, H. Hendin, C. P. O'Brien, M. E. P. Seligman, & B. T. Walsh (eds.). *Treating and preventing adolescent mental health disorders* (1st ed., pp. 532–543). New York: Oxford University Press.

Penn, D. L., Kohlmaier, J., & Corrigan, P. W. (2000). Interpersonal factors contributing to the stigma of schizophrenia: Social skills, perceived attractiveness, and symptoms. *Schizophrenia Research, 45*, 37–45.

Perlick, D. A., Rosenheck, R. A., Clarkin, J. F., Sirey, J., Salahi, J., Struening, E., & Link, B. G., (2001). Stigma as a barrier to recovery: Adverse effects of perceived stigma on social adaptation of persons diagnosed with bipolar disorder. *Psychiatric Services, 52*, 1627–1632.

Pescosolido, B. A., Fettes, D. L., Martin, J. K., Monahan, J., & McLeod, J. D. (2007). Perceived dangerousness of children with mental health problems and support for coerced treatment. *Psychiatric Services, 58*(5), 619–625.

Pescosolido, B. A., Martin, J. K., Long, J. S., Medina, T. R., Phelan, J. C., & Link, B. G. (2010). "A disease like any other"? A decade of change in public reactions to schizophrenia, depression, and alcohol dependence. *American Journal of Psychiatry, 167*, 1321–1330.

Pescosolido, B. A., Monahan, J., Link, B. G., Stueve, A., & Kikuzawa, S. (1999). The public's view of the competence, dangerousness, and need for legal coercion of persons with mental health problems. *American Journal of Public Health, 89*, 1339–1345.

Pettigrew, T. F. (2016). In pursuit of three theories; authoritarianism, relative deprivation, and intergroup contact. *Annual Review of Psychology, 67*, 1–21.

Pettigrew, T. F., & Tropp, L. R. (2006). A meta-analytic test of intergroup contact theory. *Journal of Personality and Social Psychology, 90*(5), 751.

Phelan, J. C., Cruz-Rojas, R., & Reiff, M. (2002). Genes and stigma: The connection between perceived genetic etiology and attitudes and beliefs about mental illness. *Psychiatric Rehabilitation Skills, 6*(2), 159–185.

Phelan, J. C., & Link, B. G. (1999). The labeling theory of mental disorder (I): The role of social contingencies in the application of psychiatric labels. In A. V. Horwitz & T. L. Scheid (Eds.), *A handbook for the study of mental health: Social contexts, theories, and systems* (pp. 139–149). New York: Cambridge University Press.

Pidano, A., & Honigfeld, L. (2012). Pediatric psychopharmacology: Context, model programs, and considerations for care. *Psychiatric Services, 63*(9), 929–934.

Pincus, H. A., Spaeth-Rublee, B., & Watkins, K. E. (2011). The case for measuring quality in mental health and substance abuse care. *Health Affairs, 30*(4), 730–736.

Planty, M., & Truman, J. L. (2013). *Firearm violence, 1993–2011*. Report No. 241730. Washington, DC: U.S. Dept of Justice, Bureau of Justice Statistics.

Pollock, N. K., & Martin, C. S. (1999). Diagnostic orphans: Adolescents with alcohol symptoms who do not qualify for DSM-IV abuse or dependence diagnoses. *American Journal of Psychiatry, 156*(6), 897–901.

Post, R. M., Leverich, G., Xing, G., & Weiss, S. R. B. (2001). Developmental vulnerabilities to the onset and course of bipolar disorder. *Development and Psychopathology, 13*, 581–598.

Poulin, F., Dishion, T. J., & Burraston, B. (2001). 3-year iatrogenic effects associated with aggregating high-risk adolescents in cognitive-behavioral preventive interventions. *Applied Developmental Science, 5*(4), 214–224.

Pugatch, D., Bennett, L., & Patterson, D. (2002). HIV medication adherence in adolescents: A qualitative study. *Journal of HIV/AIDS Prevention and Education for Adolescents and Children, 5*, 9–29.

Rahdert, E., & Czechowicz, D. (1995). Adolescent drug abuse: Clinical assessment and therapeutic interventions. *National Institute on Drug Abuse Research Monograph 156*. Washington, DC: U.S. Government Printing Office.

Reardon, S. (2014). Teen drug use gets supersize study: US government programme will examine 10,000 adolescents to document effects on developing brains. *Nature, 512*, 123.

Reavley, N. J., & Jorm, A. F. (2011). Stigmatizing attitudes towards people with mental disorders: Findings from an Australian National Survey of Mental Health Literacy and Stigma. *Australian and New Zealand Journal of Psychiatry, 45*(12), 1086–1093.

Reiss, F. (2013). Socioeconomic inequalities and mental health problems in children and adolescents: A systematic review. *Social Science and Medicine, 90*, 24–31.

Ringwalt, C., Vincus, A. A., Ennett, S. T., Hanley, S., Bowling, J. M., Yacoubian, G. S., & Rohrbach, L. A. (2009). Responses to positive results from suspicionless random drug tests in US public school districts. *Journal of School Health, 79*(4), 177–183.

Robert Wood Johnson Foundation. (2011). *Does publicly reporting performance help improve health care quality?* Health Policy Snapshot. http://www.rwjf.org/.

Robert Wood Johnson Foundation. (2013). *Return on investments in public health: Saving lives and money.* Policy Highlight Brief.

Roberts, R. E., Roberts, C. R., & Chan, W. (2009). One-year incidence of psychiatric disorders and associated risk factors among adolescents in the community. *Journal of Child Psychology and Psychiatry, 50*(4), 405–415.

Roman, P. M., & Johnson, J. A. (2002). Adoption and implementation of new technologies in substance abuse treatment. *Journal of Substance Abuse Treatment, 22*(4), 210–218.

Romer, D., & Bock, M. (2008). Reducing the stigma of mental illness among adolescents and young adults: The effects of treatment information. *Journal of Health Communication, 13*, 742–758.

Romer, D., & McIntosh, M. (2005a). The role of primary care physicians in detection and treatment of adolescent mental health problems. In D. Evans, E. Foa, R. Gur, H. Hendin, C. O'Brien, M. Seligman, & T. Walsh (Eds.), *Treating and preventing adolescent mental health disorders* (1st ed., pp. 579–595). New York: Oxford University Press.

Romer, D., & McIntosh, M. (2005b). The roles and perspectives of school mental health professionals in promoting adolescent mental health. In D. Evans, E. Foa, R. Gur, H. Hendin, C. O'Brien, M. Seligman, & T. Walsh (Eds.), *Treating and preventing adolescent mental health disorders* (1st ed., pp. 597–615). New York: Oxford University Press.

Ryan, C. S., Robinson, D. R., & Hausmann, L. R. (2001). Stereotyping among providers and consumers of public mental health services: The role of perceived group variability. *Behavior Modification, 25*, 406–442.

Sadow, D., & Ryder, M. (2008). Reducing stigmatizing attitudes held by future health professionals: The person is the message. *Psychological Services, 5*(4), 362–372.

Saitz, R., Larson, M. J., Labelle, C., Richardson, J., & Samet, J. H. (2008). The case for chronic disease management for addiction. *Journal of Addiction Medicine, 2*, 55–65.

Saiz, J. (1992). *No hagen juego, senores* (Don't begin the game). *Interviu, 829*, 24–28.

Saldana, L., Chamberlain, P., Bradford, W. D., Campbell, M., & Landsverk, J. (2015). The cost of implementing new strategies (COINS): A method for mapping implementation resources using the stages of implementation completion. *Children and Youth Services Review* 39: 177–182.

SAMHSA. (2008). *SAMHSA awards $66 million for programs teaching early intervention techniques* *to use with patients at risk for substance abuse.* Retrieved February 21, 2016, from http://www.samhsa.gov/newsroom/press-announcements/200809080300.

SAMHSA. (2012). *Results from the 2011 National Survey on Drug Use and Health: Summary of national findings.* NSDUH Series. Rockville, MD: Substance Abuse and Mental Health Services Administration.

SAMHSA. (2015a). *Screening, brief intervention, and referral to treatment (SBIRT) grantees.* Retrieved February 21, 2016, from http://www.samhsa.gov/sbirt/grantees.

SAMHSA. (2015b). *Screening, brief intervention, and referral to treatment (SBIRT) health professions student training.* Funding Opportunity Announcement (FOA) Information; FOA Number: TI-16-002. Retrieved February 21, 2016, from http://www.samhsa.gov/grants/grant-announcements/ti-16-002

Sanders, M. R., Baker, S., & Turner, K. M. T. (2012). A randomized controlled trial evaluating the efficacy of Triple P Online with parents of children with early-onset conduct problems. *Behaviour Research & Therapy, 50*(11), 675–684.

Santelli, J., Kouzis, A., & Newcomer, S. (1996). School-based health centers and adolescent use of primary care and hospital care. *Journal of Adolescent Health, 19*(4), 267–275.

Sartorius, N. (2002). Iatrogenic stigma of mental illness. *British Medical Journal, 324*, 1470–1471.

Sarvet, B., Gold, J., Bostic, J. Q., Masek, B. J., Prince, J. B., Jeffers-Terry, M., ... Straus, J. H. (2010). Improving access to mental health care for children: The Massachusetts Child Psychiatry Access Project. *Pediatrics, 126*(6), 1191–1200.

Schoen, C., Osborn, R., Squires, D., Doty, M., Rasmussen, P., Pierson, R., & Applebaum, S. (2012). A survey of primary care doctors in ten countries shows progress in use of health information technology, less in other areas. *Health Affairs, 31*(12), 2805–2816.

Schulze, B., Richter-Werling, M., Matschinger, H., & Angermeyer, M. C. (2003). Crazy? So what! Effects of a school project on students' attitudes towards people with schizophrenia. *Acta Psychiatrica Scandinavica, 107*, 142–150.

Scott, C. K., Dennis, M. L., & Foss, M. A. (2005). Utilizing recovery management checkups to shorten the cycle of relapse, treatment reentry, and recovery. *Drug and Alcohol Dependence, 78*(3), 325–338.

Seattle Implementation Research Collaborative. (2013). *Instrument Review Project: A comprehensive review of dissemination and implementation science instruments.* Retrieved September 13, 2013, from http://www.seattleimplementation.org/sir.-projects/sirc-instrument-project/

Secker, J., Armstrong, C., & Hill, M. (1999). Young people's understanding of mental illness. *Health and Education Research, 14*, 729–739.

Segal, B., Morral, A. R., & Stevens, S. J. (2014). *Adolescent substance abuse treatment in the United States: Exemplary models from a national evaluation study.* London/New York: Routledge.

Segrin, C. (2000). Social skill deficits associated with depression. *Clinical Psychology Review, 20*, 379–403.

Sexton, T., Chamberlin, P., Landsverk, J., Ortiz, A., & Schoenwald, S. (2010). Action brief: Future directions in the implementation of evidence-based treatment and practices in child and adolescent mental health. *Administration and Policy in Mental Health and Mental Health Services Research, 37*(1-2), 132–134.

Shapiro, V. B., Hawkins, D., Oesterle, S., Monahan, K. C., Brown, E. C., & Arthur, M. W. (2013). Variation in the effect of Communities That Care on community adoption of a scientific approach to prevention. *Journal of Society for Social Work and Research, 4*(3), 154–164.

Sigel, B. A., Kramer, T. L., Conners-Burrow, N. A., Church, J. K., Worley, K. B., & Mitrani, N. A. (2013). Statewide dissemination of trauma-focused cognitive-behavioral therapy (TF-CBT). *Children and Youth Services Review, 35*(6), 1023–1029.

Signorielli, N. (2001). Television's gender role images and contribution to stereotyping: Past, present, future. In D. Singer & J. L. Singer (Eds.), *Handbook of children and the media* (pp. 341–358). Thousand Oaks, CA: Sage Publishers.

Silver, E. (2001). *Mental illness and violence: The importance of neighborhood context.* New York: LFB Scholarly Publishing LLC.

Silverman, W. K., & Hinshaw, S. P. (2008). The second special issue on evidence-based psychosocial treatments for children and adolescents: A 10-year update. *Journal of Clinical Child & Adolescent Psychology, 37*(1), 1–7.

Sirey, J., Bruce, M. L., Alexopoulos, G. S., Perlick, D A., Freidman, S. J., & Meyers, B. S. (2001a). Stigma as a barrier to recovery: Perceived stigma and patient rated severity of illness as predictors of antidepressant drug adherence. *Psychiatric Services, 52*, 1615–1620.

Sirey, J., Bruce, M. L., Alexopoulos, G. S., Perlick, D. A., Raue, P., Friedman, S. J., & Meyers, B. S.

(2001b). Perceived stigma as a predictor of treatment discontinuation in young and older outpatients with depression. *American Journal of Psychiatry, 158*, 479–481.

Solberg, L. I., Glasgow, R. E., Unützer, J., Jaeckels, N., Oftedahl, G., Beck, A., ... Crain, A. L. (2010). Partnership research: A practical trial design for evaluation of a natural experiment to improve depression care. *Medical Care, 48*(7), 576–582.

Soler, M. (1992). Interagency services in juvenile justice systems. In I. M. Schwartz (Ed.), *Juvenile justice and public policy: Toward a national agenda* (pp. 134–150). New York: Lexington Books.

Southam-Gerow, M. A., Daleiden, E. L., Chorpita, B. F., Bae, C., Mitchell, C., Faye, M., & Alba, M. (2014). MAPping Los Angeles County: Taking an evidence-informed model of mental health care to scale. *Journal of Clinical Child & Adolescent Psychology, 43*(2), 190–200.

Spirito, A., Monti, P. M., Barnett, N. P., Colby, S. M., Sindelar, H., Rohsenow, D. J., ... Myers, M. (2004). A randomized clinical trial of a brief motivational intervention for alcohol-positive adolescents treated in an emergency department. *Journal of Pediatrics, 145*, 396–402.

Squeglia, L. M., Jacobus, J., & Tapert, S. F. (2009). The influence of substance use on adolescent brain development. *Clinical EEG and Neuroscience, 40*(1), 31–38.

Squeglia, L. M., Spadoni, A. D., Infante, M. A., Myers, M. G., & Tapert, S. F. (2009). Initiating moderate to heavy alcohol use predicts changes in neuropsychological functioning for adolescent girls and boys. *Psychology of Addictive Behaviors, 23*(4), 715–722.

Sterling, S., Kline-Simon, A. H., Wibbelsman, C., Wong, A., & Weisner, C. (2012). Screening for adolescent alcohol and drug use in pediatric health-care settings: Predictors and implications for practice and policy. *Addiction Science & Clinical Practice, 7*, 13.

Sterling, S., Valkanoff, T., Hinman, A., & Weisner, C. (2012). Integrating substance use treatment into adolescent health care. *Current Psychiatry Reports, 14*, 453–461.

Sterling, S., & Weisner, C. (2007). *The role of primary care in addressing adolescent substance use: Screening, treatment, and coordination.* Symposium conducted at the meeting of the California Society of Addiction Medicine, Los Angeles, CA.

Sterling, S., Weisner, C., Hinman, A., & Parthasarathy, S. (2010). Access to treatment for adolescents with substance use and co-occurring disorders: Challenges and opportunities. *Journal of the American Academy of Child and Adolescent Psychiatry, 49*(7), 637–646.

Straus, J. H., & Sarvet, B. (2012). Programs in 26 states part of network to improve child psychiatry access. *American Academy of Pediatrics News, 33*(5), 13.

Substance Abuse and Mental Health Services Administration. (2007). *Results from the 2006 National Survey on Drug Use and Health: National findings*. Rockville, MD: Department of Health and Human Services.

Substance Abuse and Mental Health Services Administration. (2013). *Substance Abuse and Mental Health Services Administration, Results from the 2012 National Survey on Drug Use and Health: Summary Of National Findings*. Rockville, MD: Author.

Substance Abuse and Mental Health Services Administration. (2013a). Disaster Technical Assistance Center (DTAC). Retrieved November 8, 2013, from http://www.samhsa.gov/dtac

Substance Abuse and Mental Health Services Administration. (2013b). National Registry of Evidence-based Programs and Practices. Retrieved November 5, 2013, from http://nrepp.samhsa.gov/AboutNREPP.aspx

Sznitman, S. R., Reisel, L., & Romer, D. (2011). The neglected role of adolescent mental health in national educational achievement: Bridging the gap between education and mental health policies. *Journal of Adolescent Health,* 48(2), 135–142.

Tait, R. J., Hulse, G. K., Robertson, S. I., & Sprivulis, P. C. (2005). Emergency department-based intervention with adolescent substance users: 12-month outcomes. *Drug and Alcohol Dependence, 79*, 359–363.

Tanner-Smith, E. E., Wilson, S. J., & Lipsey, M. W. (2013). The comparative effectiveness of outpatient treatment for adolescent substance abuse: A meta-analysis. *Journal of Substance Abuse Treatment, 44*(2), 145–158.

Tebb, K., Sedlander, E., Pica, G., Diaz, A., Peake, K., & Brandis, C. (2014). *Protecting adolescent confidentiality under health care reform: The special care regarding explanation of benefits (EOBs).* Philips R. Lee Institute for Health Policy Studies and Division of Adolescent and Young Adult Medicine, Department of Pediatrics, University of California, San Francisco.

Terry-McElrath, Y. M., O'Malley, P. M., & Johnston, L. D. (2013). Middle and high school drug testing and student illicit drug use: A national study

1998–2011. *Journal of Adolescent Health, 52*(6), 707–715.

Thoits, P. A. (2006). Personal agency in the stress process. *Journal of Health and Social Behavior*, 47, 309–323.

Thornicroft, G., Mehta, N., Clement, S., Evans-Lacko, S., Doherty, M., Rose, D., . . . Henderson, C. (2016). Evidence for effective interventions to reduce mental-health-related stigma and discrimination. *Lancet, 387*, 1123–1132.

Torda, P., & Tinoco, A. (2013). Achieving the promise of electronic health record-enabled quality measurement: A measure developer's perspective. *eGEMs (Generating Evidence & Methods to Improve Patient Outcomes), 1*(2), Article 3.

Trudeau, K. J., Ainscough, J., & Charity, S. (2012). *Technology in treatment: Are adolescents and counselors interested in online relapse prevention?* Paper presented at Child & Youth Care Forum.

U.S. Department of Health and Human Services. (1999). *Mental health: A report of the surgeon general*. Rockville, MD: U.S. Department of Health and Human Services, Substance Abuse and Mental Health Services Administration, Center for Mental Health Services, National Institutes of Health, National Institute of Mental Health.

U.S. Public Health Service. (1999). *Mental health: A report of the Surgeon General*. Washington, DC: U.S. Department of Health and Human Services.

U.S. Public Health Service. (2000). *Report of the Surgeon General's Conference on Children's Mental Health: A national action agenda*. Washington, DC: U.S. Department of Health and Human Services.

Valuck, R. J., Anderson, H. O., Libby, A. M., Brandt, E., Bryan, C., Allen, R. R., . . . Pace, W. D. (2012). Enhancing electronic health record measurement of depression severity and suicide ideation: A Distributed Ambulatory Research in Therapeutics Network (DARTNet) study. *Journal of the American Board of Family Medicine, 25*(5), 582–593.

Van Hook, S., Harris, S. K., Brooks, T., Carey, P., Kossack, R., Kulig, J., & Knight, J. R. (2007). The "Six T's": Barriers to screening teens for substance abuse in primary care. *Journal of Adolescent Health, 40*, 456–461.

Vecchione, A. (2012). 8 Accountable Care Organizations worth closer look. *InformationWeek: Healthcare - Policy & Regulation*. Retrieved September 13, 2013, from http://www.informationweek.com/healthcare/policy/8-accountable-care-organizations-worth-c/240005118?queryText=8%20Accountable%20Care%20Organizations%20Worth%20Closer%20Look.

Wagner, E. F., Kortlander, E., & Morris, S. L. (2001). The teen intervention project: A school-based intervention for adolescents with substance abuse problems. In E. F. Wagner & H. B. Waldron (Eds.), *Innovations in adolescent substance abuse interventions* (p. 189). New York: Pergamon Press, Elsevier Science.

Wagner, E. F., & Waldron, H. B. (2001). *Innovations in adolescent substance abuse interventions*. New York: Pergamon Press, Elsevier Science.

Wagner, F. A., & Anthony, J. C. (2002). Into the world of illegal drug use: Exposure opportunity and other mechanisms linking the use of alcohol, tobacco, marijuana, and cocaine. *American Journal of Epidemiology, 155*(10), 918–925.

Wahl, O. F. (1995). *Media madness: Public images of mental illness*. New Brunswick, NJ: Rutgers University Press.

Wahl, O. F. (2002). Children's view of mental illness: A review of the literature. *Psychiatric Rehabilitation Skills, 6*, 134–158.

Wahl, O. F. (2003). Depiction of mental illnesses in children's media. *Journal of Mental Health, 12*, 249–258.

Wahl, O. F., & Roth R. (1982). Television images of mental illness: Results of a metropolitan Washington Media Watch. *Journal of Broadcasting, 26*, 599–605.

Wahl, O. F., Wood, A., Zaveri, P., Drapalski, A., & Mann, B. (2003). Mental illness depiction in children's films. *Journal of Community Psychology, 31*, 553–560.

Walker, S. C., Kerns, S. E., Lyon, A. R., Bruns, E. J., & Cosgrove, T. (2010). Impact of school-based health center use on academic outcomes. *Journal of Adolescent Health, 46*(3), 251–257.

Walton, M. A., Chermack, S. T., Shope, J. T., Bingham, C. R., Zimmerman, M. A., Blow, F. C., & Cunningham, R. M. (2010). Effects of a brief intervention for reducing violence and alcohol misuse among adolescents. *Journal of the American Medical Association, 304*, 527–535.

Wang, W., Saldana, L., Brown, C. H., & Chamberlain, P. (2010). Factors that influenced county system leaders to implement an evidence-based program: A baseline survey within a randomized controlled trial. *Implementation Science, 5*, 72.

Weiner, B. (1993). On sin and sickness: A theory of perceived responsibility and social motivation. *American Psychologist, 48*, 957–965.

Weiner, B., Perry, R. P., & Magnusson, J. (1988). An attributional analysis of reactions to stigmas.

Journal of Personality and Social Psychology, 55, 738–748.

Weisz, J. R. (2004). *Psychotherapy for children and adolescents: Evidence-based treatments and case examples*. Cambridge, UK: Cambridge University Press.

Weisz, J. R., Chorpita, B. F., Palinkas, L. A., Schoenwald, S. K., Miranda, J., Bearman, S. K., ... Research Network on Youth Mental Health. (2012). Testing standard and modular designs for psychotherapy treating depression, anxiety, and conduct problems in youth: A randomized effectiveness trial. *Archives of General Psychiatry, 69*(3), 274–282.

Wells, K. B., Jones, L., Chung, B., Dixon, E. L., Tang, L., Gilmore, J., ... Miranda, J. (2013). Community-partnered cluster-randomized comparative effectiveness trial of community engagement and planning or resources for services to address depression disparities. *Journal of General Internal Medicine, 28*(10), 1268–1278.

Werrbach, G., & DePoy, E. (1993). Social work students' interest in working with persons with serious mental illness. *Journal of Social Work Education, 29*, 200–211.

White, A. M., & Swartzwelder, H. S. (2005). Age-related effects of alcohol on memory and memory-related brain function in adolescents and adults. In M. Galanter (Ed.), *Recent developments in alcoholism, Vol. 17: Alcohol problems in adolescents and young adults* (pp. 161–176). New York: Kluwer Academic/Plenum Publishers.

White, W. L. (1998). *Chasing the dragon: A history of addiction and recovery in America*. Bloomington, IL: Lighthouse Institute Publications.

Williams, M., & Taylor, J. (1995). Mental illness: Media perpetuation of stigma. *Contemporary Nurse, 4*, 41–45.

Wilson, C., Nairn, R., Coverdale, J., & Panapa, A. (2000). How mental illness is portrayed in children's television: A prospective study. *British Journal of Psychiatry, 176*, 440–443.

Wintemute, G. J. (2015). The epidemiology of firearm violence in the twenty-first-century United States. *Annual Review of Public Health, 36*, 5–19.

Winters, K. C. (1999). Treating adolescents with substance use disorders: An overview of practice issues and treatment outcome. *Substance Abuse, 20*(4), 203–225.

Winters, K. C., Stinchfield, R. D., Opland, E., Weller, C., & Latimer, W. W. (2000). The effectiveness of the Minnesota Model approach in the treatment of adolescent drug abusers. *Addiction, 95*(4), 601–612.

Wisdom, J. P., Chor, K. H. B., Hoagwood, K., & Horwitz, S. (2014). Innovation adoption: A review of theories and constructs. *Administration and Policy in Mental Health and Mental Health Services Research, 41*(4), 480–502.

WPA. (2005). The WPA global programme to reduce the stigma and discrimination because of schizophrenia, Volume IV. Retrieved May 9, 2016, from http://www.open-the doors.com/english/media/Training_8.15.05.pdf

Wright, E. R., Gronfein, W. P., & Owens, T. J. (2000). Deinstitutionalization, social rejection, and the self-esteem of former mental patients. *Journal of Health and Social Behavior, 41*, 68–90.

Yamaguchi, R., Johnston, L. D., & O'Malley, P. M. (2003a). *Drug testing in schools: Policies, practices, and association with student drug use*. Institute for Social Research, University of Michigan.

Yamaguchi, R., Johnston, L. D., & O'Malley, P. M. (2003b). Relationship between student illicit drug use and school drug-testing policies. *Journal of School Health, 73*(4), 159–164.

Yoshikawa, H., Aber, J. L., & Beardslee, W. R. (2012). The effects of poverty on the mental, emotional, and behavioral health of children and youth: Implications for prevention. *American Psychologist, 67*(4), 272–284.

Young, D. W., Dembo, R., & Henderson, C. E. (2007). A national survey of substance abuse treatment for juvenile offenders. *Journal of Substance Abuse Treatment, 32*, 255–266.

Zeese, K. B. (2002). Drug testing fails at school and work. *Common Sense for Drug Policy*, from http://www.csdp.org

Zima, B. T., & Mangione-Smith, R. (2011). Gaps in quality measures for child mental health care: An opportunity for a collaborative agenda. *Journal of the American Academy of Child and Adolescent Psychiatry, 50*(8), 735–737.

Zima, B. T., Murphy, J. M., Scholle, S. H., Hoagwood, K. E., Sachdeva, R. C., Mangione-Smith, R., ... Jellinek, M. (2013). National quality measures for child mental health care: Background, progress, and next steps. *Pediatrics, 131*(Supplement 1), S38–S49.

Index

Page numbers followed by *b*, *f*, and *t* indicate boxes, figures, and tables, respectively.